DIABETES & THE GUT

Topical and Important Articles from the

AMERICAN DIABETES ASSOCIATION

SCHOLARLY JOURNALS

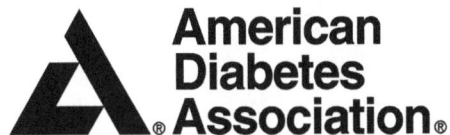

American Diabetes Association

DIABETES & THE GUT

Printed in the United States of America
1 3 5 7 9 10 8 6 4 2

ADA titles may be purchased for business or promotional use or for special sales. To purchase more than 50 copies of this book at a discount, or for custom editions of this book with your logo, contact the American Diabetes Association at the address below, at booksales@diabetes.org, or by calling 703-299-2046.

American Diabetes Association
1701 North Beauregard Street
Alexandria, Virginia 22311

DOI: 10.2337/9781580404532

DIABETES AND THE GUT

GUT HORMONES

NONALCOHOLIC FATTY LIVER DISEASE

GUT INFLAMMATION AND CELIAC DISEASE

GLUCAGON-LIKE PEPTIDE-1

Brain Glucagon-Like Peptide-1 Regulates Arterial Blood Flow, Heart Rate, and Insulin Sensitivity

Cendrine Cabou,[1,2,3] Gérard Campistron,[1,2,3] Nicolas Marsollier,[4] Corinne Leloup,[2,5]
Celine Cruciani-Guglielmacci,[4] Luc Pénicaud,[2,5] Daniel J. Drucker,[6] Christophe Magnan,[4]
and Rémy Burcelin[1,2]

OBJECTIVE—To ascertain the importance and mechanisms underlying the role of brain glucagon-like peptide (GLP)-1 in the control of metabolic and cardiovascular function. GLP-1 is a gut hormone secreted in response to oral glucose absorption that regulates glucose metabolism and cardiovascular function. GLP-1 is also produced in the brain, where its contribution to central regulation of metabolic and cardiovascular homeostasis remains incompletely understood.

RESEARCH DESIGN AND METHODS—Awake free-moving mice were infused with the GLP-1 receptor agonist exendin-4 (Ex4) into the lateral ventricle of the brain in the basal state or during hyperinsulinemic eu-/hyperglycemic clamps. Arterial femoral blood flow, whole-body insulin-stimulated glucose utilization, and heart rates were continuously recorded.

RESULTS—A continuous 3-h brain infusion of Ex4 decreased femoral arterial blood flow and whole-body glucose utilization in the awake free-moving mouse clamped in a hyperinsulinemic-hyperglycemic condition, only demonstrating that this effect was strictly glucose dependent. However, the heart rate remained unchanged. The metabolic and vascular effects of Ex4 were markedly attenuated by central infusion of the GLP-1 receptor (GLP-1R) antagonist exendin-9 (Ex9) and totally abolished in GLP-1 receptor knockout mice. A correlation was observed between the metabolic rate and the vascular flow in control and Ex4-infused mice, which disappeared in Ex9 and GLP-1R knockout mice. Moreover, hypothalamic nitric oxide synthase activity and the concentration of reactive oxygen species (ROS) were also reduced in a GLP-1R–dependent manner, whereas the glutathione antioxidant capacity was increased. Central GLP-1 activated vagus nerve activity, and complementation with ROS donor dose-dependently reversed the effect of brain GLP-1 signaling on peripheral blood flow.

CONCLUSIONS—Our data demonstrate that central GLP-1 signaling is an essential component of circuits integrating cardiovascular and metabolic responses to hyperglycemia. *Diabetes* 57:2577–2587, 2008

From the [1]Institut National de la Santé et de la Recherche Médicale (IN-SERM), U858, Institute of Molecular Medicine Rangueil, Toulouse, France; the [2]Université Toulouse III Paul-Sabatier, IFR31, Toulouse, France; the [3]Faculté des Sciences Pharmaceutiques, Toulouse, France; the [4]Université Paris 7, UMR CNRS 7059, Paris, France; [5]UMR UPS-CNRS 5241, Toulouse, France; and the [6]Banting and Best Diabetes Centre, Samuel Lunenfeld Research Institute, Mt. Sinai Hospital, University of Toronto, Toronto, Ontario, Canada.

Corresponding author: Rémy Burcelin, remy.burcelin@inserm.fr.

Received 28 January 2008 and accepted 8 July 2008.

Published ahead of print at http://diabetes.diabetesjournals.org on 15 July 2008. DOI: 10.2337/db08-0121.

There is now compelling evidence supporting the interplay between metabolic and vascular diseases (1,2) in which neuronal circuits in the central nervous system seem to play a critical role in orchestrating the control of glucose homeostasis (3). We recently demonstrated that the central infusion of insulin decreased blood pressure and increased arterial blood flow and heart rate through a molecular mechanism depending on the synthesis of nitric oxide in the hypothalamus (4). Importantly, the central regulation of nitric oxide (NO) metabolism affected whole-body glucose utilization (5). This mechanism was impaired during high-fat diet–induced insulin resistance and diabetes and reverted upon central NO supplementation (4). These findings raise the possibility that signals from peripheral tissues, which act on the brain to control glucose metabolism, could also regulate vascular function.

Enteroendocrine cells have important roles in regulating energy intake and glucose homeostasis through their actions on peripheral target organs, including the endocrine pancreas. Enteroendocrine cells secrete multiple hormones, including glucagon-like peptide (GLP)-1, which controls pancreatic endocrine secretion (6). GLP-1 is also a neuropeptide synthesized by neurons in the caudal regions of the nucleus of the solitary tract (NTS) (7,8). GLP-1 is released into the hypothalamus and controls food intake, blood pressure, and heart rate (9,10). Whereas most of the glucose-lowering actions of GLP-1 have been attributed to the direct effect of the hormone on the endocrine pancreas, i.e., to stimulation of insulin and inhibition of glucagon secretion, we demonstrated the importance of extra-pancreatic GLP-1 receptor–dependent control of insulin secretion (11) and whole-body glucose distribution (12). The infusion into the brain of the GLP-1 receptor antagonist exendin-9 (Ex9) inhibited insulin secretion induced by gut glucose (11). Conversely, central administration of the GLP-1 receptor agonist exendin-4 (Ex4) augmented intravenous glucose-stimulated insulin secretion to a level similar to that obtained during an intragastric glucose infusion (11). Our data suggested that the absorptive state was associated with the stimulation of the gut-to-brain axis leading to the activation of brain GLP-1 signaling and, consequently, to hyperinsulinemia. During the absorptive state, blood flow redistribution toward mesenteric organs is also observed, which has been proposed to favor nutrient redistribution into the liver (13). Importantly, stimulation of the central GLP-1 receptor increases blood pressure and heart rate and activates autonomic regulatory neurons (8,14,15). However, recently it has been shown that GLP-1 reduced islet blood flow after glucose administration (16). There-

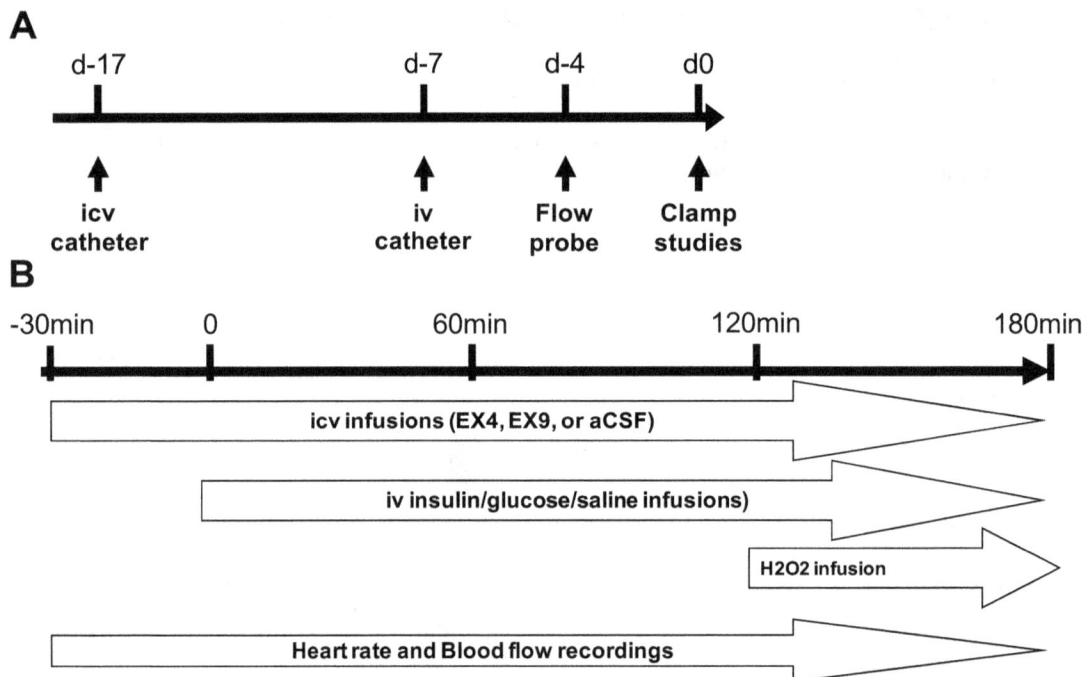

FIG. 1. Surgical and experimental procedures. *A*: Seventeen days (J-17) before infusions and clamp studies, a catheter was indwelled into the brain lateral ventricle. Seven days before the infusion (J-7), a catheter was indwelled into the left femoral vein, and the flow probe was indwelled 4 days (J-4) before the infusions (J0). *B*: Thirty minutes before the infusions, Ex4, Ex9, or aCSF was infused into the lateral ventricle of the mouse until completion of the 3-h clamp procedure. The clamp procedure was initiated by a concomitant infusion of glucose and insulin and was compared with the saline intravenous infusions.

fore, the role of brain GLP-1 signaling also in the control of cardiovascular homeostasis remains incompletely understood.

We have now pursued the importance of GLP-1 action in the central nervous system for control of cardiovascular function using studies in conscious free-moving mice. After central GLP-1 infusion, we simultaneously recorded femoral arterial blood flow, heart rate, and insulin and glucose sensitivity during hyperinsulinemic-euglycemic or hyperglycemic clamps. We now demonstrate that hypothalamic reactive oxygen and nitrogen species are controlled by brain GLP-1 and are essential for the coordinated regulation of metabolic and cardiovascular function.

RESEARCH DESIGN AND METHODS

Animals. Experiments were carried out under protocols approved by the Institutional Animal Care and Use Committee. Eleven-week-old male C57BL/6J (Janvier, Larbresle, France) and GLP-1 receptor knockout mice from our colony (in C57BL/6 background) were used, as previously described (4). Throughout the study period, the mice were housed at 21–22°C with a normal daily cycle and food and water ad libitum.

Surgical procedures. A catheter (Charles River Laboratories, L'Arbresles, France) was inserted into the lateral cerebral ventricle and secured on the top of the skull under anesthesia with isoflurane-oxygen (17). Ten days after the intracerebroventricular surgery, an intravenous catheter was introduced into the left femoral vein, sealed under the skin, and externalized at the back of the neck (Fig. 1). The mice were allowed to recover for 3 days, before an ultrasonic flow probe (Transonic System, Emka Technologies, France) was inserted surrounding the right femoral artery. The probe wire was inserted through the skin at the back of the neck, where it was secured using surgical thread. After surgery, the mice returned to their cages and allowed to recover for at least 4 days before infusions (18). At the end of the recovery period, mice that did not reach their presurgery weights were not used for subsequent experiments (i.e., 15% of the animals).

Infusions. On the day of the study (Fig. 1), the flow probe wire was connected to a Transonic model T403 flowmeter (Transonic System; Emka Technologies, Paris, France) to record the blood flow (ml/min) of the femoral artery and the heart rate (beats/min). The basal femoral arterial blood flow

and heart rate were recorded for 30 min in overnight fasted free-moving mice before starting the infusions.

Glucose clamp. A hyperinsulinemic-euglycemic (5.5 mmol/l) or hyperglycemic (20 mmol/l) clamp was performed to activate GLP-1–sensitive cells and to assess whole-body glucose utilization (18) (Table 1). Briefly, insulin was infused through the intrafemoral catheter at a rate of 18 mU · kg^{-1} · min^{-1} for 3 h. Glycemia was clamped at 5.5 or 20 mmol/l by adjusting an intrafemoral glucose infusion. A control group was infused with NaCl 0.9% (saline) for 3 h at a rate that was matched to the mean glucose infusion rate during the hyperinsulinemic clamps. This procedure did not change the hematocrit value, which remained close, ranging between 38.3 and 39.1% when considering all groups.

To ensure the filling of the tubing connected to the brain, intracerebroventricular infusions were started 30 min before the beginning of the clamp procedure and continued throughout the whole study. Briefly, a 5-µl bolus (5 µl) followed by a continuous (12 µl/h) infusion was performed with the cerebral vehicle (artificial cerebrospinal fluid [aCSF], pH 7.35, Na$^+$ 144 mmol/l, Cl$^-$ 146 mmol/l, K$^+$ 3 mmol/l, Mg^{2+} 1 mmol/l, Ca^{2+} 1.5 mmol/l, PO$_4^{2-}$ 1.2 mmol/l, pH 7.35) or with the GLP-1 receptor agonist (Ex4) or antagonist (exendin 9 [Ex9]), at a rate of 0.5 pmol · kg^{-1} · min^{-1} for 3 h, as described (11,12). This Exh infusion is expected to result in cerebral supraphysiological concentrations of GLP-1. However, this exendin infusion rate is 10 times lower than the one required to induce a physiological effect using a systemic infusion (11,12).

Measurement of autonomic nervous system activity. To assess the vagus nerve activity, a subset of mice bearing an intracerebroventricular catheter for 1 week was anesthetized with isoflurane maintained on a heating blanket at 37°C in a Faraday cage. The vagus nerve was isolated from the carotid at the level of the trachea, and one monopolar platinum electrode (Diameter: 125 µm, Phymep, Paris, France) was approximated to the vagal nerve. A second electrode was implanted directly on the skin as a reference. Both electrodes were connected to a BioAMp amplificator system (Ad Instrument; Phymep, Paris, France). The signal was filtered between 0.1 to 1,000 Hz (low and high frequency). The output signal was then directed toward a data acquisition system (PowerLab 8/30, Ad instrument). The neural activity was quantified by counting the frequency of spikes that exceeded a voltage threshold level set just above the electrical noise by using the Spike Histogram software (computer program Chart 5, Ad instrument). Baseline unit activity was recorded for 10 min before and during brain infusions. The neural activity was continuously recorded and quantified for 10 min at different time periods during the brain infusions. At completion of the recording, 600 μg acetylcholine chloride was injected intraperitoneally to demonstrate appropriate responsivity and recording of the vagus nerve activity.

Hydrogen peroxide infusions. To study the role of reactive oxygen species (ROS) in the brain on arterial blood flow, heart rate, and whole-body glucose utilization, hydrogen peroxide (H_2O_2) was infused into the lateral ventricle of the mice 120 min after the beginning of the hyperglycemic clamp. Hydrogen peroxide was extemporaneously diluted in aCSF and infused at the rates of 2 or 20 nmol/min, as previously described (19). Briefly, 2 μl H_2O_2 was followed by a continuous infusion at a rate of 12 μl/h. At the end of the infusions, the mice were decapitated and the brain was removed from the skull within <15 s. The brain was put into a frozen brain frame and the hypothalamus was dissected out and frozen at −80°C. To validate that the probe was correctly recording the blood flow, at the end of the insulin infusion, some mice were given a flash injection of a rapid NO donor (sodium nitroprusside (10 mg/kg, 25–40 μl i.v.). Upon a correct implantation of the probe, the nitroprusside injection induced at least a 100% increase in blood flow and a rapid increase in heart rate.

TABLE 1
Summary of experimental conditions

Studies protocols	n
1: Clamps	
Euglycemic clamps	
aCSF (icv)	7
Ex4 (icv)	6
Hyperglycemic clamps	
aCSF (icv)	7
aCSF (icv) (GLP-1R KO)	6
Ex4 (icv)	7
Ex9 (icv)	5
Ex4 + hydrogen peroxide (20 nmol/min) (icv)	5
2: Saline intravenous infusion	
aCSF (icv)	6
3: Basal blood flow and heart rate studies	
aCSF (icv)	7
Ex4 (icv)	12
Ex9 (icv)	8
PBS (icv)	4
Hydrogen peroxide (2 nmol/min, icv)	4
Hydrogen peroxide (20 nmol/min, icv)	5
4: Vagal activity studies	
aCSF (icv)	5
Ex4 (icv)	4
5: ROS studies	
aCSF (icv, saline iv, WT)	5
aCSF (icv, clamp 5.5 mmol/l, WT)	15
aCSF (icv, clamp 20 mmol/l, WT)	10
Ex4 (icv, clamp 5.5 mmol/l, WT)	8
Ex4 (icv, clamp 20 mmol/l, WT)	14
aCSF (icv, clamp 5.5 mmol/l, GLP-1R KO)	5
aCSF (icv, clamp 20 mmol/l, GLP-1R KO)	5
6: NOS activity studies	
aCSF (icv, clamp 20 mmol/l)	5
Ex4 (icv, clamp 20 mmol/l)	5

The number of mice studied (n) is indicated for each experimental condition. aCSF, mice infused with artificial cerebrospinal fluid into the brain (intracerebroventricular [icv]). Some mice were clamped with insulin in euglycemic or hyperglycemic conditions or underwent a saline infusion equivalent to the corresponding insulin and glucose infusion volumes and rates performed during the clamp conditions. Some mice were studied in basal conditions (no insulin, glucose, or saline infusion) only. Hydrogen peroxide was used at the concentration of 2 or 20 nmol/min icv only, as specified. The vagal activity was recorded in response to aCSF or Ex4 icv infusions in a subset of mice. ROS production was assessed in all conditions in WT or GLP-1 receptor knockout mice (GLP-1R KO) mice. The activity of the NOS was studied in a subset of mice during hyperglycemic-hyperinsulinemic clamp conditions in the presence or absence of Ex4 icv.

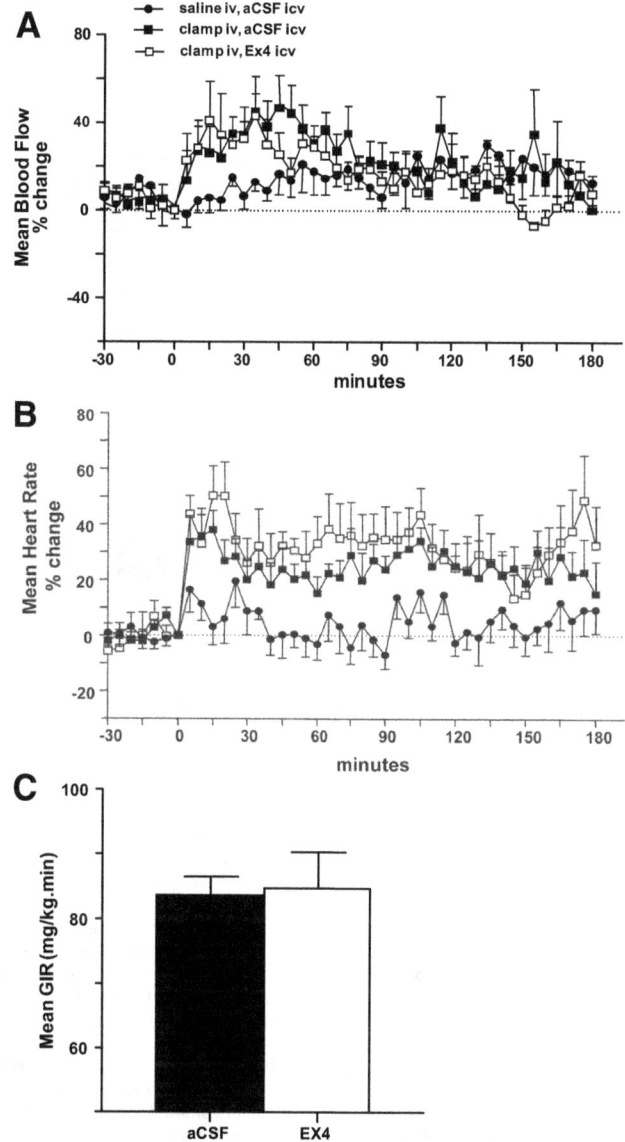

FIG. 2. Hyperinsulinemia controls arterial blood flow, heart, and whole-body glucose utilization rates in wild-type mice. Percent changes are shown from baseline of mean arterial femoral blood flow (*A*) and heart rates (*B*) during 3 h of hyperinsulinemic-euglycemic conditions where aCSF (■) or Ex4 (□) was simultaneously infused into the brain of awake free-moving C57BL/6 J wild-type mice. In a subset of wild-type mice, where aCSF was infused into the brain, intravenous saline was simultaneously infused instead of glucose or insulin (control group, ●). Data are means ± SE for six to seven mice per group and significantly different between the control group and the two other groups (*P* < 0.05). In *C*, whole-body glucose utilization rate, glucose infusion rate (GIR) (mg · kg^{-1} · min^{-1}), was calculated in steady-state euglycemic-hyperinsulinemic conditions (5.5 mmol/l) in mice infused with aCSF or Ex4 into the brain. Means ± SE are shown for six to seven mice per group.

Blood sampling. At the end of the intracerebroventricular infusions, blood was collected from the retro-orbital sinus into a tube, mixed with 1 μg/μl aprotinin/0.1 mmol/l EDTA, and centrifuged at 8,000 rpm for 5 min at 4°C. Plasma was stored at −80°C until assay. The insulin level was measured using an ELISA kit (Mercodia, Sweden). Briefly, 10 μl plasma was incubated for 2 h in the anti-insulin antibody–coated 96-well plate. Then, after washing the secondary, antibody conjugated with peroxidase was added for 30 min. The reaction was stopped by adding acid to give a colorimetric end point that is read spectrophotometrically. The interassay variation coefficient was ~8% and the intra-assay coefficient was ~4%.

Hypothalamic ROS and glutathione determinations. Tissue treatment for ROS determination was accomplished according to the method of Szabados et

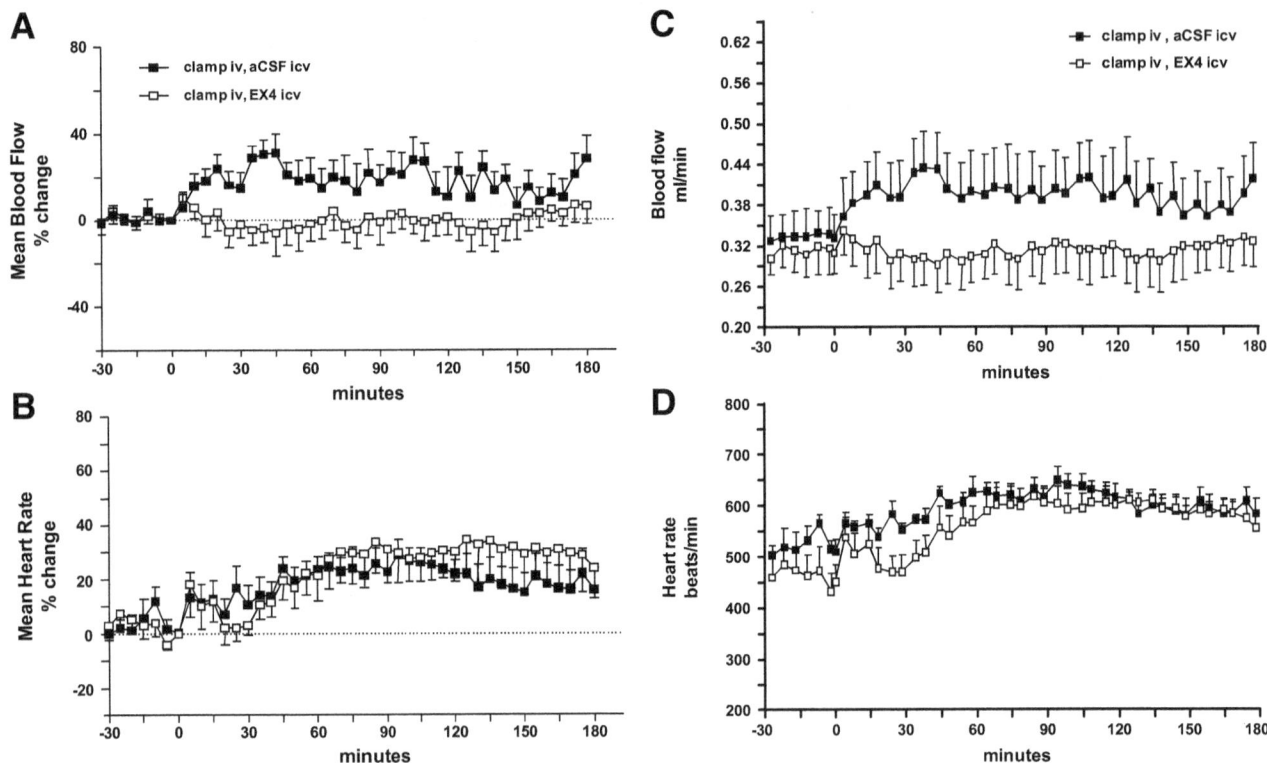

al. (20). Briefly, we used a rodent brain matrix (World Precision Instrument, Sarasota, FL) to carefully slice out the hypothalamus and the surrounding tissues. This frame allows an accurate and repeated sampling of a 1-mm-thick brain slice. Then, a second frame is used to dissect out the hypothalamus precisely and uniquely from the other part of the brain surrounding the hypothalamus. Hypothalamic pieces were carefully homogenized using a dounce and loaded with the dichlorodihydro-fluorescein diacetate probe that is oxidized to fluorescent dichlorofluorescein by H_2O_2 and classically used to monitor intracellular generation of ROS (CM-H_2DCFDA, Molecular Probes). It is noteworthy that this probe is very specific for H_2O_2 and that the background level is very low. However, the origin of the ROS produced, i.e., mitochondrial or cytoplasmic, cannot be detected. Hypothalamic homogenates were incubated with 4 μmol/l CM-H_2DCFDA in a final 0.5-ml volume for 30 min at 37°C. After centrifugation, ROS measurements (on a 200-μl supernatant) were performed in a Fluorescent Plate Reader (Perkin Elmer). Intensity of fluorescence was expressed as arbitrary units per milligram protein. Oxidized glutathione/total glutathione ratio was assessed in hypothalamic homogenates. They were immediately grounded in 1% EDTA/5% metaphosphoric acid (1:5 vol/vol). After centrifugation, supernatants were used to detect total reduced glutathione and its oxidized form (GSSG) by reverse-phase high-performance liquid chromatography with electrochemical detection as described (21).

Hypothalamic NO synthase activities. To assess hypothalamic NO synthase (NOS) activities, the tissues were collected, weighted, and homogenized in buffer (250 mmol/l Tris-HCl, 10 mmol/l EDTA and EGTA). The NOS assay kit (Calbiochem, Darmstadt, Germany) is based on the biochemical conversion of [3H]-L-arginine to [3H]-L-citrulline by NOS. The data are hence considered as an index of NOS activity. NOS catalyzes the stoichiometric conversion of L-arginine into L-citrulline in the presence of NADPH, oxygen, calmodulin, and calcium. The tissues were incubated with radiolabeled [3H]-L-arginine (1 μCi/μl) and passed through a column containing a resin that binds L-arginine but not L-citrulline. The quantification of [3H]-L-citrulline radioactivity is performed from the eluate. Results are expressed in counts per minute by milligram of tissues.

Data analysis and statistics. Data are expressed as means ± SE. Data were analyzed using the GraphPad Prism version 5.00 for Windows (GraphPad Software, San Diego, CA). Statistical significance was determined by applying, respectively, a Student's t test, a Mann-Whitney test, a Kruskal-Wallis followed by a Dunn's multiple comparison test, a Pearson test, or a two-way ANOVA test for repeated measurements with fixed factors of treatment/genotype, time, and treatment/genotype × time followed by post hoc test (Bonferroni's

multiple comparison test) when appropriate. The acceptable level of significance was defined as $P < 0.05$.

The Student's t test was used for the glucose infusion rate and NOS activities, since it is designed to compare two means together within a binomial distribution. The Kruskal Wallis followed by the Dunn post hoc test was used to compare more than two means together with single values obtained during different experiments and was used for the comparison of ROS activities. Eventually, we used the two-way ANOVA for repeated measurements with fixed factors followed by the Bonferroni post hoc test for all time courses: heart rate, blood flow, and vagal activities.

RESULTS

The activation of the central GLP-1 receptor regulates femoral arterial blood flow, heart rate, and whole-body glucose utilization under hyperglycemic conditions. The systemic infusion of insulin during a euglycemic-hyperinsulinemic clamp increased femoral blood flow and heart rate (Fig. 2A and B). The simultaneous brain infusion of the GLP-1 receptor agonist Ex4 did not affect hemodynamic parameters and whole-body glucose utilization (Fig. 2A–C) when the mice were clamped under euglycemic conditions. Because we previously demonstrated that brain GLP-1 signaling was glucose-dependent (11), the blood glucose was raised to 20 mmol/l during the hyperinsulinemic clamp. Hyperglycemia modestly diminished the relative increase in femoral arterial blood flow (compare Fig. 3A and 2A). Remarkably, coinfusion of Ex4 into the brain under hyperglycemic conditions abolished the increase in femoral artery blood flow (Fig. 3A and C). Simultaneously, hyperglycemia diminished the increase in heart rate (Fig. 3B and D) observed under euglycemic clamp conditions (compare Fig. 3B and 2B), but unlike blood flow, heart rate was not affected by Ex4. Concomitantly, the whole-body glucose utilization rate was also reduced by Ex4 (Fig. 3E). In contrast to the effects seen under conditions of systemic hyperglycemia and hyperinsulinemia, infusion of Ex4 into the lateral ventricle

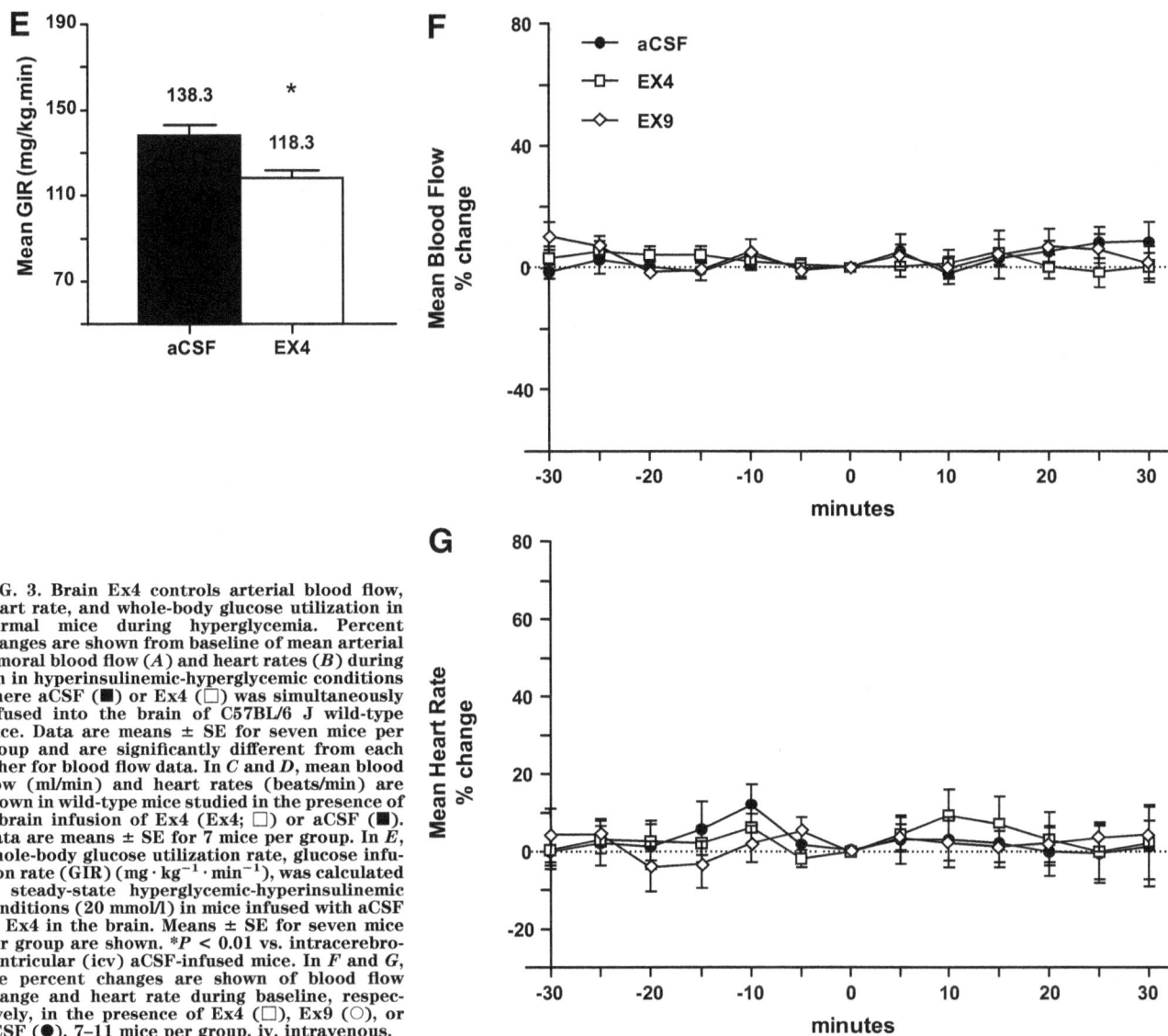

FIG. 3. Brain Ex4 controls arterial blood flow, heart rate, and whole-body glucose utilization in normal mice during hyperglycemia. Percent changes are shown from baseline of mean arterial femoral blood flow (*A*) and heart rates (*B*) during 3 h in hyperinsulinemic-hyperglycemic conditions where aCSF (■) or Ex4 (□) was simultaneously infused into the brain of C57BL/6 J wild-type mice. Data are means ± SE for seven mice per group and are significantly different from each other for blood flow data. In *C* and *D*, mean blood flow (ml/min) and heart rates (beats/min) are shown in wild-type mice studied in the presence of a brain infusion of Ex4 (Ex4; □) or aCSF (■). Data are means ± SE for 7 mice per group. In *E*, whole-body glucose utilization rate, glucose infusion rate (GIR) (mg · kg^{-1} · min^{-1}), was calculated in steady-state hyperglycemic-hyperinsulinemic conditions (20 mmol/l) in mice infused with aCSF or Ex4 in the brain. Means ± SE for seven mice per group are shown. *$P < 0.01$ vs. intracerebroventricular (icv) aCSF-infused mice. In *F* and *G*, the percent changes are shown of blood flow change and heart rate during baseline, respectively, in the presence of Ex4 (□), Ex9 (○), or aCSF (●), 7–11 mice per group. iv, intravenous.

had no effect on blood flow and heart rate in the fasting basal state (Fig. 3*F* and *G*).

To further examine the importance of endogenous GLP-1 receptor signaling for the control of femoral arterial blood flow and whole-body glucose utilization, we used *1*) GLP-1 receptor knockout and *2*) wild-type mice infused into the brain with the GLP-1 receptor antagonist Ex9 under hyperinsulinemic-hyperglycemic conditions. Remarkably, transient attenuation or genetic elimination of central GLP-1 receptor signaling markedly augmented femoral arterial blood flow (Fig. 4*A*). Similarly, heart rate was increased in GLP-1 receptor knockout mice, and whole-body glucose utilization rates were also increased by the disruption of central GLP-1 receptor signaling (Fig. 4*B* and *C*).

Femoral arterial blood flow correlates with whole-body glucose utilization in the presence of an activated GLP-1 receptor. To determine whether the control of whole-body glucose utilization by brain GLP-1 signaling is intimately related to the rate of femoral arterial blood flow, we correlated both parameters for each mouse independently, under different experimental conditions. The data show that femoral arterial blood flow and whole-body glucose utilization rates were positively correlated under hyperglycemic-hyperinsulinemic conditions (Fig. 5*A*) and the mean values of each group for both parameters exhibited a highly significant correlation (Fig. 5*B*). In contrast, no correlation between femoral blood flow and glucose utilization was observed in mice with transient central or complete genetic disruption of GLP-1 receptor signaling (Fig. 5*D*) when compared with WT control mice (Fig. 5*C*).

GLP-1 receptor activation decreases hypothalamic nitric oxide synthase activity and reactive oxygen species concentration. We previously showed that hyperinsulinemia increases femoral arterial blood flow by a mechanism requiring eNOS activation (4). Therefore, we assessed the activity of nitric oxide synthases in the hypothalamus of mice clamped in hyperglycemia and infused with Ex4 into the brain. Central Ex4 significantly reduced total nitric oxide synthase activity (Fig. 6*A*). Because ROS are also regulated by insulin and glucose in the brain (22), we assessed the impact of glucose and Ex4 in vivo on ROS production. Hyperglycemia significantly reduced ROS production, which was even more markedly

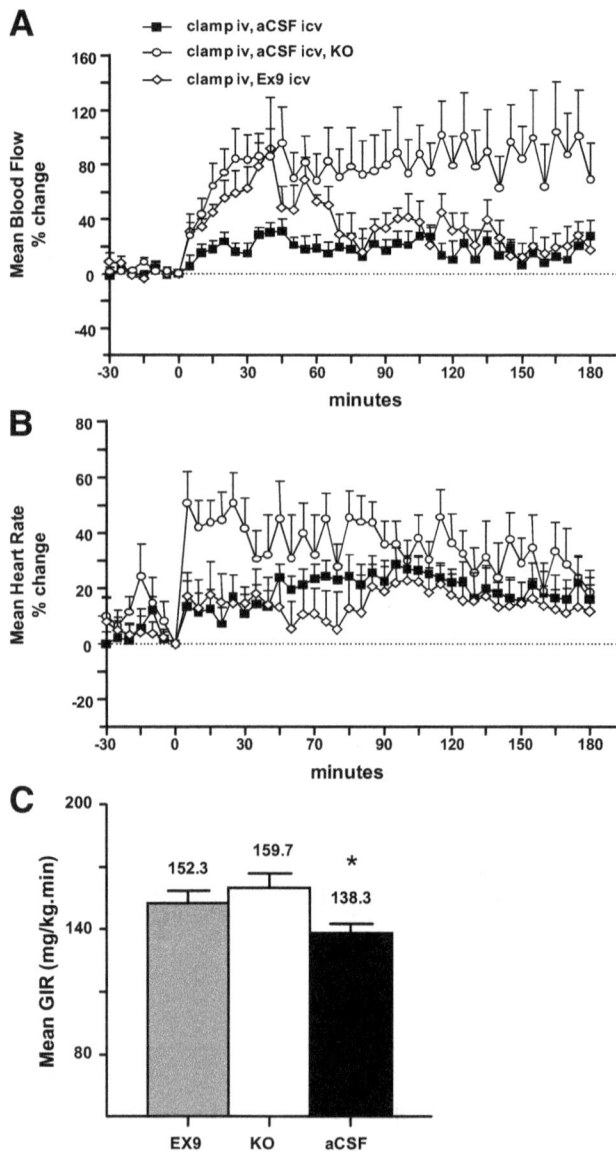

FIG. 4. Brain GLP-1 receptor inactivation modulates arterial blood flow, heart rate, and whole-body glucose utilization in mice. Percent changes from baseline of mean arterial femoral blood flow (*A*) and heart rates (*B*) during 3 h in hyperinsulinemic-hyperglycemic conditions, where aCSF was infused in the brain of wild-type (WT, ■) or GLP-1 receptor knockout mice (KO, ○), or in WT infused with Ex9 into the brain (◇). Data are means ± SE for 5–7 mice per group. Statistical significance was determined between mice infused with Ex9 or aCSF and between GLP-1R KO mice and wild-type mice infused with aCSF (*P* < 0.05 for the mean blood flow data only). In *C*, whole-body glucose utilization rate, glucose infusion rate (GIR) (mg · kg^{-1} · min^{-1}), was calculated in steady-state hyperglycemic-hyperinsulinemic conditions (20 mmol/l) in wild-type mice infused with aCSF or Ex9 in the brain and in GLP-1 receptor knockout (KO) mice. *P* < 0.05 vs. intracerebroventricular (icv) aCSF-infused KO mice. iv, intravenous.

suppressed by Ex4 in a glucose-dependent manner (Fig. 6*B*). Remarkably, the ability of glucose to diminish hypothalamic ROS was completely abrogated in GLP-1 receptor knockout mice (Fig. 6*B*). This reduced ROS concentration was associated with an increased antioxidant capacity in response to the Ex4 treatment and in hyperglycemia only, since the oxidized glutathione–to–total glutathione ratio was slightly reduced (Fig. 6*C*). However, we cannot rule out that another antioxidant mechanism could also have

controlled the ROS production in response to brain GLP-1 signaling.

ROS in the central nervous system controls femoral arterial blood flow and whole-body glucose utilization in a glucose-dependent manner. Because we previously demonstrated that the pharmacological modulation of brain NO controlled femoral arterial blood flow and whole-body glucose utilization rates (4), we focused here on the role of ROS. To determine whether changes in ROS could link GLP-1 receptor activation to the control of femoral arterial blood flow and whole-body glucose utilization rates, we performed a continuous infusion of oxygen peroxide into the lateral ventricular cavity of control mice under basal conditions. H_2O_2 induced a dose-dependent increase in femoral arterial blood flow (Fig. 7*A*). We next determined whether H_2O_2 could reverse the effects of Ex4 on blood flow. The ROS donor was injected 120 min after the beginning of the simultaneous hyperglycemic-hyperinsulinemic clamp and Ex4 infusion (Fig. 7*B*). H_2O_2 dramatically and rapidly increased the arterial blood flow in the presence of Ex4 (Fig. 7*B*). Conversely, the heart rate was reduced in the same experiments (Fig. 7*C*).

Vagus nerve activity is increased in response to brain Ex4 administration. To determine whether the autonomic nervous system is a candidate for transmission of the brain GLP-1 signal to peripheral tissues, we recorded vagus nerve activity during brain Ex4 infusion. Ex4 administration rapidly increased the firing rate of the vagus nerve within 5 min (Fig. 8*B* and *C*), which lasted for 55 min, i.e., until the end of the infusion (Fig. 8*B* and *C*).

DISCUSSION

The present data demonstrate that in the awake freemoving mouse, brain GLP-1 receptor signaling simultaneously controls femoral arterial blood flow, heart rate, and glucose utilization. We further show that reactive nitric oxide and oxygen species are regulated by brain GLP-1 signaling and likely important for the coordinated regulation of metabolic and cardiovascular function. The brain to periphery signal was associated with an increased vagus nerve activity. Notably, the action of GLP-1R signaling for control of nitric oxide and ROS was strictly glucose dependent.

We previously reported that brain GLP-1 induced insulin resistance and increased insulin secretion to favor hepatic glucose storage (11). We now extend these findings by demonstrating that brain GLP-1 signaling reduces hindlimb arterial blood flow under conditions of hyperglycemia. Hence, these new data strongly suggest that brain GLP-1 signaling may modify the metabolic activity of hindlimb muscles by a mechanism involving changes in blood flow. Consistent with this hypothesis, a strong correlation was observed between glucose utilization and blood flow rates. Importantly, this correlation was no longer present in experimental conditions where brain GLP-1 signaling was abolished in GLP-1 receptor knockout mice and, even more selectively, in mice infused with the GLP-1 receptor antagonist Ex9 into the brain. It is noteworthy that there is an important difference between the blood flow profiles obtained in the KO mice and those obtained with the GLP-1 receptor antagonist Ex9. It is suggested that either the GLP-1 receptor KO mice have adapted to the genetic mutation or that the GLP-1 receptor is also important to regulate blood flow somewhere else in the body. Recent evidence suggests that GLP-1 regulates

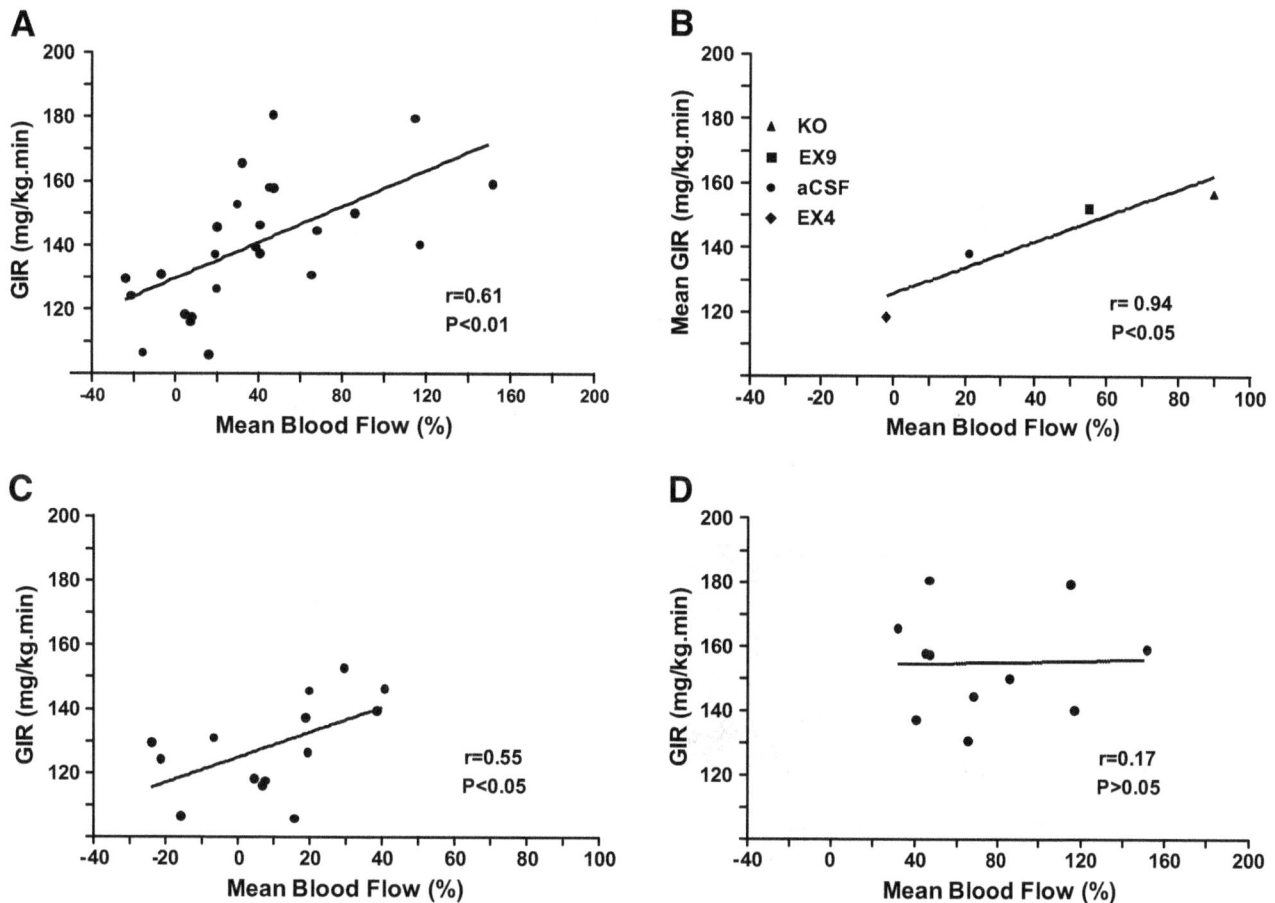

FIG. 5. Correlations between femoral arterial blood flow and whole-body glucose utilization rates under hyperglycemic conditions. The maximal blood flow rates (%) calculated during the hyperinsulinemic-hyperglycemic clamp were plotted in *A* against the glucose infusion rate (GIR, mg · $kg^{-1} \cdot min^{-1}$) for individual mice ($n = 25$). In *B*, the mean values are represented for mice infused into the brain with Ex4 (♦), aCSF (●), or Ex9 (■) or in GLP-1 receptor knockout mice (KO, ▲). In *C*, individual data are presented for mice with active brain GLP-1R signaling (wild-type aCSF or Ex4-infused mice, $n = 14$). In *D*, individual data are presented for mice where brain GLP-1 receptor signaling was blocked by Ex9 or in GLP-1R knockout mice (KO) ($n = 11$). The Pearson *r* value was calculated and a positive correlation was statistically significant when $P < 0.05$.

endothelial function. GLP-1 relaxed femoral artery in a dose-response manner (23), and GLP-1 is associated with vasodilation induced by acetylcholine (24). In humans, the systemic infusion of GLP-1 or its analogs does not induce hypertension but, rather, has protective effects (25,26). Therefore, the increased vascular resistance demonstrated by the present data seems to be specific for brain GLP-1 signaling and not observed in response to a systemic infusion. It is noteworthy that Ex4 is infused into the brain and that the rate of infusion is so low that no systemic effect could be detected (11). It is noteworthy that our animal model was designed to study the pharmacological effect of brain GLP-1 signaling on vascular and metabolic functions. We performed hyper-insulinemic-hyperglycemic clamps that do not correspond to any physiological situation.

Therefore, we conclude that brain GLP-1 signaling contributes to the regulation of both metabolic and cardiovascular functions. Importantly, we cannot directly demonstrate a causal relationship between metabolic and vascular function in response to brain GLP-1 signaling.

It has been previously shown that both intravenous and intracerebroventricular administration of GLP-1 receptor agonists increased blood pressure and heart rate (8). We do not have direct evidence of changes in blood pressure under our experimental conditions. However, because the arterial femoral blood flow was reduced in response to brain Ex4 infusion, we could suggest that our data fit previous data from the literature. We here further demonstrate that this increased blood pressure could be due to an increased peripheral vascular resistance.

Moreover, GLP-1 receptors are also expressed in the area postrema of the rat brain, which could interact with circulating GLP-1 (27,28). In our experimental procedure, hyperglycemia was induced by a systemic glucose infusion; therefore, under these conditions, GLP-1 secretion from the gut is not increased. Our data strongly support the idea that central GLP-1 is a direct regulator of peripheral cardiovascular function. Furthermore, previous studies showed that the intracerebroventricular administration of GLP-1R agonists increased arterial blood pressure and heart rate, which was blocked by previous intracerebroventricular administration of Ex9 (14). This is in agreement with our data suggesting that this increased blood pressure could be due to the reduced blood flow that we observed in the present study. Bilateral vagotomy blocked the stimulating effect of intracerebroventricular GLP-1 on arterial blood pressure and heart rate in rats (14). These findings, taken together with our current data, suggest that neural information emerging in the brain after GLP-1 receptor activation is transmitted to the periphery through the vagus nerve. We previously reported that brain insulin

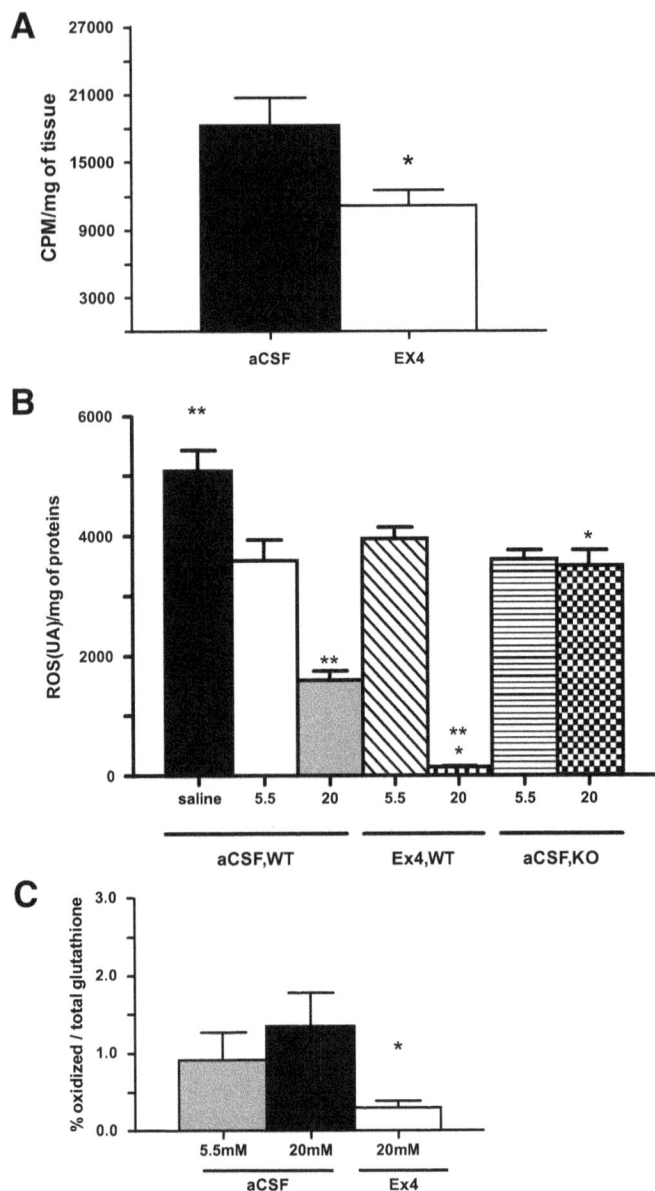

FIG. 6. NOS activity and the concentration of ROS are reduced in the hypothalamus of mice infused with Ex4 into the brain under hyperglycemic conditions. In A, hypothalamic nitric oxide activity (cpm/mg tissue) in hyperglycemic-hyperinsulinemic conditions in wild-type mice is infused with Ex4 or aCSF into the brain. The mean of five mice per group is shown. $*P < 0.05$ vs. intracerebroventricular (icv) aCSF-infused mice. B: ROS (arbitrary units [AU]/mg protein) in euglycemic (5.5 mmol/l) or hyperglycemic (20 mmol/l) conditions during a hyperinsulinemic clamp or during an intravenous saline infusion (saline) in wild-type mice simultaneously infused with aCSF or Ex4 into the brain. GLP-1 receptor knockout mice (KO) were studied in hyperinsulinemic-euglycemic or hyperglycemic conditions. Data are means ± SE for 5–14 mice per group. $*P < 0.05$ vs. icv aCSF-infused wild-type or mice in hyperglycemic conditions; $P < 0.05$ vs. 5.5 nmol/l condition. C: Oxidized glutathione–to–total glutathione ratio in hyperinsulinemic-euglycemic or hyperinsulinemic mice clamped in the presence or absence of Ex4 in the lateral ventricle of the brain. Data are means of 5–8 mice per group. $*P < 0.05$ vs. hyperglycemic icv aCSF-infused mice.

signaling increases the arterial femoral blood flow by a mechanism that does not require the cholinergic tone, since the central insulin signal was not affected by atropine (4). We suspected that noncholinergic fibers would be present in the vagus nerve. We here show that Ex4 activates the firing activity of the vagus nerve and is

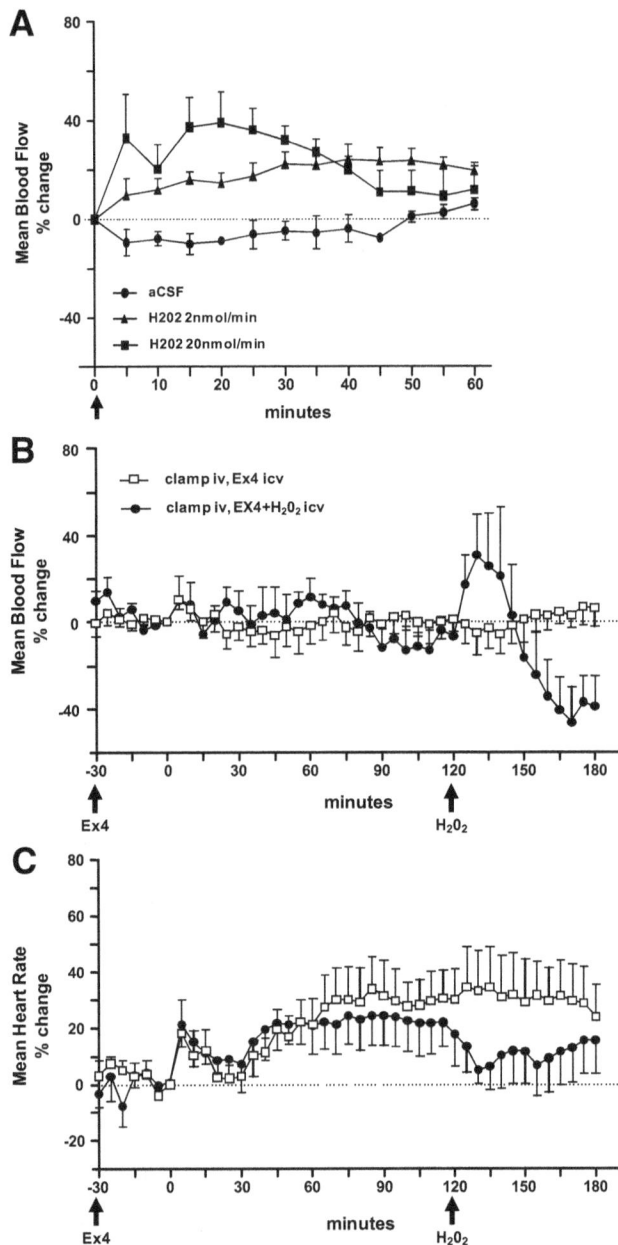

FIG. 7. A brain ROS donor increases femoral arterial blood flow and reduces heart rate in a dose-dependent manner. In A, the femoral arterial blood flow rate was recorded under basal conditions. aCSF or hydrogen peroxide (H_2O_2, low 2 nmol/min and high 20 nmol/min) were infused in the lateral ventricle at the time indicated by the arrow. Statistical significance ($P < 0.05$) was determined between mice infused with aCSF or H_2O_2. In B, the femoral arterial blood flow rate was recorded in hyperglycemic conditions and in the presence of Ex4 infused into the brain (arrow at −30 min). After 120 min, an infusion of hydrogen peroxide was performed in a separate group of mice (see arrow at 120 min, 20 nmol/min). aCSF infusion under the same experimental conditions did not modify the blood flow (not shown). In C, the mean heart rate was recorded simultaneously. Data are means ± SE for 5–7 mice per group. icv, intracerebroventricular; iv, intravenous.

associated with vasoconstriction. Therefore, in the mouse, the reduction of the arterial blood flow might be associated with an increased activity of the vagus nerve. It is noteworthy that we studied anesthetized mice in basal conditions, where Ex4 alone was infused into the brain. Therefore, more experiments should be done to validate this conclusion in awake free-moving mice in response to hyperglycemic-hyperinsulinemic clamps.

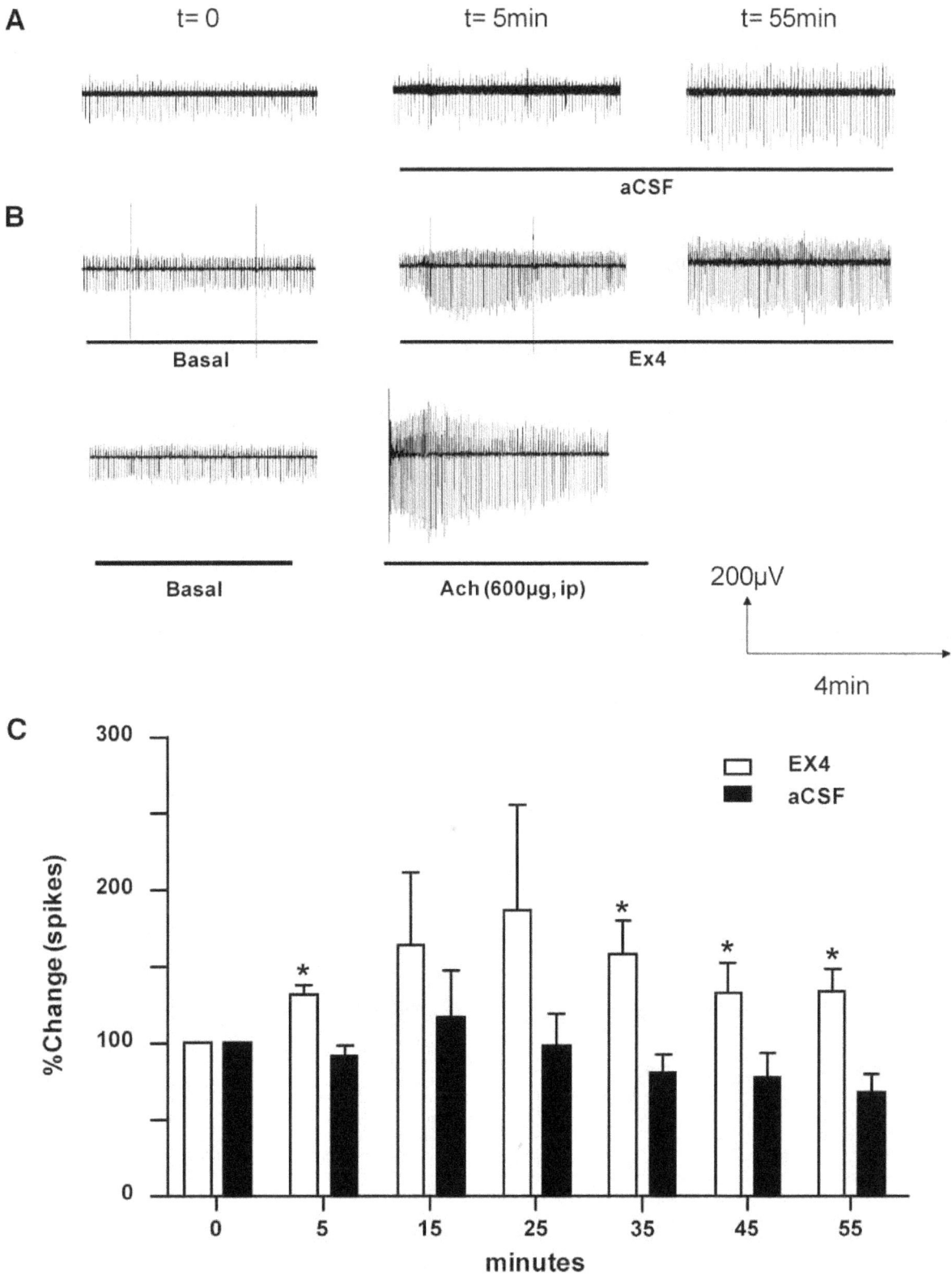

FIG. 8. Brain Ex4 infusion rapidly increases vagus nerve activity. *A*: Firing rate activity of the vagus nerve in microvolt/time shown before ($t =$ 0) and 5 ($t = 5$) and 55 ($t = 55$) min after the beginning of the intracerebroventricular (icv) aCSF (*A*) or Ex4 (*B*) infusions. At completion of the experiment, an intraperitoneal flash injection of acetylcholine chloride was performed as a positive control and compared with the basal value. In *C*, the firing rate activity was quantified by assessing the number of spikes per minute and represented in percent of change versus T0 in aCSF and Ex4-infused mice. *Significantly different from aCSF-infused mice when $P < 0.05$.

Importantly, in our experimental procedure, brain GLP-1 signaling was strictly glucose dependent. The glucose dependency of GLP-1 signaling is a main general feature. This characteristic minimizes the risk of hypoglycemia by blunting insulin secretion when glycemia returns to the basal value. Here, we suggest that the vascular effect of GLP-1 would also be blunted when the blood glucose concentration reaches euglycemia. The mechanisms responsible for the glucose dependency of GLP-1 signaling into the brain are unknown but could be related to those that we described into the portal vein (12,29). For example, the glucose transporter GLUT2 is probably a key of the brain glucose sensitivity (3,30).

Brain GLP-1 receptor signaling is activated in response to oral glucose absorption (11), such as that in the fed condition. Glucose and insulin are two other important regulators of brain signaling (31,32). We previously showed that brain insulin increases femoral arterial blood flow by a mechanism depending on the production of NO by eNOS (4) and muscle glucose utilization (17). We have now demonstrated that brain GLP-1 signaling conversely decreased NOS activity and prevented the vasodilatory effect of insulin in a glucose-dependent manner. Hyperglycemia is absolutely required for the control of GLP-1 action on glucose homeostasis (6), and recent data showed that brain glucose sensing requires ROS signaling. The transient increase from 5 to 20 mmol/l glucose increased ROS concentration in hypothalamic slices ex vivo, which is reversed by adding antioxidants (33). In our in vivo experimental condition, i.e., 3 h of hyperglycemia and hyperinsulinemia, the ROS concentration was reduced in the hypothalamus. This was associated with an increased antioxidative activity, since the oxidized glutathione/total glutathione ratio was reduced. We cannot rule out that other ROS scavenging mechanisms could have been activated in response to Ex4. Our current data extend these findings by demonstrating that *1*) exogenous GLP-1R activation markedly reduces glucose-dependent ROS generation and *2*) basal endogenous GLP-1R signaling is required for the transmission of the signal linking hyperglycemia to diminished ROS generation. However, we cannot directly demonstrate that the ROS concentration and GST activity changes were located exclusively in GLP-1 receptor–expressing cells. Recent data from our group and from the literature showed that GLP-1 receptor–expressing cells are located at a high density in the arcuate nucleus of the hypothalamus in the rats and mice. Such cells are mainly associated with pro-opiomelanocortin (POMC)– and neuropeptide Y (NPY)–expressing neurons (34,35). The interpretation would rather be that the hypothalamic GLP-1–sensitive cells would transmit the GLP-1 signal to multiple different cells in connection with the former one. In addition, we used Ex4 instead of GLP-1 in our infusion procedures to demonstrate the role of the GLP-1 receptor. We previously validated that brain Ex4 effects on glucose metabolism and insulin sensitivity specifically depended on brain GLP-1 receptors by studying GLP-1 receptor knockout mice. Although we cannot exclude any unknown Ex4-specific effect, our data strongly suggest that most if not all the effects of Ex4 mimic native brain GLP-1 signaling.

In conclusion, the central nervous system is tightly involved in the integrated control of blood glucose and cardiovascular homeostasis. We have shown that, although at a supraphysiological concentration, central GLP-1 behaves as a molecular signal linking both metabolic and cardiovascular functions. Recently, two new therapeutic strategies based on GLP-1 have been approved for the treatment of diabetes. One involves GLP-1 receptor activation using GLP-1R agonists such as Ex4. The second mechanism involves the prevention of endogenous GLP-1 degradation by the use of inhibitors of the GLP-1 degrading enzyme dipeptidyl peptidase-4. Although both strategies lead to similar reduction of A1C in patients with type 2 diabetes, it seems reasonable to postulate that GLP-1R agonists and dipeptidyl peptidase-4 inhibitors may produce different effects on brain mechanisms regulating glucose homeostasis and cardiovascular function, an issue that will be important to address in future studies.

ACKNOWLEDGMENTS

This work was supported by grants from the Agence Nationale pour la Recherche to R.B. (Nutrisens 05-PNRA-004, Mithycal, Metaprofile, brain GLP-1) and to C.M. (Nutrisens, Brain GLP-1). Support was also provided by the Programme National de Recherche sur le Diabete, Paul Sabatier University, the Club d'Etude du Système Nerveux Autonome (CESNA), and the Juvenile Diabetes Research Foundation (D.J.D.).

We would like to thank Professor J. Amar for helpful discussion and Anne Galinier for technical help with regards to the glutathione assay.

REFERENCES

1. Grundy SM: Metabolic syndrome: connecting and reconciling cardiovascular and diabetes worlds. *J Am Coll Cardiol* 47:1093–1100, 2006
2. Haffner SM, Ruilope L, Dahlof B, Abadie E, Kupfer S, Zannad F: Metabolic syndrome, new onset diabetes, and new end points in cardiovascular trials. *J Cardiovasc Pharmacol* 47:469–475, 2006
3. Marty N, Dallaporta M, Thorens B: Brain glucose sensing, counterregulation, and energy homeostasis. *Physiology (Bethesda)* 22:241–251, 2007
4. Cabou C, Cani PD, Campistron G, Knauf C, Mathieu C, Sartori C, Amar J, Scherrer U, Burcelin R: Central insulin regulates heart rate and arterial blood flow: an endothelial nitric oxide synthase-dependent mechanism altered during diabetes. *Diabetes* 56:2872–2877, 2007
5. Shankar R, Zhu J, Ladd B, Henry D, Shen H, Baron A: Central nervous system nitric oxide synthase activity regulates insulin secretion and insulin action. *J Clin Invest* 102:1403–1412, 1998
6. Holst JJ: The physiology of glucagon-like peptide 1. *Physiol Rev* 87:1409–1439, 2007
7. Jin SL, Han VK, Simmons JG, Towle AC, Lauder JM, Lund PK: Distribution of glucagonlike peptide I (GLP-I), glucagon, and glicentin in the rat brain: an immunocytochemical study. *J Comp Neurol* 271:519–532, 1988
8. Yamamoto H, Lee CE, Marcus JN, Williams TD, Overton JM, Lopez ME, Hollenberg AN, Baggio L, Saper CB, Drucker DJ, Elmquist JK: Glucagon-like peptide-1 receptor stimulation increases blood pressure and heart rate and activates autonomic regulatory neurons. *J Clin Invest* 110:43–52, 2002
9. Delzenne NM, Cani PD, Neyrinck AM: Modulation of glucagon-like peptide 1 and energy metabolism by inulin and oligofructose: experimental data. *J Nutr* 137:2547S–2551S, 2007
10. Burcelin R, Cani PD, Knauf C: Glucagon-like peptide-1 and energy homeostasis. *J Nutr* 137:2534S–2538S, 2007
11. Knauf C, Cani P, Perrin C, Iglesias M, Maury J, Bernard E, Benhamed F, Grémeaux T, Drucker D, Kahn C, Girard J, Tanti J, Delzenne N, Postic C, Burcelin R: Brain glucagon-like peptide-1 increases insulin secretion and muscle insulin resistance to favor hepatic glycogen storage. *J Clin Invest* 115:3554–3563, 2005
12. Burcelin R, Da Costa A, Drucker D, Thorens B: Glucose competence of the hepatoportal vein sensor requires the presence of an activated glucagon-like peptide-1 receptor. *Diabetes* 50:1720–1728, 2001
13. Kearney MT, Cowley AJ, Macdonald IA: The cardiovascular responses to feeding in man. *Exp Physiol* 80:683–700, 1995
14. Barragan JM, Eng J, Rodriguez R, Blazquez E: Neural contribution to the effect of glucagon-like peptide-1-(7-36) amide on arterial blood pressure in rats. *Am J Physiol* 277:E784–E791, 1999
15. Isbil-Buyukcoskun N, Gulec G: Effects of centrally injected GLP-1 in various experimental models of gastric mucosal damage. *Peptides* 25:1179–1183, 2004
16. Svensson A, Ostenson C, Efendic S, Jansson L: Effects of glucagon-like

peptide-1-(7-36)-amide on pancreatic islet and intestinal blood perfusion in Wistar rats and diabetic GK rats. *Clin Sci* 345–351, 2007

17. Perrin C, Knauf C, Burcelin R: Intracerebroventricular infusion of glucose, insulin, and the adenosine monophosphate-activated kinase activator, 5-aminoimidazole-4-carboxamide-1-beta-D-ribofuranoside, controls muscle glycogen synthesis. *Endocrinology* 145:4025–4033, 2004

18. Cani P, Amar J, Iglesias M, Poggi M, Knauf C, Bastelica D, Neyrinck A, Fava F, Tuohy K, Chabo C, Waget A, Delmée E, Cousin B, Sulpice T, Chamontin B, Ferrières J, Tanti J, Gibson G, Casteilla L, Delzenne N, Alessi M, Burcelin R: Metabolic endotoxemia initiates obesity and insulin resistance. *Diabetes* 56:1761–1772, 2007

19. Maximo Cardoso L, de Almeida Colombari DS, Vanderlei Menani J, Alves Chianca D Jr, Colombari E: Cardiovascular responses produced by central injection of hydrogen peroxide in conscious rats. *Brain Res Bull* 71:37–44, 2006

20. Szabados E, Fischer G, Toth K, Csete B, Nemeti B, Trombitas K, Habon T, Endrei D, Sumegi B: Role of reactive oxygen species and poly-ADP-ribose polymerase in the development of AZT-induced cardiomyopathy in rat. *Free Radic Biol Med* 26:309–317, 1999

21. Melnyk S, Pogribna M, Pogribny I, Hine RJ, James SJ: A new HPLC method of the simultaneous determination of oxidized and reduced plasma aminothiols using coulometric electrochemical detection. *J Nutr Biochem* 10:490–497, 1999

22. Suh SW, Hamby AM, Swanson RA: Hypoglycemia, brain energetics, and hypoglycemic neuronal death. *Glia* 55:1280–1286, 2007

23. Nystrom T, Gonon AT, Sjoholm A, Pernow J: Glucagon-like peptide-1 relaxes rat conduit arteries via an endothelium-independent mechanism. *Regul Pept* 125:173–177, 2005

24. Basu A, Charkoudian N, Schrage W, Rizza RA, Basu R, Joyner MJ: Beneficial effects of GLP-1 on endothelial function in humans: dampening by glyburide but not by glimepiride. *Am J Physiol Endocrinol Metab* 293:E1289–E1295, 2007

25. Sokos GG, Bolukoglu H, German J, Hentosz T, Magovern GJ Jr, Maher TD, Dean DA, Bailey SH, Marrone G, Benckart DH, Elahi D, Shannon RP: Effect of glucagon-like peptide-1 (GLP-1) on glycemic control and left ventricular function in patients undergoing coronary artery bypass grafting. *Am J Cardiol* 100:824–829, 2007

26. Saraceni C, Broderick TL: Effects of glucagon-like peptide-1 and long-acting analogues on cardiovascular and metabolic function. *Drugs R D* 8:145–153, 2007

27. Goke R, Larsen PJ, Mikkelsen JD, Sheikh SP: Distribution of GLP-1 binding sites in the rat brain: evidence that exendin-4 is a ligand of brain GLP-1 binding sites. *Eur J Neurosci* 7:2294–2300, 1995

28. Uttenthal LO, Toledano A, Blazquez E: Autoradiographic localization of receptors for glucagon-like peptide-1 (7-36) amide in rat brain. *Neuropeptides* 21:143–146, 1992

29. Burcelin R, Dolci W, Thorens B: Glucose sensing by the hepatoportal sensor is GLUT-2 dependent: in vivo analysis in GLUT-2null mice. *Diabetes* 49:1643–1648, 2000

30. Marty N, Dallaporta M, Foretz M, Emery M, Tarussio D, Bady I, Binnert C, Beermann F, Thorens B: Regulation of glucagon secretion by glucose transporter type 2 (glut2) and astrocyte-dependent glucose sensors. *J Clin Invest* 115:3545–3553, 2005

31. Penicaud L, Leloup C, Fioramonti X, Lorsignol A, Benani A: Brain glucose sensing: a subtle mechanism. *Curr Opin Clin Nutr Metab Care* 9:458–462, 2006

32. Obici S, Feng Z, Karkanias G, Baskin DG, Rossetti L: Decreasing hypothalamic insulin receptors causes hyperphagia and insulin resistance in rats. *Nat Neurosci* 5:566–572, 2002

33. Leloup C, Magnan C, Benani A, Bonnet E, Alquier T, Offer G, Carriere A, Periquet A, Fernandez Y, Ktorza A, Casteilla L, Penicaud L: Mitochondrial reactive oxygen species are required for hypothalamic glucose sensing. *Diabetes* 55:2084–2090, 2006

34. Sandoval DA, Bagnol D, Woods SC, DA D'Alessio, Seeley RJ: Arcuate glucagon-like peptide 1 receptors regulate glucose homeostasis but not food intake. *Diabetes* 57:2046–2054, 2008

35. Knauf C, Cani PD, Kim D-H, Iglesias MA, Chabo C, Waget A, Colom A, Rastrelli S, Delzenne NM, Drucker DJ, Seeley RJ, Burcelin R: Role of central nervous system glucagon-like peptide-1 receptors in enteric glucose sensing. *Diabetes* 57:2603–2612, 2008

GPR119 Is Essential for Oleoylethanolamide-Induced Glucagon-Like Peptide-1 Secretion From the Intestinal Enteroendocrine L-Cell

Lina M. Lauffer,[1] Roman Iakoubov,[1] and Patricia L. Brubaker[1,2]

OBJECTIVE—Intestinal L-cells secrete the incretin glucagon-like peptide-1 (GLP-1) in response to ingestion of nutrients, especially long-chain fatty acids. The $G\alpha s$-coupled receptor GPR119 binds the long-chain fatty acid derivate oleoylethanolamide (OEA), and GPR119 agonists enhance GLP-1 secretion. We therefore hypothesized that OEA stimulates GLP-1 release through a GPR119-dependent mechanism.

RESEARCH DESIGN AND METHODS—Murine (m) GLUTag, human (h) NCI-H716, and primary fetal rat intestinal L-cell models were used for RT-PCR and for cAMP and GLP-1 radioimmunoassay. Anesthetized rats received intravenous or intraileal OEA, and plasma bioactive GLP-1, insulin, and glucose levels were determined by enzyme-linked immunosorbent assay or glucose analyzer.

RESULTS—GPR119 messenger RNA was detected in all L-cell models. OEA treatment (10 μmol/l) of mGLUTag cells increased cAMP levels ($P < 0.05$) and GLP-1 secretion ($P < 0.001$) in all models, with desensitization of the secretory response at higher concentrations. GLP-1 secretion was further enhanced by prevention of OEA degradation using the fatty acid amide hydrolase inhibitor, URB597 ($P < 0.05$–0.001 vs. OEA alone), and was abolished by H89-induced inhibition of protein kinase A. OEA-induced cAMP levels and GLP-1 secretion were significantly reduced in mGLUTag cells transfected with GPR119-specific small interfering RNA ($P < 0.05$). Application of OEA (10 μmol/l) directly into the rat ileum, but not intravenously, increased plasma bioactive GLP-1 levels in euglycemic animals by 1.5-fold ($P < 0.05$) and insulin levels by 3.9-fold ($P < 0.01$) but only in the presence of hyperglycemia.

CONCLUSIONS—The results of these studies demonstrate, for the first time, that OEA increases GLP-1 secretion from intestinal L-cells through activation of the novel GPR119 fatty acid derivate receptor in vitro and in vivo. *Diabetes* **58:1058–1066, 2009**

Glucagon-like peptide-1 (GLP-1) is an intestinal hormone with potent insulinotropic effects that are essential to the maintenance of normal glucose homeostasis (1). In addition to glucose-dependent stimulation of insulin secretion, GLP-1 shows other favorable effects, increasing β-cell proliferation in rodents, as well as enhancing β-cell survival in both rodent and in human islets (2,3). Additionally, GLP-1 has been shown to protect cardiomyocytes from ischemia, and GLP-1 infusion improves cardiac function in patients with heart failure (4,5). Finally, the central nervous system effects of GLP-1 include inhibition of gastric emptying, reduction of appetite, and promotion of satiety in humans (6,7) and rodents (8,9). As a result of its potent antidiabetes and anorexic effects, GLP-1 analogs and GLP-1 degradation inhibitors have been successfully introduced to the clinic for pharmacologic treatment of patients with type 2 diabetes (10).

While the biological effects of GLP-1 have been well established, the mechanisms underlying GLP-1 secretion are less well understood. GLP-1 is secreted from intestinal endocrine L-cells, localized predominantly in the distal ileum and colon (11). Rapid GLP-1 release after food intake (12,13) may be regulated by afferent innervation by the vagus nerve (14,15) as well as, in rodents, by proximal gut hormones, such as glucose-dependent insulinotropic peptide (GIP) from the duodenal K-cells (16). However, L-cells also release GLP-1 in response to direct stimulation by nutrients (16), such as carbohydrates and, most notably, fat (17,18). Monounsaturated long-chain fatty acids, such as oleic acid, are strong stimulators of GLP-1 secretion from the L-cells, both in vitro and in vivo, through a signaling pathway that requires protein kinase C (PKC) ζ (17,18). Additional studies have indicated roles for the orphan G-protein–coupled receptors, GPR40 and GPR120, in the response of the L-cell to saturated fat and α-linolenic acid, respectively (19,20). Very recently, the fatty acid derivate receptor, GPR119, was also found to be expressed in a highly tissue-specific fashion by the intestinal L-cell and the pancreatic β-cell (21,22). Furthermore, a GPR119-specific pharmacological agonist was demonstrated to increase the plasma levels of both GLP-1 and insulin in mice. However, the relevance of physiological ligands of GPR119 to GLP-1 secretion by the L-cell currently remains unknown.

Oleoylethanolamide (OEA) and lysophosphatidylcholine (LPC) are endogenously occurring fatty acid derivates that are specific ligands of GPR119 (23,24). While LPC is often associated with pathophysiological processes such as atherosclerosis (25), OEA is found in a variety of tissues, including the intestinal epithelium, under physiological conditions (26). OEA is synthesized in vivo from membrane phospholipids through an *N*-acylphosphatidylethanolamine (NAPE)-phospholipase D (PLD)-dependent pathway (27); OEA can also be degraded into oleic acid and ethanolamine by the naturally occurring enzyme fatty acid amide hydrolase (FAAH), which is also expressed by the intestinal epithelium (28,29). Intestinal OEA levels are known to decrease during fasting and

From the [1]Department of Physiology, University of Toronto, Toronto, Ontario, Canada; and the [2]Department of Medicine, University of Toronto, Toronto, Ontario, Canada.

Corresponding author: Patricia L. Brubaker, p.brubaker@utoronto.ca.

Received 5 September 2008 and accepted 5 February 2009.

Published ahead of print at http://diabetes.diabetesjournals.org on 17 February 2009. DOI: 10.2337/db08-1237.

TABLE 1
PCR primers

Gene (GenBank accession no.)	Primers (5′–3′)	Position	Amplicon (bp)
m/rGPR119 (NM_181751)	TGATGGTGTTGGCCTTTGCTTCAC	328–351	666
	TGGTAAAGGCAGCATTTGTGGCAG	993–970	
hGPR119 (NM_178471)	TCTCGGCCCACACAGAAGA	208–226	62
	GCTGCGGAGGAAGTGACAAA	269–250	
mGPR40 (NM_194057)	TCTGATCTCCTACTGGCCATCACT	151–175	608
	AGGTCCGGGTTTATGAAACTAGCC	734–758	
hGPR40 (NM_005303)	TTCAGCCTCTCTCTCCTGCTCTTT	550–573	328
	TTCTTGCCGCACACACTGTCTTCA	877–854	
mGPR120 (NM_181748)	TTTCTTCTCGGATGTCAAGGGCGA	126–149	638
	TCCGCGATGCTTTCGTGATCTGTA	763–740	
hGPR120 (NM_181745)	TCGATTTGCACACTGATTTGGCCC	630–653	408
	AAATGTGAAGGCCACCACCCAGAA	1,037–1,014	

increase upon refeeding, and OEA administration to rats reduces food intake, suggesting a role for OEA in the regulation of satiety (26,30–32). As OEA was first identified as a ligand for the intranuclear peroxisome proliferator–activated receptor (PPAR) α, it has been generally assumed that the appetite reduction is dependent on PPARα activation (33). However, as GLP-1 is known to induce satiety, we hypothesized that OEA may also stimulate GLP-1 secretion from the intestinal L-cells in a GPR119-dependent fashion.

RESEARCH DESIGN AND METHODS

Cell models. The murine (m) GLUTag L-cell line was cultured in Dulbecco's modified Eagle's medium (DMEM) containing 25 mmol/l glucose and supplemented with 10% FBS; the medium was changed every 2–3 days and cells were passaged by trypsinization and reseeding at a 1:3 dilution (17,34,35). The human (h) NCI-H716 L-cell line was obtained from the American Type Culture Collection (Manassas, VA). Cells were grown in suspension in RPMI-1640 supplemented with 10% FBS (35,36). Fetal rat intestinal cultures (FRICs) were prepared by enzymatic dispersal of term fetal intestines from 19 to 20 days' pregnant Wistar rats, and cells were maintained overnight in DMEM containing 25 mmol/l glucose, 10% FBS, and penicillin-streptomycin, as previously reported (15,17,35,37). All three models of the intestinal L-cell have been validated with respect to the regulation of GLP-1 secretion, such that GLP-1 is secreted in response to known secretagogues, including muscarinic/cholinergic agonists, leptin and long-chain fatty acids in all models, as well as glucose-dependent insulinotropic peptide (GIP) in the rodent cells (17,34–38).
In vitro experiments. mGLUTag cells were plated in poly-D-lysine–coated 24-well culture plates and grown to 80% confluence. For experiments with hNCI-H716 cells, adhesion of the cells was initiated by plating on Matrigel matrix (Becton Dickinson, Bedford, MA) in DMEM medium, supplemented with 10% FBS, 2 days before the experiment, as described (35,38). FRIC cells were investigated the day after cell dispersal and plating. Adenosine 3′,5′-cyclic monophosphate (cAMP) responses to OEA were determined by washing mGLUTag cells with Hanks' balanced salt solution followed by treatment for 30 min with FBS-free medium containing 1% DMSO alone (negative control), 10 μmol/l forskolin (positive control), or 10–15 μmol/l OEA, as previously described (39). To prevent cAMP degradation, all media contained 10 μmol/l 3-isobutyl-1-methylxanthine (Sigma-Aldrich, Oakville, ON, Canada). Cells were then extracted in ethanol for radioimmunoassay (RIA) of cAMP content. Secretion experiments were performed as described (17,34–36). In brief, mGLUTag, hNCI-H716, and FRIC cells were washed and then incubated for 2 h with FBS-free DMEM containing 1% DMSO alone (negative control), 10 μmol/l forskolin (Sigma-Aldrich), or 1 μmol/l GIP (positive controls) (Bachem, Torrance, CA) or with different concentrations of OEA, palmitoylethanolamide (PEA), or LPC (all from Sigma-Aldrich). Some cells were preincubated for 30 min with 10 μmol/l or 30 μmol/l H89 (Sigma-Aldrich) to inhibit protein kinase A (PKA) or with 1 μmol/l URB597 (Calbiochem, Mississauga, ON, Canada), an FAAH inhibitor (29). DMSO was used as a solvent to prepare stock solutions of fatty acid derivates and inhibitors. For secretion experiments, medium and cells were collected separately and peptides were extracted by reversed-phase adsorption using C_{18} silica cartridges (Sep-Pak; Waters Scientific, Mississauga, ON, Canada), as previously

described (17,34–36), for RIA of GLP-1 content. GLP-1 secretion was calculated as total GLP-1 content of medium normalized for the total amount of GLP-1 in the medium plus cells. Average basal secretion of mGLUTa, hNCI-H716, and FRIC cells was 3.4 ± 0.3% (n = 31), 2.7 ± 0.4% (n = 28), and 2.86 ± 0.6% (n = 4), respectively, of total GLP-1. No changes in total GLP-1 content were found under any of the experimental conditions (data not shown).
Small interfering RNA transfection. mGLUTag cells were plated in a 24-well plate, as described above. Scrambled small interfering RNA (siRNA) (control) and two siRNAs targeting murine GPR119 coding sequences were purchased from Ambion (Austin, TX). Transfection was performed by 5-h incubation in Opti-Mem medium using 20 pmol/l siRNA and 1 μl Lipofectamine 2000 (Invitrogen, Burlington, ON, Canada) as instructed by the manufacturer. Cells were allowed to recover for 2 days before cAMP and/or secretion experiments. Transfection efficiency was quantified by real-time RT-PCR. In brief, total RNA was extracted from mGLUTag cells using an RNeasy kit as instructed by the manufacturer (Qiagen, Mississauga, ON, Canada) and subjected to reverse transcription using SuperScript II and random hexamers (Invitrogen), followed by real-time PCR using TaqMan gene expression assays (Applied Biosystems, Foster City, CA) for GPR119 (Mm00731497_s1) and 18S (Hs99999901_s1; endogenous control). Relative quantification of GPR119 mRNA expression was calculated using the $\Delta\Delta$ cycle threshold method (40).
In vitro assays. Viability of the mGLUTag cells after treatment was determined using the 3-(4,5-dimethylthiazol-2-yl)-2,5-diphenyltetrazolium bromide (MTT) (Sigma-Aldrich) assay, as reported (17). Cells were plated in poly-D-lysine–coated 96-well plates and treated for 2 h with medium containing 1% DMSO alone (control), 5 mmol/l H_2O_2 (positive control), or fatty acid derivates or inhibitors at concentrations used for the secretion experiment, after which the MTT reaction was carried out. The resulting absorbance was measured at 570 nm; higher absorbance correlates with cell viability and lower absorbance with cell death. cAMP was measured by RIA of ethanol extracts as described (39) (Biomedical Technologies, Stoughton, MA). RIA for COOH-terminal GLP-1 immunoreactivity was conducted using an established lab assay (17,34–36).
As there is currently no good GPR119 antiserum commercially available, GPR119 expression was determined by RT-PCR. Human jejunum and colon total RNA was purchased from Ambion, and human placental RNA was a kind gift from Dr. J.R. Challis (University of Toronto, Toronto, ON, Canada). Total RNA from mGLUTag, hNCI-H716, and FRIC cells, as well as from rodent tissues, was extracted as described above. The primer pairs used for amplification of human GPR119 were described by Soga et al. (23) and for mouse GPR40 and GPR120 by Iakoubov et al. (17); all other primer pairs were designed using PrimerQuest (IDT, Coralville, IA) (sequences are shown in Table 1). PCR were carried out at 57°C for 35 cycles, and PCR without RNA template was used as the negative control. Products were analyzed by agarose gel electrophoresis and visualized with ethidium bromide.
In vivo experiments. In vivo animal protocols were approved by the University of Toronto Animal Care Committee. Male Wistar rats (200–300 g) were obtained from Charles River Laboratories (St. Constant, QC, Canada) and maintained on a standard laboratory diet with free access to water under a 12-h light-dark schedule. Following an overnight fast, rats were anesthetized with isoflurane (Baxter, Mississauga, ON, Canada). One hour before blood sampling, some rats were intraperitoneally injected with 3 mg/kg URB597 to inhibit FAAH (29,41). URB597 alone did not affect the levels of glucose,

insulin, or bioactive GLP-1 in these studies; therefore, data from rats with and without URB597 injection were combined. The carotid artery was cannulated for blood sampling and the jugular vein for injections. To prevent bioactive GLP-1 degradation by dipeptidylpeptidase (DPP) IV, rats received 5 mg/kg Sitagliptin (Januvia; MSD Sharp & Dohme, Haar, Germany), a selective inhibitor of DPP-IV (10,42), intravenously 30 min before blood collection. Some rats also received a femoral vein cannula for continuous infusion of 37.5% glucose to maintain glycemia at 13 mmol/l for at least 30 min. The glucose infusion rate was adjusted based on frequent (every 5–10 min) blood glucose measurements, as described in Goh et al. (43). Rats undergoing a hyperglycemic clamp were not pretreated with Sitagliptin in order to reduce the number of variables that might affect glycemia. The abdominal cavity of all rats was then opened and a 10-cm section of the distal ileum was cleansed by perfusion with saline and tied off to create a luminally distinct compartment that retained vascular perfusion. Subsequent to collection of the basal blood sample at $t = 0$ min, either the luminal compartment was filled with 2 ml of 10 μmol/l OEA or vehicle (0.9% saline/10% Tween 80; Sigma-Aldrich), or 5 mg/kg OEA or vehicle (0.9% saline/10% Tween 80) was administered intravenously, and additional blood samples were collected at 5, 15, 30, and 60 min. All samples (1 ml each) were collected into 10% (vol/vol) Trasylol (5,000 Kalikrein inactivating units/ml; Bayer, Toronto, ON, Canada), EDTA (12 mg/ml), and diprotin A (a DPP-IV inhibitor, 68 mg/ml; Sigma-Aldrich), and plasma was stored at −80°C until analysis. Plasma glucose levels were analyzed on a Beckman Analyzer II (Beckman, Fullerton, CA), and plasma insulin levels were measured by enzyme-linked immunosorbent assay (Crystal Chem, Downers Grove, IL) in normoglycemic animals and by RIA (Millipore, Billerica, MA) in hyperglycemic animals due to the wider insulin detection range. Plasma levels of bioactive GLP-1 were determined by electrochemiluminescence-based detection assay (Meso Scale Discovery, Gaithersburg, MD).

Statistical analyses. All results are expressed as means ± SE. Area under the curve (AUC) was determined using the trapezoidal rule, and the data are expressed per min. Statistical analysis was performed using SAS software (SAS Institute, Cary, NC). One- and two-way ANOVA was followed by Student's t test or n-1 custom hypotheses post hoc tests, as appropriate. To reduce interassay variations, some data were normalized to basal levels. Significance was assumed at $P < 0.05$.

RESULTS

Expression of GPR40, GPR119, and GPR120. RT-PCR for rodent GPR119 mRNA transcripts was performed on total RNA extracted from mGLUTag and FRIC cells, as well as from mouse ileum and rat colon tissue. As shown in Fig. 1A, GPR119 mRNA was detected in both rodent L-cell models, as well as in the intestinal samples. Additionally, GPR119 mRNA was detected in the hNCI-H716 cells and in human colon and placental tissue (Fig. 1B). In contrast to previous reports (22), we did not detect GPR119 mRNA in human jejunum, possibly due to a low number of L-cells in this tissue (11). Consistent with our previous findings (17), mRNA transcripts for both GPR40 and GPR120 were detected in the mGLUTag cells, and both receptor mRNAs were also found to be expressed in the hNCI-H716 cells (Fig. 1C).

OEA induces GLP-1 secretion in vitro. Possible effects of GPR119 receptor activation on GLP-1 secretion were first investigated in mGLUTag cells. Release of GLP-1 was increased to 3.1 ± 0.4–fold of basal values by treatment with forskolin, a direct activator of adenylyl cyclase and strong L-cell secretagogue (34). OEA (5–20 μmol/l), a known ligand of GPR119 (24), significantly increased GLP-1 secretion to a maximum of 2.1 ± 0.2–fold of basal levels at 10 μmol/l ($P < 0.001$) (Fig. 2A). The same concentrations of PEA, a saturated fatty acid ethanolamide (16:0) that is a very weak agonist of GPR119 (23,24), did not increase GLP-1 secretion from mGLUTag cells. Importantly, OEA treatment did not affect the viability of the GLUTag cells (Fig. 2B). In contrast, although LPC treatment of mGLUTag cells at concentrations reported to activate GPR119 (10–15 μmol/l) also enhanced GLP-1 release (to a maximum of 10.4 ± 0.5–fold of control values;

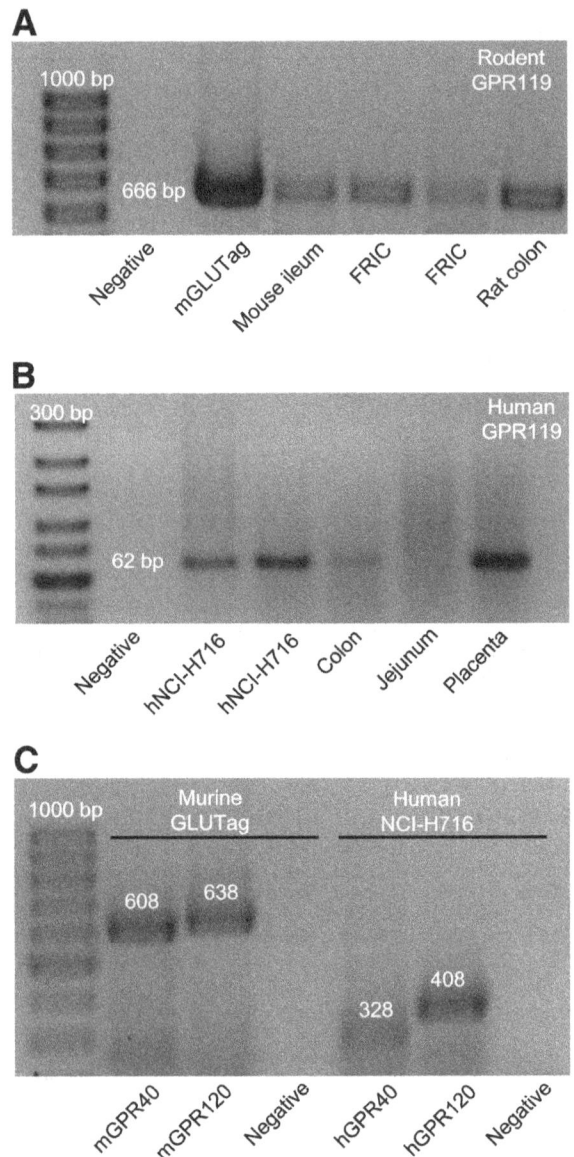

FIG. 1. Expression of GPR119 mRNA in L-cell models. **A:** Total RNA from mGLUTag cells, FRICs, and murine intestinal tissues was analyzed for expression of GPR119 mRNA by RT-PCR. **B:** Total RNA from hNCI-H716 cells, human intestinal tissues, and human placenta was analyzed for expression of GPR119 mRNA by RT-PCR. **C:** Total RNA from mGLUTag cells and hNCI-H716 cells was analyzed for expression of GPR40 and GPR120 mRNA by RT-PCR. All products were separated on agarose gels and visualized with ethidium bromide, with the molecular-size ladder on the left. Negative controls did not include RNA template. The anticipated band sizes of products are indicated in base pairs (bp).

data not shown), LPC was found to markedly reduce cell viability by up to 60.0 ± 6.8% compared with control cells ($P < 0.05$ and $P < 0.001$) (Fig. 2B); LPC was, therefore, not used in further experiments. The effects of OEA on GLP-1 secretion were also confirmed in hNCI-H716 and FRIC cells (Fig. 2C and D), wherein OEA treatment significantly increased GLP-1 secretion to 2.6 ± 0.2– and 5.8 ± 2.5–fold of basal levels at 10 μmol/l ($P < 0.001$ and $P < 0.01$), respectively. Interestingly, higher concentrations of OEA were associated with diminished GLP-1 release in all cell models, suggestive of desensitization.

To verify the activity of GPR119 in the L-cell, mGLUTag and hNCI-H716 cells were treated with a specific GPR119

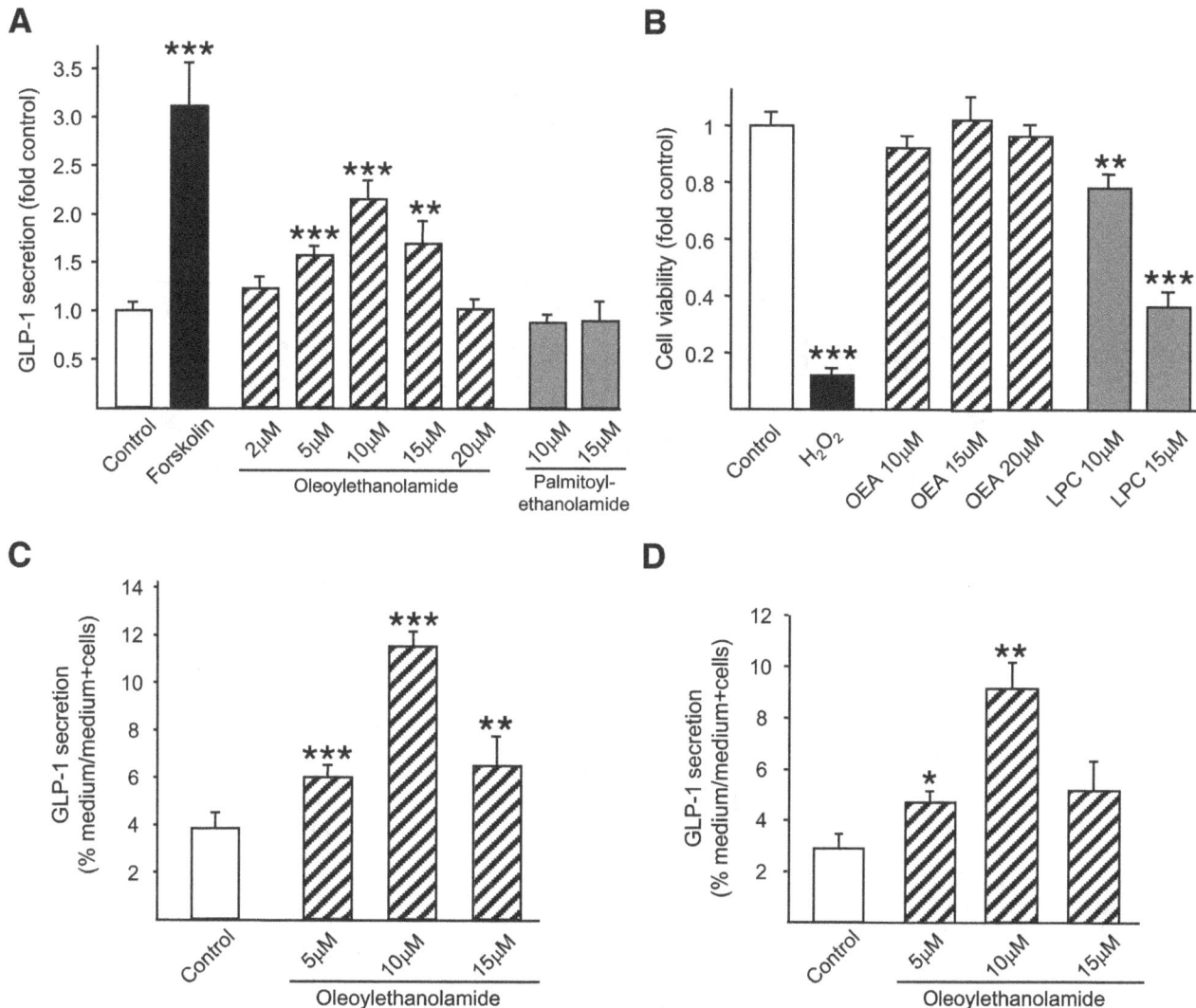

FIG. 2. Effects of OEA on GLP-1 secretion. mGLUTag cells ($n = 9–12$) (*A*), hNCI-H716 cells ($n = 8$) (*C*), and FRIC cells ($n = 4$) (*D*) were incubated with medium alone (1% DMSO, negative control), forskolin (10 μmol/l, positive control), OEA (2–20 μmol/l), or PEA (10–15 μmol/l, negative control) for 2 h. GLP-1 content of media and cells was determined by RIA. *B*: To determine potential effects on cell viability, mGLUTag cells were incubated with medium alone (1% DMSO, negative control), H_2O_2 (5 mmol/l, positive control), OEA (10–20 μmol/l), or LPC (10–15 μmol/l) for 2 h, followed by MTT assay ($n = 8–16$). *$P < 0.05$; **$P < 0.01$; ***$P < 0.001$ vs. control.

agonist, PSN632408 (10 μmol/l) (24). PSN632408 increased GLP-1 secretion by both cell lines to 2.1 ± 0.2– and 2.9 ± 0.5–fold of basal values ($P < 0.01$ for mGLUTag and $P < 0.05$ for hNCI-H716 cells) (Fig. 3), demonstrating that GPR119 is functional and can initiate GLP-1 secretion in these cells. To determine possible function of the other fatty acid receptors expressed in the L-cell lines GPR40 and GPR120 (Fig. 1*C*), both mGLUTag and hNCI-H716 cells were also treated with the combined GPR40/GPR120 agonist GW9508 (10 μmol/l) (24). Consistent with previous findings from our group (17), GPR40 and GPR120 were not found to be involved in GLP-1 secretion from mGLUTag cells, as treatment with GW9508 did not increase GLP-1 secretion (Fig. 3). In contrast, GW9508 increased GLP-1 secretion by hNCI-H716 cells to 4.5 ± 0.6–fold of basal values ($P < 0.01$), providing indication for a role of GPR40 and/or GPR120 in human L-cells.

Prevention of OEA degradation with URB597 significantly increased OEA-induced GLP-1 secretion to 3.2 ± 0.4– and 3.3 ± 0.3–fold of control values at 10 and 15 μmol/l

OEA in mGLUTag cells ($P < 0.001$ compared with URB597 alone and $P < 0.01–0.001$ compared with OEA treatment without URB597) (Fig. 4*A*), as well as in hNCI-H716 cells (to 3.5 ± 0.2– and 5.5 ± 0.7–fold of control values at 10 and 15 μmol/l OEA ($P < 0.001$ compared with URB597 alone and $P < 0.05–0.001$ compared with OEA treatment without URB597) (Fig. 4*B*). These findings indicate that degradation by FAAH limits the effects of OEA on GLP-1 secretion in both of the intestinal L-cell lines utilized.

OEA signals through a PKA- and GPR119-dependent mechanism. As ligand binding to GPR119 leads to activation of adenylyl cyclase, increased production of cAMP, and enhanced PKA activity (24), mGLUTag cells were first examined for cAMP responses to OEA (10–15 μmol/l) and GIP, which is known to signal through cAMP- and PKA-dependent pathways (positive control) (44). OEA treatment alone caused a small but significant increase in intracellular cAMP to 1.11 ± 0.03 – and 1.12 ± 0.04–fold of control values at 10 and 15 μmol/l, respectively ($P < 0.05$) (Fig. 5*A*). This effect was enhanced when OEA degradation

A

B

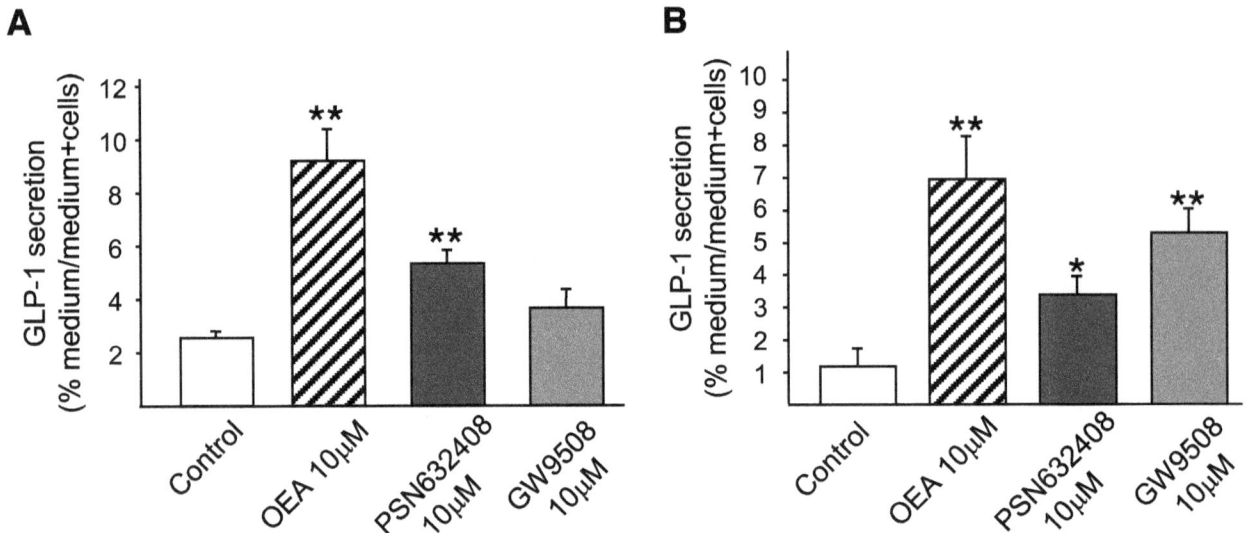

FIG. 3. Effects of GPR119 and GPR40/120 agonists on GLP-1 secretion. mGLUTag ($n = 4$) (A) and hNCI-H716 ($n = 4$) (B) cells were incubated with medium alone (1% DMSO, negative control), OEA (10 μmol/l), the GPR119 agonist PSN632408 (10 μmol/l), or the combined GPR40/GPR120 agonist GW9508 (10 μmol/l) for 2 h. GLP-1 content of media and cells was determined by RIA. *$P < 0.05$; **$P < 0.01$ vs. control.

was prevented with URB597, such that cAMP levels increased by an additional 1.3 ± 0.04 – and 1.3 ± 0.03–fold, respectively ($P < 0.001$ compared with URBB597 alone and $P < 0.05$–0.01 compared with OEA treatment without URB597). Furthermore, pretreatment of the mGLUTag cells with the PKA inhibitor H89 (10 μmol/l) completely abolished OEA (10–15 μmol/l)-induced GLP-1 secretion (Fig. 5B). Similar results were found in hNCI-H716 cells, although an increased concentration of H89 (30 μmol/l) was required to abrogate OEA-induced GLP-1 release (Fig. 5C). H89 treatment did not affect GPR40/120-induced GLP-1 secretion (Fig. 5C, $inset$), demonstrating the specificity of this inhibitor for PKA-mediated signaling.

To determine whether the effects of OEA on cAMP production and GLP-1 secretion are dependent upon GPR119, mGLUTag cells were transfected with specific GPR119 siRNA or scrambled siRNA (control), resulting in 23% knockdown of GPR119 mRNA, as determined by real-time RT-PCR (Fig. 6A, $inset$). Despite the relatively low level of GPR119 knockdown, OEA (10 μmol/l) failed to enhance cAMP levels in cells treated with GPR119 siRNA, whereas the cAMP response to OEA treatment was preserved in the control cells ($P < 0.05$) (Fig. 6A). Furthermore, GPR119 knockdown led to a 45% reduction in the GLP-1 secretory response to OEA ($P < 0.05$) (Fig. 5B). These data therefore provide support for a role of GPR119 and the PKA signaling pathway in OEA-induced GLP-1 secretion.

OEA enhances GLP-1 secretion in vivo. To establish the effects of OEA on the L-cell in vivo, rats were treated with OEA either intraluminally or intravenously. Intraluminal application of OEA (10 μmol/l; e.g., 20 nmol/rat) to euglycemic rats significantly increased plasma bioactive GLP-1 concentrations to 1.5 ± 0.2–fold of basal values ($P < 0.05$) within 5 min of administration, and this stimulation was maintained throughout the entire 60-min time course of the experiment (Fig. 7A). Thus, the AUC for the bioactive GLP-1 response was significantly increased to 1.6 ± 0.1–fold of vehicle-infused rats ($P < 0.001$) (Fig. 7B). In contrast, intravenous administration of OEA at a 200-fold–higher dose (e.g., 4 μmol/250 g rat) than that

used intraluminally demonstrated no effect on bioactive GLP-1 concentrations compared with rats treated with vehicle alone. Throughout the 60-min experiment, the plasma levels of glucose (Fig. 7C) and insulin (Fig. 7D) remained stable at basal levels and did not differ between treatment and control groups.

As GLP-1 is known to lose its insulinotropic effects under normoglycemic conditions, changes in insulin levels upon OEA treatment were also measured under hyperglycemic conditions. Glycemia was maintained at 13 mmol/l, the upper physiological level in rats, for at least 30 min before the start of OEA application and throughout the remainder of the procedure. The basal concentration of insulin before OEA application was 1.4 ± 0.4 pg/ml and did not differ between the groups. Intraluminal application of OEA caused a 3.9 ± 0.7–fold increase in insulin plasma levels within 5 min of application (11.2 ± 2.1 vs. 2.8 ± 2.0 pg/ml in the control group; $P < 0.01$) (Fig. 7D, $inset$). In contrast, intravenous infusion of OEA did not affect insulin levels during the entire treatment period in the hyperglycemic rats.

DISCUSSION

Previous studies have indicated that the fatty acid derivate receptor GPR119 is present on pancreatic β-cells and intestinal L-cells, and its stimulation by a GPR119 agonist increases insulin and GLP-1 secretion, respectively (21,22,24). However, the role of physiologically occurring ligands of GPR119, such as OEA, and the intracellular mechanisms underlying GPR119-dependent GLP-1 secretion from the intestinal L-cell have remained undefined. The results of the present study demonstrate, for the first time, that OEA stimulates GLP-1 secretion from both mouse and human intestinal L-cell lines, as well as from primary rat L-cells in vitro. Additionally, application of OEA directly into the intestinal lumen in rats induced a significant and persistent increase in bioactive GLP-1 levels over 1 h, supporting the in vitro findings and demonstrating a role for OEA as a GLP-1 secretagogue in vivo.

A

B

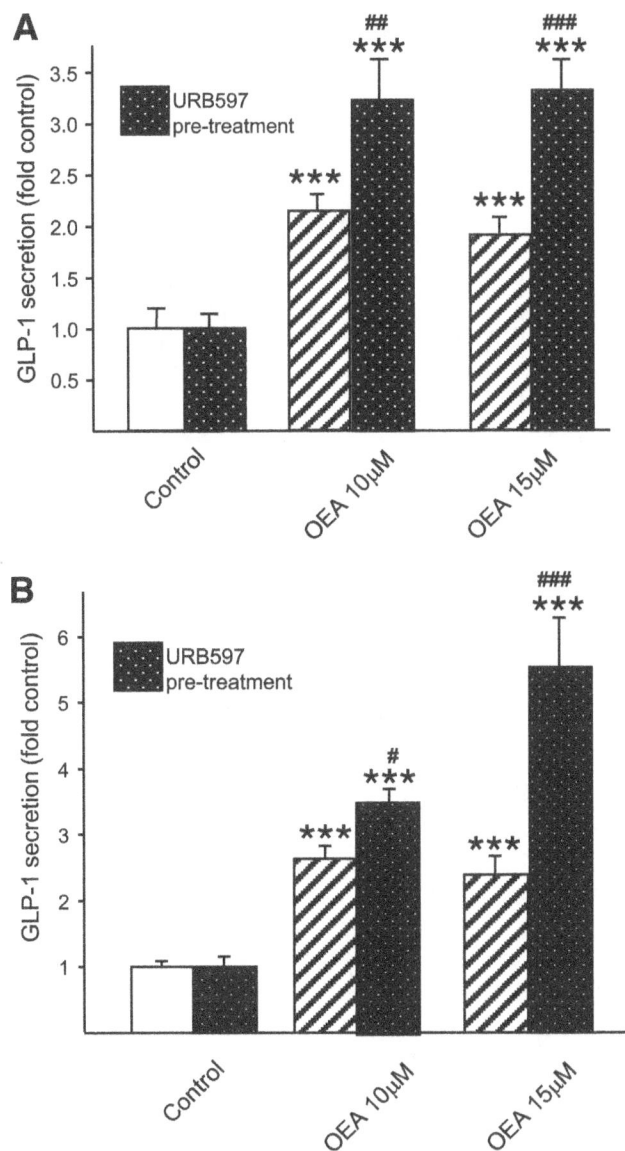

FIG. 4. Effect of inhibition of OEA degradation on OEA-induced GLP-1 secretion. mGLUTag ($n = 6$–18) (*A*) and hNCI-H716 ($n = 12$) (*B*) cells were pretreated for 30 min with URB597 (1 μmol/l) to inhibit FAAH and prevent OEA degradation before incubation with medium alone (1%DMSO, negative control) or OEA (10–15 μmol/l) for 2 h. GLP-1 content of media and cells was determined by RIA. ***$P < 0.001$ vs. control; #$P < 0.05$; ##$P < 0.01$; ###$P < 0.001$ vs. OEA treatment alone.

To further establish the role of OEA in GLP-1 secretion, the intracellular signaling mechanisms underlying its effects on the L-cell were investigated. OEA induced a small, but significant, increase in intracellular cAMP concentration in both the mGLUTag and hNCI-H716 cells, comparable with findings in OEA-treated RINm5 and MIN6 pancreatic β-cell lines (45). Furthermore, GLP-1 secretion in OEA-treated cells was strictly dependent on PKA in both the human and mouse L-cells, as indicated by complete abrogation of the response in H89-treated cells. These findings are consistent with studies by our lab and others showing that increased cAMP levels, in response to cAMP analogs as well as to secretagogues such as GIP, stimulate GLP-1 release by the intestinal L-cell (16,34,46). Furthermore, while initial studies on OEA identified the intranuclear receptor PPARα and transient receptor po-

tential vanilloid type 1 (TRPV1) as targets for OEA (27,33,47), neither of these receptors has been reported to stimulate the cAMP/PKA signaling pathway. In contrast, the deorphanization of GPR119 as a cAMP-linked OEA receptor (24) implicated GPR119 as more likely target for OEA in the intestinal L-cell. Consistent with this hypothesis, treatment of human and mouse intestinal L-cells with a GPR119-specific agonist PSN632408 significantly increased GLP-1 secretion in both cell lines. Furthermore, transfection of mGLUTag cells with GPR119 siRNA significantly diminished both the cAMP and GLP-1 responses to OEA. When taken together, these findings provide support for both the presence of functional GPR119 in the intestinal L-cell and the requirement for this novel G-protein–coupled receptor in OEA-induced GLP-1 secretion.

We have previously reported that oleic acid is a strong L-cell secretagogue, increasing GLP-1 secretion both in vivo and in vitro (17,18,48). It is therefore interesting that OEA is rapidly degraded to oleic acid and ethanolamide via FAAH-dependent hydrolysis (29), thereby providing a possible GPR119-independent mechanism underlying OEA-induced GLP-1 secretion. Therefore, to exclude the possible effects of oleic acid on the actions of OEA, L-cells were pretreated with the FAAH inhibitor URB597 to reduce OEA hydrolysis and resultant oleic acid accumulation. The increase in OEA-induced GLP-1 secretion found with URB597 treatment provides support for a direct role of OEA, and not of oleic acid, in OEA-induced GLP-1 secretion.

While intraluminal application of OEA in vivo significantly increased GLP-1 secretion in normal rats, intravenous injection of OEA at a 200-fold–higher dose failed to increase circulating levels of bioactive GLP-1. Additionally, while intraluminal OEA application clearly increased insulin levels in hyperglycemic rats, intravenous injection of OEA did not affect insulin levels in these animals under either euglycemic or hyperglycemic conditions. Taken together, this data suggests that circulating OEA does not cause significant increases in hormone release from either of its known target tissues (the intestinal L-cell and the pancreatic β-cell). There are several possible explanations for these findings. First, the volume of distribution for OEA as a lipophilic substance should be high, therefore increasing the concentration of OEA required for administration into the jugular vein to reach distant target tissues at stimulatory concentrations. However, higher levels of OEA cannot be achieved in the circulation of the rat due to the limited solubility of OEA in solvents. Furthermore, whether OEA is cleared through the liver and/or lungs is unknown and may be significant.

The actions of both OEA and a GRP119 agonist on insulin secretion have previously been reported to be glucose dependent (21,45), as further confirmed in the present study. Previous studies have also demonstrated that ~45% of the glucose-lowering effect of an oral GPR119 agonist given concurrently with oral glucose is mediated through enhancement of GLP-1 release (22), suggesting that the insulinotropic effect of GPR119 activation is mediated both directly, through GPR119 expressed on the β-cell, and indirectly, through enhanced release of GLP-1. Nonetheless, although both the L-cell and the β-cell are responsive to OEA, the glucose sensitivity of the β-cell response, compared with the glucose insensitivity of the L-cell response that we have observed, suggests that oral administration of this fatty acid derivate alone to enhance GLP-1 secretion, without influencing insulin release, will

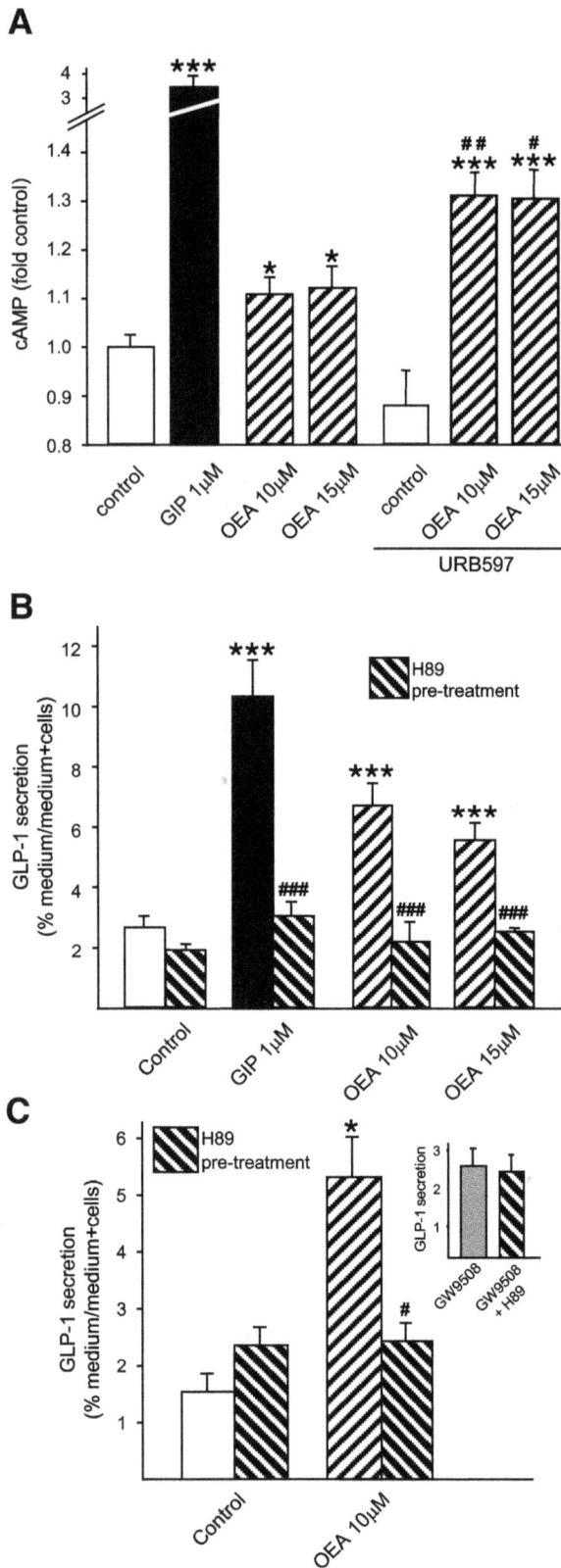

FIG. 5. Effect of PKA inhibition on OEA-induced GLP-1 secretion. mGLUTag ($n = 6$–9) (A and B) and hNCI-H716 ($n = 4$–6) (C) cells were pretreated for 30 min with medium alone (1% DMSO, negative control), H89 (10 µmol/l for mGLUTag and 30 µmol/l for hNCI-H716), or URB597 (1 µmol/l) to inhibit PKA or FAAH, respectively, followed by incubation with medium alone (1% DMSO, negative control), GIP (1 µmol/l, positive control), or OEA (10–15 µmol/l) for 2 h. C, inset: hNCI-H716 cells were pretreated for 30 min with media alone (1%

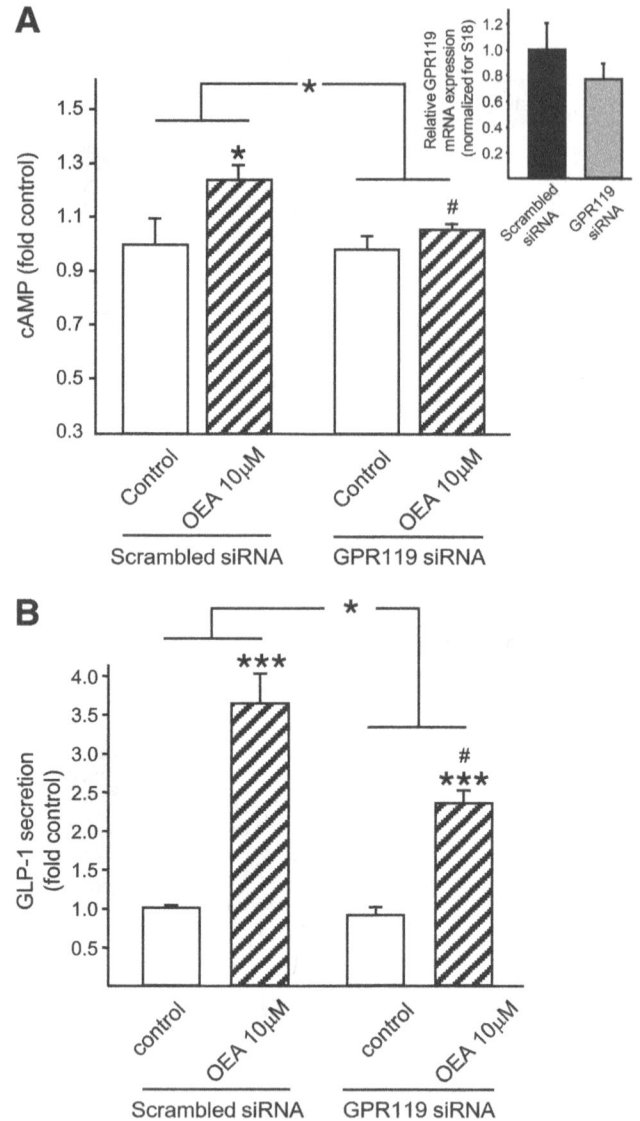

FIG. 6. Effect of GPR119 knockdown on OEA-induced GLP-1 secretion. mGLUTag cells were transfected with scrambled siRNA (20 pmol/l, control) or GPR119 siRNA (20 pmol/l) 2 days before the experiment. Cells were then incubated with medium alone (1% DMSO, negative control) or OEA (10–15 µmol/l) for 2 h. cAMP content of cells ($n = 6$) (A) and GLP-1 content of media and cells ($n = 9$) (B) were determined by RIA. A, inset: GPR119 mRNA transcript levels were determined by quantitative RT-PCR relative to 18S transcript levels. *$P < 0.05$; ***$P < 0.001$ vs. control or vs. the Δ change in control cells, as indicated by the lines. #$P < 0.05$ vs. OEA treatment with scrambled siRNA.

permit the insulin-independent biological actions of GLP-1. In contrast, administration of OEA in the setting of a glucose-containing meal would facilitate release of both GLP-1 and insulin, thereby also modulating glycemic responses (22,49).

The observation of apparent desensitization in all of the dose-response curves was unexpected, as this has not previously been reported for GPR119. However, Gαs-coupled receptors are well established to undergo homol-

DMSO) or with H89 (30 µmol/l), followed by incubation with the GPR40/120 agonist GW9508 (10 µmol/l). cAMP content of cells and GLP-1 content of media and cells were determined by RIA. *$P < 0.05$; ***$P < 0.001$ vs. appropriate control; #$P < 0.05$; ##$P < 0.01$; ###$P < 0.001$ vs. paired treatment alone.

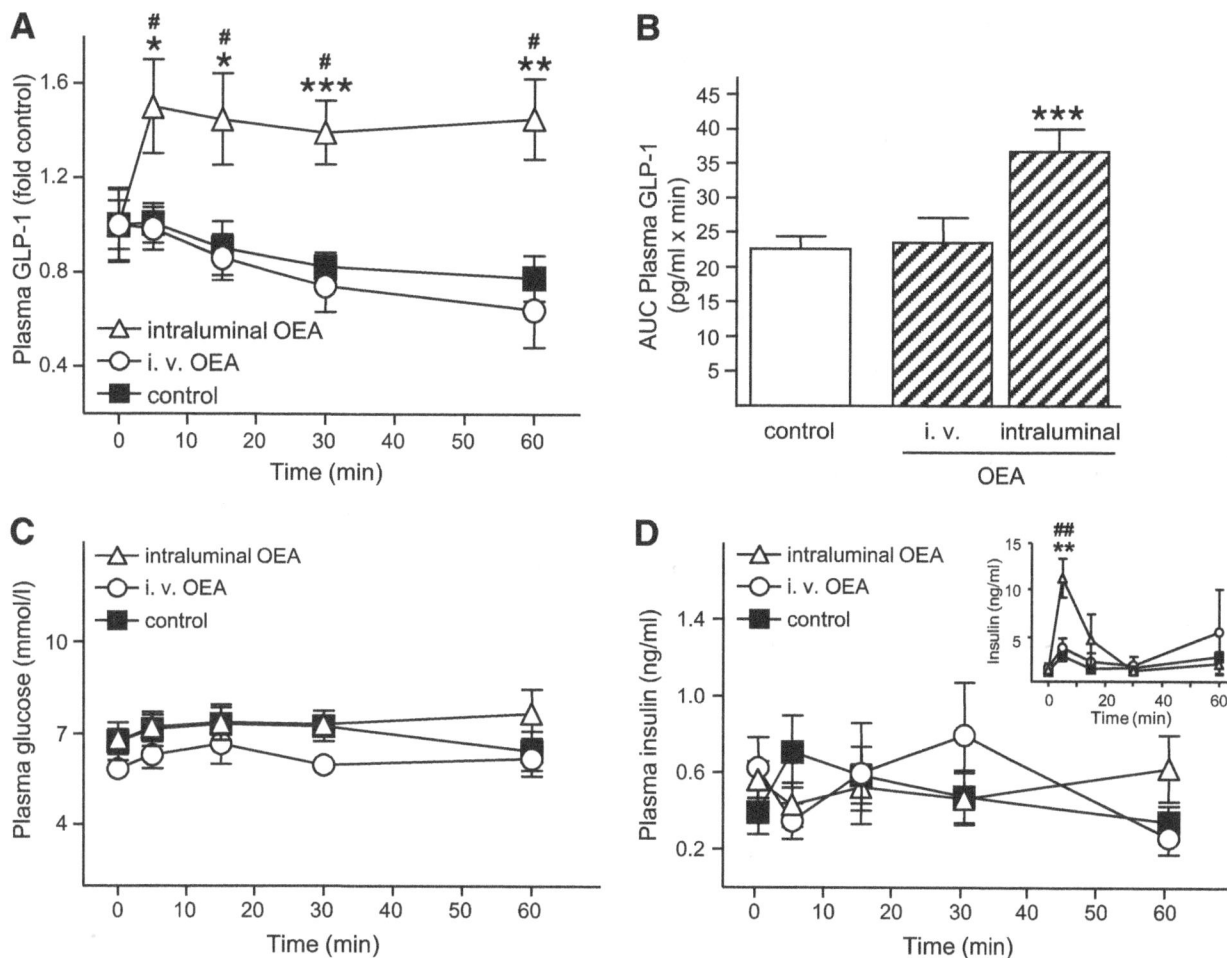

FIG. 7. In vivo effect of OEA on GLP-1 secretion. Anesthetized rats received intraluminal or intravenous injections of vehicle (saline/10% Tween 80; combined controls), intraluminal OEA (2 ml of 10 μmol/l), or intravenous OEA (5 mg/kg), and blood samples were collected over a 1-h period. Plasma concentrations of bioactive GLP-1 (*A*), glucose (*C*), and insulin (*D*) were determined by ELISA and glucose analyzer, as appropriate (*n* = 5–11). *B*: AUC for the absolute plasma bioactive GLP-1 concentrations was determined using the trapezoidal rule and is expressed per min. *D*, *inset*: Rats (*n* = 4–5) were maintained at 13 mmol/l plasma glucose (hyperglycemic clamp) for a minimum of 30 min, and this was maintained throughout the OEA treatment procedure. Plasma insulin levels were determined by RIA. *A*: To reduce interassay variations due to use of separate kits, bioactive GLP-1 concentrations were calculated as fold increase over basal GLP-1 levels (control: 29.4 ± 8.6 pg/ml; intraluminal OEA: 18.9 ± 4.9 pg/ml; and intravenous OEA: 32.7 ± 3.4 pg/ml; *P* = NS between the basal values). *$P < 0.05$ vs. control; **$P < 0.01$ vs. control; ***$P < 0.001$ vs. control; #$P < 0.05$ and ##$P < 0.01$ vs. basal values.

ogous desensitization (50); indeed, preliminary studies in which hNCI-716 cells were pretreated with the GPR119 agonist PSN632408 (10 μmol/l for 6 h) demonstrated a 70.9 ± 4.6% and 50.7 ± 11.7% decrease in subsequent OEA- and PSN632408-induced GLP-1 secretion, respectively (data not shown). Collectively, these findings indicate that GPR119 may undergo homologous desensitization, a phenomenon that clearly warrants further investigation.

In summary, the results of this study establish, for the first time, the role of GPR119 in OEA-induced GLP-1 secretion and add GPR119 to the growing list of fatty acid–responsive pathways that function to modulate release of GLP-1, including GPR40, GPR120, and PKCζ. When combined with the reported insulinotropic effects of GPR119 agonists, these findings implicate GPR119 as a potential pharmacological target, as well as OEA as a nutriceutical approach to enhance GLP-1 in patients with type 2 diabetes.

ACKNOWLEDGMENTS

L.M.L. was supported by postdoctoral fellowships from the European Foundation for the Study of Diabetes (EFSD; Albert Renold and EFSD/Lilly Research Fellowships). R.I. was supported by postdoctoral fellowships from the Banting and Best Diabetes Centre, University of Toronto (Toronto, ON, Canada), and from Deutsche Forschungsgemeinschaft (DFG; the German Research Foundation). P.L.B. was supported by the Canada Research Chairs Program. This work was supported by an operating grant from the Canadian Diabetes Association (no. 2374). No other potential conflicts of interest relevant to this article were reported.

The authors are grateful to J.R. Challis (University of Toronto, Toronto, ON, Canada) for the gift of placental RNA.

REFERENCES

1. Drucker DJ. The biology of incretin hormones. Cell Metab 2006;3:153–165
2. Wang Q, Brubaker PL. Glucagon-like peptide-1 treatment delays the onset of diabetes in 8 week-old db/db mice. Diabetologia 2002;45:1263–1273
3. Farilla L, Bulotta A, Hirshberg B, Li Calzi S, Khoury N, Noushmehr H, Bertolotto C, Di Mario U, Harlan DM, Perfetti R. Glucagon-like peptide 1 inhibits cell apoptosis and improves glucose responsiveness of freshly isolated human islets. Endocrinology 2003;144:5149–5158
4. Sokos GG, Nikolaidis LA, Mankad S, Elahi D, Shannon RP. Glucagon-like peptide-1 infusion improves left ventricular ejection fraction and func-

tional status in patients with chronic heart failure. J Card Fail 2006;12: 694–699

5. Ban K, Noyan-Ashraf MH, Hoefer J, Bolz SS, Drucker DJ, Husain M. Cardioprotective and vasodilatory actions of glucagon-like peptide 1 receptor are mediated through both glucagon-like peptide 1 receptor-dependent and -independent pathways. Circulation 2008;117:2340–2350

6. Flint A, Raben A, Ersboll AK, Holst JJ, Astrup A. The effect of physiological levels of glucagon-like peptide-1 on appetite, gastric emptying, energy and substrate metabolism in obesity. Int J Obes Relat Metab Disord 2001;25: 781–792

7. Meier JJ, Gallwitz B, Salmen S, Goetze O, Holst JJ, Schmidt WE, Nauck MA. Normalization of glucose concentrations and deceleration of gastric emptying after solid meals during intravenous glucagon-like peptide 1 in patients with type 2 diabetes. J Clin Endocrinol Metab 2003;88:2719–2725

8. Tang-Christensen M, Larsen PJ, Goke R, Fink-Jensen A, Jessop DS, Moller M, Sheikh SP. Central administration of GLP-1-(7–36) amide inhibits food and water intake in rats. Am J Physiol 1996;271:R848–R856

9. Talsania T, Anini Y, Siu S, Drucker DJ, Brubaker PL. Peripheral exendin-4 and peptide YY(3–36) synergistically reduce food intake through different mechanisms in mice. Endocrinology 2005;146:3748–3756

10. Drucker DJ, Nauck MA. The incretin system: glucagon-like peptide-1 receptor agonists and dipeptidyl peptidase-4 inhibitors in type 2 diabetes. Lancet 2006;368:1696–1705

11. Eissele R, Goke R, Willemer S, Harthus HP, Vermeer H, Arnold R, Goke B. Glucagon-like peptide-1 cells in the gastrointestinal tract and pancreas of rat, pig and man. Eur J Clin Invest 1992;22:283–291

12. Elliott RM, Morgan LM, Tredger JA, Deacon S, Wright J, Marks V. Glucagon-like peptide-1 (7–36)amide and glucose-dependent insulinotropic polypeptide secretion in response to nutrient ingestion in man: acute post-prandial and 24-h secretion patterns. J Endocrinol 1993;138:159–166

13. Schirra J, Katschinski M, Weidmann C, Schafer T, Wank U, Arnold R, Goke B. Gastric emptying and release of incretin hormones after glucose ingestion in humans. J Clin Invest 1996;97:92–103

14. Rocca AS, Brubaker PL. Role of the vagus nerve in mediating proximal nutrient-induced glucagon-like peptide-1 secretion. Endocrinology 1999; 140:1687–1694

15. Anini Y, Hansotia T, Brubaker PL. Muscarinic receptors control postprandial release of glucagon-like peptide-1: in vivo and in vitro studies in rats. Endocrinology 2002;143:2420–2426

16. Roberge JN, Brubaker PL. Regulation of intestinal proglucagon-derived peptide secretion by glucose-dependent insulinotropic peptide in a novel enteroendocrine loop. Endocrinology 1993;133:233–240

17. Iakoubov R, Izzo A, Yeung A, Whiteside CI, Brubaker PL. Protein kinase Czeta is required for oleic acid-induced secretion of glucagon-like peptide-1 by intestinal endocrine L cells. Endocrinology 2007;148:1089–1098

18. Rocca AS, LaGreca J, Kalitsky J, Brubaker PL. Monounsaturated fatty acid diets improve glycemic tolerance through increased secretion of glucagon-like peptide-1. Endocrinology 2001;142:1148–1155

19. Hirasawa A, Tsumaya K, Awaji T, Katsuma S, Adachi T, Yamada M, Sugimoto Y, Miyazaki S, Tsujimoto G. Free fatty acids regulate gut incretin glucagon-like peptide-1 secretion through GPR120. Nat Med 2005;11:90–94

20. Edfalk S, Steneberg P, Edlund H. Gpr40 is expressed in enteroendocrine cells and mediates free fatty acid stimulation of incretin secretion. Diabetes 2008;57:2280–2287

21. Chu ZL, Jones RM, He H, Carroll C, Gutierrez V, Lucman A, Moloney M, Gao H, Mondala H, Bagnol D, Unett D, Liang Y, Demarest K, Semple G, Behan DP, Leonard J. A role for beta-cell-expressed G protein-coupled receptor 119 in glycemic control by enhancing glucose-dependent insulin release. Endocrinology 2007;148:2601–2609

22. Chu ZL, Carroll C, Alfonso J, Gutierrez V, He H, Lucman A, Pedraza M, Mondala H, Gao H, Bagnol D, Chen R, Jones RM, Behan DP, Leonard J. A role for intestinal endocrine cell-expressed g protein-coupled receptor 119 in glycemic control by enhancing glucagon-like peptide-1 and glucose-dependent insulinotropic peptide release. Endocrinology 2008;149:2038–2047

23. Soga T, Ohishi T, Matsui T, Saito T, Matsumoto M, Takasaki J, Matsumoto S, Kamohara M, Hiyama H, Yoshida S, Momose K, Ueda Y, Matsushime H, Kobori M, Furuichi K. Lysophosphatidylcholine enhances glucose-dependent insulin secretion via an orphan G-protein-coupled receptor. Biochem Biophys Res Commun 2005;326:744–751

24. Overton HA, Babbs AJ, Doel SM, Fyfe MC, Gardner LS, Griffin G, Jackson HC, Procter MJ, Rasamison CM, Tang-Christensen M, Widdowson PS, Williams GM, Reynet C. Deorphanization of a G protein-coupled receptor for oleoylethanolamide and its use in the discovery of small-molecule hypophagic agents. Cell Metab 2006;3:167–175

25. Kougias P, Chai H, Lin PH, Lumsden AB, Yao Q, Chen C. Lysophosphatidylcholine and secretory phospholipase A2 in vascular disease: mediators of endothelial dysfunction and atherosclerosis. Med Sci Monit 2006;12:RA5–16

26. Fu J, Astarita G, Gaetani S, Kim J, Cravatt BF, Mackie K, Piomelli D. Food intake regulates oleoylethanolamide formation and degradation in the proximal small intestine. J Biol Chem 2007;282:1518–1528

27. Lo Verme J, Gaetani S, Fu J, Oveisi F, Burton K, Piomelli D. Regulation of food intake by oleoylethanolamide. Cell Mol Life Sci 2005;62:708–716

28. Cravatt BF, Giang DK, Mayfield SP, Boger DL, Lerner RA, Gilula NB. Molecular characterization of an enzyme that degrades neuromodulatory fatty-acid amides. Nature 1996;384:83–87

29. Fegley D, Gaetani S, Duranti A, Tontini A, Mor M, Tarzia G, Piomelli D. Characterization of the fatty acid amide hydrolase inhibitor cyclohexyl carbamic acid 3′-carbamoyl-biphenyl-3-yl ester (URB597): effects on anandamide and oleoylethanolamide deactivation. J Pharmacol Exp Ther 2005;313:352–358

30. Rodriguez de Fonseca F, Navarro M, Gomez R, Escuredo L, Nava F, Fu J, Murillo-Rodriguez E, Giuffrida A, LoVerme J, Gaetani S, Kathuria S, Gall C, Piomelli D. An anorexic lipid mediator regulated by feeding. Nature 2001;414:209–212

31. Oveisi F, Gaetani S, Eng KT, Piomelli D. Oleoylethanolamide inhibits food intake in free-feeding rats after oral administration. Pharmacol Res 2004; 49:461–466

32. Astarita G, Di Giacomo B, Gaetani S, Oveisi F, Compton TR, Rivara S, Tarzia G, Mor M, Piomelli D. Pharmacological characterization of hydrolysis-resistant analogs of oleoylethanolamide with potent anorexiant properties. J Pharmacol Exp Ther 2006;318:563–570

33. Fu J, Gaetani S, Oveisi F, Lo Verme J, Serrano A, Rodriguez De Fonseca F, Rosengarth A, Luecke H, Di Giacomo B, Tarzia G, Piomelli D. Oleylethanolamide regulates feeding and body weight through activation of the nuclear receptor PPAR-alpha. Nature 2003;425:90–93

34. Brubaker PL, Schloos J, Drucker DJ. Regulation of glucagon-like peptide-1 synthesis and secretion in the GLUTag enteroendocrine cell line. Endocrinology 1998;139:4108–4114

35. Anini Y, Brubaker PL. Role of leptin in the regulation of glucagon-like peptide-1 secretion. Diabetes 2003;52:252–259

36. Anini Y, Brubaker PL. Muscarinic receptors control glucagon-like peptide 1 secretion by human endocrine L cells. Endocrinology 2003;144:3244–3250

37. Brubaker PL. Control of glucagon-like immunoreactive peptide secretion from fetal rat intestinal cultures. Endocrinology 1988;123:220–226

38. Reimer RA, Darimont C, Gremlich S, Nicolas-Metral V, Ruegg UT, Mace K. A human cellular model for studying the regulation of glucagon-like peptide-1 secretion. Endocrinology 2001;142:4522–4528

39. Shin ED, Estall JL, Izzo A, Drucker DJ, Brubaker PL. Mucosal adaptation to enteral nutrients is dependent on the physiologic actions of glucagon-like peptide-1 in mice. Gastroenterology 2005;128:1340–1353

40. Pfaffl MW. A new mathematical model for relative quantification in real-time RT-PCR. Nucleic Acid Res 2001;29:e45

41. Kathuria S, Gaetani S, Fegley D, Valino F, Duranti A, Tontini A, Mor M, Tarzia G, La Rana G, Calignano A, Giustino A, Tattoli M, Palmery M, Cuomo V, Piomelli D. Modulation of anxiety through blockade of anandamide hydrolysis. Nat Med 2003;9:76–81

42. Beconi MG, Reed JR, Teffera Y, Xia YQ, Kochansky CJ, Liu DQ, Xu S, Elmore CS, Ciccotto S, Hora DF, Stearns RA, Vincent SH. Disposition of the dipeptidyl peptidase 4 inhibitor sitagliptin in rats and dogs. Drug Metab Dispos 2007;35:525–532

43. Goh TT, Mason TM, Gupta N, So A, Lam TK, Lam L, Lewis GF, Mari A, Giacca A. Lipid-induced beta-cell dysfunction in vivo in models of progressive beta-cell failure. Am J Physiol Endocrinol Metab 2007;292:E549–E560

44. Usdin TB, Mezey E, Button DC, Brownstein MJ, Bonner TI. Gastric inhibitory polypeptide receptor, a member of the secretin-vasoactive intestinal peptide receptor family, is widely distributed in peripheral organs and the brain. Endocrinology 1993;133:2861–2870

45. Ning Y, O'Neill K, Lan H, Pang L, Shan LX, Hawes BE, Hedrick JA. Endogenous and synthetic agonists of GPR119 differ in signalling pathways and their effects on insulin secretion in MIN6c4 insulinoma cells. Br J Pharmacol 2008;155:1056–1065

46. Simpson AK, Ward PS, Wong KY, Collord GJ, Habib AM, Reimann F, Gribble FM. Cyclic AMP triggers glucagon-like peptide-1 secretion from the GLUTag enteroendocrine cell line. Diabetologia 2007;50:2181–2189

47. Ahern GP. Activation of TRPV1 by the satiety factor oleoylethanolamide. J Biol Chem 2003;278:30429–30434

48. Rocca AS, Brubaker PL. Stereospecific effects of fatty acids on proglucagon-derived peptide secretion in fetal rat intestinal cultures. Endocrinology 1995;136:5593–5599

49. Lauffer L, Iakoubov R, Brubaker PL. GPR119: "double-dipping" for better glycemic control. Endocrinology 2008;149:2035–2037

50. Kelly E, Bailey CP, Henderson G. Agonist-selective mechanisms of GPCR desensitization. Br J Pharmacol 2008;153 (Suppl)1:S379–S388

Glucagon-Like Peptide-1 Protects β-Cells Against Apoptosis by Increasing the Activity of an Igf-2/Igf-1 Receptor Autocrine Loop

Marion Cornu,[1] Jiang-Yan Yang,[2] Evrim Jaccard,[2] Carine Poussin,[1] Christian Widmann,[2] and Bernard Thorens[1]

OBJECTIVE—The gluco-incretin hormones glucagon-like peptide (GLP)-1 and gastric inhibitory peptide (GIP) protect β-cells against cytokine-induced apoptosis. Their action is initiated by binding to specific receptors that activate the cAMP signaling pathway, but the downstream events are not fully elucidated. Here we searched for mechanisms that may underlie this protective effect.

RESEARCH DESIGN AND METHODS—We performed comparative transcriptomic analysis of islets from control and $GipR^{-/-};Glp-1-R^{-/-}$ mice, which have increased sensitivity to cytokine-induced apoptosis. We found that IGF-1 receptor expression was markedly reduced in the mutant islets. Because the IGF-1 receptor signaling pathway is known for its antiapoptotic effect, we explored the relationship between gluco-incretin action, IGF-1 receptor expression and signaling, and apoptosis.

RESULTS—We found that GLP-1 robustly stimulated IGF-1 receptor expression and Akt phosphorylation and that increased Akt phosphorylation was dependent on IGF-1 but not insulin receptor expression. We demonstrated that GLP-1–induced Akt phosphorylation required active secretion, indicating the presence of an autocrine activation mechanism; we showed that activation of IGF-1 receptor signaling was dependent on the secretion of IGF-2. We demonstrated, both in MIN6 cell line and primary β-cells, that reducing IGF-1 receptor or IGF-2 expression or neutralizing secreted IGF-2 suppressed GLP-1–induced protection against apoptosis.

CONCLUSIONS—An IGF-2/IGF-1 receptor autocrine loop operates in β-cells. GLP-1 increases its activity by augmenting IGF-1 receptor expression and by stimulating secretion; this mechanism is required for GLP-1–induced protection against apoptosis. These findings may lead to novel ways of preventing β-cell loss in the pathogenesis of diabetes. *Diabetes* **58:1816–1825, 2009**

The number of pancreatic islet β-cells as well as their capacity to secrete insulin is modulated in normal physiological conditions to respond to the metabolic demand of the organism (1). A failure of the endocrine pancreas to maintain an adequate insulin secretory capacity due to reduced β-cell number and function underlies the pathogenesis of both type 1 and type 2 diabetes. In type 1 diabetes, β-cells are destroyed by an autoimmune mechanism in which cytokine-induced apoptosis is thought to play an important role (2). In the pathogenesis of type 2 diabetes, hyperglycemia appears when β-cell mass and insulin secretory capacity are no longer sufficient to compensate for insulin resistance. The reduction in β-cell mass results from increased apoptosis, most probably caused by the combined action of cytokines and increased plasma glucose and free fatty acid levels (3,4). Therefore, finding means to protect β-cell against apoptosis may be useful for the treatment or prevention of diabetes.

The gluco-incretin hormones GLP-1 and GIP can protect β-cells against apoptosis induced by cytokines or glucose and free fatty acids (5). Both hormones bind to specific stimulatory G-protein (Gs)–coupled receptors, which trigger cAMP formation (6,7). In β-cells, basal cAMP levels control glucose competence (8), i.e., the magnitude of the insulin secretion response to a given increase in extracellular glucose concentration. Increases in cAMP levels, for instance, as stimulated by GLP-1 or GIP action, potentiate glucose-stimulated insulin secretion by both protein kinase A (PKA)-dependent and -independent mechanisms (9); they also stimulate gene transcription through PKA-dependent phosphorylation of the transcription factor CREB (cAMP-response element binding) (10).

In β-cells, increased cAMP levels also activate the mitogen-activated protein (MAP) kinase cascade, leading to rapid phosphorylation of Erk1/2 (11). An activation of the phosphatidylinositol (PI) 3-kinase/Akt pathway is also observed. PI 3-kinase may be directly activated by the βγ subunit of Gs (12), be secondary to transactivation of the EGF receptor by betacellulin (13), or follow transcriptional induction of insulin receptor substrate (IRS)-2 through the PKA/CREB pathway. The IRS-2/PI 3-kinase/Akt pathway is known to have antiapoptotic effects (14–16); however, it is unclear why increased expression of IRS-2 leads to activation of its signaling pathway. IRS-2 may be downstream of the insulin receptor (IR) or IGF-1 receptor (IGF-1R). Studies of mice with β-cell–specific inactivation of either receptor (17–19) have indicated that the insulin receptor was important for compensatory growth of the β-cells in response to insulin resistance,

From the [1]Department of Physiology and Center for Integrative Genomics, University of Lausanne, Lausanne, Switzerland; and the [2]Department of Physiology and Department of Cellular Biology and Morphology, Biology and Medicine Faculty, University of Lausanne, Lausanne, Switzerland.
Corresponding author: Bernard Thorens, bernard.thorens@unil.ch.
Received 13 January 2009 and accepted 20 April 2009.
Published ahead of print at http://diabetes.diabetesjournals.org on 28 April 2009. DOI: 10.2337/db09-0063.

23

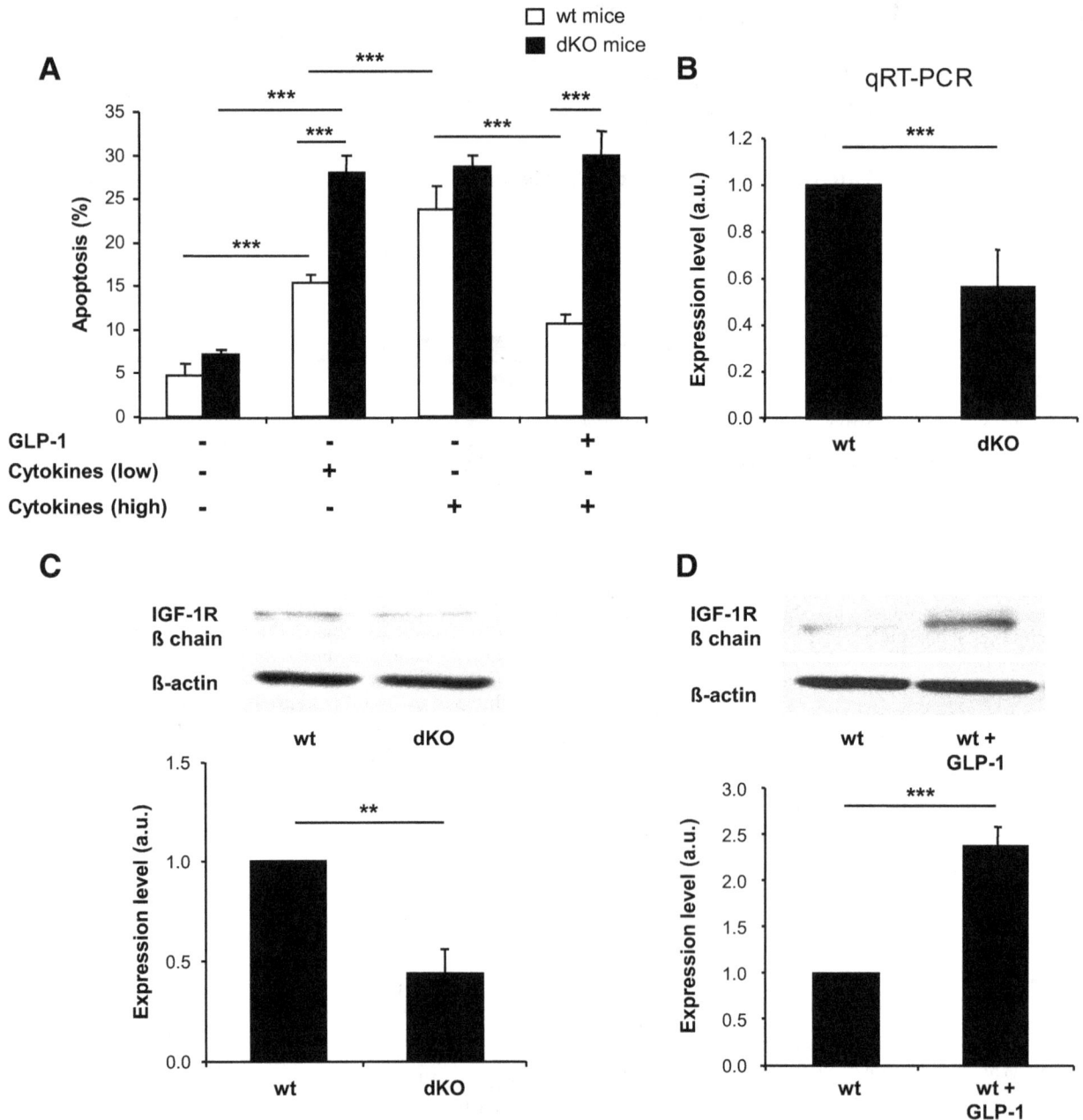

FIG. 1. Gluco-incretin signaling controls susceptibility to apoptosis and IGF-1R expression. *A*: Islets from control or $GipR^{-/-};Glp-1R^{-/-}$ mice were exposed or not to cytokines (IL-1β, TNF-α, and IFN-γ) at low or high concentrations (5, 12.5, and 5 ng/ml or 10, 25, and 10 ng/ml, respectively) and in the presence or absence of GLP-1 (100 nmol/l). *B*: Quantitative RT-PCR analysis of IGF-1R mRNA expression in islets from control (wt) and $GipR^{-/-};Glp-1R^{-/-}$ *mice (dKO)*. *C*: Reduced expression of IGF-1R expression in $GipR^{-/-};Glp-1R^{-/-}$ mouse islets as detected by Western blot analysis. *Lower panel*: Quantitation of the expression data. *D*: GLP-1 (100 nmol/l) treatment for 18 h increased IGF-1R expression as detected by Western blot analysis. *Lower panel*: Quantitation of the expression data. For all panels, data are means ± SD, $n = 3$ independent experiments. **$P < 0.01$; ***$P < 0.001$.

whereas the IGF-1 receptor was involved in the control of glucose competence.

Here we studied islets from mice with inactivation of both the GLP-1 and GIP receptor genes. We showed them to be more sensitive than control islets to cytokine-induced apoptosis. By comparative transcriptomic analysis of islets from control and mutant mice, we found that expression of the IGF-1R was markedly decreased in the mutant islets. In control islets, GLP-1–activated IGF-1R expression and signaling and GLP-1–induced IGF-1R signaling required autocrine secretion of IGF-2. We provided

evidence that increasing the activity of this autocrine loop was required for GLP-1 to protect β-cells against apoptosis. These data provide an integrated description of the interaction between the GLP-1 and IGF-1 receptor signaling pathways that operate to protect β-cells against apoptosis.

RESEARCH DESIGN AND METHODS

Mice. Male C57BL/6 and $GipR^{-/-};Glp-1-R^{-/-}$ mice backcrossed for seven generations into the C57BL/6 background were used between 8 and 10 weeks

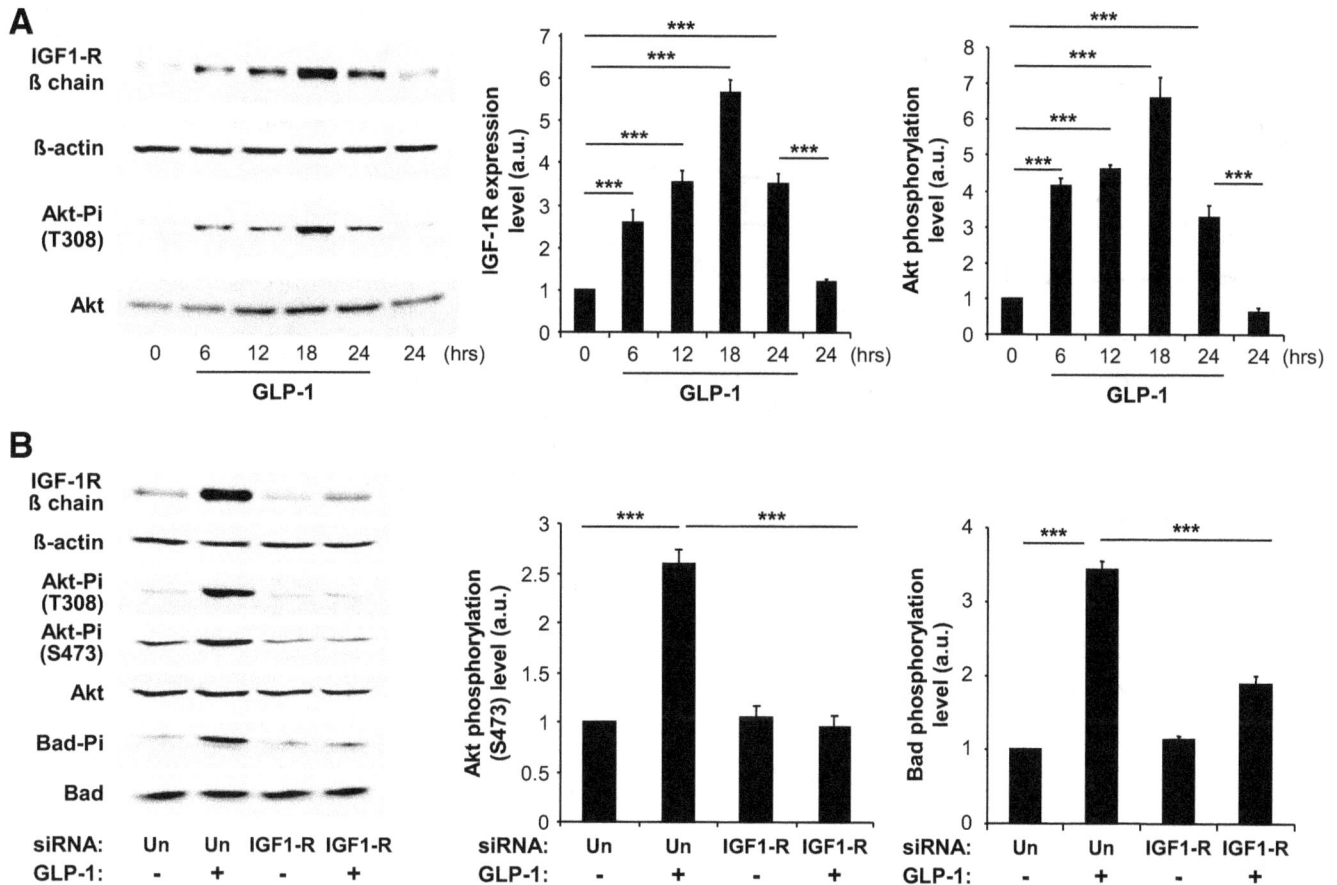

FIG. 2. GLP-1 increased IGF-1R expression and signaling in MIN6 cells. *A*: MIN6 cells were treated with GLP-1 for the indicated periods of time, and IGF-1R expression and Akt phosphorylation were analyzed by Western blot analysis. *B*: MIN6 cells were transfected with a control (Un) or an IGF-1R siRNA and treated for 18 h with GLP-1. GLP-1 induced IGF-1 receptor expression, Akt phosphorylation on both T308 and S473, and Bad phosphorylation. Preventing IGF-1R expression suppressed GLP-1–induced Akt and Bad phosphorylation. For all panels, data are means ± SD, $n = 3$ independent experiments. ***$P < 0.001$.

of age. All experimental procedures received approval from the Service Vétérinaire du Canton de Vaud.

Antibodies. Rabbit polyclonal antibody against actin was purchased from Sigma (St. Louis, MO); rabbit polyclonal antibodies against the IGF-1R (C20; sc-713), the insulin receptor (C19; sc-711), and total Akt ([H-136]: sc-8312) were from Santa Cruz Biotechnology (Nunningen, Switzerland); rabbit monoclonal antibody against phosphorylated Akt (pAktThr-308) (no. 4056), rabbit polyclonal antibodies against phosphorylated Akt (pAktSer-473) (no. 9271), phosphorylated Bad (pBadSer-112) (no. 9291), and total Bad (no. 9292) were from Cell Signaling (Danvers, MA); and goat polyclonal antibody against IGF-2 (ab10731) was purchased from Abcam (Cambridge, U.K.).

Pancreatic islet isolation. Islets were isolated according to published procedures (20) using a Histopaque density gradient. Islets were cultured overnight at 37°C in 5% CO_2 in RPMI-1640, 10% FCS, 2 mmol/l glutamax, 100 units/ml penicillin, and 100 µg/ml streptomycin. β-Cells were purified by cell sorter as described (21).

Microarray and quantitative PCR analyses. Islets were isolated from 8-to 10-week-old mice and kept in culture overnight before RNA extraction. Total islet RNA was extracted using RNeasy Mini kit (Qiagen); purity and quality were assessed by an Agilent bioanalyzer. After linear amplification with T7 polymerase, the RNA was reverse transcribed and labeled with Cy3 or Cy5 and hybridized to cDNA arrays containing 17,664 different probes, prepared by the University of Lausanne DNA Array Facility (www.unil.ch/dafl). Hybridization, data acquisition, and quality control were performed as previously described (22). Differentially expressed genes were identified using linear models implemented in the Limma package from Bioconductor (http://www.bioconductor.org). All statistical analyses were performed using the R software (http://www.r-project.org). Real-time quantitative PCR was performed using Light Cycler Technology (Roche, France). Primers sets were chosen to amplify products of ~200 bp. cDNAs were obtained from 2.5 µg total RNA with SuperScript II RNAse H- Reverse Transcriptase (Invitrogen, Carlsbad,

CA) and 50 pmol random hexamer (Applied Biosystem). cDNA amplification was performed in a 20-µl reaction mixture including 1× QuantiTect SYBR Green PCR Master Mix (Qiagen) and 10 pmol of each primer. Primers for mouse IGF-1 (sense, 5′-GGCATTGTGGATGAGTGTTG-3′; antisense, 5′-AGT-TGCCTCCGTTACCTCCT-3′), mouse IGF-2 (sense, 5′-GTCGATGTTGGTGCT-TCTCA-3′; antisense, 5′-AAGCAGCACTCTTCCACGAT-3′), and mouse cyclophilin (sense, 5′-TCCATCGTGTCATCAAGGAC-3′; antisense, 5′-CTTGC-CATCCAGCCAGGAG-3′) were used. All measurements were normalized to cyclophilin.

MIN6 cell culture and secretion tests. MIN6 cells were grown in Dulbecco's modified Eagle's medium, 15% FCS, 2 mmol/l glutamine, and 50 µmol/l β-mercaptoethanol and used between passages 19 and 30. For pharmacological treatments, 10^6 MIN6 cells were plated in 6-cm-diameter tissue culture dishes for 4 days, the medium was replaced, and cells were incubated for 2 h at 37°C before addition of various reagents at the concentrations and for the periods of time indicated in the figure legends.

For gene silencing, MIN6 cells were transfected 1 day after plating with 0.5 µg of a green fluorescent protein (GFP) expression plasmid and siRNAs at a final concentration of 100 nmol/l using lipofectamine (Invitrogen, Carlsbad, CA). After 6 h at 37°C, the growth medium was replaced, and the cells were used 48 h later.

For secretion tests, MIN6 cells were seeded at 10^6 cells in sixwell plates. Three days later, cells were washed and preincubated for 2 h in Krebs-Ringer bicarbonate HEPES buffer (120 mmol/l NaCl, 4 mmol/l KH_2PO_4, 20 mmol/l HEPES, 1 mmol/l $MgCl_2$, 1 mmol/l $CaCl_2$, 5 mmol/l $NaHCO_3$, and 0.5% BSA, pH 7.4) supplemented with 2 mmol/l glucose. Then, the medium was replaced with Krebs-Ringer bicarbonate HEPES buffer containing 2 or 20 mmol/l glucose for an additional hour. Secretion and cellular IGF-2 (extracted in PBS-Tween 5%) was assessed by ELISA (no. DY702, R&D; Minneapolis, MN).

Gel electrophoresis and immunoblotting. MIN6 cells were placed on ice, washed twice with PBS, and lysed for 30 min on ice in 50 mmol/l Tris (pH 7.5)

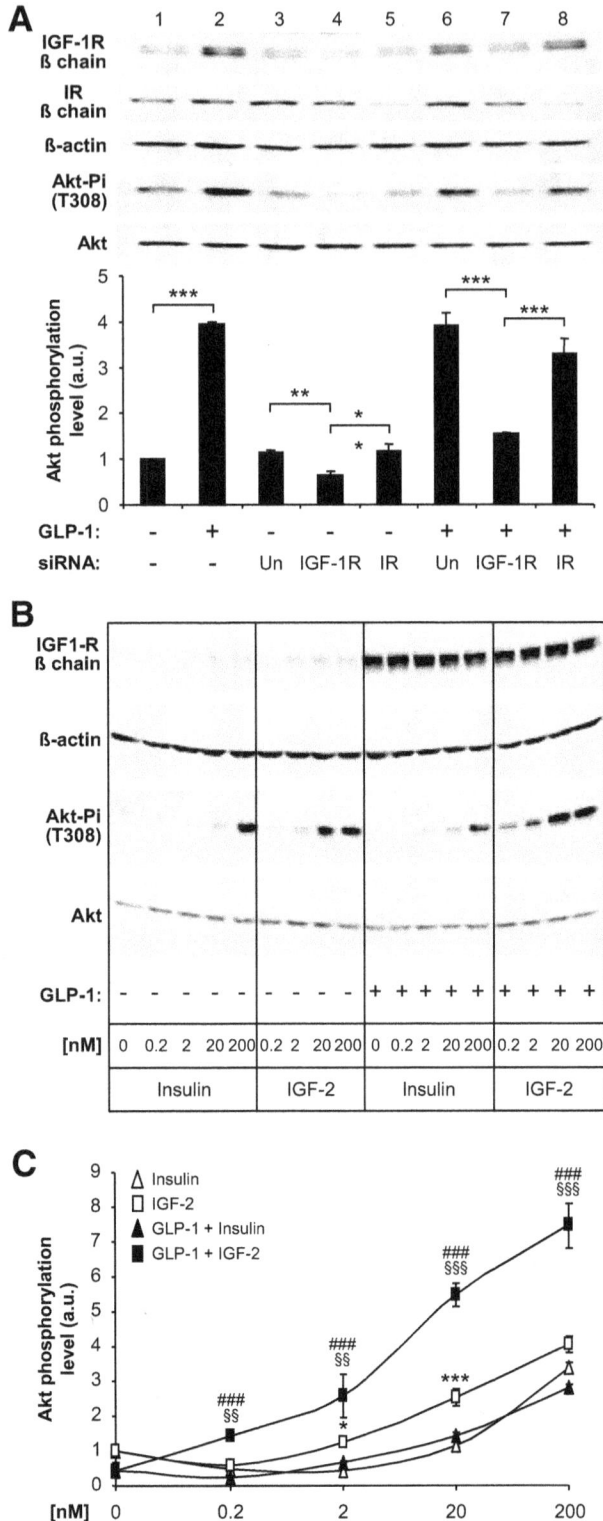

FIG. 3. GLP-1–induced Akt phosphorylation depends on IGF-1R but not IR expression. *A*: MIN6 cells were transfected with control (Un, *lanes 3* and *6*), IGF-1R (*lanes 4* and *7*), or IR-specific (*lanes 5* and *8*) siRNAs and exposed (+) or not (−) to GLP-1 for 18 h before Western analysis. *Lanes 1* and *2* show the induction by GLP-1 of IGF-1R expression in nontransfected cells. *Lane 3* shows the basal level of IGF-1R and IR expression in transfected cells; reducing IGF-1R expression (*lane 4*) but not the IR (*lane 5*) reduced Akt phosphorylation. *Lane 6*: GLP-1–treated cells showed higher expression of the IGF-1R but not of the IR; reducing IGF-1R expression (*lane 7*) but not IR (*lane 8*) reduced Akt

containing 1 mmol/l EDTA, 1 mmol/l EGTA, 1% Triton, 10 mmol/l β-glycerol-phosphate, 1 mmol/l Na_3VO_4, 50 mmol/l NaF, 5 mmol/l phenylmethylsulfonyl fluoride, 10 μg/ml aprotinin, leupeptin, and pepstatin. The lysates were centrifuged for 15 min at 13,000 rpm at 4°C.

Mouse islets were washed twice with PBS and lysed in 160 mmol/l Tris (pH 6.8) containing 5 mmol/l EDTA, 20% glycerol, 10% β-mercaptoethanol, 10% SDS, 1 mmol/l Na_3VO_4, 50 mmol/l NaF, 5 mmol/l phenylmethylsulfonyl fluoride, and 10 μg/ml aprotinin. Lysates were sonicated for 15 s before protein determination. Western blot analysis was performed as described (21) with antibodies diluted in Tris-buffered saline–5% nonfat dry milk (1/500 dilution for IGF-1R, IR and phosphorylated Akt [Thr308 and Ser473], and phosphorylated Bad and 1/1,000 for actin, total Akt, total Bad, and IGF-2) and revealed using horseradish peroxidase–conjugated donkey anti-rabbit IgG or horseradish peroxidase–conjugated sheep anti-mouse IgG as secondary antibodies (Amersham, Buckinghamshire, U.K.). Band intensities were determined using a Bio-Rad densitometer (Strasbourg, France).

Apoptosis assay. Apoptosis was induced by exposing the MIN6 cells or islets to cytokines at the indicated concentrations for 24 h; GLP-1(7–36)amide (100 nmol/l) was added 4 h before the cytokines and was present for the entire cytokine incubation period (24 h). Apoptosis was assessed by scoring the number of cells expressing GFP and displaying pyknotic nuclei labeled with Hoechst 33342 (10 μg/ml) (23). Islets were first dissociated in 100 μl dissociation buffer (Gibco, product number 13151-014) for 15 min at 37°C before apoptosis was assessed.

Adenovirus. Recombinant adenoviruses expressing enhanced GFP alone (Ad-GFP) or together with IGF-1R (Ad-IGF-1R) were generated using the AdEasy system (24). Islets were infected with a multiplicity of infection of 40 in 500 μl of medium for 3 h at 37°C and then cultured for 48 h before insulin secretion tests, as described above. Preliminary experiments showed that ~85% of islet cells were infected and that infection did not affect glucose-induced insulin secretion.

Statistical analysis. All experiments were performed at least three times. Results are expressed as means ± SD. Comparisons were performed using unpaired Student's t test or one-way or two-way ANOVA for the different groups followed by post hoc pair-wise multiple-comparison procedures (Tukey test or Bonferroni, respectively).

RESULTS

Increased susceptibility to apoptosis of islets from $GipR^{-/-};Glp-1R^{-/-}$ mice. To evaluate whether absence of both gluco-incretin hormone receptor expression led to increased susceptibility to cytokine-induced apoptosis, islets from $GipR^{-/-};Glp-1-R^{-/-}$ mice were exposed to low or high concentrations of cytokines (interleukin [IL]-1β, tumor necrosis factor [TNF]-α, and interferon [IFN]-γ), and the percent of apoptotic cells was determined. Figure 1*A* shows that islets from mutant mice were significantly more sensitive than control islets to apoptosis induced by the low dose of cytokine; at the high dose, apoptosis was similar in both types of islets. As expected, GLP-1 protected control but not mutant islets against cytokine-induced apoptosis.

Gluco-incretins control IGF-1R expression and signaling. To search for genes differentially expressed in control and mutant islets and that could be involved in the increased susceptibility to cytokine-induced apoptosis, we performed microarray analysis of transcripts expressed in control and mutant islets. We found that the IGF-1R mRNA was downregulated in the mutant islets (Fig. 1*B*) and that IGF-1R protein expression was also markedly decreased (Fig. 1*C*). This suggested that expression of the IGF-1R

phosphorylation. *Bottom panel*: Quantitation of the data. Data are means ± SD, $n = 3$ independent experiments. **$P < 0.01$; ***$P < 0.001$. *B*: MIN6 cells were treated or not for 18 h with GLP-1 to increase IGF-1R expression, then incubated with 2 mmol/l glucose for 2 h, and exposed for 15 min to the indicated concentrations of insulin or IGF-2. IGF-1R and total and phosphorylated Akt were determined by Western blot analysis. *C*: Quantification of the data in *B*. *$P < 0.05$, ***$P < 0.001$ for IGF-2 vs. insulin; §§$P < 0.01$, §§§$P < 0.001$ for IGF-2 in control vs. GLP-1–treated cells; ###$P < 0.001$ for IGF-2 vs. insulin in GLP-1–treated cells. a.u., arbitrary units.

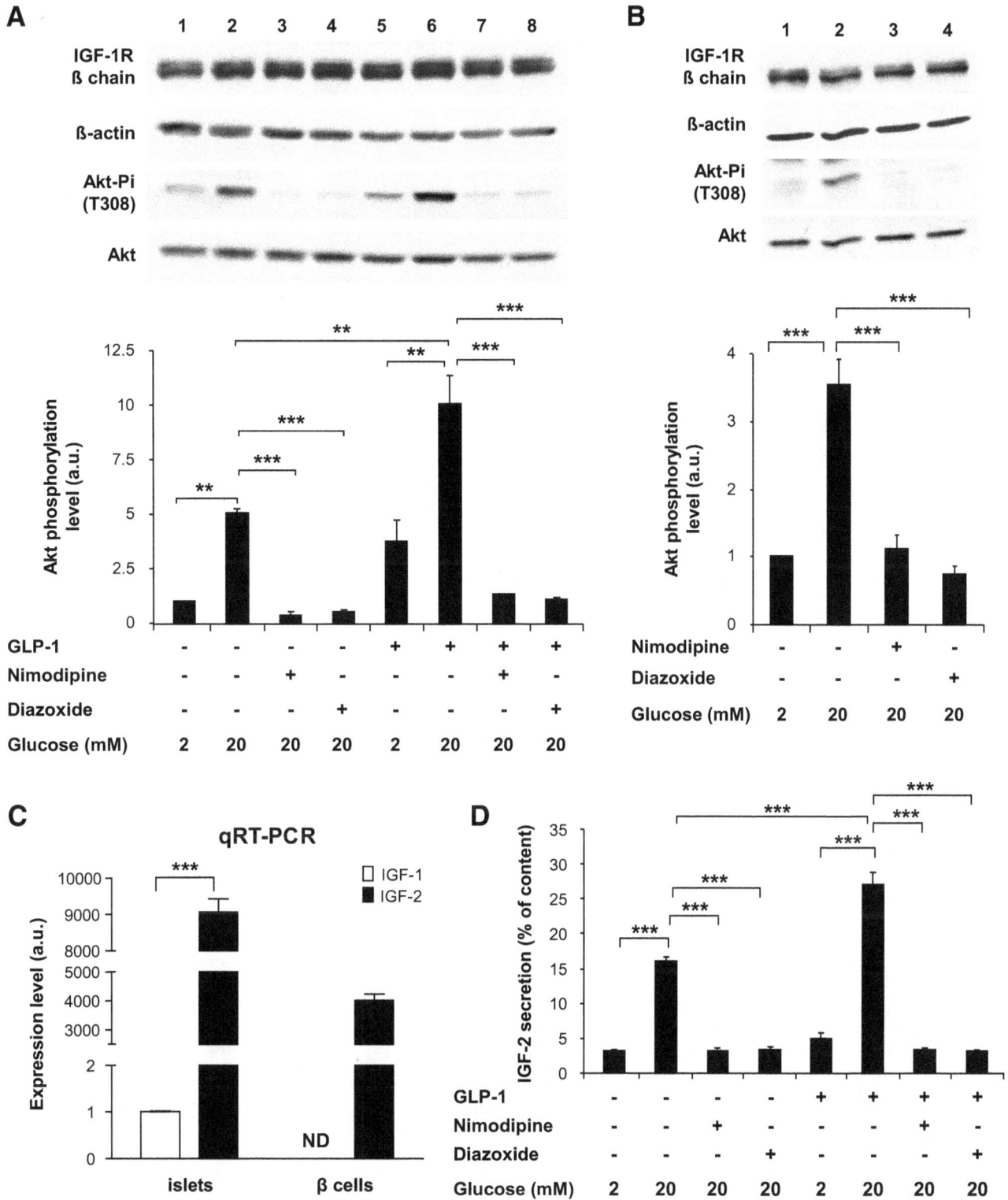

FIG. 4. Activation of Akt phosphorylation by GLP-1 depends on glucose-induced secretion. *A*: MIN6 cells were incubated for 18 h with GLP-1 to induce IGF-1R expression, then with 2 mmol/l glucose for 2 h, and finally for 1 h with 2 or 20 mmol/l glucose with or without GLP-1 and nimodipine (1 μmol/l) or diazoxide (200 μmol/l). *Bottom panel*: Quantitation of the data. *B*: Pancreatic islets were treated as the MIN6 cells in *A*. *C*: qRT-PCR analysis of IGF-1 and IGF-2 mRNA expression in mouse islets and cell sorter–purified β-cells. *D*: Secretion of IGF-2 by MIN6 cells incubated to 2 or 20 mmol/l glucose and in the presence of nimodipine, diazoxide, or GLP-1, as indicated. Total IGF-2 content was 10 ng/4 × 10^6 cells. *A–D*: Data are means ± SD, $n = 3$ independent experiments. **$P < 0.01$; ***$P < 0.001$. a.u., arbitrary units.

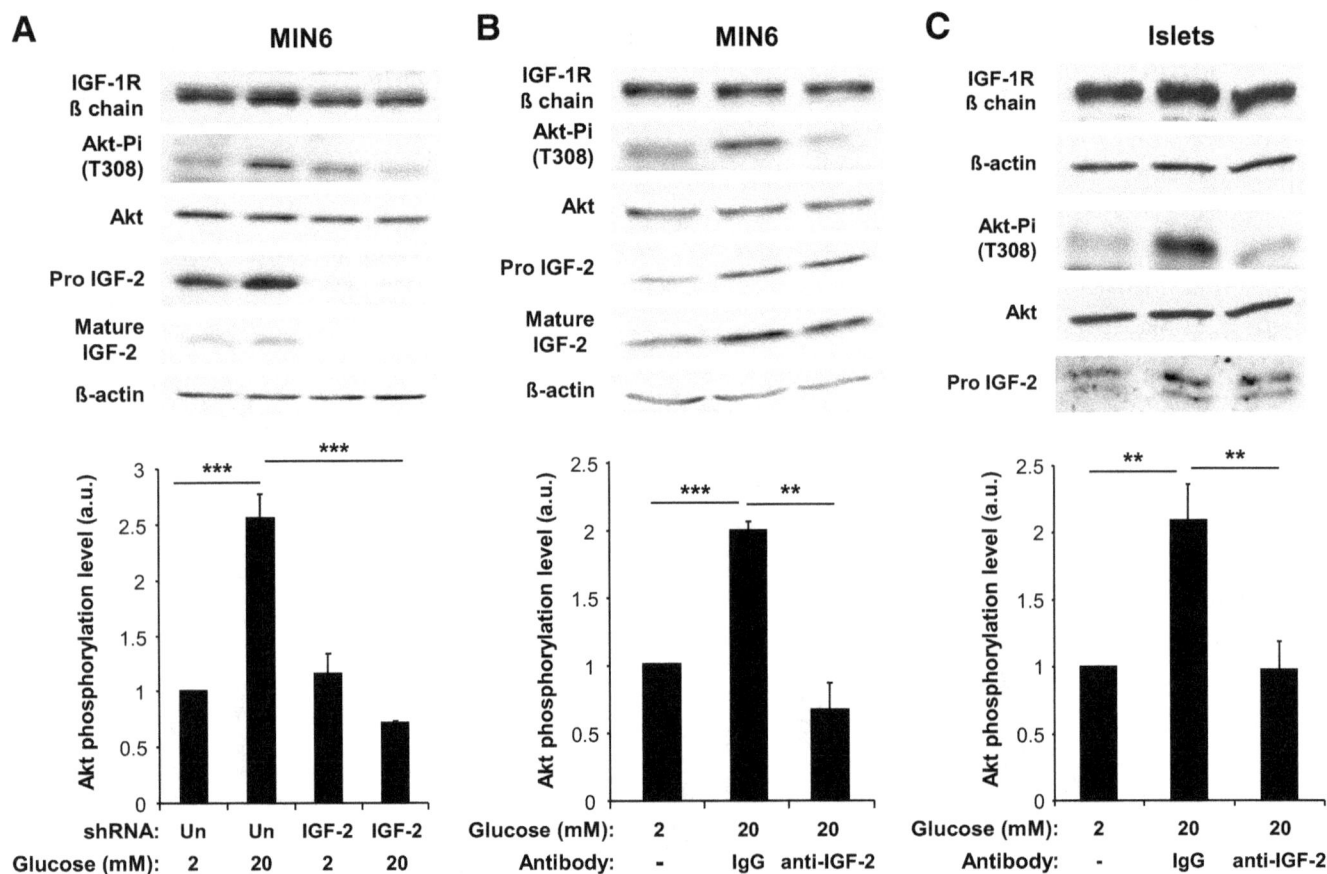

FIG. 5. GLP-1–increased Akt phosphorylation depends on secreted IGF-2. *A*: MIN6 cells were transfected with an unrelated (Un) or an IGF-2–specific shRNA. Forty-eight hours later, they were stimulated with GLP-1 for 18 h to increase IGF-1R expression and then incubated with 2 mmol/l glucose for 2 h and for 1 h in either 2 or 20 mmol/l glucose. *B*: MIN6 cells were stimulated with GLP-1 for 18 h and then incubated with 2 mmol/l glucose for 2 h and for 1 h in either 2 or 20 mmol/l glucose and with nonspecific IgGs or an IGF-2 blocking antibody. *C*: Pancreatic islets were stimulated with GLP-1 for 18 h and then incubated with 2 mmol/l glucose for 2 h and for 1 h in either 2 or 20 mmol/l glucose and with nonspecific IgGs or an IGF-2 blocking antibody. *A–C*: Data are means ± SD, $n = 3$ independent experiments. **$P < 0.01$; ***$P < 0.001$. a.u., arbitrary units.

could be regulated by gluco-incretin hormones. Figure 1*D* shows that GLP-1 indeed induced a marked increase in IGF-1 receptor expression in control islets.

To investigate in more detail the regulation by gluco-incretins of IGF-1R expression and signaling, we used MIN6 cells as a model system and concentrated our study on the effect of GLP-1, since GLP-1 and GIP use the same signaling pathway. We first demonstrated that, as in primary islets, GLP-1 increased IGF-1R expression with maximal induction reached after ~18 h of treatment (Fig. 2*A*). In addition, we found that induction of IGF-1R expression was associated with a corresponding increase in Akt phosphorylation on Thr308 (Fig. 2*A*). We then showed that GLP-1 treatment also induced Akt phosphorylation on Ser473 and the phosphorylation of Bad, a proapoptotic protein inactivated by phosphorylation by IGF-1R signaling (25,26) (Fig. 2*B*). We also determined that preventing IGF-1R expression by transfecting the cells with an IGF-1R–specific siRNA suppressed GLP-1–induced Akt phosphorylation on both sites and the phosphorylation of Bad (Fig. 2*B*). GLP-1 treatment of the cells induced an approximately threefold increase in IRS-2 expression (see Fig. S1 in an online-only appendix, available at http://diabetes. diabetesjournals.org/cgi/content/full/db09-0063/DC1).

Because β-cells also express the IR and secrete insulin, we searched for direct evidence that the IGF-1R, and not the IR, was responsible for the induction of Akt phosphorylation. First, we transfected MIN6 cells with IGF-1R– or IR-specific siRNAs before treating the cells with GLP-1 for 18 h and analyzing Akt phosphorylation. Figure 3*A* (*lanes 1 and 2*) shows that GLP-1 induced expression of the IGF-1R but not the IR. The receptor-specific, but not the unrelated, siRNAs led to a reduction of either IGF-1R or IR expression in the basal state (in the absence of GLP-1 stimulation; Fig. 2*A*, *lanes 3–5*) or after GLP-1 treatment (Fig. 2*A*, *lanes 6–8*). Importantly, Akt phosphorylation in the basal state or after GLP-1 treatment was reduced only when the IGF-1R, but not the IR expression, was decreased (*lanes 4 and 7* vs. *lanes 5 and 8*).

To further evaluate the respective roles of the IGF-1R and IR in activating the Akt pathway, we measured the efficiency of insulin and IGF-2 to activate Akt phosphorylation in MIN6 cells. Indeed, insulin binds to the IR with high affinity (K_d ~1 nmol/l) and to IGF-1R with an ~100-fold lower affinity, whereas IGF-2 binds to the IGF-1R with high affinity (~1 nmol/l) and with much lower affinity to the IR (27). MIN6 cells were thus pretreated or not with GLP-1 for 18 h and kept in the presence of 2 mmol/l glucose for 2 h to prevent insulin secretion. The cells were then exposed to different concentrations of each hormone for 15 min, and IGF-1R expression and Akt phosphorylation were determined (Fig. 3*B*). The data show that in the

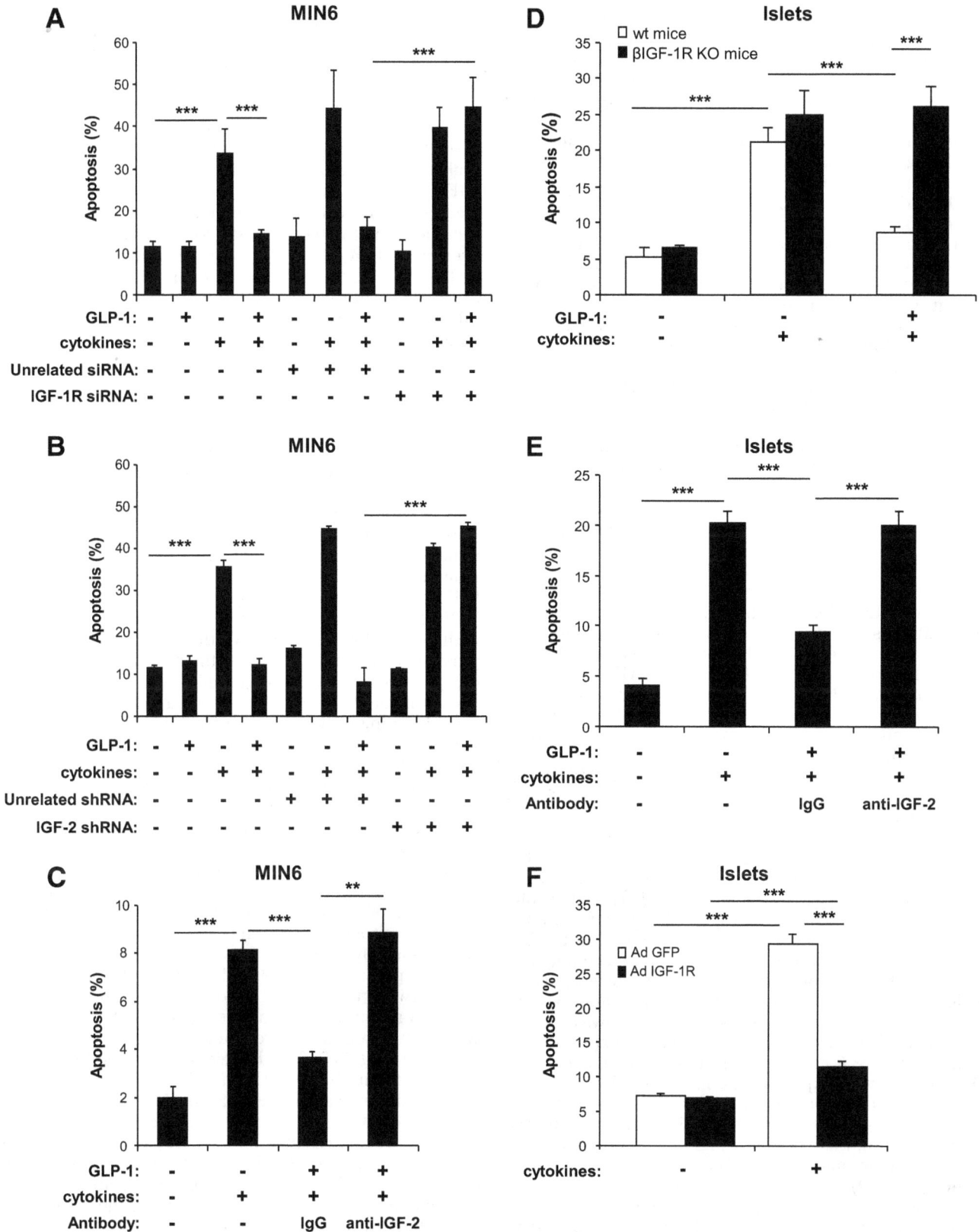

FIG. 6. GLP-1–induced protection against cytokine-induced apoptosis depends on activation of an IGF-2/IGF-1R autocrine loop. *A*: MIN6 cells were transfected with an unrelated or an IGF-1R siRNA, and 48 h later they were incubated in the presence or absence of GLP-1 for 4 h before addition of cytokines (IL-1β, 10 ng/ml; TNF-α, 25 ng/ml; IFN-γ, 10 ng/ml); the incubations were continued for 24 h in the continuous presence of GLP-1. *B*: MIN6 cells were transfected with an unrelated or an IGF-2 shRNA and then treated as described for *A*. *C*: MIN6 cells were incubated in the presence or absence of GLP-1 and in the presence of a nonspecific IgG fraction or an IGF-2 blocking antibody for 4 h before addition of cytokines (see above). *D*: Islets from β-cell–specific *Igf-1R*[−/−] mice or from their control littermates were incubated in the presence or absence of GLP-1

absence of GLP-1 pretreatment, IGF-2 was significantly more efficient in inducing Akt phosphorylation than insulin (Fig. 3B and C). After GLP-1 treatment, IGF-1R expression was markedly augmented and IGF-2 induced Akt phosphorylation with a greater efficacy than in nontreated cells; insulin-induced Akt phosphorylation, however, was not increased.

Together, the above data indicated that GLP-1–induced Akt phosphorylation was dependent on IGF-1R upregulation and independent of IR expression.

IGF-1R activation is triggered by autocrine secretion of IGF-2. To determine whether activation of the IGF-1R signaling pathway was dependent on secretion, we evaluated the level of Akt phosphorylation in cells, which had previously been treated for 18 h with or without GLP-1 to increase IGF-1R expression, then exposed for 2 h to a low glucose concentration, and then exposed to low or high glucose concentrations in the presence or absence of secretion inhibitors. We first evaluated Akt phosphorylation in cells pretreated or not pretreated with GLP-1. In the absence of pretreatment, high glucose induced an approximately threefold increase in Akt phosphorylation, whereas this increase was ~12-fold in GLP-1–treated cells (see Fig. S2 in the online appendix and Fig. 4A). The increased phosphorylation at 20 mmol/l glucose was suppressed by the ATP-sensitive K$^+$ (K$_{ATP}$) channel opener diazoxide or the Ca^{2+} channel inhibitor nimodipine (Fig. 4A). When the cells were exposed to GLP-1 during the last incubation period, Akt phosphorylation was higher than in the absence of GLP-1 but equally suppressed by the secretion inhibitors. To determine if the same regulation of Akt phosphorylation was observed in primary β-cells, mouse islets were similarly treated with GLP-1 for 18 h and then exposed to 2 or 20 mmol/l glucose in the presence or absence of nimodipine and diazoxide. As for MIN6 cells, phosphorylation of Akt was very low at 2 mmol/l glucose, increased at 20 mmol/l glucose, and suppressed by the secretion inhibitors (Fig. 4B). Thus, these observations indicated that activation of Akt phosphorylation was dependent on active secretion.

Three ligands can potentially activate the IGF-1R: insulin, IGF-1, and IGF-2. Because the data of Fig. 3 indicated that activation of Akt phosphorylation was through the IGF-1R but not the IR, it was highly unlikely that insulin was the ligand activating Akt phosphorylation. On the other hand, IGF-1 was not detectable by RT-PCR in MIN6 cells (not shown) and was expressed at an extremely low level in islets and not detectable in cell sorter–purified β-cells (Fig. 4C); IGF-1 was therefore not a candidate for activating the IGF-1 receptor signaling pathway in our experiments. Previous reports described the expression of IGF-2 in mature β-cells (28,29), and we confirmed that IGF-2 mRNA was expressed at high level in islets and purified β-cells (Fig. 4C). Furthermore, incubation of MIN6 cells at high glucose triggered IGF-2 secretion in the culture medium; this secretion was blocked by diazoxide and nimodipine and was increased when GLP-1 was present (Fig. 4D).

We thus tested whether IGF-2 was involved in activation of Akt phosphorylation in MIN6 cells exposed to

GLP-1. MIN6 cells were first transfected with an IGF-2–specific or an unrelated shRNA, then exposed to GLP-1 for 18 h to induce IGF-1R expression, and finally exposed to 2 or 20 mmol/l glucose before analysis of Akt phosphorylation. Figure 5A shows that expression of pro–IGF-2 and mature IGF-2 was strongly decreased by transfection of the specific shRNA, and this suppressed the induction of Akt phosphorylation in cells exposed to high glucose. As a second test for an autocrine role of IGF-2 secretion in Akt phosphorylation, MIN6 cells were treated as in the previous experiment but the final incubation with 20 mmol/l glucose was conducted in the presence of an IGF-2 blocking antibody or an unrelated IgG fraction. Figure 5B shows that the IGF-2 blocking antibody suppressed Akt phosphorylation. The same inhibition of Akt phosphorylation by the IGF-2 neutralizing antibody was made using primary islets (Fig. 5C). Thus, both in MIN6 cells and primary islets, activation of Akt phosphorylation by GLP-1 requires secretion of IGF-2 under these conditions. These data also indicated that an IGF-2/IGF-1R autocrine loop operated in β-cells, and its activity could be increased by GLP-1 by enhancing IGF-1R expression and by stimulating secretion in the presence of high glucose.

GLP-1 signaling protects β-cells against apoptosis by increasing the IGF-2/IGF-1R autocrine loop. To determine whether the protective effect of GLP-1 against cytokine-induced apoptosis was dependent on activation of the IGF-2/IGF-1R autocrine loop, we measured apoptosis in MIN6 cells exposed to cytokines and treated or not treated with GLP-1. Figure 6A shows that cytokine-induced apoptosis was suppressed by treatment with GLP-1 and that this protective effect was blunted when IGF-1R expression was prevented by transfection of a specific siRNA. The same blunting of the GLP-1 protective effect was obtained when the cells were transfected with an shRNA that specifically suppressed IGF-2 expression (Fig. 6B) or when the cells were incubated in the presence of an IGF-2 blocking antibody (Fig. 6C).

To determine whether GLP-1 protected primary islets using the same IGF-2/IGF-1R autocrine loop, we performed three sets of experiments. First, we tested whether GLP-1 protected islets from mice with a β-cell–specific IGF-1R gene inactivation against cytokine-induced apoptosis. As shown in Fig. 6D, apoptosis was not suppressed by GLP-1 in these islets—in contrast to the marked protection observed in control islets. Second, we showed that GLP-1 protection against cytokine-induced apoptosis was also suppressed when the islets were incubated in the presence of the neutralizing IGF-2 antibody (Fig. 6E). Third, we overexpressed the IGF-1R in islets from $GipR^{-/-};Glp-1R^{-/-}$ mice using a recombinant adenovirus (see Fig. S3 in the online appendix). Cytokine-induced apoptosis was markedly reduced in IGF-1R–overexpressing islets compared with control-infected cells (Fig. 6F). Thus, both in MIN6 cells and in primary islets, GLP-1 protected β-cells against cytokine-induced apoptosis by modulating the activity of the IGF-2/IGF-1R autocrine loop.

for 4 h before addition of cytokines (see above). E: Control islets were incubated for 4 h in the presence or absence of GLP-1 and with a nonspecific or an IGF-2 blocking antibody before cytokines treatment. F: Islets from $GipR^{-/-};Glp-1R^{-/-}$ mice were infected with a control adenovirus (Ad-GFP) or an IGF-1R–expressing adenovirus (Ad-IGF1-R) and 1 day later exposed to cytokines, as described in A. A–F: Data are means ± SD, $n = 3$ independent experiments. **$P < 0.01$; ***$P < 0.001$.

DISCUSSION

GLP-1 has previously been demonstrated to protect β-cells against apoptosis by increasing IRS-2 expression (14,16), PI 3-kinase activity (30), Akt phosphorylation (31) and Foxo1 phosphorylation, and nuclear exclusion (32). Our data are in agreement with these previous studies but present an integrated view of the operation of the GLP-1 and IGF-1R signaling pathways by providing novel findings on *1*) the regulation of IGF-1R expression by GLP-1, *2*) the predominant role of the IGF-1R compared with the IR in GLP-1–induced Akt phosphorylation, *3*) the role of IGF-2 as an autocrine regulator of this signaling pathway, and *4*) the modulation of this autocrine loop by GLP-1 as a basis for this hormone antiapoptotic effect.

Induction of IGF-1R expression by GLP-1 follows relatively slow kinetics, with a peak expression at ~18 h. This is in contrast with the induction of immediate early genes, whose expression peaks between 30 and 60 min after initiation of GLP-1 treatment (21). Thus, increased expression of the IGF-1 receptor after GLP-1 treatment may be due to transcriptional or posttranscriptional regulations that are secondary to the initial wave of GLP-1–mediated transcriptional events. A detailed understanding of these mechanisms will, however, need further investigation. The slow induction of IGF-1R expression is thus an adaptive process, which, in vivo, may link the amount of GLP-1 secreted daily to the β-cell susceptibility to apoptosis. Because there is a link between feeding and GLP-1 secretion (33), reduced susceptibility to apoptosis may also participate in the increased β-cell mass observed in obesity. This slow induction kinetics should also be considered when using GLP-1 to protect β-cells from apoptosis after islet transplantation (34). To be efficacious, this treatment may need to be started before transplanting the islets to ensure full expression of the IGF-1R and maximal antiapoptotic protection.

A question that had not previously been addressed is the mechanism by which GLP-1–induced IRS-2 expression leads to activation of its downstream signaling pathway. Our data show that GLP-1–induced Akt phosphorylation was suppressed by knocking-down IGF-1R but not IR expression; furthermore, the relative efficacy of insulin and IGF-2 induction of Akt phosphorylation in cells stimulated by GLP-1 supported a primary role of the IGF-1R. Thus, our data indicate that the IGF-1R but not the IR lies upstream of activated Akt in our experimental conditions.

Phosphorylation of Akt in GLP-1–treated cells required secretion of IGF-2, as supported by several data. First, the IR is not involved in GLP-1–induced Akt phosphorylation, and insulin is therefore unlikely to be responsible for the autocrine activation of the IGF-1R; second, IGF-1 is not expressed in MIN6 cells nor in cell sorter–purified β-cells and is present at extremely low levels in isolated islets, which is in agreement with the reported expression of IGF-1 in non–β-cells (35); third, IGF-2 mRNA is detected at relatively high levels in primary islets and in cell sorter–purified β-cells, and its secretion can be stimulated by glucose, which is in agreement with previous data showing the presence of IGF-2 in insulin granules (29,36).

The importance of secreted IGF-2 in activating IGF-1R signaling was further demonstrated by showing that IGF-2 downregulation or neutralization with a specific antibody suppressed GLP-1–induced Akt phosphorylation. Furthermore, we showed that IGF-2 was responsible for GLP-1–induced protection against apoptosis, since this protective effect was suppressed by IGF-2 knockdown, by antibody-mediated blocking of secreted IGF-2, or by suppressing IGF-1R expression. This was observed both in MIN6 cells and in pancreatic islets.

This proposed autocrine role of IGF-2 in protecting β-cells against apoptosis is in agreement with previous data suggesting a role of this hormone in the physiological regulation of β-cells during embryonic development (36) and with the reported link between reduced IGF-2 expression by the pancreas during the fetal life and impaired β-cell function in the adult GK rat (37,38). Also, in the neonatal period, when the endocrine pancreas goes through a wave of β-cell apoptosis, there is a decreased expression of IGF-2 in the islets (39). This wave of apoptosis can, however, be prevented by transgenic expression of IGF-2 in peripheral tissues, which leads to elevated circulating plasma levels of this hormone (40). Also, transgenic expression of IGF-2 in β-cells leads to increased β-cell mass in adult mice (41). However, a role for IGF-2 in the control of adult islet function has not been previously established.

Therefore, several lines of evidence support an autocrine role for secreted IGF-2 in the control of β-cell mass both during embryonic development and after birth. Interestingly, recent genome-wide association studies have identified *Igf2bp2* as a gene associated with increased incidence of type 2 diabetes (42). IGF2BP2 is an IGF-2 mRNA binding protein that regulates the translation of this mRNA (43), suggesting that the control of IGF-2 expression may also participate in regulating β-cell physiology.

Together, our studies provide an integrated view of the GLP-1 and IGF-1R signaling pathways. They show that an IGF-2/IGF-1R autocrine loop operates in β-cells and that GLP-1 increases its activity by augmenting IGF-1R expression, a long-term effect, and also by acutely stimulating IGF-2 secretion. These results therefore have important pathophysiological implications, since they can lead to alternative ways of preventing β-cell mass decrease: by modulating IGF-1R expression and/or expression and secretion of IGF-2.

ACKNOWLEDGMENTS

This work was supported by grants to B.T. from the Swiss National Science Foundation (3100A0-113525), the Juvenile Diabetes Research Foundation (Program Project 7-2005-1158), and the European Union (Integrated Project Eurodia LSHM-CT-2006-518153, Framework Programme 6 [FP6] of the European Community).

No potential conflicts of interest relevant to this article were reported.

We thank the University of Lausanne DNA Array Facility for help with cDNA microarray experiments, D. Accili and A. Efstratiadis for β-IGF1-R knockout mice, and C.B. Wollheim for helpful comments on the manuscript.

REFERENCES

1. Bouwens L, Rooman I. Regulation of pancreatic beta-cell mass. Physiol Rev 2005;85:1255–1270
2. Eizirik DL, Mandrup-Poulsen T. A choice of death: the signal-transduction of immune-mediated beta-cell apoptosis. Diabetologia 2001;44:2115–2133
3. Prentki M, Nolan CJ. Islet beta cell failure in type 2 diabetes. J Clin Invest 2006;116:1802–1812
4. Butler AE, Janson J, Bonner-Weir S, Ritzel R, Rizza RA, Butler PC. Beta-cell deficit and increased β-cell apoptosis in humans with type 2 diabetes. Diabetes 2003;52:102–110
5. Drucker DJ. The biology of incretin hormones. Cell Metab 2006;3:153–165
6. Thorens B. Expression cloning of the pancreatic beta cell receptor for the

gluco-incretin hormone glucagon-like peptide I. Proc Natl Acad Sci U S A 1992;89:8641–8645

7. Usdin TB, Mezey E, Button DC, Brownstein MJ, Bonner TI. Gastric inhibitory polypeptide receptor, a member of the secretin-vasoactive intestinal peptide receptor family, is widely distributed in peripheral organs and the brain. Endocrinology 1993;133:2861–2870

8. Schuit FC, Pipeleers DG. Regulation of adenosine 3′,5′-monophosphate levels in the pancreatic B cell. Endocrinology 1985;117:834–840

9. Ozaki N, Shibasaki T, Kashima Y, Miki T, Takahashi K, Ueno H, Sunaga Y, Yano M, Matsura Y, Iwanaga T, Takai Y, Seino S. cAMP-GEFII is a direct target of cAMP in regulated exocytosis. Nat Cell Biol 2000;2:805–811

10. Dyachok O, Isakov Y, Sagetorp J, Tengholm A. Oscillations of cyclic AMP in hormone-stimulated insulin-secreting beta-cells. Nature 2006;439:349–352

11. Gomez E, Pritchard C, Herbert TP. cAMP-dependent protein kinase and Ca^{2+} influx through L-type voltage-gated calcium channels mediate raf-independent activation of extracellular regulated kinase in response to glucagon-like peptide-1 in pancreatic β-cells. J Biol Chem 2002;277:48146–48151

12. Kerchner KR, Clay RL, McCleery G, Watson N, McIntire WE, Myung CS, Garrison JC. Differential sensitivity of phosphatidylinositol 3-kinase p110gamma to isoforms of G protein betagamma dimers. J Biol Chem 2004;279:44554–44562

13. Buteau J, Foisy S, Joly E, Prentki M. Glucagon-like peptide 1 induces pancreatic β-cell proliferation via transactivation of the epidermal growth factor receptor. Diabetes 2003;52:124–132

14. Jhala US, Canettieri G, Screaton RA, Kulkarni RN, Krajewski S, Reed J, Walker J, Lin X, White M, Montminy M. cAMP promotes pancreatic beta-cells survival via CREB-mediated induction of IRS2. Genes Dev 2003;17:1575–1580

15. Hennige AM, Burks DJ, Ozcan U, Kulkarni RN, Ye J, Park S, Schubert M, Fisher TL, Dow MA, Leshan R, Zakaria M, Mossa-Basha M, White MF. Upregulation of insulin receptor substrate-2 in pancreatic beta cells prevents diabetes. J Clin Invest 2003;112:1521–1532

16. Park S, Dong X, Fisher TL, Dunn S, Omer AK, Weir G, White MF. Exendin-4 uses Irs2 signaling to mediate pancreatic beta cell growth and function. J Biol Chem 2006;281:1159–1168

17. Xuan S, Kitamura T, Nakae J, Politi K, Kido Y, Fisher PE, Morroni M, Cinti S, White MF, Herrera PL, Accili D, Efstratiadis A. Defective insulin secretion in pancreatic β cells lacking type 1 IGF receptor. J Clin Invest 2002;110:1011–1019

18. Kulkarni RN, Holzenberger M, Shih DQ, Ozcan U, Stoffel M, Magnuson MA, Kahn CR. Beta-cell-specific deletion of the Igf1 receptor leads to hyperinsulinemia and glucose intolerance but does not alter beta-cell mass. Nat Genet 2002;31:111–115

19. Ueki K, Okada T, Hu J, Liew CW, Assmann A, Dahlgren GM, Peters JL, Shackman JG, Zhang M, Artner I, Satin LS, Stein R, Holzenberger M, Kennedy RT, Kahn CR, Kulkarni RN. Total insulin and IGF-I resistance in pancreatic beta cells causes overt diabetes. Nat Genet 2006;38:583–588

20. Gotoh M, Maki T, Satomi S, Porter J, Bonner-Weir S, O'Hara CJ, Monaco AP. Reproducible high yield of rat islets by stationary in vitro digestion following pancreatic ductal or portal venous collagenase injection. Transplantation 1987;43:725–730

21. Klinger S, Poussin C, Debril MB, Dolci W, Halban PA, Thorens B. Increasing GLP-1–induced β-cell proliferation by silencing the negative regulators of signaling cAMP response element modulator-α and DUSP14. Diabetes 2008;57:584–593

22. de Fourmestraux V, Neubauer H, Poussin C, Farmer P, Falquet L, Burcelin R, Delorenzi M, Thorens B. Transcript profiling suggests that differential metabolic adaptation of mice to a high fat diet is associated with changes in liver to muscle lipid fluxes. J Biol Chem 2004;279:50743–50753

23. Yang JY, Widmann C. Antiapoptotic signaling generated by caspase-induced cleavage of RasGAP. Mol Cell Biol 2001;21:5346–5358

24. He TC, Zhou S, da Costa LT, Yu J, Kinzler KW, Vogelstein B. A simplified system for generating recombinant adenoviruses. Proc Natl Acad Sci U S A 1998;95:2509–2514

25. Gao Y, Ordas R, Klein JD, Price SR. Regulation of caspase-3 activity by insulin in skeletal muscle cells involves both PI3-kinase and MEK-1/2. J Appl Physiol 2008;105:1772–1778

26. Liu W, Chin-Chance C, Lee EJ, Lowe WL Jr: Activation of phosphatidylinositol 3-kinase contributes to insulin-like growth factor I-mediated inhibition of pancreatic beta-cell death. Endocrinology 2002;143:3802–3812

27. Frasca F, Pandini G, Scalia P, Sciacca L, Mineo R, Costantino A, Goldfine ID, Belfiore A, Vigneri R. Insulin receptor isoform A, a newly recognized, high-affinity insulin-like growth factor II receptor in fetal and cancer cells. Mol Cell Biol 1999;19:3278–3288

28. Hoog A, Hu W, Abdel-Halim SM, Falkmer S, Qing L, Grimelius L. Ultrastructural localization of insulin-like growth factor-2 (IGF-2) to the secretory granules of insulin cells: a study in normal and diabetic (GK) rats. Ultrastruct Pathol 1997;21:457–466

29. Hoog A, Kjellman M, Nordqvist AC, Hoog CM, Juhlin C, Falkmer S, Schalling M, Grimelius L. Insulin-like growth factor-II in endocrine pancreatic tumours: immunohistochemical, biochemical and in situ hybridization findings. APMIS 2001;109:127–140

30. Buteau J, Roduit R, Susini S, Prentki M. Glucagon-like peptide-1 promotes DNA synthesis, activates phosphatidylinositol 3-kinase and increases transcription factor pancreatic and duodenal homeobox gene 1 (PDX-1) DNA binding activity in beta (INS-1)-cells. Diabetologia 1999;42:856–864

31. Wang Q, Li L, Xu E, Wong V, Rhodes C, Brubaker PL. Glucagon-like peptide-1 regulates proliferation and apoptosis via activation of protein kinase B in pancreatic INS-1 beta cells. Diabetologia 2004;47:478–487

32. Buteau J, Spatz ML, Accili D. Transcription factor FoxO1 mediates glucagon-like peptide-1 effects on pancreatic β-cell mass. Diabetes 2006;55:1190–1196

33. Vilsboll T, Krarup T, Sonne J, Madsbad S, Volund A, Juul AG, Holst JJ. Incretin secretion in relation to meal size and body weight in healthy subjects and people with type 1 and type 2 diabetes mellitus. J Clin Endocrinol Metab 2003;88:2706–2713

34. Crutchlow MF, Yu M, Bae YS, Deng S, Stoffers DA. Exendin-4 does not promote beta-cell proliferation or survival during the early post-islet transplant period in mice. Transplant Proc 2008;40:1650–1657

35. Smith FE, Rosen KM, Villa-Komaroff L, Weir GC, Bonner-Weir S. Enhanced insulin-like growth factor I gene expression in regenerating rat pancreas. Proc Natl Acad Sci U S A 1991;88:6152–6156

36. Portela-Gomes GM, Hoog A. Insulin-like growth factor II in human fetal pancreas and its co-localization with the major islet hormones: comparison with adult pancreas. J Endocrinol 2000;165:245–251

37. Calderari S, Gangnerau MN, Thibault M, Meile MJ, Kassis N, Alvarez C, Portha B, Serradas P. Defective IGF2 and IGF1R protein production in embryonic pancreas precedes beta cell mass anomaly in the Goto-Kakizaki rat model of type 2 diabetes. Diabetologia 2007;50:1463–1471

38. Serradas P, Goya L, Lacorne M, Gangnerau MN, Ramos S, Alvarez C, Pascual-Leone AM, Portha B. Fetal insulin-like growth factor-2 production is impaired in the GK rat model of type 2 diabetes. Diabetes 2002;51:392–397

39. Petrik J, Reusens B, Arany E, Remacle C, Coelho C, Hoet JJ, Hill DJ. A low protein diet alters the balance of islet cell replication and apoptosis in the fetal and neonatal rat and is associated with a reduced pancreatic expression of insulin-like growth factor-II. Endocrinology 1999;140:4861–4873

40. Hill DJ, Strutt B, Arany E, Zaina S, Coukell S, Graham CF. Increased and persistent circulating insulin-like growth factor II in neonatal transgenic mice suppresses developmental apoptosis in the pancreatic islets. Endocrinology 2000;141:1151–1157

41. Devedjian JC, George M, Casellas A, Pujol A, Visa J, Pelegrin M, Gros L, Bosch F. Transgenic mice overexpressing insulin-like growth factor-II in beta cells develop type 2 diabetes. J Clin Invest 2000;105:731–740

42. Zeggini E, Weedon MN, Lindgren CM, Frayling TM, Elliott KS, Lango H, Timpson NJ, Perry JR, Rayner NW, Freathy RM, Barrett JC, Shields B, Morris AP, Ellard S, Groves CJ, Harries LW, Marchini JL, Owen KR, Knight B, Cardon LR, Walker M, Hitman GA, Morris AD, Doney AS, McCarthy MI, Hattersley AT. Replication of genome-wide association signals in UK samples reveals risk loci for type 2 diabetes. Science 2007;316:1336–1341

43. Nielsen J, Christiansen J, Lykke-Andersen J, Johnsen AH, Wewer UM, Nielsen FC. A family of insulin-like growth factor II mRNA-binding proteins represses translation in late development. Mol Cell Biol 1999;19:1262–1270

Effect of Endogenous GLP-1 on Insulin Secretion in Type 2 Diabetes

Marzieh Salehi,[1] Benedict Aulinger,[1] Ronald L. Prigeon,[2] and David A. D'Alessio[1]

OBJECTIVE—The incretins glucagon-like peptide-1 (GLP-1) and glucose-dependent insulinotropic polypeptide (GIP) account for up to 60% of postprandial insulin release in healthy people. Previous studies showed a reduced incretin effect in patients with type 2 diabetes but a robust response to exogenous GLP-1. The primary goal of this study was to determine whether endogenous GLP-1 regulates insulin secretion in type 2 diabetes.

METHODS—Twelve patients with well-controlled type 2 diabetes and eight matched nondiabetic subjects consumed a breakfast meal containing D-xylose during fixed hyperglycemia at 5 mmol/l above fasting levels. Studies were repeated, once with infusion of the GLP-1 receptor antagonist, exendin-(9–39) (Ex-9), and once with saline.

RESULTS—The relative increase in insulin secretion after meal ingestion was comparable in diabetic and nondiabetic groups ($44 \pm 4\%$ vs. $47 \pm 7\%$). Blocking the action of GLP-1 suppressed postprandial insulin secretion similarly in the diabetic and nondiabetic subjects ($25 \pm 4\%$ vs. $27 \pm 8\%$). However, Ex-9 also reduced the insulin response to intravenous glucose ($25 \pm 5\%$ vs. $26 \pm 7\%$; diabetic vs. nondiabetic subjects), when plasma GLP-1 levels were undetectable. The appearance of postprandial ingested D-xylose in the blood was not affected by Ex-9.

CONCLUSIONS—These findings indicate that in patients with well-controlled diabetes, the relative effects of enteral stimuli and endogenous GLP-1 to enhance insulin release are retained and comparable with those in nondiabetic subjects. Surprisingly, GLP-1 receptor signaling promotes glucose-stimulated insulin secretion independent of the mode of glucose entry. Based on rates of D-xylose absorption, GLP-1 receptor blockade did not affect gastric emptying of a solid meal. *Diabetes* **59:1330–1337, 2010**

Glucagon-like peptide 1 (GLP-1) is a gut-brain peptide that is a major component of the incretin effect and is essential for normal glucose tolerance (1). Based on studies in which synthetic GLP-1, or GLP-1 receptor (GLP-1r) agonists, is administered to humans, GLP-1 has a broad range of actions that promote glucose homeostasis, including stimulating insulin secretion (2), suppressing glucagon release (3–4), delaying gastric emptying (5), and increasing hepatic glucose balance (6–7). Importantly, and unlike other insulinotropic gut peptides, the effects of GLP-1 on glucose metabolism are retained in people with diabetes (8–10). This has led to the development of novel therapeutic compounds for use in diabetic patients that are based on GLP-1r signaling (11).

The physiologic role of GLP-1 in individuals with diabetes has not been determined. However, there are several reasons to question whether the GLP-1 system is fully functional in this patient group. First, there is some evidence that GLP-1 secretion in response to meal ingestion in type 2 diabetes is impaired (12–15), although this finding has not been uniform (16–17). Second, the sensitivity of insulin secretion to exogenous GLP-1 is reduced in diabetic individuals (18). Finally, it has long been believed that the augmentation of glucose-stimulated insulin secretion during enteral glucose absorption, the incretin effect, is severely attenuated in type 2 diabetes, implying that incretins such as GLP-1 are not normally active in this group of subjects.

In this study, we tested the hypothesis that the effect of endogenous GLP-1 to promote insulin secretion after meal ingestion is reduced in people with diabetes. Diabetic subjects and age- and weight-matched nondiabetic subjects were studied with and without infusion of the specific GLP-1r antagonist, exendin-(9–39) (Ex-9), during fixed hyperglycemia before and after a breakfast meal.

RESEARCH DESIGN AND METHODS

Subjects. Twelve subjects with established type 2 diabetes (five females and seven males) and eight age- and BMI-matched nondiabetic subjects (six females and two males) were studied on two separate days (Table 1). All subjects were weight stable for 3 months prior to the experiments. Diabetic patients had good glycemic control with a mean A1C level of $6.3 \pm 0.1\%$ (range 5.9–7.6%). Normal glucose tolerance was confirmed in the nondiabetic subjects by a 2-h venous plasma glucose level of <7.8 mmol/l after a 75-g oral glucose tolerance test. The control subjects had no family history of type 2 diabetes, were free of any chronic medical conditions such as coronary artery disease, uncontrolled dyslipidemia, or hypertension, and received no medications for any of these conditions. The studies were approved by the institutional review board of the University of Cincinnati, and all participants provided written informed consent prior to the studies.

Peptides. Synthetic exendin-(9–39) (Clinalfa; Merck Biosciences AG, Läufelfingen, Switzerland) was greater than 95% pure, sterile, and free of pyrogens. Lyophilized peptide was prepared in 0.25% human serum albumin on the day of study. The use of synthetic Ex-9 is approved under the U.S. Food and Drug Administration Investigational New Drug 65,837.

Experimental procedures. Subjects were instructed to consume greater than 200 g of carbohydrate for 3 days before each visit and not to engage in vigorous physical activity. Subjects with diabetes withheld their oral antidiabetic medication for 3 days before each study. They were admitted to the General Clinical Research Center at Cincinnati Children's Hospital on separate occasions after an overnight fast. Intravenous catheters were placed in each forearm for the withdrawal of blood and the infusion of glucose and Ex-9; the arm used for blood sampling was continuously warmed using a heating pad to arterialize the venous blood. After removal of fasting blood samples, a primed continuous infusion of 20% glucose was started to achieve and maintain a target blood glucose concentration of 5 mmol/l greater than fasting levels (19). At 30 min, subjects received either *1*) an intravenous bolus of synthetic Ex-9 (7,500 pmol/kg) for 1 min followed by a continuous infusion

From the [1]University of Cincinnati, Department of Internal Medicine, Cincinnati, Ohio; and the [2]University of Maryland, Department of Medicine, Division of Gerontology, Baltimore, Maryland.

Corresponding author: Marzieh Salehi, salehim@uc.edu.

Received 26 August 2009 and accepted 24 February 2010. Published ahead of print at http://diabetes.diabetesjournals.org on 9 March 2010. DOI: 10.2337/db09-1253.

TABLE 1
Characteristics of the study participants

	Patients with type 2 diabetes	Nondiabetic subjects
Age (year)	54 (41–63)	49 (34–60)
BMI (kg/m^2)	34 (26–44)	32 (24–41)
Sex (F/M)	5/7	6/2
Duration of diabetes (month)	50 (1–200)	
Sulfonylurea/metformin/diet	4/9/3	

Data are presented as mean (range) unless otherwise noted.

(750 pmol/kg/min) for the remainder of the study, or 2) saline, as a control (19). The order of the infusions was balanced so that half the subjects received saline or Ex-9 as their first infusion, and the two experiments were separated by an interval of at least 1 week. At 90 min, subjects consumed a mixed nutrient breakfast (300 kcal with a calorie distribution of 40% carbohydrate, 20% protein, and 40% fat) consisting of scrambled eggs, English muffin, margarine, chocolate pudding mixed with 10 g D-xylose, and milk that was eaten within 10 min. Subjects were instructed to consume the pudding in the middle of the meal. The rate of intravenous glucose infusion was adjusted to maintain the blood glucose at the target rate throughout the meal and for the remainder of the study. Blood samples were drawn at −10, −5, 0, 15, 30, 45, 60, 70, 75, 80, 85, 90, 95,100, 105, 110, 120, 130, 140, 150, 160, 170, 180, 190, 200, 210, 220, 230, 240, 250, 255, 260, 265, and 270 min; the plasma was separated within 60 min of blood withdrawal and stored at −80°C until assay. Blood samples were collected in tubes containing heparin, 50 mmol/l EDTA, and 500 kallikrein inhibitory units per milliliter of aprotinin.

Assays. Blood glucose concentrations were determined by a glucose oxidase method using a glucose analyzer (YSI 2300 STAT Plus; Yellow Springs Instruments, Yellow Springs, OH). Insulin, glucagon, total GLP-1, and C-peptide were measured by radioimmunoassays as described previously (19). D-xylose was measured by colorimetric assay (20), and total glucose-dependent insulinotropic polypeptide (GIP) was measured by ELISA (Linco Research, St. Charles, MO).

Calculations and analysis. Insulin secretion rates (ISRs) were derived from plasma C-peptide concentrations using deconvolution with population estimates of C-peptide clearance (21–22). Fasting concentrations of blood glucose, hormones, and ISR were taken as the mean of the three samples drawn at −10, −5, and 0 min. Preprandial insulin secretory responses were computed as the mean increments above fasting values of ISR from 60 to 90 min; these were used to determine the responses to intravenous glucose–induced hyperglycemia. Postprandial insulin secretory responses were calculated as the mean increments above the 60–90 min values of ISR from 95 to 270 min. This measure of postprandial insulin secretion reflects the augmentation of ISR, beyond 5 mmol/l hyperglycemia, by meal-induced stimuli, and has been used previously as a surrogate for the incretin effect (23–25). The D-xylose, GLP-1, and GIP concentrations from 80 to 90 min were taken as baseline, and levels after meal consumption (95–270 min for D-xylose and GLP-1; 95–240 min for GIP) were used to compute postprandial areas under the curve (AUC) above baseline. The glucagon levels from 80 to 90 min (preprandial) were compared with fasting as well as values of glucagon from 250 to 260 min. The stability of the glucose clamps was computed as the mean of coefficients of variation for each study from 60 to 270 min. The reproducibility of the clamps was computed as the difference in mean glucose from 60 to 270 for each subject.

The contribution of endogenous GLP-1 to insulin secretion was determined by comparing the mean values of ISR for each subject during infusion of saline or Ex-9. Separate comparisons were made for the preprandial and postprandial periods.

The parameters obtained from each subject in the two studies and from the diabetic and nondiabetic groups were compared using one- and two-way ANOVA with repeated measures. Spearman correlation was used to seek relationships between measured outcomes and subject characteristics such as A1C, and paired t test was used to compare measured variables within each study. Data are presented as the mean ± SEM.

RESULTS

Fasting glucose was significantly higher in the diabetic than in the nondiabetic subjects ($P < 0.001$), but fasting insulin and C-peptide concentrations were comparable, and the values for each subject were similar on the days of the saline and Ex-9 studies (Table 2). Blood glucose concentrations were raised by ~5 mmol/l from fasting values to hyperglycemic levels from 60 to 270 min that were comparable during the Ex-9 and saline studies (Fig. 1, Table 2). The average clamped glucose levels (60–270 min) for nondiabetic subjects during the saline and Ex-9 studies were 9.3 ± 0.2 and 9.3 ± 0.2 mmol/l, respectively, with a mean difference of 0.02 ± 0.03 mmol/l. For the diabetic subjects, the mean glucose concentrations (60–270 min) were 12.0 ± 0.4 and 12.1 ± 0.4 mmol/l for the control and Ex-9 clamps, respectively, and the mean difference was 0.09 ± 0.07 mmol/l. The average coefficient of variation of the glucose concentrations during the hyperglycemic clamp control studies was 4.4 ± 0.4% for the nondiabetic and 4.9 ± 0.5% for the diabetic subjects.

The glucose infusion rates needed to reach target glycemia were higher in the nondiabetic compared with diabetic subjects during the preprandial (60–90 min; $P < 0.01$) and postprandial (95–270 min; $P < 0.05$) periods. Infusion of Ex-9 was associated with a significant reduction of the glucose infusion rates necessary to maintain target glycemia from 60 to 90 min in both groups ($P < 0.05$ for both comparisons). After ingestion of the breakfast meal, the glucose infusion rate was initially reduced in some subjects to compensate for glucose influx from the gut, but was significantly higher than preprandial infusions by the end of the study (Fig. 1, Table 2).

In both the diabetic and nondiabetic groups, β-cell secretion rose in response to intravenous glucose administration to a plateau from 60 to 90 min (Fig. 2, Table 2); preprandial insulin, C-peptide, and ISR were greater in the nondiabetic than the diabetic group ($P < 0.05$). Among the diabetic subjects, there were significant inverse correlations between the preprandial insulin secretory response and fasting glucose ($r = −0.7$, $P < 0.01$) and A1C ($r = −0.8$, $P < 0.05$). Compared with the study with saline infusion, GLP-1r blockade with Ex-9 caused a significant reduction of insulin secretion before meal ingestion (60–90 min), as indicated by significantly lower mean values of insulin, C-peptide, and ISR (Table 2). The GLP-1 effect on intravenous glucose–stimulated insulin secretion, taken as the percentage difference in mean ISR from 60 to 90 min with and without Ex-9, was 25 ± 5% in diabetic subjects and 26 ± 7% in the nondiabetic group (Fig. 3).

After meal consumption (95–270 min), β-cell secretion increased significantly over preprandial (60–90 min) values in both the nondiabetic ($P < 0.01$) and diabetic ($P < 0.05$) subjects; although the absolute responses were significantly lower in the diabetic group ($P < 0.05$; Fig. 2, Table 2). Among the diabetic subjects, there were significant inverse correlations between postprandial insulin secretory responses and A1C ($r = −0.6$, $P < 0.05$). During the saline infusion study, meal ingestion significantly enhanced ISR, by 47 ± 7% in the nondiabetic and 44 ± 4% for diabetic subjects, above preprandial ISR. During the Ex-9 infusion, postprandial ISR was 44 ± 6% and 45 ± 4% higher than preprandial ISR in the nondiabetic and diabetic groups, respectively. Blocking endogenous GLP-1 with Ex-9 diminished postprandial ISR by 27 ± 8% in nondiabetic and 25 ± 4% in diabetic subjects, compared with the studies with saline infusion (Fig. 3).

Fasting glucagon concentrations in the diabetic subjects were similar during the saline and Ex-9 studies (Table 2). During both the saline and Ex-9 infusions, the hyperglycemic clamp suppressed glucagon levels from 80 to 90 min ($P < 0.05$). Glucagon values at the conclusion of the experiments remained suppressed during the saline infu-

TABLE 2

Effect of meal ingestion during hyperglycemic clamp on β-cell hormonal response and gastrointestinal peptides in studies with and without intravenous Ex-9 in subjects with and without diabetes

Time interval (min)	Diabetic subjects		Nondiabetic subjects		Statistical effects (P values)		
	Saline	Ex-9	Saline	Ex-9	Ex-9 vs. Saline	Diabetic vs. nondiabetic subjects	Interaction
Glucose (mmol/l)							
Fasting	6.7 ± 0.3	6.5 ± 0.3	4.8 ± 0.2	4.9 ± 0.1	NS	<0.001	NS
60–90	12.3 ± 0.3	12.2 ± 0.3	9.3 ± 0.2	9.5 ± 0.2	NS	<0.001	NS
95–270	12.0 ± 0.4	12.1 ± 0.4	9.3 ± 0.2	9.3 ± 0.2	NS	<0.001	NS
GINF (mg/kg/min)							
60–90	3.9 ± 0.4	3.5 ± 0.4	6.0 ± 0.5	5 ± 0.5	<0.05	<0.01	NS
95–270	6.1 ± 1.6	4.6 ± 1.4	11.5 ± 0.7	9.6 ± 0.9	<0.01	<0.05	NS
Insulin (pmol/l)							
Fasting	128 ± 22	142 ± 28	111 ± 20	116 ± 21	NS	NS	NS
60–90	363 ± 69	207 ± 32	719 ± 134	490 ± 107	<0.001	<0.01	NS
95–270	894 ± 220	577 ± 94	2,243 ± 365	1,531 ± 287	<0.001	<0.01	<0.05
C-peptide (nmol/l)							
Fasting	1.2 ± 0.1	1.0 ± 0.1	0.9 ± 0.1	0.9 ± 0.2	0.09	NS	NS
60–90	2.1 ± 0.3	1.8 ± 0.2	3.2 ± 0.4	2.6 ± 0.4	<0.001	<0.05	NS
95–270	4.6 ± 1.1	3.4 ± 0.6	7.6 ± 0.9	5.9 ± 1.1	<0.01	<0.05	NS
ISR (nmol/min)							
Fasting	0.34 ± 0.03	0.35 ± 0.04	0.47 ± 0.11	0.49 ± 0.13	NS	NS	NS
60–90	0.71 ± 0.1	0.53 ± 0.08	1.20 ± 0.17	0.95 ± 0.2	<0.001	<0.05	NS
95–270	1.43 ± 0.32	1.03 ± 0.18	2.42 ± 0.32	1.83 ± 0.36	<0.01	<0.05	NS
Glucagon (pg/ml)							
Fasting	48 ± 4	49 ± 4	46 ± 4	51 ± 5	NS	NS	NS
80–90	41 ± 3	41 ± 4	43 ± 2	42 ± 3	NS	NS	NS
250–260	43 ± 4	58 ± 8	40 ± 4	41 ± 5	<0.05	NS	0.06
GLP-1 (pmol/l)							
80–90	3.6 ± 0.3	3.6 ± 0.2	3.1 ± 0.1	3.0 ± 0.0	NS	NS	NS
AUC$_{GLP-1}$ (pmol/l/min)							
95–270	438 ± 92	1,423 ± 340	154 ± 73	560 ± 230	<0.05	0.08	NS
GIP (μmol/l)							
80–90	0.07 ± 0.0	0.06 ± 0.0	0.05 ± 0.0	0.04 ± 0.0	NS	NS	NS
AUC$_{GIP}$ (μmol/l/min)							
95–240	12.7 ± 1.4	17.1 ± 1.4	7.9 ± 1.9	7.7 ± 2.3	NS	<0.05	NS

GINF, glucose infusion rate; NS, not significant.

sion, but were significantly higher when Ex-9 was given ($P < 0.05$). In nondiabetic subjects, plasma glucagon concentrations decreased slightly, but not significantly, between the fasting and preprandial periods, and did not change further after the meal, with either saline or Ex-9.

Plasma concentrations of D-xylose increased steadily after meal intake and peaked at 60 min after meal consumption in both diabetic and nondiabetic subjects during both saline and Ex-9 studies (Fig. 4). The area under plasma D-xylose curve in the studies with saline and Ex-9 infusion, respectively, were 105 ± 8.2 and 102 ± 9.1 mmol/l/min in diabetic and 71 ± 8.5 and 70 ± 8 mmol/l/min in nondiabetic subjects, indicating that GLP-1 receptor blockade had minimal effects on the passage of D-xylose from the stomach to the intestine. D-xylose AUC was significantly greater in the diabetic compared with the nondiabetic group ($P < 0.05$).

Fasting plasma GIP levels were comparable before meal ingestion in the studies with saline and Ex-9 infusion in the diabetic (16 ± 1 and 16 ± 2 pmol/l) and nondiabetic (20 ± 1 and 20 ± 2 pmol/l) subjects. In both the nondiabetic and diabetic groups, meal consumption caused a similar rise of GIP concentrations in the saline and Ex-9 studies (Fig. 4, Table 2), suggesting that GLP-1r blockade had no effect on GIP secretion. The GIP response was significantly greater in the diabetic compared with nondiabetic group ($P < 0.05$). Fasting plasma GLP-1 were not different in the diabetic (3.6 ± 0.3 and 3.6 ± 0.2 pmol/l) and nondiabetic (3.1 ± 0.1 and 3.0 ± 0.0 pmol/l) groups, during the saline and Ex-9 studies, but levels were undetectable in ~80% of the subjects. Plasma GLP-1 increased after meal ingestion in both groups (Fig. 4, Table 2), and Ex-9 infusion significantly increased these responses in the nondiabetic and diabetic subjects ($P < 0.05$).

Subjects tolerated the experiments without notable problems, and there were no adverse events associated with Ex-9 infusion.

DISCUSSION

The current study investigated the role of endogenous GLP-1 on islet hormone secretion and gastric emptying in patients with type 2 diabetes. Although previous studies have demonstrated that diabetic patients respond to pharmacologic amounts of GLP-1, the effect of endogenous GLP-1 has not been previously demonstrated. Our results indicate that in diabetic subjects with good glycemic control, there is an enhancement of glucose-stimulated insulin secretion after meal ingestion that is similar on a relative basis to nondiabetic individuals. Moreover, the

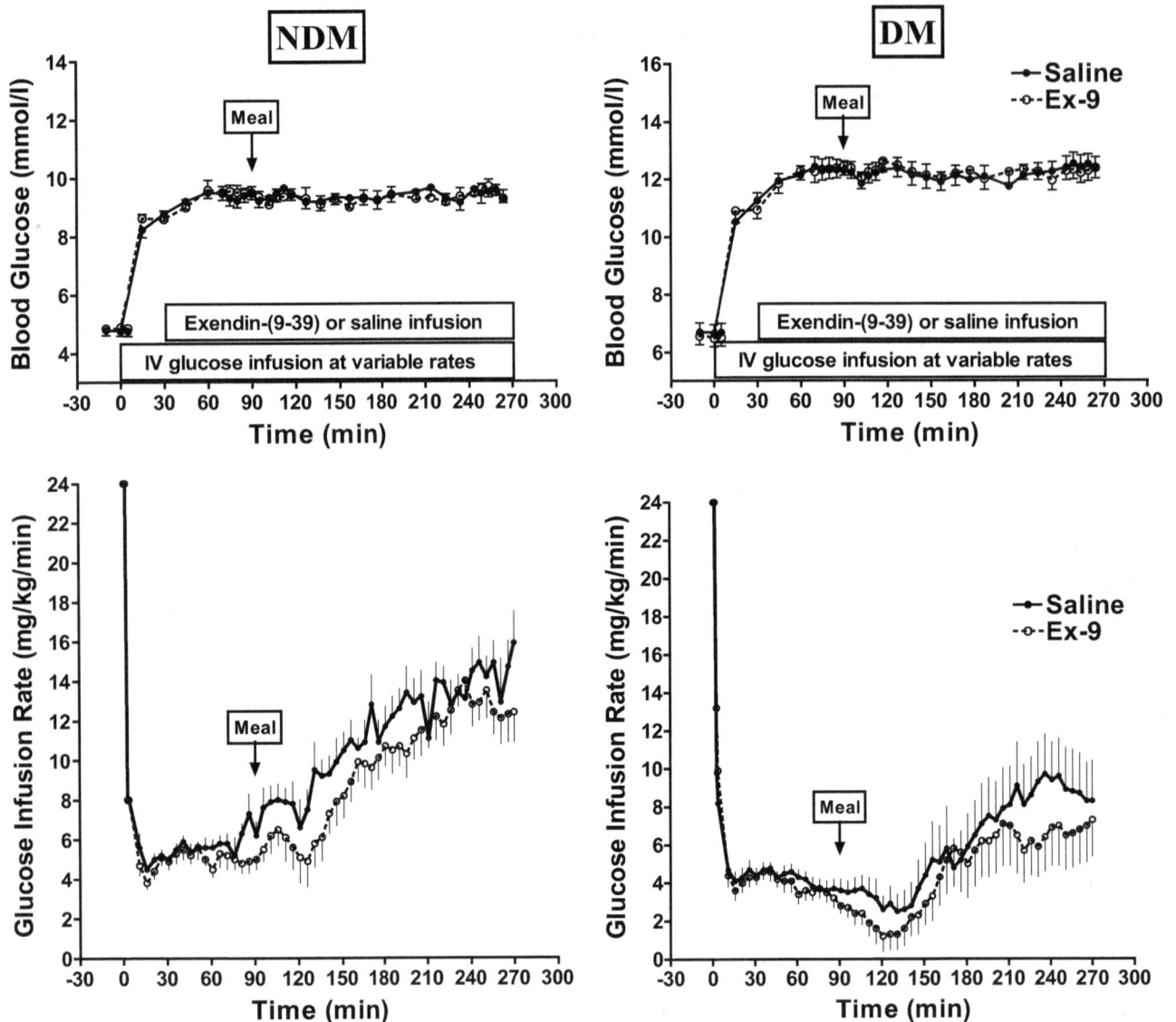

FIG. 1. Blood glucose concentrations and glucose infusion rates during intravenous-meal clamps with Ex-9 or saline infusions in nondiabetic (*left*) and diabetic (*right*) subjects. Data are presented as mean ± SEM.

impact of GLP-1r blockade was also comparable in the groups, indicating that endogenous GLP-1 contributes significantly to postprandial insulin secretion in diabetic subjects. Surprisingly, GLP-1r blockade reduced insulin secretion in response to intravenous glucose alone, and the magnitude of this effect was as great as that on postprandial β-cell responses. Gastric emptying, as reflected by D-xylose uptake, was not affected by blocking GLP-1r. These findings support an important physiologic role for GLP-1 to amplify glucose-stimulated insulin secretion, and demonstrate that this effect is retained in at least a subset of type 2 diabetic patients.

Our group and others (4,19,26–27) have previously used Ex-9 to demonstrate the effects of GLP-1r signaling in human subjects. In our previous report, we demonstrated that doses of Ex-9 identical to those used in the present study were effective for blocking supraphysiologic infusions of GLP-1 nearly completely, and for reducing postprandial insulin secretion by ~30%. Although no one has established definitively a dose of Ex-9 beyond which no

further inhibition of GLP-1 action can be detected, based on previously published results (4,19,26) we believe that the dose used in this study was near maximal for what can be achieved in an acute infusion.

The classic method for determining the incretin effect is a 2-day method with an oral glucose tolerance test on day 1 followed on day 2 by an intravenous glucose infusion isoglycemic to arterialized venous glucose levels after glucose ingestion (28). Using this method, Nauck et al. demonstrated a severe impairment of the incretin effect in subjects with type 2 diabetes (29), a much cited finding that has been very influential in shaping the understanding of enteroinsular physiology. We elected to use an alternative method, the hyperglycemic clamp-meal test, as a means of comparing the relative increase in insulin secretion when carbohydrate is absorbed enterally, because the test can be performed in a single morning, reducing day-to-day variability and the time commitment of research subjects. Variations of this method have been used previously by a number of investigators (23–25). Our

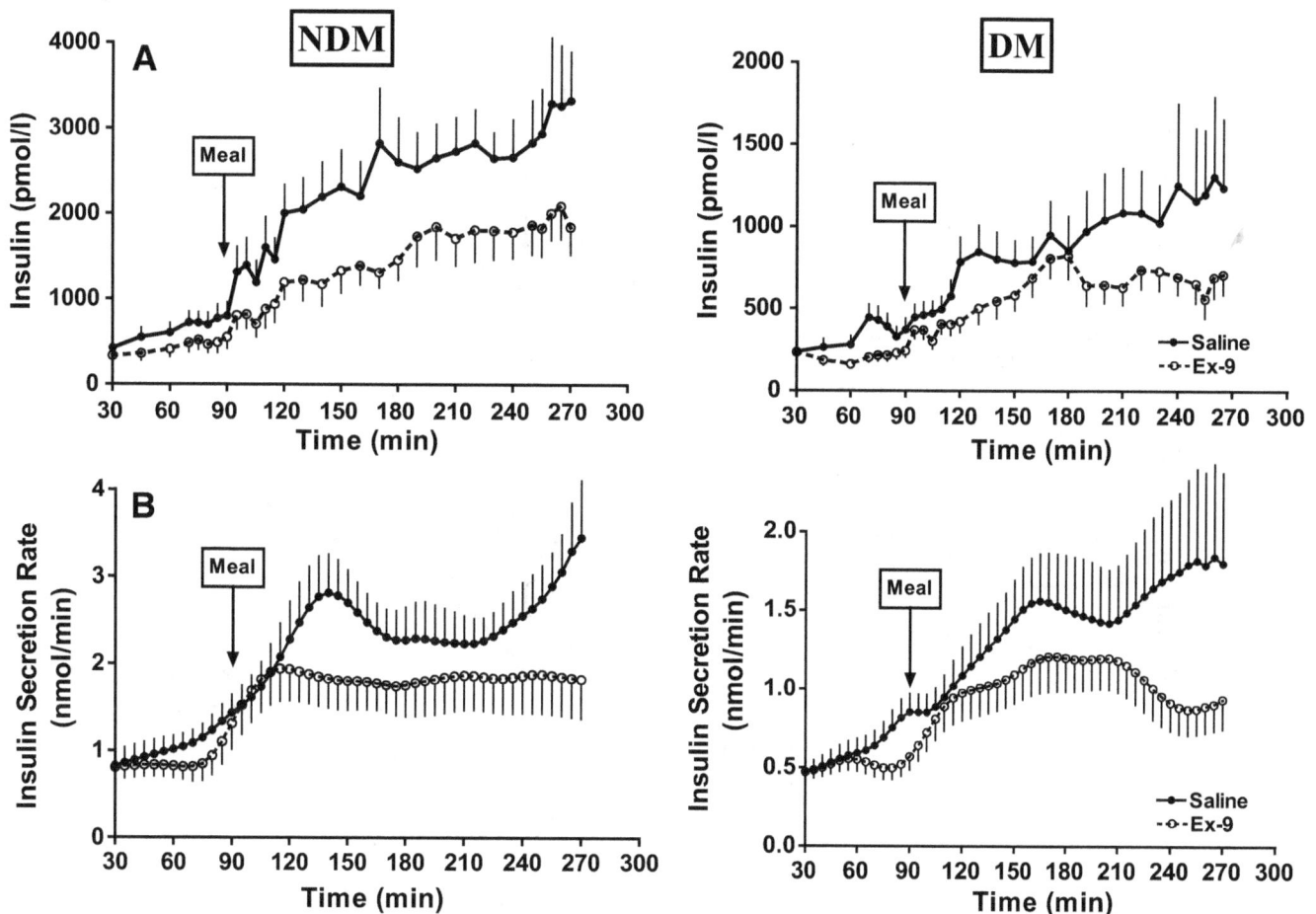

FIG. 2. β-cell secretion in response to hyperglycemia and meal ingestion with and without Ex-9 infusion. Plasma insulin concentrations (*A*) and insulin secretion rates (*B*) for nondiabetic (*left*) and diabetic (*right*) subjects. Data are presented as mean ± SEM.

preliminary data for normal glucose-tolerant subjects demonstrate that the estimation of the incretin effect using the 1-day and 2-day methods is comparable with a strong and significant within-subject correlation (30). In the present study, we used a mixed nutrient meal as the enteral stimulus during the hyperglycemic clamp to assess the nutrient, incretin, and neural responses activated by typical food consumption. We targeted the clamp as 5 mmol/l

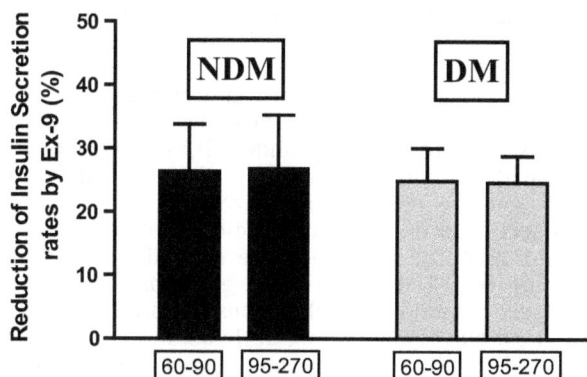

FIG. 3. The contribution of GLP-1 to preprandial and postprandial insulin secretion. The percentage reduction of insulin secretion rates by Ex-9 is shown for the preprandial (60–90 min) and postprandial (95–270 min) periods in the nondiabetic (black bars) and diabetic (gray bars) groups. Data are presented as mean ± SEM.

above fasting glucose to achieve levels that were slightly greater than what we expected as a result of meal ingestion alone. Overall, this design permitted a measure of the enhancement of insulin secretion by meal ingestion, and the GLP-1 component of it. Without further validation, this measure cannot be equated to the classically derived incretin effect, although we believe that the two methods assess similar physiologic processes.

In contrast to what was described originally by Nauck et al. (29), and confirmed in more recent studies (13), the cohort of diabetic subjects described here had a comparable degree of meal enhancement of insulin secretion to the nondiabetic group. Although β-cell secretion was clearly abnormal in diabetic compared with the nondiabetic subjects, relative to the ISR or plasma insulin levels achieved during stimulation with intravenous glucose alone, meal ingestion caused equivalent augmentation in the diabetic and nondiabetic groups (Table 2). This finding is consistent with the results reported by Perley and Kipnis more than three decades ago (31), showing that obese subjects with mild type 2 diabetes had preserved stimulation of insulin secretion by alimentary factors relative to nondiabetic control subjects. In contrast to the findings of Nauck et al. (29), the plasma GIP responses were increased in our diabetic compared with nondiabetic subjects. Increased GIP secretion has been reported previously in some studies of diabetic subjects (reviewed

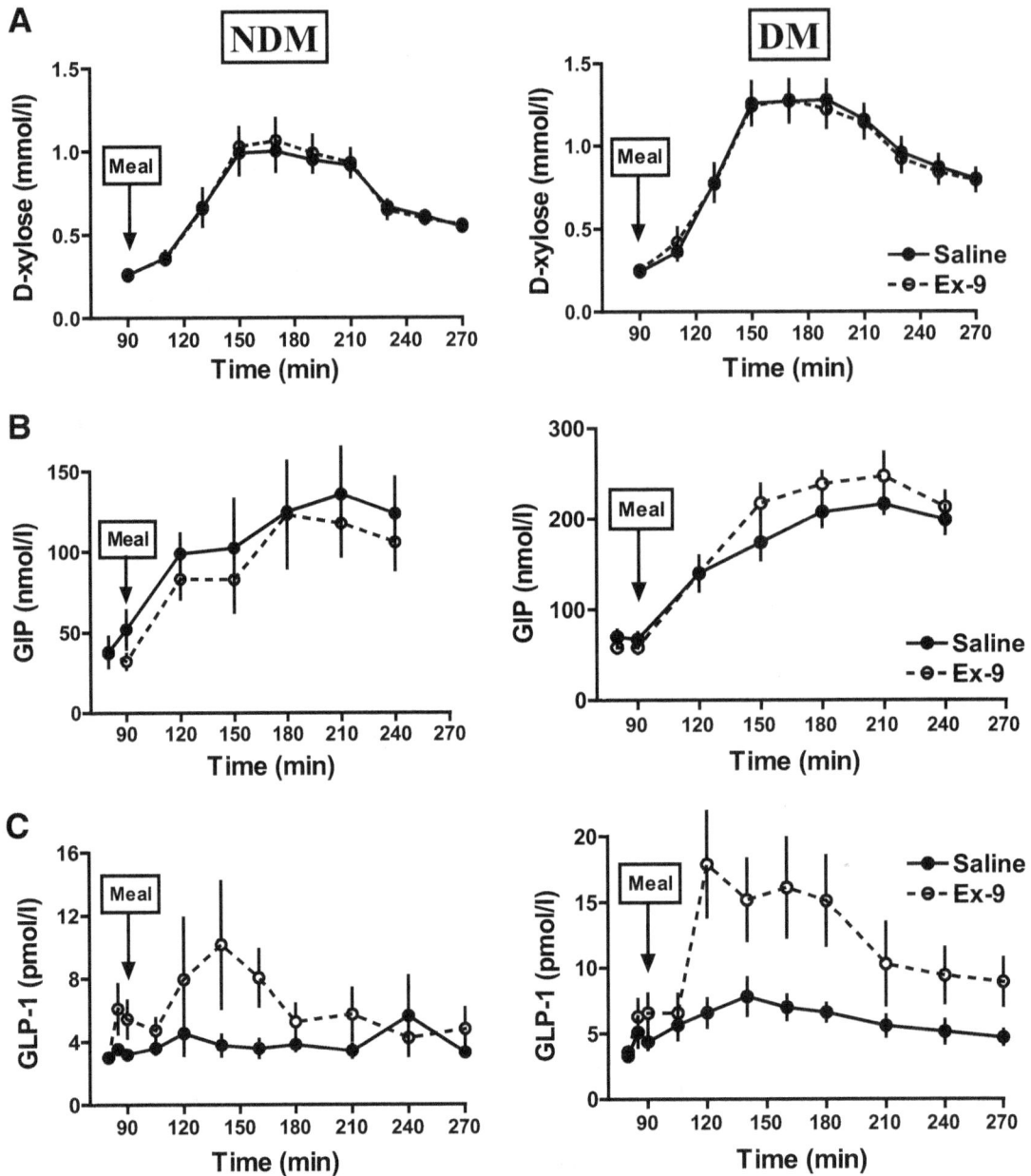

FIG. 4. Postprandial concentrations of D-xylose (*A*), GIP (*B*), and GLP-1 (*C*) in nondiabetic (*left*) and diabetic (*right*) subjects. Data are presented as mean ± SEM.

in [32]). Although an increased effect of GIP could account for a bigger augmentation of insulin secretion by meal ingestion in our diabetic subjects, most previous studies indicate that GIP has very modest effects on insulin secretion in type 2 diabetes (8).

Just as the relative increase of ISR with meal ingestion was similar in the diabetic and nondiabetic subjects, so too was the contribution of GLP-1 action to postprandial β-cell responses. Based on the effects of Ex-9, GLP-1 accounted for ~25% of the insulin response to the mixed meal at a fixed level of hyperglycemia. This is consistent with what we reported recently as the GLP-1 effect in healthy lean subjects during an oral glucose tolerance test (19). The finding of intact effects of GLP-1 in the diabetic group was unexpected, in that previous work had indicated that type 2 diabetic subjects have a blunted response

to exogenous GLP-1 infused to supraphysiologic levels (18). Although there was a weak trend toward the diabetic group having a greater postprandial GLP-1 response, there was considerable heterogeneity in the AUC among the subjects and no correlation between this measure and insulin secretion or the magnitude of insulin suppression by GLP-1 receptor blockade. These results suggest that circulating GLP-1 may not be a good predictor of the physiologic response to endogenous peptide.

The most surprising finding in this study was that Ex-9 diminished insulin secretion in response to intravenous glucose–induced hyperglycemia before meal consumption, at a time when circulatory levels of GLP-1 were often undetectable. In fact, the relative effect of GLP-1r blockade on preprandial and postprandial ISR was nearly identical. These findings indicate that GLP-1r effects on the β-cell are not restricted to the potentiation of insulin secretion after enteral nutrient absorption when circulating levels of GLP-1 increase. It is important to note that in previous studies blockade of the GLP-1 receptor did not affect fasting plasma insulin levels (4,27,33), but that Schirra et al. noted a reduction in plasma insulin, similar to what we describe here, during a hyperglycemic clamp when Ex-9 was infused (27). Thus, when considered together, the current evidence supports a role for GLP-1r signaling to potentiate glucose-stimulated but not basal insulin secretion in humans. This is consistent with studies in mice with engineered deletion of the GLP-1r gene in which similar degrees of glucose intolerance have been described to both oral and intraperitoneal glucose challenges (34), conditions with elevated and basal plasma GLP-1 levels, respectively. The mechanism whereby Ex-9 affects insulin secretion in the absence of elevated circulating levels of GLP-1 is unclear. However, recent studies raise the possibility of neural (35–36) and paracrine (37) modes of GLP-1 signaling, either of which could be affected by GLP-1r blockade. In addition, in vitro work suggests that Ex-9 can act as an inverse agonist in isolated mouse islets (38). Overall, our findings fit with an expanded model of β-cell regulation by GLP-1 that stretches beyond endocrine effects after eating.

Although several investigators have suggested that the predominant effect of GLP-1 on glucose control is based on its effect on gastric emptying (39–40), this conjecture is based on the results of studies using exogenous administration of GLP-1. Given the identical pattern of postprandial plasma D-xylose in our subjects with and without Ex-9, endogenous GLP-1 has no detectable effect on the rate of passage of nutrients from the stomach to the intestine. Appearance of ingested D-xylose followed a similar time course in diabetic and nondiabetic subjects, but D-xylose reached higher concentrations in the diabetic group, suggesting more rapid gastric emptying in patients with early or mild diabetes, compatible with previous reports (41–42). The lack of effect of Ex-9 to alter D-xylose appearance is similar to what we have reported previously in studies with GLP-1 blockade in healthy humans and nonhuman primates given liquid glucose solution (19,33). We have extended these findings in this study by using a solid meal, and our data stand against an important physiologic role for GLP-1 in the regulation of prandial gastric motility in humans. However, Deane et al. have recently published evidence that endogenous GLP-1 delays gastric emptying in healthy subjects after a solid carbohydrate meal (43). Because these investigators used scintigraphy, the gold standard for measuring gastric emptying, our findings must be interpreted cautiously. Nonetheless, our results are consistent with a recent report that gastric emptying in diabetic patients was not affected by administration of a dipeptidyl peptidase-4 inhibitor that enhanced endogenous GLP-1 by threefold (44).

In previous studies, we and others (4,19) have found that infusion of Ex-9 during oral or intestinal glucose administration increases postprandial plasma glucagon, supporting an important role for GLP-1 to regulate the α-cell. This effect was seen here, but only in the diabetic group. The diabetic subjects had equivalent suppression of glucagon in response to intravenous glucose during the Ex-9 and control experiments, but after the meal there was a significant rise in plasma levels when the GLP-1r was blocked. Interestingly, we did not see this latter effect in the nondiabetic subjects. Although this outcome could indicate differential regulation of prandial α-cell secretion in diabetes, this conclusion needs more rigorous confirmation.

In summary, we report here that administration of Ex-9 reduces insulin secretion proportionately in response to intravenous glucose and enteral stimuli, and that this effect is similar in diabetic and nondiabetic subjects. These findings indicate that the effect of endogenous GLP-1 on postprandial insulin release is preserved in patients with well-controlled type 2 diabetes. Moreover, GLP-1r signaling is important for stimulated insulin secretion independent of the mode of glucose entry. Based on these results, it appears that the function of the enteroinsular axis is intact, at least in some people with type 2 diabetes, and that the role of endogenous GLP-1 to regulate islet function is not mediated entirely by an endocrine mechanism.

ACKNOWLEDGMENTS

These studies were supported by grants from the National Institutes of Health, DK-57900 (D.A.D.) and M01-RR-08084 (Cincinnati Children's Hospital General Clinical Research Center), and the Medical Research Service of the Department of the Veterans Administration.

No potential conflicts of interest relevant to this article were reported.

Parts of this study were presented in abstract form at the 67th Scientific Sessions of the American Diabetes Association, Chicago, Illinois, 22–26 June 2007.

We thank Kay Ellis, Clinton Elfers, Ron Bitner, and Brianne Paxton for their technical support and Suzanne Summers, R.D., for assistance with the design and preparation of test meals. We also thank the nursing staff from Clinical Research Center of Cincinnati Children's Hospital for their expert technical assistance.

REFERENCES

1. Drucker DJ. The biology of incretin hormones. Cell Metab 2006;3:153–165
2. Kreymann B, Williams G, Ghatei MA, Bloom SR. Glucagon-like peptide-1 7–36: a physiological incretin in man. Lancet 1987;2:1300–1304
3. Creutzfeldt WO, Kleine N, Willms B, Orskov C, Holst JJ, Nauck MA. Glucagonostatic actions and reduction of fasting hyperglycemia by exogenous glucagon-like peptide I(7–36) amide in type I diabetic patients. Diabetes Care 1996;19:580–586
4. Schirra J, Nicolaus M, Roggel R, Katschinski M, Storr M, Woerle HJ, Göke B. Endogenous glucagon-like peptide 1 controls endocrine pancreatic secretion and antro-pyloro-duodenal motility in humans. Gut 2006;55:243–251
5. Delgado-Aros S, Kim DY, Burton DD, Thomforde GM, Stephens D, Brinkmann BH, Vella A, Camilleri M. Effect of GLP-1 on gastric volume, emptying, maximum volume ingested, and postprandial symptoms in humans. Am J Physiol Gastrointest Liver Physiol 2002;282:G424–G431
6. Prigeon RL, Quddusi S, Paty B, D'Alessio DA. Suppression of glucose production by GLP-1 independent of islet hormones: a novel extrapancreatic effect. Am J Physiol Endocrinol Metab 2003;285:E701–E707
7. Dardevet D, Moore MC, Neal D, DiCostanzo CA, Snead W, Cherrington AD. Insulin-independent effects of GLP-1 on canine liver glucose metabolism: duration of infusion and involvement of hepatoportal region. Am J Physiol Endocrinol Metab 2004;287:E75–E81
8. Nauck MA, Heimesaat MM, Orskov C, Holst JJ, Ebert R, Creutzfeldt W. Preserved incretin activity of glucagon-like peptide 1 [7–36 amide] but not of synthetic human gastric inhibitory polypeptide in patients with type-2 diabetes mellitus. J Clin Invest 1993;91:301–307
9. Nauck MA, Kleine N, Orskov C, Holst JJ, Willms B, Creutzfeldt W. Normalization of fasting hyperglycaemia by exogenous glucagon-like peptide 1 (7–36 amide) in type 2 (non-insulin-dependent) diabetic patients. Diabetologia 1993;36:741–744
10. Rachman J, Gribble FM, Barrow BA, Levy JC, Buchanan KD, Turner RC. Normalization of insulin responses to glucose by overnight infusion of glucagon-like peptide 1 (7–36) amide in patients with NIDDM. Diabetes 1996;45:1524–1530

11. Ahrén B, Schmitz O. GLP-1 receptor agonists and DPP-4 inhibitors in the treatment of type 2 diabetes. Horm Metab Res 2004;36:867–876

12. Vilsbøll T, Krarup T, Deacon CF, Madsbad S, Holst JJ. Reduced postprandial concentrations of intact biologically active glucagon-like peptide 1 in type 2 diabetic patients. Diabetes 2001;50:609–613

13. Muscelli E, Mari A, Casolaro A, Camastra S, Seghieri G, Gastaldelli A, Holst JJ, Ferrannini E. Separate impact of obesity and glucose tolerance on the incretin effect in normal subjects and type 2 diabetic patients. Diabetes 2008;57:1340–1348

14. Toft-Nielsen MB, Damholt MB, Madsbad S, Hilsted LM, Hughes TE, Michelsen BK, Holst JJ. Determinants of the impaired secretion of glucagon-like peptide-1 in type 2 diabetic patients. J Clin Endocrinol Metab 2001;86:3717–3723

15. Rask E, Olsson T, Söderberg S, Johnson O, Seckl J, Holst JJ, Ahrén B, Northern Sweden Monitoring of Trends and Determinants in Cardiovascular Disease (MONICA). Impaired incretin response after a mixed meal is associated with insulin resistance in nondiabetic men. Diabetes Care 2001;24:1640–1645

16. Vollmer K, Holst JJ, Baller B, Ellrichmann M, Nauck MA, Schmidt WE, Meier JJ. Predictors of incretin concentrations in subjects with normal, impaired, and diabetic glucose tolerance. Diabetes 2008;57:678–687

17. Meier JJ, Nauck MA. Is secretion of glucagon-like peptide-1 reduced in type 2 diabetes mellitus? Nat Clin Pract Endocrinol Metab 2008;4:606–607

18. Kjems LL, Holst JJ, Vølund A, Madsbad S. The influence of GLP-1 on glucose-stimulated insulin secretion: effects on beta-cell sensitivity in type 2 and nondiabetic subjects. Diabetes 2003;52:380–386

19. Salehi M, Vahl TP, D'Alessio DA. Regulation of islet hormone release and gastric emptying by endogenous glucagon-like peptide 1 after glucose ingestion. J Clin Endocrinol Metab 2008;93:4909–4916

20. Eberts TJ, Sample RH, Glick MR, Ellis GH. A simplified, colorimetric micromethod for xylose in serum or urine, with phloroglucinol. Clin Chem 1979;25:1440–1443

21. Van Cauter E, Mestrez F, Sturis J, Polonsky KS. Estimation of insulin secretion rates from C-peptide levels. Comparison of individual and standard kinetic parameters for C-peptide clearance. Diabetes 1992;41:368–377

22. Tillil H, Shapiro ET, Miller MA, Karrison T, Frank BH, Galloway JA, Rubenstein AH, Polonsky KS. Dose-dependent effects of oral and intravenous glucose on insulin secretion and clearance in normal humans. Am J Physiol 1988;254:E349–E357

23. Andersen DK, Elahi D, Brown JC, Tobin JD, Andres R. Oral glucose augmentation of insulin secretion. Interactions of gastric inhibitory polypeptide with ambient glucose and insulin levels. J Clin Invest 1978;62:152–161

24. Ferrannini E, Katz LD, Glickman MG, Defronzo RA. Influence of combined intravenous and oral glucose administration on splanchnic glucose uptake in man. Clin Physiol 1990;10:527–538

25. Henchoz E, D'Alessio DA, Gillet M, Halkic N, Matzinger O, Goy JJ, Chioléro R, Tappy L, Schneiter P. Impaired insulin response after oral but not intravenous glucose in heart- and liver-transplant recipients. Transplantation 2003;76:923–929

26. Edwards CM, Todd JF, Mahmoudi M, Wang Z, Wang RM, Ghatei MA, Bloom SR. Glucagon-like peptide 1 has a physiological role in the control of postprandial glucose in humans: studies with the antagonist exendin 9–39. Diabetes 1999;48:86–93

27. Schirra J, Sturm K, Leicht P, Arnold R, Göke B, Katschinski M. Exendin(9–39)amide is an antagonist of glucagon-like peptide-1(7–36)amide in humans. J Clin Invest 1998;101:1421–1430

28. Nauck MA, Homberger E, Siegel EG, Allen RC, Eaton RP, Ebert R, Creutzfeldt W. Incretin effects of increasing glucose loads in man calculated from venous insulin and C-peptide responses. J Clin Endocrinol Metab 1986;63:492–498

29. Nauck M, Stöckmann F, Ebert R, Creutzfeldt W. Reduced incretin effect in type 2 (non-insulin-dependent) diabetes. Diabetologia 1986;29:46–52

30. Tong J, Aulinger B, Salehi M, D'Alessio DA. Comparison of one- and two-day methods for measuring the incretin effect. Poster presented at 69th Scientific Sessions of The American Diabetes Association, June 2009, New Orleans, Louisiana

31. Perley MJ, Kipnis DM. Plasma insulin responses to oral and intravenous glucose: studies in normal and diabetic subjects. J Clin Invest 1967;46:1954–1962

32. Ebert R, Creutzfeldt W. Gastrointestinal peptides and insulin secretion. Diabetes Metab Rev 1987;3:1–26

33. D'Alessio DA, Vogel R, Prigeon R, Laschansky E, Koerker D, Eng J, Ensinck JW. Elimination of the action of glucagon-like peptide 1 causes an impairment of glucose tolerance after nutrient ingestion by healthy baboons. J Clin Invest 1996;97:133–138

34. Baggio L, Kieffer TJ, Drucker DJ. Glucagon-like peptide-1, but not glucose-dependent insulinotropic peptide, regulates fasting glycemia and nonenteral glucose clearance in mice. Endocrinology 2000;141:3703–3709

35. Vahl TP, Tauchi M, Durler TS, Elfers EE, Fernandes TM, Bitner RD, Ellis KS, Woods SC, Seeley RJ, Herman JP, D'Alessio DA. Glucagon-like peptide-1 (GLP-1) receptors expressed on nerve terminals in the portal vein mediate the effects of endogenous GLP-1 on glucose tolerance in rats. Endocrinology 2007;148:4965–4973

36. Sandoval DA, Bagnol D, Woods SC, D'Alessio DA, Seeley RJ. Arcuate glucagon-like peptide 1 receptors regulate glucose homeostasis but not food intake. Diabetes 2008;57:2046–2054

37. Masur K, Tibaduiza EC, Chen C, Ligon B, Beinborn M. Basal receptor activation by locally produced glucagon-like peptide-1 contributes to maintaining beta-cell function. Mol Endocrinol 2005;19:1373–1382

38. Serre V, Dolci W, Schaerer E, Scrocchi L, Drucker D, Efrat S, Thorens B. Exendin-(9–39) is an inverse agonist of the murine glucagon-like peptide-1 receptor: implications for basal intracellular cyclic adenosine 3′,5′-monophosphate levels and beta-cell glucose competence. Endocrinology 1998;139:4448–4454

39. Nauck MA. Is glucagon-like peptide 1 an incretin hormone? Diabetologia 1999;42:373–379

40. Nauck MA, Niedereichholz U, Ettler R, Holst JJ, Orskov C, Ritzel R, Schmiegel WH. Glucagon-like peptide 1 inhibition of gastric emptying outweighs its insulinotropic effects in healthy humans. Am J Physiol 1997;273:E981–E988

41. Schwartz JG, Green GM, Guan D, McMahan CA, Phillips WT. Rapid gastric emptying of a solid pancake meal in type II diabetic patients. Diabetes Care 1996;19:468–471

42. Bertin E, Schneider N, Abdelli N, Wampach H, Cadiot G, Loboguerrero A, Leutenegger M, Liehn JC, Thiefin G. Gastric emptying is accelerated in obese type 2 diabetic patients without autonomic neuropathy. Diabete Metab 2001;27:357–364

43. Deane AM, Nguyen NQ, Stevens JE, Fraser RJ, Holloway RH, Besanko LK, Burgstad C, Jones KL, Chapman MJ, Rayner CK, Horowitz M. Endogenous glucagon-like peptide-1 slows gastric emptying in healthy subjects, attenuating postprandial glycemia. J Clin Endocrinol Metab 2010;95:215–221

44. Vella A, Bock G, Giesler PD, Burton DB, Serra DB, Saylan ML, Dunning BE, Foley JE, Rizza RA, Camilleri M. Effects of dipeptidyl peptidase-4 inhibition on gastrointestinal function, meal appearance, and glucose metabolism in type 2 diabetes. Diabetes 2007;56:1475–1480

The Possible Protective Role of Glucagon-Like Peptide 1 on Endothelium During the Meal and Evidence for an "Endothelial Resistance" to Glucagon-Like Peptide 1 in Diabetes

Antonio Ceriello, md[1]
Katherine Esposito, md[2]
Roberto Testa, md[3]
Anna Rita Bonfigli, phd[3]
Maurizio Marra, phd[3]
Dario Giugliano, md[2]

OBJECTIVE—Glucagon-like peptide 1 (GLP-1) stimulates insulin secretion. However, GLP-1 also improves endothelial function in diabetes.

RESEARCH DESIGN AND METHODS—Sixteen type 2 diabetic patients and 12 control subjects received a meal, an oral glucose tolerance test (OGTT), and two hyperglycemic clamps, with or without GLP-1. The clamps were repeated in diabetic patients after 2 months of strict glycemic control.

RESULTS—During the meal, glycemia, nitrotyrosine, and plasma 8-iso prostaglandin F2α (8-iso-PGF2a) remained unchanged in the control subjects, whereas they increased in diabetic patients. Flow-mediated vasodilation (FMD) decreased in diabetes, whereas GLP-1 increased in both groups. During the OGTT, an increase in glycemia, nitrotyrosine, and 8-iso-PGF2a and a decrease in FMD were observed at 1 h in the control subjects and at 1 and 2 h in the diabetic patients. In the same way, GLP-1 increased in both groups at the same levels of the meal. During the clamps, in both the control subjects and the diabetic patients, a significant increase in nitrotyrosine and 8-iso-PGF2a and a decrease in FMD were observed, effects that were significantly reduced by GLP-1. After improved glycemic control, hyperglycemia during the clamps was less effective in producing oxidative stress and endothelial dysfunction and the GLP-1 administration was most effective in reducing these effects.

CONCLUSIONS—Our data suggest that during the meal GLP-1 can simultaneously exert an incretin effect on insulin secretion and a protective effect on endothelial function, reasonably controlling oxidative stress generation. The ability of GLP-1 in protecting endothelial function seems to depend on the level of glycemia, a phenomenon already described for insulin secretion.

Diabetes Care 34:697–702, 2011

Oral administration of glucose is a more potent secretory stimulus for insulin than its intravenous infusion (1). This observation gave rise to the "incretin effect" concept, i.e., stimulation of insulin secretion as a response to food before an increase in blood glucose levels. An incretin hormone is the glucagon-like peptide 1 (GLP-1).

Type 2 diabetes mellitus is increasing all over the world. Patients with diabetes have an increased risk of cardiovascular disease. Recently, much attention has been paid to evidence that abnormalities of the postprandial state are important contributing factors to the development of atherosclerosis, even in diabetes (2). In diabetic subjects, the combination of postprandial hyperglycemia and postprandial hypertriglyceridemia has been recently proposed as an independent risk factor for cardiovascular disease (2).

The response-to-injury hypothesis of atherosclerosis states that the initial damage affects the arterial endothelium, leading to endothelial dysfunction (3). Indeed, endothelial dysfunction has been demonstrated in patients with diabetes, and hyperglycemia has been implicated as a cause of endothelial dysfunction in normal and diabetic subjects (2). It has been suggested that hyperglycemia induces an endothelial dysfunction through the production of an oxidative stress (2).

GLP-1 is now being used in clinics to enhance insulin secretion and reduce body weight in patients with type 2 diabetes mellitus (4), in whom a defect of GLP-1 secretion/action in response to the meal has often been reported (5). GLP-1 has been shown to lower postprandial and fasting glucose and HbA1c, to suppress the elevated glucagon level, and to stimulate glucose-dependent insulin synthesis and secretion (4).

Apart from the well-documented incretin effect of GLP-1, its role in the cardiovascular system also arouses interest. GLP-1 effects on the cardiovascular system may include a direct action on the endothelium, where the presence of specific receptors for GLP-1 has been demonstrated (6). GLP-1 has been demonstrated to improve endothelial function in diabetes (7). However, the explanation of why GLP-1 may have such a relevant physiologic role on cardiovascular system still remains unknown. A possible explanation would be to consider GLP-1 as an endogenous protective factor for the vascular system when this protection is especially needed: during a meal. As pointed out by Zilversmit (8) many years ago, atherosclerosis could be considered to be a prandial phenomenon. Therefore, it is clearly plausible that GLP-1, on the one hand, can help during a meal (glucose homeostasis, appetite control, fat metabolism), and on the other, can protect the endothelium against the possible damaging effect of the meal. This protective effect should be

From the [1]Insitiut d'Investigacions Biomèdiques August Pi i Sunyer, Barcelona, Spain; the [2]Division of Metabolic Diseases, Center of Excellence for Cardiovascular Diseases, Second University of Naples, Naples, Italy; and the [3]Metabolic and Nutrition Research Centre on Diabetes, INRCA, Ancona, Italy.
Corresponding author: Antonio Ceriello, aceriell@clinic.ub.es.
Received 14 October 2010 and accepted 21 December 2010.
DOI: 10.2337/dc10-1949

exerted improving the antioxidant defenses of the endothelium (9), thereby protecting the vascular system against the oxidative stress that increases after ingesting a meal (2).

The aim of this study is to prove that GLP-1 physiologically protects the endothelial function during a meal and, more specifically, protects the endothelial function from the hyperglycemia-induced alterations, and that this effect is mediated by lowering oxidative stress. Moreover, a further aim is to explore this aspect in diabetes.

RESEARCH DESIGN AND

METHODS—Sixteen type 2 diabetic patients and 12 matched healthy control subjects participated in the study. Baseline characteristics of the study groups are shown in Table 1.

The study was approved by the ethics committee of Institut d'Investigacions Biomèdiques August Pi i Sunyer (IDIBAPS), and written consent from the study subjects was obtained.

Ten patients were on diet alone, and the other six patients were on metformin, which was discontinued at least 4 weeks before the study. None of the type 2 diabetic patients had retinopathy, nephropathy, or neuropathy. Five patients had hypertension treated with an angiotensin-converting enzyme inhibitor, which was withheld on the study days. None of the subjects were receiving statin or antioxidant supplementation.

Synthetic GLP-1 (7–36) amide was purchased from PolyPeptide Laboratories

(Wolfenbuttel, Germany), and the same lot number was used in all studies.

Study design

Both healthy control subjects and type 2 diabetic patients underwent the following studies: a standard meal according to Vollmer et al. (10) and an oral glucose tolerance test (OGTT; 75 g glucose in 300 mL water) in randomized order, on different days. These tests were followed in a randomized order and on different days by two hyperglycemic clamps (11) with or without GLP-1. GLP-1 was infused at a rate aiming to have the same plasma concentration reached during the OGTT (0.4 pmol · kg^{-1} · min^{-1}) according to Nauck et al. (12). During the hyperglycemic clamp, the level of glycemia was settled at the same level as that of mean glycemia reached at 1 h (control subjects 8.5 mmol/L; diabetic patients 15 mmol/L) and 2 h (control subjects 5 mmol/L; diabetic patients 12.8 mmol/L) during the OGTT.

At the end of these studies, diabetic patients were treated intensively with insulin for 2 months to improve glycemic control. The clamp studies were then repeated randomly with the same levels of glycemia and GLP-1 infusion rate.

At baseline and at 1 and 2 h, during the meal test and the OGTT, and during each clamp, glycemia, insulin, endothelial function (flow-mediated vasodilation [FMD]), plasma nitrotyrosine and plasma 8-iso prostaglandin F2α (8-iso-PGF2a) (both markers of oxidative stress), and

GLP-1 (active 7–36) plasma levels were measured.

Biochemical measurements

Cholesterol and triglycerides were measured enzymatically (Roche Diagnostics, Basel, Switzerland). HDL cholesterol was estimated after the precipitation of apolipoprotein B with phosphotungstate/ magnesium (13). LDL cholesterol was calculated after lipoprotein separation (13). Plasma glucose was measured by the glucose-oxidase method, HbA$_{1c}$ was measured by high-performance liquid chromatography, and insulin was measured by microparticle enzyme immunoassay (Abbott Laboratories, Wiesbaden, Germany). Nitrotyrosine plasma concentration was assayed by enzyme-linked immunosorbent assay, recently validated by our laboratory (13).

A commercially available kit was used to measure 8-iso-PGF2a (Cayman Chemical, Ann Arbor, MI). GLP-1 (active 7–36) was measured by a radioimmunoassay kit (Peninsula Laboratories, Belmont, CA). The detection limit is 10 pg/mL, and the intra- and interassay coefficient of variation are 8 and 18% at 50 pg/mL and 5 and 13% at 300 pg/mL, respectively.

Endothelial function

FMD was evaluated (14). At the end of each test, sublingual nitroglycerin (0.3 mg) was administered, and 3 min later the last measurements were performed to measure endothelium-independent vasodilation.

Statistical analysis

Data are expressed as mean ± SE. The sample size was selected according to previous studies (7,10). The Kolmogorov–Smirnov algorithm was used to determine whether each variable had a normal distribution. Comparisons of baseline data among the groups were performed using unpaired Student t test or Mann-Whitney U test, where indicated. The changes in variables during the tests were assessed by two-way ANOVA with repeated measures or Kolmogorov–Smirnov test, where indicated. If differences reached statistical significance, post hoc analyses with paired, two-tailed t test or Wilcoxon signed rank test for paired comparisons were used to assess differences at individual time periods in the study. Statistical significance was defined as $P < 0.05$.

RESULTS—As expected, basal glycemia, insulin, HbA$_{1c}$, nitrotyrosine, and

Table 1—*Baseline characteristics of the control and type 2 diabetic subjects*

	Control subjects ($n = 12$)	Type 2 diabetic subjects ($n = 16$)
Sex	6M/6F	9M/7F
Age, years	50.5 ± 2.5	51.3 ± 2.6
BMI, kg/m^2	28.5 ± 3.1	29.5 ± 3.3
Duration of diabetes, years		5.5 ± 1.3
Fasting plasma glucose, mmol/L	4.5 ± 0.3	7.8 ± 2.2*
HbA$_{1c}$, %	4.8 ± 0.2	8.4 ± 0.3*
Resting systolic blood pressure, mmHg	117.3 ± 5.5	123.4 ± 6.4
Resting diastolic blood pressure, mmHg	77.5 ± 2.2	80.2 ± 3.6
Total cholesterol, mmol/L	4.5 ± 0.6	5.1 ± 0.8
Triglycerides, mmol/L	0.9 ± 0.2	1.2 ± 0.4
HDL cholesterol, mmol/L	1.4 ± 0.2	1.2 ± 0.3
LDL cholesterol, mmol/L	2.5 ± 0.3	2.6 ± 0.4
FMD, %	11.7 ± 0.7	5.9 ± 0.6*
Nitrotyrosine, μmol/L	0.24 ± 0.05	0.52 ± 0.03*
8-iso-PGF2a, pg/mL	32.6 ± 4.6	65.0 ± 4.5*
Fasting insulin, pmol/L	73.3 ± 4.4	107.3 ± 15.2*

Data are expressed as means ± SE. *$P < 0.001$ vs. control subjects.

8-iso-PGF2a were increased in diabetes, and FMD was decreased (Table 1). Basal, fasting level of GLP-1 was not different between control subjects and diabetic patients (Table 1).

During the meal, all test parameters, except those for GLP-1 and insulin, remained unchanged in the control subjects, whereas a significant increase at 1 and 2 h of glycemia, insulin, nitrotyrosine, and 8-iso-PGF2a and a decrease in FMD were observed in type 2 diabetic patients compared with their basal values. In both control subjects and diabetic patients, GLP-1 increased at 1 and 2 h in a similar manner (Fig. 1).

In the control subjects, during the OGTT, an increase of glycemia, insulin, nitrotyrosine, and 8-iso-PGF2a and a decrease of FMD were observed at 1 h, whereas at 2 h all the parameters returned to the basal values (Fig. 1). In the diabetic patients, at both 1 and 2 h, a significant

increase of glycemia, insulin, nitrotyrosine, and 8-iso-PGF2a and a decrease of FMD were observed compared with the basal values (Fig. 1). In both control subjects and diabetic patients, during the OGTT, GLP-1 increased at 1 and 2 h in a similar manner (Fig. 1), and the values were not different from those reached during the meal test (Fig. 1).

In diabetic patients, at both 1 and 2 h, a significant increase in glycemia ($P < 0.01$), insulin ($P < 0.01$), nitrotyrosine ($P < 0.05$), and 8-iso-PGF2a ($P < 0.05$), and a decrease in FMD ($P < 0.05$) were observed compared with the values reached during the OGTT, whereas no difference was found for GLP-1 (Fig. 1).

According to the values observed during the OGTT, during the clamps glycemia was maintained for the first hour at 8.5 mmol/L in control subjects and at 15 mmol/L 1 h in diabetic patients, whereas for the second hour glycemia

was maintained at 5 mmol/L in control subjects and at 13 mmol/L in diabetic patients. During the clamps, performed with placebo, GLP-1 concentration remained unchanged during the study period in both control subjects and diabetic patients, whereas its concentration was almost equivalent to that observed during the meal test and the OGTT when it was constantly infused (Fig. 2). Insulin concentration increased in both control subjects and diabetic patients during the hyperglycemic clamp, and its increase was significantly higher during GLP-1 infusion (Fig. 2). During both the clamps, with or without GLP-1, in the control subjects, an increase in nitrotyrosine and 8-iso-PGF2a and a decrease in FMD were observed at 1 h, whereas at 2 h, all the parameters returned to their basal values (Fig. 2). Similarly, in diabetic patients, at both 1 and 2 h during both the clamps, a significant increase in nitrotyrosine and 8-iso-PGF2a and a decrease in FMD were observed compared with the basal values (Fig. 2). However, in the control subjects, at 1 h, the values of nitrotyrosine and 8-iso-PGF2a significantly increased, and the values of FMD significantly decreased in the clamp with placebo compared with the values observed during the clamp with GLP-1 (Fig. 2). Similarly, in diabetic patients at both 1 and 2 h, the values of nitrotyrosine and 8-iso-PGF2a significantly increased, and the values of FMD significantly decreased in the clamp with placebo compared with the values observed during the clamp with GLP-1 (Fig. 2).

Two months of insulin treatment resulted in a significant decrease in HbA$_{1c}$ (8.4 ± 0.3 vs. $7.2 \pm 0.4\%$, $P < 0.01$) and an improvement of fasting glycemia (8.2 ± 2.0 vs. 6.4 ± 1.8 mmol/L, $P < 0.01$), insulin (110.3 ± 17.2 vs. 86.2 ± 13.2 pmol/L, $P < 0.01$), nitrotyrosine (0.52 ± 0.03 vs. 0.39 ± 0.06 μmol/L, $P < 0.05$), 8-iso-PGF2a (65.0 ± 4.5 vs. 44.2 ± 2.5 pg/mL, $P < 0.05$), and FMD (5.9 ± 0.6 vs. $7.8 \pm 0.7\%$, $P < 0.05$) in diabetic patients.

During the two clamps, in diabetic patients, at 1 and 2 h, a significant increase in nitrotyrosine and 8-iso-PGF2a and a decrease in FMD ($P < 0.01$) were observed compared with the basal values (Fig. 3). As before the improvement of glycemic control, at both 1 and 2 h, the values of nitrotyrosine and 8-iso-PGF2a significantly increased and the values of FMD significantly decreased in the clamp with placebo compared with the values observed during the clamp with GLP-1

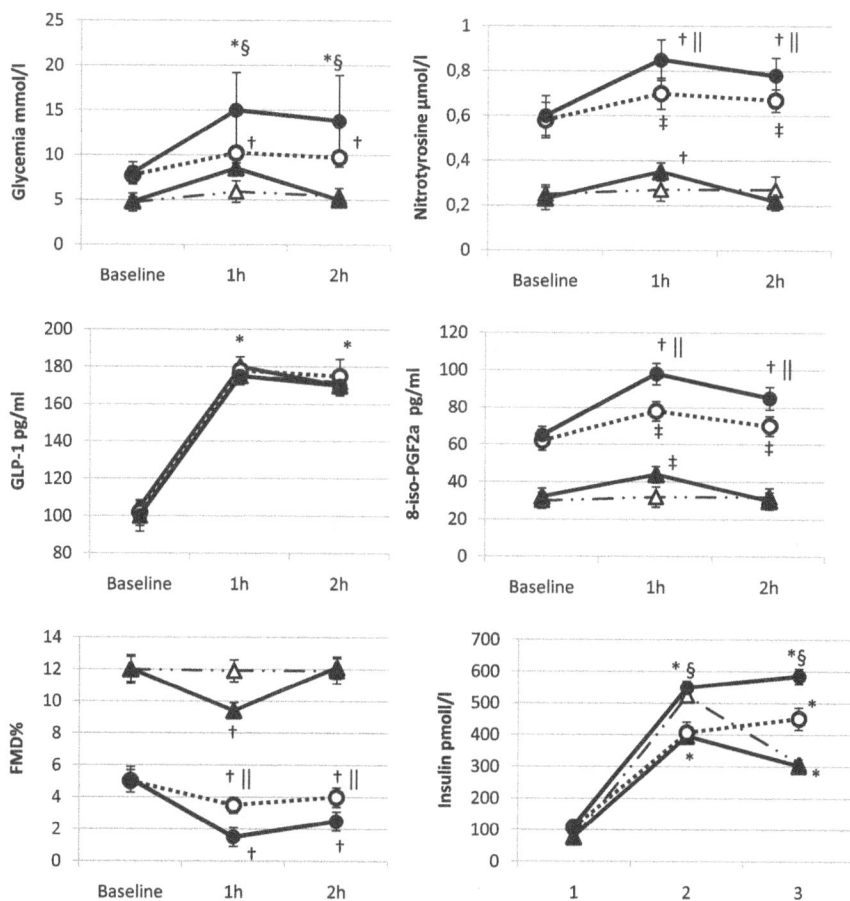

Figure 1—*Changes of glycemia, GLP-1, FMD, plasma nitrotyrosine, 8-iso-PGF2a, and insulin during the meal and the OGTT in normal healthy control subjects and type 2 diabetic patients. Data are expressed as mean ± SE;* △*, meal test controls;* ▲*, OGTT controls;* ○*, meal test type 2 diabetes;* ●*, OGTT type 2 diabetes;* *P < 0.001 vs. basal; †P < 0.01 vs. basal; ‡P < 0.05 vs. basal; §P < 0.01 vs. OGTT; ‖P < 0.05 vs. OGTT.*

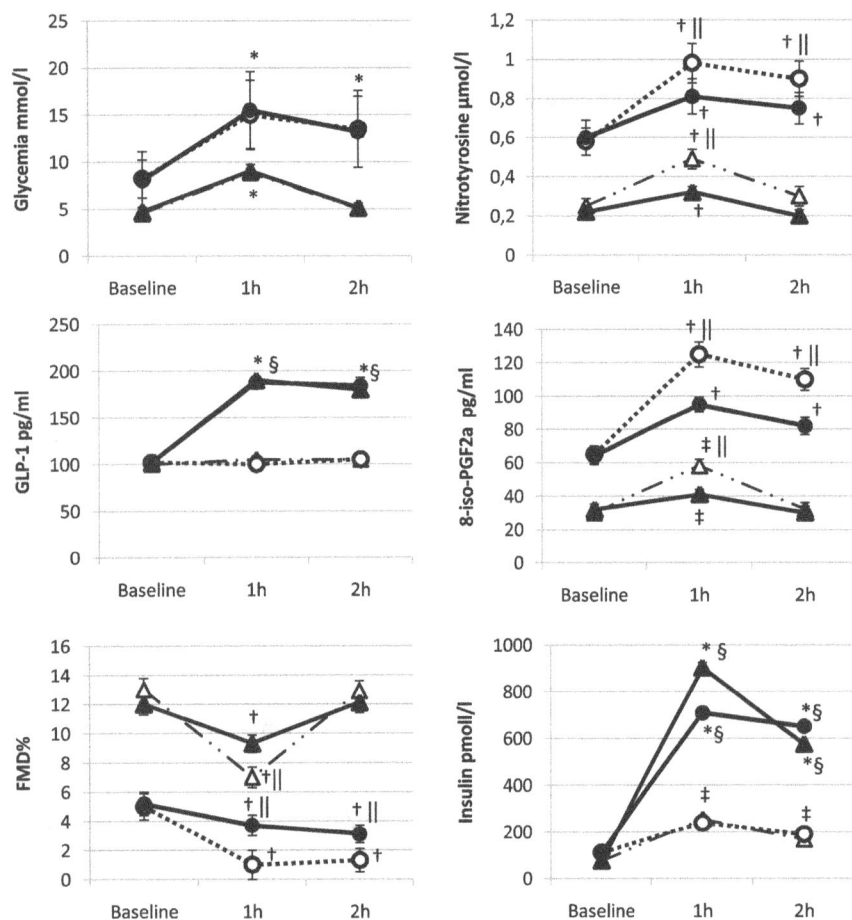

Figure 2—*Changes of glycemia, GLP-1, FMD, plasma nitrotyrosine, 8-iso-PGF2a, and insulin during the hyperglycemic clamp with or without GLP-1 infusion in normal healthy control subjects and type 2 diabetic patients. Data are expressed as mean ± SE; △, hyperglycemic clamp + placebo control subjects; ▲, hyperglycemic clamp + GLP-1 control subjects; ○, hyperglycemic clamp + placebo type 2 diabetes; ●, hyperglycemic clamp + GLP-1 type 2 diabetes; *P < 0.001 vs. basal; †P < 0.01 vs. basal; ‡P < 0.05 vs. basal; §P < 0.01 vs. placebo; ||P < 0.05 vs. placebo.*

(Fig. 3). However, the same values of glycemia were less effective in producing oxidative stress and endothelial dysfunction after 2 months of improved glycemic control. Because the basal values before and after tight glycemic control were significantly different, we have compared the Δ between the basal value and the value at 1 and 2 h, during each clamp, respectively: Δnitrotyrosine 1 h 0.42 ± 0.04 vs. 0.20 ± 0.05, P < 0.01; Δnitrotyrosine 2 h 0.32 ± 0.03 vs. 0.15 ± 0.05, P < 0.01; Δ 8-iso-PGF2a 1 h 68.9 ± 4.1 vs. 30.3 ± 3.2, P < 0.05; Δ 8-iso-PGF2a 2 h 50.5 ± 3.1 vs. 20.3 ± 1.2, P < 0.01; Δ FMD 1 h 4.1 ± 0.5 vs. 2.3 ± 0.2, FMD, P < 0.05; Δ FMD 2 h 3.7 ± 0.5 vs. 2.2 ± 0.2, FMD, P < 0.05 in the study performed with placebo, compared with that in the previous clamp. Of particular interest is that GLP-1 administration was most effective in

this condition of improved metabolic control than in previous experiments: Δnitrotyrosine 1 h 0.21 ± 0.02 vs. 0.08 ± 0.02, P < 0.01; Δnitrotyrosine 2 h 0.15 ± 0.04 vs. 0.03 ± 0.02, P < 0.01; Δ 8-iso-PGF2a 1 h 31.5 ± 4.1 vs. 15.3 ± 3.7, P < 0.05; Δ 8-iso-PGF2a 2 h 20.3 ± 2.1 vs. 10.2 ± 1.5, P < 0.05; Δ FMD 1 h 1.5 ± 0.4 vs. 0.6 ± 0.2, FMD, P < 0.05; Δ FMD 2 h 2.1 ± 0.3 vs. 0.3 ± 0.2, FMD, P < 0.05 in the study performed with placebo, compared with the previous clamp. GLP-1 infusion after optimized glycemic control was accompanied by a significant increase in insulin secretion at both 1 and 2 h (Fig. 3). No difference was found in endothelium-independent vasodilatation in all the studies.

CONCLUSIONS—This study demonstrated that the presence of GLP-1

during hyperglycemia significantly protects endothelial function and decreases hyperglycemia-induced oxidative stress generation. This evidence clearly emerges when we compare the effect of hyperglycemia during the clamps in both normal and diabetic patients. In the absence of GLP-1, hyperglycemia induces endothelial dysfunction and oxidative stress, whereas the concomitant infusion of GLP-1 significantly prevents this effect. It has already been largely demonstrated that hyperglycemia induces endothelial dysfunction through the generation of an oxidative stress (2) and that GLP-1 can reduce oxidative stress (9). GLP-1 also improves endothelial dysfunction in diabetes (7). Therefore, our data suggest that GLP-1 may protect endothelia function during hyperglycemia, reducing oxidative stress generation.

Our data also support a possible physiologic protective role of GLP-1 on endothelial function. However, the effect of GLP-1 on endothelial function seems to be dependent on the level of hyperglycemia. The same plasma levels of GLP-1 have a different effect on the endothelial function and oxidative stress in normal subjects during the test meal and the OGTT. Consistent with a previous study, in normal control subjects the levels of GLP-1 are almost superimposable during the meal and the OGTT (9). However, during the meal test, when glycemia remains constantly in the normal range, endothelial function and oxidative stress remain unaltered. However, at 1 h, during the OGTT, as already reported (15), when hyperglycemia appears, endothelial function and oxidative stress also appear. These data suggest that in the presence of hyperglycemia, GLP-1 partly loses its protective effect on endothelial function and oxidative stress.

This finding is also supported by the data in diabetic patients. As previously reported (10), the plasma levels of GLP-1 were not different between the meal test and the OGTT. As expected, the levels of glycemia were significantly different between the meal test and the OGTT, and this was accompanied by a parallel worsening of both oxidative stress and endothelial function.

The possibility that hyperglycemia may condition the protective effects of GLP-1 on endothelial function and oxidative stress is also supported by the data with clamps in type 2 diabetic patients after a period of improved glycemic control.

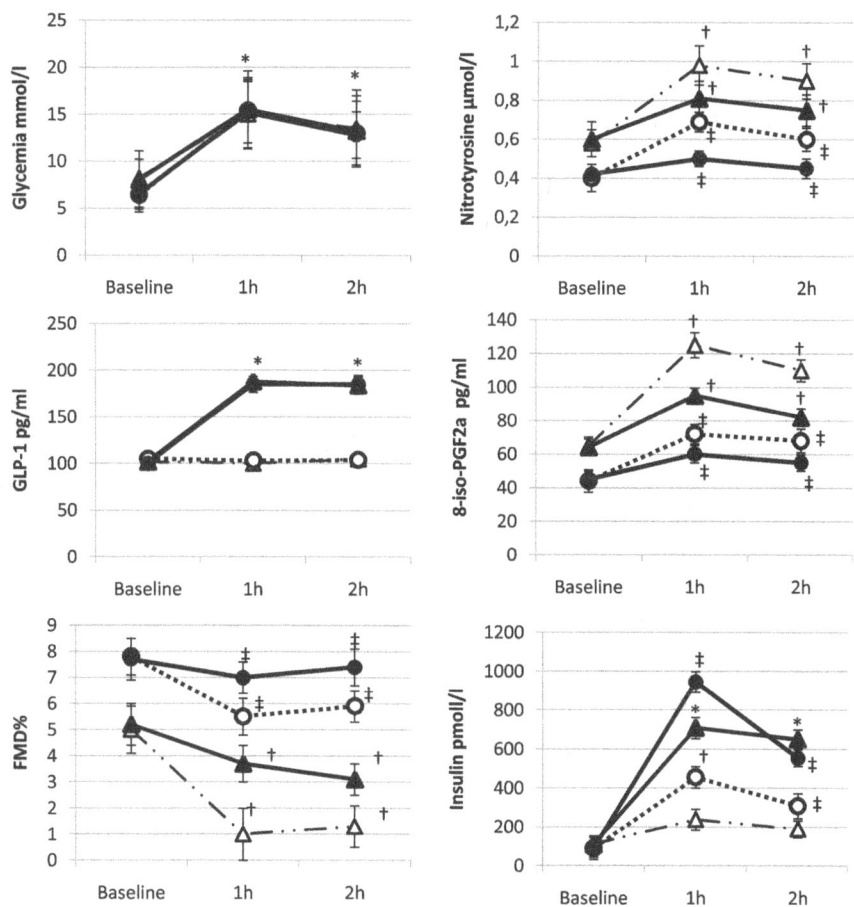

Figure 3—*Changes of glycemia, GLP-1, FMD, plasma nitrotyrosine, 8-iso-PGF2a, and insulin during the hyperglycemic clamp with or without GLP-1 infusion in normal healthy control subjects and type 2 diabetic patients at baseline and after 2 months of optimized glycemic control. For the comparisons between baseline and after 2 months of optimized glycemic control, see the* RESULTS *section. Data are expressed as mean ± SE; △, hyperglycemic clamp + placebo; ○, hyperglycemic clamp + placebo after 2 months of optimized glycemic control; ▲, hyperglycemic clamp + GLP-1; ●, hyperglycemic clamp + GLP-1 after 2 months of optimized glycemic control; *P < 0.001 vs. basal; †P < 0.01 vs. basal; ‡P < 0.05 vs. basal.*

reduced compared with 1 h (Fig. 3). In addition, insulin can induce an endothelial dysfunction (20,21), evidence that supports the possibility that GLP-1 has a direct beneficial effect on endothelial function.

In conclusion, our data suggest that during the meal, GLP-1 can simultaneously exert an incretin effect on insulin secretion and have a protective effect on the endothelial function, reasonably controlling oxidative stress generation. As for insulin secretion, the ability of GLP-1 in protecting endothelial function seems to be dependent on the level of glycemia (5). Hyperglycemia may induce at the endothelial level, as well as at the level of the β-cells, a resistance to the GLP-1 action.

Acknowledgments—No potential conflicts of interest relevant to this article were reported.

A.C. and K.E. researched data, wrote the article, and researched and reviewed the article. R.T. researched and reviewed the article. A.R.B. and M.M. reviewed the article. D.G. researched data, wrote the article, and researched and reviewed the article.

References
1. Drucker DJ. Minireview: the glucagon-like peptides. Endocrinology 2001;142:521–527
2. Ceriello A. Postprandial hyperglycemia and diabetes complications: is it time to treat? Diabetes 2005;54:1–7
3. Ross R. The pathogenesis of atherosclerosis: a perspective for the 1990s. Nature 1993;362:801–809
4. Peters A. Incretin-based therapies: review of current clinical trial data. Am J Med 2010;123(Suppl.):S28–S37
5. Meier JJ, Nauck MA. Is the diminished incretin effect in type 2 diabetes just an epi-phenomenon of impaired beta-cell function? Diabetes 2010;59:1117–1125
6. Mudaliar S, Henry RR. Effects of incretin hormones on beta-cell mass and function, body weight, and hepatic and myocardial function. Am J Med 2010;123(Suppl.):S19–S27
7. Nyström T, Gutniak MK, Zhang Q, et al. Effects of glucagon-like peptide-1 on endothelial function in type 2 diabetes patients with stable coronary artery disease. Am J Physiol Endocrinol Metab 2004;287:E1209–E1215
8. Zilversmit DB. Atherogenesis: a postprandial phenomenon. Circulation 1979;60:473–485
9. Oeseburg H, de Boer RA, Buikema H, van der Harst P, van Gilst WH, Silljé HH. Glucagon-like peptide 1 prevents reactive oxygen species–induced endothelial cell senescence through the activation of

As previously reported, improving glycemic control partly restored basal endothelial function and oxidative stress (16), as well as the response to the same level of glycemia during the clamp in terms of oxidative stress and endothelial function. However, the protective effect of infused GLP-1 was more pronounced in this situation of improved glycemic control compared with the previous study.

These data together support the hypothesis that the endothelium became less sensitive to GLP-1 in hyperglycemia, more than GLP-1 itself loses its activity.

This concept has already been proposed for insulin secretion, where evidence suggests that the impaired GLP-1 incretin effect is mostly related to an impairment of β-cell function than to an impairment of incretin secretion (5). Højberg et al. (17) reported that a near-normalization of blood glucose has no effect on postprandial GLP-1 secretion, but it augments β-cell responsiveness, similar to our data for endothelial function.

A possible direct influence of insulin concentration on our results cannot be excluded. Insulin by itself has antioxidant and vasodilatory effects (18), and GLP-1 infusion during any clamp was accompanied by a significant increase of insulin concentration compared with the placebo. However, it has been reported that acute hyperglycemia during a clamp, as in our case, blunts the vasodilatory effect of insulin (19). Moreover, at 2 h during the clamps the effect of GLP-1 on FMD was almost similar to that at 1 h; even at 2 h, insulin concentration was significantly

protein kinase A. Arterioscler Thromb Vasc Biol 2010;30:1407–1414

10. Vollmer K, Holst JJ, Baller B, et al. Predictors of incretin concentrations in subjects with normal, impaired, and diabetic glucose tolerance. Diabetes 2008;57: 678–687

11. DeFronzo RA, Tobin JD, Andres R. Glucose clamp technique: a method for quantifying insulin secretion and resistance. Am J Physiol 1979;237:E214–E223

12. Nauck MA, Heimesaat MM, Orskov C, Holst JJ, Ebert R, Creutzfeldt W. Preserved incretin activity of glucagon-like peptide 1 [7-36 amide] but not of synthetic human gastric inhibitory polypeptide in patients with type-2 diabetes mellitus. J Clin Invest 1993;91:301–307

13. Ceriello A, Mercuri F, Quagliaro L, et al. Detection of nitrotyrosine in the diabetic plasma: evidence of oxidative stress. Diabetologia 2001;44:834–838

14. Corretti MC, Anderson TJ, Benjamin EJ, et al.; International Brachial Artery Reactivity Task Force. Guidelines for the ultrasound assessment of endothelial-dependent flow-mediated vasodilation of the brachial artery: a report of the International Brachial Artery Reactivity Task Force. J Am Coll Cardiol 2002;39:257–265

15. Kawano H, Motoyama T, Hirashima O, et al. Hyperglycemia rapidly suppresses flow-mediated endothelium-dependent vasodilation of brachial artery. J Am Coll Cardiol 1999;34:146–154

16. Ceriello A, Kumar S, Piconi L, Esposito K, Giugliano D. Simultaneous control of hyperglycemia and oxidative stress normalizes endothelial function in type 1 diabetes. Diabetes Care 2007;30:649–654

17. Højberg PV, Vilsbøll T, Zander M, et al. Four weeks of near-normalization of blood glucose has no effect on postprandial GLP-1 and GIP secretion, but augments pancreatic

B-cell responsiveness to a meal in patients with type 2 diabetes. Diabet Med 2008;25: 1268–1275

18. Dandona P, Chaudhuri A, Ghanim H, Mohanty P. Insulin as an anti-inflammatory and antiatherogenic modulator. J Am Coll Cardiol 2009;53(Suppl.):S14–S20

19. Srinivasan M, Herrero P, McGill JB, et al. The effects of plasma insulin and glucose on myocardial blood flow in patients with type 1 diabetes mellitus. J Am Coll Cardiol 2005;46:42–48

20. Arcaro G, Cretti A, Balzano S, et al. Insulin causes endothelial dysfunction in humans: sites and mechanisms. Circulation 2002;105:576–582

21. Campia U, Sullivan G, Bryant MB, Waclawiw MA, Quon MJ, Panza JA. Insulin impairs endothelium-dependent vasodilation independent of insulin sensitivity or lipid profile. Am J Physiol Heart Circ Physiol 2004;286:H76–H82

INCRETINS

Original Article

Downregulation of GLP-1 and GIP Receptor Expression by Hyperglycemia

Possible Contribution to Impaired Incretin Effects in Diabetes

Gang Xu,[1] Hideaki Kaneto,[1] D. Ross Laybutt,[1,2] Valerie F. Duvivier-Kali,[1] Nitin Trivedi,[1] Kiyoshi Suzuma,[3] George L. King,[3] Gordon C. Weir,[1] and Susan Bonner-Weir[1]

Stimulation of insulin secretion by the incretin hormones glucagon-like peptide 1 (GLP-1) and glucose-dependent insulinotropic peptide (GIP) has been found to be diminished in type 2 diabetes. We hypothesized that this impairment is due to a defect at the receptor level induced by the diabetic state, particularly hyperglycemia. Gene expression of incretin receptors, GLP-1R and GIPR, were significantly decreased in islets of 90% pancreatectomized (Px) hyperglycemic rats, with recovery when glucose levels were normalized by phlorizin. Perifused islets isolated from hyperglycemic Px rats showed reduced insulin responses to GLP-1 and GIP. To examine the acute effect of hyperglycemia on incretin receptor expression, a hyperglycemic clamp study was performed for 96 h with reduction of GLP-1 receptor expression but increase in GIP receptor expression. Similar findings were found when islets were cultured at high glucose concentrations for 48 h. The reduction of GLP-1 receptor expression by high glucose was prevented by dominant-negative protein kinase C (PKC)α overexpression, whereas GLP-1 receptor expression was reduced with wild-type PKCα overexpression. Taken together, GLP-1 and GIP receptor expression is decreased with chronic hyperglycemia, and this decrease likely contributes to the impaired incretin effects found in diabetes. *Diabetes* **56:1551–1558, 2007**

From the [1]Section on Islet Transplantation and Cell Biology, Joslin Diabetes Center, Harvard Medical School, Boston, Massachusetts; the [2]Diabetes and Obesity Research Program, Garvan Institute of Medical Research, St. Vincent's Hospital, Sydney, Australia; and the [3]Section of Vascular Cell Biology, Joslin Diabetes Center, Harvard Medical School, Boston, Massachusetts.

Address correspondence and reprint requests to Susan Bonner-Weir, PhD, Section of Islet Transplantation and Cell Biology, Joslin Diabetes Center, Harvard Medical School, One Joslin Place, Boston, MA 02215. E-mail: susan-.bonner-weir@joslin.harvard.edu.

Received for publication 25 July 2006 and accepted in revised from 19 February 2007.

Published ahead of print at http://diabetes.diabetesjournals.org on 14 March 2007. DOI: 10.2337/db06-1033.

Ad-GFP, adenovirus-expressing green fluorescent protein; cAMP, cyclic AMP; DN-PKCα, dominant-negative PKCα; dNTP, deoxynucleotide triphosphate; GIP, glucose-dependent insulinotropic peptide; GLP-1, glucagon-like peptide 1; GSIS, glucose-stimulated insulin secretion; TPA, 12-*O*-tetradecanoylphorbol-13-acetate.

The incretin effect causes more insulin to be secreted when glucose is taken orally than when given intravenously, even when blood glucose levels have the same profile (1,2). This effect is thought to be very important for maximizing insulin responses during meals, thereby limiting postprandial glucose excursions. Two incretins have been identified: glucagon-like peptide 1 (GLP-1) (3,4) and glucose-dependent insulinotropic peptide (GIP) (2,5). It is thought that incretins play an important role in glucose homeostasis by promoting insulin secretion immediately on meal ingestion. Their physiological importance has been demonstrated by the finding of glucose intolerance both in GLP-1 (6,7) and GIP (8) receptor knockout mice.

The incretin effect has been extensively studied in type 2 diabetes. Plasma GIP levels after meals have been found in most studies to be normal in type 2 diabetes while GLP-1 levels have been found to be modestly reduced (9,10). Striking abnormalities, however, have been found in the action of incretin hormones in type 2 diabetes, particularly GIP, which, when infused, has almost no effect on insulin secretion (11,12). In contrast, the effects of GLP-1 are partially preserved, which is important for its therapeutic potential, but insulin responses are substantially reduced, especially when studies are done at comparable glucose levels (13,14). When studied in the rat partial pancreatectomized (Px) model of hyperglycemia, GLP-1 effect on insulin secretion was similarly reduced (15). As expected, GLP-1 and GIP receptors are expressed in pancreatic β-cells (16), which raises questions about whether some of the impairment of the incretin effect occurs at the receptor level. An earlier study found a modest reduction of GLP-1 gene expression in rat islets cultured in high glucose concentrations (17). In the present study, this hypothesis is further examined with in vivo and in vitro experiments.

RESEARCH DESIGN AND METHODS

Px model. Male Sprague-Dawley rats (Taconic Farms, Germantown, NY), weighing 90–100 g were submitted to 85–95% Px or sham surgery as described previously (18). Briefly, tissue was removed by gentle abrasion with cotton applicators leaving the pancreas within 1–2 mm of the common pancreatic bile duct and extending from the duct to the first part of the duodenum. The proportion removed was varied to generate 85–95% Px rats that develop different degrees of hyperglycemia. For sham surgery, the pancreatic tissue was only lightly rubbed instead of being removed. Animals were kept under conventional conditions with free access to water and standard food. All animal procedures were approved by the Joslin Diabetes Center Animal Care Committee.

Animals were weighed, and blood was obtained in heparinized microcapillary tubes from snipped tails of fed rats (9:00–10:00 A.M.) weekly. Whole blood glucose levels were measured with a portable Medisense Precision QID glucometer (Abbott Laboratories, Bedford, MA). Rats were classified according to their averaged blood glucose levels from 3 weeks after surgery; low Px was assigned to Px rats with blood glucose levels <100 mg/dl, moderate Px between 100 and 150 mg/dl, and high Px >150 mg/dl as described previously (19,20). To reverse hyperglycemia, Px rats were treated with phlorizin for the final 2 weeks of the 4-week study period. Phlorizin was dissolved in 1, 2-propanediol and injected intraperitoneally twice a day (9:00 A.M. and 9:00 P.M.) at a dose of 0.8 g · kg^{-1} · day^{-1}. At 4 weeks after the surgery, rats were anesthetized, and their islets from the pancreatic remnant or sham pancreas were isolated by distending the pancreas duct with collagenase. After digestion, the islets were separated on a Histopaque density gradient (Histopaque 1077; Sigma-Aldrich, St. Louis, MO) and further purified by handpicking under a stereomicroscope. Islets of similar size were used for extraction of RNA. In several cases, it was necessary to pool islets from two Px rats with similar glycemic levels to obtain an islet yield sufficient for RNA extraction. Gene expression data for other genes in these animals were previously published (21).

Hyperglycemic clamp study. Catheterized Sprague-Dawley rats (~250 g) were infused for 4 days with glucose (500 g/l hydrated glucose; McGaw, Irvine, CA) or saline (4.5 g/l) as previously described (22,23). The glucose infusion rate was regularly adjusted to maintain the blood glucose level at ~200 mg/dl. At the end of the infusion period, islets were isolated and RNA extracted for RT-PCR analysis; genetic expression data for other genes in these animals were previously published (23).

Islet isolation and culture. Islets isolated from normal Sprague-Dawley rats as above were cultured in RPMI-1640 medium (Cell-gro; Mediatech) containing 11.1 mmol/l glucose supplemented with 10% fetal bovine serum, penicillin (100 units/ml), and streptomycin (100 μg/ml) in standard humidified culture conditions of 5% CO_2 and 95% O_2 air at 37°C. After overnight culture, batches of 200 islets were further cultured in six-well dishes for 48 h under various glucose concentrations.

Immunostaining. Under anesthesia, the pancreas or pancreatic remnant was excised, fixed in 4% paraformaldehyde, and processed for paraffin embedding. Sections (5 μm) were immunostained using rabbit anti–protein kinase C (PKC) isoform antibodies (Santa Cruz) and rabbit anti–GLP-1 receptor (HM-316) (24) and anti-GIP receptor (25) antibodies (kindly provided by Dr. Joel F. Habener, Massachusetts General Hospital, and by Dr. Timothy J. Kieffer, University of British Columbia) and fluorochromes as previously described (26). No signal was present if the primary antibodies were omitted. Images were taken at the same settings for all groups of the same experiment for comparison on a Zeiss 410 LSM confocal microscope in the confocal mode.

Semiquantitative radioactive multiplex PCR. After quantification of total RNA extracted from the rat islets, 500 ng RNA was heated at 85°C for 3 min and then reverse transcribed into cDNA in a final reaction solution of 25 μl containing the following: 1X (5 μl) Superscript first-strand buffer (50 mmol/l Tris-HCl, 75 mmol/l KCl, and 3 mmol/l $MgCl_2$) (Invitrogen), 160 umol/l deoxynucleotide triphosphate (dNTP), 40 units RNAsin (Promega, Madison, WI), 10 mmol/l dithiothreitol, 50 ng random hexamers, and 200 units Superscript II Rnase H- reverse transcriptase (Invitrogen). Reverse transcription reactions were incubated for 10 min at 25°C, 60 min at 42°C, and 10 min at 95°C. Resultant cDNA products were diluted to a concentration corresponding to 10 ng of starting RNA per 1.5 μl. PCRs were carried out in a volume of 25 μl consisting of 10 ng cDNA (1.5 μl), 1 μl GeneAmp PCR Gold buffer (Applied Biosystems, Foster City, CA), 1–2 mmol/l $MgCl_2$, 80–160 μmol/l dNTP, 80–600 nmol oligonucleotide primers (Sigma-Aldrich), 1.25 μCi of [α-^{32}P] dCTP (3,000 Ci/mmol; Perkin-Elmer Life Sciences), and 2.5 units AmpliTaq Gold DNA Polymerase (Applied Biosystems). Reactions were performed in a 9700 Thermocycler (Applied Biosystems) in which samples underwent a 10-min initial denaturing step, followed by the number of amplification cycles (1 min denaturation at 94°C, 1 min at the annealing temperature, and 1 min extension at 72°C). The final extension step was 10 min at 72°C. Amplimers were resolved by 6% PAGE in Tris borate EDTA buffer. The amount of [α-^{32}P] dCTP incorporated into amplimers was measured with a Storm 840 PhosphorImager and quantified with ImageQuant software (Molecular Dynamics, Sunnyvale, CA). The average intensity of each product was expressed as relative to the internal control gene. These ratios were then used to calculate the percentage of control expression for each sample in the same RT-PCR. We verified that the multiplex PCR products for each set of primers were linearly amplified. Control experiments were performed to adjust the PCR conditions so that the number of cycles used was

in the exponential phase of amplification for all products and that each PCR product in a multiplex reaction increased linearly with the amount of starting material. Thirty cycles were used for both GLP-1 and GIP receptors.

Real-time PCR. Islet RNA samples from obese diabetic db/db and littermate lean nondiabetic db/+ mice were analyzed by real-time PCR; genetic expression data for other genes in these animals were previously published (27). Reactions were carried out in a volume of 10 μl consisting of 1 μl cDNA, 1x LightCycler enzyme and reaction mix (SYBR Green I dye, TaqDNA polymerase, dNTP; Roche), 1.5 mmol/l $MgCl_2$, and 600 nmol oligonucleotide primers. All reactions were performed in a LightCycler (Roche) in which samples underwent 40 cycles of PCR with an annealing temperature of 55°C. The following primers were used (forward and reverse, respectively): GGGTCTCT GGCTACATAAGGACAAC and AAGGATGGCTGAAGCGATGAC (GLP-1 receptor), GCGTGCTCTACTGCTTCATCAAC and AACTTTCCAAGACCTCATCCCC (GIP receptor), and TGTGCCAGGGTGGTGACTTTAC and TGGGAACCGTT TGTGTTTGG (cyclophilin). The value obtained for each specific product was normalized to a control gene (cyclophilin) and expressed as a percentage of the value in control db/+ extracts.

Assessment of insulin secretion by islet perifusion. Insulin secretion from islets in response to GLP-1 was assessed by perifusion in RPMI-1640 with 10% newborn calf serum at a flow rate of 0.5 ml/min at 37°C. At 4–6 weeks after surgery, 50–100 handpicked islets from sham and Px rats were loaded into chambers (Swinnex 13; Millipore, Bedford, MA) and perifused for 1 hour with 2.8 mmol/l glucose, followed by 15 min with 16.7 mmol/l glucose, 25 min with 16.8 mmol/l glucose plus 100 nmol/l GLP-1 or 10 nmol/l GIP (Sigma-Aldrich), and then 20 min at 2.8 mmol/l glucose. Islets from five sham and Px animals each were used as separate samples; the size of the islets was visually measured with an eyepiece micrometer for normalization to islet equivalents (150 μm diameter). Samples were taken at 10-min intervals, except for 1-min intervals during stimulation, and stored at −20°C until radioimmunoassay. Insulin concentrations were measured by radioimmunoassay in the Joslin Diabetes Endocrine Research Center Specialized Assay Core. Stimulation index was calculated as the area under the curve during GLP-1 or GIP stimulation and normalized per islet equivalent.

Preparation of recombinant adenoviruses containing the cDNA encoding each PKC isoform (α, β2, δ, ε, and ζ). Recombinant adenoviruses containing the cDNA encoding each PKC isoform (α, β2, δ, ε, and ζ) were prepared using the AdEasy system (kindly provided by Dr. Bert Vogelstein, Johns Hopkins Oncology Center) (28). In brief, the encoding region of each PKC isoform (α, β2, δ, ε, and ζ) was cloned into a shuttle vector pAdTrack-CMV. To produce homologous recombination, 1.0 μg linearized plasmid containing each PKC isoform and 0.1 μg of the adenoviral backbone plasmid pAdEasy-1 were introduced into electrocompetent Escherichia coli BJ5183 cells with electroporation (2,500 V, 200 Ohms). The resultant plasmids were re-transformed into E. coli XL-Gold Ultracompetent Cells (Stratagene, La Jolla, CA), linearized with PacI, and then transfected into the adenovirus packaging cell line 293 using LipofectAMINE (Life Technologies, Grand Island, NY). Ten days after transfection, cell lysates were obtained from the 293 cells. The cell lysates were added to 293 cells again, and when most of the cells were killed by the adenovirus infection and detached, cell lysates were again obtained (this process was repeated three times). Control adenovirus-expressing green fluorescent protein (Ad-GFP) was prepared in the same manner. Isolated rat islets (~200 islets) were infected with adenovirus-expressing PKC isoforms (α, β2, δ, ε, or ζ) (with green fluorescent protein) or control Ad-GFP (without PKC isoform), using a 1-h exposure to 30 μl of the adenovirus (1 × 10^8 plaque forming units/ml). One hour after infection, the islets were cultured for 3 days in 3 ml RPMI-1640 medium.

Statistical analysis. Results were expressed as means ± SE. One-way ANOVA was used for the first determination. Unpaired Student's t test (two tailed) followed if there was significance. P value <0.05 was considered statistically significant.

RESULTS

Decreased GLP-1 and GIP receptor expression in islets of 90% Px diabetic rats and obese diabetic db/db mice.

We first examined the expression of GLP-1 and GIP receptors in islets isolated from 85 to 95% Px diabetic rats that had been exposed to chronic hyperglycemia for 4 weeks. The animals were divided into the following groups according to blood glucose levels by the end of 4 weeks after surgery: Low Px (<100 mg/dl), moderate Px (100–150 mg/dl), and high Px (>150 mg/dl) rats. As shown in Fig. 1A, GLP-1 receptor mRNA expression was decreased in a glucose-dependent manner, and

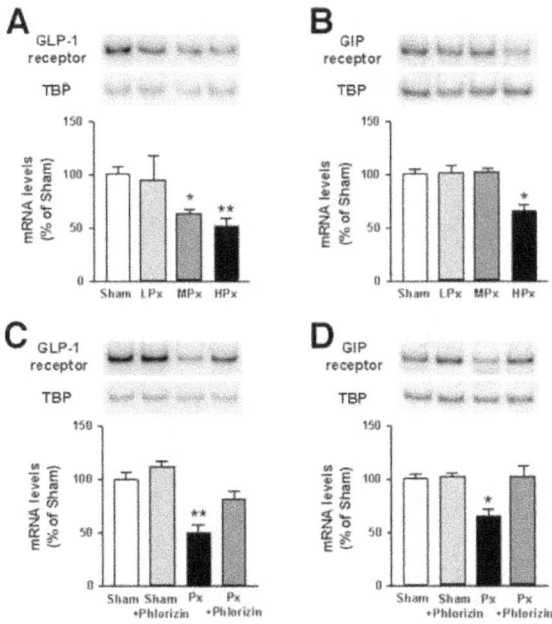

FIG. 1. Decreased GLP-1 and GIP receptor mRNA expression in islets of 85–95% Px diabetic rats. *A* and *B*: Pancreatic islets were isolated from Px rats that were exposed to chronic hyperglycemia for 4 weeks, and GLP-1 and GIP receptor mRNA expression was evaluated. Rats were classified according to their averaged blood glucose levels from 3 weeks after surgery; low Px was assigned to Px rats with blood glucose levels <100 mg/dl, moderate Px between 100 and 150 mg/dl, and high Px >150 mg/dl. *C* and *D*: Phlorizin is known to lower blood glucose levels by preventing reabsorption of glucose from the glomerular filtrate. To examine the effects of hyperglycemia, we treated some high Px rats with phlorizin and evaluated its effect on GLP-1 and GIP receptor mRNA levels. *P < 0.05; **P < 0.01. n = 4–6 in each group.

phlorizin treatment prevented this decrease (Fig. 1*C*). Phlorizin lowers blood glucose levels by preventing glucose reabsorption from the glomerular filtrate in the kidney. These data suggest that hyperglycemia per se leads to decreased GLP-1 receptor expression. In contrast, GIP receptor expression was decreased only in the high Px group (Fig. 1*B*), suggesting that GIP receptor expression is less sensitive to hyperglycemia than that of the GLP-1 receptor. The decrease of GIP receptor expression was also prevented by phlorizin treatment (Fig. 1*D*).

This reduction of receptor expression was confirmed in another well-characterized model of type 2 diabetes, the *db/db* mouse. Islets from obese diabetic *db/db* mice and lean nondiabetic *db/+* littermates show a similar pattern of incretin receptor downregulation: both GLP-1 and GIP receptor mRNA levels were decreased in the islets of long-term diabetic *db/db* mice (GLP-1 receptor mRNA levels: control 100 ± 10 vs. *db/db* $52 \pm 7\%$, $P < 0.01$; GIP receptor: control 100 ± 7 vs. *db/db* $55 \pm 15\%$, $P < 0.01$). Thus, data from the *db/db* mouse model confirm the Px data of downregulation of incretin receptors with long-term diabetes. The *db/db* mouse also shows a similar pattern of β-cell dedifferentiation, which is induced by time-dependent exposure to hyperglycemia (27).

Next, to examine the effect of hyperglycemia on GLP-1 and GIP receptor protein expression in β-cells, we performed double staining for insulin and the GLP-1 or GIP receptor on pancreatic tissue from sham and diabetic Px rats 4 weeks after surgery. As shown in Fig. 2, GLP-1 receptor was mainly localized in β-cells with strong expression in islets from sham-operated rats. The intensity of GLP-1 receptor staining was dramatically decreased in islets from high Px rats compared with those from sham rats; this decrease of intensity was prevented by phlorizin

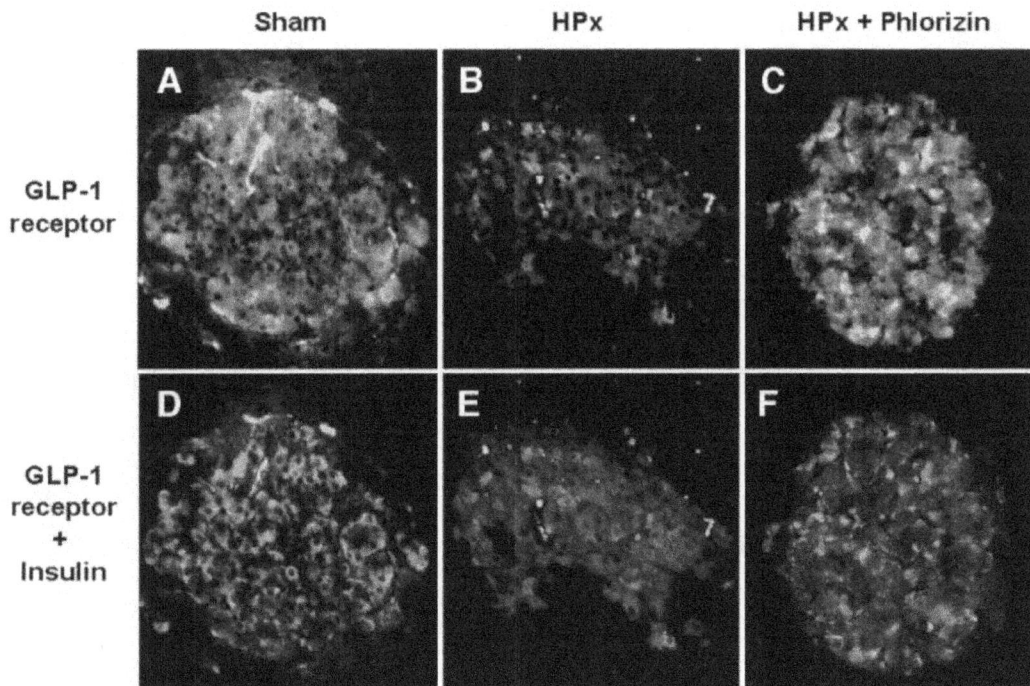

FIG. 2. Decreased GLP-1 receptor protein expression in islets of hyperglycemic Px rats. Sections of pancreas from sham (*A* and *D*) and Px (high Px) (*B* and *E*) rats were immunostained with GLP-1R and insulin antibodies. To examine the effects of hyperglycemia, we treated some high Px rats with phlorizin and evaluated its effect on GLP-1R expression (*C* and *F*). In *A–C*, only GLP-1 staining (green channel) is shown; in *D–F*, the same image with both the red (insulin) and green (GLP-1 receptor) channels is shown. Representative of three evaluations. Magnification bar = 50 μm.

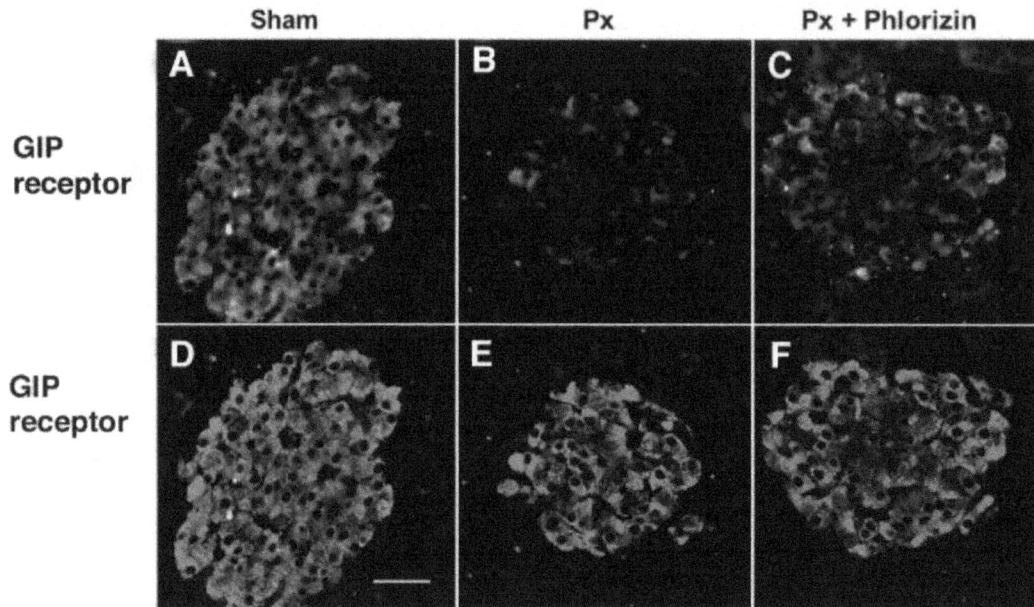

FIG. 3. Decreased GIP receptor protein expression in islets of hyperglycemic Px rats. Sections of pancreas from sham (*A* and *D*) and Px (high Px) (*B* and *E*) rats were immunostained with GIPR and insulin antibodies. To examine the effects of hyperglycemia, we treated some high Px rats with phlorizin and evaluated its effect on GIPR expression (*C* and *F*). In *A–C*, only GIPR (green channel) is shown; in *D–F*, the same image with both the red (insulin) and green (GIPR) channels are shown. Representative of three evaluations. Magnification bar = 50 μm.

treatment associated with normalization of hyperglycemia. As shown in Fig. 3, GIP receptor expression was mainly localized in β-cells with strong expression in islets from sham rats, but the intensity of GIP receptor staining was only moderately decreased in islets from high Px rats compared with those from sham rats.

Impaired insulin secretion in response to GLP-1 or GIP in islets isolated from hyperglycemic Px rats. To assess the possible functional consequence of reduction in GLP-1 and GIP receptor expression, we perifused islets isolated from Px and sham rats 4–6 weeks after surgery. As seen in Fig. 4, the insulin response to GLP-1 was markedly reduced in islets isolated from high Px rats compared with those from sham rats. Similarly, the insulin response to GIP was also reduced in islets isolated from high Px rats compared with those from sham rats (Fig. 5).

These results indicate that decreased GLP-1 and GIP receptor expression leads to reduction of β-cell function. **Decreased GLP-1 receptor expression, but not that of GIP receptor, in islets after exposure to high glucose.** To further examine the role of hyperglycemia on incretin receptor expression, glucose infusions were performed in conscious rats for 4 days. Intravenous infusion of 50% glucose resulted in blood glucose levels of 150–250 mg/dl throughout the experiment, while the saline-infused controls varied from 117 to 125 mg/dl. As shown in Fig. 6*A*, GLP-1 receptor mRNA levels 4 days after glucose infusion were lower compared with those of saline-infused rats. By contrast, however, GIP receptor mRNA levels 4 days after glucose infusion were higher compared with saline-infused rats (Fig. 6*B*). To further examine the effect of glucose concentration on GLP-1 and GIP receptor expres-

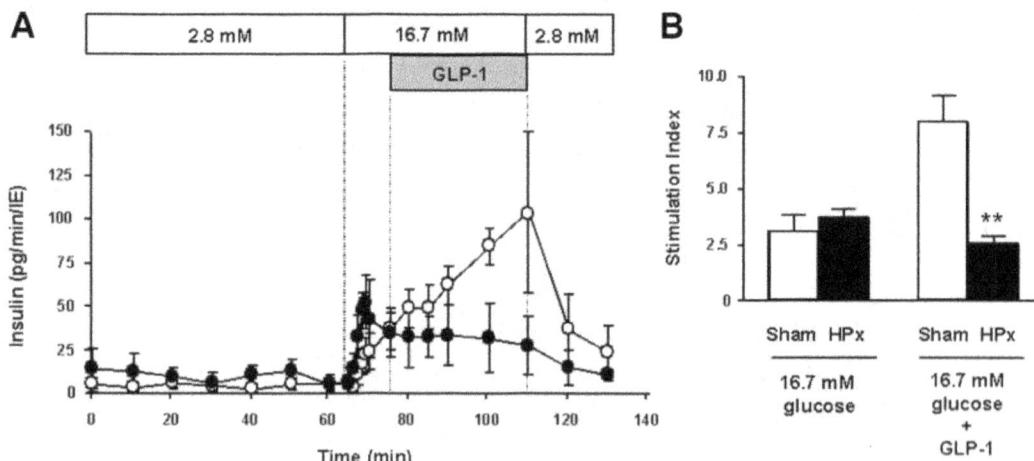

FIG. 4. Impaired insulin secretion in response to GLP-1 in islets isolated from hyperglycemic Px rats. To assess the possible functional consequence of a reduction in expression of GLP-1 receptor, islet perifusion studies were performed using islets isolated from sham and high Px rats. We evaluated the effect of GLP-1 (100 nmol/l) on insulin secretion (*A*) and estimated stimulation index by calculating the area over basal (*B*); *n* = 5 animals per group. Data are means ± SE. ○, sham; ●, high Px.

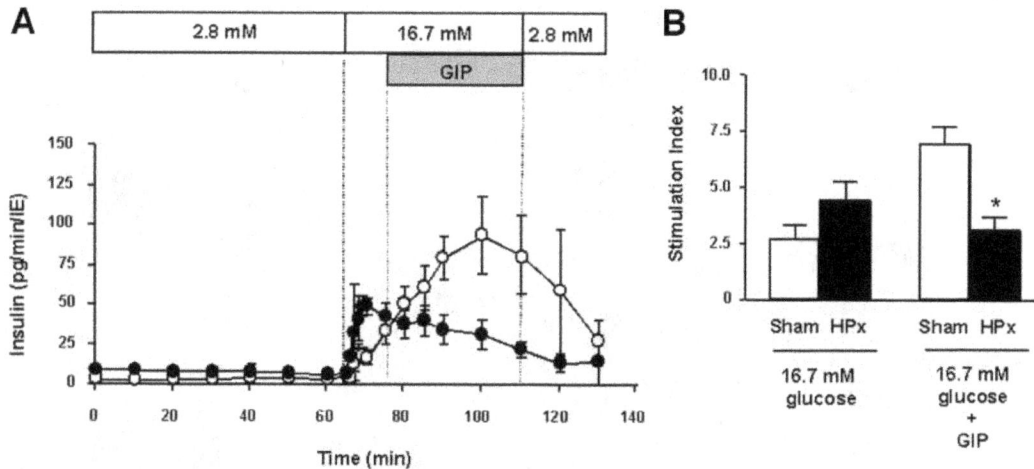

FIG. 5. Impaired insulin secretion in response to GIP in islets isolated from hyperglycemic Px rats. To assess the possible functional consequence of the reduction in expression of GLP-1 receptor, we performed islet perifusion study using islets isolated from sham and high Px rats. We evaluated the effect of GIP (10 nmol/l) on insulin secretion (*A*) and estimated stimulation index by calculating the area over basal (*B*); *n* = 5 animals per group. Data are means ± SE. ○, sham; ●, high Px.

sion, we exposed isolated rat islets to various concentrations of glucose (5–30 mmol/l) for 2 days. Isolated islets were placed in six-well culture plates with 2 ml media containing 5, 10, 20, or 30 mmol/l glucose. In cultured islets, high glucose resulted in decreased GLP-1 receptor expression but increased GIP receptor expression (Fig. 6*C* and *D*).

Involvement of PKCα in decreased GLP-1 receptor by high glucose. Since PKC is activated by high glucose in various cell types, including pancreatic islets (29,30), we

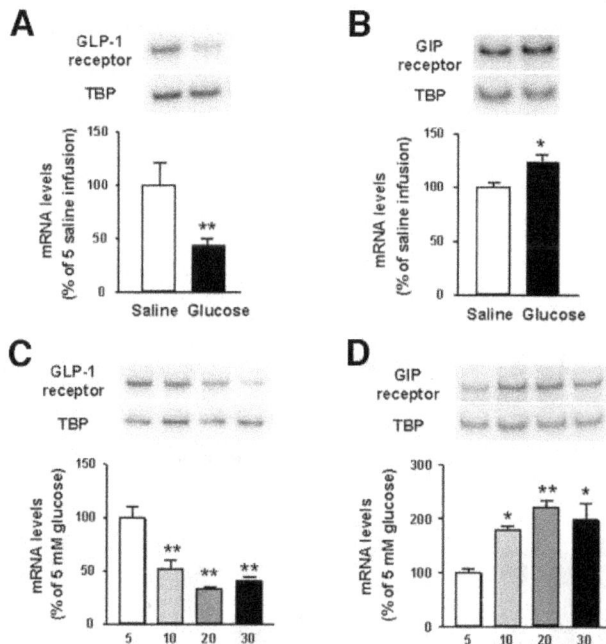

FIG. 6. Decreased GLP-1 receptor expression in islets after exposure to high glucose. *A* and *B*: Glucose or saline was infused in conscious rats for 4 days. GLP-1 and GIP receptor mRNA levels for each animal were examined 4 days after infusion. *C* and *D*: Isolated rat islets were exposed to various concentrations of glucose (5–30 mmol/l) for 2 days, and GLP-1 and GIP receptor mRNA levels were examined (*n* = 4 independent experiments). Representative gels show the receptor and internal control (TBP [TATA-binding protein]) to which the values were normalized in the graphs. *$P < 0.05$; **$P < 0.01$.

hypothesized that PKC activation is involved in the reduction of GLP-1 receptor expression by high glucose. Indeed, GLP-1 receptor expression was decreased after treatment with 100 nmol/l 12-*O*-tetradecanoylphorbol-13-acetate (TPA), an activator of the PKC pathway (control 100 ± 12 vs. 6 h TPA 72 ± 7%, $P < 0.01$; 12 h TPA 85 ± 9%, $P < 0.05$), indicating an involvement of PKC activation in reduction of GLP-1 receptor expression. PKCα, -β2, -δ, -ε, and -ζ have been detected in pancreatic islets (29,30), and PKCα, -β2, -δ, and -ε are activated by high glucose (29,30). First, we examined the distribution of PKC isoforms (PKCα, -β2, -δ, -ε, and -ζ) in rat pancreatic islets by immunostaining (Fig. 7). PKCα, -β2, and -δ were clearly expressed in rat β-cells, but PKCε and -ζ were not detected. Next, we examined the effect of each PKC isoform on GLP-1R mRNA expression in isolated rat islets by adenovirus-mediated overexpression. Three days after exposure to each adenovirus, we examined GLP-1 receptor expression levels. Figure 8*A* shows representative islets 3 days after exposure to control Ad-GFP; many cells in islets were infected with the adenovirus. We have previously found that Ad-GFP infects >50% of the islet cells but does not penetrate to the center of the islet and that glucose-stimulated insulin secretion (GSIS) was not affected by such adenoviral infection (31). GLP-1 receptor mRNA levels were markedly reduced by PKCα overexpression but not by overexpression of the other PKC isoforms (PKCβ2, -δ, -ε, and -ζ) (Fig. 8*B*). To examine an involvement of PKCα in the downregulation of GLP-1 receptor by high glucose, we prepared dominant-negative PKCα (DN-PKCα)-expressing adenovirus (K368R). As shown in Fig. 8*C*, overexpression of DN-PKCα did not result in reduced GLP-1 receptor expression. Together, these results suggest that PKCα is involved in downregulation of GLP-1 receptor by high glucose.

DISCUSSION

In this study, it was found that exposure of β-cells to high blood glucose concentrations in vivo and in vitro led to downregulation of the GLP-1 receptor both at the gene expression and protein levels. The gene expression changes were found in rat islets 4 weeks after partial Px, after 4 days of an in vivo glucose clamp, and in isolated

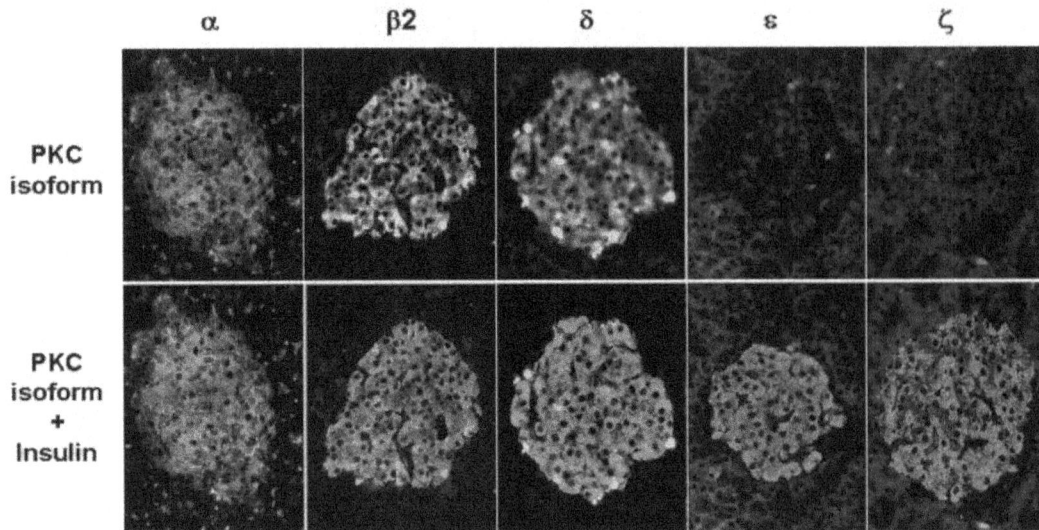

FIG. 7. Immunostaining for PKC isoforms (α, $\beta2$, δ, ε, and ζ) in rat pancreatic islets. Pancreatic sections of normal rats were immunostained with each PKC isoform antibody (PKCα, -$\beta2$, -δ, -ε, and -ζ) (green; *upper panels*) and insulin (red; *lower panels*). Magnification bar = 50 μm.

islets cultured in the presence of high glucose for 48 h. Supporting the concept that the changes are caused by reversible glucotoxicity effect, the gene expression changes were prevented when glucose levels were normalized with phlorizin, as has previously been found with various other expression changes seen in the Px model (19,21,32). With regard to insulin secretion, in agreement with observations in humans (13,14) and perfused pancreas studies in partially Px rats (15), reduced insulin responses to GLP-1 were found with perifused isolated islets. These findings are consistent with the hypothesis that the unresponsiveness to GLP-1 is in part due to the receptor changes. It would be important to examine whether GLP-1 receptor gene transcription or its mRNA stability is decreased by hyperglycemia, but practically it is very difficult to perform luciferase assay and/or run-off assay with freshly isolated rat islets. It has been reported, however, that GLP-1 receptor mRNA stability is not af-

fected by TPA, an activator of PKC, in β-cell line RINm5F (20). Thus, although not examined in this study, we assume that decrease of GLP-1 receptor mRNA expression was presumably due to decrease of GLP-1 receptor gene transcription itself rather than decrease of its mRNA stability.

There are interesting questions about the relationship of the reduced responsiveness to GLP-1 and the impairment of GSIS consistently found in humans and in animal models of diabetes (33). Earlier studies in the neonatal streptozocin rat model showed that treatment with theophylline, which raises cyclic AMP (cAMP) levels, partially restored defective GSIS secretion (34), raising questions about the degree to which defective cAMP generation from reduction of GLP-1 signaling might contribute to abnormalities in GSIS. It has been postulated that GLP-1 acts as a glucose sensitizer on β-cells (2), which fits with this concept.

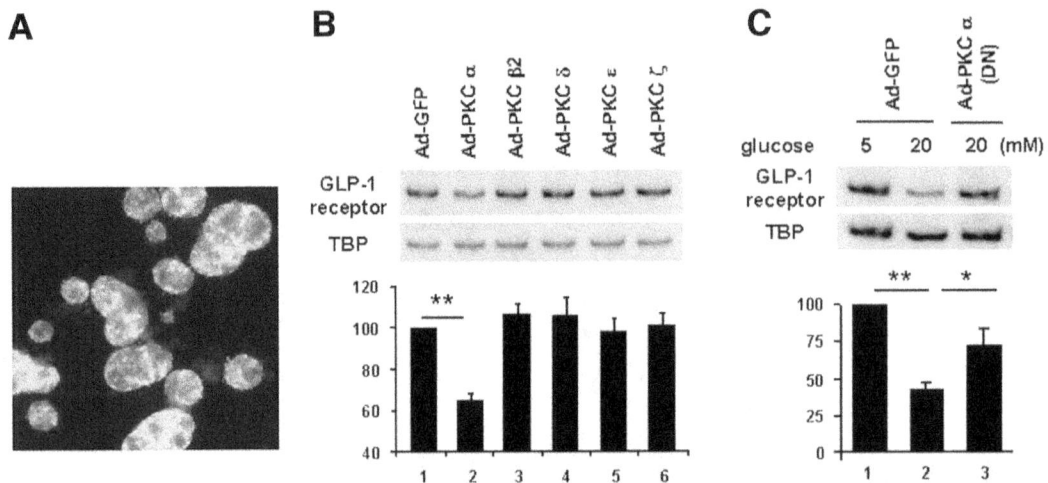

FIG. 8. Involvement of PKCα in downregulation of GLP-1 receptor by high glucose in isolated rat islets. *A*: Isolated rat islets infected with Ad-GFP were cultured for 3 days in RPMI medium. Panel shows representative islets 3 days after exposure to control Ad-GFP. As seen in this fluorescent micrograph, many cells in islets are infected with the adenovirus. Representative of five evaluations. *B*: Isolated rat islets were infected with an adenovirus-expressing PKC isoform (α, $\beta2$, δ, ε, or ζ), and 3 days after the infection, GLP-1 mRNA levels were evaluated. *C*: Isolated rat islets were infected with Ad-GFP– or DN-PKCα–expressing adenovirus, and 3 days after the infection the islets were exposed to 5 or 20 mmol/l glucose for 2 days; then GLP-1 mRNA levels were evaluated. *$P < 0.05$; **$P < 0.01$ ($n = 4$ independent experiments). TBP, TATA-binding protein.

The changes in GIP receptor gene expression are somewhat different than those found with the GLP-1 receptor. Reduction in expression was found in the Px model, but in the shorter-term glucose infusion model and cultured islets with exposure to high glucose, increases in GIP receptor gene expression were found. These differences in the GIP and GLP-1 receptor gene expression appear to be due to timing and raise interesting questions about the mechanisms underlying these major differing outcomes. It was surprising to find no impairment in the first-phase insulin response in the perifused islets and to find such similarly reduced insulin responses to GIP and GLP-1, considering the studies in humans showing profound reductions in responsiveness to GIP and partially preserved responses to GLP-1 (11,12,14). It is possible that a more complete dose-response study might have brought out differences between GIP and GLP-1 receptors—or perhaps this is a species difference.

The results for GIP receptor are discrepant between the partial Px rats (hyperglycemia for 4 weeks) and the glucose infusion for 4 days. In the first model, GIP receptor expression was reduced, as was in vitro insulin secretion in response to GIP, whereas in the second model, GIP receptor gene expression was increased. The duration of hyperglycemia (acute versus chronic) may account for the difference in the receptor expression. We have previously shown that short-term (4-day) hyperglycemia maintained by glucose clamp induced very little change in β-cell gene expression (22), whereas long-term hyperglycemia after Px induced global alterations (35). These data establish a relationship between the duration of hyperglycemia and the deterioration of the β-cell phenotype with diabetes. The rapid increase in GIP receptor could contribute to the maintenance of insulin output during the elevated metabolic demand induced by hyperglycemia. In fact, the overall capacity of insulin secretion is not diminished after acute hyperglycemia. In contrast, the reduction of the incretin receptors may be, at least partially, due to the dedifferentiation or loss of the specific phenotype of β-cells in Px rats as a result of chronic exposure to hyperglycemia (35). Indeed, when we examined the expression of these genes in another long-term model of type 2 diabetes, the *db/db* mouse, we observed a similar alteration in the pattern of incretin receptor expression: both GLP-1 and GIP receptor expression were decreased in islets of hyperglycemic *db/db* mice.

While GLP-1 is known to stimulate the generation of cAMP and activate protein kinase A, it has recently been appreciated that it can also work through the cAMP-regulated guanine nucleotide exchange factor II (also known as Epac2), which has a variety of targets (36). Stimulation with phorbol esters causing PKC activation has been shown to phosphorylate the GLP-1 receptor with a resultant rapidly diminished signaling (37,38). Since high glucose can activate PKC, hyperglycemia was suggested to act through the PKC pathway to desensitize the GLP-1 receptor without change in expression (38). The present study suggests that the PKCα isoform, which is clearly present in β-cells, is involved and actually decreases the GLP-1 message. Overexpression of PKCα following adenoviral infection led to decrease of GLP-1 message that was comparable with the infection efficiency of β-cells. Then, even more convincing, treatment with an adenovirus containing a dominant-negative form of PKCα partially protected islets against the reduction of GLP-1 receptor

expression seen when islets were cultured in a high-glucose concentration.

Taken together, our results show that GLP-1 receptor expression is decreased by hyperglycemia. We suggest that the downregulation of the GLP-1 receptor by hyperglycemia is largely responsible for the impaired incretin effects and thus in part explains the β-cell dysfunction found in diabetes. These findings have important implications for the design of new therapies based on activation of the GLP-1 receptor.

ACKNOWLEDGMENTS

This work was supported by grants from the National Institutes of Health (DK-44523 to S.B.-W.); the Joslin DERC Animal, Media and Advanced Microscopy Cores (DK36836); the Diabetes Research and Wellness Foundation; and an important group of private donors. H.K. was a recipient of a fellowship and grant from the Japan Society for the Promotion of Science. D.R.L. and V.F.D.-K. were recipients of Juvenile Diabetes Research Center postdoctoral fellowships.

We thank Sharon Lee for her secretarial assistance and Jennifer Hollister-Lock for her technical support.

REFERENCES

1. McIntyre N, Holdsworth CD, Turner DS: Intestinal factors in the control of insulin secretion. *J Clin Endocrinol Metab* 25:1317–1324, 1965
2. Holst JJ, Gromada J: Role of incretin hormones in the regulation of insulin secretion in diabetic and nondiabetic humans. *Am J Physiol Endocrinol Metab* 287:E199–E206, 2004
3. Mojsov S, Weir GC, Habener JF: Insulinotropin: glucagon-like peptide I (7–37) co-encoded in the glucagon gene is a potent stimulator of insulin release in the perfused rat pancreas. *J Clin Invest* 79:616–619, 1987
4. Kreymann B, Williams G, Ghatei MA, Bloom SR: Glucagon-like peptide-1 7–36: a physiological incretin in man. *Lancet* 2:1300–1303, 1987
5. Brown JC, Dryburgh JR, Ross SA, Dupré J: Identification and actions of gastric inhibitory polypeptide. *Recent Prog Horm Res* 31:487–532, 1975
6. Scorcchi LA, Brown TJ, MaClusky N, Brubaker PL, Auerbach AB, Joyner AL, Drucker DJ: Glucose intolerance but normal satiety in mice with a null mutation in the glucagon-like peptide 1 receptor gene. *Nat Med* 2:1254–1258, 1996
7. Baggio L, Kieffer TJ, Drucker DJ: Glucagon-like peptide-1, but not glucose-dependent insulinotropic peptide, regulates fasting glycemia and nonenteral glucose clearance in mice. *Endocrinology* 141:3703–3709, 2000
8. Miyawaki K, Yamada Y, Yano H, Niwa H, Ban N, Ihara Y, Kubota A, Fujimoto S, Kajikawa M, Kuroe A, Tsuda K, Hashimoto H, Yamashita T, Jomori T, Tashiro F, Miyazaki J, Seino Y: Glucose intolerance caused by a defect in the entero-insular axis: a study in gastric inhibitory polypeptide receptor knockout mice. *Proc Natl Acad Sci U S A* 96:14843–14847, 1999
9. Toft-Nielsen MB, Damholt MB, Madsbad S, Hilsted LM, Hughes TE, Michelsen BK, Holst JJ: Determinants of the impaired secretion of glucagon-like peptide-1 in type 2 diabetic patients. *J Clin Endocrinol Metab* 86:3717–3723, 2001
10. Forbes S, Moonan M, Robinson S, Anyaoku V, Patterson M, Murphy KG, Ghatei MA, Bloom SR, Johnston DG: Impaired circulating glucagon-like peptide-1 response to oral glucose in women with previous gestational diabetes. *Clin Endocrinol (Oxf)* 62:51–55, 2005
11. Nauck MA, Heimesaat MM, Orskov C, Holst JJ, Ebert R, Creutzfeldt W: Preserved incretin activity of glucagon-like peptide 1 [7–36 amide] but not of synthetic human gastric inhibitory polypeptide in patients with type-2 diabetes mellitus. *J Clin Invest* 91:301–307, 1993
12. Elahi D, McAloon-Dyke M, Fukagawa NK, Meneilly GS, Sclater AL, Minaker KL, Habener JF, Andersen DK: The insulinotropic actions of glucose-dependent insulinotropic polypeptide (GIP) and glucagon-like peptide-1 (7–37) in normal and diabetic subjects. *Regul Pept* 51:63–74, 1994
13. Fritsche A, Stefan N, Hardt E, Haring H, Stumvoll M: Characterisation of beta-cell dysfunction of impaired glucose tolerance: evidence for impairment of incretin-induced insulin secretion. *Diabetologia* 43:852–858, 2000
14. Kjems LL, Holst JJ, Volund A, Madsbad S: The influence of GLP-1 on glucose-stimulated insulin secretion: effects on β-cell sensitivity in type 2 and nondiabetic subjects. *Diabetes* 52:380–386, 2003
15. Hosokawa YA, Hosokawa H, Chen C, Leahy JL: Mechanism of impaired

glucose-potentiated insulin secretion in diabetic 90% pancreatectomy rats: study using glucagonlike peptide-1 (7–37). *J Clin Invest* 97:180–186, 1996

16. Moens K, Heimberg H, Flamez D, Huypens P, Quartier E, Ling Z, Pipeleers D, Gremlich S, Thorens B, Schuit F: Expression and functional activity of glucagon, glucagon-like peptide 1, and glucose-dependent insulinotropic peptide receptors in rat pancreatic islet cells. *Diabetes* 45:257–261, 1996

17. Abrahamsen N, Nishimura E: Regulation of glucagon and glucagon-like peptide-1 receptor messenger ribonucleic acid expression in cultured rat pancreatic islets by glucose, cyclic adenosine 3′,5′-monophosphate, and glucocorticoids. *Endocrinol* 136:1572–1578, 1995

18. Bonner-Weir S, Trent DF, Weir GC: Partial pancreatectomy in the rat and subsequent defect in glucose-induced insulin release. *J Clin Invest* 71: 1544–1553, 1983

19. Laybutt DR, Sharma A, Sgroi DC, Gaudet J, Bonner-Weir S, Weir GC: Genetic regulation of metabolic pathways in beta-cells disrupted by hyperglycemia. *J Biol Chem* 277:10912–10921, 2002

20. Fehmann HC, Schweinfurth J, Jiang J, Goke B: Regulation of glucagon-like peptide-I receptor expression and transcription by the protein kinase C pathway. *Res Exp Med (Berl)* 196:219–225, 1996

21. Jonas JC, Sharma A, Hasenkamp W, Ilkova H, Patane G, Laybutt R, Bonner-Weir S, Weir GC: Chronic hyperglycemia triggers loss of pancreatic beta cell differentiation in an animal model of diabetes. *J Biol Chem* 274:14112–14121, 1999

22. Steil GM, Trivedi N, Jonas JC, Hasenkamp WM. Sharma A, Bonner-Weir S, Weir GC: Adaptation of beta-cell mass to substrate oversupply: enhanced function with normal gene expression. *Am J Physiol Endocrinol Metab* 280:E788–E796, 2001

23. Jonas JC, Laybutt DR, Steil GM, Trivedi N, Pertusa JG, Van de Casteele M, Weir GC, Henquin JC: High glucose stimulates early response gene c-Myc expression in rat pancreatic beta cells. *J Biol Chem* 276:35375–35381, 2001

24. Heller RS, Kieffer TJ, Habener JF: Insulinotrophic glucagon-like peptide I receptor expression in glucagon-producing α cells of the rat endocrine pancreas. *Diabetes* 46:785–791, 1997

25. Lewis, JT, Dayanandan B, Habener JF, Kieffer TJ: Glucose-dependent insulinotrophic peptide confers early phase insulin release to oral glucose in rats: demonstration by a receptor antagonist. *Endocrinology* 141:3710–3716, 2000

26. Xu G, Stoffers DA, Habener JF, Bonner-Weir S: Exendin-4 stimulates both β-cell replication and neogenesis, resulting in increased β-cell mass and improved glucose tolerance in diabetic rats. *Diabetes* 48:2270–2276, 1999

27. Kjorholt C, Akerfeldt MC, Biden TJ, Laybutt DR: Chronic hyperglycemia, independent of plasma lipid levels, is sufficient for the loss of β-cell differentiation and secretory function in the *db/db* mouse model of diabetes. *Diabetes* 54:2755–2763, 2005

28. He TC, Zhou S, Da Costa LT, Yu J, Kinzler KW, Vogelstein B: A simplified system for generating recombinant adenoviruses. *Proc Natl Acad Sci U S A* 95:2509–2514, 1998

29. Kaneto H, Suzuma K, Sharma A, Bonner-Weir S, King GL, Weir GC: Involvement of protein kinase C beta 2 in c-myc induction by high glucose in pancreatic beta-cells. *J Biol Chem* 277:3680–3685, 2002

30. Hoy M, Berggren PO, Gromada J: Involvement of protein kinase C-epsilon in inositol hexakisphosphate-induced exocytosis in mouse pancreatic beta-cells. *J Biol Chem* 278:35168–35171, 2003

31. Kaneto H, Sharma A, Suzuma K, Laybutt DR, Xu G, Bonner-Weir S, Weir GC: Induction of c-Myc expression suppresses insulin gene transcription by inhibiting NeuroD/BETA2-mediated transcriptional activation. *J Biol Chem* 277:12998–13006, 2002

32. Laybutt DR, Kaneto H, Hasenkamp W, Grey S, Jonas JC, Sgroi DC, Groff A, Ferran C, Bonner-Weir S, Sharma A, Weir GC: Increased expression of antioxidant and antiapoptotic genes in islets that may contribute to β-cell survival during chronic hyperglycemia. *Diabetes* 51:413–423, 2002

33. Weir GC, Bonner-Weir S: Five stages of evolving β-cell dysfunction during progression to diabetes. *Diabetes* 53 (Suppl 3):S16–S21, 2004

34. Weir GC, Clore ET, Zmachinski CJ, Bonner-Weir S: Islet secretion in a new experimental model for non-insulin-dependent diabetes. *Diabetes* 30:590–595, 1981

35. Laybutt DR, Glandt M, Xu G, Ahn YB, Trivedi N, Bonner-Weir S, Weir GC: Critical reduction in beta-cell mass results in two distinct outcomes over time: adaptation with impaired glucose tolerance or decompensated diabetes. *J Biol Chem* 278:2997–3005, 2003

36. Holz GG: Epac: A new cAMP-binding protein in support of glucagon-like peptide-1 receptor–mediated signal transduction in the pancreatic β-cell. *Diabetes* 53:5–13, 2004

37. Widmann C, Dolci W, Thorens B: Heterologous desensitization of the glucagon-like peptide-1 receptor by phorbol esters requires phosphorylation of the cytoplasmic tail at four different sites. *J Biol Chem* 271:19957–19963, 1996

38. Widmann C, Dolci W, Thorens B: Internalization and homologous desensitization of the GLP-1 receptor depend on phosphorylation of the receptor carboxyl tail at the same three sites. *Mol Endocrinol* 11:1094–1102, 1997

Original Article

Reduced Incretin Effect in Type 2 Diabetes
Cause or Consequence of the Diabetic State?

Filip K. Knop,[1,2] Tina Vilsbøll,[1] Patricia V. Højberg,[1] Steen Larsen,[3] Sten Madsbad,[4] Aage Vølund,[5] Jens J. Holst,[2] and Thure Krarup[1]

We aimed to investigate whether the reduced incretin effect observed in patients with type 2 diabetes is a primary event in the pathogenesis of type 2 diabetes or a consequence of the diabetic state. Eight patients with chronic pancreatitis and secondary diabetes (A1C mean [range] of 6.9% [6.2–8.0]), eight patients with chronic pancreatitis and normal glucose tolerance (NGT; 5.3 [4.9–5.7]), eight patients with type 2 diabetes (6.9 [6.2–8.0]); and eight healthy subjects (5.5 [5.1–5.8]) were studied. Blood was sampled over 4 h on 2 separate days after a 50-g oral glucose load and an isoglycemic intravenous glucose infusion, respectively. The incretin effect (100% × [β-cell secretory response to oral glucose tolerance test − intravenous β-cell secretory response]/β-cell secretory response to oral glucose tolerance test) was significantly ($P < 0.05$) reduced (means ± SE) in patients with chronic pancreatitis and secondary diabetes (31 ± 4%) compared with patients with chronic pancreatitis and NGT (68 ± 3) and healthy subjects (60 ± 4), respectively. In the type 2 diabetes group, the incretin effect amounted to 36 ± 6%, significantly ($P < 0.05$) lower than in chronic pancreatitis patients with NGT and in healthy subjects, respectively. These results suggest that the reduced incretin effect is not a primary event in the development of type 2 diabetes, but rather a consequence of the diabetic state. *Diabetes* 56: 1951–1959, 2007

The phenomenon that oral glucose elicits a higher insulin response than intravenous glucose at identical plasma glucose (PG) profiles (isoglycemia) is called the incretin effect. The incretin effect is conveyed by the two incretin hormones glucagon-like peptide (GLP-1) 1 and glucose-dependent insulinotropic polypeptide (GIP) (1). Both hormones are secreted from the small intestine in response to ingestion of nutrients (1,2). They are highly insulinotropic in a strictly glucose-dependent fashion (1). In type 2 diabetes, the incretin effect has been shown to be markedly reduced (3). This incretin defect is accompanied by a reduced GLP-1 response to a mixed meal (4,5), a decreased insulinotropic potency of GLP-1 (6), and an almost complete loss of late-phase insulin secretion in response to GIP (7). In addition, we have recently shown that the suppression of glucagon secretion is impaired during oral glucose tolerance tests (OGTTs) as opposed to isoglycemic intravenous glucose infusion in patients with type 2 diabetes (8). The pathophysiological background for the reduced incretin effect observed in patients with type 2 diabetes is unclear. In the current study we exploited the fact that patients with chronic pancreatitis eventually develop diabetes secondary to their inflammatory condition in the pancreas (9–12). If patients with chronic pancreatitis and secondary diabetes exhibit reduced incretin effect and patients with chronic pancreatitis and normal glucose tolerance (NGT) are normal in that regard, it is likely that the reduced incretin effect is a consequence of the diabetic state. On the other hand, if the incretin effect is preserved independently of the diabetic state of patients with chronic pancreatitis, the incretin defect in type 2 diabetes could be a primary pathogenetic defect. Therefore, in the current study, the classical isoglycemic technique was applied to gauge the incretin effect in patients with chronic pancreatitis and NGT and in patients with chronic pancreatitis and secondary diabetes. Healthy subjects and patients with type 2 diabetes were studied for comparison.

From the [1]Department of Internal Medicine F, Gentofte Hospital, Hellerup, Denmark; the [2]Department of Medical Physiology, The Panum Institute, University of Copenhagen, Copenhagen, Denmark; the [3]Department of Internal Medicine M, Glostrup Hospital, Hellerup, Denmark; the [4]Department of Endocrinology, Hvidovre Hospital, Hvidovre, Denmark; and the [5]Department of Biostatistics, Novo Nordisk, Copenhagen, Denmark.

Address correspondence and reprint requests to Filip Krag Knop, MD, Department of Internal Medicine, Gentofte Hospital, University of Copenhagen, Niels Andersens Vej 65, DK-2900 Hellerup, Denmark. E-mail: filipknop@dadlnet.dk.

Received for publication 23 January 2007 and accepted in revised form 3 May 2007.

Published ahead of print at http://diabetes.diabetesjournals.org on 18 May 2007. DOI: 10.2337/db07-0100.

AUC, area under the curve; FPG, fasting plasma glucose; GIP, glucose-dependent insulinotropic polypeptide; GLP, glucagon-like peptide; HOMA, homeostasis model assessment; HOMA-IR, HOMA for insulin resistance; ICA, islet cell autoantibody; ISR, insulin secretion rate; NGT, normal glucose tolerance; OGTT; oral glucose tolerance test; PG, plasma glucose.

RESEARCH DESIGN AND METHODS

Group 1 consisted of eight patients with chronic pancreatitis and secondary diabetes diagnosed according to criteria of the World Health Organization (13). Subject characteristics are shown in Table 1. In group 1 subjects, diabetes developed after the diagnosis of chronic pancreatitis had been established, and none of the patients had first-degree relatives with diabetes. Five were treated with diet alone, two with a sulfonylurea, and one with metformin and a sulfonylurea. Five patients in this group suffered from exocrine pancreatic insufficiency and were treated with pancreatic enzyme supplementation to alleviate steatorrhea. The etiology of chronic pancreatitis was judged to be alcoholism in seven patients and idiopathic in one patient.

Group 2 consisted of eight patients with chronic pancreatitis and NGT (PG concentration at 120 min after 75-g OGTT [$PG_{120\ min}$] of <7.8 mmol/l) without any family history of diabetes. Three patients in this group suffered from exocrine pancreatic insufficiency and were treated with pancreatic enzyme supplementation on a daily basis. The etiology of chronic pancreatitis was judged to be alcoholism in four patients and idiopathic in the rest.

All patients with chronic pancreatitis (groups 1 and 2) were without clinical and/or biochemical signs (amylase, C-reactive protein, and leukocyte

TABLE 1

Anthropometric data for patients with chronic pancreatitis and secondary diabetes, patients with chronic pancreatitis and NGT, patients with type 2 diabetes, and healthy subjects

	Patients with chronic pancreatitis and secondary diabetes	Patients with chronic pancreatitis and NGT	Patients with type 2 diabetes	Healthy subjects
n (F/M)	2/6	2/6	2/6	2/6
Age (years)	56 (44–65)	50 (45–59)	62 (51–75)	57 (44–69)
BMI (kg/m^2)	22 (15–29)	22 (18–29)	24 (21–26)	22 (20–26)
Waist-to-hip ratio	1.0 (0.9–1.1)	1.0 (0.9–1.0)	1.0 (0.9–1.0)	1.0 (0.9–1.0)
FPG (mmol/l)	8.0 (4.8–13.5)	5.2 (4.9–5.6)	8.1 (6.2–10.4)	5.2 (4.9–5.6)
A1C (%)	6.9 (6.2–8.0)	5.5 (5.1–5.6)	6.8 (6.2–8.7)	5.5 (5.1–5.8)

Data are means (range).

counts within normal limits) of acute inflammatory activity in the pancreas. None of the patients drank alcohol on a daily basis, and there were no clinical or biochemical signs (albumin, aspartate aminotransferase/alanine aminotransferase, alkaline phosphatase, and international normalized ratio within normal limits × 1.5) of affected liver function. The diagnostic criteria of chronic pancreatitis were according to Layer et al. (12), and all chronic pancreatitis subjects had unequivocal morphological changes of the pancreas evident by ultrasonography, computed tomography scan, magnetic resonance cholangiopancreatography, or endoscopic retrograde cholangiopancreatography according to the Cambridge classification (14).

Group 3 consisted of eight patients with type 2 diabetes diagnosed according to the criteria of the World Health Organization (13). Four were treated with diet, three with a sulfonylurea, and one with a sulfonylurea in combination with metformin.

Group 4 consisted of eight healthy subjects without a family history of diabetes. All had NGT according to a 75-g OGTT performed immediately before inclusion in the study.

All participants were negative with regard to islet cell autoantibodies (ICAs) and GAD-65 autoantibodies, except for one subject in group 2 and one subject in group 4, both of whom had elevated GAD-65 autoantibodies (23.0 and 27.3 IU/l, respectively; normal: <9.5). Both had NGT (PG$_{120 min}$ 6.4 and 4.3 mmol/l), normal fasting plasma glucose (FPG) (5.8 and 5.3 mmol/l), normal A1C (5.9 and 5.3%), and normal ICA. Otherwise, all subjects had normal clinical and biochemical parameters. None of the subjects took drugs likely to

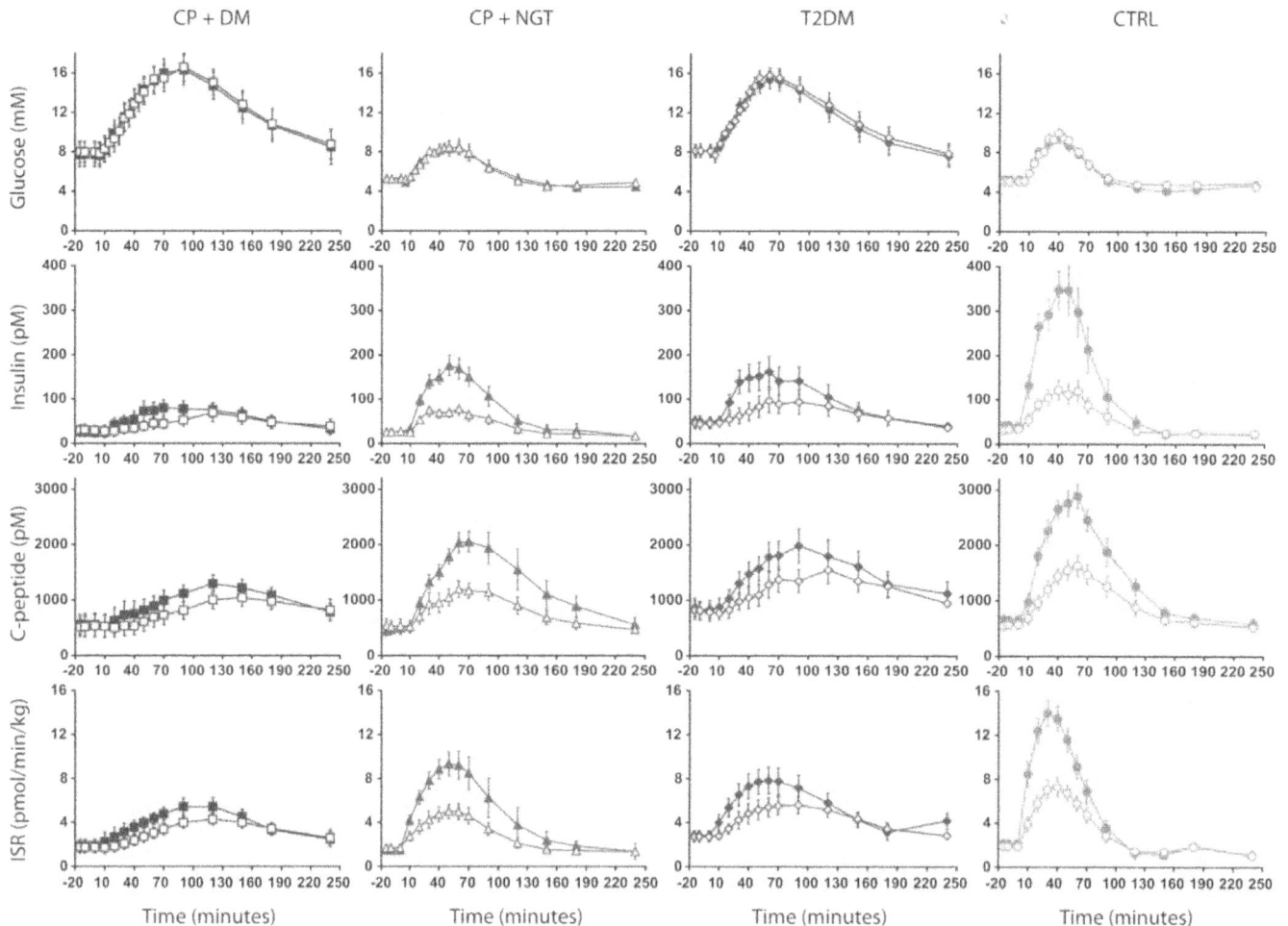

FIG. 1. PG, plasma insulin, plasma C-peptide, and ISR in patients with chronic pancreatitis and NGT (triangles), patients with chronic pancreatitis and secondary diabetes (squares), healthy subjects (circles), and patients with type 2 diabetes (diamonds) after 50-g OGTT (filled symbols) and isoglycemic intravenous glucose infusion (open symbols), respectively. *Significant differences ($P < 0.05$) between the individual OGTT and isoglycemic intravenous glucose infusion curves (repeated-measures ANOVA). CP, chronic pancreatitis; CTRL, control; T2DM, type 2 diabetes.

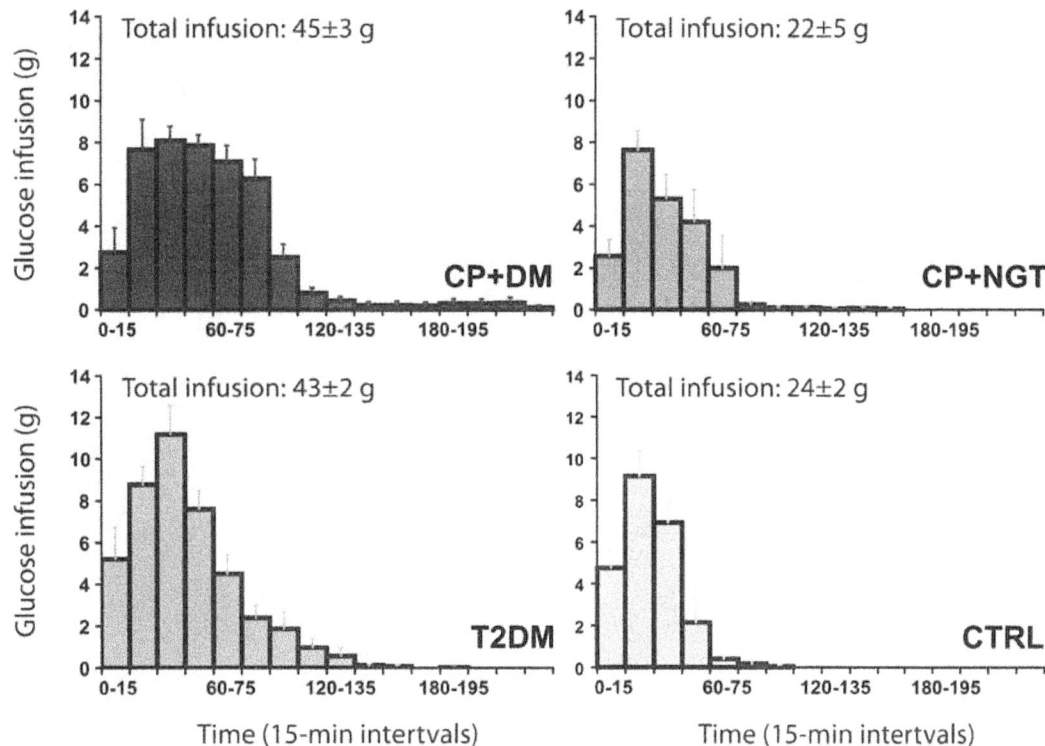

FIG. 2. Mean glucose infusion rates per 15 min used during the isoglycemic intravenous glucose infusion in the four groups. Total amounts of glucose needed to copy the 50-g OGTT curves are indicated. CP, chronic pancreatitis; CTRL, control; T2DM, type 2 diabetes.

differentially affect the responses of insulin, glucagon, or incretin hormones, respectively, to oral compared with intravenous glucose, and none had impaired renal function (they had normal plasma creatinine levels and no albuminuria). Seven of the healthy control subjects and the eight patients with type 2 diabetes had also participated in a recently published study and were reanalyzed for the current study.

All subjects agreed to participate after receiving oral and written information. The study design was approved by the scientific-ethical committee of the County of Copenhagen in March 2004 (registration no. KA 04034), and the study was conducted according to the principles of the Helsinki Declaration II.
Methods. All subjects were studied on two occasions separated by at least 24 h. Before each occasion the patients with diabetes had not taken their oral antidiabetic therapy, if any, for a period of no less than 1 week. Otherwise, the participants continued their normal lifestyle. On both occasions the subjects were studied in a recumbent position after an overnight (10-h) fast.

On day 1 a cannula was inserted in the retrograde direction in a dorsal hand vein. The cannulated hand was placed in a heating box (42°C) throughout the experiment for collection of arterialized blood samples. The subjects ingested 50 g of water-free glucose dissolved in 400 ml water over 5 min (0–5 min). Arterialized blood was drawn at time −15, −10, 0, 15, 30, 45, 60, 90, 120, 150, 180, and 240 min and distributed into chilled tubes containing EDTA plus aprotinin (Trasylol at 500 kIU/ml blood; Bayer, Leverkusen, Germany) and a specific dipeptidyl peptidase IV inhibitor (valine-pyrrolidide, final concentration of 0.01 mmol/l; a gift from Dr. R.B. Carr, Novo Nordisk, Bagsværd, Denmark) for analysis of glucagon, GLP-1, and GIP. For analysis of insulin and C-peptide, blood was distributed into chilled tubes containing heparin plus aprotinin (500 KIU/ml blood). All tubes were immediately cooled on ice and then centrifuged for 20 min at 4,000 rounds per min (rpm) and 4°C. Plasma for GLP-1 and GIP analysis was stored at −20°C, and plasma for insulin and C-peptide analysis was stored at −80°C until analysis. For bedside measurement of PG, blood was distributed into fluoride tubes and centrifuged immediately for 2 min at 10,000 rpm at room temperature.

On day 2 we inserted a retrograde cannula in a dorsal hand vein for blood sampling (42°C) and a cannula in the contralateral cubital vein for glucose infusion. An isoglycemic intravenous glucose infusion (20% wt/vol) was performed, aiming at a duplication of the PG profile determined on day 1. Blood was sampled as on day 1, except for more frequent PG sampling.
Analyses. PG concentrations were measured by the glucose oxidase method, using a glucose analyzer (2300 Stat Plus analyzer; YSI, Yellow Springs, OH). Plasma samples were assayed for total GLP-1 immunoreactivity, as previously

described (15), using a radioimmunoassay (antiserum no. 89390) that is specific for the COOH terminus of the GLP-1 molecule and that reacts equally with intact GLP-1 and the primary (NH$_2$-terminally truncated) metabolite. Intact GLP-1 was measured using an enzyme-linked immunosorbent assay (16). The assay was a two-site sandwich assay using two monoclonal antibodies: GLP-1F5 as a catching antibody (COOH-terminally directed) and Mab26.1 as a detecting antibody (NH$_2$-terminally directed) (17).

Total GIP was measured using the COOH-terminally directed antiserum R65 (18,19), which reacts fully with intact GIP and the NH$_2$-terminally truncated metabolite. Intact, biologically active GIP was measured using antiserum no. 98171 (20).

The glucagon assay was directed against the COOH terminus of the glucagon molecule (antibody code no. 4305) and, therefore, measured glucagon of mainly pancreatic origin (21). Neither glicentin nor oxyntomodulin cross-react, but proglucagon 1-61, which is mainly formed in the pancreas, did react fully in this assay (22,23). Plasma insulin and C-peptide concentrations were measured using AutoDelfia time-resolved fluoroimmunoassay (Wallac Oy, Turku, Finland) (24).
Calculations and statistical analyses. All results are means ± SE. Area under the curve (AUC) values were calculated using the trapezoidal rule and are presented as the incremental values (baseline levels subtracted) if nothing else is stated. Incretin effect values were calculated by relating the difference in integrated β-cell secretory responses (insulin, C-peptide, and insulin secretion rate [ISR]) between stimulation with oral and isoglycemic intravenous glucose to the response after oral glucose, which was taken as 100% (3). The following formula was used: 100% × (integrated response to OGTT − intravenous integrated response)/integrated response to OGTT. ISR was calculated by deconvolution of measured C-peptide concentrations and application of population-based parameters for C-peptide kinetics as described previously (24–26). ISR is expressed as picomoles of insulin secreted per minute per kilogram body weight. The homeostatic model assessment (HOMA) was used to assess insulin resistance (HOMA-IR) (27). Comparisons of experiments in which the data were distributed normally were made with two-tailed Student's t test (paired within groups, unpaired between groups). For data that did not follow a normal distribution, the significance of differences between groups was tested using the Mann-Whitney U test, and for within-subject comparisons, the Wilcoxon test for paired differences was used. Within-group comparisons of oral and intravenous profiles were made using a mixed-model ANOVA for repeated measures (SAS/STAT Proc Mixed, version 8.2; SAS Institute, Cary, NC). Differences between the groups, with

TABLE 2
Integrated β-cell secretory responses (insulin, C-peptide, and ISR) to oral glucose (50 g in 400 ml H_2O) and adjustable (isoglycemic) intravenous glucose infusion (20% wt/vol), and calculated incretin effects (percent of the β-cell secretory response after oral glucose) in patients with chronic pancreatitis and secondary diabetes, patients with chronic pancreatitis and NGT, patients with type 2 diabetes, and healthy subjects

	Patients with chronic pancreatitis and secondary diabetes*	Patients with chronic pancreatitis and NGT†	Patients with type 2 diabetes‡	Healthy subjects§
n (F/M)	2/6	2/6	2/6	2/6
Integrated β-cell secretory responses				
Insulin (nmol/l per 4 h)				
Oral	8.8 ± 1.7§	10.9 ± 1.8	12.1 ± 2.3	18.4 ± 3.1†
Intravenous	5.5 ± 1.3	3.0 ± 0.7	6.8 ± 1.8	5.2 ± 1.7
Oral-intravenous	3.4 ± 1.0†§¶	7.8 ± 1.5*¶	5.3 ± 1.6§¶	13.1 ± 3.0*‡¶
C-peptide (nmol/l per 4 h				
Oral	127 ± 20	186 ± 37	154 ± 28	186 ± 21
Intravenous	87 ± 13	62 ± 14	96 ± 14	88 ± 11
Oral-intravenous	40 ± 11*†§	124 ± 29*‡¶	58 ± 18†¶	98 ± 20*¶
ISR (nmol/l per kg)				
Oral	687 ± 110	698 ± 169	783 ± 127	649 ± 61
Intravenous	455 ± 61†	222 ± 53*‡	511 ± 114†	305 ± 39
Oral-intravenous	166 ± 63*†§	476 ± 135*‡	272 ± 68¶	345 ± 55*¶
Relative incretin effects (%)				
Insulin	36 ± 7†	68 ± 7*‡	44 ± 9†	73 ± 6*‡
C-peptide	26 ± 7†	67 ± 6*‡	31 ± 9†	52 ± 7*‡
ISR	31 ± 5†	68 ± 6*‡	34 ± 7†	53 ± 5*‡
Average	31 ± 4†	68 ± 3*‡	36 ± 6†	60 ± 4*‡

Data are means ± SE. Significant differences ($P < 0.05$) between responses to oral glucose and isoglycemic intravenous glucose infusion within each group (¶) and significant differences ($P < 0.05$) in integrated β-cell secretory responses and incretin effects, respectively, between the four groups are indicated. *Compared with patients with chronic pancreatitis and secondary diabetes. †Compared with patients with chronic pancreatitis and NGT. ‡Compared with patients with type 2 diabetes. §Compared with healthy subjects.

respect to incretin effects, were calculated using a one-way ANOVA with post hoc analysis. $P < 0.05$ was considered to be statistically significant.

RESULTS
Glucose. No significant differences in FPG between days 1 and 2 were observed in any of the four groups. No significant differences between FPG in the two diabetic groups or between the two glucose-tolerant groups were evident, whereas mean FPG in both diabetic groups were higher ($P < 0.0001$) than the corresponding values in both glucose-tolerant groups. As illustrated in Fig. 1 the PG responses to oral glucose displayed the characteristic differences between normal glucose-tolerant subjects and diabetic subjects. The oral glucose curves were mimicked during the adjustable intravenous glucose infusions (with no significant differences between the two glucose curves in any of the groups) using glucose infusion rates as illustrated in Fig. 2.
Insulin, C-peptide ISR, incretin effect, and HOMA. There were no significant differences between fasting values on days 1 and 2 for plasma insulin or C-peptide in any of the four groups, and no differences between the groups were observed. Significant differences in the dynamic time courses for insulin, C-peptide, and ISR (Fig. 1), respectively, between day 1 and day 2 were observed in all groups ($P < 0.0014$). As shown in Table 2, integrated β-cell secretory responses (incremental AUC values for insulin, C-peptide, and ISR, respectively) were greater in all four groups during the OGTT compared with isoglycemic intravenous infusion ($P < 0.05$). Significant differences in integrated β-cell secretory responses (and in integrated responses to oral − integrated responses to intravenous glucose) between the groups are indicated in Table 2. Incretin effects calculated from the three integrated β-cell

secretory responses are shown in Table 2. As indicated, no differences in incretin effects between the two groups of diabetic patients or between the two groups of glucose-tolerant subjects were observed, whereas each value for the individual diabetic group differed significantly from the corresponding value of each glucose-tolerant group ($P < 0.05$). No differences in HOMA-IR were observed between days 1 and 2 in any of the four groups.
GLP-1. Time courses for total and intact GLP-1 are shown in Fig. 3. No significant differences in basal values between days 1 and 2 were observed in any of the four groups. Basal levels in the chronic pancreatitis plus diabetes group and in the type 2 diabetes group were significantly higher compared with the control group. In all groups significant increases in both total and intact forms were observed after the OGTT. During the isoglycemic intravenous glucose infusion, no significant responses occurred in any of the groups. The AUC for total GLP-1 was significantly bigger during the OGTT compared with the isoglycemic intravenous infusion in all four groups, but with respect to the AUC for intact GLP-1, significant differences were only observed for the chronic pancreatitis plus diabetes group and the control group (Table 3). No differences in AUC between the four groups were observed.
GIP. Time courses for total and intact GIP are shown in Fig. 3. No significant differences in basal values between days 1 and 2 were observed in any of the four groups. In all groups significant increases in both total and intact forms were observed after the OGTT. During the isoglycemic intravenous glucose infusion, no significant responses occurred in any of the groups. The AUCs for total and intact GIP were significantly larger during the OGTT compared with isoglycemic intravenous infusion in all four groups (Table 3). Patients with chronic

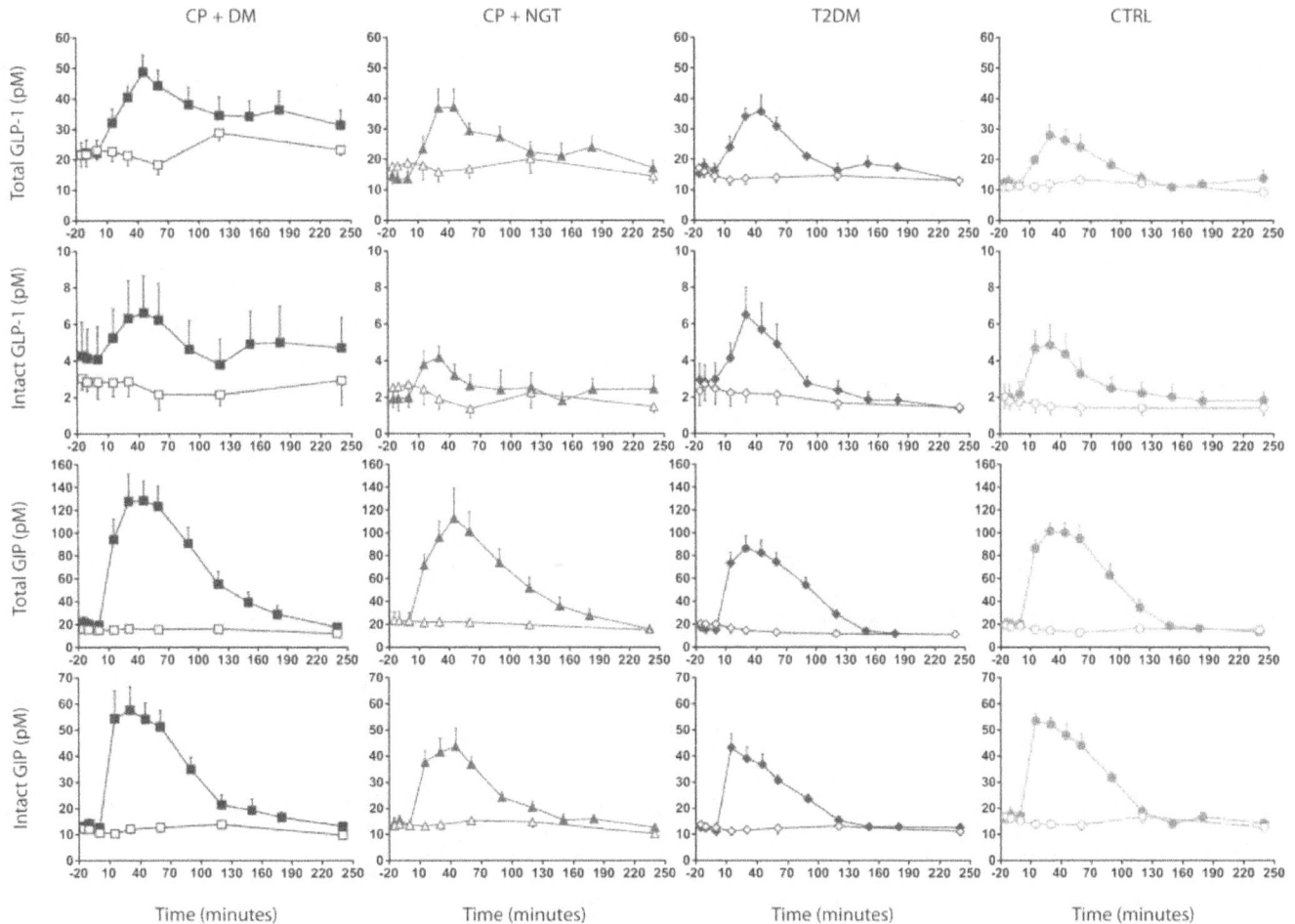

FIG. 3. Total GLP-1, intact GLP-1, total GIP, and intact GIP in patients with chronic pancreatitis and NGT (triangles), patients with chronic pancreatitis and secondary diabetes (squares), healthy subjects (circles), and patients with type 2 diabetes (diamonds) after 50-g OGTT (filled symbols), and isoglycemic intravenous glucose infusion (open symbols), respectively. *Significant differences ($P < 0.05$) between the individual OGTT and isoglycemic intravenous glucose infusion curves (repeated-measures ANOVA). CP, chronic pancreatitis; CTRL, control; T2DM, type 2 diabetes.

pancreatitis plus diabetes displayed significantly larger responses during OGTT compared with the other groups. Otherwise, no differences between the groups were observed.

Glucagon. Time courses for plasma glucagon are presented in Fig. 4. Similar basal values on the two experimental days were observed in all of the four groups ($P =$ NS). As expected, patients with type 2 diabetes exhibited significantly higher basal levels compared with the control group (9.5 ± 0.9 vs. 7.6 ± 0.6 pmol/l, $P = 0.01$). Otherwise no significant differences between the groups were observed. In the control group equal suppression of plasma glucagon concentrations was observed on both experimental days with similar nadirs of 5.4 ± 0.4 and 5.3 ± 0.5 pmol/l. As illustrated in Fig. 4, decremental AUC values during the 1st hour of the two experimental days in the control group amounted to -67 ± 19 and -92 ± 28 pmol/l per 1 h, respectively ($P =$ NS). In the remaining three groups (chronic pancreatitis plus diabetes, chronic pancreatitis plus NGT, and type 2 diabetes), complete lack of suppression of plasma glucagon was observed during the initial 60 min after the OGTT (23 ± 34, -13 ± 30, and -3 ± 18 pmol/l per 1 h; $P =$ NS), but normal suppression was observed during the isoglycemic intravenous glucose

infusion (-43 ± 22, -88 ± 26, and -75 ± 22 pmol/l per 1 h; $P =$ NS) compared with the control group (Fig. 4).

DISCUSSION

With the current study, we confirm the observation made by Nauck et al. (3) in 1986 that the incretin effect is reduced in patients with type 2 diabetes, and we conclude that this deficiency is most likely a consequence of the diabetic state and not a primary pathogenic trait leading to type 2 diabetes.

Until now, the incretin defect in patients with type 2 diabetes has been considered a possible candidate for a primary deficiency in type 2 diabetes. However, Nauck et al. (28) estimated the incretin effect in first-degree relatives of patients with type 2 diabetes and found it to be similar to that of matched healthy subjects, suggesting the deficiency to be a consequence of the diabetic state. In support of this, the incretin effect has been found to be reduced in individuals with type 1 diabetes (positive ICA) and normal fasting glucose levels (29). Recently, the incretin effect was shown to be affected in subjects who had impaired glucose tolerance and who were therefore at high risk for developing type 2 diabetes (30). This obser-

TABLE 3
Integrated incretin hormone responses (total and intact GLP-1 and total and intact GIP) to oral glucose (50 g in 400 ml H_2O) and adjustable (isoglycemic) intravenous glucose infusion (20% wt/vol) in patients with chronic pancreatitis and secondary diabetes, patients with chronic pancreatitis and NGT, patients with type 2 diabetes, and healthy subjects

Integrated incretin hormone responses	Patients with chronic pancreatitis and diabetes	Patients with chronic pancreatitis and NGT	Patients with type 2 diabetes	Healthy subjects
n (F/M)	8/6	8/6	8/6	8/6
Total GLP-1 (nmol/l × 4 h)				
Oral	3.3 ± 0.4	2.6 ± 0.6	1.1 ± 0.5	1.0 ± 0.3
Intravenous	0.5 ± 0.4	−0.1 ± 1.0	−0.5 ± 0.1	0.1 ± 0.1
Oral-intravenous	3.0 ± 0.8*	2.7 ± 1.2*	1.6 ± 0.4*	0.9 ± 0.3*
Intact GLP-1 (pmol/l × 4 h)				
Oral	211 ± 138	161 ± 60	11 ± 130	138 ± 39
Intravenous	−103 ± 58	−176 ± 213	−167 ± 157	−98 ± 28
Oral-intravenous	314 ± 144*	336 ± 207	177 ± 129	235 ± 53*
Total GIP (nmol/l × 4 h)				
Oral	10.6 ± 2.0†	7.7 ± 2.3	5.4 ± 0.5‡	6.3 ± 1.1‡
Intravenous	−0.2 ± 0.3	−1.0 ± 0.5	−1.8 ± 0.7	−0.8 ± 0.3
Oral-intravenous	10.8 ± 2.0*	8.7 ± 2.1*	7.2 ± 0.8*	7.1 ± 1.0*
Intact GIP (pmol/l × 4 h)				
Oral	4.0 ± 0.7§	2.2 ± 0.5‡	2.2 ± 0.3‡	2.5 ± 0.5‡
Intravenous	0.1 ± 0.2	0.0 ± 0.3	−0.2 ± 0.3	−0.8 ± 0.5
Oral-intravenous	3.8 ± 0.7*	2.2 ± 0.5*	2.4 ± 0.3*	3.2 ± 0.3*

Data are means ± SE. Significant differences between incretin responses to oral glucose and isoglycemic intravenous glucose infusion within each group ($P < 0.05$) and significant differences in incretin responses between the four groups are indicated . *$P < 0.05$; †$P < 0.05$ compared with patients with type 2 diabetes and healthy subjects; ‡$P < 0.05$ compared with patients with chronic pancreatitis and diabetes; §$P < 0.05$ compared with patients with chronic pancreatitis and NGT, patients with type 2 diabetes, and healthy subjects.

vation could imply a primary role for the reduced incretin effect in type 2 diabetes, but on the other hand, the finding could also represent an early consequence of the chronic mild hyperglycemia of impaired glucose tolerance. Thus, no firm conclusion can be drawn from the existing literature.

Type 2 diabetes is characterized by a severely reduced insulinotropic effect of GIP, especially on the late-phase insulin response, compared with healthy control subjects. The effect of GIP has also been evaluated in first-degree relatives of patients with type 2 diabetes (31) and found to be reduced compared with healthy subjects, pointing toward an early, possibly genetic defect. On the other hand, we found a similar lack of GIP effect in patients with chronic pancreatitis and secondary diabetes (32), and Meier et al. (33) showed that the GIP effect was preserved in women who had a history of gestational diabetes and who were therefore at high risk of developing type 2 diabetes. It was therefore of interest to investigate whether patients with secondary diabetes exhibit a similar loss of incretin effect as patients with type 2 diabetes, which would indicate that the loss might be a secondary rather than a primary event in the pathogenesis of type 2 diabetes. Furthermore, we sought to investigate whether our recent finding that the regulation of α-cell secretion in patients with type 2 diabetes is different during an OGTT and isoglycemic intravenous glucose infusion (8) could be demonstrated in patients with chronic pancreatitis (with and without secondary diabetes).

Chronic pancreatitis is a chronic inflammatory condition in the pancreas that results in a progressive destruction of the pancreatic cells, with subsequent development of exocrine and endocrine pancreatic insufficiency (12). No good estimates for the time from diagnosis of chronic pancreatitis to the onset of secondary diabetes have been published, but in a large Danish cohort, one-third of the patients with chronic pancreatitis had NGT, one-third had impaired glucose tolerance or non–insulin-dependent dia-

betes, and one-third had insulin-dependent diabetes (11), in accordance with other published findings (34–36). These data suggest that the development of secondary glucose intolerance represents a continuum, worsening with the duration of chronic pancreatitis.

In the current study, the two groups of patients with chronic pancreatitis differed with respect to glucose tolerance, but they were very similar with regard to other chronic pancreatitis–related pathologies. All patients in the chronic pancreatitis plus diabetes group had relatively well-regulated glucose homeostasis on diet and/or oral antidiabetic drugs, suggesting the preservation of a substantial number of functional β-cells on which the incretin hormones could exert their actions. Therefore, a difference in incretin effect between the two groups of patients with chronic pancreatitis is most likely to be attributed to their different glycemic control. No matter how the incretin effect was calculated, a lower incretin effect was seen in patients with chronic pancreatitis plus diabetes (decreased to the level of patients with type 2 diabetes or even lower) compared with patients with chronic pancreatitis plus NGT, who exhibited an incretin effect similar to that of healthy subjects (Table 2). The abnormality is not likely to be explained by a decrease in β-cell mass. This notion is supported by the observation that the insulin and C-peptide responses to isoglycemic intravenous glucose challenges were similar in the four groups, indicating that all groups have a number of β-cells sufficient to respond equally to intravenous glucose. Furthermore, in a previous study, we found that insulin and C-peptide responses to a 15-mmol/l hyperglycemic clamp could be completely normalized in patients with type 2 diabetes (compared with matched healthy control subjects) after intravenous infusion of a supraphysiological amount of GLP-1 (7), and preliminary data from our group suggest that the same is true for patients with chronic pancreatitis and secondary diabetes compared with patients with chronic pancreatitis

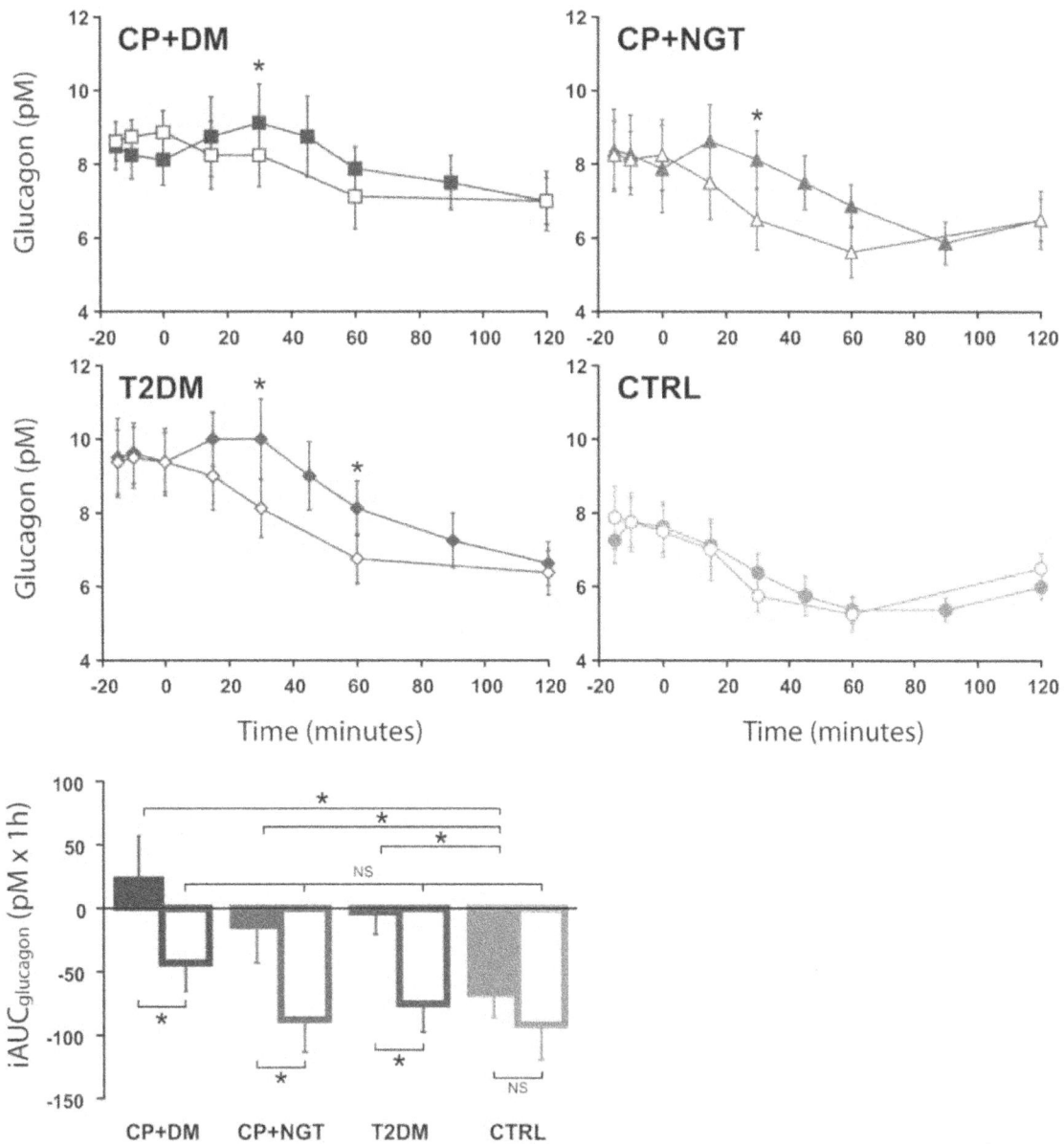

FIG. 4. Plasma glucagon in patients with chronic pancreatitis and NGT (triangles), patients with chronic pancreatitis and secondary diabetes (squares), healthy subjects (circles), and patients with type 2 diabetes (diamonds) after a 50-g OGTT (filled symbols) and isoglycemic intravenous glucose infusion (open symbols), respectively. Lower panel: Incremental AUC values for plasma glucagon ($iAUC_{glucagon}$) during the first hour of 50-g OGTT (filled bars) and isoglycemic intravenous glucose infusion (open bars), respectively, in the four groups. *Significant differences ($P < 0.05$). CP, chronic pancreatitis; CTRL, control; T2DM, type 2 diabetes.

and NGT (F.K.K., T.V., P.V.H., S.L., S.M., J.J.H., T.K., personal communication).

These observations suggest that patients with type 2 diabetes and patients with chronic pancreatitis and secondary diabetes do have a substantial residual β-cell secretory capacity that only needs the right stimulus to be recruited. Because the diabetes resulting from chronic pancreatitis is secondary, and therefore presumably nongenetic, we propose that the diabetic state results in a dysfunction of the β-cells, making them resistant to the insulinotropic effects of the incretin hormones. One might speculate whether it is possible to reestablish the incretin effect in patients with diabetes by near-normalization of PG for a longer period. That this notion might be feasible is supported by our recent finding that in patients with

type 2 diabetes, 4 weeks of strict glycemic control during insulin treatment improved β-cell responsiveness to GLP-1 (37).

To further evaluate mechanisms underlying the reduced incretin effect, we measured intact (indicators of the endocrine impact on the β-cells) and total (indicators of the overall levels of secretion) plasma concentrations of GIP and GLP-1, respectively, during both experimental days. Baseline levels of GLP-1 were found to be increased in diabetic patients (chronic pancreatitis plus diabetes group and type 2 diabetes group) compared with healthy control subjects (Fig. 3). This supports the notion of a feed-forward cycle where high PG enhances GLP-1 secretion (4,38). In all groups the responses (AUC) of the total forms were significantly higher during oral glucose compared with isoglycemic intravenous glucose infusion, as were the responses of intact GIP. Responses of intact GLP-1 were significantly greater during oral glucose compared with isoglycemic intravenous glucose only in the chronic pancreatitis plus diabetes group and in the control group. The corresponding differences in the remaining groups failed to reach statistical significance. The latter observation is probably attributable to the fact that because GLP-1 is subject to degradation by dipeptidyl peptidase IV almost immediately on its release (39), only 10–15% of intact GLP-1 actually reaches the systemic circulation (40), thereby reducing the possibility of detecting the response in the peripheral circulation. Interestingly, no differences in incretin hormone responses between the four groups could explain the different magnitude of the incretin effect in glucose-tolerant and -intolerant subjects, respectively. Therefore, studies investigating possible differences in the effects of the incretin hormones in patients with chronic pancreatitis plus NGT and chronic pancreatitis plus diabetes are warranted.

Finally, with regard to our recent results showing that the regulation of α-cell secretion in patients with type 2 diabetes is different during oral glucose and isoglycemic intravenous glucose infusion, we investigated whether this finding could be reproduced in patients with chronic pancreatitis and diabetes and therefore could be attributed to the diabetic state per se or whether it might be a primary event leading to type 2 diabetes. Interestingly, we observed that glucagon secretion was differentially regulated during oral glucose and isoglycemic intravenous glucose infusion, respectively, in patients with chronic pancreatitis and secondary diabetes and, to a lesser extent, in patients with chronic pancreatitis and NGT. This suggests that the inflammatory condition in the pancreas blunts the glucagon suppression during the OGTT independently of normal insulin secretion and normal glucose homeostasis. Thus, we suspect that (as indicated in studies of patients with acute pancreatitis) (41,42) the α-cells are very sensitive to inflammation (more sensitive than the β-cells) and that hyperglycemia worsens the ability of the α-cells to further suppress glucagon during the OGTT. However, the phenomenon that different glucagon responses are elicited by the OGTT and isoglycemic intravenous glucose infusion, respectively, in patients with type 2 diabetes and in those with chronic pancreatitis is currently unclear, and further studies are clearly needed to establish the underlying mechanisms.

In conclusion, the current study suggests that reduced incretin effect in type 2 diabetes is a consequence of the diabetic state rather than a primary event leading to type 2 diabetes.

ACKNOWLEDGMENTS

This study was supported by grants from the Danish Diabetes Association, Novo Nordisk, the Danish Medical Research Council, the Else and Svend Madsen's Foundation, and the Chief Physician Johan Boserup and Lise Boserup's Foundation.

We are grateful to our volunteers, whose availability made this work possible, and to Birgitte Bischoff, Nina Kjeldsen, Jytte Purtoft, Charlotte Rasmussen, Susanne Reimer, and Lone B. Thielsen for technical assistance.

REFERENCES

1. Holst JJ: On the physiology of GIP and GLP-1. *Horm Metab Res* 36:747–754, 2004
2. Dube PE, Brubaker PL: Nutrient, neural and endocrine control of glucagon-like peptide secretion. *Horm Metab Res* 36:755–760, 2004
3. Nauck M, Stockmann F, Ebert R, Creutzfeldt W: Reduced incretin effect in type 2 (non-insulin-dependent) diabetes. *Diabetologia* 29:46–52, 1986
4. Toft-Nielsen MB, Damholt MB, Madsbad S, Hilsted LM, Hughes TE, Michelsen BK, Holst JJ: Determinants of the impaired secretion of glucagon-like peptide-1 in type 2 diabetic patients. *J Clin Endocrinol Metab* 86:3717–3723, 2001
5. Vilsboll T, Krarup T, Deacon CF, Madsbad S, Holst JJ: Reduced postprandial concentrations of intact biologically active glucagon-like peptide 1 in type 2 diabetic patients. *Diabetes* 50:609–613, 2001
6. Kjems LL, Holst JJ, Volund A, Madsbad S: The influence of GLP-1 on glucose-stimulated insulin secretion: effects on beta-cell sensitivity in type 2 and nondiabetic subjects. *Diabetes* 52:380–386, 2003
7. Vilsboll T, Krarup T, Madsbad S, Holst JJ: Defective amplification of the late phase insulin response to glucose by GIP in obese type II diabetic patients. *Diabetologia* 45:1111–1119, 2002
8. Knop FK, Vilsboll T, Madsbad S, Krarup T, Holst JJ: Lack of suppression of glucagon during OGTT but not during isoglycemic IVGTT in patients with type 2 diabetes (Abstract). *Diabetes* 55 (Suppl. 1): 2006
9. Nyboe Andersen B, Krarup T, Thorsgaard Pedersen NT, Faber OK, Hagen C, Worning H: B cell function in patients with chronic pancreatitis and its relation to exocrine pancreatic function. *Diabetologia* 23:86–89, 1982
10. Domschke S, Stock KP, Pichl J, Schneider MU, Domschke W: Beta-cell reserve capacity in chronic pancreatitis. *Hepatogastroenterology* 32:27–30, 1985
11. Larsen S, Hilsted J, Tronier B, Worning H: Metabolic control and B cell function in patients with insulin-dependent diabetes mellitus secondary to chronic pancreatitis. *Metabolism* 36:964–967, 1987
12. Layer P, Yamamoto H, Kalthoff L, Clain JE, Bakken LJ, Dimagno EP: The different courses of early-onset and late-onset idiopathic and alcoholic chronic pancreatitis. *Gastroenterology* 107:1481–1487, 1994
13. The Expert Committee on the Diagnosis and Classification of Diabetes Mellitus: Report of the Expert Committee on the Diagnosis and Classification of Diabetes Mellitus. *Diabetes Care* 25 (Suppl. 1):S5–S20, 2002
14. Axon AT, Classen M, Cotton PB, Cremer M, Freeny PC, Lees WR: Pancreatography in chronic pancreatitis: international definitions. *Gut* 25:1107–1112, 1984
15. Orskov C, Rabenhoj L, Wettergren A, Kofod H, Holst JJ: Tissue and plasma concentrations of amidated and glycine-extended glucagon-like peptide I in humans. *Diabetes* 43:535–539, 1994
16. Vilsboll T, Krarup T, Sonne J, Madsbad S, Volund A, Juul AG, Holst JJ: Incretin secretion in relation to meal size and body weight in healthy subjects and people with type 1 and type 2 diabetes mellitus. *J Clin Endocrinol Metab* 88:2706–2713, 2003
17. Wilken M, Larsen FS, Buckley D, Holst JJ: New highly specific immunoassays for glucagon-like peptide-1 (GLP-1) (Abstract). *Diabetologia* 42 (Suppl. 1):A196 1999
18. Krarup T, Holst JJ: The heterogeneity of gastric inhibitory polypeptide in porcine and human gastrointestinal mucosa evaluated with five different antisera. *Regul Pept* 9:35–46, 1984
19. Krarup T, Madsbad S, Moody AJ, Regeur L, Faber OK, Holst JJ, Sestoft L: Diminished immunoreactive gastric inhibitory polypeptide response to a meal in newly diagnosed type I (insulin-dependent) diabetics. *J Clin Endocrinol Metab* 56:1306–1312, 1983
20. Deacon CF, Nauck MA, Meier J, Hucking K, Holst JJ: Degradation of endogenous and exogenous gastric inhibitory polypeptide in healthy and in type 2 diabetic subjects as revealed using a new assay for the intact peptide. *J Clin Endocrinol Metab* 85:3575–3581, 2000
21. Orskov C, Jeppesen J, Madsbad S, Holst JJ: Proglucagon products in plasma of noninsulin-dependent diabetics and nondiabetic controls in the fasting state and after oral glucose and intravenous arginine. *J Clin Invest* 87:415–423, 1991
22. Baldissera FGA, Holst JJ: Glucagon-related peptides in the human gastrointestinal mucosa. *Diabetologia* 26:223–228, 1984
23. Holst JJ, Pedersen JH, Baldissera F, Stadil F: Circulating glucagon after total pancreatectomy in man. *Diabetologia* 25:396–399, 1983
24. Kjems LL, Christiansen E, Volund A, Bergman RN, Madsbad S: Validation of methods for measurement of insulin secretion in humans in vivo. *Diabetes* 49:580–588, 2000
25. Kjems LL, Volund A, Madsbad S: Quantification of beta-cell function during IVGTT in Type II and non-diabetic subjects: assessment of insulin secretion by mathematical methods. *Diabetologia* 44:1339–1348, 2001

26. Van Cauter E, Mestrez F, Sturis J, Polonsky KS: Estimation of insulin secretion rates from C-peptide levels: comparison of individual and standard kinetic parameters for C-peptide clearance. *Diabetes* 41:368–377, 1992

27. Matthews DR, Hosker JP, Rudenski AS, Naylor BA, Treacher DF, Turner RC: Homeostasis model assessment: insulin resistance and beta-cell function from fasting plasma glucose and insulin concentrations in man. *Diabetologia* 28:412–419, 1985

28. Nauck MA, El Ouaghlidi A, Gabrys B, Hucking K, Holst JJ, Deacon CF, Gallwitz B, Schmidt WE, Meier JJ: Secretion of incretin hormones (GIP and GLP-1) and incretin effect after oral glucose in first-degree relatives of patients with type 2 diabetes. *Regul Pept* 122:209–217, 2004

29. Greenbaum CJ, Prigeon RL, D'Alessio DA: Impaired beta-cell function, incretin effect, and glucagon suppression in patients with type 1 diabetes who have normal fasting glucose. *Diabetes* 51:951–957, 2002

30. Muscelli E, Mari A, Natali A, Astiarraga BD, Camastra S, Frascerra S, Holst JJ, Ferrannini E: Impact of incretin hormones on beta-cell function in subjects with normal or impaired glucose tolerance. *Am J Physiol Endocrinol Metab* 291:E1144–E1150, 2006

31. Meier J, Hucking K, Holst J, Deacon C, Schmiegel W, Nauck M: Reduced insulinotropic effect of gastric inhibitory polypeptide in first-degree relatives of patients with type 2 diabetes. *Diabetes* 50:2497–2504, 2001

32. Vilsboll T, Knop FK, Krarup T, Johansen A, Madsbad S, Larsen S, Hansen T, Pedersen O, Holst JJ: The pathophysiology of diabetes involves a defective amplification of the late-phase insulin response to glucose by glucose-dependent insulinotropic polypeptide-regardless of etiology and phenotype. *J Clin Endocrinol Metab* 88:4897–4903, 2003

33. Meier JJ, Gallwitz B, Askenas M, Vollmer K, Deacon CF, Holst JJ, Schmidt WE, Nauck MA: Secretion of incretin hormones and the insulinotropic effect of gastric inhibitory polypeptide in women with a history of gestational diabetes. *Diabetologia* 48:1872–1881, 2005

34. James O, Agnew JE, Bouchier IA: Chronic pancreatitis in England: changing picture? *Br Med J* 2:34–38, 1974

35. Lankisch PG, Otto J, Erkelenz I, Lembcke B: Pancreatic calcifications: no indicator of severe exocrine pancreatic insufficiency. *Gastroenterology* 90:617–621, 1986

36. Linde J, Nilsson LH, Barany FR: Diabetes and hypoglycemia in chronic pancreatitis. *Scand J Gastroenterol* 12:369–373, 1977

37. Hojberg PV, Zander M, Vilsboll T, Knop FK, Krarup T, Holst JJ, Madsbad S: Effect of 4 weeks of near-normalization of blood glucose on beta-cell sensitivity to glucose and GLP-1 in type 2 diabetic patients. *Diabetes* 54 (Suppl. 1):A362, 2005

38. Hansen L, Hartmann B, Mineo H, Holst JJ: Glucagon-like peptide-1 secretion is influenced by perfusate glucose concentration and by a feedback mechanism involving somatostatin in isolated perfused porcine ileum. *Regul Pept* 118:11–18, 2004

39. Hansen L, Deacon CF, Orskov C, Holst JJ: Glucagon-like peptide-1-(7–36)amide is transformed to glucagon-like peptide-1-(9–36)amide by dipeptidyl peptidase IV in the capillaries supplying the L cells of the porcine intestine. *Endocrinology* 140:5356–5363, 1999

40. Holst JJ, Deacon CF: Glucagon-like peptide-1 mediates the therapeutic actions of DPP-IV inhibitors. *Diabetologia* 48:612–615, 2005

41. Donowitz M, Hendler R, Spiro HM, Binder HJ, Felig P: Glucagon secretion in acute and chronic pancreatitis. *Ann Intern Med* 83:778–781, 1975

42. Solomon SS, Duckworth WC, Jallepalli P, Bobal MA, Iyer R: The glucose intolerance of acute pancreatitis: hormonal response to arginine. *Diabetes* 29:22–26, 1980

Insulin Action in the Double Incretin Receptor Knockout Mouse

Julio E. Ayala,[1] Deanna P. Bracy,[1] Tanya Hansotia,[2] Grace Flock,[2] Yutaka Seino,[3] David H. Wasserman,[1] and Daniel J. Drucker[2]

OBJECTIVE—The incretins glucagon-like peptide 1 and glucose-dependent insulinotropic polypeptide have been postulated to play a role in regulating insulin action, although the mechanisms behind this relationship remain obscure. We used the hyperinsulinemic-euglycemic clamp to determine sites where insulin action may be modulated in double incretin receptor knockout (DIRKO) mice, which lack endogenous incretin action.

RESEARCH DESIGN AND METHODS—DIRKO and wild-type mice were fed regular chow or high-fat diet for 4 months. Clamps were performed on 5-h–fasted, conscious, unrestrained mice using an arterial catheter for sampling.

RESULTS—Compared with wild-type mice, chow and high fat–fed DIRKO mice exhibited decreased fat and muscle mass associated with increased energy expenditure and ambulatory activity. Clamp rates of glucose infusion (GIR), endogenous glucose production (endoR$_a$), and disappearance (R_d) were not different in chow-fed wild-type and DIRKO mice, although insulin levels were lower in DIRKO mice. Liver Akt expression was decreased but Akt activation was increased in chow-fed DIRKO compared with wild-type mice. High-fat feeding resulted in fasting hyperinsulinemia and hyperglycemia in wild-type but not in DIRKO mice. GIR, suppression of endoR$_a$, and stimulation of R_d were inhibited in high fat–fed wild-type mice but not in DIRKO mice. High-fat feeding resulted in impaired tissue glucose uptake (R_g) in skeletal muscle of wild-type mice but not of DIRKO mice. Liver and muscle Akt activation was enhanced in high fat–fed DIRKO compared with wild-type mice.

CONCLUSIONS—In summary, DIRKO mice exhibit enhanced insulin action compared with wild-type mice when fed a regular chow diet and are protected from high-fat diet–induced obesity and insulin resistance. *Diabetes* **57:288–297, 2008**

From the [1]Department of Molecular Physiology and Biophysics and National Institutes of Health Mouse Metabolic Phenotyping Center, Vanderbilt University School of Medicine, Nashville, Tennessee; the [2]Banting and Best Diabetes Centre, Departments of Medicine and Laboratory Medicine and Pathobiology, Samuel Lunenfeld Research Institute, Mount Sinai Hospital, University of Toronto, Toronto, Ontario, Canada; and the [3]Kansai Electric Power Hospital, Osaka, Japan.

Address correspondence and reprint requests to Julio E. Ayala, PhD, Vanderbilt University Medical Center, 2200 Pierce Ave., 702 Light Hall, Nashville, TN 37232. E-mail: julio.ayala@vanderbilt.edu.

Received for publication 25 May 2007 and accepted in revised form 26 October 2007.

Published ahead of print at http://diabetes.diabetesjournals.org on 31 October 2007. DOI: 10.2337/db07-0704.

2[14C]DG, 2[14C]deoxyglucose; 2[14C]DGP, 2[14C]deoxyglucose-6-phosphate; DIRKO, double incretin receptor knockout; endoR$_a$, endogenous glucose production; GAPDH, glyceraldehyde-3-phosphate dehydrogenase; GIP, glucose-dependent insulinotropic polypeptide; GIPR, G-protein–coupled receptor for GIP; GIR, glucose infusion rate; GLP-1, glucagon-like peptide 1; GLP-1R, G-protein–coupled receptor for GLP-1; LBM, lean body mass; NEFA, nonesterified fatty acid; RER, respiratory exchange ratio; SVL, superficial vastus lateralis.

After ingestion of a meal, multiple hormones are secreted from specialized enteroendocrine cells in the gut epithelium that coordinate events necessary for proper absorption and storage of nutrients. One such event is the control of glucose excursions and maintenance of glucose homeostasis after nutrient ingestion. Two gut-derived incretin hormones, glucose-dependent insulinotropic polypeptide (GIP) and glucagon-like peptide-1 (GLP-1), play a significant role in this process by enhancing insulin secretion from pancreatic β-cells in response to oral nutrient intake (1,2). This incretin effect is mediated via activation of distinct G-protein–coupled receptors for GIP (GIPR) and GLP-1 (GLP-1R) in β-cells, which initiates signaling cascades necessary for glucose-dependent insulin secretion (1).

GIP and GLP-1 also regulate glucose homeostasis via actions independent of insulin secretion. Activation of the incretin receptors stimulate pathways that enhance β-cell proliferation and inhibit β-cell apoptosis (3–7). GLP-1 inhibits glucagon secretion from pancreatic α-cells and delays gastric emptying, thus preventing large excursions in blood glucose levels (8–10). GLP-1 may also exert control on hepatic glucose production and peripheral glucose clearance independent of its effects on insulin secretion (11,12). GIP has been shown to stimulate insulin-mediated glucose uptake and lipoprotein lipase activity in cultured adipocytes (13).

Mice lacking either GIPR or GLP-1R exhibit only mild glucose intolerance due to impaired glucose-stimulated insulin secretion (14–19). The absence of a more severe phenotype is likely due to compensatory increases in the circulating levels of and/or sensitivity to the remaining incretin hormone. For example, disruption of GLP-1R results in increased circulating levels of and enhanced sensitivity to GIP (20). Similarly, although GLP-1 levels do not increase in mice lacking GIPR, these mice exhibit enhanced sensitivity to GLP-1 action (21).

To understand the consequences of complete loss of incretin receptor signaling, double incretin receptor knockout (DIRKO) mice have been generated. Despite a complete absence of endogenous GIP and GLP-1 action, DIRKO mice exhibit only moderate glucose intolerance compared with single incretin receptor knockout mice (22,23). Despite the metabolic stress imposed by chronic high-fat feeding, DIRKO mice chronically fed a high-fat diet exhibit only a modest deterioration in glucose tolerance, together with resistance to diet-induced obesity and increased energy expenditure and locomotor activity (24). The aims of the present studies are *1*) to assess the effects of a complete disruption of incretin signaling on insulin action in regular chow-fed mice and *2*) to determine whether the lack of incretin signaling impairs the normal compensatory mechanisms arising in high fat–fed mice. These aims were addressed using the hyperinsulinemic-euglycemic clamp, a technique that allows for the assessment of insulin action in conscious, unrestrained mice.

RESEARCH DESIGN AND METHODS

Mouse maintenance and genotyping. All procedures were approved by the Vanderbilt Animal Care and Use Committee. DIRKO mice on a CD1 background were backcrossed onto a C57BL/6 background (at least 10 generations) and bred to C57BL/6 mice (The Jackson Laboratories) to obtain double incretin receptor heterozygous founder mice. A heterozygous breeding pair was then used to generate wild-type and DIRKO breeding pairs, such that all subsequent wild-type and DIRKO mice used in these studies originated from the same heterozygous founder breeding pair. Littermates were weaned and separated by sex at 3 weeks of age. Genotyping was done by PCR of genomic DNA obtained from a tail biopsy. All mice were fed either regular chow (Purina 5001; Purina Mills) or high-fat diet (F-3282; Bio-Serv) ad libitum, were handled at least once per week, and were studied at ~4 months of age. Regular chow diet contains 12.1% calories from fat, whereas high-fat diet contains 59.4% calories from fat.

Assessment of body composition, feeding, and energy expenditure. Body composition was determined at ~4 months of age using an mq10 NMR analyzer (Bruker Optics). For food intake assessment, mice were placed in individual cages with measured amounts of food and bedding. The remaining food was weighed 48 h later, excluding fecal matter and bedding. Oxygen consumption (Vo_2) and carbon dioxide production (Vco_2) were measured using an Oxymax indirect calorimetry system (Columbus Instruments) as described previously (25). Energy expenditure was calculated as described previously (25,26). Respiratory exchange ratio (RER) was calculated as Vco_2/Vo_2. Ambulatory activity was estimated by the number of infrared beams broken in both X and Y directions.

Assessment of fat absorption. After 8 weeks of high-fat feeding, 20-week-old male wild-type and DIRKO mice ($n = 5$/group) were placed in individual cages with no bedding and provided with a preweighed amount of high-fat food. Every 24 h for 3 days, cages were changed, food was weighed, and total feces were collected. On completion of the collection phase, feces were completely dried to constant weight using a speed-vac at 60°C for 1 h. The mass of excreted feces was measured, and fat extraction was conducted on equal amounts of feces for both groups following the Nelson and O'Hopp method (27) with minor modifications. Briefly, feces were rigorously mixed in 1 volume of chloroform:methanol (1:2) and 2 volumes of 5 N HCl and incubated overnight in the dark at room temperature. After centrifugation for 30 min at 4,000 rpm, the organic phase was collected into preweighed tubes. The chloroform was evaporated, and tubes were reweighed to calculate fecal fat content.

Hyperinsulinemic-euglycemic clamps. Mice were catheterized at least 5 days before experimentation as described previously (28). Hyperinsulinemic-euglycemic clamps were performed on 5-h–fasted mice (28). A 5-µCi bolus of [3-³H]glucose was given at $t = -90$ min before insulin infusion, followed by a 0.05 µCi/min infusion for 90 min. Blood samples were obtained via an arterial catheter (28). Basal glucose specific activity was determined from blood samples at $t = -15$ and -5 min. Fasting insulin levels were determined from blood samples taken at $t = -5$ min. The clamp was begun at $t = 0$ min with a continuous infusion of human insulin (4 mU · kg⁻¹ · min⁻¹, Humulin R; Eli Lilly). The [3-³H]glucose infusion was increased to 0.2 µCi/min for the remainder of the experiment. Euglycemia (~150–160 mg/dl) was maintained by measuring blood glucose every 10 min starting at $t = 0$ min and infusing 50% dextrose as necessary. Mice received saline-washed erythrocytes from donors throughout the clamp (5–6 µl/min) to prevent a fall of >5% hematocrit. A 12-µCi bolus of 2[¹⁴C]deoxyglucose (2[¹⁴C]DG) was given at $t = 78$ min. Blood samples (80–240 µl) were taken every 10 min from $t = 80$ to 120 min and processed to determine plasma [3-³H]glucose and 2[¹⁴C]DG. Clamp insulin

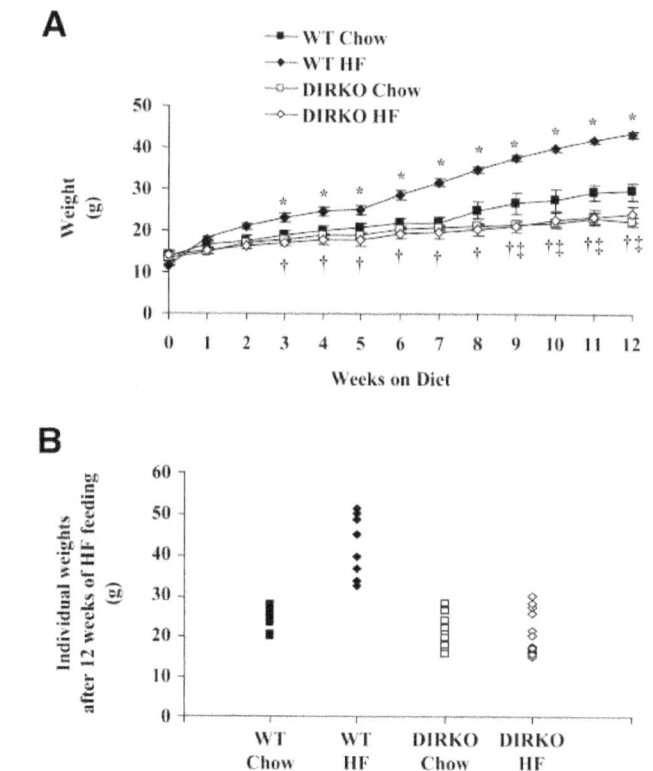

FIG. 1. Weight gain in chow-fed and high fat–fed C57BL/6 (wild-type) and DIRKO mice. Chow-fed wild type (■), high fat–fed wild type (♦), chow-fed DIRKO (□), high-fat-fed DIRKO (◇). A: Growth curve during the 12-week feeding period. B: Individual weights at the end of the 12-week feeding period. Data are mean ± SE for 8–15 mice/group. *P < 0.05 vs. chow; †P < 0.05 DIRKO high fat vs. wild-type high fat; ‡P < 0.05 DIRKO chow vs. wild-type chow.

was determined at $t = 100$ and 120 min. At $t = 120$ min, mice were anesthetized with sodium pentobarbital. The soleus, gastrocnemius, superficial vastus lateralis (SVL), liver, diaphragm, heart, and brain were excised, immediately frozen, and stored at -80°C until analyzed.

Processing of plasma and muscle samples. Insulin levels were determined by ELISA (Linco). Nonesterified fatty acids (NEFAs) were measured spectrophotometrically by an enzymatic colorimetric assay (Wako NEFA HR2 kit; Wako Chemicals). After deproteinization with barium hydroxide [Ba(OH)₂, 0.3 N] and zinc sulfate [ZnSO₄, 0.3 N], plasma [3-³H]glucose and 2[¹⁴C]DG radioactivity was determined by liquid scintillation counting (Packard TRI-CARB 2900TR) with Ultima Gold (Packard) as scintillant. Muscle samples were weighed and homogenized in 0.5% perchloric acid. Homogenates were centrifuged and neutralized with KOH. One aliquot was counted directly to determine 2[¹⁴C]DG and 2[¹⁴C]DG-6-phosphate (2[¹⁴C]DGP) radioactivity. A second aliquot was treated with Ba(OH)₂ and ZnSO₄ to remove 2[¹⁴C]DGP and any tracer incorporated into glycogen and then counted to determine 2[¹⁴C]DG radioactivity. 2[¹⁴C]DGP is the difference between the two aliquots. In all experiments, the accumulation of 2[¹⁴C]DGP was normalized to tissue weight.

Isolation of whole-cell extracts and immunoblotting. Liver and muscle (gastrocnemius) tissue (20–40 mg) was homogenized in 10 µl/mg tissue extraction buffer (50 mmol/l Tris, 1 mmol/l EDTA, 1 mmol/l EGTA, 10% glycerol, and 1% Triton-X 100, pH 7.5) supplemented with protease (Pierce)

TABLE 1
Body composition in chow-fed and high fat–fed C57BL/6 (wild-type) and DIRKO mice

	Wild-type chow fed	Wild-type high-fat fed	DIRKO chow fed	DIRKO high-fat fed
n (males/females)	12 (6/6)	8 (5/3)	13 (6/7)	15 (9/6)
Weight (g)	23.6 ± 0.8	41.9 ± 2.7*	21.1 ± 1.0†	22.1 ± 1.3†
Fat (g)	2.0 ± 0.1	14.2 ± 2.1	2.1 ± 0.1	3.8 ± 0.7
Muscle (g)	18.2 ± 0.6	24.5 ± 1.0	16.2 ± 0.8†	15.9 ± 0.6

Data are means ± SE. *P < 0.05 vs. chow; †P < 0.05 vs. wild type.

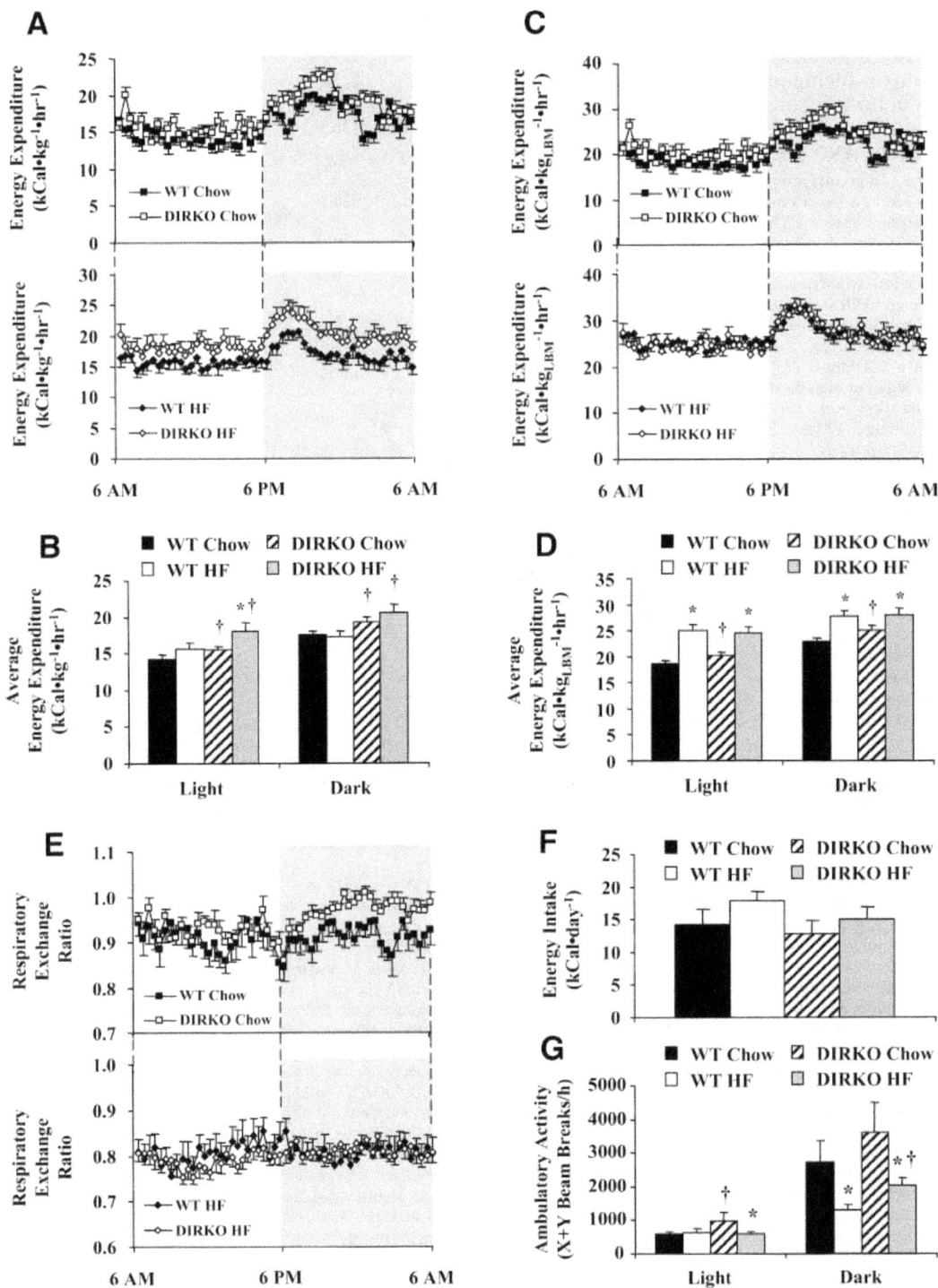

FIG. 2. Energy expenditure and intake measurements in chow-fed and high fat–fed C57BL/6 (wild-type) and DIRKO mice. Black squares and black bars, chow-fed wild type; black diamonds and white bars, high fat–fed wild type; white squares and striped bars, chow-fed DIRKO; white diamonds and gray bars, high fat–fed DIRKO. *A*: Energy expenditure normalized to total body weight. *B*: Average energy expenditure normalized to total body weight. *C*: Energy expenditure normalized to total LBM. *D*: Average energy expenditure normalized to LBM. *E*: RER. *F*: Average energy intake. *G*: Average ambulatory activity estimated as X+Y beam breaks over a 24-h period. Data are means ± SE for 6–15 mice/group. *$P < 0.05$ vs. chow; †$P < 0.05$ vs. wild type.

and phosphatase (Sigma) inhibitor cocktails. Homogenates were centrifuged (20 min, 4,500*g*, 4°C), pellets were discarded, and supernatants were retained for protein determination. Protein content was determined using a BCA protein assay kit (Bio-Rad). Whole-cell (20-μg) extracts were separated on 10% Bis-Tris SDS-PAGE gels (Invitrogen), followed by electrophoretic transfer to polyvinylidine fluoride membranes. Primary antibodies were

incubated with the membranes overnight at 4°C. Secondary antibodies were incubated at room temperature for 1 h. Imaging and densitometry were performed using the Odyssey imaging system (Li-Cor). Rabbit anti-Akt (1:1,000) and anti-phospho(Ser473)-Akt (1:1,000) were from Cell Signaling. Mouse anti-glyceraldehyde-3-phosphate dehydrogenase (anti-GAPDH) (1:2,000) was from Abcam.

A

□ WT HF
■ DIRKO HF

B

□ WT HF
■ DIRKO HF

C

□ WT HF
■ DIRKO HF

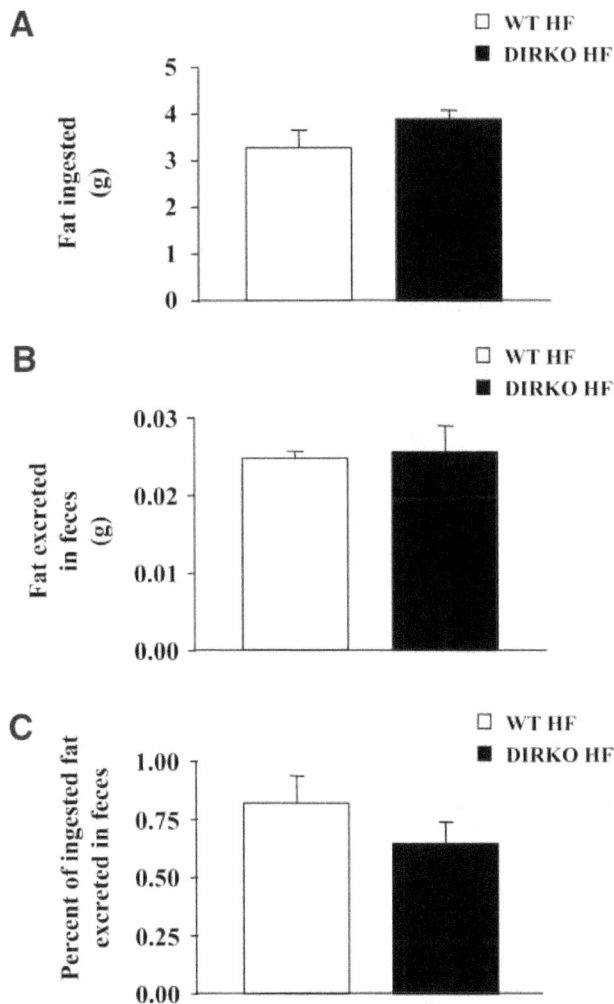

FIG. 3. Ingestion and fecal excretion of fat in high fat–fed C57BL/6 (wild-type) and DIRKO mice. □, high fat–fed wild type; ▤, high fat–fed DIRKO. A: Total fat ingested over a 72-h period. B: Total fat excreted in feces over a 72-h period. C: Percent of total fat ingested excreted in feces over a 72-h period. Data are means ± SE for five mice/group.

Calculations. Glucose appearance (R_a) and disappearance (R_d) were determined using Steele nonsteady-state equations (29). Endogenous glucose production (endoR$_a$) was determined by subtracting the glucose infusion rate (GIR) from total R_a. Glucose metabolic index (R_g) was calculated as previously described (25,30,31). R_g for all tissues was normalized to brain R_g.

Statistical analysis. Data are presented as means ± SE. Differences between groups were determined by two-way ANOVA followed by Tukey's post hoc tests or by one-tailed t test as appropriate. The significance level was $P < 0.05$.

RESULTS

DIRKO mice exhibit decreased weight gain and fat mass due to increased energy expenditure and activity. DIRKO mice on a C57BL/6 background and wild-type mice were placed on a regular chow or a high-fat diet for 12 weeks beginning at 3 weeks of age. DIRKO mice had decreased weight gain associated with reduced muscle mass compared with wild-type mice on a chow diet (Fig. 1; Table 1). High-fat feeding resulted in increased weight gain in wild-type mice (Fig. 1) associated with increased fat and muscle mass (Table 1). In contrast, high-fat feeding did not affect weight gain in DIRKO mice (Fig. 1) and resulted in only a small increase in fat mass (Table 1).

Energy expenditure normalized to total body weight

was increased in DIRKO mice compared with wild type on both chow and high-fat diets (Fig. 2A and B). DIRKO mice on high-fat diet also exhibited higher light-cycle energy expenditure than DIRKO mice on chow diet. When normalized to lean body mass, energy expenditure was increased in DIRKO mice compared with wild-type mice on chow but not on high-fat diet (Fig. 2D). RER was also not different between wild-type and DIRKO mice on either diet (Fig. 2E). Energy intake was not different between wild-type and DIRKO mice on either diet (Fig. 2F). Light-cycle ambulatory activity was increased in chow-fed, but not high fat–fed, DIRKO mice compared with wild-type mice (Fig. 2G). Conversely, dark-cycle ambulatory activity was higher in high fat–fed, but not chow-fed, DIRKO mice compared with wild-type mice (Fig. 2G). High-fat–fed DIRKO mice did not exhibit defective fat absorption, because fat intake and excretion were normal compared with high fat–fed wild-type mice (Fig. 3).

Chow- and high fat–fed DIRKO mice exhibit enhanced whole-body insulin action. Insulin action was assessed in chow-fed, conscious, unrestrained wild-type and DIRKO mice using the hyperinsulinemic (4 mU · kg^{-1} · min^{-1})-euglycemic clamp. Fasting (5-h fast) glucose and insulin levels were not different between wild-type and DIRKO mice (Fig. 4A, top panel; Table 2). Fasting NEFAs were lower in DIRKO mice (Table 2). Arterial glucose was clamped at similar levels in both groups (Fig. 4A, top panel). The GIR necessary to maintain euglycemia was not different between groups (Fig. 4A, bottom panel). However, clamp insulin levels were lower in DIRKO mice (Table 2). Thus, normalizing GIR to clamp insulin levels, an index of insulin sensitivity, shows enhanced insulin action in DIRKO mice (Table 2). Insulin-mediated suppression of endoR$_a$ and stimulation of R_d were not different between wild-type and DIRKO mice (Fig. 5), although insulin levels were lower in the latter. Clamp NEFAs were significantly lower in DIRKO mice (Table 2). The ability of insulin to suppress NEFAs was not different between wild-type and DIRKO mice, as shown by the change in NEFAs normalized to the change in insulin from fasting to clamp levels (Table 2).

Insulin action was also assessed in high fat–fed wild-type and DIRKO mice. Fasting glucose and insulin levels were markedly higher in high fat–fed wild-type than DIRKO mice (Fig. 4B, top panel; Table 2). Compared with chow-fed mice, fasting insulin and glucose levels were higher in high fat–fed wild-type mice, indicative of fasting insulin resistance. By contrast, high-fat feeding had no effect on fasting glucose in DIRKO mice but resulted in markedly lower fasting insulin levels (Table 2). As in chow-fed mice, fasting NEFAs were lower in high fat–fed DIRKO mice, even though fasting insulin levels were markedly lower in this group (Table 2). Arterial glucose was clamped at similar levels in both high fat–fed wild-type and DIRKO mice (Fig. 4B, top panel). The GIR necessary to maintain euglycemia was significantly lower in wild-type mice (Fig. 4B, bottom panel), even as clamp insulin levels were higher in this group (Table 2). Thus, normalizing GIR to clamp insulin levels shows high fat–fed DIRKO mice to have a more than threefold higher index of insulin sensitivity than wild-type mice (Table 2). Furthermore, DIRKO mice are protected from high-fat diet–induced insulin resistance, because high-fat feeding resulted in a more than threefold decrease in insulin sensitivity in wild-type mice, whereas insulin sensitivity was insignificantly decreased in DIRKO mice (Table 2).

A

B

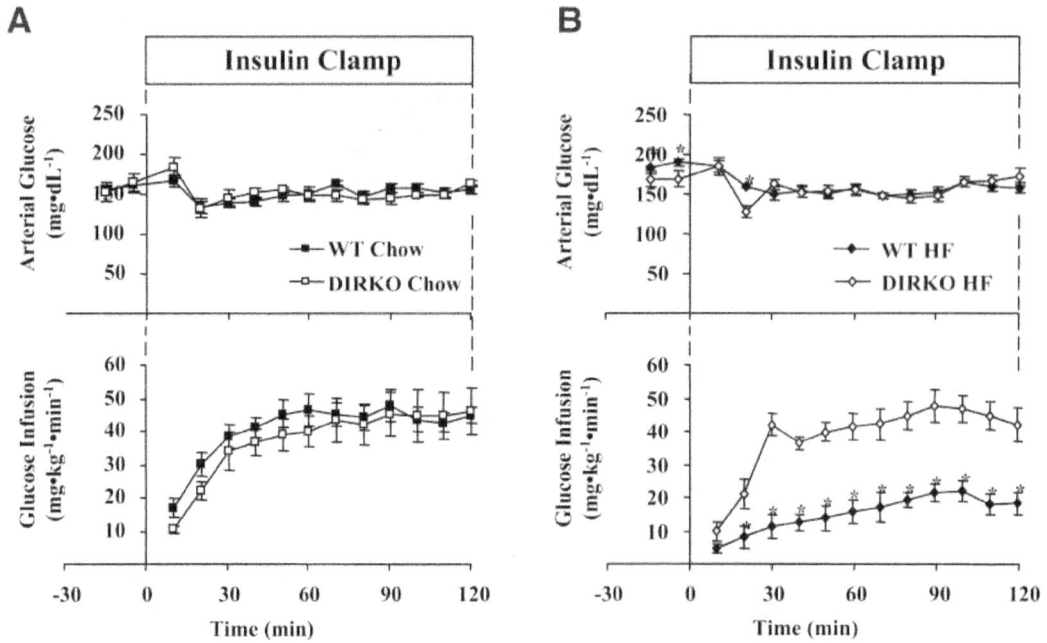

FIG. 4. Hyperinsulinemic-euglycemic clamps on 5-h–fasted, conscious, unrestrained chow-fed and high fat–fed C57BL/6 (wild-type) and DIRKO mice. *A*: Arterial glucose levels (*top panel*) and GIRs (*bottom panel*) during hyperinsulinemic-euglycemic clamps in chow-fed wild-type (■) and DIRKO (□) mice. *B*: Arterial glucose levels (*top panel*) and GIRs (*bottom panel*) during hyperinsulinemic-euglycemic clamps in high fat–fed wild-type (♦) and DIRKO (◇) mice. Data are means ± SE for 8–10 mice/group. *$P < 0.05$ vs. DIRKO.

Clamp NEFAs were also significantly lower in DIRKO mice (Table 2). As in chow-fed mice, suppression of NEFAs by insulin was not different between high fat–fed wild-type and DIRKO mice (Table 2).

Insulin-mediated suppression of endoR_a was not significantly different between high fat–fed wild-type and DIRKO mice, although insulin levels were drastically lower in the latter group (Fig. 5*A* and *B*). Compared with chow feeding, high-fat feeding resulted in impaired suppression of endoR_a in wild-type mice but not in DIRKO mice (Fig. 5*B*). Despite lower clamp insulin levels in DIRKO mice, stimulation of R_d was significantly higher in this group (Fig. 5*C* and *D*). Furthermore, whereas the stimulation of R_d was inhibited in high fat–fed wild-type mice, this inhibition did not occur in DIRKO mice.

Cardiac glucose uptake is enhanced in chow-fed DIRKO mice. A bolus of 2[^{14}C]DG was administered during the clamp to determine the glucose metabolism index (R_g), a measure of tissue glucose uptake. Absolute R_g in skeletal muscle was lower in chow-fed DIRKO mice compared with wild-type mice, as shown in gastrocnemius and SVL muscles (Fig. 6*A*). However, when normalized to clamp insulin levels, R_g in these muscles was not different between groups (Fig. 6*C*). Absolute R_g was not affected in oxidative muscles, such as soleus, diaphragm, and heart (Fig. 6*A* and *B*). When normalized to clamp insulin levels, R_g in the heart was increased in DIRKO compared with wild-type mice (Fig. 6*D*).

DIRKO mice are protected from high-fat diet–induced impairments in insulin-stimulated muscle glu-

TABLE 2
Fasting and clamp parameters in chow-fed and high fat–fed C57BL/6 (wild-type) and DIRKO mice

	Wild-type chow fed	Wild-type high-fat fed	DIRKO chow fed	DIRKO high-fat fed
n (males/females)	10 (6/4)	8 (4/4)	10 (5/5)	8 (4/4)
Glucose (mg/dl)				
Fasting	159 ± 5	185 ± 6*	159 ± 3	167 ± 6†
Clamp	154 ± 2	155 ± 3	150 ± 1	157 ± 5
Insulin (μU/ml)				
Fasting	42 ± 10	93 ± 22*	36 ± 7	16 ± 4*†
Clamp	85 ± 11	148 ± 25*	63 ± 4†	81 ± 8*†
NEFAs (mmol/l)				
Fasting	1.3 ± 0.1	1.4 ± 0.2	1.1 ± 0.1†	1.0 ± 0.1†
Clamp	0.6 ± 0.1	0.7 ± 0.1	0.4 ± 0.03†	0.5 ± 0.1†
GIR (mg · kg^{-1} · min^{-1})	45 ± 3	20 ± 7	45 ± 2	45 ± 4
Insulin sensitivity for glucose [mg · ml^{-1} · (kg · min^{-1} · mU^{-1})$^{-1}$]	546 ± 115	169 ± 79*	745 ± 79†	587 ± 92†
Insulin sensitivity for NEFA (Δmmol/l:ΔμU/ml)	1.7 ± 0.3	0.8 ± 0.3*	2.5 ± 0.4	0.8 ± 0.2*

Data are for 5-h–fasted, conscious, unrestrained mice at least 5 days after surgical catheterization. Data are means ± SE. *$P < 0.05$ vs. chow; †$P < 0.05$ vs. wild type.

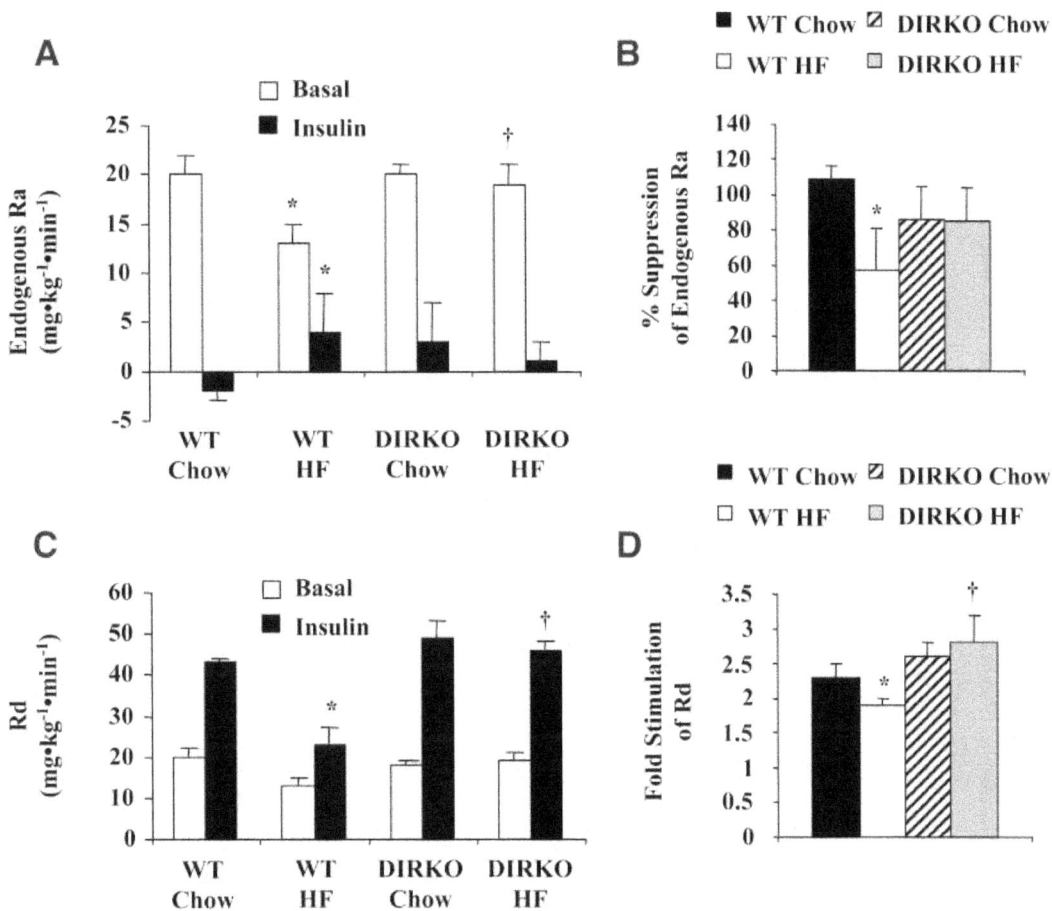

FIG. 5. Whole-body glucose turnover during hyperinsulinemic-euglycemic clamps on 5-h–fasted, conscious, unrestrained chow-fed and high fat–fed C57BL/6 (wild-type) and DIRKO mice. *A*: Basal and insulin-stimulated endoR_a. *B*: Insulin-mediated percent suppression of endoR_a. *C*: Basal and insulin-stimulated R_d. *D*: Insulin-mediated fold stimulation of R_d. *A* and *C*: Basal (white bars) and insulin (black bars). *B* and *D*: wild-type chow (black bars), wild-type high fat (white bars), DIRKO chow (striped bars), DIRKO high fat (gray bars). Data are means ± SE for 8–10 mice/group. *$P < 0.05$ vs. chow; †$P < 0.05$ vs. wild type.

cose uptake. Absolute R_g was significantly higher in all muscles analyzed from high fat–fed DIRKO compared with wild-type mice, except for soleus and gastrocnemius (Fig. 6*A* and *B*). However, when normalized to clamp insulin levels, R_g was higher in all muscles from high fat–fed DIRKO mice (Fig. 6*C* and *D*). The lack of incretin receptors also prevented the high-fat diet–induced decrease in muscle R_g observed in wild-type mice. High-fat feeding did result in decreased heart R_g normalized to clamp insulin levels in DIRKO mice, although not to the degree observed in wild-type mice (Fig. 6*D*).

DIRKO mice exhibit enhanced liver and muscle insulin signaling. To determine whether the enhanced insulin action in both chow- and high fat–fed DIRKO mice was associated with enhanced insulin signaling, Akt activation, defined as the ratio between phosphorylated (Ser473) Akt and total Akt, was assessed in liver and gastrocnemius muscle. Total gastrocnemius Akt protein levels were not different between wild-type and DIRKO mice on either chow or high-fat diets (Fig. 7*A* and *B*). Gastrocnemius Akt activation was significantly higher in DIRKO mice on high-fat diet but not on chow diet (Fig. 7*C*). Total liver Akt protein was significantly lower in DIRKO mice on chow or high-fat diet compared with wild-type mice (Fig. 7*D* and *E*). However, liver Akt activation was significantly en-

hanced in DIRKO mice fed either diet compared with their wild-type counterparts (Fig. 7*F*).

DISCUSSION

In the present studies, the hyperinsulinemic-euglycemic clamp was used to delineate specific sites where insulin action may be affected by deletion of the receptors for the incretin hormones GLP-1 and GIP. Furthermore, high-fat feeding for 12 weeks was used to precipitate phenotypes associated with the lack of incretin receptor signaling that would otherwise be silent in chow-fed mice. Compared with wild-type mice, DIRKO mice exhibit increased energy expenditure when fed either a chow or a high-fat diet due, at least in part, to increased locomotor activity. Consequently, chow-fed DIRKO mice have reduced weight gain due to decreased muscle mass. High-fat–fed DIRKO mice have reduced weight gain due to decreased fat mass compared with high fat–fed wild-type mice. Here, we show that DIRKO mice exhibit enhanced insulin sensitivity on either chow or high-fat diets. Chow-fed DIRKO mice have decreased insulin levels but demonstrate equal GIR, suppression of endoR_a, and stimulation of R_d during a hyperinsulinemic-euglycemic clamp. Moreover, DIRKO mice are protected from high-fat diet–induced insulin resistance as

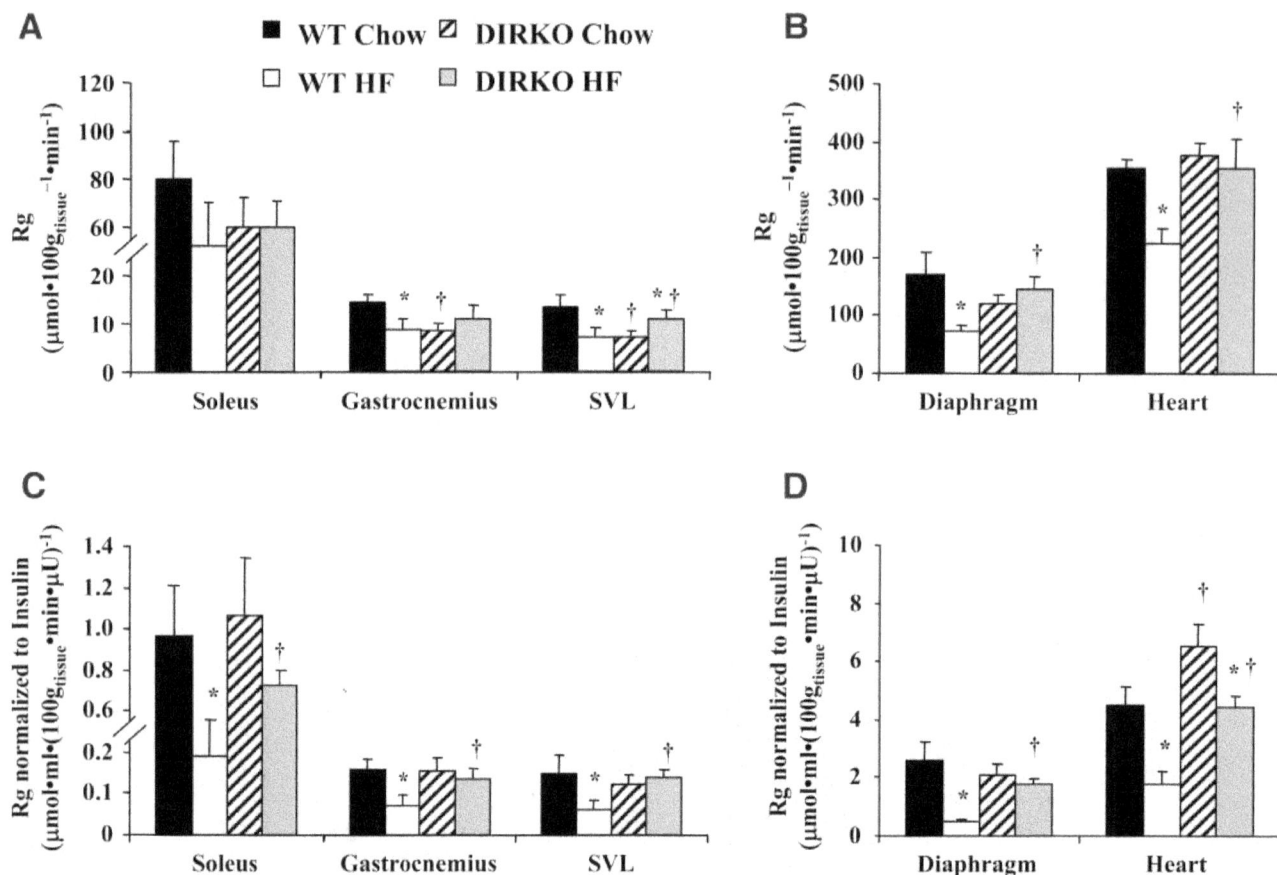

A ■ WT Chow ◪ DIRKO Chow   □ WT HF ▨ DIRKO HF

FIG. 6. R_g after hyperinsulinemic-euglycemic clamps on 5-h–fasted, conscious, unrestrained chow-fed and high fat–fed C57BL/6 (wild-type) and DIRKO mice. Wild-type chow (black bars), wild-type high fat (white bars), DIRKO chow (striped bars), and DIRKO high fat (gray bars). A: R_g in soleus, gastrocnemius, and SVL. B: R_g in diaphragm and heart. C: R_g normalized to clamp insulin levels in soleus, gastrocnemius, and SVL. D: R_g normalized to clamp insulin levels in diaphragm and heart. Data are means ± SE for 8–10 mice/group. *$P < 0.05$ vs. chow; †$P < 0.05$ vs. wild type.

shown by lower fasting glycemia and insulinemia, higher GIR, and suppression of endoR_a, R_d, and R_g during a clamp than high fat–fed wild-type mice. This effect on insulin action was associated with enhanced insulin signaling at both the liver and muscle. Thus, these results demonstrate a role for incretin receptor signaling in the control of insulin action.

A recent study by Hansotia et al. (24) showed increased energy expenditure associated with increased *ucp-1* gene transcription and greater locomotor activity in both DIRKO mice and mice lacking GLP-1R. GLP-1R knockout mice have decreased weight gain on a high-fat diet, although this was only observed in female mice (18). GIPR knockout mice are also protected from high-fat diet–induced obesity due to increased fat oxidation and energy expenditure (13). This was also observed in a model of genetic obesity, the *ob/ob* mouse, crossed with GIPR knockout mice (13). In the present studies, increased energy expenditure in both chow- and high fat–fed DIRKO mice was associated with increased locomotor activity, but the lack of an effect on the RER suggests that fat oxidation was not increased in DIRKO mice. However, NEFA levels were lower in DIRKO mice on either chow or high-fat diets, even as insulin levels were also lower. Thus, an effect of disrupted incretin signaling on increased fat oxidation cannot be ruled out. Fat absorption was also not impaired in high fat–fed DIRKO mice, because the percent

of ingested fat excreted in the feces was not different compared with wild-type mice.

The results obtained from the present studies are interesting in that a mutation that impairs β-cell function also preserves insulin sensitivity. This is especially evident in the presence of a metabolic stressor, such as high-fat feeding. Wild-type mice respond to chronic high-fat feeding by significantly increasing β-cell area, islet number, and pancreatic insulin content and are more insulin resistant. Hansotia et al. (24) showed that, in response to chronic high-fat feeding, β-cell area and islet number are increased in DIRKO mice, although not to the degree observed in wild-type mice. Unlike wild-type mice on a high-fat diet, pancreatic insulin content in high fat–fed DIRKO mice is not increased (24), resulting in significantly lower fasting insulin levels, as shown in the present studies. However, this impaired morphological and functional pancreatic response to high-fat feeding in DIRKO mice is offset by preservation of hepatic and peripheral insulin sensitivity.

Obesity is a significant risk factor associated with the development of insulin resistance and type 2 diabetes (32,33). Thus, decreased obesity is likely associated with protection from high-fat diet–induced insulin resistance in DIRKO mice. Consistent with this, chemical ablation of GIPR with (Pro^3)GIP, a GIPR antagonist, has been shown to decrease adiposity, improve glucose tolerance, and

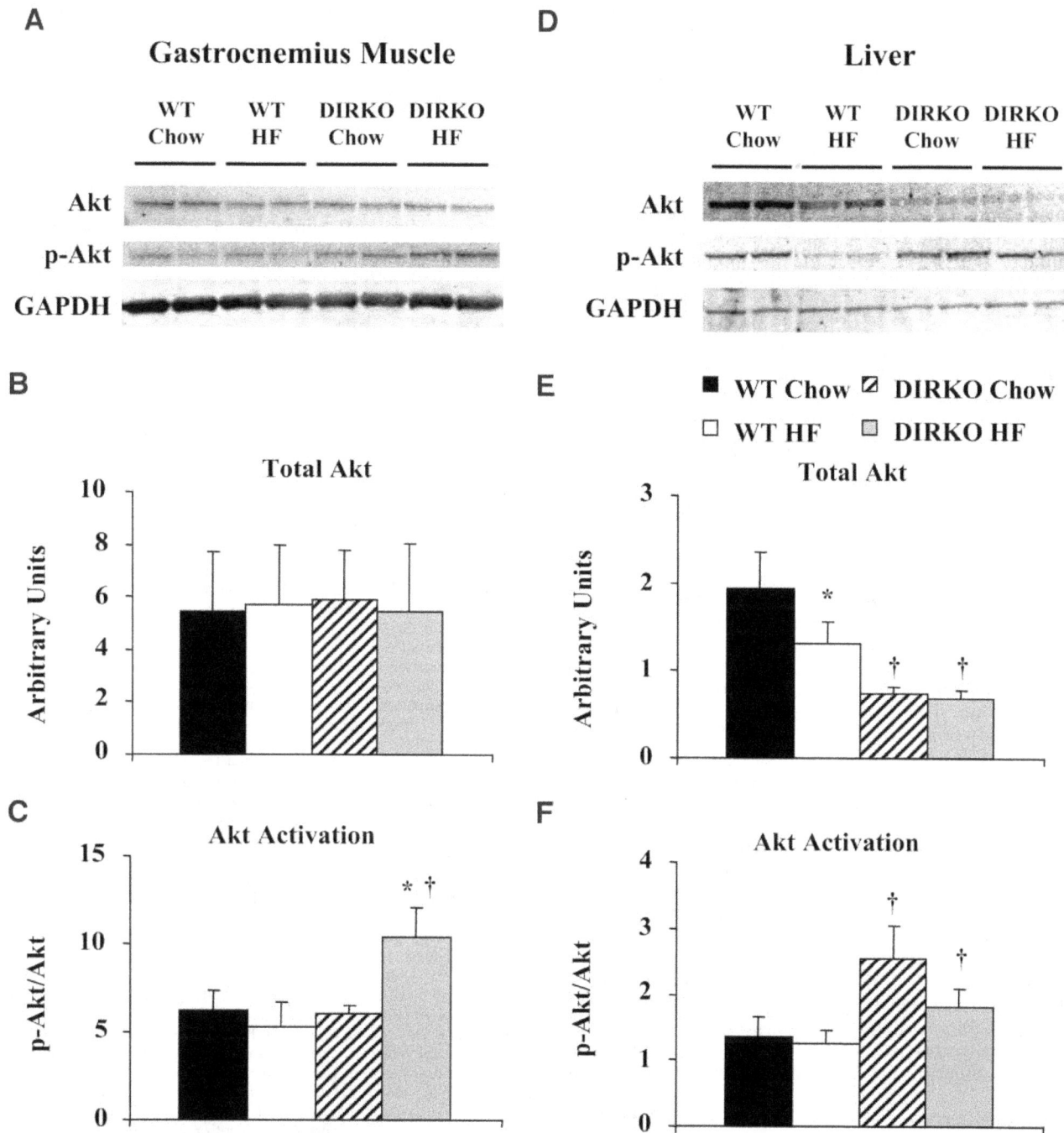

FIG. 7. Immunoblots after hyperinsulinemic-euglycemic clamps on 5-h–fasted, conscious, unrestrained chow-fed and high fat–fed C57BL/6 (wild-type) and DIRKO mice. Wild-type chow (black bars), wild-type high fat (white bars), DIRKO chow (striped bars), DIRKO high fat (gray bars). *A*: Representative images of immunoblots from gastrocnemius extracts for total Akt (Akt), phosphorylated Akt (*p*-Akt), and GAPDH. *B*: Total Akt normalized to GAPDH in gastrocnemius. *C*: Akt activation (*p*-Akt/total Akt) in gastrocnemius. *D*: Representative images of immunoblots from liver extracts for total Akt, *p*-Akt, and GAPDH. *E*: Akt normalized to GAPDH in liver. *F*: Akt activation in liver. Data are means ± SE for 8–10 mice/group. *$P < 0.05$ vs. chow; †$P < 0.05$ vs. wild type.

modestly enhance the response to intraperitoneal insulin in *ob/ob* mice (34). Similarly, tissue lipid accumulation is reduced and the glucose response to an intraperitoneal insulin injection is preserved in high fat–fed GLP-1R knockout and DIRKO mice compared with high fat–fed wild-type mice (24). To directly address the effect of a disruption in incretin signaling on insulin action, the present studies used the hyperinsulinemic-euglycemic clamp in conscious, unrestrained mice. This technique is

generally considered the "gold standard" for assessment of in vivo insulin action. The addition of isotopic glucose tracers with this technique allows for the determination of specific sites where insulin action is affected. Whereas high-fat feeding impairs insulin-mediated suppression of endoR$_a$ and stimulation of R_d in wild-type mice, these impairments do not occur in high fat–fed DIRKO mice. DIRKO mice on a high-fat diet have a more than threefold higher index of insulin sensitivity (GIR/[insulin]) than high fat–fed wild-type mice. Furthermore, R_g is impaired in wild-type mice fed a high-fat diet, whereas DIRKO mice do not exhibit such a diet-induced impairment. This protection from high fat diet–induced insulin resistance in DIRKO mice is associated with enhanced insulin signaling, because hepatic and muscle Akt activation is greater in high fat–fed DIRKO mice compared with their wild-type counterparts.

Recent evidence indicates that GLP-1 action in the brain can acutely regulate peripheral insulin sensitivity. Knauf et al. (35) showed that glucose requirements during a hyperinsulinemic-hyperglycemic clamp are higher in mice receiving an intracerebroventricular infusion of the GLP-1R antagonist exendin 9-39. Conversely, mice receiving the GLP-1R agonist exendin 4 directly into the brain showed decreased glucose requirements. 2-Deoxyglucose uptake into skeletal muscle was increased in mice receiving intracerebroventricular exendin 9-39 and decreased in mice receiving exendin 4 under hyperinsulinemic-hyperglycemic conditions. These studies suggest that endogenous GLP-1 action in the brain inhibits muscle insulin action. Thus, in agreement with the present studies, the disruption of central GLP-1 action enhances peripheral insulin sensitivity.

Phenotypes associated with insulin action were also observed in chow-fed DIRKO mice. Absolute R_g in three different skeletal muscles was lower in DIRKO than wild-type mice. However, when normalized to clamp insulin levels, there was no difference in muscle R_g between these two groups. Interestingly, Akt protein expression in the gastrocnemius was lower in DIRKO mice, but Akt activation was higher. This was evident even as clamp insulin levels were lower in DIRKO mice. R_g in the heart was also higher in DIRKO compared with wild-type mice. This is likely due to loss of GLP-1R signaling, because this incretin receptor, and not GIPR, is expressed in the heart (36,37).

DIRKO mice exhibited lower fasting NEFA levels on both chow and high-fat diets, even as fasting insulin levels were insignificantly lower in chow-fed mice and significantly lower in high fat–fed mice. Activation of GIPR in cultured 3T3-L1 adipocytes stimulates heparin-releasable lipoprotein lipase activity, increasing NEFA levels (13). Thus, disruption of GIPR signaling in adipocytes likely results in decreased fasting NEFA levels in DIRKO mice. Although insulin-mediated suppression of NEFA levels was equal in wild-type and DIRKO mice, we cannot rule out a direct effect of disrupting incretin signaling on lipid turnover.

Taken together, these studies demonstrate that although complete disruption of incretin receptor signaling results in impaired β-cell function and adaptation to chronic high-fat feeding (24), this is overcome by preservation of insulin action. This is likely secondary to effects on energy expenditure, activity, and adiposity associated with the lack of incretin receptor signaling. Although disruption of GIPR results in impaired β-cell function, it also results in increased energy expenditure and decreased adiposity. Similarly, the deleterious effects of ablating GLP-1R signaling on β-cell function are overcome by increased activity-dependent energy expenditure. Thus, the absence of incretin receptor signaling results in a metabolic status capable of responding to impaired β-cell function and the stress of high-fat feeding. These results extend the importance of incretin action in regulating glucose homeostasis beyond the pancreas and demonstrate how incretin receptor signaling can modulate insulin action by mechanisms other than stimulation of insulin secretion.

ACKNOWLEDGMENTS

This work has received support from grants U24-DK-59637, RO1-DK-54902, and RO1-DK-50277 from the National Institute of Diabetes and Digestive and Kidney Diseases.

We thank Dr. Owen McGuinness, Carlo Malabanan, Tasneem Ansari, and Anna Wilson of the Metabolic Pathophysiology Core, Vanderbilt Mouse Metabolic Phenotyping Center, for the body composition, energy expenditure, and activity measurements.

REFERENCES

1. Drucker DJ: The biology of incretin hormones. *Cell Metab* 3:153–165, 2006
2. Drucker DJ: The role of gut hormones in glucose homeostasis. *J Clin Invest* 117:24–32, 2007
3. Drucker DJ: Glucagon-like peptides: regulators of cell proliferation, differentiation, and apoptosis. *Mol Endocrinol* 17:161–171, 2003
4. Kim SJ, Winter K, Nian C, Tsuneoka M, Koda Y, McIntosh CH: Glucose-dependent insulinotropic polypeptide (GIP) stimulation of pancreatic beta-cell survival is dependent upon phosphatidylinositol 3-kinase (PI3K)/protein kinase B (PKB) signaling, inactivation of the forkhead transcription factor Foxo1, and down-regulation of bax expression. *J Biol Chem* 280:22297–22307, 2005
5. Li Y, Hansotia T, Yusta B, Ris F, Halban PA, Drucker DJ: Glucagon-like peptide-1 receptor signaling modulates beta cell apoptosis. *J Biol Chem* 278:471–478, 2003
6. Xu G, Stoffers DA, Habener JF, Bonner-Weir S: Exendin-4 stimulates both β-cell replication and neogenesis, resulting in increased β-cell mass and improved glucose tolerance in diabetic rats. *Diabetes* 48:2270–2276, 1999
7. Hui H, Nourparvar A, Zhao X, Perfetti R: Glucagon-like peptide-1 inhibits apoptosis of insulin-secreting cells via a cyclic 5′-adenosine monophosphate-dependent protein kinase A- and a phosphatidylinositol 3-kinase-dependent pathway. *Endocrinology* 144:1444–1455, 2003
8. Komatsu R, Matsuyama T, Namba M, Watanabe N, Itoh H, Kono N, Tarui S: Glucagonostatic and insulinotropic action of glucagonlike peptide I-(7-36)-amide. *Diabetes* 38:902–905, 1989
9. Dupre J, Behme MT, Hramiak IM, McFarlane P, Williamson MP, Zabel P, McDonald TJ: Glucagon-like peptide I reduces postprandial glycemic excursions in IDDM. *Diabetes* 44:626–630, 1995
10. Nauck MA, Niedereichholz U, Ettler R, Holst JJ, Orskov C, Ritzel R, Schmiegel WH: Glucagon-like peptide 1 inhibition of gastric emptying outweighs its insulinotropic effects in healthy humans. *Am J Physiol* 273:E981–E988, 1997
11. Prigeon RL, Quddusi S, Paty B, D'Alessio DA: Suppression of glucose production by GLP-1 independent of islet hormones: a novel extrapancreatic effect. *Am J Physiol Endocrinol Metab* 285:E701–E707, 2003
12. Burcelin R, Da Costa A, Drucker D, Thorens B: Glucose competence of the hepatoportal vein sensor requires the presence of an activated glucagon-like peptide-1 receptor. *Diabetes* 50:1720–1728, 2001
13. Miyawaki K, Yamada Y, Ban N, Ihara Y, Tsukiyama K, Zhou H, Fujimoto S, Oku A, Tsuda K, Toyokuni S, Hiai H, Mizunoya W, Fushiki T, Holst JJ, Makino M, Tashita A, Kobara Y, Tsubamoto Y, Jinnouchi T, Jomori T, Seino Y: Inhibition of gastric inhibitory polypeptide signaling prevents obesity. *Nat Med* 8:738–742, 2002
14. Baggio L, Kieffer TJ, Drucker DJ: Glucagon-like peptide-1, but not glucose-dependent insulinotropic peptide, regulates fasting glycemia and nonenteral glucose clearance in mice. *Endocrinology* 141:3703–3709, 2000
15. Edwards CM, Todd JF, Mahmoudi M, Wang Z, Wang RM, Ghatei MA, Bloom SR: Glucagon-like peptide 1 has a physiological role in the control of postprandial glucose in humans: studies with the antagonist exendin 9-39. *Diabetes* 48:86–93, 1999
16. Miyawaki K, Yamada Y, Yano H, Niwa H, Ban N, Ihara Y, Kubota A, Fujimoto S, Kajikawa M, Kuroe A, Tsuda K, Hashimoto H, Yamashita T, Jomori T, Tashiro F, Miyazaki J, Seino Y: Glucose intolerance caused by a defect in the entero-insular axis: a study in gastric inhibitory polypeptide receptor knockout mice. *Proc Natl Acad Sci USA* 96:14843–14847, 1999
17. Scrocchi LA, Brown TJ, MaClusky N, Brubaker PL, Auerbach AB, Joyner AL, Drucker DJ: Glucose intolerance but normal satiety in mice with a null mutation in the glucagon-like peptide 1 receptor gene. *Nat Med* 2:1254–1258, 1996

18. Scrocchi LA, Drucker DJ: Effects of aging and a high fat diet on body weight and glucose tolerance in glucagon-like peptide-1 receptor −/− mice. *Endocrinology* 139:3127–3132, 1998
19. Scrocchi LA, Marshall BA, Cook SM, Brubaker PL, Drucker DJ: Identification of glucagon-like peptide 1 (GLP-1) actions essential for glucose homeostasis in mice with disruption of GLP-1 receptor signaling. *Diabetes* 47:632–639, 1998
20. Pederson RA, Satkunarajah M, McIntosh CH, Scrocchi LA, Flamez D, Schuit F, Drucker DJ, Wheeler MB: Enhanced glucose-dependent insulinotropic polypeptide secretion and insulinotropic action in glucagon-like peptide 1 receptor −/− mice. *Diabetes* 47:1046–1052, 1998
21. Pamir N, Lynn FC, Buchan AM, Ehses J, Hinke SA, Pospisilik JA, Miyawaki K, Yamada Y, Seino Y, McIntosh CH, Pederson RA: Glucose-dependent insulinotropic polypeptide receptor null mice exhibit compensatory changes in the enteroinsular axis. *Am J Physiol Endocrinol Metab* 284:E931–E939, 2003
22. Preitner F, Ibberson M, Franklin I, Binnert C, Pende M, Gjinovci A, Hansotia T, Drucker DJ, Wollheim C, Burcelin R, Thorens B: Gluco-incretins control insulin secretion at multiple levels as revealed in mice lacking GLP-1 and GIP receptors. *J Clin Invest* 113:635–645, 2004
23. Hansotia T, Drucker DJ: GIP and GLP-1 as incretin hormones: lessons from single and double incretin receptor knockout mice. *Regul Pept* 128:125–134, 2005
24. Hansotia T, Maida A, Flock G, Yamada Y, Tsukiyama K, Seino Y, Drucker DJ: Extrapancreatic incretin receptors modulate glucose homeostasis, body weight, and energy expenditure. *J Clin Invest* 117:143–152, 2007
25. Ayala JE, Bracy DP, Julien BM, Rottman JN, Fueger PT, Wasserman DH: Chronic treatment with sildenafil improves energy balance and insulin action in high fat–fed conscious mice. *Diabetes* 56:1025–1033, 2007
26. Obici S, Wang J, Chowdury R, Feng Z, Siddhanta U, Morgan K, Rossetti L: Identification of a biochemical link between energy intake and energy expenditure. *J Clin Invest* 109:1599–1605, 2002
27. Nelson WR, O'Hopp SJ: A semiquantitative screening test and quantitative assay for total fecal fat. *Clin Chem* 15:1062–1071, 1969
28. Ayala JE, Bracy DP, McGuinness OP, Wasserman DH: Considerations in the design of hyperinsulinemic-euglycemic clamps in the conscious mouse. *Diabetes* 55:390–397, 2006
29. Altszuler N, De Bodo RC, Steele R, Wall JS: Measurement of size and turnover rate of body glucose pool by the isotope dilution method. *Am J Physiol* 187:15–24, 1956
30. Fueger PT, Bracy DP, Malabanan CM, Pencek RR, Granner DK, Wasserman DH: Hexokinase II overexpression improves exercise-stimulated but not insulin-stimulated muscle glucose uptake in high-fat-fed C57BL/6J mice. *Diabetes* 53:306–314, 2004
31. Kraegen EW, James DE, Jenkins AB, Chisholm DJ: Dose-response curves for in vivo insulin sensitivity in individual tissues in rats. *Am J Physiol* 248:E353–E362, 1985
32. Laakso M, Edelman SV, Brechtel G, Baron AD: Decreased effect of insulin to stimulate skeletal muscle blood flow in obese man: a novel mechanism for insulin resistance. *J Clin Invest* 85:1844–1852, 1990
33. DeFronzo RA, Ferrannini E: Insulin resistance: a multifaceted syndrome responsible for NIDDM, obesity, hypertension, dyslipidemia, and atherosclerotic cardiovascular disease. *Diabetes Care* 14:173–194, 1991
34. Gault VA, Irwin N, Green BD, McCluskey JT, Greer B, Bailey CJ, Harriott P, O'Harte FP, Flatt PR: Chemical ablation of gastric inhibitory polypeptide receptor action by daily (Pro3)GIP administration improves glucose tolerance and ameliorates insulin resistance and abnormalities of islet structure in obesity-related diabetes. *Diabetes* 54:2436–2446, 2005
35. Knauf C, Cani PD, Perrin C, Iglesias MA, Maury JF, Bernard E, Benhamed F, Gremeaux T, Drucker DJ, Kahn CR, Girard J, Tanti JF, Delzenne NM, Postic C, Burcelin R: Brain glucagon-like peptide-1 increases insulin secretion and muscle insulin resistance to favor hepatic glycogen storage. *J Clin Invest* 115:3554–3563, 2005
36. Bullock BP, Heller RS, Habener JF: Tissue distribution of messenger ribonucleic acid encoding the rat glucagon-like peptide-1 receptor. *Endocrinology* 137:2968–2978, 1996
37. Wei Y, Mojsov S: Tissue-specific expression of the human receptor for glucagon-like peptide-I: brain, heart and pancreatic forms have the same deduced amino acid sequences. *FEBS Lett* 358:219–224, 1995

Separate Impact of Obesity and Glucose Tolerance on the Incretin Effect in Normal Subjects and Type 2 Diabetic Patients

Elza Muscelli,[1] Andrea Mari,[2] Arturo Casolaro,[1] Stefania Camastra,[1] Giuseppe Seghieri,[3] Amalia Gastaldelli,[1] Jens J. Holst,[4] and Ele Ferrannini[1]

OBJECTIVE—To quantitate the separate impact of obesity and hyperlycemia on the incretin effect (i.e., the gain in β-cell function after oral glucose versus intravenous glucose).

RESEARCH DESIGN AND METHODS—Isoglycemic oral (75 g) and intravenous glucose administration was performed in 51 subjects (24 with normal glucose tolerance [NGT], 17 with impaired glucose tolerance [IGT], and 10 with type 2 diabetes) with a wide range of BMI (20–61 kg/m^2). C-peptide deconvolution was used to reconstruct insulin secretion rates, and β-cell glucose sensitivity (slope of the insulin secretion/glucose concentration dose-response curve) was determined by mathematical modeling. The incretin effect was defined as the oral-to-intravenous ratio of responses. In 8 subjects with NGT and 10 with diabetes, oral glucose appearance was measured by the double-tracer technique.

RESULTS—The incretin effect on total insulin secretion and β-cell glucose sensitivity and the GLP-1 response to oral glucose were significantly reduced in diabetes compared with NGT or IGT ($P \leq 0.05$). The results were similar when subjects were stratified by BMI tertile ($P \leq 0.05$). In the whole dataset, each manifestation of the incretin effect was inversely related to both glucose tolerance (2-h plasma glucose levels) and BMI (partial r = 0.27–0.59, $P \leq 0.05$) in an independent, additive manner. Oral glucose appearance did not differ between diabetes and NGT and was positively related to the GLP-1 response ($r = 0.53$, $P < 0.01$). Glucagon suppression during the oral glucose tolerance test was blunted in diabetic patients.

CONCLUSIONS—Potentiation of insulin secretion, glucose sensing, glucagon-like peptide-1 release, and glucagon suppression are physiological manifestations of the incretin effect. Glucose tolerance and obesity impair the incretin effect independently of one another. *Diabetes* **57:1340–1348, 2008**

From the [1]Department of Internal Medicine and Consiglio Nazionale delle Ricerche (CNR) Institute of Clinical Physiology, University of Pisa, Italy; the [2]CNR Institute of Biochemical Engineering, Padova, Italy; the [3]Division of Internal Medicine, Spedali Riuniti, Pistoia, Italy; and the [4]Department of Medical Physiology, Panum Institute, Copenhagen, Denmark.

Corresponding author: Ele Ferrannini, MD, Department of Internal Medicine, Via Roma, 67, 56122 Pisa, Italy. E-mail: ferranni@ifc.pi.cnr.it.

Received for publication 14 September 2007 and accepted in revised form 17 December 2007.

Published ahead of print at http://diabetes.diabetesjournals.org on 27 December 2007. DOI: 10.2337/db07-1315.

AUC, area under the time concentration curve; FFM, fat-free mass; GIP, glucose-dependent insulinotropic polypeptide; GLP, glucagon-like peptide; IGT, impaired glucose tolerance; NGT, normal glucose tolerance; OGTT, oral glucose tolerance test; TTR, tracer-to-tracee ratio.

Type 2 diabetes results from the interaction of insulin insensitivity and β-cell dysfunction (1). The relative contribution of reduced β-cell mass and β-cell dysfunction to hyperglycemia is still debated (2,3), but mounting evidence indicates that gastrointestinal factors play an important role. In fact, it has long been known that oral glucose stimulates insulin secretion over and above the stimulus that is provided by rising glucose levels (4,5). This potentiation of β-cell function by the route of nutrient administration has been termed the incretin effect (6). Among a host of factors and signals originating from the absorptive process, concentrations of glucagon-like peptide (GLP)-1 and glucose-dependent insulinotropic polypeptide (GIP) have received special attention (7). These hormones are released in parallel with insulin following oral glucose or meals, and each has been shown to potentiate glucose-dependent insulin release. The key observation that the GLP-1 response is blunted and that the β-cell response to GIP is grossly impaired in diabetes (7–11) has led to the notion that an impaired incretin effect contributes to the β-cell incompetence of diabetes (11). In recent years, the clinical data showing that GLP-1 analogs can normalize glycemia by stimulating insulin secretion in diabetic patients (12,13) has strengthened the incretin theory.

The impact of obesity on the incretin effect is uncertain. Obese subjects, especially those with visceral fat accumulation, frequently are insulin resistant and insulin hypersecretors, in proportion to the degree of overweight (14). The incretin effect has been reported to be increased in obese adolescents (15) but normal in obese adults (16). In some studies, the GLP-1 response of obese subjects has been found to be normal, whereas the GIP response was increased in the fasting state and early after a meal (17,18). In others studies (19–21), however, GLP-1 levels in response to oral carbohydrate or a meal were reduced in obese patients. Because diabetes is strongly associated with obesity, the question of the separate impact of obesity and hyperglycemia on the incretin effect has full pathophysiologic relevance. The primary aim of the present work was to answer this question.

Previous work from our laboratory has shown that the incretin effect, as tested with the use of the isoglycemic protocol (22), can be quantitated by measuring not only the plasma insulin response, as per the original definition (6), but also the two main parameters describing β-cell function, namely, absolute insulin secretion and β-cell glucose sensitivity (i.e., insulin secretion in relation to the concomitant plasma glucose concentration). We therefore set forth to measure β-cell function and hormones in response to oral glucose and isoglycemic intravenous glucose in a large group of volunteers, including subjects with normal glucose tolerance (NGT), impaired glucose tolerance (IGT), or diabetes over a wide range of body mass. Because gastrointestinal hormone responses are linked with the rate of nutrient absorption (23), a secondary aim of the study was to measure the rate of appearance of ingested glucose in the systemic circulation in subjects with different incretin effect (i.e., NGT and diabetes).

RESEARCH DESIGN AND METHODS

Fifty-one subjects, selected from the outpatient clinic, volunteered for the study. None of them had lost weight or changed dietary habits during the 3 months preceding the study. Three diabetic patients were on treatment with metformin alone and one with acarbose, and both were withheld 3 weeks before the study. All subjects had resting arterial blood pressure ≤140/90 mmHg and normal results for liver and renal function tests. Fat-free mass (FFM) was measured by electrical bioimpedance using a body composition analyzer model TB-300 (Tanita, Tokyo, Japan) (24); fat mass was then obtained as the difference between body weight and FFM. On the oral glucose tolerance test (OGTT) (Table 1), 24 had NGT, 17 had IGT, and 10 had type 2 diabetes according to American Diabetes Association criteria (25). Partial data from 11 subjects with NGT and 10 with IGT have been published previously (22). The study was approved by an institutional review board, and all subjects gave informed, written consent to the study.

Two studies were carried out in each subject after an overnight (12- to 14-h) fast at 1-week intervals. In the first study, subjects underwent a 3-h OGTT (75 g), with measurements of plasma glucose concentrations at 10-min intervals. In the second study (isoglycemic test), the plasma glucose profile was reproduced by a variable intravenous glucose (20% dextrose) infusion by using an ad hoc–developed algorithm. In both studies, venous blood was sampled at −30, 0, 10, 20, 30, 40, 60, 90, 120, 150, and 180 min for plasma insulin, C-peptide, glucagon, GLP-1, and GIP measurements.

In a subgroup of 18 participants (8 with NGT and 10 with diabetes), glucose fluxes were measured by the double-tracer technique (26). With this protocol, a primed-constant infusion of [6,6-^{2}H$_2$]-glucose (Cambridge Isotype Laboratories, Boston, MA) ([28 μmol/kg × [fasting glycemia/5] − prime followed by a 0.28 μmol/kg infusion) was administered throughout the basal period (−180 to 0 min) and during the OGTT (0–180 min). At time 0, subjects drank a 75-g glucose solution containing 1.5 g [1-^{2}H]-glucose.

Assays. Plasma glucose was measured by the glucose oxidase technique (Beckman Glucose Analyzers; Beckman, Fullerton, CA). Plasma insulin was measured in duplicate by radioimmunoassay using a kit for human insulin with negligible cross-reactivity with proinsulin and its split products (Linco Research, St. Louis, MO). Glucagon and C-peptide were measured by radioimmunoassay (Linco Research). Plasma triglyceride and serum HDL cholesterol were assayed in duplicate by standard spectrophotometric methods on a Synchron Clinical System CX4 (Beckman). Total COOH-terminal amidated GLP-1 was assayed by radioimmunoassay using the polyclonal antiserum no. 89390 (raised in rabbits), which has an absolute requirement for the amidated C-terminus of GLP-1 and does not cross-react with C-terminally truncated metabolites or with the glycine-extended forms. The assay cross-reacts <0.01% with GLP-1 (7–35) and GLP-1 (7–37), 83% with GLP-1 (9–36) amide, and 100% with GLP-1 (1–36) amide, GLP-1 (7–36) amide, and GLP-1 (8–36) amide. The assay has a detection limit of ~1 pmol/l and an ED$_{50}$ of 25 pmol/l. Intra- and interassay coefficients of variation are <6 and <15%, respectively (27,28). The active (NH$_2$-terminal) GIP was assayed by radioimmunoassay using polyclonal antiserum 98171 (raised in rabbits) that is NH$_2$-terminally directed and does not recognize NH$_2$-terminally truncated peptides. It has a cross-reactivity of 100% with human GIP 1–42 and <0.1% with human GIP 3–42, GLP-1 (7–36) amide, GLP-1 (9–36) amide, GLP-2 (1–33), GLP-2 (3–33), and glucagon. Detection limit is ~ 5 pmol/l with an ED$_{50}$ of 48 pmol/l. Intra- and interassay coefficients of variation were <6 and <15%, respectively (29). 6,6-[^{2}H$_2$]glucose and [1-^{2}H]-glucose enrichment were measured by gas chromatography/mass spectrometry.

Calculations. Insulin sensitivity was estimated from the plasma glucose and insulin responses to oral glucose loading by calculating the oral glucose insulin sensitivity index, which has previously been shown to be well correlated with the *M* value from the euglycemic-hyperinsulinemic clamp (30). Areas under the time concentration curves (AUCs) were calculated by the trapezium rule. To estimate the size of the incretin effect, we used the ratio of oral to intravenous measures (6). This calculation cancels the impact of glucose levels, per se, which were matched by protocol.

All glucose fluxes were expressed per kilogram of FFM, since this

normalization has been shown to minimize differences due to sex, obesity, and age (26). During the last 20 min of the basal tracer equilibration period, plasma glucose concentrations and 6,6-[^{2}H]glucose enrichment were stable in all subjects. Therefore, endogenous glucose production was calculated as the ratio of the 6,6-[^{2}H$_2$]glucose infusion rate to the plasma tracer enrichment (tracer-to-tracee ratio [TTR]$_{6,6}$, mean of three determinations). After glucose ingestion, the total glucose rate of appearance was calculated from TTR$_{6,6}$ using Steele's equation, as previously described (26). Before applying Steele's equation, plasma TTR$_{6,6}$ data were smoothed using a spline-fitting approach to stabilize the calculation of the derivative of enrichment. The plasma glucose concentration resulting from the absorption of ingested glucose (exogenous glucose concentration) was calculated from the product of total plasma glucose concentration and the ratio of plasma [1-^{2}H]-glucose TTR to the [1-^{2}H]-glucose TTR of the ingested glucose. The plasma glucose concentration resulting from endogenous glucose release was obtained as the difference between total and exogenous glucose concentration. TTR$_{end}$ of endogenous glucose and oral glucose rate of appearance were calculated as described (26). The tracer-determined rate of glucose disappearance (R_d) provided a measure of insulin-mediated total-body glucose disposal.

β-Cell function modeling. The model used to reconstruct insulin secretion and its control by glucose has been previously described (31). In brief, the model consists of three blocks: *1*) a model for fitting the glucose concentration profile, the purpose of which is to smooth and interpolate plasma glucose concentrations; *2*) a model describing the dependence of insulin (or C-peptide) secretion on glucose concentration; and *3*) a model of C-peptide kinetics (i.e., the two-exponential model proposed by Van Cauter et al. [32]), in which the model parameters are individually adjusted to the subject's anthropometric data. In particular, with regard to the insulin secretion block (block 2), the relationship between insulin release and plasma glucose concentrations is modeled as the sum of two components: *1*) The first component is the relationship between insulin secretion and glucose concentration (i.e., a dose-response function). The dose-response function is modulated by a time-varying factor, expressing a potentiation effect on insulin secretion, which was calculated as the ratio of the 2-h to zero time value. The mean slope of the dose-response function is taken to represent β-cell glucose sensitivity, and *2*) the second insulin secretion component represents a dynamic dependence of insulin secretion on the rate of change of glucose concentration. This component, termed rate sensitivity, accounts for anticipation of insulin secretion as glucose levels rise (data not reported here). Total insulin secretion is the sum of the two components described above, and is calculated every 10 min for the whole 3-h period.

Statistical analysis. Data are given as means ± SD or median (interquartile range) for nonnormally distributed variables. The latter were transformed into their natural logarithms for use in statistical testing. Group differences were analyzed by ANOVA; individual group differences were analyzed by the Bonferroni-Dunn test. Paired group values were compared by the Wilcoxon test. Differences in time course between groups were analyzed by 2-way ANOVA for repeated measures. Linear regression models were tested by standard techniques. Adjustment for covariates was carried out by ANCOVA. A *P* value ≤0.05 was considered statistically significant; when post hoc performing multiple comparisons; the *P* value was divided by the number of comparisons.

RESULTS

The groups with NGT, IGT, and diabetes had similar age and sex distribution, BMI, and fat mass. A1C and serum triglycerides were higher in diabetes, and insulin sensitivity was reduced in both IGT and diabetes (Table 1). The fasting and post-OGTT plasma glucose concentrations were higher in IGT and diabetes than in NGT and by design were virtually identical during OGTT and the isoglycemic test in each group (Fig. 1). The plasma insulin response to oral glucose was higher in IGT and lower in diabetes compared with NGT. Fasting insulin secretion rates were increased in diabetes (median 115 [interquartile range 53]) versus subjects with NGT (86 [81] pmol · min^{-1} · m^{-2}; *P* < 0.05). The insulin secretory response to oral glucose was similar in NGT, IGT, and diabetes (60 [27] nmol/m^2 vs. 67 [21] nmol/m^2 vs. 67 [38] nmol/m^2) but delayed in diabetes (*P* < 0.0001 by repeated-measures ANOVA). The total secretory response to intravenous glucose was significantly lower than to oral glucose in NGT and IGT but not in diabetes. In contrast, β-cell glucose sensitivity was progres-

TABLE 1
Anthropometric and metabolic characteristics of the study subjects by glucose tolerance status

	NGT	IGT	Diabetes	$P*$
n	24	17	10	
Male/female	10/14	5/12	9/1	NS
Age (years)	41 ± 11	47 ± 13	50 ± 9	NS
BMI (kg/m^2)	33.1 ± 10.5	35.9 ± 8.0	35.5 ± 11.5	NS
Waist circumference (cm)	98 ± 20	102 ± 12	112 ± 19	NS
Fat mass (%)	35 ± 13	42 ± 6	38 ± 15	NS
A1C (%)	5.3 ± 0.4	5.5 ± 0.1	6.8 ± 0.6†	<0.0001
LDL cholesterol (mmol/l)	2.90 ± 0.83	3.37 ± 0.74	3.00 ± 0.73	NS
HDL cholesterol (mmol/l)	1.35 ± 0.47	1.19 ± 0.29	1.19 ± 0.22	NS
Triglycerides (mmol/l)	1.26 ± 0.69	1.32 ± 0.68	1.99 ± 0.97†	<0.02
Insulin sensitivity (ml · min^{-1} · m^{-2})	380 ± 51	319 ± 49†	305 ± 32†	<0.0001

Data are means ± SD. *ANOVA. †$P \leq 0.05$ vs. NGT by Bonferroni-Dunn test. NS, not significant.

sively impaired in IGT and diabetes compared with NGT on both the OGTT and isoglycemic test. However, β-cell glucose sensitivity was better with oral than intravenous glucose in NGT and IGT but not in diabetes (Fig. 2). Rate sensitivity was significantly higher during the oral than intravenous study in all groups (all $P < 0.001$) and was impaired in diabetes (749 [671] pmol · min^{-1} · m^{-2} · mmol^{-1} · l, $P = 0.03$, vs. 1,482 [1,589] pmol · min^{-1} · m^{-2} · mmol^{-1} · l for NGT); however, the incretin effect (ratio of oral to intravenous values) did not differ across glucose tolerance status. Likewise, the incretin effect on potentiation (as a single value at 2 h versus baseline) was similar across groups.

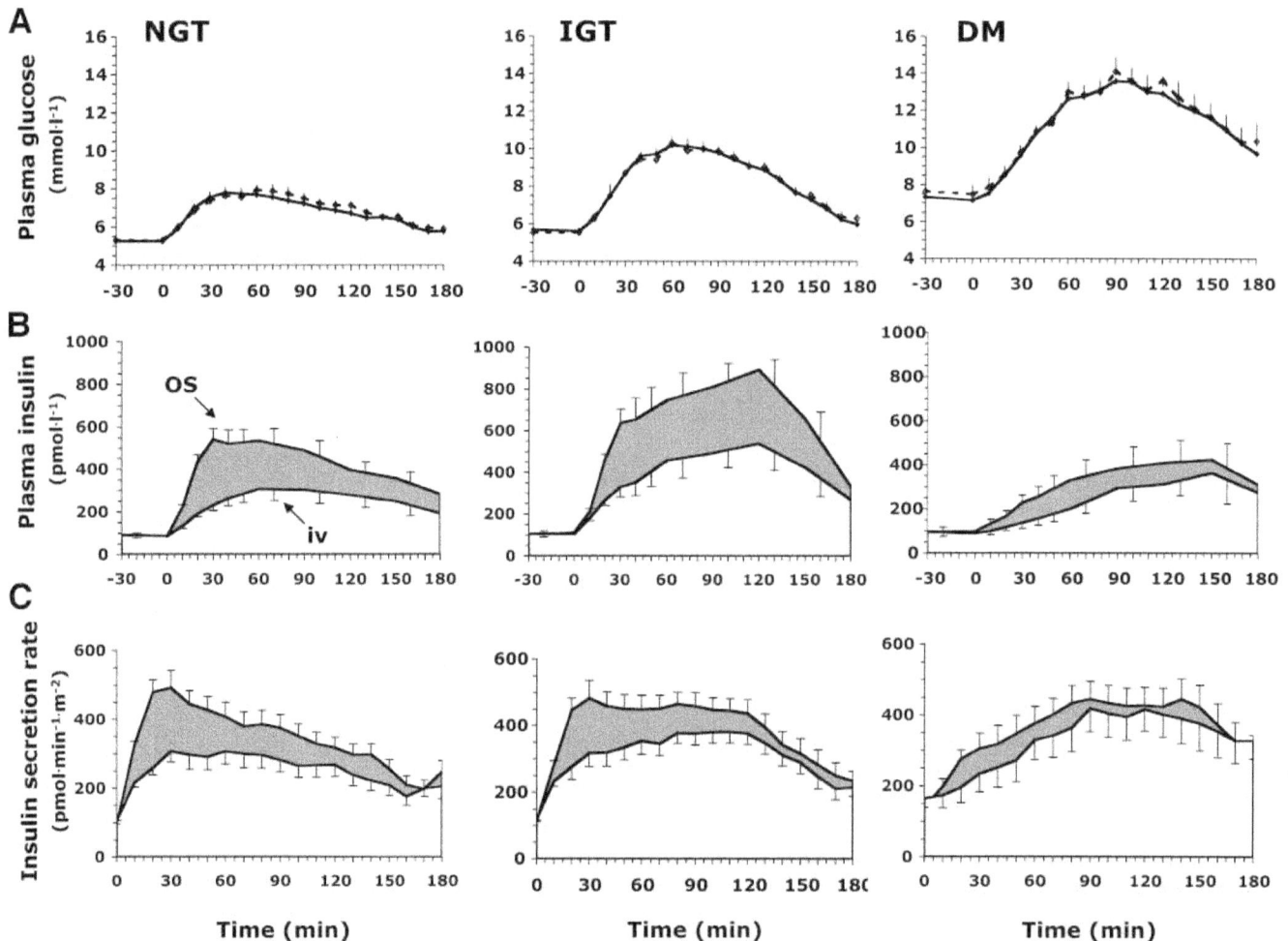

FIG. 1. Time-course of plasma glucose (A), insulin concentrations (B), and insulin secretion rates (C), as reconstructed from C-peptide deconvolution, in nondiabetic patients (NGT) and patients with IGT and type 2 diabetes (DM), following oral glucose (continuous line) and isoglycemic intravenous glucose administration (dashed line). The plasma glucose profiles are significantly higher in both IGT and diabetes than in NGT ($P < 0.0001$ for the time × group interaction by two-way ANOVA). Compared with NGT, the plasma insulin concentration and secretion responses to oral glucose were higher in IGT ($P < 0.0001$ and $P = 0.08$, respectively) and lower in diabetes ($P < 0.0001$ for both). The stippled areas visualize the incretin effect. Data are means ± SE.

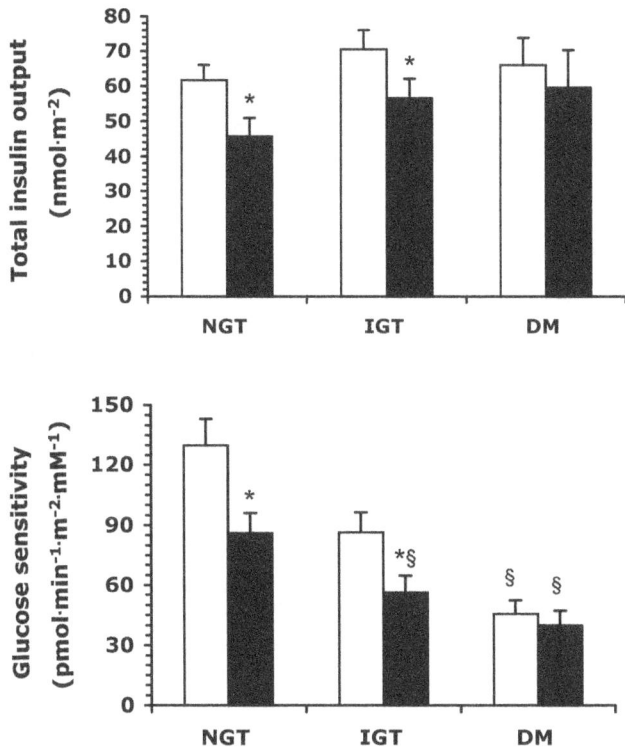

FIG. 2. Total insulin secretion and β-cell glucose sensitivity in response to oral (□) and intravenous (■) glucose in the three groups. *$P \leq 0.05$ for the difference between oral and intravenous (Wilcoxon test). §$P \leq 0.05$ for the difference from the group with NGT (Bonferroni-Dunn test).

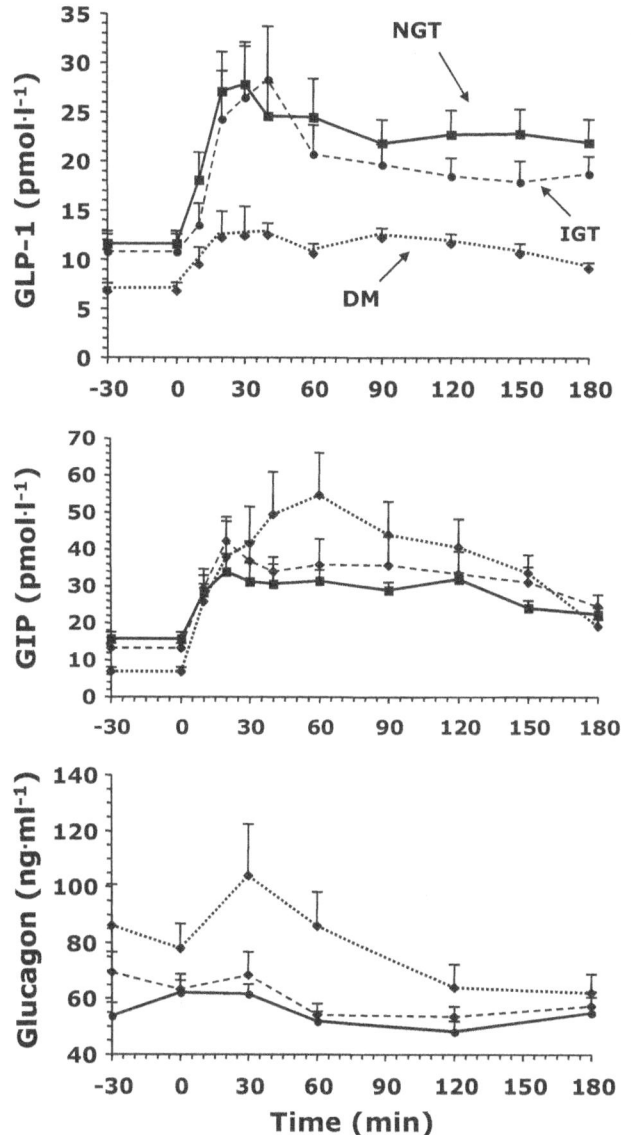

FIG. 3. Time-course of plasma GLP-1, GIP, and glucagon concentrations in response to oral glucose in the three groups. The GLP-1 response is significantly ($P < 0.01$) reduced, and the GIP and glucagon responses are significantly higher in diabetes versus NGT ($P = 0.03$ and $P = 0.002$, respectively).

With the OGTT, plasma GLP-1 levels were similar in IGT and NGT but markedly reduced in diabetes, whereas plasma GIP concentrations were higher in diabetes than in either NGT or IGT, with a prompt response and a delayed peak. Plasma glucagon levels were similar in NGT and IGT but were significantly higher in diabetes, which showed a paradoxical rise 30 min into the OGTT (Fig. 3). Neither GLP-1 nor GIP changed significantly during the intravenous test, whereas glucagon was equally suppressed in all groups (data not shown). The analysis of the hormonal AUCs is reported in Table 2.

In the subgroup receiving the double-tracer protocol, oral glucose was still appearing in the systemic circulation at 180 min at sizeable rates (averaging 16 ± 10 μmol · min^{-1} · kg_{FFM}^{-1}). The amount of oral glucose appearing over the 3 h of the OGTT totaled 43 ± 7 g in diabetes and 47 ± 11 g in NGT ($P = NS$); over the same time period, plasma glucose clearance was markedly reduced in diabetes (2.3 ± 0.4 vs. 4.2 ± 1.4 ml · min^{-1} · kg_{FFM}^{-1}; $P < 0.001$). Oral glucose appearance was positively related to the GLP-1 incremental AUC ($r = 0.53$, $P < 0.01$).

When the study population was stratified into BMI tertiles, groups had similar A1C levels and glucose AUCs and an approximately equal proportion of diabetic subjects ($\chi^2 = 5.6$, $P = 0.2$) (Table 3). As expected, insulin sensitivity was progressively lower and insulin levels and secretion rates (fasting and postglucose) were progressively higher with increasing BMI (Table 4). However, β-cell glucose sensitivity was similar across BMI tertiles with oral glucose and increased somewhat with intravenous glucose. Rate sensitivity and potentiation were sim-

ilar in BMI groups. The GLP-1 response, but not the GIP or glucagon response, was impaired with increasing BMI.

Incretins and the incretin effect. The incretin effect was analyzed separately for total insulin secretion and β-cell glucose sensitivity. For both parameters, the incretin effect was markedly attenuated in association with diabetes (Fig. 2). When analyzed by BMI tertiles, the incretin effect on total insulin secretion was progressively lower with higher BMI (oral-to-intravenous ratio = 1.8 ± 0.6 vs. 1.4 ± 0.3 vs. 1.1 ± 0.2; $P = 0.0002$); the same was true of the incretin effect on β-cell glucose sensitivity (2.1 ± 1.0 vs. 1.6 ± 0.8 vs. 1.3 ± 0.5; $P = 0.02$). In bivariate analysis, the impact of BMI and glucose tolerance were independent of each other. Using continuous variables, the incretin effect on total insulin secretion was a simultaneous function of BMI (partial $r = -0.59$, $P < 0.0001$) and 2-h plasma glucose levels (partial $r = -0.36$, $P < 0.01$). Likewise, the incretin effect on β-cell glucose sensitivity

TABLE 2
Hormone AUC by glucose tolerance status

	NGT	IGT	Diabetes	$P*$
AUC_I (nmol $\cdot$ l^{-1} $\cdot$ h)				
OGTT	75 ± 40	118 ± 64†	59 ± 42	0.007
Intravenous	45 ± 36	73 ± 53†	40 ± 29	0.05
P‡	<0.0001	0.0003	0.005	
AUC_{CP} (nmol $\cdot$ l^{-1} $\cdot$ h)				
OGTT	441 ± 159	494 ± 159	450 ± 177	NS
Intravenous	330 ± 186	401 ± 166	409 ± 247	NS
P‡	<0.0001	0.003	NS	
AUC_{Glg} (ng $\cdot$ l^{-1} $\cdot$ h)				
OGTT	10.3 ± 4.1	9.5 ± 2.7	13.9 ± 5.9*	<0.03
Intravenous	9.2 ± 2.6	8.7 ± 3.0	11.1 ± 5.0	NS
P‡	0.02	NS	0.008	
AUC_{GLP-1} (nmol $\cdot$ l^{-1} $\cdot$ h)				
OGTT	4.1 ± 2.3	3.4 ± 1.5	2.0 ± 0.5†	0.01
Intravenous	2.4 ± 1.4	2.3 ± 1.3	1.0 ± 0.3†	0.02
P‡	<0.0001	0.0005	0.005	
AUC_{GIP} (nmol $\cdot$ l^{-1} $\cdot$ h)				
OGTT	5.9 ± 4.2	5.0 ± 1.9	7.4 ± 4.0	NS
Intravenous	2.5 ± 1.4	2.8 ± 1.4	1.3 ± 0.7†	0.02
P‡	<0.0001	0.0003	0.005	

Data are means ± SD. *ANOVA. †$P \leq 0.05$ vs. NGT by Bonferroni-Dunn test. ‡Wilcoxon's signed-rank test, OGTT versus intravenous. NS, not significant.

was reciprocally related to both BMI (partial $r = -0.41$, $P = 0.003$) and 2-h glucose levels (partial $r = -0.27$, $P = 0.05$). In both these models, sex and age were not significant covariates; furthermore, replacing 2-h plasma glucose levels with the glucose AUC did not change the results, and there was no evidence of interaction between BMI and glucose levels.

Using the regression coefficients of the above models, incretin effects (in percent) were calculated for BMIs of 25, 30, and 45 kg/m^2 and for 2-h plasma glucose levels corresponding to the median of the groups with NGT, IGT, and diabetes. The predicted values clearly illustrate the additive effect of obesity and IGT on the incretin effects on total insulin secretion and β-cell glucose sensitivity (Fig. 4).

The GLP-1, but not the GIP, response to oral glucose was independently related to both BMI and 2-h plasma glucose levels (Fig. 5). The GLP-1, but not the GIP, AUC was directly related to the incretin effect on both insulin output and β-cell glucose sensitivity ($r = 0.51$, $P < 0.001$ and $r = 0.28$, $P = 0.05$). The incretin effect on glucagon, on

the other hand, was unrelated to BMI but was significantly ($P = 0.02$) higher in diabetes (1.4 ± 0.3) than in IGT (1.1 ± 0.3) or NGT (1.1 ± 0.3) when using the oral-to-intravenous ratio of the 0- to 60-min AUC.

DISCUSSION
The main finding of the present study is that obesity and glucose tolerance each attenuate the incretin effect on β-cell function and GLP-1 response independently of one another. The incretin effect, assessed as the plasma insulin response gradient during an isoglycemic protocol, is blunted in diabetes as previously demonstrated (11). Our results specify the mechanisms of this defect. First, the oral-to-intravenous ratio in total insulin output was narrower in diabetes compared with control subjects (Fig. 2). Of note, the insulin secretory response to intravenous glucose was, if anything, greater in diabetic patients than subjects with NGT, on account of the higher plasma glucose levels. Therefore, in diabetes the incretin defect consisted of an inability to increment insulin release when

TABLE 3
Anthropometric and metabolic characteristics of the study subjects by BMI tertile

	OB 1	OB 2	OB 3	$P*$
n	17	17	17	
Male/female	8/9	9/8	7/10	NS
NGT/IGT/diabetes	11/2/4	6/8/3	7/7/3	NS
Age (years)	46 ± 11	50 ± 13	46 ± 10	0.02
BMI (kg/m^2)	25.1 ± 2.7	32.1 ± 2.7†	46.3 ± 6.5†	—
Waist circumference (cm)	84 ± 10	104 ± 9†	121 ± 15†	<0.0001
Fat mass (%)	27 ± 10	38.7 ± 8†	47 ± 5†	<0.0001
A1C (%)	5.7 ± 0.8	5.7 ± 0.7	6.0 ± 0.8	NS
LDL cholesterol (mmol/l)	2.85 ± 0.57	3.28 ± 0.99	3.00 ± 0.72	NS
HDL cholesterol (mmol/l)	1.55 ± 0.55	1.18 ± 0.22†	1.17 ± 0.26†	0.03
Triglycerides (mmol/l)	1.12 ± 0.86	1.61 ± 0.76	1.40 ± 0.73	NS
Insulin sensitivity (ml $\cdot$ min^{-1} $\cdot$ m^{-2})	381 ± 47	328 ± 58†	327 ± 52†	0.005

Data are means ± SD. *ANOVA. †$P \leq 0.05$ vs. OB 1 by Bonferroni-Dunn test. NS, not significant; OB, obese subject.

TABLE 4
Hormone AUC and β-cell function parameters by BMI tertile

	OB 1	OB 2	OB 3	$P*$
AUC_G ($\mu mol \cdot l^{-1} \cdot h^{-1}$)				
OGTT	$1{,}447 \pm 436$	$1{,}583 \pm 402$	$1{,}425 \pm 216$	NS
Intravenous	$1{,}478 \pm 435$	$1{,}594 \pm 403$	$1{,}438 \pm 203$	NS
$P\dagger$	0.02	NS	NS	
AUC_I ($nmol \cdot l^{-1} \cdot h^{-1}$)				
OGTT	51 ± 23	$86 \pm 47\ddagger$	$122 \pm 62\ddagger$	0.0003
Intravenous	24 ± 10	$48 \pm 28\ddagger$	$88 \pm 51\ddagger$	<0.0001
$P\dagger$	0.0003	0.0003	0.003	
AUC_{CP} ($nmol \cdot l^{-1} \cdot h^{-1}$)				
OGTT	324 ± 81	$471 \pm 133\ddagger$	$585 \pm 143\ddagger$	<0.0001
Intravenous	204 ± 79	$358 \pm 129\ddagger$	$546 \pm 176\ddagger$	<0.0001
$P\dagger$	0.0004	0.007	0.04	
AUC_{Glg} ($ng \cdot l^{-1} \cdot h^{-1}$)				
OGTT	10.1 ± 3.4	9.8 ± 2.5	12.3 ± 6.2	NS
Intravenous	8.6 ± 2.6	8.8 ± 2.2	$10.9 \pm 4.5\ddagger$	NS
$P\dagger$	0.009	NS	0.06	
AUC_{GLP-1} ($nmol \cdot l^{-1} \cdot h^{-1}$)				
OGTT	4.7 ± 2.3	$3.5 \pm 1.5\ddagger$	$2.2 \pm 0.8\ddagger$	0.0002
Intravenous	2.9 ± 1.4	$2.1 \pm 1.1\ddagger$	$1.3 \pm 1.1\ddagger$	0.001
$P\dagger$	0.0004	0.0003	0.005	
AUC_{GIP} ($nmol \cdot l^{-1} \cdot h^{-1}$)				
OGTT	6.5 ± 2.8	5.8 ± 2.1	5.2 ± 5.1	NS
Intravenous	3.0 ± 2.8	2.6 ± 1.5	$1.5 \pm 0.8\ddagger$	0.004
$P\dagger$	0.0003	0.0003	0.003	
Fasting ISR ($pmol \cdot min^{-1} \cdot m^{-2}$)				
OGTT	65 ± 25	$108 \pm 41\ddagger$	$160 \pm 57\ddagger$	<0.0001
Intravenous	70 ± 31	$111 \pm 42\ddagger$	$183 \pm 82\ddagger$	<0.0001
$P\dagger$	NS	NS	NS	
Total IS ($nmol/m^2$)				
OGTT	48 ± 13	$69 \pm 20\ddagger$	$80 \pm 21\ddagger$	<0.0001
Intravenous	30 ± 13	$51 \pm 18\ddagger$	$75 \pm 25\ddagger$	<0.0001
$P\dagger$	0.0004	0.0007	0.04	
β-Cell glucose sensitivity ($pmol \cdot min^{-1} \cdot m^{-2} \cdot mmol^{-1} \cdot l$)				
OGTT	101 ± 82	101 ± 49	95 ± 46	NS
Intravenous	48 ± 26	$77 \pm 60\ddagger$	$78 \pm 36\ddagger$	NS
$P\dagger$	0.0006	0.05	0.04	

Data are means ± SD. *By ANOVA. †Wilcoxon's signed-rank test, OGTT versus intravenous. ‡$P \leq 0.05$ vs. OB 1 by Bonferroni-Dunn test. NS, not significant; OB, obese subject.

the plasma glucose profile was the result of glucose ingestion. In addition, β-cell glucose sensitivity was progressively worse in IGT and diabetes on both intravenous and oral glucose, but subjects with NGT and IGT retained the ability to enhance β-cell glucose sensitivity when the stimulus came by mouth, whereas diabetic patients failed to do so. There was no major impact of IGT or diabetes on the incretin effect on rate sensitivity or potentiation.

As previously reported (8,9), the GLP-1 secretory response was depressed in diabetes and the GIP response was enhanced (at least early during absorption) (Fig. 3). By pooling data from all groups, we found a positive correlation between the GLP-1 response and the incretin effect (insulin output and β-cell glucose sensitivity). Of note, the GLP-1 response accounted for a relatively small fraction (~25%) of the variance of these incretin effects, suggesting that other factors contribute to the incretin effect or that circulating GLP-1 concentrations are a distant reflection of its biological activity. Like others (11), we found no correlation between the GIP response and incretin effects. In summary, each aspect of the incretin effect (quantitative insulin response, β-cell glucose sensing, and GLP-1 secretory response) was impaired in dia-

betes. Whether this defect is inherent in the diabetic state or secondary to diabetic hyperglycemia is still somewhat uncertain. The weight of available evidence, however, favors the view that the defective incretin function is a secondary phenomenon. Thus, one or the other aspect of incretin function has been reported to be normal in first-degree relatives of subjects with diabetes (33,34), in nondiabetic twins of diabetic probands (9), and in nondiabetic patients with chronic pancreatitis (while a reduced incretin effect is demonstrable in patients with chronic pancreatitis and secondary diabetes) (35). Furthermore, preliminary data suggest that normalization of glycemia in patients with diabetes with insulin treatment improves insulin secretion in response to GLP-1 infusion (36). Whether correction of chronic hyperglycemia reverses all manifestations of the incretin effect as measured by the isoglycemic protocol remains to be proven.

When the study population was stratified by obesity, the incretin effect (on insulin output, β-cell glucose sensitivity, and GLP-1 response) was gradely depressed across increasing degrees of overweight despite the fact that the clinical (Table 3) and metabolic (Table 4) features of BMI groupings were different from those of the glucose toler-

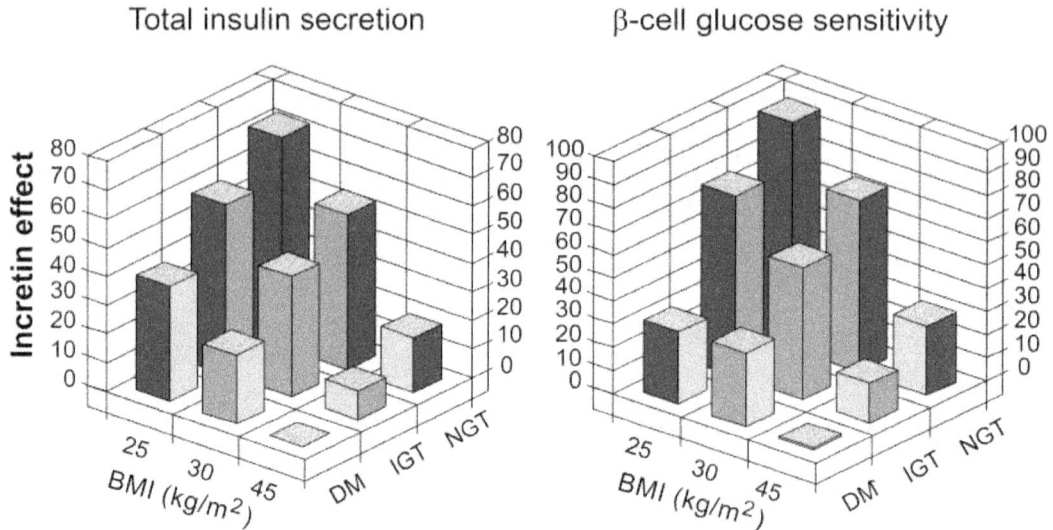

FIG. 4. Predicted percent changes in the incretin effect on total insulin secretion and β-cell glucose sensitivity as a simultaneous function of BMI and 2-h plasma glucose levels in the whole study group.

ance groupings. Thus, fasting and total insulin release rose markedly across BMI tertiles, whereas β-cell glucose sensitivity did not change (Table 4) (i.e., the opposite of the glucose tolerance ranking). As a consequence, bivariate analysis of the whole dataset convincingly showed an independent contribution of BMI and 2-h glucose levels on all manifestations of incretin function (insulin release and β-cell glucose sensitivity [Fig. 4] and GLP-1 response [Fig. 5]). Previous studies (15,16,20,21) of incretin function in obesity have been largely inconclusive. In obese diabetic patients undergoing gastric bypass surgery (37), GLP-1 and GIP release and insulin secretion were enhanced early postoperatively at a time when body weight was unchanged but glycemia was improved. In nondiabetic obese subjects, dietary-induced weight reduction was associated with a small (~9%), albeit statistically significant, increase in the GLP-1 response to a mixed meal (21). All in all, previous studies have not separated out the impact of obesity, per se, from that of hyperglycemia on the incretin effect. Which feature of the obese state is causally related to the incretin defect

remains unknown. Circulating free fatty acids have been suggested to inhibit GLP-1 release and stimulate GIP secretion (19). However, Verdich et al. (21) and Toft-Nielsen et al. (8) did not find a correlation between plasma free fatty acids and GLP-1 response. In pancreatectomized, hyperglycemic rats, both GLP-1 and GIP receptor expression in islets was downregulated (38). Whether a similar phenomenon occurs in spontaneous human diabetes or as a result of obesity is unknown.

Short of changes in splanchnic glucose uptake, the pattern of appearance of orally derived glucose is the integrated result of gastric emptying and intestinal glucose absorption (39), the former being rate limiting. If the release of GLP-1 were delaying gastric emptying (40), as occurs when exogenously GLP-1 is given by constant infusion (41,42), a defective incretin effect should be manifested as accelerated gastric transfer of ingested glucose. However, in the current study, appearance of ingested glucose in the systemic circulation occurred at similar rates and in similar time course in NGT and diabetes despite the largely different incretin effect. There-

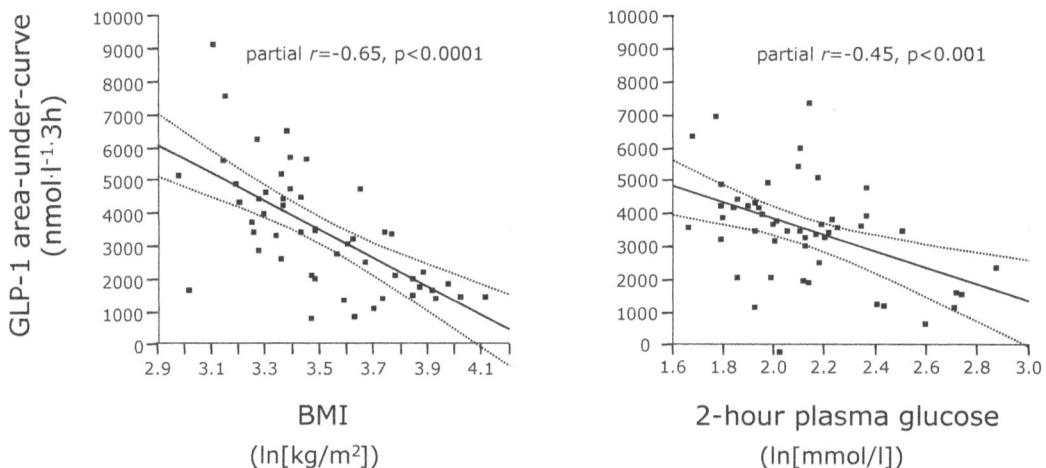

FIG. 5. Dual dependence of plasma GLP-1 response on BMI and 2-h plasma glucose concentrations. The graphs plot the residuals of one independent variable against the other.

fore, we can conclude that during an OGTT, changes in oral glucose appearance (or, at least major detectable differences) are not part of the incretin effect. The positive relation of GLP-1 response to oral glucose appearance (also found by others [23]) is best explained by the fact that the rate of glucose transfer across the intestinal mucosa is a quantitative determinant of the release of gastrointestinal hormones (43). This conclusion is indirectly supported by the observation that dipeptidyl-peptidase intravenous inhibitors, which cause modest increments in endogenous GLP-1 levels, have been shown not to alter gastric emptying (44), whereas the use of GLP-1 analogs delays gastric emptying (45).

In contrast to oral glucose appearance, the observed changes in plasma glucagon concentrations between oral and intravenous glucose administration do imply an incretin effect. In fact, during the early phase of glucose absorption, the oral-to-intravenous ratio of glucagon level was significantly higher in diabetes than in either IGT or NGT. A paradoxical, short-lived rise in glucagon levels following oral glucose has been documented in diabetic patients long ago (46) and has been held responsible for the inappropriately high rate of endogenous glucose production that is seen in diabetes following oral glucose (47) or mixed meals (48). Thus, in agreement with previous data (49), a defective incretin effect on glucagon release may explain, at least in part, the paradoxical hyperglucagonemia of diabetes and participate in the genesis of postprandial hyperglycemia in these patients.

In summary, using the isoglycemic protocol the incretin effect can be described as the glucose-independent stimulation of total insulin secretion, β-cell glucose sensitivity, and GLP-1 and glucagon release induced by oral glucose administration. This complex response is significantly impaired in association with both obesity, per se, and glucose intolerance in an independent and additive manner.

ACKNOWLEDGMENTS

We thank Sara Burchielli and Silvia Pinnola for their technical assistance. Parts of this study were presented in abstract form at the 43rd annual meeting of the European Association for the Study of Diabetes, Amsterdam, the Netherlands, 17–21 September 2007.

REFERENCES

1. Ferrannini E: Insulin resistance versus insulin deficiency in non-insulin-dependent diabetes mellitus: problems and prospects. *Endocr Rev* 19:477–490, 1998
2. Butler AE, Janson J, Bonner-Weir S, Ritzel R, Rizza RA, Butler PC: β-Cell deficit and increased β-cell apoptosis in humans with type 2 diabetes. *Diabetes* 52:102–110, 2003
3. Kahn SE: The relative contributions of insulin resistance and beta-cell dysfunction to the pathophysiology of type 2 diabetes. *Diabetologia* 46:3–19, 2003
4. McIntyre N, Holdsworth CD, Turner DS: Intestinal factors in the control of insulin secretion *J Clin Endocrinol Metab* 25:1317–1324, 1965
5. Perley MJ, Kipnis DM: Plasma insulin responses to oral and intravenous glucose: studies in normal and diabetic subjects. *J Clin Invest* 46:1954–1962, 1967
6. Nauck MA, Homberger E, Eberhard GS, Allen RC, Eaton RP, Ebert R, Creutzfeldt W: Incretin effects of increasing glucose loads in man calculated from venous insulin and C-peptide responses. *J Clin Endocrinol Metab* 63:492–498, 1986
7. Vilsbøll T, Holst JJ: Incretins, insulin secretion and type 2 diabetes mellitus. *Diabetologia* 47:357–366, 2004
8. Toft-Nielsen MB, Damholt MB, Madsbad S, Hilsted LM, Hughes TE, Michelsen BK, Holst JJ: Determinants of the impaired secretion of glucagon-like peptide-1 in type 2 diabetic patients. *J Clin Endocrinol Metab* 86:3717–3723, 2001
9. Vaag AA, Holst JJ, Volund A, Beck-Nielsen HB: Gut incretin hormones in identical twins discordant for non-insulin-dependent diabetes mellitus (NIDDM): evidence for decreased glucagon-like peptide 1 secretion during oral glucose ingestion in NIDDM twins. *Eur J Endocrinol* 135:425–432, 1996
10. Nauck M, Heimesaat MM, Orskov C, Holst JJ, Ebert R, Creutzfeldt W: Preserved incretin activity of glucagon-like peptide 1 [7–36 amide] but not of synthetic human gastric inhibitory polypeptide in patients with type-2 diabetes mellitus. *J Clin Invest* 91:301–307, 1993
11. Nauck M, Stöckmann F, Ebert R, Creutzfeldt W: Reduced incretin effect in type 2 (non-insulin-dependent) diabetes. *Diabetologia* 29:46–52, 1986
12. Zander Mette, Madsbad S, Madsen JL, Holst JJ: Effect of 6-week course of glucagon-like peptide 1 on glycaemic control, insulin sensitivity, and beta-cell function in type 2 diabetes: a parallel-group study. *Lancet* 359:824–830, 2002
13. Creutzfeldt W: The entero-insular axis in type 2 diabetes: incretins as therapeutic agents. *Exp Clin Endocrinol Diabetes* 109 (Suppl. 2):S288–S303, 2001
14. Ferrannini E, Natali A, Bell P, Cavallo-Perin P, Lalic N, Mingrone G: Insulin resistance and hypersecretion in obesity: European Group for the Study of Insulin Resistance (EGIR). *J Clin Invest* 100:1166–1173, 1997
15. Heptulla RA, Tamborlane WV, Cavaghan M, Bronson M, Limb C, Ma YZ, Sherwin RS, Caprio S: Augmentation of alimentary insulin secretion despite similar gastric inhibitory peptide (GIP) responses in juvenile obesity. *Pediatr Res* 47:628–633, 2000
16. Lauritsen KB, Christensen KC, Stokholm KH: Gastric inhibitory polypeptide (GIP) release and incretin effect after oral glucose in obesity and after jejunoileal bypass. *Scand J Gastroenterol* 15:489–495, 1980
17. Vilsbøll T, Krarup J, Sonne S, Madsbad A, Vølund A, Juul AG, Holst JJ: Incretin secretion in relation to meal size and body weight in healthy subjects and people with type 1 and type 2 diabetes mellitus. *J Clin Endocrinol Metab* 88:2706–2713, 2005
18. Salera M, Giacomoni P, Cornia G, Capelli M, Marini A, Benfenatti F, Miglioli M, Barbara LG: Gastric inhibitory polypeptide release after oral glucose: relationship to glucose intolerance, diabetes mellitus, and obesity. *J Clin Endocrinol Metab* 55:329–336, 1982
19. Ranganath LR, Beety JM, Morgan LM, Wright JW, Howland R, Marks V: Attenuated GLP-1 secretion in obesity: cause or consequence? *Gut* 38:916–919, 1996
20. Lugari R, Dei Cas A, Ugolotti D, Barilli AL, Camellini C, Ganzerla GC, Luciani A, Salerni B, Mittenperger F, Nodari S, Gnudi A, Zandomeneghi R: Glucagon-like peptide 1 (GLP-1) secretion and plasma dipeptidyl peptidase IV (DPP-IV) activity in morbidly obese patients undergoing biliopancreatic diversion. *Horm Metab Res* 36:111–115, 2004
21. Verdich C, Toubro S, Buemann B, Madsen JL, Holst JJ, Astrup A: The role of postprandial releases of insulin and incretin hormones in meal-induced satiety-effect of obesity and weight reduction. *Int J Obes Relat Metab Disord* 25:1206–1214, 2001
22. Muscelli E, Mari A, Natali A, Astiarraga BD, Camastra S, Frascerra S, Holst JJ, Ferrannini E: Impact of incretin hormones on beta-cell function in subjects with normal or impaired glucose tolerance. *Am J Physiol Endocrinol Metab* 291:E1144–E1150, 2006
23. Watchers-Hagedoorn RE, Priebe MG, Heimweg JAJ, Heiner AM, Englyst KN, Holst JJ, Stellaard F: The rate of intestinal glucose absorption is correlated with plasma glucose-dependent insulinotropic polypeptide concentrations in healthy men. *J Nutr* 136:1511–1516, 2006
24. Jebb SA, Cole TJ, Doman D, Murgatroyd PR, Prentice AM: Evaluation of the Tanita body-fat analyser to measure body composition by comparison with a four-compartment model. *Br J Nutr* 83:115–122, 2000
25. American Diabetes Association: Report of the Expert Committee on Diagnosis and Classification of Diabetes Mellitus (Position Statement). *Diabetes Care* 20:1183–1197, 1997
26. Gastaldelli A, Casolaro A, Pettiti M, Nannipieri M, Ciociaro D, Frascerra S, Buzzigoli E, Baldi S, Mari A, Ferrannini E: Effect of pioglitazone on the metabolic and hormonal response to a mixed meal in type II diabetes. *Clin Pharmacol Ther* 81:205–212, 2007
27. Hvidberg A, Nielsen MT, Hilstead J, Ørskov C, Holst JJ: Effect of glucagon-like peptide-1 (proglucagon 78–107 amide) on hepatic glucose production in healthy man. *Metabolism* 43:104–108, 1994
28. Ørskov C, Rabenhøj L, Wettergren A, Kofod H, Holst JJ: Tissue and plasma concentrations of amidated and glycine-extended glucagon-like peptide 1 in humans. *Diabetes* 43:535–539, 1994
29. Deacon CF, Nauck MA, Meier J, Hücking J, Holst JJ: Degradation of endogenous and exogenous gastric inhibitory polypeptide in healthy and in

type 2 diabetic subjects as revealed using a new assay for the intact peptide. *J Clin Endocrinol Metab* 85:3575–3581, 2000

30. Mari A, Pacini G, Murphy E, Ludvik B, Nolan JJ: A model-based method for assessing insulin sensitivity from the oral glucose tolerance test. *Diabetes Care* 24:539–548, 2001

31. Mari A, Schmitz O, Gastaldelli A, Oestergaard T, Nyholm B, Ferrannini E: Meal and oral glucose tests for assessment of β-cell action: modeling analysis in normal subjects. *Am J Physiol Endocrinol Metab* 283:E1159–E1166, 2002

32. Van Cauter E, Mestrez F, Sturis J, Polonsky KS: Estimation of insulin secretion rates from C-peptide levels: comparison of individual and standard kinetic parameters for C-peptide clearance. *Diabetes* 41:368–377, 1992

33. Nyholm B, Walker M, Gravholt CH, Shearing PA, Sturis J, Alberti KG, Holst JJ, Schmitz O: Twenty-four-hour insulin secretion rates, circulating concentrations of fuel substrates and gut incretin hormones in healthy offspring of type II (non-insulin-dependent) diabetic parents: evidence of several aberrations. *Diabetologia* 42:1314–1323, 1999

34. Nauck MA, El-Ouaghlidi A, Gabris B, Hücking K, Holst JJ, Deacon CF, Gallwitz B, Schmidt WE, Meier JJ: Secretion of incretin hormones (GIP and GLP-1) and incretin effect after oral glucose in first-degree relatives of patients with type 2 diabetes. *Regul Pept* 122:209–217, 2004

35. Knop FK, Visboll T, Hojberg PV, Larsen S, Madsbad S, Volund A, Holst JJ, Krarup T: Reduced incretin effect in type 2 diabetes: cause or consequence of the diabetic state? *Diabetes* 56:1951–1959, 2007

36. Hojberg PV, Zander M, Vilsboll T, Knop FK, Krarup T, Holst JJ, Madsbad S: Effect of 4 weeks of near normalization of blood glucose on β-cell sensitivity to glucose and GLP-1 in type 2 diabetic patients (Abstract). *Diabetes* 54 (Suppl. 1):A362, 2005

37. Laferrère B, Hesha S, Wang K, Khan Y, McGinty J, Teixeira J, Hart AB, Olivan B: Incretin levels and effect are markedly enhanced 1 month after Roux-en-Y gastric bypass surgery in obese patients with type 2 diabetes. *Diabetes Care* 30:1709–1716, 2007

38. Hu G, Kaneto H, Laybutt DR, Duvivier-Kali VF, Trivedi N, Suzuma K, King GL, Weir GC, Bonner-Weir S: Downregulation of GLP-1 and GIP receptor expression by hyperglycemia: possible contribution to impaired incretin effects in diabetes. *Diabetes* 56:1551–1558, 2007

39. DeFronzo RA, Ferrannini E: Regulation of hepatic glucose metabolism in humans. *Diabetes Metab Rev* 3:415–459, 1987

40. Wishart JM, Horowitz M, Morris AH, Jones KL, Nauck MA: Relation between gastric emptying of glucose and plasma concentrations of glucagon-like peptide-1. *Peptides* 19:1049–1053, 1998

41. Naslund E, Bogefors J, Skogar S, Gryback P, Jacobsson H, Holst JJ, Hellstrom PM: GLP-1 slows solid gastric emptying and inhibits insulin, glucagon, and PYY release in humans. *Am J Physiol* 277:R910–R916, 1999

42. Meier JJ, Gethmann A, Götze O, Gallwitz B, Holst JJ, Schmidt WE, Nauck MA: Glucagon-like peptide 1 abolishes the postprandial rise in triglyceride concentrations and lowers levels of non-esterified fatty acids in humans. *Diabetologia* 49:452–458, 2006

43. Schirra J, Katschinski M, Weidmann C, Schäfer T, Wank U, Arnold R, Göke B: Gastric emptying and release of incretin hormones after glucose ingestion in humans. *J Clin Invest* 97:92–10, 1996

44. Vella A, Bock G, Giesler PD, Burton DB, Serra DB, Saylan ML, Dunning BE, Foley JE, Rizza RA, Camilleri M: Effects of dipeptidyl peptidase-4 inhibition on gastrointestinal function, meal appearance, and glucose metabolism in type 2 diabetes. *Diabetes* 56:1475–1480, 2007

45. Kolterman OG, Buse JB, Fineman MS, Gaines E, Heintz S, Bicsak TA, Taylor K, Kim D, Aisporna M, Wang Y, Baron AD: Synthetic exendin-4 (exenatide) significantly reduces postprandial and fasting plasma glucose in subjects with type 2 diabetes. *J Clin Endocrinol Metab* 88:3082–3089, 2003

46. Muller WA, Faloona GR, Aguilar-Parada E, Unger RH: Abnormal alpha-cell function in diabetes: response to carbohydrate and protein ingestion. *N Engl J Med* 283:109–115, 1970

47. Ferrannini E, Simonson DC, Katz LD, Reichard G Jr, Bevilacqua S, Barrett EJ, Olsson M, DeFronzo RA: The disposal of an oral glucose load in patients with non-insulin-dependent diabetes. *Metabolism* 37:79–85, 1988

48. Firth RG, Bell PM, Marsh HM, Hansen I, Rizza RA: Postprandial hyperglycemia in patients with noninsulin-dependent diabetes mellitus: role of hepatic and extrahepatic tissues. *J Clin Invest* 77:1525–1532, 1986

49. Knop FK, Vilsbøll T, Madsbad S, Holst JJ, Krarup T: Inappropriate suppression of glucagon during OGTT but not during isoglycaemic i.v. glucose infusion contributes to the reduced incretin effect in type 2 diabetes mellitus. *Diabetologia* 50:797–805, 2007

Gpr40 Is Expressed in Enteroendocrine Cells and Mediates Free Fatty Acid Stimulation of Incretin Secretion

Sara Edfalk, Pär Steneberg, and Helena Edlund

OBJECTIVE—The G-protein–coupled receptor *Gpr40* is expressed in β-cells where it contributes to free fatty acid (FFA) enhancement of glucose-stimulated insulin secretion (1–4). However, other sites of *Gpr40* expression, including the intestine, have been suggested. The transcription factor IPF1/PDX1 was recently shown to bind to an enhancer element within the 5′-flanking region of *Gpr40* (5), implying that IPF1/PDX1 might regulate *Gpr40* expression. Here, we addressed whether *1)* *Gpr40* is expressed in the intestine and *2)* *Ipf1/Pdx1* function is required for *Gpr40* expression.

RESEARCH DESIGN AND METHODS—In the present study, *Gpr40* expression was monitored by X-gal staining using *Gpr40* reporter mice and by in situ hybridization. *Ipf1/Pdx1*-null and β-cell specific mutants were used to investigate whether *Ipf1/Pdx1* controls *Gpr40* expression. Plasma insulin, glucose-dependent insulinotropic polypeptide (GIP), glucagon-like peptide-1 (GLP-1), and glucose levels in response to acute oral fat diet were determined in *Gpr40* mutant and control mice.

RESULTS—Here, we show that *Gpr40* is expressed in endocrine cells of the gastrointestinal tract, including cells expressing the incretin hormones GLP-1 and GIP, and that *Gpr40* mediates FFA-stimulated incretin secretion. We also show that *Ipf1/Pdx1* is required for expression of *Gpr40* in β-cells and endocrine cells of the anterior gastrointestinal tract.

CONCLUSIONS—Together, our data provide evidence that *Gpr40* modulates FFA-stimulated insulin secretion from β-cells not only directly but also indirectly via regulation of incretin secretion. Moreover, our data suggest a conserved role for *Ipf1/Pdx1* and Gpr40 in FFA-mediated secretion of hormones that regulate glucose and overall energy homeostasis. ***Diabetes* 57:2280–2287, 2008**

Mature β-cells respond to elevated glucose levels by secreting insulin in a tightly controlled manner. The physiological response of the β-cell to elevated blood glucose levels is critical for maintenance of normoglycemia, and impaired glucose-stimulated insulin secretion (GSIS) is a prominent feature of overt type 2 diabetes. Although glucose is recognized as the major stimulator of insulin secretion from β-cells, other stimuli, such as amino acids, hormones, and free fatty acids (FFAs), also influence insulin secretion (6,7). Thus, under normal settings, insulin secretion from β-cells in response to food intake is evoked by the collective stimuli of nutrients, such as glucose, amino acids, and FFAs, and hormones like the incretins glucagon-like peptide-1 (GLP-1) and glucose-dependent insulinotropic polypeptide (GIP) (6,7).

FFAs are known to influence insulin secretion from β-cells primarily by enhancing GSIS. The FFA receptor Gpr40 is preferentially expressed in β-cells and is activated by medium- to long-chain FFAs, thereby triggering a signaling cascade that results in increased levels of $[Ca^{2+}]_i$ in β-cell lines and subsequent stimulation of insulin secretion (1,3,8). *Gpr40*-deficient β-cells secrete less insulin in response to FFAs, providing evidence that Gpr40 mediates part of the FFA stimulatory effect on insulin secretion (2,4). However, loss of *Gpr40* protects mice from obesity-induced hyperglycemia, glucose intolerance, hyperinsulinemia, fatty liver development, increased hepatic glucose output, and hypertriglyceridemia (2). These data provide evidence that FFA stimulation of insulin secretion via Gpr40 contributes to obesity-induced hyperinsulinemia, which in turn is linked to fatty liver development and hepatic insulin resistance.

Lipids and FFAs also stimulate the secretion of several gut "satiety" hormones, including cholocystokinine (CCK), GLP1, and peptide YY (PYY), and the related FFA receptor Gpr120 has been suggested to mediate FFA-stimulated secretion of GLP-1 from L-cells (9). In addition, stimulation of the G-protein–coupled receptor Gpr119, the ligands of which are phospholipids and fatty acid amides, have also been shown to result in increased GLP-1 and GIP secretion (10). RT-PCR analyses have suggested that *Gpr40* is expressed in the intestine, leaving open a potential role also for Gpr40 in FFA stimulation of gut hormones (1,11).

The transcription factor IPF1/PDX1 is highly expressed in β-cells and controls key aspects of β-cell function by regulating the expression of genes involved in glucose sensing, insulin gene expression, and insulin secretion (12–14). Loss or perturbation of *Ipf1/Pdx1* function in β-cells leads to impaired GSIS and consequently diabetes or glucose intolerance in both mice and humans (12,15), highlighting the central role for *Ipf1/Pdx1* in ensuring β-cell function. Recently, IPF1/PDX1 has been shown to bind to an enhancer element within the 5′-flanking region of *Gpr40* (5), implying that *Ipf1/Pdx1* might regulate *Gpr40* expression in β-cells and thus FFA-mediated stimulation of insulin secretion.

To determine whether *Gpr40* is expressed in the intestine and whether *Ipf1/Pdx1* function is required for *Gpr40* expression, we investigated the expression of *Gpr40* in

From the Umeå Center for Molecular Medicine, University of Umeå, Umeå, Sweden.
Corresponding author: Helena Edlund, helena.edlund@ucmm.umu.se.
Received 3 March 2008 and accepted 27 May 2008.
Published ahead of print at http://diabetes.diabetesjournals.org on 2 June 2008. DOI: 10.2337/db08-0307.
P.S. and H.E. are joint senior authors of this work.

wild-type and *Ipf1/Pdx1* mutant mice. Here, we show that *Gpr40* is expressed in endocrine cells of gastrointestinal tract, including cells expressing the incretin hormones GLP-1 and GIP. We also show that *Ipf1/Pdx1* is required for *Gpr40* expression in β-cells and endocrine cells of the anterior gastrointestinal tract. Moreover, we show that secretion of GLP-1 and GIP is diminished in *Gpr40*-null mutant mice. Together, these data raise the possibility that *Gpr40* modulates FFA-stimulated insulin secretion from β-cells not only directly but also indirectly via regulation of incretin secretion.

RESEARCH DESIGN AND METHODS

The animal studies were approved by the Institutional Animal Care and Use Committee of Umeå University and conducted in accordance with the Guidelines for the Care and Use of Laboratory Animals. The generation of *Gpr40*⁺/ᴸᵃᶜᶻ, *Ipf1/Pdx1*⁻/⁻, and *Rip1/Ipf1*Δ have been previously described (2,12,16). Briefly, *Gpr40*⁺/ᴸᵃᶜᶻ mice were generated by replacing the *Gpr40* open reading frame with the *lacZ* gene encoding β-galactosidase (β-gal). In *Ipf1/Pdx1*⁻/⁻-null mice, exon 2, encoding the DNA-binding homeodomain, was deleted. The *Rip1/Ipf1*Δ mice are generated by breeding mice in which exon 2 of the *Ipf1/Pdx1* gene is flanked by two loxP sites with mice where the Cre-recombinase is under the control of *Rat insulin 1* (*Rip1*) promoter. In the resulting *Rip1/Ipf1*Δ mice, exon 2 of *Ipf1/Pdx1* becomes out-recombined specifically in β-cells as a consequence of Cre-recombinase expression and activity.

Glucose, insulin, GIP, GLP-1, glucagon, FFA, and triglyceride measurements. Intraperitoneal glucose tolerance tests were performed on overnight-fasted, sedated mice essentially as previously described (2). For oral glucose tolerance test, 300 μl 20% glucose solution was administered to overnight-fasted, sedated mice. For the acute, high-fat diet experiments, a paste was generated by mixing 7.5 g diet D12309 (58% kcal fat content; Research Diets) with 3 ml tap water, and 300 mg paste was then administered by oral gavage to overnight-fasted, sedated mice. Blood glucose levels were measured using a Glucometer Elite (Bayer), serum insulin levels were measured using ELISA (Mercodia), and total plasma GIP and GLP-1 concentrations were determined according to the manufacturer's instructions for the GIP-ELISA (EZRMGIP-55K; Linco Research) and the GLP-1-RIA (GLP1T-36HK; Linco Research) kit. Plasma glucagon levels were determined using the Glucagon RIA kit (GL-32K; Linco Research). FFA and triglyceride measurements were done according to the manufacturer's instructions using FFAs, Half-micro test (Roche), and Accutrend GCT Triglycerides (Roche).

In situ hybridizations, X-gal staining, and immunohistochemistry. In situ hybridization using DIG-labeled probes specific for the mouse *Gpr40* transcript was carried out on embryonic day (e) 17 embryos as previously described (2). Immunohistochemical localization of antigens, double-label immunohistochemistry, and X-gal staining on tissues and confocal microscopy were carried out as previously described (2). Primary antibodies used were rabbit anti–β-gal (Cappel), chicken anti–β-gal (AbCam), rabbit anti-GIP (Peninsula), rabbit anti–GLP-1 (Peninsula), guinea pig anti-gastrin (Euro Diagnostics), goat anti-ghrelin (Santa Cruz Biotechnology), rabbit anti-CCK (Chemicon), rabbit anti-secretin, rabbit anti-substance P, rabbit anti-PYY, rabbit anti-neuropeptide 4 (NPY), rabbit anti-serotonin (Euro-Diagnostica), rabbit anti-somatostatin (Dako), and rabbit anti-Ipf1 (17). Secondary antibodies used were Alexa 488 anti-goat, Alexa 488 anti–guinea pig, Alexa 594 anti–guinea pig, Alexa 594 anti-rabbit, Alexa 594 anti-goat (all from Molecular Probe), Cy3 anti-rabbit, and fluorescein isothiocyanate (FITC) anti-chicken (The Jackson Laboratories). The gut hormone and *Gpr40* expression analyses were performed on 2- to 3-month-old mice. For the antibody cocktail experiment, we made a two-step staining procedure: The tissue sections was first incubated with a mixture of antibodies directed against GIP, GLP-1, ghrelin, CCK, and gastrin, and for these, the corresponding Alexa 594-fluorochrome secondary antibodies were used. Next, the tissue sections were incubated with antibodies directed against β-gal for which a FITC-conjugated secondary antibody was used.

Cell counting. Pylorus and the three proximal centimetres of small intestine corresponding to the duodenum and part of the jejunum were isolated from wild-type, *Gpr40*⁺/ᴸᵃᶜᶻ, and *Gpr40*ᴸᵃᶜᶻ/ᴸᵃᶜᶻ (*n* = 3) nonfasted mice, fixed in 4% paraformaldehyde at 4°C for 1–2 h, cryoprotected in 30% sucrose at 4°C overnight, frozen in Tissue-Tek (Sakura), and kept at −80°C. Three 8-μm-thick sections where collected on every slide with ~160 μm between sections. The sections of pylorus/duodenum were stained with antibodies against GIP, GLP-1, ghrelin, CCK, gastrin, PYY, secretin, serotonin, substance P, and β-gal and manually analyzed for distribution and colocalization of the different

markers. Colocalization between β-gal and GLP-1 was also determined in the distal 3 cm of the ileum, i.e., close to the appendix, in *Gpr40*⁺/ᴸᵃᶜᶻ mice.

Quantification of mRNA expression levels. cDNA was prepared from total RNA isolated from islets (18) and from e16 pylorus/duodenum and the distal part of the ileum using NucleoSpin RNAII-kit (635990; Machery-Nagel) and Super SMART PCR (635000; Clontech). Quantitative real-time PCR analysis was performed using the ABI PRISM 7000 Sequence Detection System and SYBR Green PCR Master Mix (ABI) according to the manufacturer's recommendations. Expression of the β-2-microglobulin (*β2M*), TATA-box–binding protein (*TBP*), *β-actin*, and glyceraldehyde-3-phosphate dehydrogenase (*Gapdh*) genes was used to normalize expression levels. Primer sequences were as follows: *β-actin*, 5′-GCTCTGGCTCCTAGCACCAT-3′ and 5′-GCCACCGATCCACACAGAGT-3′; *Gapdh*, 5′-CGTGTTCCTACCCCCAATGT-3′ and 5′-TGTCATCATACTTGGCAG GTTTCT-3′; *β2M*, 5′-GCTATCCAGAAAACCCCTCAAA-3′ and 5′-CTGTGTTAC GTAGCAGTTCAGTATGTTC-3′; *TBP*, 5′-GAATTGTACCGCAGCTTCAAAA-3′ and 5′-AGTGCAATGGTCTTTAGGTCAAGTT; *Ipf1/Pdx1*, 5′-TAGGACTCTTTCCTG GGACCAA-3′ and 5′-AATAAAAAGGGTACAAACTTGAGCGT-3′; and *Gpr40*, 5′-TTTCATAAACCCGGACCTAGGA-3′ and 5′-CCAGTGACCAGTGGGTTGAGT-3′.

Statistical analyses were performed by an unpaired Student's *t* test.

RESULTS

***Gpr40* is expressed in cells of the gastrointestinal tract.** *Gpr40* has been suggested to be expressed at other sites than β-cells, including in the intestine (1,11). However, these *Gpr40* expression studies build on RT-PCR analyses, and because the coding region of *Gpr40* lacks an intron, contaminating genomic DNA might give false positives in PCR analyses. To avoid such problems, we previously made use of the *lacZ* reporter gene insertion into the *Gpr40* locus of targeted *Gpr40*⁺/ᴸᵃᶜᶻ mice and showed that *Gpr40* is not expressed in brain, liver, muscle, or adipose tissue (2). We therefore extended our analyses of *Gpr40* expression using the *Gpr40*⁺/ᴸᵃᶜᶻ mice to elucidate whether *Gpr40* is expressed in the gastrointestinal tract. Distinct X-gal staining was evident in scattered epithelial cells of the gastric pylorus, duodenum, jejunum, ileum, and colon (Fig. 1*A*). The expression of *Gpr40* in the epithelium of the stomach and intestine was evident from e14.5–e15 (data not shown), i.e., coincident with the appearance of differentiated endocrine cells of the gastrointestinal tract. The expression of *Gpr40* in pylorus and duodenum was confirmed by in situ hybridization analyses using a *Gpr40* riboprobe (Fig. 1*B*). Together, these data demonstrate that *Gpr40* is expressed in scattered cells distributed throughout the gastrointestinal tract.

The *Gpr40*⁺ cells of the gastrointestinal tract represent enteroendocrine cells. To determine the identity of the gastrointestinal cells expressing *Gpr40*, we next performed double immunohistochemical analyses of the epithelium of the gastric pylorus, duodenum, and ileum in 2- to 3-month-old mice using anti–β-gal antibodies and antibodies specific for different gastrointestinal hormones. The β-gal⁺, i.e., *Gpr40*⁺, cells were shown to express a wide variety of endocrine hormones. In the pylorus and duodenum, β-gal/*Gpr40* expression colocalized with gastrin, GIP, GLP-1, ghrelin, CCK, PYY, secretin, serotonin, and substance P expression; and in the ileum, β-gal/*Gpr40* expression colocalized predominantly with that of GLP-1 (Fig. 1*C*; data not shown). In contrast, no coexpression of β-gal/*Gpr40* and somatostatin or NPY was observed (data not shown). The degree of β-gal/*Gpr40* expression varied between ~20 and 55% for the different gastrin, GIP, GLP-1, ghrelin, CCK, PYY, secretin, and serotonin hormone-expressing cells (Table 1), and <1% of the substance P⁺ cells expressed β-gal/*Gpr40* (data not shown). However, immunohistochemical analyses using a cocktail of gut hormone antibodies, including GIP, GLP-1, ghrelin, CCK, and gastrin and β-gal antibodies, revealed that virtually all β-gal/

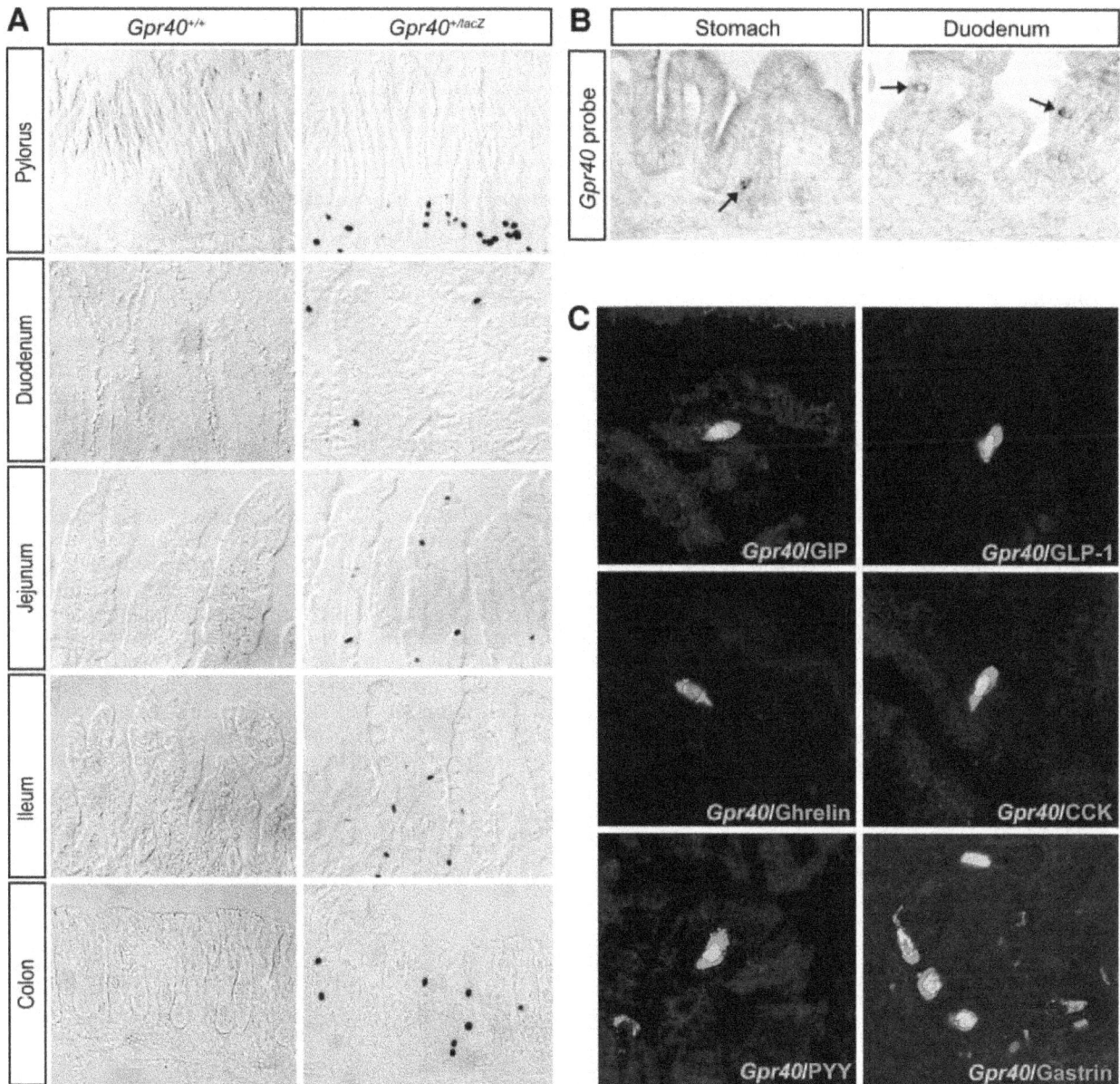

FIG. 1. *Gpr40* is expressed in gut enteroendocrine cells. *A*: X-gal staining of sections of pylorus, duodenum, jejunum, ileum, and colon in 2-month-old *Gpr40*[+/+] and *Gpr40*[+/lacZ] mice. *B*: In situ hybridization using *Gpr40*-specific probes on sections of neonatal epithelium in stomach and duodenum. Arrows indicate cells expressing *Gpr40* mRNA. *C*: Confocal sections of 2- to 3-month-old adult *Gpr40*[+/lacZ] pylorus and duodenum stained with anti–β-gal antibodies (green) to indicate *Gpr40* expression and antibodies specific for the indicated enteroendocrine hormones (red). (Please see http://dx.doi.org/10.2337/db08-0307 for a high-quality digital representation of this figure.)

Gpr40-expressing cells were hormone positive (data not shown). The distribution and number of enteroendocrine cells were normal in *Gpr40*[lacZ/lacZ] mice (Table 2; data not shown). Thus, *Gpr40* is expressed both in insulin-producing β-cells and hormone-producing cells of the gastrointestinal tract.

Impaired secretion of GIP and GLP-1 in *Gpr40*-null mutants. GIP and GLP-1 hormones are secreted from the intestinal K- and L-cells, respectively (19), and the secretion of GIP and GLP-1 hormones can be stimulated both by glucose and FFAs (20,21). The secretion of GLP-1 and GIP hormones into the circulation positively influences insulin

TABLE 1
Coexpression of gut hormones and *Gpr40*

Gastrin	GIP	GLP-1	Ghrelin	CCK	PYY	Secretin	Serotonin
52 ± 0.6	50 ± 5	55 ± 5	34 ± 3	50 ± 1	21 ± 2	30 ± 4	19 ± 3

Data are percentage of hormone-expressing cells coexpressing β-gal/*Gpr40*. Sections of pylorus (gastrin) and duodenum (GIP, GLP-1, ghrelin, CCK, PYY, secretin, and serotonin) from 2- to 3-month-old *Gpr40*[+/lacZ] mice ($n = 3$) were double stained for gut hormones and β-gal.

TABLE 2
Gut hormone-expressing cells in $Gpr40^{lacZ/lacZ}$ mice

	GIP	GLP-1	Ghrelin	CCK	Gastrin
$Gpr40^{+/+}$	490 ± 113	279 ± 38	1,114 ± 249	492 ± 40	689 ± 20
$Gpr40^{lacZ/lacZ}$	530 ± 45	246 ± 36	1,040 ± 171	383 ± 81	754 ± 52
t test	0.63	0.18	0.29	0.87	0.46

Data are n. Hormone-expressing cells were counted on sections from pylorus (gastrin) and duodenum (GIP, GLP-1, ghrelin, and CCK) in 2- to 3-month-old $Gpr40^{+/+}$ ($n = 3$) and $Gpr40^{lacZ/lacZ}$ ($n = 3$) mice.

secretion. This so-called incretin effect is evident when comparing oral and intravenous or intraperitoneal administration of glucose; oral glucose administration triggers a more robust insulin secretory response (19). The expression of *Gpr40* in both GIP-and GLP-1–expressing cells leaves open the possibility that Gpr40 may affect insulin secretion not only directly by virtue of its expression in β-cells, but also indirectly via regulation of incretin secretion. Consistent with the FFA but not glucose responsiveness of Gpr40, no difference in glucose clearance rates or insulin secretion was observed between $Gpr40^{lacZ/lacZ}$ and wild-type mice, regardless of whether glucose was administered orally or injected in the peritoneum (Fig. 2A–D).

We next explored the glucose and insulin response to acute, oral administration of high-fat diet in $Gpr40^{lacZ/lacZ}$ and wild-type mice. Plasma levels of FFAs, triglycerides, and glucagon were similar in oral high-fat diet–treated $Gpr40^{lacZ/lacZ}$ and wild-type mice (Supplementary Fig. 1 available in an online appendix at http://dx.doi.org/10.2337/db08-0307). In contrast, plasma insulin levels were reduced and blood glucose levels were increased at 60 min

in $Gpr40^{lacZ/lacZ}$ compared with that of wild-type mice in response to oral high-fat diet (Fig. 3A and B), suggesting that incretin secretion in response to fat might be impaired in $Gpr40^{lacZ/lacZ}$ mice. Analyses of incretin levels after oral high-fat diet showed that total plasma GIP levels were reduced at 30 and 60 min and total plasma GLP-1 levels were reduced at 60 min compared with that of wild types (Fig. 3C and D). In contrast, no difference in total GIP or GLP-1 levels were observed at 30 or 60 min after oral glucose administration (Supplementary Fig. 2). Taken together, these data provide evidence for a role for Gpr40 in FFA-mediated secretion of the incretins GIP and GLP-1.

Ipf1/Pdx1 is required for the expression of *Gpr40* in β-cells. Recent data show that the transcription factor IPF1/PDX1 can bind to an enhancer element within the *Gpr40* 5′-flanking region (5), leaving open the possibility that IPF1/PDX1 might regulate *Gpr40* expression. *Ipf1/Pdx1*-null mutant mice fail to form a pancreas and thus die at the neonatal stage (16), precluding any analyses of a role for IPF1/PDX1 in the regulation of *Gpr40* expression in β-cells. We have, however, previously generated β-cell–

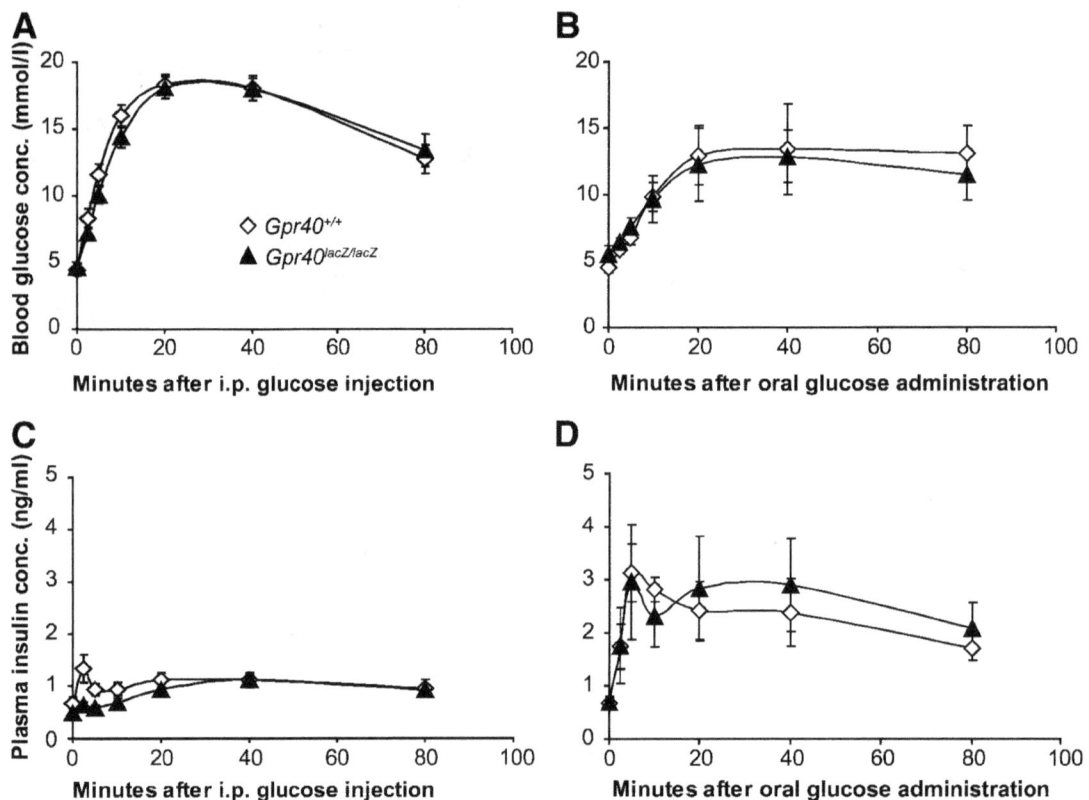

FIG. 2. Oral glucose tolerance is normal in $Gpr40^{lacZ/lacZ}$ mice. Blood glucose (*A* and *B*) and plasma insulin (*C* and *D*) levels in 2- to 3-month-old $Gpr40^{+/+}$ (◇) and $Gpr40^{lacZ/lacZ}$ (▲) mice after intraperitoneal glucose injections (*A* and *C*) and oral glucose administration (*B* and *D*). $Gpr40^{+/+}$ ($n = 16$) and $Gpr40^{lacZ/lacZ}$ ($n = 16$) for the intraperitoneal glucose injections. $Gpr40^{+/+}$ ($n = 6$) and $Gpr40^{lacZ/lacZ}$ ($n = 5$) for the oral glucose administration test.

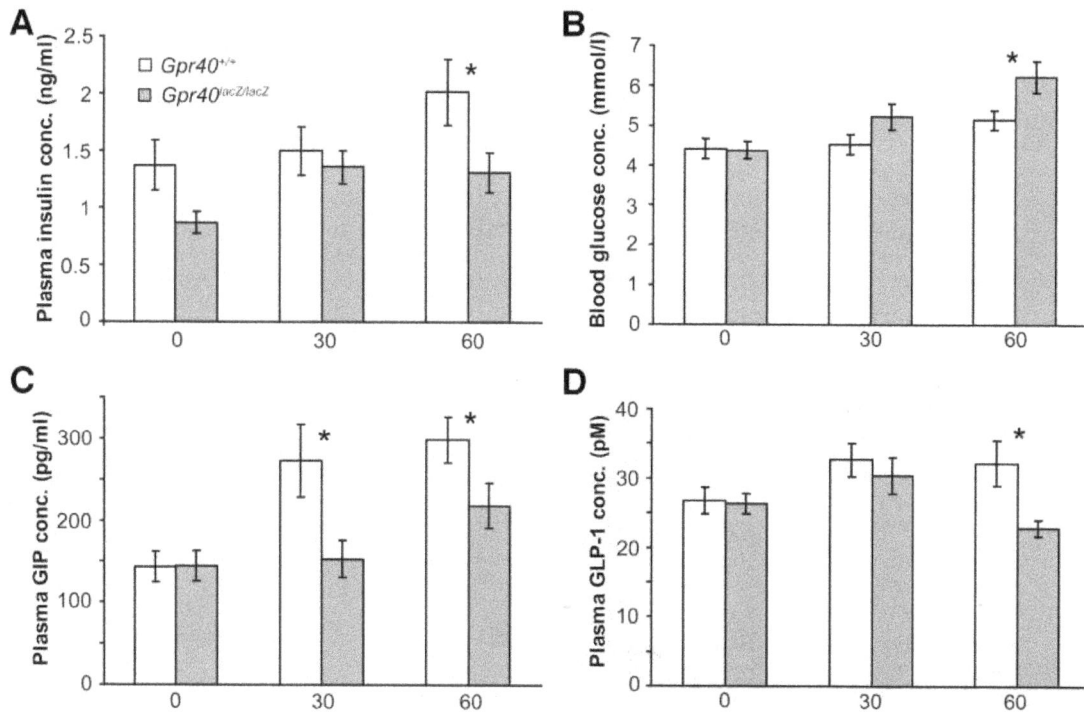

FIG. 3. Reduced plasma levels of GIP and GLP-1 in *Gpr40^{lacZ/lacZ}* mice in response to fat diet. Plasma insulin, GIP (total), GLP-1 (total), and blood glucose levels (*A–D*) were determined in 2- to 3-month-old *Gpr40^{+/+}* (*n* = 10–16, □) and *Gpr40^{lacZ/lacZ}* (*n* = 8–20, ▧) mice after oral high-fat diet administration. *x*-axis indicates minutes after oral gavage. Data are means ± SE. *$P < 0.05$ for *Gpr40^{+/+}* vs. *Gpr40^{lacZ/lacZ}*.

specific *Ipf1/Pdx1* mutants, denoted *RIP/Ipf1^Δ* mice, using the Cre-LoxP system (12). The conditional inactivation of *Ipf1/Pdx1* in β-cells of *RIP/Ipf1^Δ* mice results in β-cell dysfunction due to reduced expression of key β-cell components, including insulin, glucose transporter type 2, and PC1/3, and the mice consequently show severely impaired insulin secretion and develop diabetes (12). To elucidate whether *Gpr40* expression was regulated by *Ipf1/Pdx1* in adult β-cells, we bred the *Gpr40^{+/lacZ}* allele into the *RIP/Ipf1^Δ* background. The *Gpr40^{+/lacZ}* mice carry the *lacZ* gene targeted into the *Gpr40* locus, thus allowing monitoring of *Gpr40* expression by X-gal staining. In *RIP/Ipf1^Δ* mice, the conditional inactivation of the *Ipf1/Pdx1* gene in β-cells occurs progressively after birth, and the mice develop overt diabetes when *Ipf1/Pdx1* has been inactivated in ~80% of the β-cells (12).

In 5-week-old *Ipf1/Pdx1^{+/+}*;*Gpr40^{+/lacZ}* control mice, strong, uniform X-gal staining was observed in the β-cells (Fig. 4*A*). In contrast, the majority of the β-cells in islets of age-matched, glucose-intolerant but not overt diabetic *RIP/Ipf1^Δ*;*Gpr40^{+/lacZ}* mice were X-gal⁻, providing evidence that conditional inactivation of *Ipf1/Pdx1* in β-cells results in a loss of *Gpr40* expression (Fig. 4*A*). Quantitative RT-PCR of cDNA prepared from islets confirmed the decreased expression of *Gpr40* in β-cells of *RIP/Ipf1^Δ* mice and showed that *Gpr40* expression was reduced to a similar extent to that of *Ipf1/Pdx1* in isolated islets (Fig. 4*B*). Together, these data provide evidence that *Ipf1/Pdx1* (directly or indirectly) is required for *Gpr40* expression in β-cells.

Gpr40 expression in endocrine cells of the anterior gastrointestinal tract requires *Ipf1/Pdx1*. Apart from β-cells, IPF1/PDX1 is expressed also in hormone-producing cells of the gastric pylorus and duodenum, where it has been shown to be required for the expression of several hormones (22). The similar expression profiles observed

for IPF1/PDX1 and *Gpr40* raised the possibility that the expression of *Gpr40* in endocrine cells of the anterior gastrointestinal tract, like that in β-cells, is dependent on *Ipf1/Pdx1*. To explore a potential role for IPF1/PDX1 in regulating *Gpr40* expression, we bred the *Gpr40^{+/lacZ}* allele into the *Ipf1/Pdx1*-null mutant (16) background and analyzed the intestinal expression of *Gpr40* by X-gal staining. Because *Ipf1/Pdx1*-null mutants die at the neonatal stage, *Gpr40* expression analyses were performed on late-stage, embryonic gastrointestinal tissue. In contrast to control *Ipf1/Pdx1^{+/+}*;*Gpr40^{+/lacZ}* mice, no X-gal⁺, i.e., *Gpr40*-expressing, cells were observed in the gastric pylorus and duodenum of *Ipf1/Pdx1^{-/-}*;*Gpr40^{+/lacZ}* embryos (Fig. 5*A*). Quantitative RT-PCR on cDNA isolated from the gastric pylorus and duodenum of wild-type and *Ipf1/Pdx1^{-/-}* embryos confirmed that expression of *Gpr40* in these regions of the gastrointestinal tract is dependent on *Ipf1/Pdx1* (Fig. 5*B*). In the more distal regions of gastrointestinal tract, including the ileum, where IPF1/PDX1 is not expressed, β-gal/*Gpr40* expression was unaffected in *Ipf1/Pdx1*-null mice (data not shown). Together, these data provide evidence for a conserved role for *Ipf1/Pdx1* in regulating *Gpr40* expression in pancreatic β-cells and endocrine cells of the gastric pylorus and duodenum.

DISCUSSION

The FFA-responsive G-protein–coupled receptor Gpr40 is expressed in pancreatic β-cells where it contributes to FFA-mediated enhancement of glucose-induced insulin secretion (1–4), and *Gpr40* mutant mice do not develop hyperinsulinemia on a high-fat diet (2). Here, we show that *Gpr40* is expressed also in hormone-producing cells of the gastrointestinal tract, including GIP⁺ and GLP-1⁺ cells. FFAs are known to stimulate the secretion of both GIP and GLP-1 incretin hormones (20,21), and other G-protein–

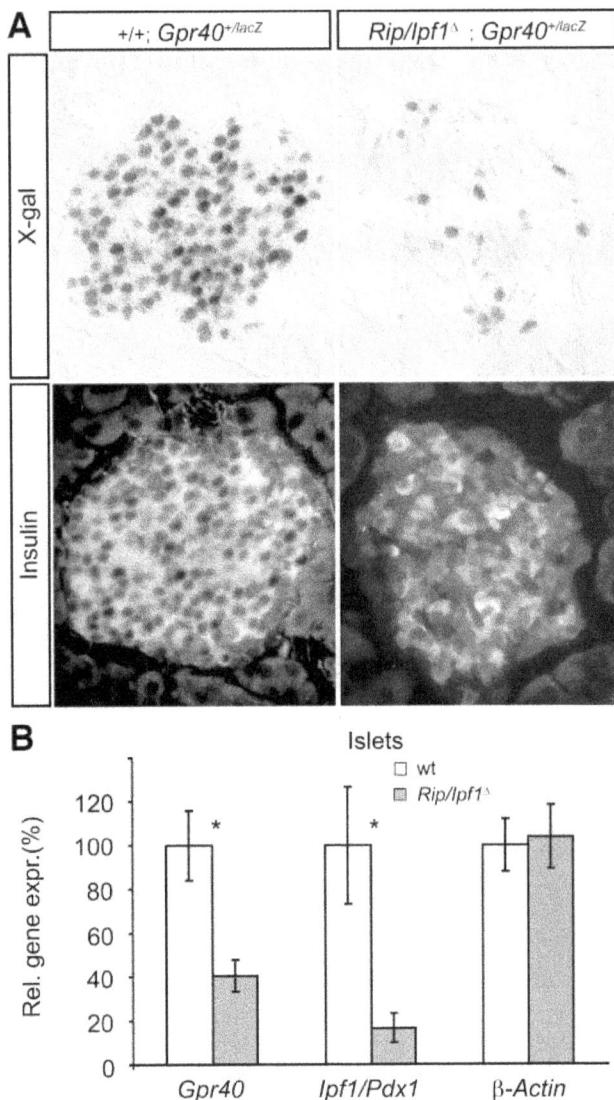

FIG. 4. *Gpr40* expression in β-cells cells requires *Ipf1/Pdx1*. *A*: X-gal–stained sections (*top panel*) of 5-week-old adult islets from *Ipf1/Pdx1*[+/+];*Gpr40*[+/lacZ] and *RIP/Ipf1*[Δ];*Gpr40*[+/lacZ] mice counterstained with anti-insulin antibodies (*bottom panel*). *B*: Quantitative real-time RT-PCR expression analyses of islet cDNA from *Ipf1/Pdx1*[+/+] (□, *n* = 4) and *RIP/Ipf1*[Δ] (▨, *n* = 6) mice. Data are means ± SE. **P* < 0.05 for *Ipf1/Pdx1*[+/+] vs. *RIP/Ipf1*[Δ] islets.

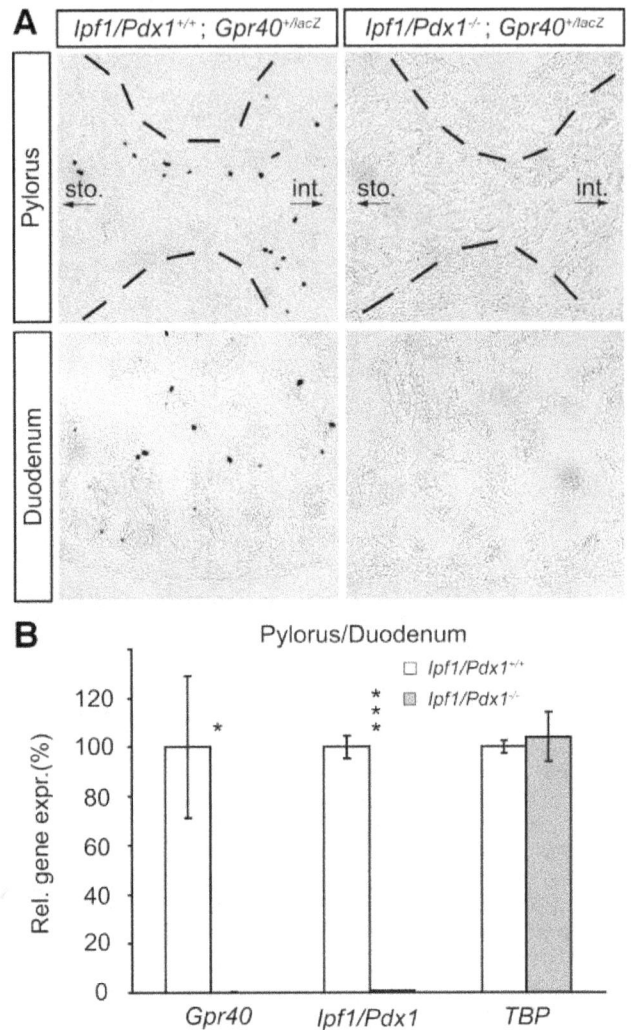

FIG. 5. *Gpr40* expression in enteroendocrine cells requires *Ipf1/Pdx1*. *A*: X-gal–stained sections of the pyloric sphincter and in duodenum of e17 *Ipf1/Pdx1*[+/+];*Gpr40*[+/lacZ] and *Ipf1/Pdx1*[−/−];*Gpr40*[+/lacZ] embryos. *B*: Quantitative real-time RT-PCR expression analysis of cDNA isolated from pylorus/duodenum of *Ipf1/Pdx1*[+/+] (□, *n* = 3) and *Ipf1/Pdx1*[−/−] embryos (▨, *n* = 3). Data are means ± SE. **P* < 0.05 and ****P* < 0.001 for *Ipf1/Pdx1*[+/+] vs. *Ipf1/Pdx1*[−/−]. Brackets in *A* indicate the border of the smooth muscle layer surrounding the lumen of the gut tube. sto., stomach; int., intestine.

coupled receptors, such as Gpr120 and Gpr119, have been implicated in the secretion of incretin hormones (9,10). Activation of Gpr120 by α-linolenic acid, docosahexaoienic, or palmitoleic acid in STC-1 cells promoted GLP-1 secretion (9), and upon an oral load of the Gpr119 agonist AR231453, plasma concentrations of GLP-1 and GIP increased in control animals but not in *Gpr119*-deficient mice (10). In this study, we found that *Gpr40*-null mice show impaired secretion of both GIP and GLP-1 in response to acute, oral fat diet administration with a concomitant reduction in insulin secretion and glucose clearance. Together, these findings provide evidence for a role for Gpr40 in FFA stimulation of incretin secretion. The expression of *Gpr40* in endocrine cells of gastrointestinal tract leaves open the possibility that Gpr40, as a component of the entero-insular axis, may regulate insulin secretion in response to fatty acids at several levels. Thus, apart from directly influencing insulin secretion from

β-cells via circulating FFAs, Gpr40 may indirectly stimulate GSIS from β-cells by modulating the secretion of the incretin hormones GIP and GLP-1 in response to FFAs present in the gastrointestinal lumen (23,24).

The gut hormones ghrelin and CCK play important and opposing roles in regulating food intake; ghrelin is considered to be an appetite hormone, and CCK a satiety hormone. The release of these two hormones is regulated by food intake, especially fat. Ghrelin levels in blood circulation are reduced by long-chain fatty acids (25), whereas CCK levels are increased by medium- to long-chain fatty acids (26). However, *Gpr40* mutant mice show a normal growth rate on both control and high-fat diet and do not present with any apparent signs of perturbed food intake patterns (2,4). Ghrelin has also been suggested to influence insulin secretion, but the data are conflicting; both stimulatory and inhibitory effects on insulin secretion have been reported (27–31). The role, if any, for Gpr40 in mediating secretion of ghrelin and CCK in response to FFAs will have to await future analyses.

In β-cells, IPF1/PDX1 regulates the expression of several genes that ultimately ensure proper GSIS and thus β-cell function (12–14,17). Relatively little is known about the regulation of *Gpr40* expression in β-cells. A recent study suggests, however, that IPF1/PDX1 and the basic-helix-loop-helix transcription factor NeuroD/β2, which also is expressed in β-cells, bind to an enhancer element within the 5′-flanking region of *Gpr40* (5). Here, we show in vivo that loss of *Ipf1/Pdx1* in β-cells impairs *Gpr40* expression, providing evidence not only that IPF1/PDX1 can bind to the *Gpr40* 5′-flanking region (5) but that IPF1/PDX1 is required for *Gpr40* expression in β-cells. IPF1/PDX1 is expressed also in endocrine cells of the gastric pyloric antrum and duodenum (22,32). In *Ipf1/Pdx1*-null mutant mice, the expression profile of several gut hormones is changed; fewer gastrin[+] but more serotonin[+] cells were, for example, observed in the antrum of these mice (22). In this study, we show that the expression of *Gpr40* in endocrine cells of the anterior gastrointestinal tract is lost in *Ipf1/Pdx1*[−/−] mice. Thus, like *Ipf1/Pdx1*, *Gpr40* is expressed in both β-cells and endocrine cells of the anterior gastrointestinal tract, and *Ipf1/Pdx1* function is essential for *Gpr40* expression in both of these cell types. Taken together, these data suggest a conserved role for *Ipf1/Pdx1* in cells that secrete hormones in response to food intake. However, IPF1/PDX1 is not expressed in the more distal part of the gastrointestinal tract, and *Gpr40* expression at these sites is not affected in *Ipf1/Pdx1*-null mice. Thus, *Gpr40* expression in posterior enteroendocrine cells is *Ipf1/Pdx1* independent. However, the identity of transcription factors regulating *Gpr40* expression in endocrine cells of the posterior gastrointestinal tract remains unknown.

Like other cells of the gastrointestinal epithelium, enteroendocrine cells undergo constant renewal involving stem cell division, differentiation, and cell death. *Gpr40*[+] cells are more abundant in the gastric pyloric antrum and duodenum than in the more posterior ileum and colon. In the gastric pyloric antrum, *Gpr40* is predominantly expressed in gastrin[+] cells close to the crypts of pyloric pits. In the intestine, *Gpr40* expression was evident in endocrine cells expressing ghrelin, GIP, GLP-1, CCK, PYY, substance P, serotonin, and secretin. Although virtually all *Gpr40*-expressing cells were hormone positive, only ~20–55% of the individual hormone expressing cells also expressed *Gpr40*. Whether this reflects the maturation process of the cycling enteroendocrine cells, i.e., that *Gpr40* is expressed only at a specific stage of differentiation or that only a subpopulation of the individual enteroendocrine cells expresses *Gpr40*, which in turn would indicate functional differences, remains an open question.

By virtue of its contribution to FFA-enhanced insulin secretion from β-cells, GPR40 is a link between obesity and type 2 diabetes. FFA stimulation of insulin secretion from β-cells is reduced in *Gpr40* mutant mice, and these mice do not develop hyperinsulinemia on a high-fat diet (2). The expression of *Gpr40* in GLP-1[+] and GIP[+] cells and the impaired secretion of these hormones in Gpr40-null mice in response to acute, oral fat diet leaves open the possibility that the difference in insulin levels in control and *Gpr40*-null mice on high-fat diet results from combined direct, i.e., β-cells, and indirect, i.e., incretin cells, effects of FFA on insulin secretion. The expression of *Gpr40* in endocrine cells expressing hormones that control food intake is suggestive of a role for Gpr40 in the secretion of also these hormones. Increased knowledge of the role for Gpr40 in β-cells and endocrine cells of the gastrointestinal tract may therefore be of great therapeutic relevance not only for obesity-associated diabetes but also for obesity itself but will have to await the generation of β-cell– and enteroendocrine cell–specific *Gpr40* mutant mice.

ACKNOWLEDGMENTS

H.E. has received grants from the Swedish Research Council, the European Union (Integrated Project EuroDia LSHM-CT-2006-518153 in the Framework Program 6 of the European Community), the Kempe Foundations, and the Swedish Diabetes Association.

We thank members of our laboratory for technical instructions, suggestions, and helpful discussions; Dr. Michael Walker for helpful discussions and valuable advice; and Drs. Kelly Loffler and Thomas Edlund for critical reading and helpful discussions.

REFERENCES

1. Itoh Y, Kawamata Y, Harada M, Kobayashi M, Fujii R, Fukusumi S, Ogi K, Hosoya M, Tanaka Y, Uejima H, Tanaka H, Maruyama M, Satoh R, Okubo S, Kizawa H, Komatsu H, Matsumura F, Noguchi Y, Shinohara T, Hinuma S, Fujisawa Y, Fujino M: Free fatty acids regulate insulin secretion from pancreatic beta cells through GPR40. *Nature* 422:173–176, 2003
2. Steneberg P, Rubins N, Bartoov-Shifman R, Walker MD, Edlund H: The FFA receptor GPR40 links hyperinsulinemia, hepatic steatosis, and impaired glucose homeostasis in mouse. *Cell Metab* 1:245–258, 2005
3. Shapiro H, Shachar S, Sekler I, Hershfinkel M, Walker MD: Role of GPR40 in fatty acid action on the beta cell line INS-1E. *Biochem Biophys Res Commun* 335:97–104, 2005
4. Latour MG, Alquier T, Oseid E, Tremblay C, Jetton TL, Luo J, Lin DC, Poitout V: GPR40 is necessary but not sufficient for fatty acid stimulation of insulin secretion in vivo. *Diabetes* 56:1087–1094, 2007
5. Bartoov-Shifman R, Ridner G, Bahar K, Rubins N, Walker MD: Regulation of the gene encoding GPR40, a fatty acid receptor expressed selectively in pancreatic beta cells. *J Biol Chem* 282:23561–23571, 2007
6. Easom RA: Beta-granule transport and exocytosis. *Semin Cell Dev Biol* 11:253–266, 2000
7. Rutter GA: Nutrient-secretion coupling in the pancreatic islet beta-cell: recent advances. *Mol Aspects Med* 22:247–284, 2001
8. Schnell S, Schaefer M, Schofl C: Free fatty acids increase cytosolic free calcium and stimulate insulin secretion from beta-cells through activation of GPR40. *Mol Cell Endocrinol* 263:173–180, 2007
9. Hirasawa A, Tsumaya K, Awaji T, Katsuma S, Adachi T, Yamada M, Sugimoto Y, Miyazaki S, Tsujimoto G: Free fatty acids regulate gut incretin glucagon-like peptide-1 secretion through GPR120. *Nat Med* 11:90–94, 2005
10. Chu ZL, Carroll C, Alfonso J, Gutierrez V, He H, Lucman A, Pedraza M, Mondala H, Gao H, Bagnol D, Chen R, Jones RM, Behan DP, Leonard J: A role for intestinal endocrine cell-expressed GPR119 in glycemic control by enhancing GLP-1 and GIP release. *Endocrinology* 149:2038–2047, 2008
11. Briscoe CP, Tadayyon M, Andrews JL, Benson WG, Chambers JK, Eilert MM, Ellis C, Elshourbagy NA, Goetz AS, Minnick DT, Murdock PR, Sauls HR Jr, Shabon U, Spinage LD, Strum JC, Szekeres PG, Tan KB, Way JM, Ignar DM, Wilson S, Muir AI: The orphan G protein-coupled receptor GPR40 is activated by medium and long chain fatty acids. *J Biol Chem* 278:11303–11311, 2003
12. Ahlgren U, Jonsson J, Jonsson L, Simu K, Edlund H: Beta-cell-specific inactivation of the mouse Ipf1/Pdx1 gene results in loss of the beta-cell phenotype and maturity onset diabetes. *Genes Dev* 12:1763–1768, 1998
13. Hart AW, Baeza N, Apelqvist A, Edlund H: Attenuation of FGF signalling in mouse beta-cells leads to diabetes. *Nature* 408:864–868, 2000
14. Li Y, Cao X, Li LX, Brubaker PL, Edlund H, Drucker DJ: β-Cell Pdx1 expression is essential for the glucoregulatory, proliferative, and cytoprotective actions of glucagon-like peptide-1. *Diabetes* 54:482–491, 2005
15. Stoffers DA, Ferrer J, Clarke WL, Habener JF: Early-onset type-II diabetes mellitus (MODY4) linked to IPF1. *Nat Genet* 17:138–139, 1997
16. Jonsson J, Carlsson L, Edlund T, Edlund H: Insulin-promoter-factor 1 is required for pancreas development in mice. *Nature* 371:606–609, 1994

17. Ohlsson H, Karlsson K, Edlund T: IPF1, a homeodomain-containing transactivator of the insulin gene. *EMBO J* 12:4251–4259, 1993

18. Ahren B, Simonsson E, Scheurink AJ, Mulder H, Myrsen U, Sundler F: Dissociated insulinotropic sensitivity to glucose and carbachol in high-fat diet-induced insulin resistance in C57BL/6J mice. *Metabolism* 46:97–106, 1997

19. Holst JJ, Orskov C: Incretin hormones: an update. *Scand J Clin Lab Invest Suppl* 234:75–85, 2001

20. Adachi T, Tanaka T, Takemoto K, Koshimizu TA, Hirasawa A, Tsujimoto G: Free fatty acids administered into the colon promote the secretion of glucagon-like peptide-1 and insulin. *Biochem Biophys Res Commun* 340:332–337, 2006

21. Yip RG, Wolfe MM: GIP biology and fat metabolism. *Life Sci* 66:91–103, 2000

22. Larsson LI, Madsen OD, Serup P, Jonsson J, Edlund H: Pancreatic-duodenal homeobox 1: role in gastric endocrine patterning. *Mech Dev* 60:175–184, 1996

23. MacDonald PE, El-Kholy W, Riedel MJ, Salapatek AM, Light PE, Wheeler MB: The multiple actions of GLP-1 on the process of glucose-stimulated insulin secretion. *Diabetes* 51 (Suppl. 3):S434–S442, 2002

24. Yamada Y, Miyawaki K, Tsukiyama K, Harada N, Yamada C, Seino Y: Pancreatic and extrapancreatic effects of gastric inhibitory polypeptide. *Diabetes* 55 (Suppl. 2):S86–S91, 2006

25. Feinle-Bisset C, Patterson M, Ghatei MA, Bloom SR, Horowitz M: Fat digestion is required for suppression of ghrelin and stimulation of peptide YY and pancreatic polypeptide secretion by intraduodenal lipid. *Am J Physiol Endocrinol Metab* 289:E948–E953, 2005

26. Liddle RA, Goldfine ID, Rosen MS, Taplitz RA, Williams JA: Cholecystokinin bioactivity in human plasma: molecular forms, responses to feeding, and relationship to gallbladder contraction. *J Clin Invest* 75:1144–1152, 1985

27. Broglio F, Arvat E, Benso A, Gottero C, Muccioli G, Papotti M, van der Lely AJ, Deghenghi R, Ghigo E: Ghrelin, a natural GH secretagogue produced by the stomach, induces hyperglycemia and reduces insulin secretion in humans. *J Clin Endocrinol Metab* 86:5083–5086, 2001

28. Date Y, Nakazato M, Hashiguchi S, Dezaki K, Mondal MS, Hosoda H, Kojima M, Kangawa K, Arima T, Matsuo H, Yada T, Matsukura S: Ghrelin is present in pancreatic α-cells of humans and rats and stimulates insulin secretion. *Diabetes* 51:124–129, 2002

29. Lee HM, Wang G, Englander EW, Kojima M, Greeley GH Jr: Ghrelin, a new gastrointestinal endocrine peptide that stimulates insulin secretion: enteric distribution, ontogeny, influence of endocrine, and dietary manipulations. *Endocrinology* 143:185–190, 2002

30. Reimer MK, Pacini G, Ahren B: Dose-dependent inhibition by ghrelin of insulin secretion in the mouse. *Endocrinology* 144:916–921, 2003

31. Dezaki K, Sone H, Koizumi M, Nakata M, Kakei M, Nagai H, Hosoda H, Kangawa K, Yada T: Blockade of pancreatic islet-derived ghrelin enhances insulin secretion to prevent high-fat diet-induced glucose intolerance. *Diabetes* 55:3486–3493, 2006

32. Offield MF, Jetton TL, Labosky PA, Ray M, Stein RW, Magnuson MA, Hogan BL, Wright CV: PDX-1 is required for pancreatic outgrowth and differentiation of the rostral duodenum. *Development* 122:983–995, 1996

Incretin-Based Therapies for the Treatment of Type 2 Diabetes: Evaluation of the Risks and Benefits

Daniel J. Drucker, md[1]
Steven I. Sherman, md[2]
Fred S. Gorelick, md[3]

Richard M. Bergenstal, md[4]
Robert S. Sherwin, md[3]
John B. Buse, md, phd[5]

Type 2 diabetes is a complex metabolic disorder characterized by hyperglycemia arising from a combination of insufficient insulin secretion together with resistance to insulin action. The incidence and prevalence of type 2 diabetes are rising steadily, fuelled in part by a concomitant increase in the worldwide rates of obesity. As longitudinal studies of type 2 diabetes provide evidence linking improved glycemic control with a reduction in the rates of diabetes-associated complications, there is considerable interest in the therapy of type 2 diabetes (Fig. 1), with a focus on the development and use of new agents that exhibit improved efficacy and safety relative to current available medicines.

Although the number of patients with type 2 diabetes that successfully achieve target levels of A1C is steadily improving, a substantial number of subjects continue to fall short of acceptable treatment goals, leaving them at high risk for development of diabetes-associated complications (1). More importantly, a large number of subjects with type 2 diabetes fail to achieve target values for glucose, lipids, and blood pressure, with only 12.2% of patients meeting target values despite recent improvements in therapeutic agents targeting hyperglycemia, dyslipidemia, and hypertension (2). The development of multiple new agents for the treatment of type 2 diabetes has broadened the options for patient-specific therapy. However, no currently available agents exhibit the ideal profile of exceptional glucose-lowering efficacy to safely achieve target levels of glycemia in a broad range of patients. Hence, highly efficacious agents that exhibit unimpeachable safety, excellent tolerability, and ease of administration to ensure long-term adherence and that also clearly reduce common comorbidities and complications of diabetes are clearly needed (Fig. 1). Furthermore, most patients require combination therapy to achieve effective control of their disease (3). Recommended initial therapy generally includes comprehensive lifestyle management and patient education combined with metformin therapy. Although metformin is widely accepted as the preferred agent for the initial treatment of type 2 diabetes, there remains considerable uncertainty and lack of consensus in regard to choice of additional agents that need to be added to metformin to optimize glycemic control.

Recent recommendations have highlighted the use of insulin, sulfonylureas, and thiazolidinediones as second-line therapies because of their proven efficacy in long-term outcome studies. Nevertheless, more recent studies involving intensive use of these therapies in patients with clinical cardiovascular disease or multiple risk factors to achieve lower target glucose levels were associated with hypoglycemia, bone fractures, hospitalization for congestive heart failure, weight gain, and, in some analyses, increased mortality with modest benefit on rates of myocardial infarction. This has led to a re-examination of treatment recommendations to minimize the risk of cardiovascular morbidity and mortality (3,4) and specifically an interest in incretin-based therapies in this regard.

Incretin-based therapies: mechanisms of action and benefits

The two most recently approved classes of therapeutic agents for the treatment of type 2 diabetes, glucagon-like peptide-1 (GLP-1) receptor (GLP-1R) agonists and dipeptidyl peptidase-4 inhibitors (DPP-4i), exert their actions through potentiation of incretin receptor signaling. Incretins are gut-derived hormones, principally GLP-1 and glucose-dependent insulinotropic peptide (GIP), that are secreted at low basal levels in the fasting state. Circulating levels increase rapidly and transiently following food ingestion. As native GLP-1 displays a very short circulating half-life due to renal clearance and NH_2-terminal degradation by the enzyme DPP-4, degradation-resistant GLP-1R agonists have been developed. Exendin-4, a GLP-1R agonist structurally related to the native gut peptide, was approved for the treatment of type 2 diabetes in the U.S. in April 2005 and is currently administered as a subcutaneous injection (10 μg twice daily) for use as monotherapy in subjects not achieving adequate glycemic control on lifestyle modification alone or one or more oral agents. Liraglutide is an investigational human acylated GLP-1R agonist approved in Europe that binds noncovalently to albumin and exhibits a more prolonged duration of action suitable for once daily administration. A longer-acting microsphere preparation of exenatide suitable for once weekly administration, exenatide (once weekly), has also been studied in controlled clinical trials and appears to be somewhat more effective compared with exenatide twice daily (5).

Sitagliptin was the first DPP-4i approved in the U.S. in October 2006. It exerts its glucoregulatory actions through

From the [1]Department of Medicine, Samuel Lunenfeld Research Institute, University of Toronto, Toronto, Ontario; [2]The University of Texas M.D. Anderson Cancer Center, Houston, Texas; the [3]Department of Internal Medicine, Yale University School of Medicine, New Haven, Connecticut; the [4]International Diabetes Center, Minneapolis, Minnesota; and the [5]Division of Endocrinology, University of North Carolina School of Medicine, Chapel Hill, North Carolina.
Corresponding author: Daniel J. Drucker, d.drucker@utoronto.ca.
Received 20 August 2009 and accepted 17 October 2009.
DOI: 10.2337/dc09-1499

See accompanying editorial, p. 453.

Antihyperglycemic Agents in Type 2 Diabetes

Class	A1C Reduction	Hypo-Glycemia	Weight Change	CVD Risk Factors	Dosing (times/day)	Diabetes Comorbidity Contraindications
Metformin	1.5	No	Neutral	Minimal	2	Kidney, liver
Insulin, Long-acting	1.5 - 2.5	Yes	Gain	TG	1, Injected	None
Insulin, Rapid-acting	1.5 - 2.5	Yes	Gain	TG	1-4, Injected	None
Sulfonylureas	1.5	Yes	Gain	None	1	Essentially none
Thiazolidinediones	0.5 - 1.4	No	Gain	Variable	1	CHF, liver
Repaglinide	1 - 1.5	Yes	Gain	None	3	Essentially none
Nateglinide	0.5 - 0.8	Rare	Gain	None	3	Essentially none
Alpha-glucosidase Inhibitors	0.5 - 0.8	No	Neutral	Minimal	3	Essentially none
Amylin-mimetics	0.5 - 1.0	No	Loss	With weight loss	3, Injected	None
GLP-1R Agonist	0.5 - 1.0	No	Loss	With weight loss	2, Injected	Kidney
DPP-4 Inhibitor	0.6 - 0.8	No	Neutral	None	1	None
Bile acid sequestrant	0.5	No	Neutral	LDL	1-2	Severe TGs
Bromocriptine	0.7	No	Neutral	Minimal	1	Essentially none

Figure 1—Relative comparison of properties exhibited by different classes of agents approved for the treatment of type 2 diabetes. CVD, cardiovascular disease; TG, triglycerides; CHF, congestive heart failure. A1C reduction depends on starting A1C.

prevention of incretin degradation, leading to potentiation of GLP-1 and GIP action (6). Sitagliptin is administered as a single 100-mg daily tablet either as monotherapy or in combination therapy with oral antidiabetic agents. Sitagliptin is well tolerated and is not associated with nausea or vomiting as the levels of endogenous intact GLP-1 achieved following DPP-4 inhibition are at the upper limit of the normal physiological range; hence, it is not sufficient to induce an aversive response. Conversely, DPP-4i therapy is not associated with inhibition of gastric emptying or weight loss, and the available data suggest that long-acting GLP-1R agonists achieve more potent control of glycemia, relative to DPP-4i, due to more potent and sustained GLP-1R activation. Vildagliptin, a second DPP-4i, is approved in Europe and other countries, while saxagliptin has recently been approved in the U.S. and several other DPP-4i are under regulatory review.

GLP-1R agonists control blood glucose through regulation of islet function, principally with the stimulation of insulin and inhibition of glucagon secretion (7). Notably, these GLP-1R–dependent actions are glucose dependent, thereby minimizing the risk of hypoglycemia in the absence of concomitant sulfonylurea therapy. GLP-1R activation also inhibits

gastric emptying and reduces food intake, leading to weight loss in the majority of treated subjects (8). The GLP-1R is expressed in cardiomyocytes and endothelial cells, and preclinical studies demonstrate that GLP-1R activation is associated with substantial cardioprotection and reduced infarct size in experimental models of coronary artery ischemia (9,10). Limited evidence suggests that GLP-1 may also preserve ventricular function and improve outcomes in human subjects with heart failure or myocardial infarction (11,12). Moreover, both exenatide and liraglutide reduce blood pressure, body weight, and plasma lipid profiles in subjects with type 2 diabetes (13), raising the hope that long-term treatment with these agents may reduce the incidence of cardiovascular events. Intriguingly, the GLP-1 metabolite, GLP-1 (9–36), also exerts cardioprotective actions in preclinical studies through mechanisms independent of the known GLP-1R (14); hence, ongoing research is directed at understanding the complexity of incretin biology in the cardiovascular system and the potential for incretin-based therapies to differentially modulate cardioprotective signals in the diabetic heart and blood vessel in vivo (15). The principal treatment-related adverse events associated with exenatide

and liraglutide therapy are nausea and vomiting, which generally diminish over time (13). Analysis of the antidiabetic actions pursuant to GLP-1 administration has demonstrated that activation of the GLP-1R for 24 h provides more sustained and potent control of glycemia relative to shorter periods of GLP-1R agonism (16). In contrast, sustained GLP-1R activation may be associated with a modest reduction in control of postprandial glycemia (5,13), observations of interest to scientists studying the link between postprandial glucose and the development of cardiovascular morbidity and mortality. As exenatide requires twice daily administration and does not provide 24-h GLP-1R activation, there has been considerable interest in development of GLP-1R analogues with more prolonged durations of action (Fig. 2) suitable for once-daily or once-weekly administration (17). Consistent with the notion that continuous GLP-1R activation is required for optimal glucoregulation, liraglutide administered once daily and exenatide administered once weekly appear to be more potent glucose-lowering agents, relative to twice-daily exenatide (5,13). Furthermore, they seem to be associated with better tolerability and patient-reported outcomes as well as trends toward greater benefit on cardiovascular disease risk factors (Fig.

Exenatide and Long-Acting GLP-1 Agonists: *Similarities and Differences*

Properties/Effect	Exenatide[1]	Investigational >24 hr agonists[2,3]
Glucose-dependent insulin secretion and glucagon	Yes	Yes
Slows gastric emptying	Yes	Little or no
Effect on body weight	Weight loss	Weight loss
Effect on A1C	Reduction ~1%	Reduction ~1.5%
Effect on fasting glucose	Modest	Good
Effect on postprandial glucose	Good	Modest
Effect on CVD risk factors	Improve (with weight loss)	Improve
Common side effects	Nausea	Less nausea
Pancreatitis	Rare	Rare
Administration	Twice-daily	Daily or weekly
Rodent medullary thyroid cancer	Little to no signal	Signal

1. Amori RE, et al. *JAMA*. 2007; 298:194-206.
2. Exenatide LAR (once weekly): Drucker DJ, et al. *Lancet*. 2008; 372:1240-1250.
3. Liraglutide: Blonde L, et al. *Can J Diabetes*. 2008;32(suppl): A107.

Figure 2—*Comparison of features associated with exenatide twice daily versus the properties of the emerging class of long-acting GLP-1R agonists that achieve more prolonged and sustained GLP-1R activation. CVD, cardiovascular disease.*

2). There are now over a dozen long-acting investigational GLP-1R agonists being developed for the treatment of type 2 diabetes (8). Several recent reviews have emphasized the mechanisms of action and clinical results obtained in trials examining the efficacy of incretin-based therapies (8,17). Herein we examine adverse events and safety concerns associated with these agents.

Adverse events associated with GLP-1R agonists

Acute pancreatitis. Pancreatitis has been reported as a rare side effect of exenatide therapy principally through postmarketing surveillance. There are many risk factors and predisposing causes for acute pancreatitis, as well as over 200 drugs linked to the development of acute pancreatitis. The incidence of pancreatitis varies considerably among drugs, being relatively common for individuals taking 6-mercaptopurine and azathioprine (2–5%), but very uncommon for steroids and thiazide diuretics. The severity of the disease also varies; pancreatitis induced by 6-mercaptopurine is often quite severe, while that caused by cholinesterase inhibitors is usually mild. There are only two circumstances in which the mechanism of drug-induced disease is understood, drugs that cause hypertriglyceridemia (e.g., some HIV-protease inhibitors, estrogens, isotrentinoin) and drugs that are mitochondrial toxins. Drugs are not thought to cause chronic pancreatitis

(with the exception of alcohol and smoking), although they have the theoretical potential to do so. Numerous animal models for pancreatitis have been developed; however, drugs that are associated with pancreatitis in humans rarely cause disease in rodents. Whether these species-specific observations reflect differences in drug metabolism, pancreatitis responses including inflammation, or the fact that some drugs may act as sensitizers and require other factors to cause disease, remains unclear.

Clinical data relating GLP-1R agonists and DPP-4i to pancreatitis come from a limited number of case reports, the U.S. Food and Drug Administration's (FDA) adverse event reporting system, and clinical trial records from pharmaceutical companies. A summary of initial 30 cases of individuals taking exenatide who developed acute pancreatitis was published in 2008 (18). The authors noted that in least 90% of these subjects, there were other factors that could predispose the individuals to pancreatitis. Rechallenge, a standard measure for assigning causality in drug-induced pancreatitis, was performed in only three patients but associated with recurrence of symptoms in each. However, the recurrence of symptoms with rechallenge was reported to occur only after weeks in some patients. In most patients with drug-induced pancreatitis, rechallenge usually causes disease within days. Subsequently, hemorrhagic pancreatitis and several deaths have been

reported to the FDA in patients who previously used exenatide and similar cases but no deaths have been reported in patients treated with sitagliptin (19). A recent study used insurance records to determine that the risk of pancreatitis for subjects followed up to a year was 0.12% and 0.13% with sitagliptin and exenatide, respectively (20). These relative risks did not differ from a control cohort treated with metformin or glyburide. Data from the manufacturer of liraglutide reported a low incidence of acute pancreatitis (0.8 cases/1,000 patient-years). Notably, analysis of pancreatitis in subjects with type 2 diabetes suggests that their risk is increased threefold over nondiabetic subjects (21). Since only a fraction of this risk could be attributed to biliary pancreatitis, it seems likely that other factors such as obesity and hypertriglyceridemia might contribute to the increased risk in this population.

Several experimental studies have examined the effects of incretin-based agents on the pancreas in animal models. Koehler et al. (22) found no evidence of pancreatitis in mice treated with the GLP-1R agonist exendin-4 alone and no GLP-1R–dependent enhancement of pancreatitis responses in the caerulein-hyperstimulation model. In contrast, Nachnani et al. (23) detected histological evidence for acinar inflammation, cell drop-out and possible fibrosis and increased levels of serum lipase in Sprague-Dawley rats treated with exendin-4 for 75 days. A study by Matveyenko et al. (24) examined the effects of sitagliptin in human islet amyloid polypeptide (HIP) transgenic diabetic rats. The investigators reported that one of eight HIP rats receiving the drug developed acute pancreatitis and noted extensive pancreatic ductal proliferation and metaplasia and accompanying fibrosis in three HIP rats treated with sitagliptin. Some of the histological findings from the latter two studies were very similar, and reminiscence of changes was seen with chronic pancreatitis. The animal studies raise several confounding issues, namely might there be differences in pancreatitis responses between GLP-1R agonists and DPP-4i in humans versus rodents and in specific diabetic versus nondiabetic preclinical models? Though the relevance of the HIP transgenic rat model to human disease remains unclear, that study does suggest that DPP-4i might induce pancreatic metaplasia under specific experimental conditions. In summary, the clinical and experimental data linking GLP-1R agonists and DPP-4i to pancreatitis are still incomplete. More information is required to allow one to determine whether these agents substantially increase the risk of acute pancreatitis and whether such disease tends to be severe. However, patients receiving these medications will need to undergo continued surveillance for pancreatitis and clinicians should carefully exclude other causes of acute pancreatitis when it occurs in subjects receiving these drugs. Although the diagnosis of drug-induced pancreatitis would ideally be associated with confirmatory clinical data following drug rechallenge, physicians should exercise caution before considering a trial of drug rechallenge. As GLP-1R agonists may also affect smooth muscle responses and may regulate cholangiocyte function (25), their effects on the biliary tract and gallstone formation should also be examined.

Issues linking these agents with pancreatic metaplasia and chronic pancreatitis, as now suggested by two experimental studies, present a different challenge. Longer-term experimental studies using different GLP-1R agonists and DPP-4i in several species and experimental models of diabetes need to be undertaken to help clarify the importance of these findings. Hence, monitoring of pancreatic function and pancreatic disease in humans treated with GLP-1R agonists and DPP-4i in ongoing long-term prospective controlled clinical trials seems prudent.

Medullary thyroid cancer. Medullary thyroid carcinoma (MTC) is an uncommon neuroendocrine malignancy with an estimated U.S. annual incidence of fewer than 1,000 persons and a lifetime risk of development of 0.013% (26). When diagnosed early and still confined to the thyroid gland, the long-term survival of MTC is nearly 100% (27). About 25% of MTCs occur as part of an inherited autosomal dominant syndrome, either multiple endocrine neoplasia type II or familial MTC, and virtually all familial tumors are caused by inherited mutations in the RET proto-oncogene. Of sporadic MTCs, at least 40% are associated with somatic mutations and RET, and prognosis is worse in those mutated tumors.

The histological precursors to MTC in the inherited syndromes are well described, beginning with C-cell hyperplasia, leading to nodular C-cell hyperplasia, and then eventually to MTC. However, among the sporadically occurring MTCs, the role of this histological sequence is not defined, and the exact distinction between neoplastic and non-neoplastic C-cell hyperplasia is controversial (28,29). As a tumor derived from C-cells, MTCs generally secrete calcitonin, and high serum levels of calcitonin (>100 pg/ml) are nearly 100% specific for the presence of MTC (30,31). Nonetheless, the specificity of serum calcitonin concentrations between the upper end of the reference range and 100 pg/ml is considerably more limited. Other etiologies of mild degrees of hypercalcitoninemia include lymphocytic thyroiditis, chronic renal insufficiency, pancreatitis, hypercalcemia, hypergastrinemia (of any etiology), and even the postprandial state (31,32). Stimulation of calcitonin release with pentagastrin infusion has long been used to distinguish neoplastic from non-neoplastic causes of mild hypercalcitoninemia; however, pentagastrin is no longer available for human use in the U.S., and the diagnostic accuracy of testing with alternative stimulants such as calcium infusion remains to be established (31).

Animal models of MTC have limitations in regard to the biology and epidemiology of human MTC. Rats develop spontaneous age-related C-cell lesions at remarkably high frequency, especially nodular C-cell hyperplasia. Sporadic MTC occurs in 0.5–1% of most rat species evaluated, with increased frequency in males and with advancing age; spontaneous RET mutations have not been re-

ported, and some typical histological features of human MTC are generally lacking. Mice develop spontaneous MTC less frequently, and most animal models in use are either transgenic or xenografts of the well-characterized TT cell line.

Food intake links incretin secretion with stimulation of calcitonin secretion in rodents, potentially via GLP-1 receptors expressed on rodent MTC cell lines, and GLP-1 stimulates calcitonin release in rodents in vivo (33–35). Analysis of data reported at the 2 April 2009 FDA Advisory Committee review of liraglutide revealed that preclinical toxicology studies with liraglutide reported C-cell hyperplasia and MTC with increasing exposure to liraglutide. At the highest drug exposures, MTC was reported in 14% of male and 6% of female Sprague-Dawley rats, which was above the rates observed in untreated rat controls. C-cell lesions were also reported to be more common with liraglutide in CD-1 mice, albeit at much lower frequencies; no C-cell lesions were described in the cynomologous monkey. In contrast, once-daily administration of exenatide in rodents is associated with a high frequency of nodular C-cell lesions but no carcinomas were reported (36). In safety monitoring of multiple liraglutide clinical trials, many patients with undetectable calcitonin levels before initiation of investigational (liraglutide, placebo, or active comparator) therapy were found to have levels that rose into the mid-reference normal range; rare patients developed mild hypercalcitoninemia during therapy. Across the trials, six patients were found to have C-cell findings at thyroidectomy following therapy (36). Of these patients, four were in liraglutide treatment arms, but three of these had elevated calcitonin levels before initiation of treatment. The remaining two patients were in the active comparator arms of trials, and one had an elevated calcitonin level before treatment. This single patient had MTC and was treated with an active non-GLP-1–based comparator; the patient had a markedly elevated calcitonin level before initiating non-GLP-1–based comparator therapy. All of the remaining patients who underwent thyroidectomy for hypercalcitoninemia were reported to have C-cell hyperplasia. According to the FDA briefing documents, no cases of C-cell lesions have been documented by histology in patients treated with exenatide. Several cases of papillary thyroid cancer have also been reported in the liraglutide clinical development program; however, the small number of cases, the incidental histopathologic identification of the lesions, together with the lack of biological plausibility, suggest that this is an incidental finding not directly related to therapy with GLP-1R agonists.

In summary, rodents exposed to liraglutide and exenatide develop C-cell lesions at relatively high frequency, although the currently available data suggest that rodent MTC may be specific to long-acting GLP-1R agonists, likely due to sustained GLP-1R activation. Because of the historic difficulty of distinguishing neoplastic and non-neoplastic forms of C-cell hyperplasia in both rodents and humans, the diagnostic significance of C-cell hyperplasia is unclear. Minimal elevations of calcitonin levels are very nonspecific, and available methods of dynamic testing add little to clarify the etiologies. Given the extreme rarity of MTC in humans, the numbers of patients who would need to be treated for 10 years to yield one additional case of MTC may be extremely high (35–55,000 if risk is doubled; 10–15,000 if risk is quintupled). Moreover, the differences in rodent versus human C-cell biology with regard to responsivity to GLP-1R activation raise important questions about the suitability of mice and rats as models for understanding the effects of GLP-1R agonists on human C-cells.

Summary and conclusions

Incretin-based therapies provide new options for the treatment of type 2 diabetes and enable intensification of therapy while controlling body weight through mechanisms associated with a low rate of hypoglycemia. Investigational long-acting GLP-1R agonists require less frequent administration and appear to be more potent with respect to A1C reduction than twice-daily exenatide or once-daily sitagliptin with respect to A1C reduction. These long-acting GLP-1R agonists have considerable potential as antidiabetic therapies as they not only lower glucose as or more effectively than other noninsulin antihyperglycemic therapies, they do so in concert with weight loss, improvement in cardiovascular disease risk factors, and with very low risk of hypoglycemia. However, two safety issues have been raised—pancreatitis and medullary carcinoma of the thyroid.

The relationship between the use of incretin therapy and the development of pancreatitis remains unclear. These agents may not substantially increase the

risk of acute pancreatitis in humans and might not affect the risk at all. The relevance to humans of the pancreatic metaplasia observed with these agents in two of the rodent studies is unknown. Continued clinical monitoring and more research are required to clarify the actions of GLP-1R agonists and DPP-4i on the normal and diabetic exocrine pancreas.

GLP-1R activation stimulates calcitonin secretion and promotes the development of C-cell hyperplasia and medullary thyroid cancer in rodents but not in monkeys, and the actions of GLP-1R agonists on human C-cells remain uncertain. Because of the rarity of medullary carcinoma of the thyroid and the lack of specificity of clinical markers, screening strategies, except in the setting of familial syndromes, almost certainly would be associated with an increase in morbidity and perhaps mortality as a result of false positives.

Taken together, the available evidence supports the use of incretin-based therapies for patients requiring effective control of glycemia and body weight while minimizing the risk of hypoglycemia. Ongoing scrutiny and further studies are required to clarify the potential significance of reports of pancreatic injury, including pancreatitis and metaplasia, and rodent medullary thyroid cancer for human subjects treated with GLP-1R agonists and DPP-4i.

Acknowledgments— R.M.B.'s employer, Park Nicollet Institute, has contracted with a variety of companies since 2002 for his services as an investigator or consultant (with no personal income from these services going directly to R.M.B.) including Abbott, Amylin, Bayer, Eli Lilly, Hygieia, Intuity, LifeScan, MannKind, Medtronic, Novo Nordisk, National Institutes of Health, Pfizer, ResMed, Roche, sanofi-aventis, United Health Group, and Valeritas. RMB holds stock in Merck (family inheritance). J.B.B. is a shareholder in Insulet. His employer, the University of North Carolina, has contracted with a variety of companies since 2005 for his services as an investigator and/or consultant including Amylin, Bristol-Myers Squibb, Eli Lilly, GlaxoSmithKline, Hoffman-La Roche, Merck, Novartis, Novo Nordisk, Pfizer, sanofi-aventis, and Wyeth. D.J.D. is a consultant to Amylin, GlaxoSmithKline, Eli Lilly, Merck, Novo Nordisk, and Roche and receives research support for preclinical studies from Arena, Merck, Metabolex, Novo Nordisk, and Roche. S.I.S. receives research support from Amgen, AstraZeneca, Eisai, Genzyme, the National Cancer Institute, and The V Foundation for

Cancer Research; is a consultant to Bayer, Celgene, Exelixis, Eli Lilly, Oxigene, Plexxikon, and Semafore; is on a speaker's bureau for Genzyme; and has received honoraria from Genzyme and Exelixis. R.S.S. has stock options for Insulet; serves on the scientific advisory boards or as a consultant for Amylin, Boehringer Ingelheim, Biodel, Johnson & Johnson, MannKind, Medtronic, Merck, and Novartis.

No other potential conflicts of interest relevant to this article were reported.

References

1. Hoerger TJ, Segel JE, Gregg EW, Saaddine JB. Is glycemic control improving in U.S. adults? Diabetes Care 2008;31:81–86
2. Cheung BM, Ong KL, Cherny SS, Sham PC, Tso AW, Lam KS. Diabetes prevalence and therapeutic target achievement in the United States, 1999 to 2006. Am J Med 2009;122:443–453
3. Nathan DM, Buse JB, Davidson MB, Ferrannini E, Holman RR, Sherwin R, Zinman B, American Diabetes Association, European Association for Study of Diabetes. Medical management of hyperglycemia in type 2 diabetes: a consensus algorithm for the initiation and adjustment of therapy: a consensus statement of the American Diabetes Association and the European Association for the Study of Diabetes. Diabetes Care 2009;32:193–203
4. Bergenstal RM, Bailey CJ, Kendall DM. Therapeutic decision-making in type 2 diabetes: assessing the relative risks and benefits of glucose lowering medications. Am J Med. In press
5. Drucker DJ, Buse JB, Taylor K, Kendall DM, Trautmann M, Zhuang D, Porter L, DURATION-1 Study Group. Exenatide once weekly versus twice daily for the treatment of type 2 diabetes: a randomised, open-label, non-inferiority study. Lancet 2008;372:1240–1250
6. Hansotia T, Baggio LL, Delmeire D, Hinke SA, Yamada Y, Tsukiyama K, Seino Y, Holst JJ, Schuit F, Drucker DJ. Double incretin receptor knockout (DIRKO) mice reveal an essential role for the enteroinsular axis in transducing the glucoregulatory actions of DPP-IV inhibitors. Diabetes 2004;53:1326–1335
7. Drucker DJ. The biology of incretin hormones. Cell Metab 2006;3:153–165
8. Lovshin JA, Drucker DJ. Incretin-based therapies for type 2 diabetes mellitus. Nat Rev Endocrinol 2009;5:262–269
9. Timmers L, Henriques JP, de Kleijn DP, Devries JH, Kemperman H, Steendijk P, Verlaan CW, Kerver M, Piek JJ, Doevendans PA, Pasterkamp G, Hoefer IE. Exenatide reduces infarct size and improves cardiac function in a porcine model of ischemia and reperfusion injury. J Am Coll Cardiol 2009;53:501–510

10. Noyan-Ashraf MH, Momen MA, Ban K, Sadi AM, Zhou YQ, Riazi AM, Baggio LL, Henkelman RM, Husain M, Drucker DJ. GLP-1R agonist liraglutide activates cytoprotective pathways and improves outcomes after experimental myocardial infarction in mice. Diabetes 2009;58:975–983

11. Nikolaidis LA, Mankad S, Sokos GG, Miske G, Shah A, Elahi D, Shannon RP. Effects of glucagon-like peptide-1 in patients with acute myocardial infarction and left ventricular dysfunction after successful reperfusion. Circulation 2004;109:962–965

12. Sokos GG, Nikolaidis LA, Mankad S, Elahi D, Shannon RP. Glucagon-like peptide-1 infusion improves left ventricular ejection fraction and functional status in patients with chronic heart failure. J Card Fail 2006;12:694–699

13. Buse JB, Rosenstock J, Sesti G, Schmidt WE, Montanya E, Brett JH, Zychma M, Blonde L, LEAD-6 Study Group. Liraglutide once a day versus exenatide twice a day for type 2 diabetes: a 26-week randomised, parallel-group, multinational, open-label trial (LEAD-6). Lancet 2009;374:39–47

14. Ban K, Noyan-Ashraf MH, Hoefer J, Bolz SS, Drucker DJ, Husain M. Cardioprotective and vasodilatory actions of glucagon-like peptide 1 receptor are mediated through both glucagon-like peptide 1 receptor-dependent and -independent pathways. Circulation 2008;117:2340–2350

15. Ban K, Hui S, Drucker DJ, Husain M. Cardiovascular consequences of drugs used for the treatment of diabetes: potential promise of incretin-based therapies. J Am Soc Hypertens 2009;3:245–259

16. Rachman J, Barrow BA, Levy JC, Turner RC. Near normalisation of diurnal glucose concentrations by continuous administration of glucagon-like peptide 1 (GLP-1) in subjects with NIDDM. Diabetologia 1997;40:205–211

17. Drucker DJ, Nauck MA. The incretin system: glucagon-like peptide-1 receptor agonists and dipeptidyl peptidase-4 inhibitors in type 2 diabetes. Lancet 2006;368:1696–1705

18. Ahmad SR, Swann J. Exenatide and rare adverse events. N Engl J Med 2008;358:1970–1971

19. U.S. Federal Drug Administration. Medwatch Sitagliptin Reports of acute pancreatitis [Internet], 2009. Available from http://www.fda.gov/Safety/MedWatch/SafetyInformation/SafetyAlertsforHumanMedicalProducts/ucm183800.htm.

20. Dore DD, Seeger JD, Arnold Chan K. Use of a claims-based active drug safety surveillance system to assess the risk of acute pancreatitis with exenatide or sitagliptin compared to metformin or glyburide. Curr Med Res Opin 2009;25:1019–1027

21. Noel RA, Braun DK, Patterson RE, Bloomgren GL. Increased risk of acute pancreatitis and biliary disease observed in patients with type 2 diabetes: a retrospective cohort study. Diabetes Care 2009;32:834–838

22. Koehler JA, Baggio LL, Lamont BJ, Ali S, Drucker DJ. Glucagon-like peptide-1 receptor activation modulates pancreatitis-associated gene expression but does not modify the susceptibility to experimental pancreatitis in mice. Diabetes 2009;58:2148–2161

23. Nachnani JS, Bulchandani DG, Nookala A, Herndon B, Molteni A, Pandya P, Taylor R, Quinn T, Weide L, Alba LM. Biochemical and histological effects of exendin-4 (exenatide) on the rat pancreas. Diabetologia. 13 September 2009 [Epub ahead of print]

24. Matveyenko AV, Dry S, Cox HI, Moshtaghian A, Gurlo T, Galasso R, Butler AE, Butler PC. Beneficial endocrine but adverse exocrine effects of sitagliptin in the human islet amyloid polypeptide transgenic rat model of type 2 diabetes: interactions with metformin. Diabetes 2009;58:1604–1615

25. Marzioni M, Alpini G, Saccomanno S, Candelaresi C, Venter J, Rychlicki C, Fava G, Francis H, Trozzi L, Glaser S, Benedetti A. Glucagon-like peptide-1 and its receptor agonist exendin-4 modulate cholangiocyte adaptive response to cholestasis. Gastroenterology 2007;133:244–255

26. Horner MJ, Ries LAG, Krapcho M, Neyman N, Aminou R, Howlader N, Altekruse SF, Feuer EJ, Huang L, Mariotto A, Miller BA, Lewis DR, Eisner MP, Stinchcomb DG, Edwards BK (Eds). *SEER Cancer Statistics Review, 1975–2006* [Internet], 2009. Bethesda, MD, National Cancer Institute. Available from http://seer.cancer.gov/csr/1975_2006/, based on November 2008 SEER data submission

27. Roman S, Lin R, Sosa JA. Prognosis of medullary thyroid carcinoma: demographic, clinical, and pathologic predictors of survival in 1252 cases. Cancer 2006;107:2134–2142

28. LiVolsi VA. C cell hyperplasia/neoplasia. J Clin Endocrinol Metab 1997;82:39–41

29. Verga U, Ferrero S, Vicentini L, Brambilla T, Cirello V, Muzza M, Beck-Peccoz P, Fugazzola L. Histopathological and molecular studies in patients with goiter and hypercalcitoninemia: reactive or neoplastic C-cell hyperplasia? Endocr Relat Cancer 2007;14:393–403

30. Costante G, Meringolo D, Durante C, Bianchi D, Nocera M, Tumino S, Crocetti U, Attard M, Maranghi M, Torlontano M, Filetti S. Predictive value of serum calcitonin levels for preoperative diagnosis of medullary thyroid carcinoma in a cohort of 5817 consecutive patients with thyroid nodules. J Clin Endocrinol Metab 2007;92:450–455

31. Elisei R. Routine serum calcitonin measurement in the evaluation of thyroid nodules. Best Pract Res Clin Endocrinol Metab 2008;22:941–953

32. Baloch Z, Carayon P, Conte-Devolx B, Demers LM, Feldt-Rasmussen U, Henry JF, LiVosli VA, Niccoli-Sire P, John R, Ruf J, Smyth PP, Spencer CA, Stockigt JR, the Guidelines Committee, the National Academy of Clinical Biochemistry. Laboratory medicine practice guidelines: laboratory support for the diagnosis and monitoring of thyroid disease. Thyroid 2003;13:3–126

33. Crespel A, De Boisvilliers F, Gros L, Kervran A. Effects of glucagon and glucagon-like peptide-1-(7–36) amide on C cells from rat thyroid and medullary thyroid carcinoma CA-77 cell line. Endocrinology 1996;137:3674–3680

34. Körner M, Stöckli M, Waser B, Reubi JC. GLP-1 receptor expression in human tumors and human normal tissues: potential for in vivo targeting. J Nucl Med 2007;48:736–743

35. Lamari Y, Boissard C, Moukhtar MS, Jullienne A, Rosselin G, Garel JM. Expression of glucagon-like peptide 1 receptor in a murine C cell line: regulation of calcitonin gene by glucagon-like peptide 1. FEBS Lett 1996;393:248–252

36. Parola A. FDA Advisory Committee Nonclinical Briefing Document. NDA 2009;22–341

Is the Diminished Incretin Effect in Type 2 Diabetes Just an Epi-Phenomenon of Impaired β-Cell Function?

Juris J. Meier[1] and Michael A. Nauck[2]

Type 2 diabetes is characterized by a deficit in β-cell mass, impaired insulin secretion in response to various stimuli (1–3), as well as a variable extent of insulin resistance (4). More specifically, regarding β-cell function, a significant reduction of the incretin effect, i.e., the postprandial augmentation of insulin secretion by gut hormones, has been described in patients with type 2 diabetes (5). Thus, while the two incretin hormones gastric inhibitory polypeptide (glucose-dependent insulinotopic polypeptide [GIP]) and glucagon-like peptide 1 (GLP-1) are held responsible for ~50–70% of the postprandial insulin responses in healthy individuals (6), their contribution to the overall insulin responses after oral glucose ingestion may amount to <20% in patients with type 2 diabetes (5,7). The reasons underlying the loss of incretin activity in type 2 diabetes are still incompletely understood. The present article reviews the available evidence regarding disturbances in the enteroinsular axis in patients with type 2 diabetes and provides possible explanations for their etiologies, focusing on the personal experience of the authors.

Secretion of incretin hormones in patients with type 2 diabetes. Because the incretin effect has been related to the secretion and insulinotropic action of GIP and GLP-1 (8,9), it was obvious to compare these parameters between patients with type 2 diabetes and healthy control subjects: Regarding the secretion of GIP, elevated, normal, and reduced plasma levels have been described in patients with type 2 diabetes (10–15). However, taking together all the evidence available, the secretion of GIP appears to be relatively unchanged in type 2 diabetic patients. For GLP-1 release, the case is even more complex. Several studies have reported significant reductions in GLP-1 levels after mixed meal ingestion in patients with type 2 diabetes (10,16,17). In addition, one study has found minor impairments in GLP-1 levels in individuals with impaired glucose tolerance (IGT) (16). However, upon more careful evaluation, the defects in GLP-1 secretion in these patients with type 2 diabetes were only found ~2–3 h after meal ingestion, whereas GLP-1 levels were rather unaltered in the immediate postprandial period. Thus, the observed impairments in GLP-1 release do not seem to coincide with the alterations in insulin secretion typically found in patients with type 2 diabetes. Furthermore, these reports are contrasted by a number of other studies showing normal GLP-1 responses in type 2 diabetic patients compared with healthy individuals (11,18–20). Overall, GLP-1 concentrations appear to be highly variable between individuals, both with and without type 2 diabetes, mean values being relatively normal in most groups with type 2 diabetes (18), suggesting that impaired GLP-1 release is not a typical prerequisite for the development of the disease (21). Figure 1 depicts the integrated GLP-1 levels after oral glucose ingestion in relation to the respective glucose concentrations in the fasting state and 120 min after oral glucose ingestion in 48 individuals with different degrees of oral glucose tolerance (11).

Insulinotropic effect of incretin hormones in type 2 diabetes. The relatively normal secretion of GIP and GLP-1 is contrasted by their diminished activity in patients with type 2 diabetes. In the case of GLP-1, the insulinotropic activity is usually referred to as being largely preserved in patients with type 2 diabetes, which has led to the broad utilization of its glucose-lowering potential in the pharmacotherapy of type 2 diabetes (22). However, upon careful examination, the amount of insulin released in response to a supra-physiological GLP-1 infusion during hyperglycemic clamp conditions has also been found to be reduced by ~29% compared with healthy control subjects (23). Furthermore, studies applying a graded glucose infusion protocol have demonstrated a significant impairment in the β-cell responsiveness to the combined administration of GLP-1 and glucose (24). However, the extent to which the insulinotropic activity of GLP-1 is reduced in patients with type 2 diabetes appears to be less pronounced than the defects found in response to intravenous glucose (25) and can almost be fully compensated for by raising GLP-1 plasma concentrations to higher levels (24). By these means, the hyperglycemia in patients with type 2 diabetes can readily be normalized by the intravenous administration of GLP-1 (26), even at relatively low doses (27). Taken together the available evidence, there does not seem to be a severe impairment in GLP-1 action in patients with type 2 diabetes. The modest impairments in insulin release found during GLP-1 administration are most likely a consequence of the general impairment in β-cell function in patients with type 2 diabetes (2).

For GIP, a marked impairment in the insulinotropic activity has uniformly been described in all studies administering the hormone to patients with type 2 diabetes (23,28–31). Thus, during hyperglycemic clamp conditions, an intravenous infusion of GIP in patients with type 2 diabetes elicited only 46% of the insulin responses found in healthy control subjects (23). Unlike with GLP-1, this lack of insulinotropic efficacy cannot be offset by raising GIP doses even to highly supra-physiological concentrations (30). Interestingly, the loss of GIP activity seems to be more pronounced during its continuous infusion than after an intravenous

From the [1]Department of Medicine I, St. Josef-Hospital, Ruhr-University Bochum, Bochum, Germany; and the [2]Diabeteszentrum Bad Lauterberg, Bad Lauterberg, Germany.
Corresponding author: Juris J. Meier, juris.meier@rub.de.
Received 28 December 2009 and accepted 28 January 2010.
DOI: 10.2337/db09-1899

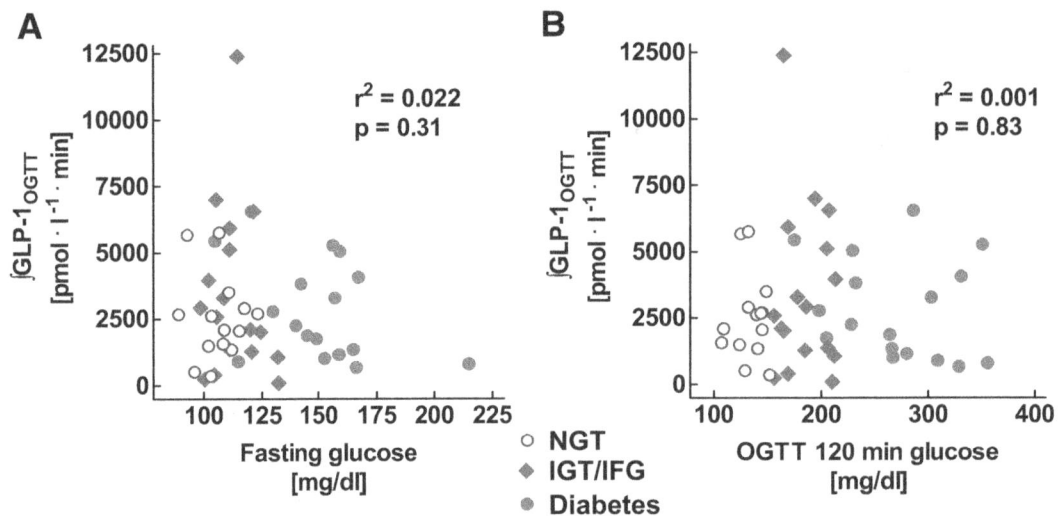

FIG. 1. Relationship between the glucose concentrations at fasting (*A*) and 120 min after the ingestion of 75 g oral glucose (*B*) and the respective integrated GLP-1 levels measured over 240 min after oral glucose ingestion in 14 nondiabetic individuals (blue), 17 people with impaired glucose tolerance or impaired fasting glucose (green), and 17 patients with type 2 diabetes (red). Individual data were taken from ref. 11. r^2 and *P* values were calculated by linear regression analyses. NGT, normal glucose tolerance; OGTT, oral glucose tolerance test.

bolus administration of the peptide (30–32). Consistent with the reduction of its insulinotropic activity, infusing GIP to hyperglycemic patients with type 2 diabetes has no significant glucose-lowering effect (33). The lack of glucose-lowering activity of GIP in type 2 diabetes may also partly be related to its stimulation of glucagon release (34), which counteracts its residual glucose-lowering actions.

Does the reduction of the incretin effect predispose the development of type 2 diabetes? To address whether the diminished incretin effect is a primary, possibly genetically determined, defect predisposing the development of type 2 diabetes, we have undertaken a series of studies in nondiabetic individuals at high risk for the disease: In initial experiments, first-degree relatives of patients with type 2 diabetes, patients with overt type 2 diabetes, and healthy control subjects were examined with the intravenous infusion of GIP during a hyperglycemic clamp experiment (29). Under these conditions, the amount of insulin released in response to GIP was markedly impaired in the type 2 diabetic patients and intermediate in the first-degree relatives, suggesting an early impairment in GIP action in ~50% of these individuals. However, upon further analysis it became obvious that these first-degree relatives also exhibited a similar impairment in insulin secretion after intravenous glucose administration, thereby suggesting that the reduced insulin levels found during GIP and glucose co-administration were secondary to a more general impairment in insulin secretion rather than a specific defect in GIP action. Interestingly, when we tested the effects of GIP administered as an intravenous bolus at normal fasting glucose levels in a larger cohort of first-degree relatives, we were unable to detect any impairment in the insulinotropic activity of GIP (32). Consistent with these findings, the relative size of the incretin effect, as well as the secretion of GIP and GLP-1 after oral glucose ingestion, were completely normal in first-degree relatives (35); furthermore, the same cohort studied previously did not develop disturbances of oral glucose tolerance during 4 years of follow-up, as expected for a high-risk population, and insulin sensitivity in those with a lesser insulinotropic response to GIP was higher, making the

lower insulin secretory response still adequate for the prevailing degree of insulin resistance (36). Taken together, these studies did not reveal any evidence for the existence of a specific defect in GIP action in first-degree relatives of patients with type 2 diabetes.

Women with a history of gestational diabetes are another group at high risk for developing type 2 diabetes. Because the typical metabolic abnormalities in these women may be different from those in the first-degree relatives, we decided to examine the potential disturbances in the incretin system in these women as well. Thus, the group of women included in this study was predominantly characterized by insulin resistance rather than by β-cell dysfunction (37). Interestingly, there were no differences in insulin secretion in response to GIP administered by continuous infusion during a hyperglycemic clamp or as an intravenous bolus in the fasting state between the women with previous gestational diabetes and control subjects. Likewise, GLP-1 and GIP levels after oral glucose ingestion were normal in the women with previous gestational diabetes (37). Taken together, the findings in the first-degree relatives of patients with type 2 diabetes and the women with a history of gestational diabetes seemed to refute the hypothesis that the loss of GIP activity and the impaired incretin effect in patients with type 2 diabetes are due to a primary defect predisposing the development of the disease (21,38). Rather, the loss of incretin activity seems to go along with the other metabolic abnormalities in type 2 diabetes.

In support of this concept, Vilsbøll et al. (39) were able to demonstrate that a reduced insuliotropic effect of GIP is not only present in patients with "typical" type 2 diabetes, but that it can also be found in patients with other types of diabetes, such as maturity-onset diabetes of the young or diabetes secondary to pancreatitis. Subsequent studies determining the percentage contribution of the incretin effect in such patients were able to confirm these initial findings (40).

Potential factors responsible for the reduced incretin effect in type 2 diabetes. The importance of the diminished incretin effect for the dysregulation of postprandial glucose control in type 2 diabetes becomes

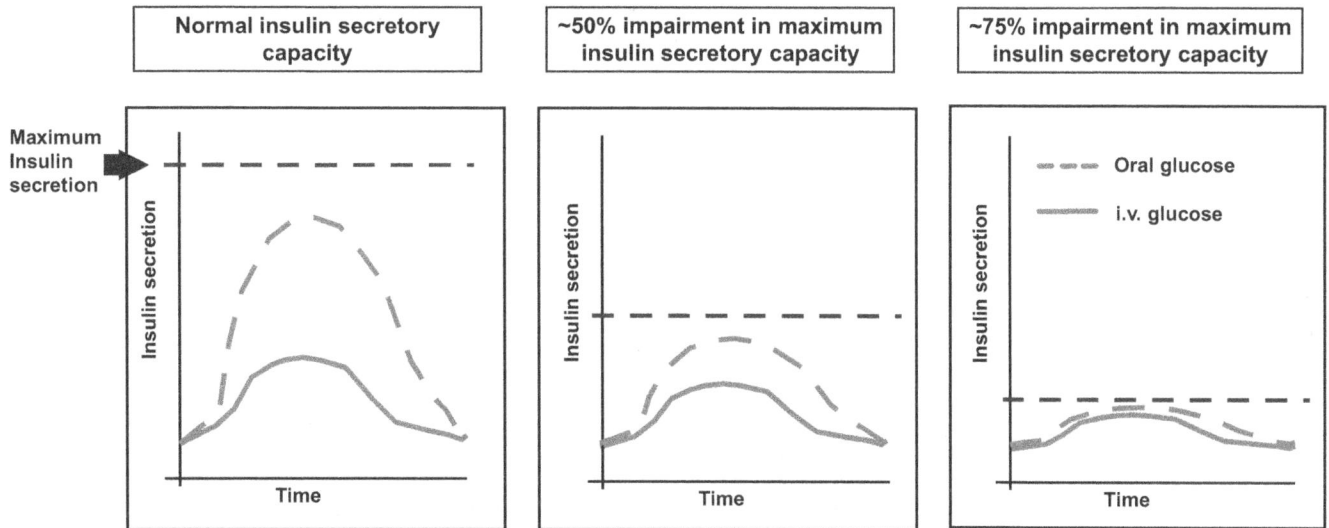

FIG. 2. Hypothetical impact of a general impairment in β-cell function on the incretin effect: In individuals with a normal insulin secretory capacity, an oral glucose load elicits a much greater insulin secretory response than an intravenous (i.v.) glucose load. With a decreasing β-cell secretory capacity, the insulin response to the oral glucose load is relatively more diminished than the insulin response to intravenous glucose infusion. By these means, the incretin effect, i.e., the difference in the insulin responses to oral and intravenous glucose, diminishes with declining β-cell function. For details, see text.

evident from experiments in animals with a genetic knockout of the GIP or GLP-1 receptor as well as from earlier experiments with GIP immune-neutralization (41–43).

The reasons underlying this phenomenon are less well established, and three possible factors appear possible: *Diminished maximum insulin secretory capacity.* The incretin effect is defined by the differences in the insulin secretory responses elicited by oral glucose administration and intravenous glucose infusion (6,8). Of course, in terms of β-cell stimulation the oral glucose load represents a much more potent stimulus, because it combines the insulinotropic effects of circulating glucose, the incretin hormones GIP and GLP-1 (and potentially other ones), as well as some minor effects of afferent vagal nerves (8). In contrast, the insulinotropic effect of the intravenous glucose infusion is restricted to the direct stimulatory effects of circulating glucose. By these means, comparing the insulinotropic activity of oral and intravenous glucose does not only examine the efficacy of the incretin hormones GIP and GLP-1, but it also compares the effects of a relatively modest activator of insulin release (i.e., hyperglycemia) with a relatively potent stimulus of insulin release (i.e., oral glucose). Given the limited maximum secretory capacity of the β-cells in patients with type 2 diabetes (44), it is obvious that the insulinotropic response to a larger stimulus would be relatively more impaired that that of a less potent secretagogue. In other words, the difference between the insulin responses elicited by a potent secretagogue and a weaker secretagogue would be expected to shrink down with diminishing β-cell function (and perhaps mass). Furthermore, the total amount of glucose administered via the oral route (~50 g) typically exceeds the amount of glucose infused intravenously (~20 g) during isoglycemic clamp experiments. Because the insulin response to glucose is usually markedly impaired in patients with type 2 diabetes, this might further contribute to the diminished incretin effect in such patients. On that basis, the diminished incretin effect in patients with type 2 diabetes may simply reflect the reduced maximum secretory capacity of the β-cells in

such patients rather than a specific problem in incretin secretion or action. The hypothetical consequences of a reduction in β-cell mass and/or function for the incretin effect are demonstrated in Fig. 2. Consistent with this view, we observed a linear inverse relationship between fasting glucose concentrations and the "size" of the incretin effect (percentage difference in the insulin responses between oral and intravenous glucose stimulation) in 48 individuals with and without diabetes (Fig. 3). This interpretation is further supported by the finding that a diminished incretin effect can also readily be observed in patients with other types of diabetes (45), and by the fact that it can be restored through pancreas transplantation in patients with type 1 diabetes (46). However, further studies will be required to substantiate this hypothesis.
Reduced GLP-1 secretion. One popular explanation for the diminished incretin effect in type 2 diabetes has been a reduction of GLP-1 secretion (47). This hypothesis has been based on studies demonstrating reductions in meal-

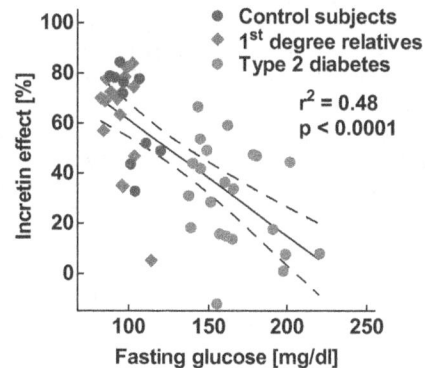

FIG. 3. Relationship between the relative percentage contribution of the incretin effect on the overall insulin responses after oral glucose ingestion and to the respective fasting glucose concentrations in 48 individuals with and without diabetes. Individual data were taken from refs. 35 and 7. The solid line denotes the regression line calculated by regression analyses in relation to the upper and lower 95% CIs.

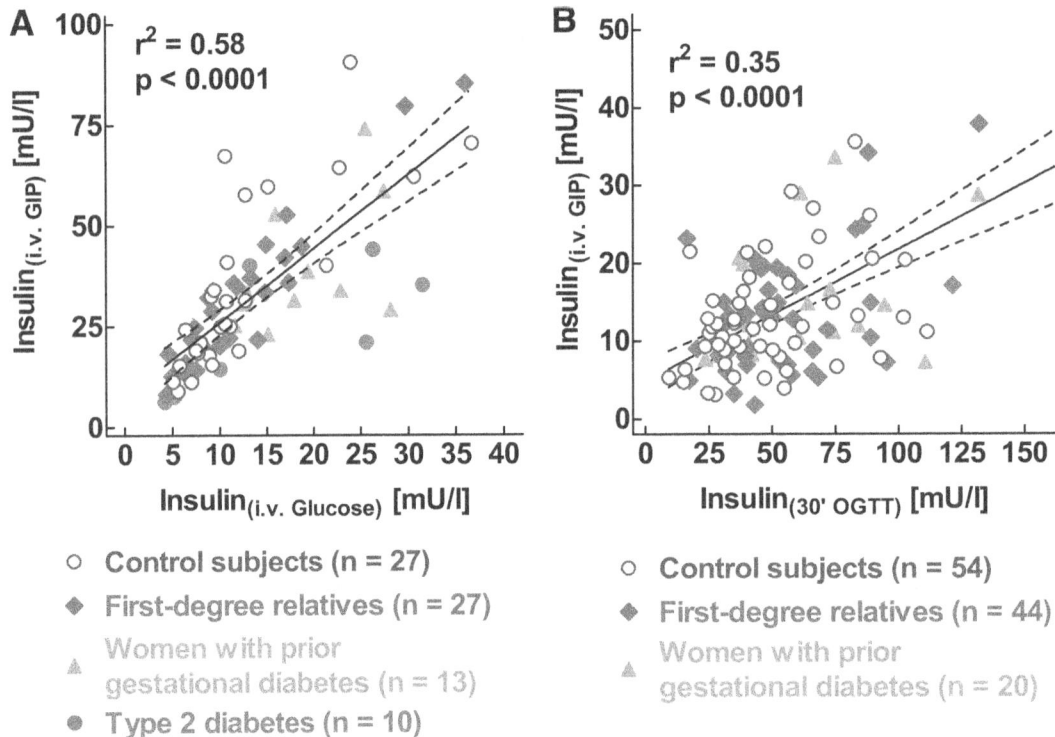

FIG. 4. *A*: Relationship between the plasma insulin levels during the intravenous (i.v.) administration of glucose alone and the insulin levels during the combined administration of i.v. glucose and GIP in 27 healthy control subjects, 27 first-degree relatives of patients with type 2 diabetes, 13 women with previous gestational diabetes, and 10 patients with type 2 diabetes. Individual data were taken from refs. 29, 35, and 37. *B*: Relationship between the plasma insulin levels during the intravenous administration of GIP and glucose and the insulin levels measured 30 min after oral ingestion of 75 g glucose in 54 healthy control subjects, 44 first-degree relatives of patients with type 2 diabetes, and 20 women with previous gestational diabetes. Individual data were taken from refs. 32 and 37. The solid line denotes the regression line calculated by regression analyses in relation to the upper and lower 95% CIs.

induced GLP-1 concentrations in patients with long-standing type 2 diabetes and subjects with impaired glucose tolerance (10,16,17). However, because the timing of the impairments in GLP-1 concentrations (~2–4 h after meal ingestion) does not coincide with the typical defects in meal-induced insulin release (~30–60 min after meal ingestion), such impairment in GLP-1 release cannot plausibly explain the loss of incretin activity in patients with type 2 diabetes. Furthermore, the majority of studies in patients with type 2 diabetes have failed to show similar impairments in GLP-1 concentrations (18), suggesting that in the vast majority of diabetic patients defects in GLP-1 release do not explain the diminished incretin effect. It is, however, possible that changes in the level of glycemia have an impact on the individual GIP and GLP-1 responses after meal ingestion. Along these lines, the postprandial concentrations of GIP and GLP-1 were found significantly lower during hyperglycemic clamp conditions compared with euglycemia, probably driven by a glucose-induced delay in gastric emptying (48). It is therefore conceivable that acute elevations in circulating glucose levels may partly blunt postprandial incretin responses. By this reasoning, the increased GLP-1 levels that have been reported after the administration of metformin may simply be due to the glucose-lowering effect of the drug (49). However, even though hyperglycemia appears to acutely lower GLP-1 secretion, it is completely unclear whether chronic hyperglycemia has a negative impact on GLP-1 levels as well. Correlation analyses did not reveal a significant association between fasting or postchallenge glucose concentrations and GLP-1 release (Fig. 1). Taken together,

changes in GLP-1 secretion may occur under different conditions, but a general reduction in GLP-1 release fails to explain the reduced incretin effect in type 2 diabetes.

Specific loss of GIP activity. A number of studies have compared the insulinotropic effect of GIP in patients with type 2 diabetes and healthy control subjects. Uniformly, a relative reduction of GIP activity has been described in these studies (23,28–31). However, while this may certainly suggest a defect in GIP signaling, one should not forget that the efficacy of other secretagogues, especially glucose, is also severely impaired in these patients (3,44,50). Thus, in a direct comparison between patients with type 2 diabetes and healthy control subjects, the insulinotropic effect of an intravenous glucose bolus was found to be reduced by ~85% in the diabetic patients (51), and other studies have clearly shown a reduction in first-phase insulin release in response to glucose with increasing fasting glucose levels (52). The magnitude of the impairment in glucose-induced insulin secretion therefore seems to be comparable to the respective defect in GIP-induced insulin secretion described in other studies (23,30). To address this point, we have correlated the insulin secretory responses to GIP administration with the respective responses to intravenous glucose administration in a large group of individuals (n = 77), including patients with type 2 diabetes, first-degree relatives of patients with type 2 diabetes, women with a history of gestational diabetes, and healthy subjects (Fig. 4). Indeed, there was a tight correlation between the insulin responses to GIP and to glucose administration in these studies, consistent with the idea that the impairment in

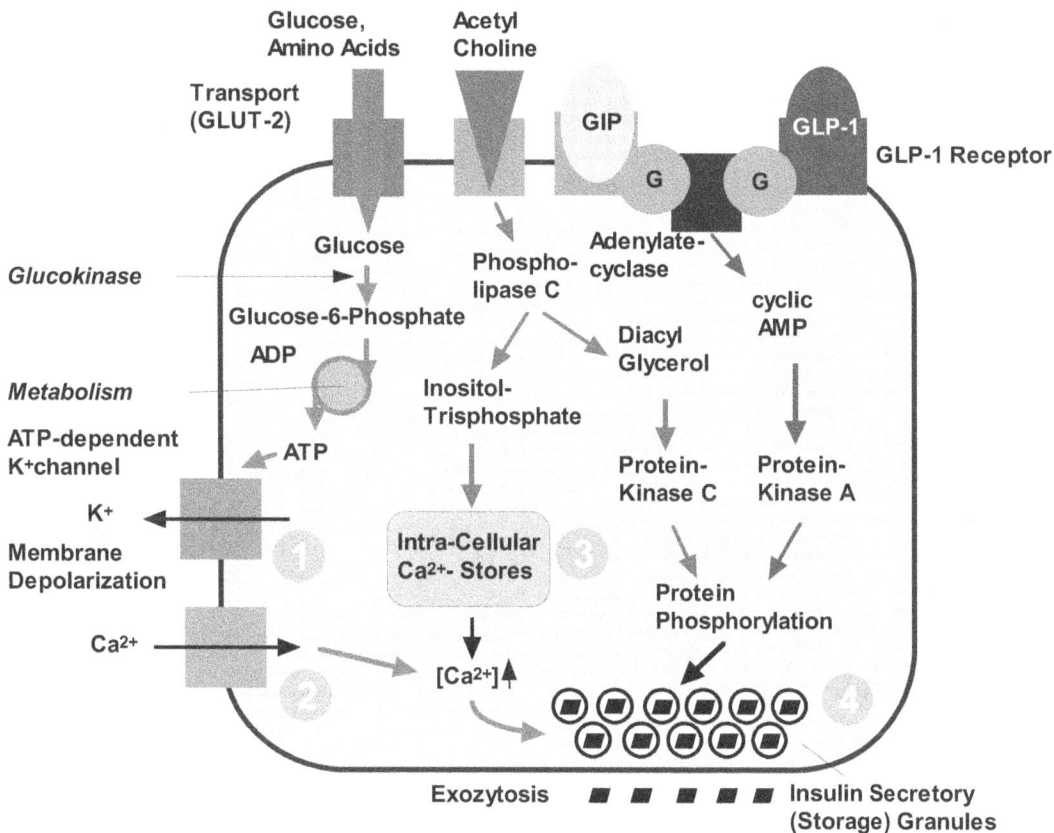

FIG. 5. Intracellular actions of GIP and GLP-1 on the β-cell. Several cellular functions are affected: closing of the ATP-dependent potassium channel (*1*); calcium influx in response to action potentials (*2*); release of calcium from intracellular stores (*3*); and the readiness with which insulin storage granules are released (*4*), probably depending on protein phosphorylation. These effects are tightly linked to the glucose-dependent generation of ATP, meaning that GLP-1 and GIP augment insulin release only in the presence of hyperglycemia. For details, see ref. 74.

GIP-induced insulin secretion goes along with a defect in glucose-induced insulin secretion. A less close relationship was observed between the insulin release elicited by the intravenous bolus administration of GIP at normal fasting glucose levels and the insulin concentrations 30 min after oral glucose ingestion (Fig. 4). Given that GIP acts in concert with glucose to enhance insulin secretion (Fig. 5), it is possible that the inability of GIP to augment insulin secretion during hyperglycemia is primarily due to the lack of glucose-potentiation of insulin release in patients with diabetes. However, while such an argument may seem to plausibly explain the loss of GIP action in patients with type 2 diabetes, one striking phenomenon still remains unexplained: Why does GLP-1 still potently stimulate insulin release during hyperglycemia in patients with type 2 diabetes? Possibly, the unequal insulinotropic efficacy of GIP and GLP-1 in patients with type 2 diabetes is due to an additional (and yet unexplored) mechanism of action rather than due to a specific defect in GIP signaling. In fact, both GIP and GLP-1 have been shown to exert their actions through binding to G-protein–coupled receptors on the β-cells, activation of adenylate cyclase, and subsequent cAMP generation (53). In addition, PI 3-kinase activation has been reported for both GIP and GLP-1. However, while these downstream signaling mechanisms are rather similar for both incretin hormones, recent studies have suggested a preferential upregulation of insulin receptor substrate 2 (IRS-2) through epidermal growth factor receptor activation by GLP-1 (54). This and

other yet unexplored mechanisms may therefore contribute to the unequal efficacy of GIP and GLP-1 in patients with type 2 diabetes.

Working models for the loss of GIP activity in type 2 diabetes. Assuming that a specific problem in GIP signaling in patients with type 2 diabetes does indeed exist, the obvious question arising is: What are the reasons underlying such defect? In fact, the loss of insulinotropic GIP effects in type 2 diabetes despite the relatively well preserved activity of GLP-1 is quite surprising because both incretins are structurally similar, are released under almost identical conditions, and share similar signaling pathways inside the β-cell (53,55). Thus, both hormones bind to similar but distinct seven–membrane spanning G-protein–coupled surface receptors leading to intracellular cAMP generation and intracellular calcium release (53,55). However, this does not exclude alterations in the function or quantitative expression of the GIP receptor in patients with type 2 diabetes (56).

Considering the loss of GIP efficacy in type 2 diabetes in light of the available evidence from clinical studies as well as from animal and tissue culture based experiments, two different working models seem to arise:

Genetic defects in GIP signaling. The lack of GIP effect in type 2 diabetes has given rise to try and link polymorphisms in the GIP receptor with the type 2 diabetic phenotype. Two earlier studies from Europe and Japan have failed to establish an association between type 2 diabetes and GIP receptor polymorphisms (57,58). A more recent study found a slightly impaired action of GLP-1, but not GIP in carriers of the T allele of rs7903146 TCF7L2 (59). Likewise, Schäfer and colleagues found a reduced insulinotropic effect of GLP-1 in carriers of the rs10010131 polymorphism of the WFS1 gene (60) as well as in carriers of TCF7L2 polymorphisms (61). These studies therefore suggest that genetic alterations in GLP-1 action may play a role in type 2 diabetes (62), which is surprising, given the relatively well preserved efficacy of GLP-1 in such patients (23). However, a genetic defect in GIP action predisposing to type 2 diabetes has not yet been established. Clearly, further studies in this area will be required.

Down-regulation/desensitization of the GIP receptor in response to hyperglycemia. The idea of a reduced expression of GIP receptors in patients with type 2 diabetes has already been expounded in 1997 (56), but until now no data regarding GIP receptor expression on islets from humans with and without type 2 diabetes have become available, owing to the limited accessibility of human pancreatic tissue. However, a couple of experimental studies have lent support to this concept: Lynn et al. (63) found reduced GIP receptor mRNA and protein levels in islets from Vancouver diabetic fatty rats, suggesting an impaired receptor expression in response to hyperglycemia. Subsequent experiments from the same group found a down-regulation of the GIP receptor in a transfected β-cell line (INS-cells) (64). More recently, Xu et al. (65) found reduced GIP mRNA levels in hyperglycemic rats after a 90% partial pancreatectomy. Interestingly, these effects could be reversed by glucose-normalization using phlorizin treatment. However, in the same study the expression of the GLP-1 receptor was regulated by hyperglycemia in a similar manner (65), which is rather inconsistent with the clinical findings on GIP and GLP-1 efficacy in patients with type 2 diabetes (23). In addition to this downregulation of the GIP receptor in response to hyperglycemia, a desensitization of the GIP receptor in response to chronically elevated GIP concentrations has also been described in GIP receptor–transfected cell lines (66). However, since elevations in GIP plasma concentrations are not a typical finding in most patients with type 2 diabetes (67), this mechanism is less likely to contribute to the impairment of GIP efficacy in type 2 diabetes.

To examine the impact of chronic hyperglycemia on GIP-induced insulin release, we have compared the relative stimulation of insulin secretion during the intravenous administration of GIP at hyperglycemic clamp conditions in a total of 93 individuals with the respective fasting glucose concentrations at the day of the experiment (Fig. 6). The insulin responses to GIP were found relatively normal in the individuals presenting with fasting glucose concentrations of less than ~100 mg/dl. However, as glucose concentrations exceeded this level, there was a progressive decline in GIP activity on insulin secretion, with an almost complete loss of efficacy in patients with overt hyperglycemia of 150–250 mg/dl. Thus, even though the association between the insulinotropic effect of GIP and the respective fasting glucose levels cannot serve to prove any causality, these analyses are very consistent with the concept of a GIP receptor downregulation in response to high glucose concentrations. The potential factors contributing to the diminished incretin effect in type 2 diabetes have been summarized as a working model in Fig. 7.

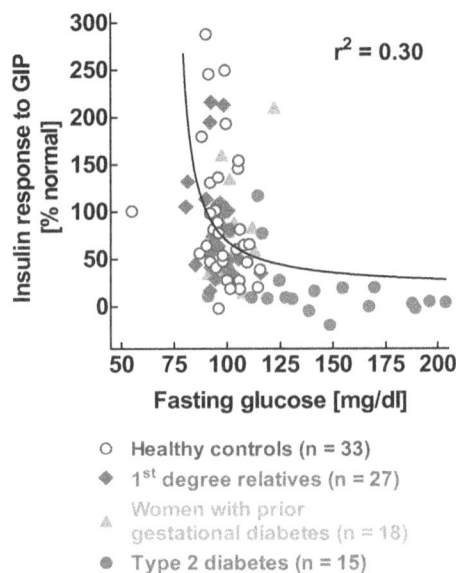

FIG. 6. Relationship between the relative increase in insulin secretion during the intravenous administration of GIP at hyperglycemic clamp conditions and the respective fasting glucose concentrations in 93 individuals with and without diabetes. The relative increments in insulin secretion were expressed in relation to the mean values obtained in the individuals with normal glucose concentrations (fasting glucose levels <100 mg/dl). Individual data were taken from refs. 29, 30, and 35. The solid line denotes the regression line calculated by nonlinear regression analyses using an exponential decay function.

Can the incretin effect be restored by normalizing hyperglycemia? Assuming that the relative impairment of the incretin effect and the loss of GIP activity in patients with type 2 diabetes are secondary to the chronic hyperglycemia, the clinical implication would be that normalizing the hyperglycemia in these patients should also restore the insulinotropic effect of GIP. Højberg and colleagues (68–70) set out to address this point by subjecting eight patients with type 2 diabetes in poor glycemic control (A1C levels 8.6 ± 1.3%) to a 4-week intensive insulin treatment with the aim of completely normalizing glycemia in these patients. The insulin responses to GIP and GLP-1 were determined before and after the intervention during a hyperglycemic clamp experiment. There was indeed a significant improvement in insulin secretion in response to both GIP and GLP-1 after glucose lowering (68), whereas no effects were found with regards to the secretion of both hormones after meal ingestion (69). However, a complete regain of GIP activity to the levels found in healthy subjects was not accomplished in this study (68). Furthermore, the observed improvements in insulin secretion were not specific to the actions of GIP but also affected the insulinotropic effect of GLP-1 as well as the overall β-cell responses to meal ingestion (69). It is therefore difficult to fully ascribe these phenomena to the reversal of a specific defect in incretin signaling. In fact, a number of previous studies have demonstrated that lowering hyperglycemia in patients with type 2 diabetes can also lead to marked improvements of insulin secretion in response to intravenous glucose and other secretagogues, probably mediated by the mechanism of β-cell rest (71–73). In addition, although glucose control was significantly improved by the insulin treatment in this study, complete normoglycaemia was not achieved in these patients at the end of the study (mean glucose concentrations 7.4 mmol/l [133 mg/dl]) (68). Based on the analyses of our studies

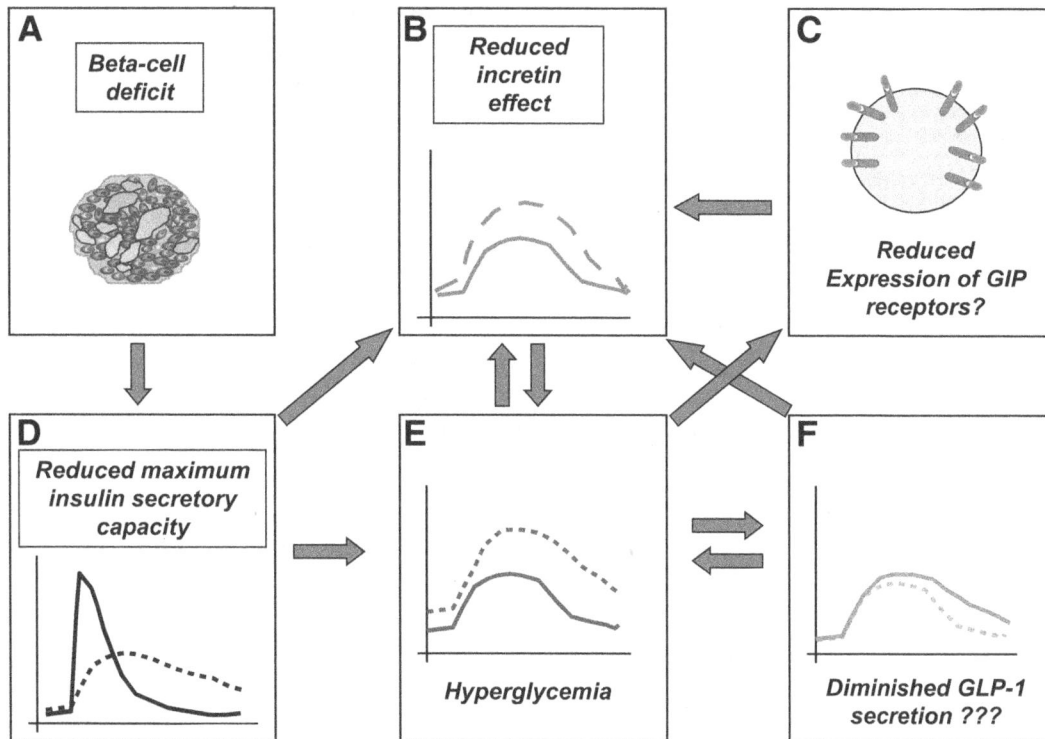

FIG. 7. Working model for the diminished incretin effect in type 2 diabetes: The reduction in β-cell mass (*A*) leads to a significant impairment in the maximum insulin secretory capacity of the β-cells (*D*). The reduced secretory capacity leads to a preferential impairment of the relative insulin response to oral glucose, whereas a relatively normal insulin response to intravenous glucose (a comparably weaker β-cell stimulus) can still be maintained. The defects in β-cell function and the impaired incretin effect (*B*) lead to chronic hyperglycemia (*E*), which may diminish GLP-1 secretion (*F*) and impair GIP action through GIP-receptor downregulation (*C*), thereby further diminishing the incretin effect. Genetic factors may independently modify β-cell mass and function as well as GLP-1 secretion. Dashed lines in *D*, *E*, and *F* indicate the respective patterns typical of patients with type 2 diabetes, solid lines show the respective normal patterns. The dashed line in *B* illustrates the insulin levels after oral glucose ingestion; the solid line shows the respective patterns after isoglycemic intravenous glucose administration.

presented herein, both the incretin effect and the relative activity of GIP were still severely impaired in individuals with similar fasting glucose concentrations. Nevertheless, the studies by Madsbad and Højberg clearly demonstrate that reducing the hyperglycemia in patients with type 2 diabetes can also elicit significant improvements in the incretin effect.

Conclusions and outlook. The diminished incretin effect in patients with type 2 diabetes was described more than 20 years ago (5), but even now the underlying causes remain elusive. Although a couple of studies have described alterations in the postprandial concentrations of GIP and GLP-1, there is little evidence to suggest that impairments in incretin secretion play a major role in the pathogenesis of type 2 diabetes (21). The insulinotropic action of the incretin hormones is clearly impaired in patients with type 2 diabetes, with GLP-1 retaining significantly more efficacy than GIP (23). However, the magnitude of the reduction in GIP efficacy in patients with type 2 diabetes appears to be comparable to the impairment in glucose-induced insulin secretion in such patients, suggesting that the impaired GIP-induced insulin secretion may largely be secondary to of a general impairment in β-cell function. In addition, there is evidence from preclinical and clinical studies that hyperglycemia further reduces the insulinotropic effect of GIP, possibly through downregulation of the GIP receptor (63). Ultimately, the diminished incretin effect in patients with type 2 diabetes may be a consequence of the inability of the β-cells to

provide an appropriate secretory response to a large stimulus (i.e., oral glucose), whereas a smaller stimulus (i.e., intravenous glucose) may still elicit a relatively normal insulin response (Fig. 2). On the basis of such reasoning, the reduction of the incretin effect in patients with diabetes may simply be an epi-phenomenon of chronic hyperglycemia, independent of any primary defect in GIP or GLP-1 action. Reducing hyperglycemia and enhancing β-cell function in general terms may therefore also improve the incretin effect, independent of specific interventions related to circulating levels of GIP or GLP-1.

ACKNOWLEDGMENTS

J.J.M. has received speaker honoraria and consulting fees from the following companies: Novo Nordisk, Eli Lilly, Merck Sharp & Dohme, Novartis, sanofi-aventis, and Astra-Zeneca. M.A.N. has received research grants from Bayer Vital Pharma, Eli Lilly & Co. Indianapolis, Menarini/Berlin-Chemie, Merck Sharp & Dohme, and Novo Nordisk; and has accepted honoraria for membership in advisory boards and consulting and has received honoraria for speaking on incretin-based antidiabetic medications from Amylin Pharmaceuticals, AstraZeneca, Menarini/Berlin-Chemie, Biovitrum, Eli Lilly & Co., Indianapolis, Glaxo-SmithKline, Hoffman La Roche, Novartis Pharma, Sanofi-aventis Pharma, and Takeda. No other potential conflicts of interest relevant to this article were reported.

REFERENCES

1. Klöppel G, Löhr M, Habich K, Oberholzer M, Heitz PU. Islet pathology and the pathogenesis of type 1 and type 2 diabetes mellitus revisited. Surv Synth Pathol Res 1985;4:110–125
2. Butler AE, Janson J, Bonner-Weir S, Ritzel R, Rizza RA, Butler PC. Beta-cell deficit and increased beta-cell apoptosis in humans with type 2 diabetes. Diabetes 2003;52:102–110
3. Meier JJ, Butler PC. Insulin secretion. In *Endocrinology*. 5th ed. DeGroot LJ, Jameson JL, Eds. Philadelphia, Elsevier Saunders, 2005, p. 961–973
4. DeFronzo RA. Lily lecture 1987: The triumvirate: β-cell, muscle, and liver: a collusion responsible for NIDDM. Diabetes 1988;37:667–687
5. Nauck M, Stöckmann F, Ebert R, Creutzfeldt W. Reduced incretin effect in type 2 (non-insulin-dependent) diabetes. Diabetologia 1986;29:46–52
6. Nauck MA, Homberger E, Siegel EG, Allen RC, Eaton RP, Ebert R, Creutzfeldt W. Incretin effects of increasing glucose loads in man calculated from venous insulin and C-peptide responses. J Clin Endocrinol Metab 1986;63:492–498
7. Foley JE, Becker l, Köthe L, Dejager S, Schweizer A, Nauck MA. Inhibition of DPP-4 with vildagliptin improved insulin secretion in response to oral as well as "isoglycaemic" glucose without numerically changing the incretin effect in patients with type 2 diabetes. Diabetologia 2008;51(Suppl. 1):367
8. Creutzfeldt W. The incretin concept today. Diabetologia 1979;16:75–85
9. Creutzfeldt W, Nauck M. Gut hormones and diabetes mellitus. Diabetes Metab Res Rev 1992;8:149–177
10. Vilsbøll T, Krarup T, Deacon CF, Madsbad S, Holst JJ. Reduced postprandial concentrations of intact biologically active glucagon-like peptide 1 in type 2 diabetic patients. Diabetes 2001;50:609–613
11. Vollmer K, Holst JJ, Baller B, Ellrichmann M, Nauck MA, Schmidt WE, Meier JJ. Predictors of incretin concentrations in subjects with normal, impaired, and diabetic glucose tolerance. Diabetes 2008;57:678–687
12. Crockett SE, Mazzaferri EL, Cataland S. Gastric inhibitory peptide (GIP) in maturity-onset diabetes mellitus. Diabetes 1976;25:931–935
13. Ross SA, Brown JC, Dupré J. Hypersecretion of gastric inhibitory polypeptide following oral glucose in diabetes mellitus. Diabetes 1977;26:525–529
14. Krarup T. Immunoreactive gastric inhibitory polypeptide. Endocrine Reviews 1988;9:122–134
15. Ebert R, Creutzfeldt W. Hypo- and hypersecretion of GIP in maturity-onset diabetics (Abstract). Diabetologia 1980;19:271–272
16. Toft-Nielsen MB, Damholt MB, Madsbad S, Hilsted LM, Hughes TE, Michelsen BK, Holst JJ. Determinants of the impaired secretion of glucagon-like peptide-1 in type 2 diabetic patients. J Clin Endocrinol Metab 2001;86:3717–3723
17. Muscelli E, Mari A, Casolaro A, Camastra S, Seghieri G, Gastaldelli A, Holst JJ, Ferrannini E. Separate impact of obesity and glucose tolerance on the incretin effect in normal subjects and type 2 diabetic patients. Diabetes 2008;57:1340–1348
18. Meier JJ, Nauck MA. Is secretion of glucagon-like peptide-1 reduced in type 2 diabetes mellitus? Nat Clin Pract Endocrinol Metab 2008;4:606–607
19. Ryskjaer J, Deacon CF, Carr RD, Krarup T, Madsbad S, Holst J, Vilsbøll T. Plasma dipeptidyl peptidase-IV activity in patients with type-2 diabetes mellitus correlates positively with HbAlc levels, but is not acutely affected by food intake. Eur J Endocrinol 2006;155:485–493
20. Orskov C, Jeppesen J, Madsbad S, Holst JJ. Proglucagon products in plasma of noninsulin-dependent diabetics and nondiabetic controls in the fasting state and after oral glucose and intravenous arginine. J Clin Invest 1991;87:415–423
21. Meier JJ. The contribution of incretin hormones to the pathogenesis of type 2 diabetes. Best Pract Res Clin Endocrinol Metab 2009;23:433–441
22. Meier JJ, Nauck MA. The potential role of glucagon-like peptide 1 in diabetes. Curr Opin Investig Drugs 2004;5:402–410
23. Nauck MA, Heimesaat MM, Orskov C, Holst JJ, Ebert R, Creutzfeldt W. Preserved incretin activity of glucagon-like peptide 1 [7–36 amide] but not of synthetic human gastric inhibitory polypeptide in patients with type-2 diabetes mellitus. J Clin Invest 1993;91:301–307
24. Kjems LL, Holst JJ, Vølund A, Madsbad S. The influence of GLP-1 on glucose-stimulated insulin secretion: effects on beta-cell sensitivity in type 2 and nondiabetic subjects. Diabetes 2003;52:380–386
25. Pfeifer MA, Halter JB, Porte D Jr. Insulin secretion in diabetes mellitus. Am J Med 1981;70:579–588
26. Nauck MA, Kleine N, Orskov C, Holst JJ, Willms B, Creutzfeldt W. Normalization of fasting hyperglycaemia by exogenous glucagon-like peptide 1 (7–36 amide) in type 2 (non-insulin-dependent) diabetic patients. Diabetologia 1993;36:741–744
27. Meier JJ, Gallwitz B, Salmen S, Goetze O, Holst JJ, Schmidt WE, Nauck MA. Normalization of glucose concentrations and deceleration of gastric emptying after solid meals during intravenous glucagon-like peptide 1 in patients with type 2 diabetes. J Clin Endocrinol Metab 2003;88:2719–2725
28. Krarup T, Saurbrey N, Moody AJ, Kühl C, Madsbad S. Effect of porcine gastric inhibitory polypeptide on β-cell function in type I and type II diabetes mellitus. Metabolism 1988;36:677–682
29. Meier JJ, Hücking K, Holst JJ, Deacon CF, Schmiegel WH, Nauck MA. Reduced insulinotropic effect of gastric inhibitory polypeptide in first-degree relatives of patients with type 2 diabetes. Diabetes 2001;50:2497–2504
30. Meier JJ, Gallwitz B, Kask B, Deacon CF, Holst JJ, Schmidt WE, Nauck MA. Stimulation of insulin secretion by intravenous bolus injection and continuous infusion of gastric inhibitory polypeptide in patients with type 2 diabetes and healthy control subjects. Diabetes 2004;53(Suppl. 2):S220–S224
31. Vilsbøll T, Krarup T, Madsbad S, Holst JJ. Defective amplification of the late phase insulin response to glucose by GIP in obese type II diabetic patients. Diabetologia 2002;45:1111–1119
32. Meier JJ, Nauck MA, Siepmann N, Greulich M, Holst JJ, Deacon CF, Schmidt WE, Gallwitz B. Similar insulin secretory response to a gastric inhibitory polypeptide bolus injection at euglycemia in first-degree relatives of patients with type 2 diabetes and control subjects. Metabolism 2003;52:1579–1585
33. Amland PF, Jorde R, Aanderud S, Burhol PG, Giercksky KE. Effects of intravenously infused porcine GIP on serum insulin, plasma C-peptide, and pancreatic polypeptide in non-insulin-dependent diabetes in the fasting state. Scand J Gastroenterol 1985;20:315–320
34. Meier JJ, Gallwitz B, Siepmann N, Holst JJ, Deacon CF, Schmidt WE, Nauck MA. Gastric inhibitory polypeptide (GIP) dose-dependently stimulates glucagon secretion in healthy human subjects at euglycaemia. Diabetologia 2003;46:798–801
35. Nauck MA, El-Ouaghlidi A, Gabrys B, Hücking K, Holst JJ, Deacon CF, Gallwitz B, Schmidt WE, Meier JJ. Secretion of incretin hormones (GIP and GLP-1) and incretin effect after oral glucose in first-degree relatives of patients with type 2 diabetes. Regul Pept 2004;122:209–217
36. Nauck MA, Baller B, Meier JJ. Gastric inhibitory polypeptide and glucagon-like peptide-1 in the pathogenesis of type 2 diabetes. Diabetes 2004;53(Suppl. 3):S190–S196
37. Meier JJ, Gallwitz B, Askenas M, Vollmer K, Deacon CF, Holst JJ, Schmidt WE, Nauck MAS. Secretion of incretin hormones and the insulinotropic effect of gastric inhibitory polypeptide in women with a history of gestational diabetes. Diabetologia 2005;48:1872–1881
38. Nauck MA, Baller B, Meier JJ. Gastric inhibitory polypeptide and glucagon-like peptide-1 in the pathogenesis of type 2 diabetes. Diabetes 2004;53(Suppl. 3):S190–S196
39. Vilsbøll T, Knop FK, Krarup T, Johansen A, Madsbad S, Larsen S, Hansen T, Pedersen O, Holst JJ. The pathophysiology of diabetes involves a defective amplification of the late-phase insulin response to glucose by glucose-dependent insulinotropic polypeptide-regardless of etiology and phenotype. J Clin Endocrinol Metab 2003;88:4897–4903
40. Knop FK, Vilsbøll T, Højberg PV, Larsen S, Madsbad S, Vølund A, Holst JJ, Krarup T. Reduced incretin effect in type 2 diabetes: cause or consequence of the diabetic state? Diabetes 2007;56:1951–1959
41. Miyawaki K, Yamada Y, Yano H, Niwa H, Ban N, Ihara Y, Kubota A, Fujimoto S, Kajikawa M, Kuroe A, Tsuda K, Hashimoto H, Yamashita T, Jomori T, Tashiro F, Miyazaki J, Seino Y. Glucose intolerance caused by a defect in the entero-insular axis: a study in gastric inhibitory polypeptide receptor knockout mice. Proc Natl Acad Sci U S A 1999;96:14843–14847
42. Scrocchi LA, Brown TJ, MaClusky N, Brubaker PL, Auerbach AB, Joyner AL, Drucker DJ. Glucose intolerance but normal satiety in mice with a null mutation in the glucagon-like peptide 1 receptor gene. Nat Med 1996;2:1254–1258
43. Ebert R, Creutzfeldt W. Influence of gastric inhibitory polypeptide anti-serum on glucose-induced insulin secretion in rats. Endocrinol 1982;111:1601–1606
44. Ward WK, Bolgiano DC, McKnight B, Halter JB, Porte D Jr. Diminished β cell secretory capacity in patients with non-insulin-dependent diabetes mellitus. J Clin Invest 1984;74:1318–1328
45. Knop FK, Vilsbøll T, Højberg PV, Larsen S, Madsbad S, Vølund A, Holst JJ, Krarup T. Reduced incretin effect in type 2 diabetes: cause or consequence of the diabetic state? Diabetes 2007;56:1951–1959
46. Nauck MA, Büsing M, Orskov C, Siegel EG, Talartschik J, Baartz A, Baartz T, Hopt UT, Becker HD, Creutzfeldt W. Preserved incretin effect in type 1 diabetic patients with end-stage nephropathy treated by combined heterotopic pancreas and kidney transplantation. Acta Diabetol 1993;30:39–45
47. Stonehouse AH, Holcombe JH, Kendall DM. Management of type 2 diabetes: the role of incretin mimetics. Expert Opin Pharmacother 2006;7:2095–2105

48. Vollmer K, Gardiwal H, Menge BA, Goetze O, Deacon CF, Schmidt WE, Holst JJ, Meier JJ. Hyperglycemia acutely lowers the postprandial excursions of glucagon-like peptide-1 and gastric inhibitory polypeptide in humans. J Clin Endocrinol Metab 2009;94:1379–1385

49. Yasuda N, Inoue T, Nagakura T, Yamazaki K, Kira K, Saeki T, Tanaka I. Enhanced secretion of glucagon-like peptide 1 by biguanide compounds. Biochem Biophys Res Commun 2002;298:779–784

50. Gerich JE. The genetic basis of type 2 diabetes mellitus: impaired insulin secretion versus impaired insulin sensitivity. Endocr Rev 1998;19:491–503

51. Pfeifer MA, Halter JB, Porte D Jr. Insulin secretion in diabetes mellitus. Am J Med 1981;70:579–588

52. Brunzell JD, Robertson RP, Lerner RL, Hazzard WR, Ensinck JW, Bierman EL, Porte D Jr. Relationship between fasting plasma glucose levels and insulin secretion during intravenous glucose tolerance tests. J Clin Endocrinol Metab 1976;42:222–229

53. Gromada J, Holst JJ, Rorsman P. Cellular regulation of islet hormone secretion by the incretin hormone glucagon-like peptide 1. Pflügers Arch/Eur J Physiol 1998;435:583–594

54. Jessen L, D'Alessio D. The incretins and β-cell health: the incretins and beta-cell health: contrasting glucose-dependent insulinotropic polypeptide and glucagon-like peptide-1 as a path to understand islet function in diabetes. Gastroenterology 2009;137:1891–1894

55. Gromada J, Bokvist K, Ding WG, Holst JJ, Nielsen JH, Rorsman P. Glucagon-like peptide 1 (7–36) amide stimulates exocytosis in human pancreatic beta-cells by both proximal and distal regulatory steps in stimulus-secretion coupling. Diabetes 1998;47:57–65

56. Holst JJ, Gromada J, Nauck MA. The pathogenesis of NIDDM involves a defective expression of the GIP receptor. Diabetologia 1997;40:984–986

57. Almind K, Ambye L, Urhammer SA, Hansen T, Echwald SM, Holst JJ, Gromada J, Thorens B, Pedersen O. Discovery of amino acid variants in the human glucose-dependent insulinotropic polypeptide (GIP) receptor: the impact on the pancreatic beta cell responses and functional expression studies in Chinese hamster fibroblast cells. Diabetologia 1998;41:1194–1198

58. Kubota A, Yamada Y, Hayami T, Yasuda K, Someya Y, Ihara Y, Kagimoto S, Watanabe R, Taminato T, Tsuda K, Seino Y. Identification of two missense mutations in the GIP receptor gene: a functional study and association analysis with NIDDM. Diabetes 1996;45:1701–1705

59. Pilgaard K, Jensen CB, Schou JH, Lyssenko V, Wegner L, Brøns C, Vilsbøll T, Hansen T, Madsbad S, Holst JJ, Vølund A, Poulsen P, Groop L, Pedersen O, Vaag AA. The T allele of rs7903146 TCF7L2 is associated with impaired insulinotropic action of incretin hormones, reduced 24 h profiles of plasma insulin and glucagon, and increased hepatic glucose production in young healthy men. Diabetologia 2009;52:1298–1307

60. Schäfer SA, Müssig K, Staiger H, Machicao F, Stefan N, Gallwitz B, Häring HU, Fritsche A. A common genetic variant in WFS1 determines impaired glucagon-like peptide-1-induced insulin secretion. Diabetologia 2009;52:1075–1082

61. Schäfer SA, Tschritter O, Machicao F, Thamer C, Stefan N, Gallwitz B,

Holst JJ, Dekker JM, 't Hart LM, Nijpels G, van Haeften TW, Häring HU, Fritsche A. Impaired glucagon-like peptide-1-induced insulin secretion in carriers of transcription factor 7-like 2 (TCF7L2) gene polymorphisms. Diabetologia 2007;50:2443–2450

62. Nauck MA, Meier JJ. The enteroinsular axis may mediate the diabetogenic effects of TCF7L2 polymorphisms. Diabetologia 2007;50:2413–2416

63. Lynn FC, Pamir N, Ng EH, McIntosh CH, Kieffer TJ, Pederson RA. Defective glucose-dependent insulinotropic polypeptide receptor expression in diabetic fatty Zucker rats. Diabetes 2001;50:1004–1011

64. Lynn FC, Thompson SA, Pospisilik JA, Ehses JA, Hinke SA, Pamir N, McIntosh CH, Pederson RA. A novel pathway for regulation of glucose-dependent insulinotropic polypeptide (GIP) receptor expression in beta cells. Faseb J 2003;17:91–93

65. Xu G, Kaneto H, Laybutt DR, Duvivier-Kali VF, Trivedi N, Suzuma K, King GL, Weir GC, Bonner-Weir S. Downregulation of GLP-1 and GIP receptor expression by hyperglycemia: possible contribution to impaired incretin effects in diabetes. Diabetes 2007;56:1551–1558

66. Tseng CC, Boylan MO, Jarboe LA, Usdin TB, Wolfe MM. Chronic desensitization of the glucose-dependent insulinotropic polypeptide receptor in diabetic rats. Am J Physiol (Endocrinol Metab) 1996;270:E661–E666

67. Meier JJ, Nauck MA. Clinical endocrinology and metabolism. Glucose-dependent insulinotropic polypeptide/gastric inhibitory polypeptide. Best Pract Res Clin Endocrinol Metab 2004;18:587–606

68. Højberg PV, Vilsbøll T, Rabøl R, Knop FK, Bache M, Krarup T, Holst JJ, Madsbad S. Four weeks of near-normalisation of blood glucose improves the insulin response to glucagon-like peptide-1 and glucose-dependent insulinotropic polypeptide in patients with type 2 diabetes. Diabetologia 2009;52:199–207

69. Højberg PV, Vilsbøll T, Zander M, Knop FK, Krarup T, Vølund A, Holst JJ, Madsbad S. Four weeks of near-normalization of blood glucose has no effect on postprandial GLP-1 and GIP secretion, but augments pancreatic β-cell responsiveness to a meal in patients with Type 2 diabetes. Diabet Med 2008;25:1268–1275

70. Højberg PV, Zander M, Vilsbøll T, Knop FK, Krarup T, Vølund A, Holst JJ, Madsbad S. Near normalisation of blood glucose improves the potentiating effect of GLP-1 on glucose-induced insulin secretion in patients with type 2 diabetes. Diabetologia 2008;51:632–640

71. Turner RC, McCarthy ST, Holman RR, Harris E. Beta-cell function improved by supplementing basal insulin secretion in mild diabetes. Br Med J 1976;1:1252–1254

72. Cusi K, Cunningham GR, Comstock JP. Safety and efficacy of normalizing fasting glucose with bedtime NPH insulin alone in NIDDM. Diabetes Care 1995;18:843–851

73. Brown RJ, Rother KI. Effects of beta-cell rest on beta-cell function: a review of clinical and preclinical data. Pediatr Diabetes 2008;9:14–22

74. Gromada J, Ding WG, Barg S, Renström E, Rorsman P. Multisite regulation of insulin secretion by cAMP-increasing agonists: evidence that glucagon-like peptide 1 and glucagon act via distinct receptors. Pflugers Arch 1997;434:515–524

Glucose Intolerance and Reduced Proliferation of Pancreatic β-Cells in Transgenic Pigs With Impaired Glucose-Dependent Insulinotropic Polypeptide Function

Simone Renner,[1] Christiane Fehlings,[1] Nadja Herbach,[2] Andreas Hofmann,[3]
Dagmar C. von Waldthausen,[1] Barbara Kessler,[1] Karin Ulrichs,[4] Irina Chodnevskaja,[4]
Vasiliy Moskalenko,[4] Werner Amselgruber,[5] Burkhard Göke,[6] Alexander Pfeifer,[3,7]
Rüdiger Wanke,[2] and Eckhard Wolf[1]

OBJECTIVE—The insulinotropic action of the incretin glucose-dependent insulinotropic polypeptide (GIP) is impaired in type 2 diabetes, while the effect of glucagon-like peptide-1 (GLP-1) is preserved. To evaluate the role of impaired GIP function in glucose homeostasis and development of the endocrine pancreas in a large animal model, we generated transgenic pigs expressing a dominant-negative GIP receptor (GIPR[dn]) in pancreatic islets.

RESEARCH DESIGN AND METHODS—GIPR[dn] transgenic pigs were generated using lentiviral transgenesis. Metabolic tests and quantitative stereological analyses of the different endocrine islet cell populations were performed, and β-cell proliferation and apoptosis were quantified to characterize this novel animal model.

RESULTS—Eleven-week-old GIPR[dn] transgenic pigs exhibited significantly reduced oral glucose tolerance due to delayed insulin secretion, whereas intravenous glucose tolerance and pancreatic β-cell mass were not different from controls. The insulinotropic effect of GIP was significantly reduced, whereas insulin secretion in response to the GLP-1 receptor agonist exendin-4 was enhanced in GIPR[dn] transgenic versus control pigs. With increasing age, glucose control deteriorated in GIPR[dn] transgenic pigs, as shown by reduced oral and intravenous glucose tolerance due to impaired insulin secretion. Importantly, β-cell proliferation was reduced by 60% in 11-week-old GIPR[dn] transgenic pigs, leading to a reduction of β-cell mass by 35% and 58% in 5-month-old and 1- to 1.4-year-old transgenic pigs compared with age-matched controls, respectively.

CONCLUSIONS—The first large animal model with impaired incretin function demonstrates an essential role of GIP for insulin secretion, proliferation of β-cells, and physiological expansion of β-cell mass. *Diabetes* 59:1228–1238, 2010

From the [1]Chair for Molecular Animal Breeding and Biotechnology and Laboratory for Functional Genome Analysis, Gene Center, Ludwig Maximilians University (LMU) Munich, Munich, Germany; the [2]Institute of Veterinary Pathology, Faculty of Veterinary Medicine, LMU Munich, Munich, Germany; the [3]Institute of Pharmacology and Toxicology, University of Bonn, Bonn, Germany; the [4]Department of Experimental Transplantation Immunology, Surgical Clinic I, University Hospital of Würzburg, Würzburg, Germany; the [5]Institute of Anatomy and Physiology, University of Stuttgart-Hohenheim, Stuttgart, Germany; the [6]Medical Clinic II, Klinikum Grosshadern, LMU Munich, Munich, Germany; and the [7]Pharma Center Bonn, University of Bonn, Bonn, Germany.
Corresponding author: Eckhard Wolf, ewolf@lmb.uni-muenchen.de.
Received 8 April 2009 and accepted 10 February 2010. Published ahead of print at http://diabetes.diabetesjournals.org on 25 February 2010. DOI: 10.2337/db09-0519.
C.F. and N.H. contributed equally to this article.

The incretin hormones glucose-dependent insulinotropic polypeptide (GIP) and glucagon-like peptide-1 (GLP-1) are secreted by enteroendocrine cells in response to nutrients like fat and glucose and enhance glucose-induced release of insulin from pancreatic β-cells (1). The effects of GIP and GLP-1 are mediated through specific receptors, GIPR and GLP-1R, respectively. Both receptors belong to the family of seven transmembrane-domain heterotrimeric G-protein–coupled receptors (2). Activation of the GIPR or GLP-1R leads to enhanced exocytosis of insulin-containing granules (3). Interestingly, variation in the *GIPR* gene influences glucose and insulin responses to an oral glucose challenge in humans (4). Furthermore, findings in insulinoma cells (5–7) and rodent models (8,9) indicate that activation of incretin receptors promotes proliferation and survival of β-cells. Type 2 diabetic patients and ~50% of their first-degree relatives show a reduced incretin effect, mainly due to an impaired insulinotropic action of GIP (10,11). Nearly sustained insulinotropic action of GLP-1 (11) in type 2 diabetic patients revealed its therapeutic potential and initiated the ongoing development of GLP-1R agonists as well as inhibitors of dipeptidyl peptidase-4 (1,12), which rapidly degrades incretin hormones in vivo. The reasons for the reduced response to GIP in type 2 diabetes are unclear (1), but impaired GIP action might be involved in the early pathogenesis of type 2 diabetes (13).

To clarify this point, a mouse model lacking functional GIPR expression was generated by gene targeting (14). *Gipr*[−/−] mice displayed only slightly impaired glucose tolerance and did not develop diabetes. Interestingly, double incretin receptor knockout mice exhibited a similar phenotype. As possible explanations for this relatively mild phenotype (rev. in 15), compensatory regulation of the GLP-1 system or other compensatory mechanisms were discussed. In contrast, transgenic mice overexpressing a dominant-negative GIPR (GIPR[dn]) displayed a severe phenotype (i.e., early-onset diabetes accompanied by a marked fasting hypoinsulinemia and severe reduction of β-cell mass associated with extensive structural alterations of the pancreatic islets) (16).

In light of these discrepant findings in mouse models, we generated a large animal model to address the question whether GIPR signaling plays a role in maintaining pancreatic islet function and structure. Efficient lentiviral vectors (17) were used to generate transgenic pigs expressing a GIPR[dn] under the control of the rat *Ins2* promoter in the pancreatic islets. This novel animal model, in contrast to GIPR^{dn} transgenic mice (16), initially only exhibits a disturbed incretin effect but develops progressive deterioration of glucose control with increasing age, associated with reduced β-cell proliferation and an impairment of physiological age-related expansion of pancreatic β-cell mass.

RESEARCH DESIGN AND METHODS

Generation of RIP II-GIPR^{dn} transgenic pigs. The expression cassette consisting of the rat *Ins2* promoter (RIP II) and the cDNA of a human *GIPR^{dn}* (16) was cloned into the lentiviral vector LV-*pGFP* (18) (supplementary Fig. 1 of the online appendix [available at http://diabetes.diabetesjournals.org/cgi/content/full/db09-0519/DC1]). Recombinant lentivirus was produced (18) and injected into the perivitelline space of zygotes from superovulated gilts (17). Embryos were transferred into synchronized recipients (19). Offspring were genotyped by PCR and Southern blot analyses using a probe directed toward the RIP II promoter sequence. Expression of GIPR^{dn} mRNA in the pancreatic islets was determined by RT-PCR. A total of 400 ng of total RNA were reverse transcribed into cDNA using SuperScriptII reverse transcriptase (Invitrogen) and random hexamer primers (Invitrogen) after digestion with DNaseI (Roche). For PCR, the following transgene specific primers were used: sense 5′-TTT TTA TCC GCA TTC TTA CAC GG-3′ and antisense 5′-ATC TTC CTC AGC TCC TTC CAG G-3′. All animal experiments were carried out according to the German animal protection law.

Oral/intravenous glucose tolerance test and GIP/exendin-4 stimulation test. For the oral glucose tolerance test (OGTT), one central venous catheter (Cavafix Certo; B. Braun) was inserted nonsurgically into the external jugular vein. After an 18-h overnight fast, animals were fed 2 g glucose/kg body weight (BW) (20) mixed with 50/100 g (11-week-old/5-month-old) commercial pig fodder. Blood samples were obtained from the jugular vein catheter at the indicated time points. For the intravenous glucose tolerance test (IVGTT) and GIP/exendin-4 stimulation test, two central venous catheters (Cavafix Certo) were surgically inserted into the external jugular vein under general anesthesia (21). For both tests, a bolus injection of 0.5 g glucose/kg BW (22) was administered through the central venous catheter after an 18-h fasting period. For the GIP/exendin-4 stimulation test, 80 pmol/kg BW of synthetic porcine GIP (Bachem) or 40 pmol/kg BW synthetic exendin-4 (Bachem) were administered intravenously in addition to glucose. Blood samples were collected at the indicated time points. Serum glucose levels were determined using an AU 400 autoanalyzer (Olympus). Serum insulin levels were measured using a porcine insulin radioimmunoassay kit (Millipore).

Pancreas preparation and islet isolation. Pancreatic islets were isolated from three 12- to 13-month-old GIPR^{dn} transgenic pigs and three littermate control animals (23). After explantation of the pancreas in toto, the left pancreatic lobe was separated from the rest of the organ (supplementary Fig. 2). The left pancreatic lobe was digested using a modification of the half-automated digestion-filtration method as previously described (24). Purification of the isolated islets was performed with the discontinuous OptiPrep density gradient (Progen) in the COBE 2991 cell processor (COBE) (25). Islet numbers were determined using dithizone-stained islet samples (26), which were counted under an Axiovert 25 microscope (Zeiss) with a calibrated grid in the eyepiece. For determination of islet vitality, fluorescein diacetate/propidium iodide (Sigma-Aldrich) staining was performed (27).

Immunohistochemistry and quantitative stereological analyses. After prefixation, the pancreas was cut into 1-cm-thick slices. Slices were tilted to their left side and covered by a 1-cm^2 point-counting grid. Tissue blocks were selected by systematic random sampling, fixed in 10% neutral buffered formalin, routinely processed, and embedded in paraffin. The volume of the pancreas [$V_{(Pan)}$] before embedding was calculated by the quotient of the pancreas weight and the specific weight of pig pancreas (1.07 g/cm^3). The specific weight was determined by the submersion method (28). Paraffin sections were routinely prepared, and insulin, glucagon, somatostatin, and pancreatic polypeptide containing cells were stained, using the indirect immunoperoxidase technique (16) and the antibodies described in the online appendix. The volume densities of α-, β-, δ-, and pp-cells in the islets [$Vv_{(α-cell/Islet)}$, $Vv_{(β-cell/Islet)}$, $Vv_{(δ-cell/Islet)}$, and $Vv_{(pp-cell/Islet)}$], the total volumes of α-, β-, δ-, and pp-cells in the islets [$V_{(α-cell, Islet)}$, $V_{(β-cell, Islet)}$, $V_{(δ-cell, Islet)}$, and $V_{(pp-cell, Islet)}$] as well as the total volume of β-cells in the pancreas [referring to β-cells in the islets and isolated β-cells, $V_{(β-cell, Pan)}$], and the total volume of isolated β-cells in the pancreas [$V_{(isoβ-cell, Pan)}$], a parameter indicative of islet neogenesis (29–31), were determined as described previously (32). Volume densities of the various endocrine cell types in the islets refer to the volume fraction of the particular endocrine cell type in relation to the cumulative

volume of the various endocrine islet cells, thus excluding capillaries and other interstitial tissues in the islets.

Proliferation/apoptosis rates of β-cells were determined by double immunohistochemical staining for insulin and the proliferation marker Ki67 (33) or the apoptosis marker cleaved caspase-3 (34) as detailed in the online appendix. A minimum of 10^4 β-cells per animal was included in the quantification of β-cell proliferation and apoptosis. Cell proliferation/apoptosis index was defined as the number of immunolabeled cell nuclei divided by the total number of cell nuclei counted and expressed as the number of immunolabeled (Ki67+/Casp-3+) cell nuclei per 10^5 nuclei. GIPR and GLP-1R were detected in pancreas sections using the streptavidin-biotin complex technique and the antibodies described in the online appendix.

Statistics. All data are presented as means ± SE. The results of glucose tolerance tests and incretin stimulation tests were statistically evaluated by ANOVA (linear mixed models; SAS 8.2; PROC MIXED), taking the fixed effects of group (wild type, transgenic), time (relative to glucose or hormone application), and the interaction group × time as well as the random effect of animal into account (35). Results of the linear mixed models analysis are shown in supplementary Table 1. The same model was used to compare body weight gain of GIPR^{dn} transgenic and control pigs. Pancreas weight and the results of quantitative stereological analyses were evaluated by the general linear models procedure (SAS 8.2) taking the effects of group (wild type, transgenic), age (11 weeks, 5 months, or 1–1.4 years), and the interaction group × age into account. Results of the general linear models analysis are shown in Table 1. Calculation of areas under the curve (AUCs) was performed using Graph Pad Prism 4 software. Statistical significance of differences between transgenic and wild-type pigs was tested using the Mann-Whitney U test in combination with an exact test procedure (SPSS 16.0, Chicago, IL). P values <0.05 were considered significant.

RESULTS

Generation of GIPR^{dn} transgenic pigs. A lentiviral vector was cloned that expresses a dominant-negative GIPR (GIPR^{dn}) under the control of the rat insulin 2 gene promoter (RIP II) (Fig. 1A). The GIPR^{dn} has an eight–amino acid deletion (positions 319–326) and an Ala→Glu exchange at amino acid position 340 in the third intracellular loop, which is essential for signal transduction (16). Lentiviral vectors were injected into the perivitelline space of pig zygotes (17). A total of 113 injected zygotes were transferred laparoscopically into the oviducts of three cycle-synchronized recipient gilts. Nineteen piglets (17% of the transferred zygotes) were born. Southern blot analysis identified nine founder animals (47% of the born animals) carrying one or two lentiviral integrants (Fig. 1B), confirming the high efficiency of lentiviral transgenesis in large animals (17).

Two male founder animals (nos. 50 and 51) were mated to nontransgenic females (Fig. 1B). The resulting offspring demonstrated germ line transmission and segregation of the integrants according to Mendelian rules (Fig. 1B). To analyze expression of GIPR^{dn} mRNA, pancreatic islets were isolated from transgenic and nontransgenic offspring and analyzed by RT-PCR. Expression of the GIPR^{dn} was detected in the islets of all transgenic animals but not in the islets of nontransgenic control animals (Fig. 1C). GIPR^{dn} transgenic pigs developed normally and did not show any deviation in body weight gain compared with controls (Fig. 2).

Normal fasting glucose and fructosamine levels in GIPR^{dn} transgenic pigs. To evaluate effects of GIPR^{dn} expression on glucose homeostasis, fasting blood glucose and serum fructosamine levels were determined in regular intervals from 1 to 7 months of age. No significant differences in blood glucose levels and serum fructosamine levels were detected between GIPR^{dn} transgenic and control pigs (supplementary Fig. 3). Fasting blood glucose levels, determined in irregular intervals up to an age of 2

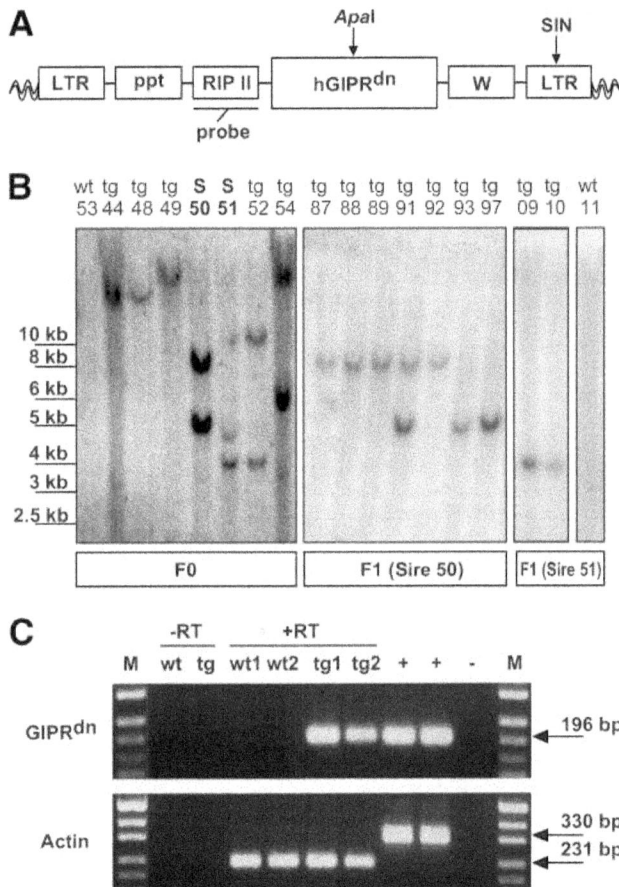

A: The lentiviral vector (LV-*GIPR^dn*) carrying the cDNA of

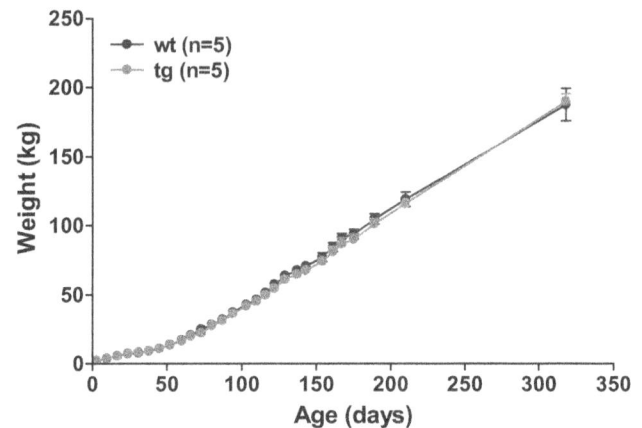

FIG. 2. Body weight gain of GIPR^dn transgenic pigs (tg) compared with control pigs (wt). Data are means ± SE. (A high-quality digital representation of this figure is available in the online issue.)

FIG. 1. Lentiviral vector, Southern blot analyses, and transgene expression. *A*: The lentiviral vector (LV-*GIPR^dn*) carrying the cDNA of the dominant-negative *GIPR* (*GIPR^dn*) under the control of the rat *Ins2* gene promoter (RIP II). *Apa*I, restriction site of *Apa*I; LTR, long terminal repeat; ppt, polypurine tract; SIN, self-inactivating mutation; W, woodchuck hepatitis posttranscriptional regulatory element; probe, probe used for Southern blot analyses; *wavy lines*, pig genome. *B*: Southern blot analyses of *Apa*I-digested genomic DNA isolated from EDTA blood of piglets generated by subzonal injection of LV-GIPR^dn (transgenic [tg]) and two nontransgenic littermates (wild type [wt]). Pigs of the F0 generation show either one or two single-copy integration sites of the transgene. Sires 50 and 51 (S 50/S 51) were selected to establish two transgenic lines. Note that pigs of the F1 generation show segregation of the integrants according to the Mendelian rules. *C*: Analysis of transgene expression (GIPR^dn) in isolated porcine islets of Langerhans of transgenic (tg) and nontransgenic littermates (wt) by RT-PCR. β-Actin RT-PCR used for confirmation of reverse transcription efficiency. Due to the use of intron-spanning primers to detect β-actin, two different-sized bands are visible differentiating cDNA and genomic DNA. M: pUC Mix Marker; −RT wt: minus RT wild-type pigs; −RT tg: minus RT GIPR^dn transgenic pigs (no signals were obtained from islets of transgenic offspring after omission of the RT step, demonstrating that expressed rather than integrated sequences were detected); +, genomic DNA of GIPR^dn transgenic pig; −, aqua bidest.

years, were unaltered in GIPR^dn transgenic pigs (data not shown).

Reduced insulinotropic effect of GIP but enhanced insulinotropic effect of exendin-4 in GIPR^dn transgenic pigs. To evaluate whether expression of a GIPR^dn specifically impairs the function of GIP, we performed stimulation tests with GIP and the GLP-1 receptor agonist exendin-4 (1). The insulinotropic effect of GIP, intravenously administered as a bolus, was significantly diminished (Fig. 3A), while insulin secretion in response to exendin-4 was increased in GIPR^dn transgenic versus control pigs (Fig. 3B), leading to a faster decrease of

serum glucose levels (Fig. 3*D*). These findings demonstrate that expression of GIPR^dn specifically reduces the insulinotropic action of GIP and does not impair the function of a related G-protein–coupled receptor, namely the GLP-1R. Further, the enhanced insulinotropic effect of exendin-4 in GIPR^dn transgenic versus control pigs indicates a compensatory hyperactivation of the GLP-1/ GLP-1R system, which has also been observed in *Gipr*^−/− mice (rev. in 15). To clarify, whether compensatory mechanisms involve altered expression of incretin receptors, we performed immunohistochemical staining of pancreas sections for GIPR (Fig. 3*E*) and GLP-1R (Fig. 3*F*), which revealed no apparent difference in the abundance and spatial distribution of both receptors comparing GIPR^dn transgenic and control pigs.

Disturbed incretin function in young GIPR^dn transgenic pigs. An OGTT (2 g glucose/kg BW) was performed in 11-week-old GIPR^dn transgenic pigs ($n = 5$) and controls ($n = 5$) originating from founder boars nos. 50 and 51. GIPR^dn transgenic pigs exhibited elevated ($P < 0.05$) serum glucose levels (Fig. 4*A*) as well as a distinct delay in insulin secretion (Fig. 4*B*) after glucose challenge. The area under the insulin curve (AUC insulin) during the first 45 min following glucose challenge was 31% ($P < 0.05$) smaller in GIPR^dn transgenic pigs than in age-matched controls (Fig. 4*B*); however, the total amount of insulin secreted during the experimental period (i.e., total AUC insulin until 120 min following glucose load) was not different between the two groups ($5,155 \pm 763$ vs. $5,698 \pm 625$; $P = 0.351$). These findings indicate that expression of a GIPR^dn in the pancreatic islets of transgenic pigs is sufficient to interfere with the incretin effect but does not initially affect the total AUC insulin. This assumption is supported by the fact that intravenous glucose tolerance was not reduced in GIPR^dn transgenic pigs (Fig. 5*A*), and the time course and amount of insulin secreted in response to an intravenous glucose load were not different between the two groups (Fig. 5*B*). Quantitative stereological investigations of the pancreas (32) revealed that the total volume of β-cells in the pancreas was not different between GIPR^dn transgenic pigs and controls (Fig. 6*A*). Further, the total volume of isolated β-cells (single insulin-positive cells and small clusters of insulin-positive cells not belonging to established islets) was equal in the two groups (49 ± 4 vs. 49 ± 6 mm^3; $P = 0.695$). These findings

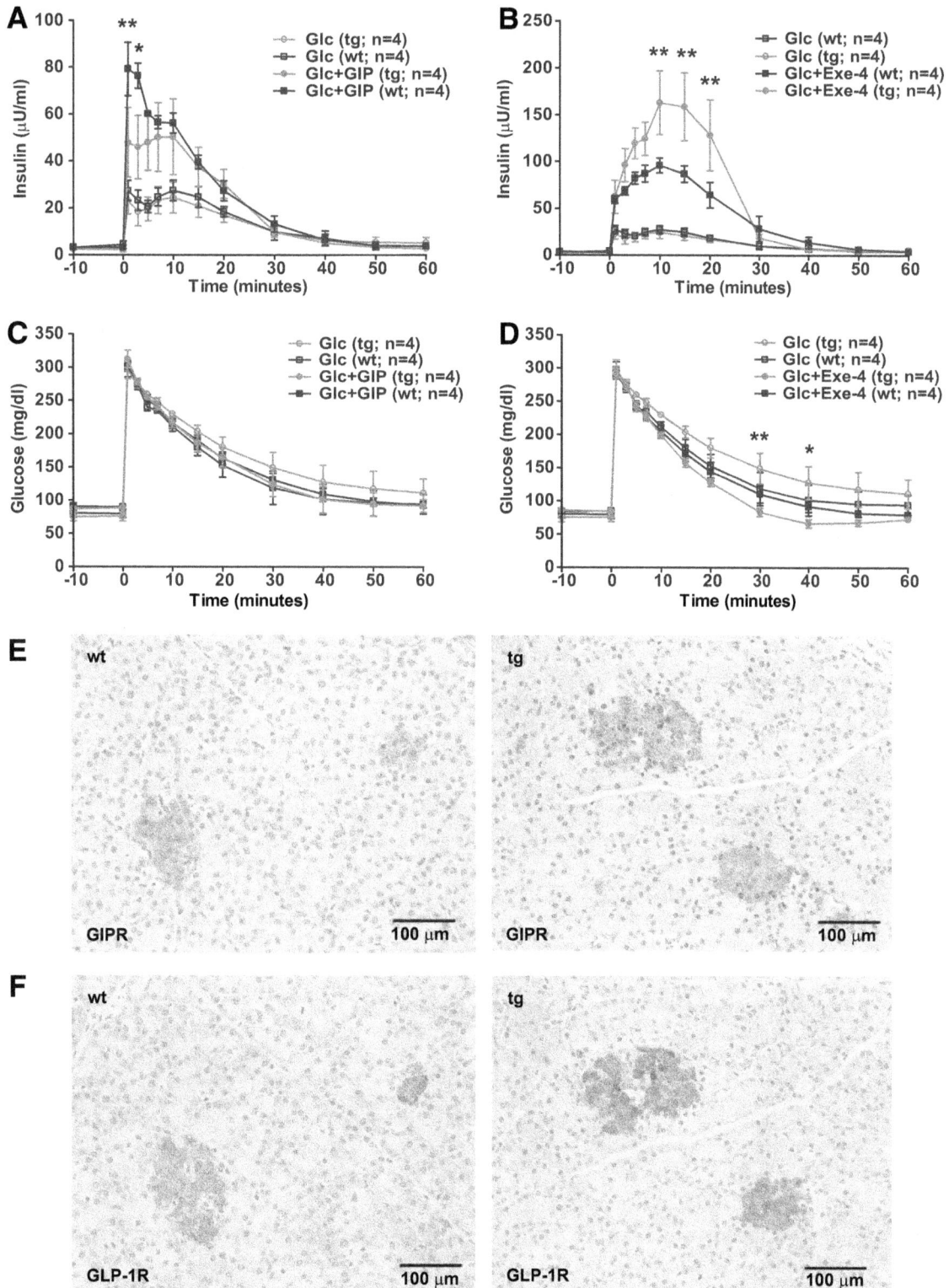

FIG. 3. Functional analysis of GIPR[dn] expression by GIP/exendin-4 stimulation test. Reduced insulinotropic action of GIP but enhanced insulinotropic action of exendin-4 in 11-week-old GIPR[dn] transgenic pigs (tg) compared with nontransgenic control animals (wt). *A*: Serum insulin levels of GIPR[dn] transgenic (tg) and control (wt) pigs after intravenous administration of glucose (Glc) ± GIP. *B*: Serum insulin levels of GIPR[dn] transgenic (tg) and control (wt) pigs after intravenous administration of glucose (Glc) ± exendin-4 (Exe-4). *C* and *D*: Corresponding serum glucose levels for the GIP (*C*) and exendin-4 (*D*) stimulation test. 0 min = point of Glc/GIP/exendin-4 administration. Data are means ± SE. *$P < 0.05$ vs. control; **$P < 0.01$ vs. control. *E* and *F*: Immunohistochemical staining of GIPR (*E*) and GLP-1R (*F*) in pancreas sections from 11-week-old GIPR[dn] transgenic pigs (tg) and nontransgenic control animals (wt) does not provide evidence for differences in receptor abundance. (A high-quality digital representation of this figure is available in the online issue.)

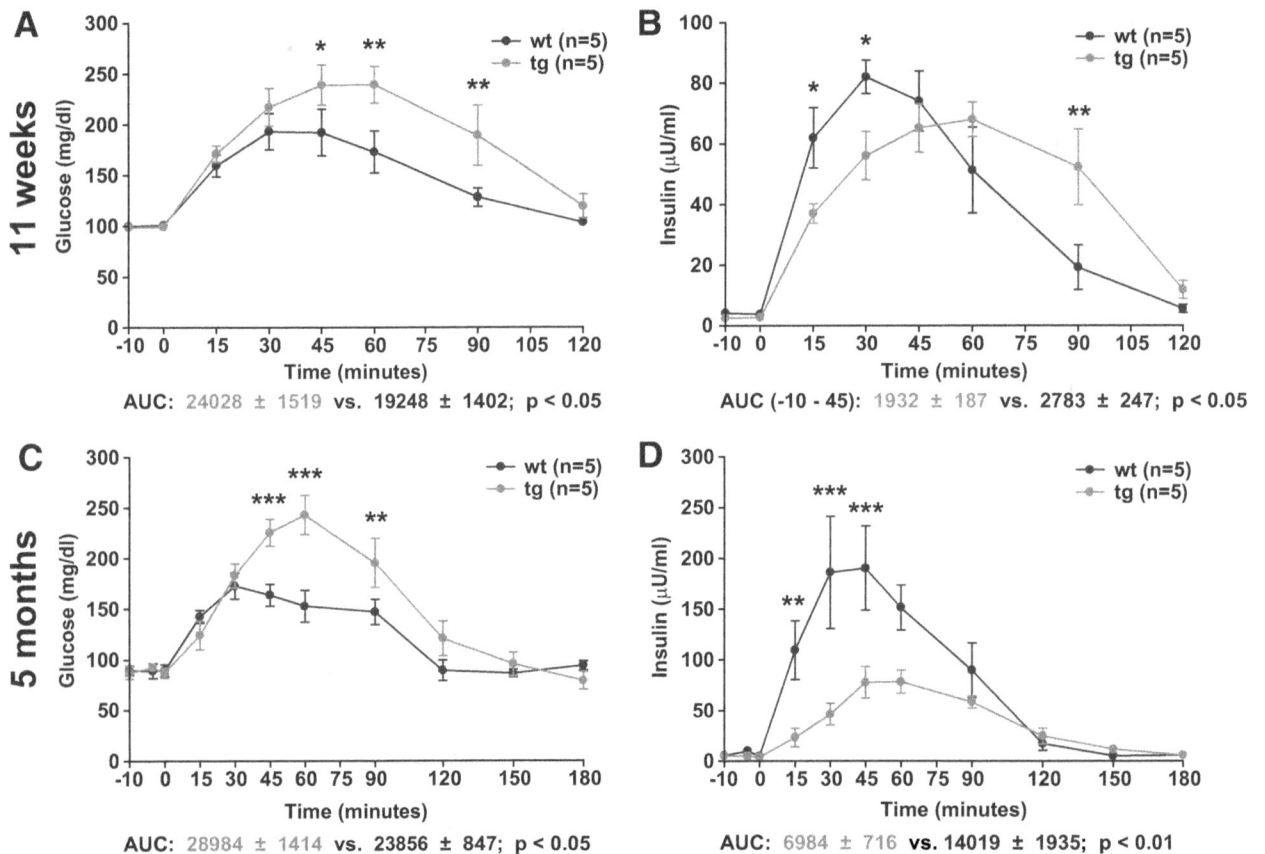

FIG. 4. Oral glucose tolerance in 11-week-old and 5-month-old GIPR^{dn} transgenic pigs (tg) compared with nontransgenic littermates (wt). A and C: Serum glucose levels; 0 min = point of glucose administration. B and D: Serum insulin levels. AUC glucose/insulin for transgenic pigs (red) and wild-type pigs (blue). Data are means ± SE. *P < 0.05 vs. control; **P < 0.01 vs. control; ***P < 0.001 vs. control. Note that in 11-week-old transgenic pigs, there is a delay in insulin secretion leading to a significant reduction of insulin secretion during the first 45 min following oral glucose load, although the total amount of insulin secreted over 120 min is not different from controls. In contrast, 5-month-old transgenic pigs display not only delayed but also reduced insulin secretion. A high-quality digital representation of this figure is available in the online issue.

clearly demonstrate that expression of a GIPR^{dn} does not exhibit a toxic effect on pancreatic islets and further suggest that pancreatic islet neogenesis is not disturbed.

Glucose control in GIPR^{dn} transgenic pigs deteriorates with increasing age. To monitor the long-term consequences of GIPR^{dn} expression, a second collective of animals was repeatedly investigated. First, an OGTT was performed in 5-month-old (20 ± 1 weeks) GIPR^{dn} transgenic pigs ($n = 5$) and littermate controls ($n = 5$) originating from founder boars nos. 50 and 51. GIPR^{dn} transgenic pigs exhibited elevated glucose levels (Fig. 4C) as well as a distinct reduction of initial insulin secretion after glucose challenge compared with their nontransgenic littermates (Fig. 4D). In addition, peak insulin levels were clearly reduced compared with controls. The AUC glucose was 26% ($P < 0.05$) larger (Fig. 4C), whereas AUC insulin was 49% ($P < 0.01$) smaller in GIPR^{dn} transgenic pigs (Fig. 4D). The latter finding suggests that, in contrast to 11-week-old animals, the overall insulin secretion following an oral glucose load is reduced in 5-month-old GIPR^{dn} transgenic pigs and that their islets may undergo progressive functional and/or structural changes. Additionally, an IVGTT was carried out in 5-month-old (22.5 ± 1.5 weeks) GIPR^{dn} transgenic and control pigs ($n = 4$ per group; different collective of animals). Intravenous glucose tolerance (Fig. 5C), as well as insulin secretion (Fig. 5D), in GIPR^{dn} transgenic pigs was similar to controls. However, a

tendency toward reduced intravenous glucose tolerance and reduced insulin secretion in GIPR^{dn} transgenic pigs was visible.

Next, we performed an IVGTT in 11-month-old (45 ± 2 weeks) GIPR^{dn} transgenic pigs ($n = 5$) and littermate controls ($n = 4$) from the same collective of animals used for OGTT at 5 months of age. GIPR^{dn} transgenic pigs exhibited a decelerated decline of blood glucose levels (10% larger AUC glucose; $P < 0.05$) (Fig. 5E), going along with significantly reduced insulin release (52% smaller AUC insulin; $P < 0.05$) (Fig. 5F). This observation corroborated the suspicion that impaired GIPR function may cause a general disturbance of insulin secretion and/or alterations in islet structure and/or islet integrity over time.

Impaired age-related expansion of pancreatic β-cell mass in GIPR^{dn} transgenic pigs. To clarify long-term effects of GIPR^{dn} expression on the islets, we performed quantitative stereological analyses of pancreata from 5-month-old and from 1- to 1.4-year-old GIPR^{dn} transgenic pigs and controls. Pancreas weight did not differ between GIPR^{dn} transgenic pigs and control animals in both age-groups (Table 1).

Qualitative histological assessment revealed that pancreatic islet profiles of 5-month-old and 1- to 1.4-year-old GIPR^{dn} transgenic pigs appeared to be smaller in size and reduced in number (Fig. 6B and C). These findings were

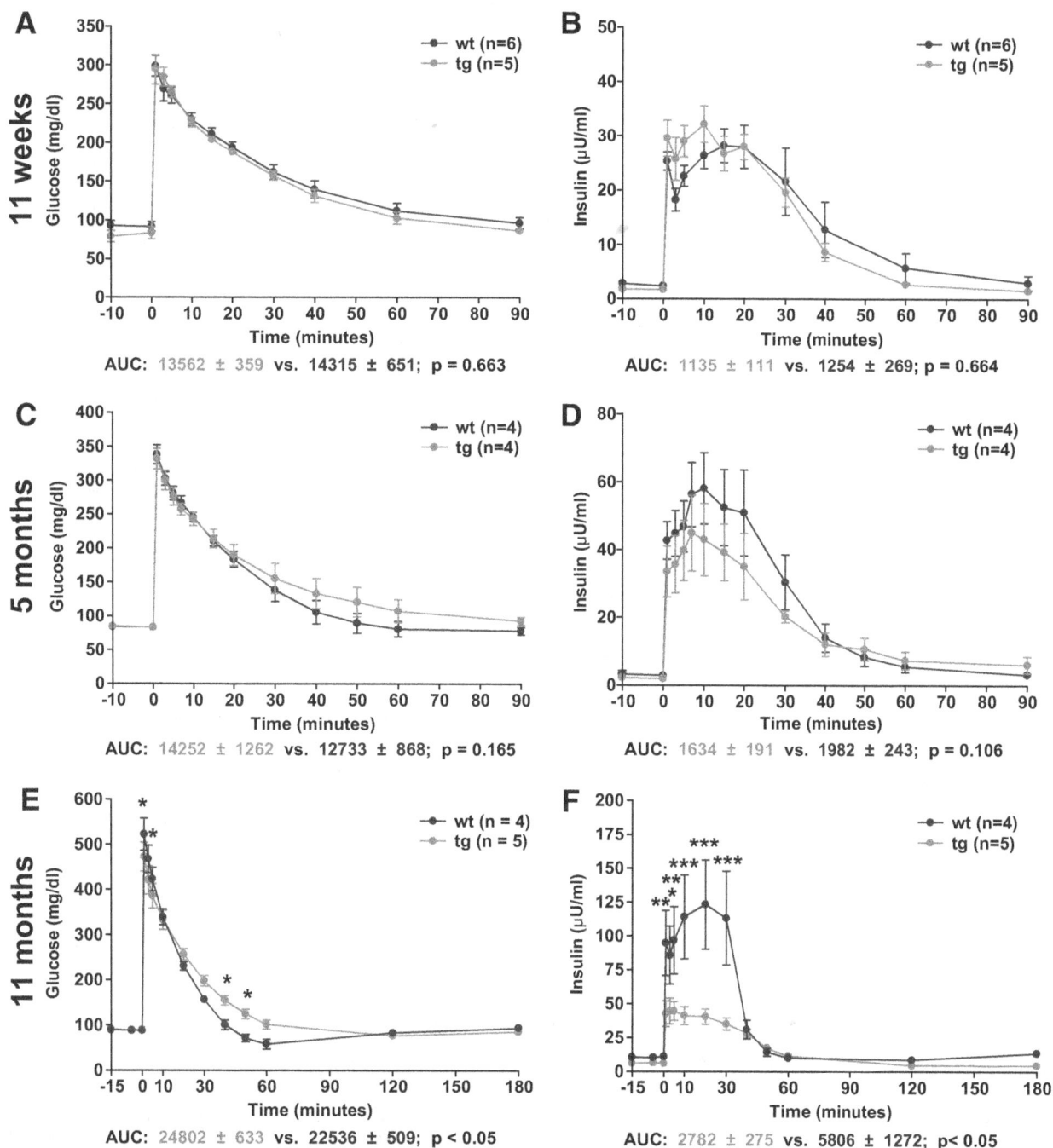

FIG. 5. Intravenous glucose tolerance in GIPR^{dn} transgenic pigs (tg) compared with nontransgenic controls (wt). *A*, *C*, and *E*: Serum glucose levels; 0 min = point of glucose administration. *B*, *D*, and *F*: Serum insulin levels. AUC glucose/insulin for transgenic pigs (red) and wild-type pigs (blue). Data are means ± SE. *$P < 0.05$ vs. control; **$P < 0.01$ vs. control; ***$P < 0.001$ vs. control. Note that intravenous glucose tolerance (*A*) and insulin secretion (*B*) are not altered in 11-week-old transgenic pigs. In 5-month-old transgenic pigs, a tendency of reduced insulin secretion (*D*) is observed, while 11-month-old transgenic pigs display a significantly reduced intravenous glucose tolerance (*E*) due to a significantly reduced insulin secretion (*F*). (A high-quality digital representation of this figure is available in the online issue.)

confirmed by quantitative stereological investigations. In 5-month-old GIPR^{dn} transgenic pigs ($n = 4$), the total volume of β-cells [$V_{(\beta\text{-cell, Pan})}$] was diminished by 35% ($P < 0.05$) versus controls ($n = 4$) (Fig. 6*B*). In 1- to 1.4-year-old GIPR^{dn} transgenic pigs ($n = 5$), the reduction of total β-cell volume compared with controls ($n = 5$) was even more pronounced (58%; $P < 0.01$) (Fig. 6*C*). Reduced β-cell mass of young adult GIPR^{dn} transgenic pigs compared with controls was confirmed by islet isolation experiments. The number of islet equivalents recovered from pancreas samples of GIPR^{dn} transgenic pigs ($n = 3$) was reduced by 93% ($P < 0.05$) as compared with littermate controls ($n = 3$) (supplementary Table 2).

In contrast, volume density (data not shown) as well as the total volume of isolated β-cells were not different between GIPR^{dn} transgenic and control pigs, neither at 5 months of age (121 ± 18 vs. 127 ± 15 mm^3; $P = 0.883$) nor at 1–1.4 years of age (77 ± 8 vs. 71 ± 5 mm^3; $P = 0.844$).

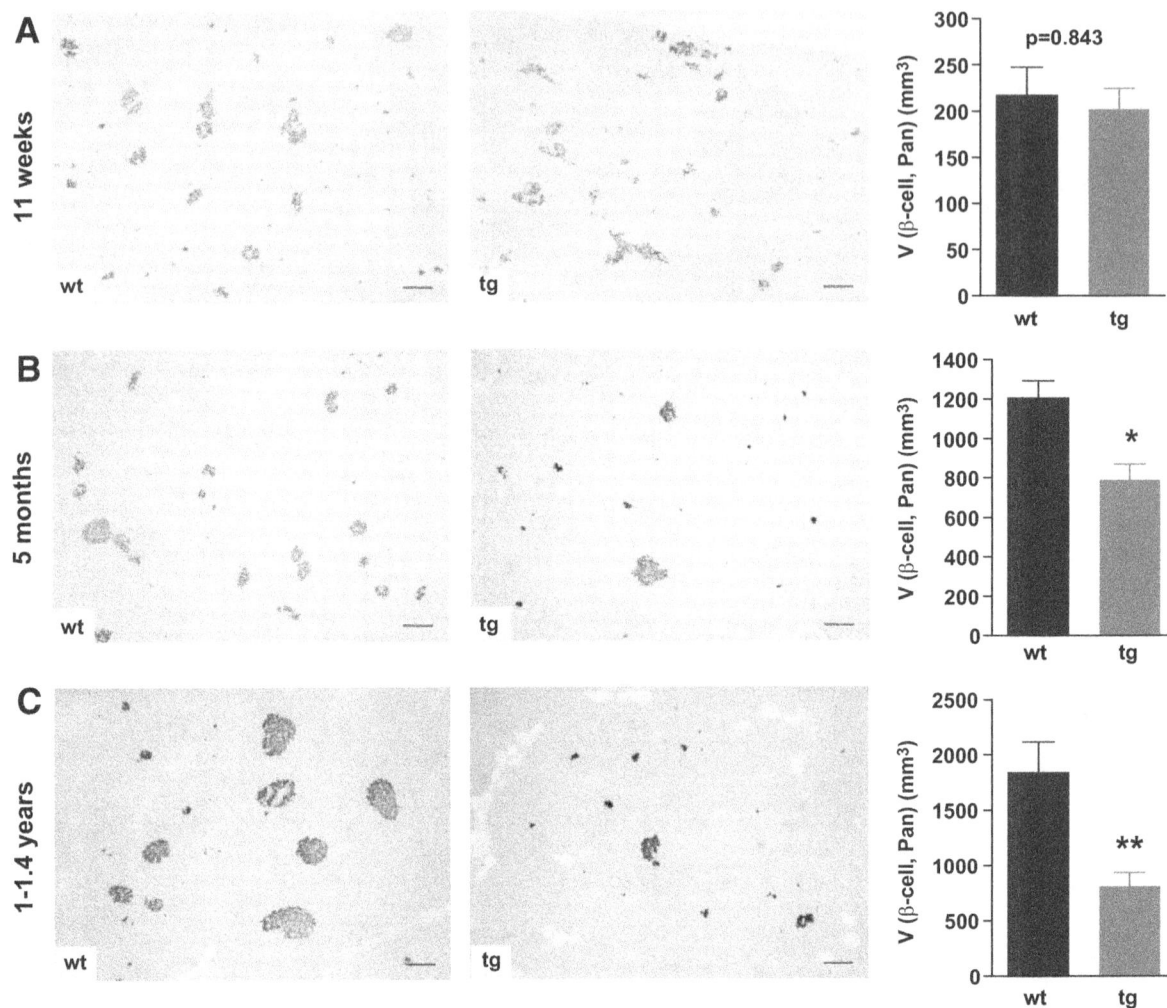

FIG. 6. Immunohistochemistry for insulin and total β-cell volume in the pancreas [$V_{(\beta\text{-cell, Pan})}$] determined with quantitative stereological methods. A–C: Representative histological sections of pancreatic tissue from a control (wt) and a GIPR^{dn} transgenic pig (tg); scale bar = 200 μm. Unaltered total β-cell volume in 11-week-old GIPR^{dn} transgenic pigs ($n = 5$ per group) (A) but reduction of the total β-cell volume in 5-month-old ($n = 4$ per group) (B) and young adult (1–1.4 years old) ($n = 5$ per group) GIPR^{dn} transgenic pigs (C) compared with controls. Data are means ± SE. *$P < 0.05$ vs. control; **$P < 0.01$ vs. control. A high-quality digital representation of this figure is available in the online issue.

These data clearly demonstrate an age-related reduction of pancreatic β-cell mass expansion in GIPR^{dn} transgenic pigs, which is in line with previous evidence for a trophic action of GIP on β-cells in vitro (5–7).

Altered cellular composition of islets in GIPR^{dn} transgenic pigs. To evaluate effects of GIPR^{dn} expression on the volume densities of the various endocrine islet cells and their total volumes, we performed detailed stereological analyses of the pancreatic islets in all three age classes investigated. In control animals, total volumes of α-, β-, δ-, and pp-cells in established islets increased significantly with age (Table 1). In GIPR^{dn} transgenic pigs, a similar age-dependent increase was seen for the total volumes of α-, δ-, and pp-cells. However, in comparison with controls, the increase of total β-cell volume of GIPR^{dn} transgenic pigs was less pronounced from 11 weeks to 5 months of age. Importantly, there was no further augmentation of total β-cell volume in 1- to 1.4-year-old GIPR^{dn} transgenic pigs, demonstrating that impaired GIPR function interferes with the physiological expansion of pancreatic β-cells. In addition, the fractional volume of β-cells in the islets was decreased, while that of α- and δ-cells was increased in 1- to 1.4-year-old GIPR^{dn} transgenic pigs. However, the total volumes of these non–β-cell populations were not different from those of age-matched control pigs (Table 1).

Reduced proliferation rate of β-cells in GIPR^{dn} transgenic pigs. To clarify the mechanism of impaired β-cell expansion in GIPR^{dn} transgenic pigs, we determined β-cell proliferation by double immunohistochemical staining for insulin and the proliferation marker Ki67 in all three age-groups. Indeed, β-cell proliferation was significantly reduced by 60% ($P < 0.05$) in 11-week-old GIPR^{dn} transgenic pigs (Fig. 7A and B). In addition, we performed double immunohistochemical staining for insulin and the apoptosis marker cleaved caspase-3 to evaluate a potential impact of GIPR^{dn} expression on cell death in the β-cell compartment. Overall, the proportion of cleaved caspase-3 positive cells was very low, with no significant difference between GIPR^{dn} transgenic pigs and controls of all age classes. However, there was a trend ($P = 0.075$) of more cleaved caspase-3 positive β-cells in 1- to 1.4-year-old GIPR^{dn} transgenic pigs as compared with age-matched controls (Fig. 7C and D).

TABLE 1
Quantitative stereological analyses of the endocrine pancreas of GIPR[dn] transgenic pigs (tg) and wild-type control pigs (wt)

Parameter	11 weeks ($n = 5$ wt, 5 tg) Means ± SE	5 months ($n = 4$ wt, 4 tg) Means ± SE	1–1.4 years ($n = 5$ wt, 5 tg) Means ± SE	ANOVA		
				Group	Age	Group × age
Pancreas weight (g)						
Wild type	34.5 ± 4.2	115.3 ± 5.6	183.4 ± 13.8	NS	<0.0001	NS
Transgenic	32.7 ± 3.1	125.7 ± 6.1	206.1 ± 4.9			
$V_{V(\beta\text{-cell/islet})}$ (%)						
Wild type	69.8 ± 2.2	89.0 ± 1.5	90.2 ± 1.2	0.0066	<0.0001	0.0024
Transgenic	70.8 ± 1.3	87.0 ± 1.2	76.4 ± 3.2*			
$V_{V(\alpha\text{-cell/islet})}$ (%)						
Wild type	14.1 ± 1.2	5.0 ± 0.8	5.0 ± 0.7	0.0122	<0.0001	0.0008
Transgenic	12.2 ± 0.7	6.5 ± 0.7	13.8 ± 2.3*			
$V_{V(\delta\text{-cell/islet})}$ (%)						
Wild type	13.5 ± 2.8	4.3 ± 0.8	2.2 ± 0.6	NS	<0.0001	NS
Transgenic	13.0 ± 1.0	5.5 ± 0.9	5.8 ± 0.9†			
$V_{V(\text{pp-cell/islet})}$ (%)						
Wild type	2.7 ± 0.7	1.8 ± 0.3	2.8 ± 0.8	NS	0.0355	NS
Transgenic	3.9 ± 0.5	1.3 ± 0.3	3.8 ± 1.1			
$V_{(\beta\text{-cell/islet})}$ (mm³)						
Wild type	168.7 ± 29.5	1,088.2 ± 82.0	1,694.6 ± 251.7	0.0002	<0.0001	0.0024
Transgenic	152.1 ± 17.1	664.1 ± 74.5†	663.7 ± 130.5*			
$V_{(\alpha\text{-cell/islet})}$ (mm³)						
Wild type	32.6 ± 8.7	58.4 ± 6.3	95.7 ± 17.4	NS	<0.0001	NS
Transgenic	24.5 ± 1.7	47.7 ± 4.5	112.8 ± 14.5			
$V_{(\delta\text{-cell/islet})}$ (mm³)						
Wild type	26.6 ± 3.9	49.5 ± 6.1	36.8 ± 6.3	NS	0.0014	NS
Transgenic	25.9 ± 1.8	39.6 ± 3.5	47.5 ± 5.2			
$V_{(\text{pp-cell/islet})}$ (mm³)						
Wild type	6.0 ± 1.8	20.7 ± 2.9	52.4 ± 12.6	NS	<0.0001	NS
Transgenic	8.2 ± 1.7	9.3 ± 2.1	30.3 ± 7.9			

Data were analyzed by the general linear models procedure (SAS Institute) taking the effects of group (wild type, transgenic), age (11 weeks, 5 months, 1–1.4 years), and the interaction group × age into account. For significant effects of these factors P values are indicated in the last three columns. In addition, significant differences between groups within age classes are marked by: *$P < 0.01$; †$P < 0.05$; NS, not significant.

DISCUSSION

This study established the first transgenic large animal model of impaired incretin function. The cDNA of the human *GIPR* was mutated at the third intracellular loop, where a deletion of eight amino acids (positions 319–326) and a point mutation at position 340 was introduced. In stably transfected Chinese hamster lymphoblast (CHL) cells, GIPR[dn] bound GIP with normal affinity but failed to increase intracellular cAMP levels. Thus, the GIPR[dn] expressed in transgenic pigs is capable of ligand binding but not of signal transduction (16) and competes with the endogenous GIPR for GIP. Consequently, the insulinotropic effect of GIP is highly reduced but not completely eliminated, mirroring the situation in human type 2 diabetes.

In view of the severe, early-onset diabetes of GIPR[dn] transgenic mice (16), we tested the oral and intravenous glucose tolerance of young (11-week-old) GIPR[dn] transgenic and control pigs and determined their pancreatic β-cell mass by quantitative stereological analyses. The finding of reduced oral glucose tolerance associated with delayed insulin secretion is in line with a disturbance of the incretin effect. Reduced oral glucose tolerance in GIPR[dn] transgenic pigs is also consistent with previous observations in *Gipr*[−/−] mice (14). Importantly, normal intravenous glucose tolerance, insulin secretion, and unchanged β-cell mass in 11-week-old GIPR[dn] transgenic pigs strongly argue against a toxic effect of GIPR[dn] expression. The reasons for different outcomes in the GIPR[dn] trans-

genic pig and the GIPR[dn] transgenic mouse model remain unclear but may be related to different methods of transgenesis (lentiviral transgenesis versus pronuclear DNA microinjection) or different copy numbers and/or integration sites leading to different expression levels of the transgene.

To evaluate long-term effects of GIPR[dn] expression in the pancreatic islets, we performed a longitudinal study of a collective of animals, involving OGTTs and IVGTTs. These revealed a progressive deterioration of glucose control in GIPR[dn] transgenic pigs, although none of our transgenic pigs has developed fasting hyperglycemia up to an age of 2 years. Quantitative stereological investigations of pancreata from 5-month-old and from 1- to 1.4-year-old GIPR[dn] transgenic pigs showed a reduced pancreatic β-cell mass, which was confirmed by quantitative islet isolation experiments.

Quantitative stereological analyses of the pancreatic islets demonstrated a marked increase of total β-cell volume from 11 weeks to 5 months (6.4-fold) and from 5 months to 1–1.4 years (1.6-fold) of age in control pigs. In contrast, the expansion of total β-cell volume in GIPR[dn] transgenic pigs was less pronounced between 11 weeks and 5 months of age (4.3-fold), with no further increase in 1- to 1.4-year-old animals. These findings are explained by a markedly reduced proliferation rate of β-cells in 11-week-old GIPR[dn] transgenic pigs, a developmental stage characterized by massive expansion of β-cells in pigs (36). Staining for cleaved caspase-3 did not show a significantly

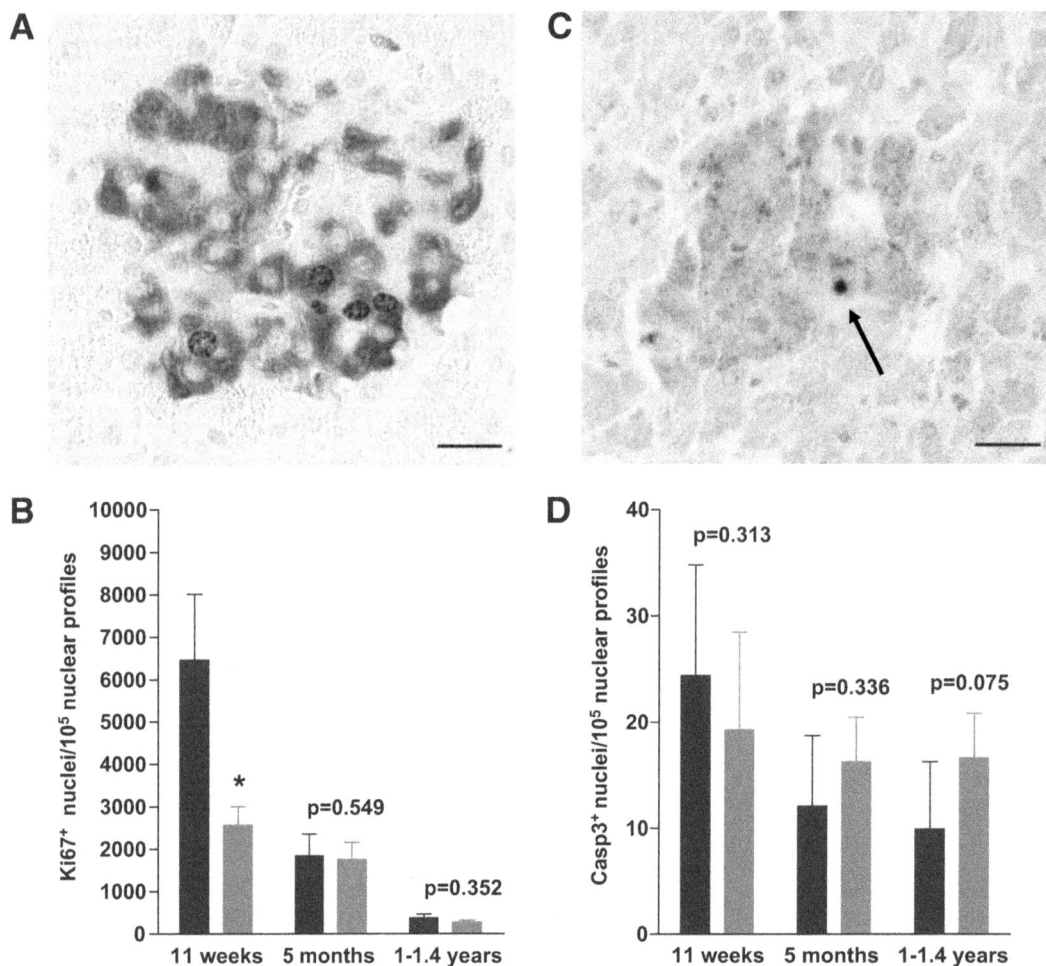

FIG. 7. β-Cell proliferation and apoptosis. *A* and *C*: Representative histological sections doublestained for insulin (blue) and Ki67 (brown) (*A*) or for insulin (light brown) plus cleaved caspase-3 (dark blue; see arrow) (*C*). *B* and *D*: Determination of the number of Ki67− (*B*) and cleaved caspase-3–positive β-cells (*D*). Wild type: blue bars, transgenic: red bars. Wild type: $n = 5$, transgenic: $n = 5$ for 11-week-old and 1- to 1.4-year-old pigs; wild type: $n = 4$, transgenic: $n = 4$ for 5-month-old pigs. Data are means ± SE. *$P < 0.05$ vs. control; scale bar = 20 μm. Note the significantly ($P < 0.05$) reduced β-cell proliferation rate in 11-week-old GIPR^{dn} transgenic pigs. (A high-quality digital representation of this figure is available in the online issue.)

increased rate of cell death in the β-cell compartment of GIPR^{dn} transgenic pigs versus controls, although a trend of higher numbers of cleaved caspase-3 positive β-cells was visible in 1- to 1.4-year-old GIPR^{dn} transgenic pigs. This may suggest a contribution of apoptosis to the reduction of total β-cell volume in mature GIPR^{dn} transgenic pigs.

Due to the reduced volume fraction of β-cells in the islets of 1- to 1.4-year-old GIPR^{dn} transgenic pigs, the relative volumes of α- and δ-cells in the islets were increased. However, since the islet volume was concomitantly reduced, the absolute volumes of α- and δ-cells were not different between GIPR^{dn} transgenic and control pigs.

The numbers of animals investigated in our study are, in part, smaller than in some rodent studies. However, due to the large size of the pig, several blood-based parameters could be measured repeatedly with short time intervals in the same animals, providing an important advantage for statistical analysis. Further, the stereological data of all animals ($n = 28$) were evaluated together by ANOVA, demonstrating significant group effects (Table 1) with P values <0.01 for many data/differences supporting our core statements.

Interestingly, $Gipr^{-/-}$ mice provided no evidence that GIPR action is required for the maintenance of islet and β-cell integrity in vivo (15,37). These mice exhibited an increase in relative β-cell area referring to pancreas area (37), leading to the conclusion that in vivo the function of GIP is primarily restricted to that of an incretin (15). However, the relatively mild phenotype of $Gipr^{-/-}$ mice may result from compensatory mechanisms (15). Although mice lacking both GIPR and GLP-1R exhibited more severe glucose intolerance than the individual mutants (38,39) these double mutant animals did not develop diabetes, raising the suspicion of the existence of compensatory mechanisms other than the GIP/GLP-1 system (38). The findings in GIPR^{dn} transgenic pigs suggest that, in addition to its role as an incretin hormone, GIP is necessary for the expansion of β-cell mass and that its partial loss of function cannot be fully compensated by hyperactivation of the GLP-1/GLP-1R system.

In conclusion, GIPR^{dn} transgenic pigs resemble characteristic features of human type 2 diabetic patients very closely in the following ways: disturbed GIP function, glucose intolerance, and reduced pancreatic β-cell mass. Moreover, GIPR^{dn} transgenic pigs may be an attractive animal model for the development and preclinical evaluation of incretin-based therapeutic strategies (40). Another potential application of GIPR^{dn} transgenic pigs is the development of novel techniques for dynamic in vivo monitoring of pancreatic islet mass (41). Due to their size and close physiological and anatomical similarities to humans (42), pigs represent attractive animal models for translating novel therapeutic and diagnostic principles into clinical practice.

ACKNOWLEDGMENTS

This study was supported by the Deutsche Forschungsgemeinschaft (GRK 1029), the Bayerische Forschungsstiftung (492/02), and the Diabetes Hilfs- und Forschungsfonds Deutschland (DHFD).

No potential conflicts of interest relevant to this article were reported.

Parts of this work were presented in abstract form at the 51st Annual Meeting of the German Society of Endocrinology, Salzburg, Austria, 7–10 March 2007; the 42nd Annual Meeting of the German Diabetes Society, Hamburg, Germany, 16–19 May 2007; the 34th Annual Conference of the International Embryo Transfer Society, Denver, Colorado, 5–9 January 2008; the 44th Annual Meeting of the German Diabetes Society, Leipzig, Germany, 20–23 May 2008; the 68th Scientific Sessions of the American Diabetes Association, San Francisco, California, 6–10 June 2008; and the 69th Scientific Sessions of the American Diabetes Association, New Orleans, Louisiana, 5–9 June 2009.

The authors thank Prof. Dr. Karl Heinritzi, Prof. Dr. Holm Zerbe, and Dr. Birgit Rathkolb for the generous support of this study; Prof. Dr. Helmut Kuechenhoff (StaBLab, Ludwig Maximilians University Munich) for expert help with the statistical analysis of longitudinal data; and Tamara Holy, Lisa Pichl, Bianca Schneiker, Elfi Holupirek, Christian Erdle, and Siegfried Elsner for excellent technical assistance and animal management.

REFERENCES

1. Baggio LL, Drucker DJ. Biology of incretins: GLP-1 and GIP. Gastroenterology 2007;132:2131–2157
2. Mayo KE, Miller LJ, Bataille D, Dalle S, Goke B, Thorens B, Drucker DJ. International Union of Pharmacology. XXXV. The glucagon receptor family. Pharmacol Rev 2003;55:167–194
3. Holst JJ, Gromada J. Role of incretin hormones in the regulation of insulin secretion in diabetic and nondiabetic humans. Am J Physiol Endocrinol Metab 2004;287:E199–E206
4. Saxena R, Hivert MF, Langenberg C, Tanaka T, Pankow JS, Vollenweider P, Lyssenko V, Bouatia-Naji N, Dupuis J, Jackson AU, Kao WH, Li M, Glazer NL, Manning AK, Luan J, Stringham HM, Prokopenko I, Johnson T, Grarup N, Boesgaard TW, Lecoeur C, Shrader P, O'Connell J, Ingelsson E, Couper DJ, Rice K, Song K, Andreasen CH, Dina C, Kottgen A, Le Bacquer O, Pattou F, Taneera J, Steinthorsdottir V, Rybin D, Ardlie K, Sampson M, Qi L, van Hoek M, Weedon MN, Aulchenko YS, Voight BF, Grallert H, Balkau B, Bergman RN, Bielinski SJ, Bonnefond A, Bonnycastle LL, Borch-Johnsen K, Bottcher Y, Brunner E, Buchanan TA, Bumpstead SJ, Cavalcanti-Proenca C, Charpentier G, Chen YD, Chines PS, Collins FS, Cornelis M, G JC, Delplanque J, Doney A, Egan JM, Erdos MR, Firmann M, Forouhi NG, Fox CS, Goodarzi MO, Graessler J, Hingorani A, Isomaa B, Jorgensen T, Kivimaki M, Kovacs P, Krohn K, Kumari M, Lauritzen T, Levy-Marchal C, Mayor V, McAteer JB, Meyre D, Mitchell BD, Mohlke KL, Morken MA, Narisu N, Palmer CN, Pakyz R, Pascoe L, Payne F, Pearson D, Rathmann W, Sandbaek A, Sayer AA, Scott LJ, Sharp SJ, Sijbrands E, Singleton A, Siscovick DS, Smith NL, Sparso T, Swift AJ, Syddall H, Thorleifsson G, Tonjes A, Tuomi T, Tuomilehto J, Valle TT, Waeber G, Walley A, Waterworth DM, Zeggini E, Zhao JH, Illig T, Wichmann HE, Wilson JF, van Duijn C, Hu FB, Morris AD, Frayling TM, Hattersley AT, Thorsteinsdottir U, Stefansson K, Nilsson P, Syvanen AC, Shuldiner AR, Walker M, Bornstein SR, Schwarz P, Williams GH, Nathan DM, Kuusisto J, Laakso M, Cooper C,

   Marmot M, Ferrucci L, Mooser V, Stumvoll M, Loos RJ, Altshuler D, Psaty BM, Rotter JI, Boerwinkle E, Hansen T, Pedersen O, Florez JC, McCarthy MI, Boehnke M, Barroso I, Sladek R, Froguel P, Meigs JB, Groop L, Wareham NJ, Watanabe RM: Genetic variation in GIPR influences the glucose and insulin responses to an oral glucose challenge. Nat Genet 2010;42:142–148
5. Ehses JA, Casilla VR, Doty T, Pospisilik JA, Winter KD, Demuth HU, Pederson RA, McIntosh CH. Glucose-dependent insulinotropic polypeptide promotes beta-(INS-1) cell survival via cyclic adenosine monophosphate-mediated caspase-3 inhibition and regulation of p38 mitogen-activated protein kinase. Endocrinology 2003;144:4433–4445
6. Trumper A, Trumper K, Horsch D. Mechanisms of mitogenic and anti-apoptotic signaling by glucose-dependent insulinotropic polypeptide in beta(INS-1)-cells. J Endocrinol 2002;174:233–246
7. Trumper A, Trumper K, Trusheim H, Arnold R, Goke B, Horsch D. Glucose-dependent insulinotropic polypeptide is a growth factor for beta (INS-1) cells by pleiotropic signaling. Mol Endocrinol 2001;15:1559–1570
8. Kim SJ, Winter K, Nian C, Tsuneoka M, Koda Y, McIntosh CH. Glucose-dependent insulinotropic polypeptide (GIP) stimulation of pancreatic beta-cell survival is dependent upon phosphatidylinositol 3-kinase (PI3K)/protein kinase B (PKB) signaling, inactivation of the forkhead transcription factor Foxo1, and down-regulation of bax expression. J Biol Chem 2005;280:22297–22307
9. Yusta B, Baggio LL, Estall JL, Koehler JA, Holland DP, Li H, Pipeleers D, Ling Z, Drucker DJ. GLP-1 receptor activation improves beta cell function and survival following induction of endoplasmic reticulum stress. Cell Metab 2006;4:391–406
10. Meier JJ, Hucking K, Holst JJ, Deacon CF, Schmiegel WH, Nauck MA. Reduced insulinotropic effect of gastric inhibitory polypeptide in first-degree relatives of patients with type 2 diabetes. Diabetes 2001;50:2497–2504
11. Nauck MA, Heimesaat MM, Orskov C, Holst JJ, Ebert R, Creutzfeldt W. Preserved incretin activity of glucagon-like peptide 1 [7–36 amide] but not of synthetic human gastric inhibitory polypeptide in patients with type-2 diabetes mellitus. J Clin Invest 1993;91:301–307
12. Drucker DJ, Nauck MA. The incretin system: glucagon-like peptide-1 receptor agonists and dipeptidyl peptidase-4 inhibitors in type 2 diabetes. Lancet 2006;368:1696–1705
13. Nauck MA, Baller B, Meier JJ. Gastric inhibitory polypeptide and glucagon-like peptide-1 in the pathogenesis of type 2 diabetes. Diabetes 2004; 53(Suppl. 3):S190–S196
14. Miyawaki K, Yamada Y, Yano H, Niwa H, Ban N, Ihara Y, Kubota A, Fujimoto S, Kajikawa M, Kuroe A, Tsuda K, Hashimoto H, Yamashita T, Jomori T, Tashiro F, Miyazaki J, Seino Y. Glucose intolerance caused by a defect in the entero-insular axis: a study in gastric inhibitory polypeptide receptor knockout mice. Proc Natl Acad Sci U S A 1999;96:14843–14847
15. Hansotia T, Drucker DJ. GIP and GLP-1 as incretin hormones: lessons from single and double incretin receptor knockout mice. Regul Pept 2005;128: 125–134
16. Herbach N, Goeke B, Schneider M, Hermanns W, Wolf E, Wanke R. Overexpression of a dominant negative GIP receptor in transgenic mice results in disturbed postnatal pancreatic islet and beta-cell development. Regul Pept 2005;125:103–117
17. Hofmann A, Kessler B, Ewerling S, Weppert M, Vogg B, Ludwig H, Stojkovic M, Boelhauve M, Brem G, Wolf E, Pfeifer A. Efficient transgenesis in farm animals by lentiviral vectors. EMBO Rep 2003;4:1054–1060
18. Pfeifer A, Ikawa M, Dayn Y, Verma IM. Transgenesis by lentiviral vectors: lack of gene silencing in mammalian embryonic stem cells and preimplantation embryos. Proc Natl Acad Sci U S A 2002;99:2140–2145
19. Klose R, Kemter E, Bedke T, Bittmann I, Kelsser B, Endres R, Pfeffer K, Schwinzer R, Wolf E. Expression of biologically active human TRAIL in transgenic pigs. Transplantation 2005;80:222–230
20. Larsen MO, Rolin B, Ribel U, Wilken M, Deacon CF, Svendsen O, Gotfredsen CF, Carr RD. Valine pyrrolidide preserves intact glucose-dependent insulinotropic peptide and improves abnormal glucose tolerance in minipigs with reduced beta-cell mass. Exp Diabesity Res 2003;4: 93–105
21. Moritz MW, Dawe EJ, Holliday JF, Elliott S, Mattei JA, Thomas AL. Chronic central vein catheterization for intraoperative and long-term venous access in swine. Lab Anim Sci 1989;39:153–155
22. Kobayashi K, Kobayashi N, Okitsu T, Yong C, Fukazawa T, Ikeda H, Kosaka Y, Narushima M, Arata T, Tanaka N. Development of a porcine model of type 1 diabetes by total pancreatectomy and establishment of a glucose tolerance evaluation method. Artif Organs 2004;28:1035–1042
23. Krickhahn M, Meyer T, Buhler C, Thiede A, Ulrichs K. Highly efficient isolation of porcine islets of Langerhans for xenotransplantation: numbers, purity, yield and in vitro function. Ann Transplant 2001;6:48–54

24. Ricordi C, Socci C, Davalli AM, Staudacher C, Baro P, Vertova A, Sassi I, Gavazzi F, Pozza G, Di Carlo V. Isolation of the elusive pig islet. Surgery 1990;107:688–694

25. van der Burg MP, Graham JM. Iodixanol density gradient preparation in university of wisconsin solution for porcine islet purification. Scientific-WorldJournal 2003;3:1154–1159

26. Latif ZA, Noel J, Alejandro R. A simple method of staining fresh and cultured islets. Transplantation 1988;45:827–830

27. Jones KH, Senft JA. An improved method to determine cell viability by simultaneous staining with fluorescein diacetate-propidium iodide. J Histochem Cytochem 1985;33:77–79

28. Scherle W. A simple method for volumetry of organs in quantitative stereology. Mikroskopie 1970;26:57–60

29. Bonner-Weir S, Baxter LA, Schuppin GT, Smith FE. A second pathway for regeneration of adult exocrine and endocrine pancreas: a possible recapitulation of embryonic development. Diabetes 1993;42:1715–1720

30. Petrik J, Reusens B, Arany E, Remacle C, Coelho C, Hoet JJ, Hill DJ. A low protein diet alters the balance of islet cell replication and apoptosis in the fetal and neonatal rat and is associated with a reduced pancreatic expression of insulin-like growth factor-II. Endocrinology 1999;140:4861–4873

31. Xu G, Stoffers DA, Habener JF, Bonner-Weir S. Exendin-4 stimulates both β-cell replication and neogenesis, resulting in increased β-cell mass and improved glucose tolerance in diabetic rats. Diabetes 1999;48:2270–2276

32. Herbach N, Rathkolb B, Kemter E, Pichl L, Klaften M, de Angelis MH, Halban PA, Wolf E, Aigner B, Wanke R. Dominant-negative effects of a novel mutated Ins2 allele causes early-onset diabetes and severe β-cell loss in Munich Ins2C95S mutant mice. Diabetes 2007;56:1268–1276

33. Iatropoulos MJ, Williams GM. Proliferation markers. Exp Toxicol Pathol 1996;48:175–181

34. Hui H, Dotta F, Di Mario U, Perfetti R. Role of caspases in the regulation of apoptotic pancreatic islet beta-cells death. J Cell Physiol 2004;200:177–200

35. Verbeke G, Molenberghs G. *Linear Mixed Models for Longitudinal Data.* New York, Springer, 2001

36. Bock T, Kyhnel A, Pakkenberg B, Buschard K. The postnatal growth of the beta-cell mass in pigs. J Endocrinol 2003;179:245–252

37. Pamir N, Lynn FC, Buchan AM, Ehses J, Hinke SA, Pospisilik JA, Miyawaki K, Yamada Y, Seino Y, McIntosh CH, Pederson RA. Glucose-dependent insulinotropic polypeptide receptor null mice exhibit compensatory changes in the enteroinsular axis. Am J Physiol Endocrinol Metab 2003;284:E931–E939

38. Hansotia T, Baggio LL, Delmeire D, Hinke SA, Yamada Y, Tsukiyama K, Seino Y, Holst JJ, Schuit F, Drucker DJ. Double incretin receptor knockout (DIRKO) mice reveal an essential role for the enteroinsular axis in transducing the glucoregulatory actions of DPP-IV inhibitors. Diabetes 2004;53:1326–1335

39. Preitner F, Ibberson M, Franklin I, Binnert C, Pende M, Gjinovci A, Hansotia T, Drucker DJ, Wollheim C, Burcelin R, Thorens B. Gluco-incretins control insulin secretion at multiple levels as revealed in mice lacking GLP-1 and GIP receptors. J Clin Invest 2004;113:635–645

40. Shaffer C. Incretin mimetics vie for slice of type 2 diabetes market. Nat Biotechnol 2007;25:263

41. Medarova Z, Moore A. MRI as a tool to monitor islet transplantation. Nat Rev Endocrinol 2009;5:444–452

42. Larsen MO, Rolin B. Use of the Gottingen minipig as a model of diabetes, with special focus on type 1 diabetes research. ILAR J 2004;45:303–313

Improved Pancreatic β-Cell Function in Type 2 Diabetic Patients After Lifestyle-Induced Weight Loss Is Related to Glucose-Dependent Insulinotropic Polypeptide

THOMAS P.J. SOLOMON, PHD[1]
JACOB M. HAUS, PHD[1,2]
KAREN R. KELLY, PHD[1,3]

MICHAEL ROCCO, MD[4]
SANGEETA R. KASHYAP, MD[5]
JOHN P. KIRWAN, PHD[1,2,3,6]

OBJECTIVE — Restoration of insulin secretion is critical for the treatment of type 2 diabetes. Exercise and diet can alter glucose-induced insulin responses, but whether this is due to changes in β-cell function per se is not clear. The mechanisms by which lifestyle intervention may modify insulin secretion in type 2 diabetes have also not been examined but may involve the incretin axis.

RESEARCH DESIGN AND METHODS — Twenty-nine older, obese (aged 65 ± 1 years; BMI 33.6 ± 1.0 kg/m^2) subjects, including individuals with newly diagnosed type 2 diabetes (obese-type 2 diabetic) and individuals with normal glucose tolerance (obese-NGT), underwent 3 months of nutritional counseling and exercise training. β-Cell function (oral glucose–induced insulin secretion corrected for insulin resistance assessed by hyperinsulinemic-euglycemic clamps) and the role of glucose-dependent insulinotropic polypeptide (GIP) were examined.

RESULTS — After exercise and diet-induced weight loss (-5.0 ± 0.7 kg), oral glucose–induced insulin secretion was increased in the obese-type 2 diabetic group and decreased in the obese-NGT group (both $P < 0.05$). When corrected for alterations in insulin resistance, the change in insulin secretion remained significant only in the obese-type 2 diabetic group (1.23 ± 0.26 vs. 2.04 ± 0.46 arbitrary units; $P < 0.01$). Changes in insulin secretion were directly related to the GIP responses to oral glucose ($r = 0.64$, $P = 0.005$), which were augmented in the obese-type 2 diabetic group and only moderately suppressed in the obese-NGT group.

CONCLUSIONS — After lifestyle-induced weight loss, improvements in oral glucose–induced insulin secretion in older, obese, nondiabetic subjects seem to be largely dependent on improved insulin sensitivity. However, in older obese diabetic patients, improved insulin secretion is a consequence of elevated β-cell function. We demonstrate for the first time that changes in insulin secretion after lifestyle intervention may be mediated via alterations in GIP secretion from intestinal K-cells.

Diabetes Care 33:1561–1566, 2010

D iet and exercise-based lifestyle interventions, such as the Diabetes Prevention Program, have been shown to successfully reduce the risk of developing diabetes (1). Insulin resistance is the major underlying defect driving hyperglycemia, the reversal of which is critical to reduce vascular complications and mortality (2). However, in addition to insulin resistance, progressive pancreatic β-cell dysfunction, marked by a decline in compensatory hyperinsulinemia across the glucose tolerance contin-uum, ultimately results in type 2 diabetes (3).

Previous work has highlighted the beneficial effects of lifestyle interventions on insulin secretion and β-cell function in obesity (4–7). However, it is rather well established that large improvements in insulin resistance occur after exercise and/or caloric restriction in obese non-diabetic and diabetic humans (8–10). Therefore, apparent changes in glucose tolerance and insulin secretion may be due to alterations in insulin resistance that expose the pancreas to less glucose, rather than intrinsic improvements in β-cell function.

Evidence suggests that postprandial insulin secretion may be partially controlled by nutrient-responsive incretin peptides released by intestinal cells. We recently reported that weight loss–induced reductions in insulin secretion in obese men and women with impaired glucose tolerance, are related to changes in secretion of the incretin hormone glucose-dependent insulinotropic polypeptide (GIP) (11). Indeed, bariatric surgery restores insulin secretory capacity in patients with type 2 diabetes via alterations in incretin secretion, including GIP (12). Further, exenatide-based incretin-mimetic pharmacological therapy also restores insulin secretion (13). These recent findings have indicated that the intravenous methods used previously to study insulin secretion, methods that bypass the incretin-releasing gastrointestinal system, may not be appropriate to study in vivo mechanisms of lifestyle-induced change in β-cell function.

In obese, insulin-resistant individuals exhibiting basal and postprandial hyperinsulinemia, an improvement in β-cell function is regarded as a reduction of insulin hypersecretion. Conversely, in type 2 diabetes the compensatory postprandial hyperinsulinemia required to correct for the severe underlying insulin resistance is absent, and therefore an increase in insulin secretion would reflect an improvement in β-cell function. However, to

From the [1]Department of Pathobiology, Cleveland Clinic, Cleveland, Ohio; the [2]Department of Physiology, Case Western Reserve University, Cleveland, Ohio; the [3]Department of Nutrition, Case Western Reserve University, Cleveland, Ohio; the [4]Department of Cardiovascular Medicine, Cleveland Clinic, Cleveland, Ohio; the [5]Department of Endocrinology, Diabetes and Metabolism, Cleveland Clinic, Cleveland, Ohio; and the [6]Department of Gastroenterology/Hepatology, Cleveland Clinic, Cleveland, Ohio.
Corresponding author: John P. Kirwan, kirwanj@ccf.org.
Received 30 October 2009 and accepted 10 February 2010. Published ahead of print at http://care.diabetesjournals.org on 3 March 2010. DOI: 10.2337/dc09-2021.

See accompanying editorial, p. 1691.

Table 1—*Subject characteristics of each of the age- and BMI-matched groups*

Subject characteristics	Obese-NGT		Obese-type 2 diabetic		ANOVA	
	Prestudy	Poststudy	Prestudy	Poststudy	Time	Time-group
Age (years)	63 ± 2		67 ± 2		—	—
Sex (male/female)	8/8		6/7		—	—
Weight (kg)	93.9 ± 3.2	88.8 ± 2.9	98.3 ± 4.6	93.4 ± 4.2	<0.0001	0.90
BMI (kg/m^2)	32.1 ± 1.1	30.4 ± 1.2	35.5 ± 1.5	33.7 ± 1.3	<0.0001	0.78
Fat (%)	41.0 ± 1.6	39.0 ± 2.1	40.8 ± 2.0	38.5 ± 2.5	0.01	0.84
VAT (cm^2)	187 ± 16	134 ± 15	202 ± 28	168 ± 27	<0.0001	0.24
Vo_{2max} (l/min)	2.11 ± 0.12	2.35 ± 0.16	1.99 ± 0.15	2.25 ± 0.15	<0.0001	0.97
Leptin (ng/ml)	25.9 ± 4.8	19.9 ± 4.4	22.3 ± 4.7	18.5 ± 4.3	0.007	0.40
TG (mg/dl)	194 ± 28	136 ± 19	181 ± 17	156 ± 19	0.003	0.15
Cholesterol (mg/dl)	199 ± 9	178 ± 8	192 ± 10	182 ± 9	0.0006	0.24
A1C (%)	5.35 ± 0.09	5.51 ± 0.08	5.86 ± 0.29	5.16 ± 0.32	0.08	0.008
FPG (mg/dl)	97.9 ± 3.5	97.2 ± 3.0	129 ± 7*	116 ± 6	0.03	0.04
2-h OGTT (mg/dl)	124 ± 3	122 ± 7	225 ± 11*	192 ± 11	0.03	0.05
FPI (μU/ml)	16.0 ± 2.0	13.7 ± 2.3	26.5 ± 7.1	17.4 ± 1.5	0.11	0.27
AUC I ($\times 10^3$ μU/ml · 0.3 h)	12.9 ± 1.6	7.6 ± 1.6	10.1 ± 2.3	11.5 ± 1.9	0.01	0.13
GDR (mg/kg/min)	2.67 ± 0.26	3.91 ± 0.38	1.85 ± 0.37*	2.34 ± 0.40	<0.0001	0.03

Data are means ± SEM. *Indicates significant difference vs. obese-NGT, $P < 0.05$. AUC I, area under the insulin response curve to the OGTT; FPI, fasting plasma insulin; GDR, glucose disposal rate during the hyperinsulinemic-euglycemic clamp; TG, triglycerides; VAT, intra-abdominal visceral adipose tissue.

demonstrate an alteration in β-cell function per se, one must account for changes in the β-cell exposure to glucose by assessing changes in insulin sensitivity. To date, the potential of nonsurgical and nonpharmacological lifestyle interventions to preserve β-cell function and increase insulin secretion in type 2 diabetes have not been fully explored. In addition, there is a paucity of data on the effects of exercise on incretin-mediated insulin secretion. In this investigation, we examined the effects of diet and exercise-induced weight loss on insulin resistance and insulin secretion in older obese type 2 diabetic individuals, compared with an age- and BMI-matched obese control group exhibiting normal glucose tolerance (NGT) and compensatory hyperinsulinemia. We hypothesized that in type 2 diabetes, in addition to relief from the underlying insulin resistance, β-cell insulin secretory function would be elevated in line with elevations in GIP secretion.

RESEARCH DESIGN AND
METHODS — Older obese men and women ($n = 29$; aged 65 ± 1 years; BMI 33.6 ± 1.0 kg/m^2) (Table 1) were recruited from the local community to participate in our ongoing obesity and diabetes studies. All participants were screened with a medical history and physical examination, blood and urine chemistry analyses, an oral glucose tolerance test (OGTT), and a resting and exercise stress test 12-lead electrocardiogram. In-

dividuals were excluded from participation if they *1*) smoked, *2*) were weight unstable (>2 kg in previous 6 months), *3*) undertook regular exercise (>30 min/ day, >3 days/week), *4*) had contraindications to elevated levels of physical activity as indicated by an electrocardiogram, *5*) demonstrated any evidence of current or previous hematological, renal, hepatic, cardiovascular, or pulmonary disease, or *6*) were taking medications known to affect our primary outcome variables. All participants also underwent resting metabolic rate testing by indirect calorimetry to calculate caloric requirements for the intervention. Participants were stratified into two age- and BMI-matched groups according to their oral glucose tolerance: those with NGT exhibiting insulin resistance with compensatory hyperinsulinemia (obese-NGT) and those with newly diagnosed type 2 diabetes (obese-type 2 diabetic) (2). Diabetic participants were only identified by our screening procedures, and their diabetes had not been previously diagnosed nor were they taking blood glucose-lowering medications. Signed informed consent was obtained before enrollment into the study, and all procedures were approved by our institutional review board.

Lifestyle intervention. All participants were entered into a 3-month diet and exercise-induced weight loss intervention. These approaches are routine in our laboratory and have been described in detail previously (8).

Diet counseling. Prestudy nutritional habits were assessed using 3-day diet records, and subjects underwent weekly counseling with a registered dietitian. Dietary habits were continuously assessed throughout the intervention. The intent of the counseling was to moderately reduce total caloric intake (−300 kcal/day) and to optimize the macronutrient composition. Nutritional analysis was performed using Nutritionist Pro (Axxya Systems, Stafford, TX).

Exercise training. Subjects also partook in fully supervised aerobic treadmill-walking exercise that was conducted for 1 h/day, 5 days/week. Initial sessions were completed at 60–65% of maximum heart rate; however, by week 4, intensity was increased and maintained at 80–85% maximum heart rate. Exercise intensity was calculated from data collected during maximal aerobic exercise tests conducted at biweekly intervals throughout the intervention (described below).

Prestudy/poststudy control period. Metabolic testing was conducted during a 3-day inpatient stay in the Clinical Research Unit. During this period, isocaloric (based on resting metabolic rate multiplied by 1.2) meals (55% carbohydrate, 30% fat, and 15% protein) were provided. Compliance with these meals was estimated by food weigh backs. Nonhabitual physical activity was also restricted during the prestudy inpatient period.

Prestudy/poststudy metabolic measures. To determine body composition, weight and height were measured by standard techniques. Whole-body fat percentage was determined using dual-energy X-ray absorptiometry (iDXA; Lunar, Madison, WI). Computed tomography scanning (Picker PQ6000 scanner; Marconi/Picker, Highland Heights, OH) was used to measure cross-sectional visceral abdominal adiposity at the fourth lumbar vertebral body, as described previously (8).

Aerobic fitness. VO_{2max} (Jaeger Oxycon Pro; Viasys, Yorba Linda, CA) measured during exhaustive exercise was used as a marker of aerobic fitness. These measurements were repeated at biweekly intervals to adjust training intensity in relation to changes in aerobic fitness. These procedures have been fully described elsewhere (8).

Oral glucose–induced insulin secretion

A 3-h 75-g OGTT was administered at 8:00 A.M., after an overnight fast. Blood samples were obtained from an intravenous antecubital line at 30-min intervals. Incremental metabolite responses (area under the curve) during the OGTT were calculated using the trapezoidal rule. Oral glucose–induced insulin secretion (referred to throughout as ΔC-Pep/ΔG) was calculated as incremental plasma C-peptide (picomoles per liter) during the first 30 min of the OGTT divided by incremental plasma glucose (millimoles per liter) during the first 30 min of the OGTT. This is a slight modification of a previous model presented by Abdul-Ghani et al. (14), based on the principle that changes in C-peptide more accurately reflect insulin secretion rates. In addition, early-phase GIP secretion was estimated as the incremental peptide response during the first 30 min of the OGTT (ΔGIP$_{0-30}$).

Insulin sensitivity

A 2-h hyperinsulinemic euglycemic (90 mg/dl) clamp was performed after an overnight fast, as described previously (15). In brief, a primed continuous 40 mU · m^{-2} · min^{-1} infusion of insulin (Humulin R U-100; Eli Lilly, Indianapolis, IN) was administered via an antecubital intravenous line, while a variable rate glucose (20% w/v) infusion was simultaneously administered to titrate fluctuations in plasma glucose. Arterialized plasma samples were obtained every 5 min from a retrograde intravenous dorsal line in a

hand warmed to ~60°C. Alterations to the glucose infusion rate were calculated as described previously (15). Peripheral tissue insulin sensitivity was estimated as the mean space-corrected glucose disposal rate over the last 30 min of the clamp.

β-Cell function

Because of the hyperbolic relationship between insulin secretion and sensitivity across the glucose tolerance continuum (3), the magnitude of the insulin response to oral glucose is influenced by the underlying state of insulin resistance. Thus, to estimate β-cell function, we corrected our measurements of insulin secretion (ΔC-Pep/ΔG) for the prevailing insulin resistance (IR) to derive an insulin secretion-to-insulin resistance index (ΔC-Pep/ΔG ÷ IR) equivalent to the disposition index of Gastaldelli et al. (16). Insulin resistance was calculated as the inverse of glucose disposal rate (micromoles per kilogram fat-free mass per minute) divided by the late-phase plasma insulin (picomoles per liter) response during the hyperinsulinemic-euglycemic clamp. In our subjects, we confirmed that baseline insulin resistance was indeed related to insulin secretion ($r = 0.78$, $P < 0.001$). In addition, hepatic insulin extraction was estimated as the incremental (area under the curve) plasma C-peptide response during the first 30 min of the OGTT divided by the incremental plasma insulin response during the first 30 min of the OGTT (17).

Analytical chemistry

Plasma glucose was measured using a glucose oxidase assay (YSI 2300 STAT Plus; YSI, Yellow Springs, OH). Plasma insulin and leptin concentrations were determined by radioimmunoassay (Millipore, Billerica, MA). Plasma triglycerides and total cholesterol were analyzed on an automated platform (Roche Modular Diagnostics, Indianapolis, IN). Total plasma GIP ($n = 10$ patients with NGT; $n = 8$ patients with type 2 diabetes) and C-peptide were assayed using an ELISA (Linco Research, St. Charles, MO). A1C was measured using nonporous ion-exchange high-pressure liquid chromatography (G7 HPLC analyzer; Tosoh Bioscience, San Francisco, CA).

Statistics

Statistical analyses were performed using Statview (SAS Institute, Cary, NC), and all data are expressed as means ± SEM. To examine differences in prestudy variables

between groups, one-way ANOVA was used to compare means. Between-group (obese-NGT vs. obese-type 2 diabetic) changes for all variables were analyzed using two-way repeated-measures ANOVA. Bonferroni post hoc tests were applied to significant group × time interactions to identify specific statistical differences between means. The addition of sex as a covariate did not reveal any group × sex × time interactions. Potential relationships between variables were analyzed using linear regression models. Statistical significance was accepted when $P < 0.05$.

RESULTS — Twenty-nine older obese adults were successfully screened into this study: $n = 16$ obese-NGT (8 men and 8 women) and $n = 13$ obese-type 2 diabetic (6 men and 7 women) individuals (Table 1). Attendance at exercise training sessions was 96.9 ± 0.6%.

Body composition and aerobic fitness

Both obese-NGT and obese-type 2 diabetic groups demonstrated significant weight loss and reductions in whole body and visceral fat ($P < 0.05$) (Table 1). VO_{2max} also improved ($P < 0.05$) (Table 1), demonstrating excellent compliance and response to the exercise training program. No group differences were observed in body composition or aerobic fitness.

Blood chemistry

All subjects exhibited significant reductions in plasma leptin, triglycerides, and cholesterol after the intervention ($P < 0.05$) (Table 1). A1C showed a nonsignificant fall in the obese-type 2 diabetic group.

Dietary intake

Compared with subjects' prestudy diet records, during the intervention total caloric intake was significantly reduced ($-342.9 ± 90.3$ kcal/day; $P < 0.05$) as was fat intake ($-4.7 ± 1.2$% kcal; $P < 0.05$). No differences were noted in dietary habits between groups.

Insulin action and β-cell function

Participants' fasting plasma glucose (FPG) and 2-h plasma glucose during the OGTT (2-h OGTT) are shown in Table 1. At baseline, the obese-type 2 diabetic group exhibited fasting and postprandial hyperglycemia compared with the obese-NGT group ($P < 0.05$). After the intervention, there were significant decreases in FPG and 2-h OGTT in the obese-type 2 dia-

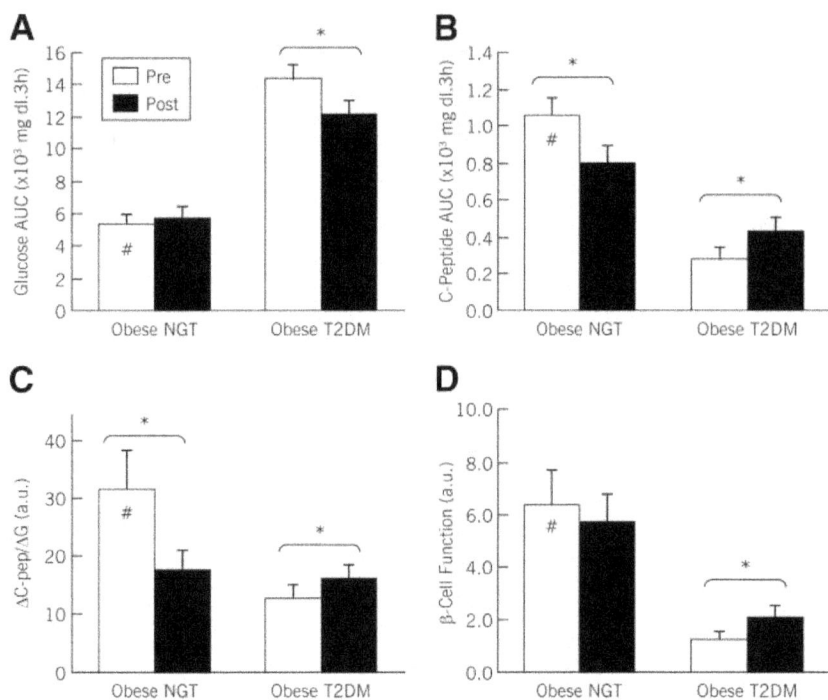

Figure 1—*Oral glucose–induced insulin secretion and β-cell function. Older obese men and women participated in a 3-month caloric restriction and exercise training–induced weight loss intervention. Participants were stratified by oral glucose tolerance: obese-NGT and obese-type 2 diabetic groups. Plasma glucose (A) and C-peptide (B) responses to OGTT were determined. After the intervention, glucose responses were reduced in the obese-type 2 diabetic group; C-peptide responses were increased in the obese-type 2 diabetic group, whereas they were reduced in the obese-NGT group. Changes in oral glucose–induced insulin secretion (ΔC-Pep/ΔG) (C) and insulin secretion corrected for the underlying insulin resistance (β-cell function) (D) were also assessed before and after the study. Insulin secretion was significantly increased in the obese-type 2 diabetic group and decreased in the obese-NGT group, whereas β-cell function significantly increased in the obese-type 2 diabetes group only, showing no change in the obese-NGT group. □, mean prestudy data; ■, mean poststudy data; errors bars represent S.E.M. *Significant prestudy vs. poststudy differences (P < 0.05). #Prestudy differences between groups (P < 0.05). a.u., arbitrary units; AUC, area under the curve.*

betic group ($P < 0.05$). These improvements were reflected in the changes in plasma glucose responses to the OGTT (area under the glucose curve) (Fig. 1*A*). Baseline plasma C-peptide responses to OGTT were markedly lower in the obese-type 2 diabetic group than in the obese-NGT group ($P < 0.05$) (Fig. 1*B*). Postintervention, C-peptide responses were significantly increased in the obese-type 2 diabetic group and decreased in the obese-NGT group (both $P < 0.05$) (Fig. 1*B*). At baseline, hepatic insulin extraction was decreased in the obese-type 2 diabetic group versus the obese-NGT group (8.96 ± 1.34 vs. 2.77 ± 0.62; $P < 0.05$). Insulin extraction was unaffected by the intervention. Changes in oral glucose–induced insulin secretion (ΔC-Pep/ΔG) are depicted in Fig. 1*C*. At baseline, insulin secretion was significantly lower in the obese-type 2 diabetic group (vs. the obese-NGT group; $P < 0.05$). After the

study, there was a significant increase in insulin secretion in the obese-type 2 diabetic group, whereas the obese-NGT group showed a significant decrease (both $P < 0.05$). Insulin-stimulated glucose disposal was lower in the obese-type 2 diabetic group than in the obese-NGT group, but the intervention induced significant elevations in both groups (Table 1). β-Cell function (ΔC-Pep/ΔG ÷ IR) is shown in Fig. 1*D*. Baseline β-cell function was significantly impaired in the obese-type 2 diabetic group compared with the obese-NGT group ($P < 0.05$). After the lifestyle intervention, β-cell function was significantly increased in the obese-type 2 diabetic group ($P < 0.05$), showing no alteration in the obese-NGT group ($P > 0.05$).

GIP responses
Figure 2*A* illustrates the changes in plasma GIP secretory responses to OGTT (ΔGIP$_{0–30}$). Baseline ΔGIP$_{0–30}$ was not dif-

ferent between the obese-type 2 diabetic and obese-NGT groups ($P > 0.05$). After the intervention, ΔGIP$_{0–30}$ increased in the obese-type 2 diabetic group ($P < 0.05$) and was nonsignificantly reduced in the obese-NGT group ($P = 0.07$). Further analysis demonstrated that ΔGIP$_{0–30}$ was not related to changes in body weight or composition in these subjects (all $P = 0.05$), whereas a significant relationship was identified between the changes in ΔGIP$_{0–30}$ and the changes in insulin secretion ($r = 0.64$, $P = 0.005$) (Fig. 2*B*).

CONCLUSIONS — After 3 months of diet- and exercise-induced weight loss, oral glucose–induced insulin secretion was increased in older obese type 2 diabetic individuals. In older obese individuals with NGT, the compensatory postprandial hyperinsulinemia was suppressed after the intervention. These changes were found to be directly related to the lifestyle-induced changes in oral glucose–induced GIP responses. When insulin secretion was corrected for the decrement in the underlying insulin resistance, it became apparent that the improvement in insulin secretion in obese individuals with NGT was driven by reduced insulin resistance. Yet, in the obese type 2 diabetic individuals, the improvement in insulin secretion appears to be a result of increased β-cell function. For the first time, using a physiological, incretin-related measure of insulin secretion corrected for the underlying rates of insulin-stimulated glucose disposal, we have demonstrated that nonsurgical and non-pharmacological weight loss can promote the restoration of insulin secretion in older obese individuals with type 2 diabetes via a mechanism related to increments in GIP secretion from intestinal K-cells.

Caloric restriction studies have previously demonstrated the potential to preserve β-cell function in diabetic individuals (4,17–19). Bogardus et al. (20) additionally found elevated insulin responses to OGTT after caloric restriction and exercise-induced weight loss, and, more recently, Dela et al. (21) and Slentz et al. (4) provided strong evidence of exercise training–induced increases in β-cell function in response to intravenous glucose in type 2 diabetic and/or obese patients. However, the nature of intravenous techniques used in several previous studies has not allowed for physiological mechanistic insight into incretin-mediated changes in insulin secretion. The assessment of insulin secretory re-

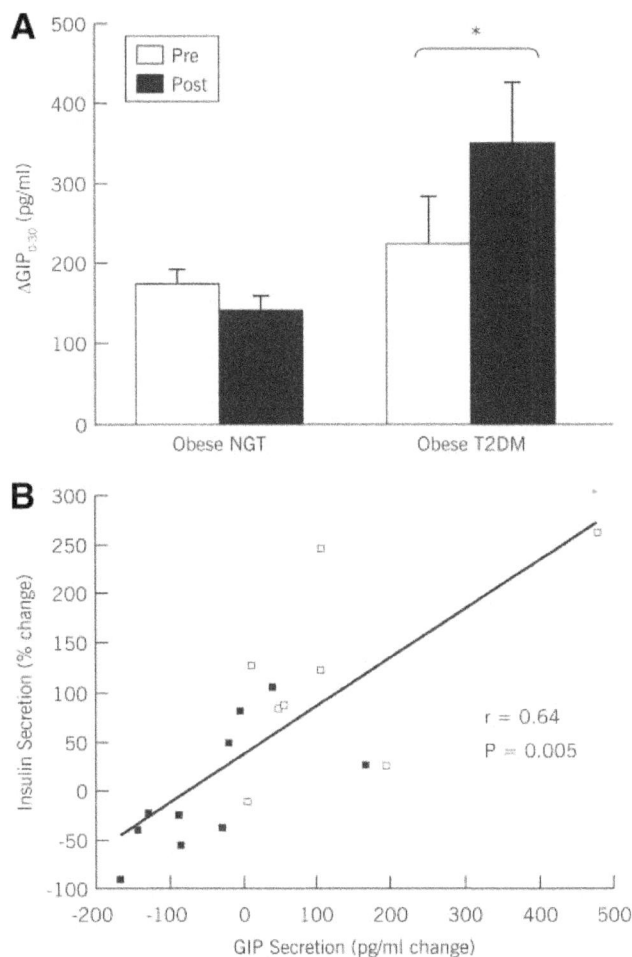

Figure 2—*Changes in plasma GIP secretion. A: Changes in total plasma GIP secretory responses to OGTT (ΔGIP_{0-30}) (obese-NGT group n = 10; obese-type 2 diabetic [T2DM] group n = 8) were assessed before and after the 3-month weight loss intervention. □, mean data before the intervention; ■, mean data after weight loss; error bars represent S.E.M. ΔGIP_{0-30} was significantly increased in the obese-type 2 diabetic group. B: Linear regression analyses revealed a significant correlation between the changes in plasma GIP responses to oral glucose and oral glucose-induced insulin secretion (r = 0.64, P = 0.005). ■, obese-NGT group; △, obese-type 2 diabetic group. *Significantly increased in obese-T2DM compared to obese-NGT (P < 0.05).*

glycemia. The restoration of insulin secretion in the diabetic state is crucial for achieving optimal glycemic control, without which uncontrolled hyperglycemia would advance vascular inflammation and oxidative stress, ultimately leading to microvascular endothelial dysfunction and macrovascular disease (3).

The dichotomy of "improved insulin secretion" in diabetic versus nondiabetic individuals is highlighted by this current study: reversal of inadequate postprandial insulinemia in diabetic individuals versus reversal of compensatory hyperinsulinemia in nondiabetic individuals. Exposure of the β-cell to chronic hyperglycemia leads to functional impairment or glucotoxicity (22). Thus, relief of extreme hyperglycemia and therefore toxicity in our diabetic population may explain the augmentation of postprandial insulin secretion. However, our diabetic subjects also demonstrate an increase in GIP secretion after the intervention. The mechanisms behind these changes are not understood, but our correlation analyses negate the effects of changes in body composition; however, it has been demonstrated that chronic hyperglycemia can downregulate pancreatic GIP receptor expression (23) and also increase GIP glycation, thus rendering the peptide dysfunctional with respect to insulinogenic capacity (24). This process may translate to the chronic hyperglycemic state in diabetes, where glucotoxicity is systemic and may therefore have the potential to impair GIP functional capacity or indeed intestinal K-cell secretion. Although caution must be used when correlative interpretations are made with low numbers of subjects, our finding that weight loss–induced changes in GIP are related to changes in insulin secretion warrants further attention. Future researchers should also examine more thoroughly the incretin axis to include the insulinogenic protein, GLP-1.

It is also interesting to note that after 3 months of lifestyle intervention neither hyperglycemia nor insulin secretion is normalized. Perhaps alternative treatment modalities are sensible. In recent years, surgical techniques and exenatide compounds have emerged (13) and received attention for their potential to initiate insulin secretion in severely obese diabetic patients. Recent data show that Roux-en-Y gastric bypass can increase pancreatic β-cell insulin secretory capacity via alteration of incretin signaling and can normalize hyperglycemia in up to

sponses to oral glucose ingestion (OGTT) is related to the incretin axis and allows clinical scientists to study β-cell function during a physiological postprandial perturbation. However, a change in the insulin secretory response may not necessarily be due to an alteration in β-cell glucose sensitivity or β-cell insulin secretory capacity per se, it may also be driven by a change in insulin sensitivity that would consequently alter the exposure of the β-cell to circulating glucose. In this respect, we applied the work of Gastaldelli et al. (16) to correct insulin secretion for the underlying peripheral tissue insulin resistance. We previously demonstrated that insulin secretion is reduced in obese impaired glucose-tolerant individuals after a similar lifestyle intervention (11).

Here we show that in subjects exhibiting insulin resistance yet normal glucose tolerance, weight loss can dramatically reverse the state of compensatory hyperinsulinemia. Although our findings do not demonstrate any alterations in β-cell function per se in such individuals, it is interesting to note that the potential progression toward impaired glucose tolerance that may occur if this group were left untreated has probably been reversed. At the other end of the glucose tolerance continuum, we demonstrate potential for exercise- and diet-induced weight loss to augment insulin secretion in type 2 diabetic patients via improvements in β-cell function, in addition to elevated rates of insulin-stimulated glucose disposal and reduced fasting and postprandial hyper-

83% of diabetic patients (12,25). Thus, the relative impact of lifestyle intervention on β-cell function may seem small. However, more prolonged interventions demonstrate even more dramatic improvements (4), and indeed the goal of clinical care is on-going dietary monitoring and physical activity. In the U.S. health care system, pharmaceutical and surgical options are a financial burden and not accessible to all, leaving low-cost lifestyle programs as a universal and valuable option.

In summary, we have furthered the work of prior investigations with intravenous methods by using an oral glucose technique to assess incretin-related insulin secretion and account for β-cell glucose exposure. We demonstrate that lifestyle intervention not only relieves the underlying insulin resistance in obesity but in older obese type 2 diabetic individuals it also has the potential to reverse β-cell dysfunction and therefore help reduce the risk of vascular disease. We also present new data demonstrating that elevations in in vivo insulin secretion in response to a physiological orally ingested glucose load is related to changes in postprandial GIP responses. This information highlights a potential mechanism to show that modification of intestinal incretin secretion after 3 months of mild caloric restriction and aerobic exercise training may explain the improvement in β-cell function in type 2 diabetic patients. A relationship between the changes in incretin secretion and β-cell function after lifestyle intervention has never before been demonstrated in type 2 diabetes.

Acknowledgments— This study was funded by National Institutes of Health (NIH) grant R01-AG-12834 (to J.P.K.), General Clinical Research Center grants M01-RR-10732, RR-00080, and RR-018390, and NIH National Center for Research Resources CTSA 1UL1-RR-024989, Cleveland, Ohio.

No potential conflicts of interest relevant to this article were reported.

We thank the research volunteers for their dedication to the lifestyle intervention. We also thank the nursing staff of the Clinical Research Unit for their contributions to this work.

References

1. Knowler WC, Barrett-Connor E, Fowler SE, Hamman RF, Lachin JM, Walker EA, Nathan DM. Reduction in the incidence of type 2 diabetes with lifestyle intervention or metformin. N Engl J Med 2002;346:393–403
2. American Diabetes Association. Diagnosis and classification of diabetes mellitus. Diabetes Care 2009;32(Suppl. 1):S62–S67
3. DeFronzo RA. Lilly Lecture 1987: The triumvirate: β-cell, muscle, liver. A collusion responsible for NIDDM. Diabetes 1988;37:667–687
4. Slentz CA, Tanner CJ, Bateman LA, Durheim MT, Huffman KM, Houmard JA, Kraus WE. Effects of exercise training intensity on pancreatic β-cell function. Diabetes Care 2009;32:1807–1811
5. Bloem CJ, Chang AM. Short-term exercise improves β-cell function and insulin resistance in older people with impaired glucose tolerance. J Clin Endocrinol Metab 2008;93:387–392
6. Kahn SE, Larson VG, Beard JC, Cain KC, Fellingham GW, Schwartz RS, Veith RC, Stratton JR, Cerqueira MD, Abrass IB. Effect of exercise on insulin action, glucose tolerance, and insulin secretion in aging. Am J Physiol 1990;258:E937–E943
7. Utzschneider KM, Carr DB, Barsness SM, Kahn SE, Schwartz RS. Diet-induced weight loss is associated with an improvement in β-cell function in older men. J Clin Endocrinol Metab 2004;89:2704–2710
8. O'Leary VB, Marchetti CM, Krishnan RK, Stetzer BP, Gonzalez F, Kirwan JP. Exercise-induced reversal of insulin resistance in obese elderly is associated with reduced visceral fat. J Appl Physiol 2006;100:1584–1589
9. Toledo FG, Menshikova EV, Ritov VB, Azuma K, Radikova Z, DeLany J, Kelley DE. Effects of physical activity and weight loss on skeletal muscle mitochondria and relationship with glucose control in type 2 diabetes. Diabetes 2007;56:2142–2147
10. Bruce CR, Kriketos AD, Cooney GJ, Hawley JA. Disassociation of muscle triglyceride content and insulin sensitivity after exercise training in patients with type 2 diabetes. Diabetologia 2004;47:23–30
11. Kelly KR, Brooks LM, Solomon TP, Kashyap SR, O'Leary VB, Kirwan JP. The glucose-dependent insulinotropic polypeptide and glucose-stimulated insulin response to exercise training and diet in obesity. Am J Physiol Endocrinol Metab 2009;296:E1269–E1274
12. Kashyap SR, Daud S, Kelly KR, Win H, Gastaldelli A, Kirwan JP, Brethauer S, Schauer PS. Acute effects of gastric bypass vs. gastric restriction on pancreatic β-cell function and insulinotropic hormones in patients with type 2 diabetes. Int J Obes (Lond) 2010;34:462–471
13. Bunck MC, Diamant M, Cornér A, Eliasson B, Malloy JL, Shaginian RM, Deng W, Kendall DM, Taskinen MR, Smith U, Yki-Järvinen H, Heine RJ. One-year treatment with exenatide improves β-cell function, compared with insulin glargine, in metformin-treated type 2 diabetic patients: a randomized, controlled trial. Diabetes Care 2009;32:762–768
14. Abdul-Ghani MA, Williams K, DeFronzo R, Stern M. Risk of progression to type 2 diabetes based on relationship between postload plasma glucose and fasting plasma glucose. Diabetes Care 2006;29:1613–1618
15. DeFronzo RA, Tobin JD, Andres R. Glucose clamp technique: a method for quantifying insulin secretion and resistance. Am J Physiol 1979;237:E214–E223
16. Gastaldelli A, Ferrannini E, Miyazaki Y, Matsuda M, DeFronzo RA. β-Cell dysfunction and glucose intolerance: results from the San Antonio metabolism (SAM) study. Diabetologia 2004;47:31–39
17. Henry RR, Brechtel G, Griver K. Secretion and hepatic extraction of insulin after weight loss in obese noninsulin-dependent diabetes mellitus. J Clin Endocrinol Metab 1988;66:979–986
18. Kelley DE, Wing R, Buonocore C, Sturis J, Polonsky K, Fitzsimmons M. Relative effects of calorie restriction and weight loss in noninsulin-dependent diabetes mellitus. J Clin Endocrinol Metab 1993;77:1287–1293
19. Gumbiner B, Polonsky KS, Beltz WF, Griver K, Wallace P, Brechtel G, Henry RR. Effects of weight loss and reduced hyperglycemia on the kinetics of insulin secretion in obese non-insulin dependent diabetes mellitus. J Clin Endocrinol Metab 1990;70:1594–1602
20. Bogardus C, Ravussin E, Robbins DC, Wolfe RR, Horton ES, Sims EA. Effects of physical training and diet therapy on carbohydrate metabolism in patients with glucose intolerance and non-insulin-dependent diabetes mellitus. Diabetes 1984;33:311–318
21. Dela F, von Linstow ME, Mikines KJ, Galbo H. Physical training may enhance β-cell function in type 2 diabetes. Am J Physiol Endocrinol Metab 2004;287:E1024–E1031
22. Rossetti L, Shulman GI, Zawalich W, DeFronzo RA. Effect of chronic hyperglycemia on in vivo insulin secretion in partially pancreatectomized rats. J Clin Invest 1987;80:1037–1044
23. Xu G, Kaneto H, Laybutt DR, Duvivier-Kali VF, Trivedi N, Suzuma K, King GL, Weir GC, Bonner-Weir S. Downregulation of GLP-1 and GIP receptor expression by hyperglycemia: possible contribution to impaired incretin effects in diabetes. Diabetes 2007;56:1551–1558
24. Mooney MH, Abdel-Wahab YH, Morgan LM, O'Harte FP, Flatt PR. Detection of glycated gastric inhibitory polypeptide within the intestines of diabetic obese (ob/ob) mice. Endocrine 2001;16:167–171
25. Schauer PR, Burguera B, Ikramuddin S, Cottam D, Gourash W, Hamad G, Eid GM, Mattar S, Ramanathan R, Barinas-Mitchel E, Rao RH, Kuller L, Kelley D. Effect of laparoscopic Roux-en Y gastric bypass on type 2 diabetes mellitus. Ann Surg 2003;238:467–484; discussion 484–485

GUT HORMONES

Can Gut Hormones Control Appetite and Prevent Obesity?

Owais B. Chaudhri, phd
Katie Wynne, phd
Stephen R. Bloom, md, dsc

The current obesity epidemic is fuelled by the availability of highly palatable, calorie-dense food, and the low requirement for physical activity in our modern environment. If energy intake exceeds energy use, the excess calories are stored as body fat. Although the body has mechanisms that act to maintain body weight over time, they primarily defend against starvation and are less robust in preventing the development of obesity. Knowledge of this homeostatic system that controls body weight has increased exponentially over the last decade and has revealed new possibilities for the treatment of obesity and its associated comorbidities. One therapeutic target is the development of agents based on the gastrointestinal hormones that control appetite. This review discusses the hormones oxyntomodulin, peptide YY, glucagon-like peptide 1, pancreatic polypeptide, and ghrelin and their emerging potential as anti-obesity treatments.

Diabetes Care 31 (Suppl. 2):S284–S289, 2008

The grave personal, societal, and economic consequences presaged by the continued worldwide rise in the prevalence of obesity are well documented (1,2). Currently, licensed non-surgical interventions are of limited efficacy (3–6). This relative failure of available therapies has imparted impetus to work directed at harnessing the physiological mechanisms of appetite control. The pursuit of the body's own satiety signals as therapeutic targets promises effective reductions in body weight with minimum disruption to other systems, avoiding the side effects that occur as an unwanted consequence of therapies targeting ubiquitous neurotransmitter and receptor complexes.

THE GUT-BRAIN AXIS

The lines of communication between the gastrointestinal (GI) tract and central nervous system (CNS) form a key component in a recently established model of appetite regulation. This gut-brain axis has both neural and humoral components that relay information to important CNS centers, including the hypothalamus and the brainstem (7). These CNS structures have extensive reciprocal connections and both receive neuronal input from the periphery, with the brainstem-vagus nerve complex being of particular significance in the control of feeding (8–10).

Neuronal activity in hypothalamic and brainstem nuclei is susceptible to influence by circulating hormones. In the hypothalamic arcuate nucleus (Arc), signals from the periphery result in changes in the relative activity of two subpopulations of neurons: an orexigenic population co-expressing the neurotransmitters neuropeptide Y and agouti-related peptide and an anorexigenic population co-expressing pro-opiomelanocortin and cocaine- and amphetamine-regulated transcript. Alterations in the release of these neuropeptides affect feeding behavior and energy expenditure, resulting in the maintenance of energy homeostasis.

The mechanisms by which hormones interact with CNS appetite centers are the subject of some contention. The proximity of both the hypothalamus and brainstem to structures with a relative deficiency of blood-brain barrier (the median eminence in the case of the hypothalamus and the area postrema in respect of the brainstem) may allow circulating factors direct access to CNS neurons. There is a growing body of evidence, however, that points to the vagus nerve as a primary site of action of some appetite-modulating hormones (11–15). From a therapeutic perspective, targeting the interaction of appetite signals with their receptors in the vagal nerve offers the potential advantage of being able to manipulate appetite at a site distant from the CNS.

GUT HORMONES

The GI-pancreatic complex is the largest endocrine organ in the body and a source of important regulatory peptides. Cholecystokinin was the first to be implicated in the short-term control of food intake (16), and other appetite-regulating hormones have subsequently been characterized. Of these, ghrelin is the only known orexigenic gut hormone, whereas a number of satiety factors exist, including glucagon-like peptide (GLP)-1, oxyntomodulin (OXM), peptide YY (PYY), and pancreatic polypeptide (PP) (7). Unlike leptin, which is thought to signal longer-term energy status, these gut hormones appear to act as meal initiators and terminators. Alterations in levels of gut hormones after bariatric surgery may contribute to the appetite suppression and sustained weight loss seen in patients undergoing this procedure and supports the development of these hormones as therapeutic targets (17,18).

Ghrelin

This 28–amino acid peptide is synthesized principally in the stomach (19). It acts via the growth hormone secretagogue receptor to increase food intake in rodents (20) and also acts to stimulate food intake in humans (21,22). Clinical studies have thus far concentrated on its use as an orexigenic agent in conditions characterized by anorexia and cachexia (23–26). Antagonists to ghrelin have been used in preclinical studies, however, paving the

From the Department of Metabolic Medicine, Imperial College London, Hammersmith Hospital, London, U.K.

Address correspondence and reprint requests to Professor S.R. Bloom, Department of Metabolic Medicine, Imperial College London, 6th Floor Commonwealth Building, Hammersmith Hospital, Du Cane Rd., London W12 0NN, U.K. E-mail: s.bloom@imperial.ac.uk.

S.R.B. is on the board of and holds stock in Thiakis. O.B.C. and K.W. declare no relevant conflict of interest.

This article is based on a presentation at the 1st World Congress of Controversies in Diabetes, Obesity and Hypertension (CODHy). The Congress and the publication of this article were made possible by unrestricted educational grants from MSD, Roche, sanofi-aventis, Novo Nordisk, Medtronic, LifeScan, World Wide, Eli Lilly, Keryx, Abbott, Novartis, Pfizer, Generx Biotechnology, Schering, and Johnson & Johnson.

Abbreviations: CNS, central nervous system; DPP-IV, dipetidyl peptidase IV; GI, gastrointestinal; GLP, glucagon-like peptide; OXM, oxyntomodulin; PYY, peptide YY.

DOI: 10.2337/dc08-s269

way for possible future evaluation as a therapy for obesity in humans (27).

GLP-1

A product of proglucagon cleavage, GLP-1 is released from the L-cells of the GI tract postprandially in proportion to the calories ingested. GLP-1 and longer-acting GLP-1 receptor agonists, such as exendin-4, reduce food intake in rodents when injected into the CNS (28) or peripherally (12,29). Given the observation of reduced circulating levels of GLP-1 and an attenuated postprandial response in the obese (30), it is not unreasonable to hypothesize that restoration of satiety through the use of exogenous GLP-1 receptor agonists might result in weight loss. To date, clinical development has focused on its strong incretin effect and its resultant use as an anti-diabetic agent: a 6-week subcutaneous infusion of GLP-1 improved blood glucose levels in poorly controlled diabetic subjects (31). However, in contrast to insulin, GLP-1 results in a tendency to reduce body weight (32). The advantages of a hypoglycemic agent that also promotes weight loss are obvious. These results may also be encouraging for the use of GLP-1 as an anti-obesity therapy.

A major hurdle to the therapeutic use of native GLP-1, and one common to many gut hormones, is its short half-life. The principle mediator of GLP-1 inactivation is the enzyme dipetidyl peptidase IV (DPP-IV). A number of DPP-IV–resistant GLP-1 receptor agonists, including liraglutide (Novo Nordisk, Denmark) and exenatide (Byetta, Amylin Pharmaceuticals, San Diego) have therefore been developed. Liraglutide has been synthesized using the GLP-1 sequence with the addition of an acyl side chain that allows for noncovalent binding to albumin and prolongs its half-life in the circulation (33). As an alternative strategy, exenatide (exendin-4) was extracted from the venom of the gila monster (*Heloderma suspectum*). It potently binds to and activates the GLP-1 receptor and is resistant to DPP-IV breakdown in the plasma.

Exenatide was recently licensed by the Food and Drug Administration for use as an adjunctive therapy for suboptimal glucose control in type 2 diabetic patients and is now undergoing further clinical trials to evaluate its utility specifically as a therapy for obesity. Initial data from open-label extension studies in diabetic patients have shown that a weight loss of 4.4 kg can be achieved by 82 weeks (34).

However, like GLP-1, dose-limiting side effects of nausea and vomiting define the maximal tolerated dose (35). The use of exenatide is also associated with hypoglycemia, although this occurs predominantly in patients receiving the drug in combination with another hypoglycemic agent (36). It has been reported that up to 30% of patients taking exenatide develop antibodies to this foreign peptide, although the clinical significance of this remains unclear (33).

Oxyntomodulin

Another product of the tissue-specific differential cleavage of proglucagon, OXM, is co-secreted with GLP-1 and PYY_{3-36} into the circulation by intestinal L-cells after nutrient ingestion (37). OXM is a satiety signal and administration reduces energy intake in both rodents and humans (38–42). Indeed, preprandial subcutaneous administration of OXM to overweight and obese humans over a 4-week period resulted in a significant reduction in body weight of 2.3 kg, compared with 0.5 kg for the placebo arm (42). In addition, OXM has been found to have a beneficial effect on energy usage, in that it increased activity levels back toward normal in overweight and obese volunteers (43). Oxyntomodulin administration was well tolerated in these studies. Longer-term trials are now required to determine whether its beneficial combination of properties can be sustained.

Although direct comparisons have not been made, OXM appears to cause less nausea than GLP-1–based treatments and thus may prove a potentially rewarding avenue of investigation. OXM is thought to act via the GLP-1 receptor (29). However, despite this common receptor, there are biological differences between the two hormones. There is evidence that OXM acts through different CNS pathways (40,44) and has a weaker incretin effect than GLP-1 (41,42,45). Its effect on food intake is more potent than that of GLP-1 in humans (41,42). In addition, the increased activity levels observed during oxyntomodulin therapy (43) have not been demonstrated with GLP-1 treatment, whose effect on energy expenditure remains controversial (46–48). The reasons for these dissimilar actions awaits elucidation but may lie in differential penetration of OXM and GLP-1 into different areas of the CNS or modification of ligand binding to the GLP-1 receptor in specific CNS regions by a receptor-associated protein. This

latter scenario is intriguing, since it offers another possible point for therapeutic intervention.

Like GLP-1, OXM is inactivated in large part by DPP-IV, and its advancement as a clinically useful treatment will be reliant on the development of a breakdown-resistant analog. Thiakis and Imperial Innovations (London, U.K.) are in the process of developing novel analogs of oxyntomodulin for the treatment of obesity.

Inhibitors of DPP-IV

In the quest for an effective anti-obesity treatment, some researchers have adopted the approach of augmenting the effectiveness of endogenous gut peptides. Multiple DPP-IV inhibitors have been tested in animals, and although they improve glucose levels in rodent models of type 2 diabetes, their effect on weight is more equivocal (49–52). A number of DPP-IV inhibitors are at various stages of development as adjuvant therapy for use in type 2 diabetic subjects with poorly controlled blood glucose levels. Of these, sitagliptin (Januvia, Merck) was granted marketing approval by the Food and Drug Administration in October 2006, and vildagliptin (Glavus, Novartis) is currently undergoing Food and Drug Administration review. The evidence from clinical trials to date suggests that these therapies were well tolerated with few adverse effects, but also have little effect on weight (53). Longer-term safety and outcome data are awaited.

Amylin

Co-secreted with insulin from the β-cells of the pancreas, the peptide amylin forms the basis of pramlintide (Symlin; Amylin Pharmaceuticals), a novel treatment for diabetes that has recently been granted Food and Drug Administration approval. In addition to favorable effects on blood glucose, pramlintide reduces food intake and has been shown to result in a 1.8-kg reduction in body weight over 26 weeks in overweight diabetic subjects (54). Phase 2 clinical trials of pramlintide for the treatment of obesity have shown weight loss of 3.5 kg over 16 weeks in 204 obese subjects (160 without diabetes and 44 with non–insulin-treated type 2 diabetes). Further evaluation of this drug as a therapy specifically for the treatment of obesity is awaited.

Peptide YY

PYY_{3-36}, the major circulating form of PYY, is co-secreted from intestinal L-cells with GLP-1 and OXM. Although there was initially some contention regarding the effects of PYY_{3-36} on energy intake in animal models (55), a number of research groups have demonstrated that peripheral PYY_{3-36} inhibits food intake and reduces body weight gain in several species (56–63). The minimization of stress, which can itself result in an inhibition of food intake, is vital to observe the anorectic effect of PYY_{3-36} in rodents (27,64). This has led some to question the utility of PYY_{3-36} as a basis for human therapy (55). However, the evidence from human studies to date is encouraging.

In the first clinical study of the intravenous administration of PYY_{3-36}, spontaneous food intake was reduced by 30% at plasma levels similar to those seen physiologically (56). A further recent study observed a dose-dependent reduction in appetite and food intake in response to intravenous PYY_{3-36} administration in normal-weight volunteers, although nausea occurred at higher doses (63).

It has been suggested that obesity is a PYY_{3-36}–deficient state, with lower basal levels and a blunted postprandial response (65). PYY_{3-36} "replacement" would therefore seem an apposite therapy for obesity, and there is evidence that obese individuals retain sensitivity to its appetite-suppressant effects (58). However, the therapeutic potential of PYY_{3-36} as an anti-obesity treatment is currently unknown, since there are limited data regarding the effect of repeated doses of PYY_{3-36} on body weight in humans.

Two drug companies are engaged in developing PYY_{3-36} for the treatment of human obesity. Amylin Pharmaceuticals has completed Phase I trials of its investigational compound AC162352, although no data are in the public domain regarding its efficacy. Nastech Pharmaceutical Company (Bothell, WA), in collaboration with Merck (Whitehouse Station, NJ), has recently completed Phase I trials of PYY_{3-36} delivered via the intranasal route. Acutely, PYY_{3-36} caused significant reductions in visual analog appetite scores, and there was a trend toward a dose-dependent reduction in food intake at a test meal (66). The most significant adverse effect noted was nausea, but this was seen in those subjects with the highest plasma levels of PYY_{3-36} after administration. Furthermore, preprandial use of the nasal spray for 6 days in 37 obese volunteers was associated with significant reductions in daily caloric intake that were sustained over the study period. Thrice-daily administration of the peptide yielded a reduction in caloric intake of 2,713 kJ and weight loss of 0.6 kg after 6 days of treatment. The results of more extensive trials are awaited.

Pancreatic polypeptide

Sharing some common structural features with PYY_{3-36}, pancreatic polypeptide is principally secreted by a population of cells located at the periphery of pancreatic islets. It is released into the circulation in a biphasic manner in response to nutrient ingestion and is subject to control by the vagus nerve and a number of other factors (67).

The role of pancreatic polypeptide in the regulation of energy balance is unclear. Studies have shown that circulating levels are reduced in the context of obesity, and there is a reduced second phase release after a meal (68), whereas in anorexic patients, levels are elevated (69). However, these findings have not been universally replicated (70,71).

PP reduces food intake when administered to rodents and humans (72–74). It remains to be evaluated whether this effect is preserved in obese humans. Work in individuals with Prader-Willi syndrome, characterized by overeating and morbid obesity, is encouraging (75), but not necessarily applicable to the more general nonsyndromic obese population. However, the observation that a single infusion of pancreatic polypeptide caused a measurable effect on food intake as long as 24 h afterward in normal-weight volunteers (74) suggests that pancreatic polypeptide may have potential as a long-term suppressor of appetite.

CONCLUSIONS — Even the modest weight loss resulting from the use of currently available therapies, such as sibutramine, rimonabant, and orlistat, can result in improvements in health and life expectancy (4,6). However, projections of future trends in the prevalence of overweight and obesity underline the urgent need for more effective treatments if the attendant socioeconomic consequences are to be lessened.

The mechanisms of postprandial satiety are still being characterized. Satiety factors secreted by the GI tract appear to occupy an important position in meal termination and the limitation of meal size. Their use as a basis for therapy in obesity therefore promises efficacy with minimal adverse effects.

Nevertheless, the therapeutic development of gut peptides is not without its difficulties. As indicated above, the short half-life of many native gut peptides necessitates unwieldy and inconvenient administration regimens (42,76). The use of stable analogs and novel methods of drug delivery, thus avoiding the need for subcutaneous injection or infusion, are two means by which this issue may be circumvented. The former is exemplified by the GLP-1 receptor agonists exenatide and liraglutide and the latter by interest in nasal delivery of PYY_{3-36}. Orally stable preparations of gut peptides remain some way off (77,78), although the development of nonpeptide receptor agonists offers a potentially fruitful alternative avenue.

Several gut hormones cause nausea in a proportion of patients receiving therapy, and this has limited the usefulness of GLP-1–based therapies to some extent (35). Satiety and nausea likely lie at different points along a spectrum of reactions to GI stimuli, and gut peptide–regulated pathways may mediate aspects of both responses (79–81). Although problematical, the application of dose-escalation regimes provides one possible solution and would not be dissimilar to the manner in which patients are commenced on other commonly used therapies such as metformin.

Perhaps a greater obstacle to the entry of GI hormone–based therapies lies in considerations of efficacy. The regulation of food intake is complex, and although its role is significant, the gut-brain axis operates alongside other components including CNS reward pathways, input from higher centers, and societal and environmental influences. The homeostatic system has developed with a high degree of in-built redundancy to guard against starvation, and this is signified by the discontinuation of development of the cholecystokinin receptor agonist 181771 by GlaxoSmithKline (Brentford, Middlesex, U.K.) after the results of clinical trials made it commercially nonviable. Similar concerns have been raised over PYY_{3-36} (55).

However, individual gut peptides are not released in isolation in response to nutrient ingestion. Rather, there is a coordinated release of a number of GI hormones, which act additively in orchestrating efficient nutrient absorption and meal termination (22). It therefore seems not unreasonable to propose that in the therapeutic targeting of appetite regulation, polypharmacy with a number of therapies might maximize clinical effect while minimizing side effects, mirroring trends in the management of other chronic conditions such as hypertension (82). Furthermore, the development of an effective gut hormone–based therapy will not absolve patients from responsibility for their own lifestyle. As with current medical therapies for obesity, the greatest weight loss is likely to be seen within the context of a multidisciplinary approach.

What then of the original question, "Can gut hormones reduce appetite and prevent obesity?" The answer at present seems to be a cautiously optimistic "yes." The etiology of obesity is complex and multifactorial. This coupled with our incomplete understanding of all the nuances and intricacies of appetite regulation will likely mean that no single treatment approach will be a panacea for the public health and economic challenges that are already starting to make themselves felt (83). Investment in a strategy that involves lifestyle, behavioral, public health, medical, and, where appropriate, surgical interventions would appear to be the most practical course to adopt. Within that framework, by exploiting the body's own satiety signals, drugs based on the actions of gut hormones will undoubtedly have a crucial role to play.

References

1. Allison DB, Saunders SE: Obesity in North America: an overview. *Med Clin North Am* 84:305–332, 2000
2. Hedley AA, Ogden CL, Johnson CL, Carroll MD, Curtin LR, Flegal KM: Prevalence of overweight and obesity among US children, adolescents, and adults, 1999–2002. *JAMA* 291:2847–2850, 2004
3. Kaplan LM: Pharmacological therapies for obesity. *Gastroenterol Clin North Am* 34: 91–104, 2005
4. Thearle M, Aronne LJ: Obesity and pharmacologic therapy. *Endocrinol Metab Clin North Am* 32:1005–1024, 2003
5. Yanovski SZ, Yanovski JA: Obesity. *N Engl J Med* 346:591–602, 2002
6. Curioni C, André C: *Rimonabant for Overweight or Obesity.* Issue 4. Art. No.: CD006162, DOI:10.1002/14651858. CD006162.pub2. Cochrane Database of Systematic Reviews, 2006
7. Stanley S, Wynne K, McGowan B, Bloom S: Hormonal regulation of food intake. *Physiol Rev* 85:1131–1158, 2005
8. Schwartz GJ: Integrative capacity of the caudal brainstem in the control of food intake. *Philos Trans R Soc Lond B Biol Sci* 361:1275–1280, 2006
9. Ellacott KL, Cone RD: The role of the central melanocortin system in the regulation of food intake and energy homeostasis: lessons from mouse models. *Philos Trans R Soc Lond B Biol Sci* 361:1265–1274, 2006
10. Schwartz MW, Woods SC, Porte D Jr, Seeley RJ, Baskin DG: Central nervous system control of food intake. *Nature* 404:661–671, 2000
11. Koda S, Date Y, Murakami N, Shimbara T, Hanada T, Toshinai K, Niiji A, Furuya M, Inomata N, Osuye K, Nakazato M: The role of the vagal nerve in peripheral PYY3–36-induced feeding reduction in rats. *Endocrinology* 146:2369–2375, 2005
12. Abbott CR, Monteiro M, Small CJ, Sajedi A, Smith KL, Parkinson JR, Ghatei MA, Bloom SR: The inhibitory effects of peripheral administration of peptide YY(3-36) and glucagon-like peptide-1 on food intake are attenuated by ablation of the vagal-brainstem-hypothalamic pathway. *Brain Res* 1044:127–131, 2005
13. Date Y, Murakami N, Toshinai K, Matsukura S, Niijima A, Matsuo H, Kangawa K, Nakazato M: The role of the gastric afferent vagal nerve in ghrelin-induced feeding and growth hormone secretion in rats. *Gastroenterology* 123:1120–1128, 2002
14. Williams DL, Grill HJ, Cummings DE, Kaplan JM: Vagotomy dissociates short- and long-term controls of circulating ghrelin. *Endocrinology* 144:5184–5187, 2003
15. Le Roux CW, Neary NM, Halsey TJ, Small CJ, Martinez-Isla AM, Ghatei MA, Theodorou NA, Bloom SR: Ghrelin does not stimulate food intake in patients with surgical procedures involving vagotomy. *J Clin Endocrinol Metab* 90:4521–4524, 2005
16. Gibbs J, Young RC, Smith GP: Cholecystokinin decreases food intake in rats. *J Comp Physiol Psychol* 84:488–495, 1973
17. Korner J, Bessler M, Cirilo LJ, Conwell IM, Daud A, Restuccia NL, Wardlaw SL: Effects of Roux-en-Y gastric bypass surgery on fasting and postprandial concentrations of plasma ghrelin, peptide YY, and insulin. *J Clin Endocrinol Metab* 90:359–365, 2005
18. Le Roux CW, Aylwin SJ, Batterham RL, Borg CM, Coyle F, Prasad V, Shurey S, Ghatei MA, Patel AG, Bloom SR: Gut hormone profiles following bariatric surgery favor an anorectic state, facilitate weight loss, and improve metabolic parameters. *Ann Surg* 243:108–114, 2006
19. Kojima M, Hosoda H, Date Y, Nakazato M, Matsuo H, Kangawa K: Ghrelin is a growth-hormone-releasing acylated peptide from stomach. *Nature* 402:656–660, 1999
20. Wren AM, Small CJ, Abbott CR, Dhillo WS, Seal LJ, Cohen MA, Batterham RL, Taheri S, Stanley SA, Ghatei MA, Bloom SR: Ghrelin causes hyperphagia and obesity in rats. *Diabetes* 50:2540–2547, 2001
21. Wren AM, Seal LJ, Cohen MA, Brynes AE, Frost GS, Murphy KG, Dhillo WS, Ghatei MA, Bloom SR: Ghrelin enhances appetite and increases food intake in humans. *J Clin Endocrinol Metab* 86:5992, 2001
22. Neary NM, Small CJ, Druce MR, Park AJ, Ellis SM, Semjonous NM, Dakin CL, Filipsson K, Wang F, Kent AS, Frost GS, Ghatei MA, Bloom SR: Peptide YY3-36 and glucagon-like peptide-17-36 inhibit food intake additively. *Endocrinology* 146: 5120–5127, 2005
23. Neary NM, Small CJ, Wren AM, Lee JL, Druce MR, Palmieri C, Frost GS, Ghatei MA, Coombes RC, Bloom SR: Ghrelin increases energy intake in cancer patients with impaired appetite: acute, randomized, placebo-controlled trial. *J Clin Endocrinol Metab* 89:2832–2836, 2004
24. Nagaya N, Itoh T, Murakami S, Oya H, Uematsu M, Miyatake K, Kangawa K: Treatment of cachexia with ghrelin in patients with COPD. *Chest* 128:1187–1193, 2005
25. Nagaya N, Moriya J, Yasumura Y, Uematsu M, Ono F, Shimizu W, Ueno K, Kitakaze M, Miyatake K, Kangawa K: Effects of ghrelin administration on left ventricular function, exercise capacity, and muscle wasting in patients with chronic heart failure. *Circulation* 110:3674–3679, 2004
26. Wynne K, Giannitsopoulou K, Small CJ, Patterson M, Frost G, Ghatei MA, Brown EA, Bloom SR, Choi P: Subcutaneous ghrelin enhances acute food intake in malnourished patients who receive maintenance peritoneal dialysis: a randomized, placebo-controlled trial. *J Am Soc Nephrol* 16:2111–2118, 2005
27. Beck B, Richy S, Stricker-Krongrad A: Feeding response to ghrelin agonist and antagonist in lean and obese Zucker rats. *Life Sci* 76:473–478, 2004
28. Turton MD, O'Shea D, Gunn I, Beak SA, Edwards CM, Meeran K, Choi SJ, Taylor GM, Heath MM, Lambert PD, Wilding JP, Smith DM, Ghatei MA, Herbert J, Bloom SR: A role for glucagon-like peptide-1 in the central regulation of feeding. *Nature* 379:69–72, 1996
29. Baggio LL, Huang Q, Brown TJ, Drucker DJ: Oxyntomodulin and glucagon-like peptide-1 differentially regulate murine food intake and energy expenditure. *Gastroenterology* 127:546–558, 2004
30. Verdich C, Toubro S, Buemann B, Lysgard MJ, Juul HJ, Astrup A: The role of postprandial releases of insulin and incretin hormones in meal-induced satiety: effect of obesity and weight reduction. *Int J*

Obes Relat Metab Disord 25:1206–1214, 2001

31. Zander M, Madsbad S, Madsen JL, Holst JJ: Effect of 6-week course of glucagon-like peptide 1 on glycaemic control, insulin sensitivity, and beta-cell function in type 2 diabetes: a parallel-group study. *Lancet* 359:824–830, 2002

32. Verdich C, Flint A, Gutzwiller JP, Naslund E, Beglinger C, Hellstrom PM, Long SJ, Morgan LM, Holst JJ, Astrup A: A meta-analysis of the effect of glucagon-like peptide-1 (7-36) amide on ad libitum energy intake in humans. *J Clin Endocrinol Metab* 86:4382–4389, 2001

33. Nauck MA, Meier JJ: Glucagon-like peptide 1 and its derivatives in the treatment of diabetes. *Regul Pept* 128:135–148, 2005

34. Blonde L, Klein EJ, Han J, Zhang B, Mac SM, Poon TH, Taylor KL, Trautmann ME, Kim DD, Kendall DM: Interim analysis of the effects of exenatide treatment on A1C, weight and cardiovascular risk factors over 82 weeks in 314 overweight patients with type 2 diabetes. *Diabetes Obes Metab* 8:436–447, 2006

35. Fineman MS, Shen LZ, Taylor K, Kim DD, Baron AD: Effectiveness of progressive dose-escalation of exenatide (exendin-4) in reducing dose-limiting side effects in subjects with type 2 diabetes. *Diabete Metab Res Rev* 20:411–417, 2004

36. Kendall DM, Riddle MC, Rosenstock J, Zhuang D, Kim DD, Fineman MS, Baron AD: Effects of exenatide (exendin-4) on glycemic control over 30 weeks in patients with type 2 diabetes treated with metformin and a sulfonylurea. *Diabetes Care* 28:1083–1091, 2005

37. Druce MR, Bloom SR: Oxyntomodulin: a novel potential treatment for obesity. *Treat Endocrinol* 5:265–272, 2006

38. Dakin CL, Gunn I, Small CJ, Edwards CM, Hay DL, Smith DM, Ghatei MA, Bloom SR: Oxyntomodulin inhibits food intake in the rat. *Endocrinology* 142:4244–4250, 2001

39. Dakin CL, Small CJ, Park AJ, Seth A, Ghatei MA, Bloom SR: Repeated ICV administration of oxyntomodulin causes a greater reduction in body weight gain than in pair-fed rats. *Am J Physiol Endocrinol Metab* 283:E1173–E1177, 2002

40. Dakin CL, Small CJ, Batterham RL, Neary NM, Cohen MA, Patterson M, Ghatei MA, Bloom SR: Peripheral oxyntomodulin reduces food intake and body weight gain in rats. *Endocrinology* 145:2687–2695, 2004

41. Cohen MA, Ellis SM, Le Roux CW, Batterham RL, Park A, Patterson M, Frost GS, Ghatei MA, Bloom SR: Oxyntomodulin suppresses appetite and reduces food intake in humans. *J Clin Endocrinol Metab* 88:4696–4701, 2003

42. Wynne K, Park AJ, Small CJ, Patterson M, Ellis SM, Murphy KG, Wren AM, Frost GS, Meeran K, Ghatei MA, Bloom SR: Subcutaneous oxyntomodulin reduces body weight in overweight and obese subjects: a double-blind, randomized, controlled trial. *Diabetes* 54:2390–2395, 2005

43. Wynne K, Park AJ, Small CJ, Meeran K, Ghatei MA, Frost GS, Bloom SR: Oxyntomodulin increases energy expenditure in addition to decreasing energy intake in overweight and obese humans: a randomised controlled trial. *Int J Obes (Lond)* 30:1729–1736, 2006

44. Chaudhri OB, Parkinson JR, Kuo YT, Druce MR, Herlihy AH, Bell JD, Dhillo WS, Stanley SA, Ghatei MA, Bloom SR: Differential hypothalamic neuronal activation following peripheral injection of GLP-1 and oxyntomodulin in mice detected by manganese-enhanced magnetic resonance imaging. *Biochem Biophys Res Commun* 350:298–306, 2006

45. Schjoldager BT, Baldissera FG, Mortensen PE, Holst JJ, Christiansen J: Oxyntomodulin: a potential hormone from the distal gut: pharmacokinetics and effects on gastric acid and insulin secretion in man. *Eur J Clin Invest* 18:499–503, 1988

46. Flint A, Raben A, Astrup A, Holst JJ: Glucagon-like peptide 1 promotes satiety and suppresses energy intake in humans. *J Clin Invest* 101:515–520, 1998

47. Flint A, Raben A, Ersboll AK, Holst JJ, Astrup A: The effect of physiological levels of glucagon-like peptide-1 on appetite, gastric emptying, energy and substrate metabolism in obesity. *Int J Obes Relat Metab Disord* 25:781–792, 2001

48. Shalev A, Holst JJ, Keller U: Effects of glucagon-like peptide 1 (7-36 amide) on whole-body protein metabolism in healthy man. *Eur J Clin Invest* 27:10–16, 1997

49. Burkey BF, Li X, Bolognese L, Balkan B, Mone M, Russell M, Hughes TE, Wang PR: Acute and chronic effects of the incretin enhancer vildagliptin in insulin-resistant rats. *J Pharmacol Exp Ther* 315:688–695, 2005

50. Sudre B, Broqua P, White RB, Ashworth D, Evans DM, Haigh R, Junien JL, Aubert ML: Chronic inhibition of circulating dipeptidyl peptidase IV by FE 999011 delays the occurrence of diabetes in male Zucker diabetic fatty rats. *Diabetes* 51:1461–1469, 2002

51. Pospisilik JA, Stafford SG, Demuth HU, McIntosh CH, Pederson RA: Long-term treatment with dipeptidyl peptidase IV inhibitor improves hepatic and peripheral insulin sensitivity in the VDF Zucker rat: a euglycemic-hyperinsulinemic clamp study. *Diabetes* 51:2677–2683, 2002

52. Reimer MK, Holst JJ, Ahren B: Long-term inhibition of dipeptidyl peptidase IV improves glucose tolerance and preserves islet function in mice. *Eur J Endocrinol* 146:717–727, 2002

53. Green BD, Flatt PR, Bailey CJ: Dipeptidyl peptidase IV (DPP IV) inhibitors: a newly emerging drug class for the treatment of type 2 diabetes. *Diab Vasc Dis Res* 3:159–165, 2006

54. Hollander P, Maggs DG, Ruggles JA, Fineman M, Shen L, Kolterman OG, Weyer C: Effect of pramlintide on weight in overweight and obese insulin-treated type 2 diabetes patients. *Obes Res* 12:661–668, 2004

55. Boggiano MM, Chandler PC, Oswald KD, Rodgers RJ, Blundell JE, Ishii Y, Beattie AH, Holch P, Allison DB, Schindler M, Arndt K, Rudolf K, Mark M, Schoelch C, Joost HG, Klaus S, Thone-Reineke C, Benoit SC, Seeley RJ, Beck-Sickinger AG, Koglin N, Raun K, Madsen K, Wulff BS, Stidsen CE, Birringer M, Kreuzer OJ, Deng XY, Whitcomb DC, Halem H, Taylor J, Dong J, Datta R, Culler M, Ortmann S, Castaneda TR, Tschop M: PYY3–36 as an anti-obesity drug target. *Obes Rev* 6:307–322, 2005

56. Batterham RL, Cowley MA, Small CJ, Herzog H, Cohen MA, Dakin CL, Wren AM, Brynes AE, Low MJ, Ghatei MA, Cone RD, Bloom SR: Gut hormone PYY(3-36) physiologically inhibits food intake. *Nature* 418:650–654, 2002

57. Chelikani PK, Haver AC, Reidelberger RD: Intravenous infusion of peptide YY(3-36) potently inhibits food intake in rats. *Endocrinology* 146:879–888, 2005

58. Batterham RL, Cohen MA, Ellis SM, Le Roux CW, Withers DJ, Frost GS, Ghatei MA, Bloom SR: Inhibition of food intake in obese subjects by peptide YY3-36. *N Engl J Med* 349:941–948, 2003

59. Pittner RA, Moore CX, Bhavsar SP, Gedulin BR, Smith PA, Jodka CM, Parkes DG, Paterniti JR, Srivastava VP, Young AA: Effects of PYY[3-36] in rodent models of diabetes and obesity. *Int J Obes Relat Metab Disord* 28:963–971, 2004

60. Sileno AP, Brandt GC, Spann BM, Quay SC: Lower mean weight after 14 days intravenous administration peptide YY(3-36) (PYY(3-36)) in rabbits. *Int J Obes (Lond)* 30:68–72, 2006

61. Koegler FH, Enriori PJ, Billes SK, Takahashi DL, Martin MS, Clark RL, Evans AE, Grove KL, Cameron JL, Cowley MA: Peptide YY(3-36) inhibits morning, but not evening, food intake and decreases body weight in Rhesus macaques. *Diabetes* 54:3198–3204, 2005

62. Challis BG, Coll AP, Yeo GS, Pinnock SB, Dickson SL, Thresher RR, Dixon J, Zahn D, Rochford JJ, White A, Oliver RL, Millington G, Aparicio SA, Colledge WH, Russ AP, Carlton MB, O'Rahilly S: Mice lacking pro-opiomelanocortin are sensitive to high-fat feeding but respond normally to the acute anorectic effects of peptide-YY(3-36). *Proc Natl Acad Sci U S A* 101:4695–4700, 2004

63. Degen L, Oesch S, Casanova M, Graf S, Ketterer S, Drewe J, Beglinger C: Effect of peptide YY3-36 on food intake in humans. *Gastroenterology* 129:1430–1436, 2005

64. Halatchev IG, Ellacott KL, Fan W, Cone RD: Peptide YY3-36 inhibits food intake in mice through a melanocortin-4 receptor-independent mechanism. *Endocrinology* 145:2585–2590, 2004

65. Le Roux CW, Batterham RL, Aylwin SJ, Patterson M, Borg CM, Wynne KJ, Kent A, Vincent RP, Gardiner J, Ghatei MA, Bloom SR: Attenuated peptide YY release in obese subjects is associated with reduced satiety. *Endocrinology* 147:3–8, 2006

66. Brandt G, Park A, Wynne K, Sileno A, Jazrawi R, Woods A, Quay S, Bloom S: Nasal peptide YY3-36: Phase 1 dose ranging and safety studies in healthy human subjects (Abstract). *86th Annual Meeting of the Endocrine Society (ENDO 2004), New Orleans, LA.* 2004

67. Katsuura G, Asakawa A, Inui A: Roles of pancreatic polypeptide in regulation of food intake. *Peptides* 23:323–329, 2002

68. Lassmann V, Vague P, Vialettes B, Simon MC: Low plasma levels of pancreatic polypeptide in obesity. *Diabetes* 29:428–430, 1980

69. Fujimoto S, Inui A, Kiyota N, Seki W, Koide K, Takamiya S, Uemoto M, Nakajima Y, Baba S, Kasuga M: Increased cholecystokinin and pancreatic polypeptide responses to a fat-rich meal in patients with restrictive but not bulimic anorexia nervosa. *Biol Psychiatry* 41:1068–1070, 1997

70. Jorde R, Burhol PG: Fasting and postprandial plasma pancreatic polypeptide (PP) levels in obesity. *Int J Obes* 8:393–397, 1984

71. Wisen O, Bjorvell H, Cantor P, Johansson C, Theodorsson E: Plasma concentrations of regulatory peptides in obesity following modified sham feeding (MSF) and a liquid test meal. *Regul Pept* 39:43–54, 1992

72. McLaughlin CL, Baile CA: Obese mice and the satiety effects of cholecystokinin, bombesin and pancreatic polypeptide. *Physiol Behav* 26:433–437, 1981

73. Asakawa A, Inui A, Ueno N, Fujimiya M, Fujino MA, Kasuga M: Mouse pancreatic polypeptide modulates food intake, while not influencing anxiety in mice. *Peptides* 20:1445–1448, 1999

74. Batterham RL, Le Roux CW, Cohen MA, Park AJ, Ellis SM, Patterson M, Frost GS, Ghatei MA, Bloom SR: Pancreatic polypeptide reduces appetite and food intake in humans. *J Clin Endocrinol Metab* 88:3989–3992, 2003

75. Zipf WB, O'Dorisio TM, Cataland S, Dixon K: Pancreatic polypeptide responses to protein meal challenges in obese but otherwise normal children and obese children with Prader-Willi syndrome. *J Clin Endocrinol Metab* 57:1074–1080, 1983

76. Naslund E, King N, Mansten S, Adner N, Holst JJ, Gutniak M, Hellstrom PM: Prandial subcutaneous injections of glucagon-like peptide-1 cause weight loss in obese human subjects. *Br J Nutr* 91:439–446, 2004

77. des Rieux A, Fievez V, Garinot M, Schneider YJ, Preat V: Nanoparticles as potential oral delivery systems of proteins and vaccines: a mechanistic approach. *J Control Release* 116:1–27, 2006

78. Mahato RI, Narang AS, Thoma L, Miller DD: Emerging trends in oral delivery of peptide and protein drugs. *Crit Rev Ther Drug Carrier Syst* 20:153–214, 2003

79. Kinzig KP, D'Alessio DA, Seeley RJ: The diverse roles of specific GLP-1 receptors in the control of food intake and the response to visceral illness. *J Neurosci* 22:10470–10476, 2002

80. Chelikani PK, Haver AC, Reidelberger RD: Dose-dependent effects of peptide YY(3-36) on conditioned taste aversion in rats. *Peptides* 27:3193–3201, 2006

81. Vrang N, Madsen AN, Tang-Christensen M, Hansen G, Larsen PJ: PYY(3-36) reduces food intake and body weight and improves insulin sensitivity in rodent models of diet-induced obesity. *Am J Physiol Regul Integr Comp Physiol* 291:R367–R375, 2006

82. Ogihara T, Matsuzaki M, Matsuoka H, Shimamoto K, Shimada K, Rakugi H, Umemoto S, Kamiya A, Suzuki N, Kumagai H, Ohashi Y, Takishita S, Abe K, Saruta T: The combination therapy of hypertension to prevent cardiovascular events (COPE) trial: rationale and design. *Hypertens Res* 28:331–338, 2005

83. Vlad I: Obesity costs UK economy 2bn pounds sterling a year. *BMJ* 327:1308, 2003

Ghrelin Infusion in Humans Induces Acute Insulin Resistance and Lipolysis Independent of Growth Hormone Signaling

Esben Thyssen Vestergaard, Lars Christian Gormsen, Niels Jessen, Sten Lund, Troels Krarup Hansen, Niels Moller, and Jens Otto Lunde Jorgensen

OBJECTIVE—Ghrelin is a gut-derived peptide and an endogenous ligand for the growth hormone (GH) secretagogue receptor. Exogenous ghrelin stimulates the release of GH (potently) and adrenocorticotropic hormone (ACTH) (moderately). Ghrelin is also orexigenic, but its impact on substrate metabolism is controversial. We aimed to study direct effects of ghrelin on substrate metabolism and insulin sensitivity in human subjects.

RESEARCH DESIGN AND METHODS—Six healthy men underwent ghrelin (5 pmol $\cdot$ kg^{-1} $\cdot$ min^{-1}) and saline infusions in a double-blind, cross-over study to study GH signaling proteins in muscle. To circumvent effects of endogenous GH and ACTH, we performed a similar study in eight hypopituitary adults but replaced with GH and hydrocortisone. The methods included a hyperinsulinemic-euglycemic clamp, muscle biopsies, microdialysis, and indirect calorimetry.

RESULTS—In healthy subjects, ghrelin-induced GH secretion translated into acute GH receptor signaling in muscle. In the absence of GH and cortisol secretion, ghrelin acutely decreased peripheral, but not hepatic, insulin sensitivity together with stimulation of lipolysis. These effects occurred without detectable suppression of AMP-activated protein kinase phosphorylation (an alleged second messenger for ghrelin) in skeletal muscle.

CONCLUSIONS—Ghrelin infusion acutely induces lipolysis and insulin resistance independently of GH and cortisol. We hypothesize that the metabolic effects of ghrelin provide a means to partition glucose to glucose-dependent tissues during conditions of energy shortage. *Diabetes* 57:3205–3210, 2008

Ghrelin, an endogenous ligand for the growth hormone (GH) secretagogue receptor (GHS-R), stimulates GH and adrenocorticotropic hormone (ACTH) secretion (1) in addition to having orexigenic and gastrokinetic effects (2,3). The observation that GHS-R is located in peripheral tissues suggests that ghrelin may exert direct effects (4). The effects of ghrelin on substrate in humans are uncertain, but insulin resistance and stimulation of lipolysis have been reported (5–7). However, it remains difficult to segregate direct effects from effects related to GH and cortisol, and we have recently demonstrated that somatostatin infusion fails to sufficiently suppress ghrelin-induced GH and cortisol secretion (8). Hormonally replaced hypopituitary patients constitute a means for studying putative GH- and cortisol-independent effects of ghrelin in human subjects in vivo.

We aimed to study potential direct effects of ghrelin on substrate metabolism and insulin sensitivity in the postabsorptive state. In one experiment in healthy adults, we assessed whether ghrelin-induced GH release translated into GH signaling in skeletal muscle, in the event of which the importance of abrogating indirect effects of ghrelin is obvious. Second, we studied the effects of ghrelin exposure on whole-body and regional substrate metabolism in the basal and insulin-stimulated state in hypopituitary patients on stable replacement with GH and hydrocortisone.

RESEARCH DESIGN AND METHODS

The studies were conducted in accordance with the Helsinki Declaration and following the approval by the local ethics committee, the Danish Medicines Agency, and the Good Clinical Practice (GCP) unit of Aarhus University Hospital. Both protocols were registered (Clinicaltrials.gov identification study 1: NCT00116025 and study 2: NCT00139945).

Preparation of synthetic ghrelin. Synthetic human acylated ghrelin (NeoMPS, Strasbourg, France) was dissolved in isotonic saline and sterilized by double passage through a 0.8/0.2-μm pore-size filter (Super Acrodisc; Gelman Sciences, Ann Arbor, MI).

Study 1: subjects and study protocol. Six healthy men (aged 23 ± 1 years, BMI 23.5 ± 0.4 kg/m^2) were examined as previously described (6). They received a constant infusion of saline or ghrelin (5 pmol $\cdot$ kg^{-1} $\cdot$ min^{-1}) starting at 0 min. At 90 min, a muscle biopsy was obtained from the lateral vastus muscle with a Bergström biopsy needle (Fig. 1).

Study 2: subjects and study protocol. Eight hypopituitary men (aged 53 ± 4 years, BMI 31.6 ± 1.0 kg/m^2) on stable replacement therapy with GH and hydrocortisone (for >3 months) participated. None of the patients had diabetes (A1C 5.7 ± 0.1% [range 4.9–6.0]) or any concomitant chronic disease. Each patient was studied on two occasions with 5-h infusions of saline or ghrelin (5 pmol $\cdot$ kg^{-1} $\cdot$ min^{-1}) in a randomized double-blind, cross-over design. Both study days commenced at 0800 h after an overnight fast (>9 h), with the subjects remaining fasting.

One intravenous cannula was inserted in the antecubital region for infusion, and one intravenous cannula was inserted in a heated dorsal hand vein for sampling of arterialized blood. At $t = 0$ min, saline or a primed-continuous ghrelin infusion (5 pmol $\cdot$ kg^{-1} $\cdot$ min^{-1}) was commenced. The bolus dose was estimated from the elimination rate constant of ghrelin (k_{01}) (6) and infused over a 20-min interval to avoid an overshoot of steady-state levels. Muscle biopsies were obtained at 120 min, as described above. A hyperinsulinemic-euglycemic clamp (insulin 0.6 mU $\cdot$ kg^{-1} $\cdot$ min^{-1}; Actrapid, Novo Nordisk, Denmark) was performed from 120 to 300 min. Plasma glucose was clamped at 5.0 mmol/l by adjusting the rate of infusion of 20% glucose according to plasma glucose measurements every 10 min. Insulin sensitivity was calculated from the glucose infusion rate (GIR) during the clamp. The period from 0 to 120 min is referred to as the basal period and the period from 120 to 300 min as the clamp period. Blood samples were obtained as indicated in Fig. 2.

From Medical Department M (Endocrinology and Diabetes), Aarhus University Hospital, Aarhus, Denmark.
Corresponding author: Esben Thyssen Vestergaard, etv@dadlnet.dk.
Received 8 January 2008 and accepted 26 August 2008.
Published ahead of print at http://diabetes.diabetesjournals.org on 5 September 2008. DOI: 10.2337/db08-0025. Clinical trial reg. nos. NCT00116025 and NCT00139945, clinicaltrials.gov.

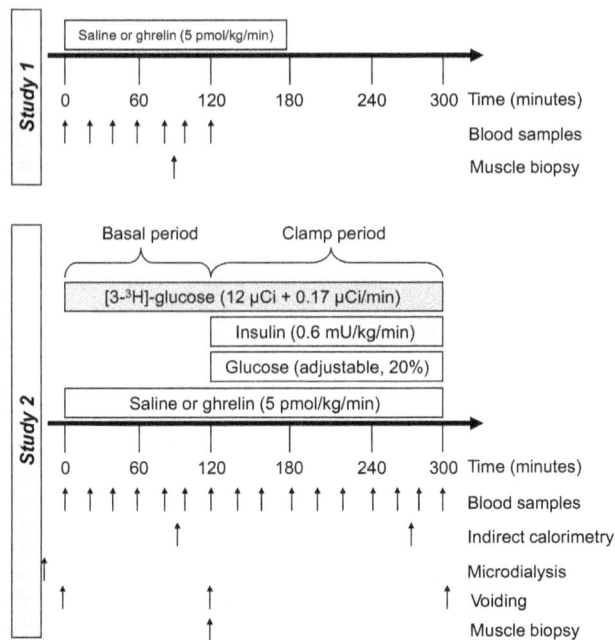

FIG. 1. Study protocol. Please refer to RESEARCH DESIGN AND METHODS **for further details.**

Tracers. A primed-continuous infusion of [3-³H]-glucose (bolus 12 μCi, 0.17 μCi/min; NEN Life Science Products, Boston, MA) was initiated at $t = 0$ min and continued throughout. Glucose rate of appearance (R_a) was calculated at 10-min intervals from 90 to 120 min and 270 to 300 min using Steele's non–steady-state equations (9). During the clamp, endogenous glucose production was calculated by subtracting the GIR from R_a. Oxidative rates of glucose (G_{OX}) and lipids were calculated from indirect calorimetry (Deltatrac; Datex Instruments, Helsinki, Finland) after correction for protein oxidation, which was estimated from the urinary excretion of urea. Nonoxidative glucose disposal was calculated as whole-body glucose disposal (R_d) minus the rate of G_{OX} (10).

Microdialysis. Microdialysis was performed and analyzed as described previously (8). Catheters (CMA 60, molecular cutoff of 20 kDa, membrane length 30 mm; CMA, Stockholm, Sweden) were placed in the lateral vastus muscle, in the subcutaneous adipose tissue, and in the femoral subcutaneous adipose tissue. The abdominal and femoral adipose tissue blood flow was estimated by Xe washout (11).

Blood samples and measurements. Plasma glucose was analyzed in duplicate using the glucose oxidase method (Beckman Instruments, Palo Alto, CA). Serum ghrelin (total levels) was measured in duplicate by an in-house assay (12). Serum GH, cortisol, and insulin were analyzed with a double monoclonal immunofluorometric assay (Delfia; Perkin Elmer, Wallac Oy, Turku, Finland). Serum free fatty acids (FFAs) were determined using a commercial kit (Wako Chemicals, Neuss, Germany). Plasma catecholamines were measured by liquid chromatography (13). Plasma glucagon was measured by radioimmunoassay (14). Glucose, glycerol, lactate, and urea in the microdialysis dialysate were measured in duplicate by an automated spectrophotometric kinetic enzymatic analyzer (CMA 600; CMA).

Western blotting and phosphatidylinositol 3-kinase assay. Muscle biopsies were homogenized as previously described (15). Aliquots of protein were resolved by SDS-PAGE, and proteins were electroblotted onto nitrocellulose membranes. Immunoblotting was performed using primary antibodies as follows: p signal transducers and activators of transcription (STAT5)a and -b, STAT5, pSTAT3, STAT3, p extracellular signal–regulated kinase (ERK)1 and -2, ERK-1 and -2, p AMP-activated protein kinase (AMPK)α, AMPKα-pan, p acetyal-CoA carboxylase (ACC), pAkt, pAkt substrate, and Akt substrate 160 (AS160). Membranes were incubated with horseradish peroxidase–coupled secondary antibodies, visualized by BioWest enhanced chemiluminescence (UVP LabWorks, Upland, CA) and quantified by the UVP BioImaging System. Densitometric measurements were adjusted to an internal control. Phosphatidylinositol 3-kinase (PI3K) activity was assessed, as previously described (15).

Statistics. Results are expressed as means ± SE. Systemic levels of hormones, metabolites, and GIR were analyzed by two-way ANOVA. The interaction between time and treatment (time × treatment) was considered the term of interest. The Bonferroni correction was used to account for multiple

comparisons when appropriate. Pairwise comparisons were carried out by Student's two-tailed paired t test when appropriate. P values <0.05 were considered significant. Statistical analysis was performed using SPSS version 14.0 for Windows.

RESULTS

Study 1. Ghrelin infusion stimulated endogenous GH secretion, which peaked at $t = 60$ min (1.1 ± 0.9 μg/l [saline] vs. 33.3 ± 8.0 μg/l [ghrelin]; $P = 0.008$). A significant elevation in serum FFA levels was recorded (0.4 ± 0.04 μg/l [saline] vs. 1.0 ± 0.1 μg/l [ghrelin]; $P = 0.003$). The levels of serum cortisol (268 ± 24 nmol/l [saline] vs. 400 ± 57 nmol/l [ghrelin]; $P = 0.06$) and plasma glucose (5.2 ± 0.1 mmol/l [saline] vs. 5.5 ± 0.1 mmol/l [ghrelin]; $P = 0.16$) were similar. Western blots performed on skeletal muscle biopsies revealed distinct STAT5 phosphorylation in all six subjects 30 min after the endogenous GH burst (Fig. 3).

Study 2. Pituitary surgery had been performed in all cases, and GH deficiency was documented by GH stimulation tests (insulin tolerance test [$n = 7$] or arginine test [$n = 1$]; means ± SE peak GH 0.3 ± 0.1 μg/l).

Hormones and metabolites. Hormones and metabolites are shown in Fig. 2. Serum ghrelin concentrations were similar at baseline on the 2 study days (0.51 ± 0.06 μg/l [saline] vs. 0.49 ± 0.06 μg/l [ghrelin]; $P = 0.38$) and correlated inversely with BMI (saline $r = -0.83$, $P = 0.01$; ghrelin $r = -0.73$, $P = 0.04$). Plasma levels of norepinephrine and epinephrine were comparable on both study days, and plasma levels of glucagon were also similar (10.9 ± 0.9 pmol/l [saline] vs. 9.3 ± 0.5 pmol/l [ghrelin], $P = 0.10$ at $t = 120$ min; and 8.6 ± 0.5 pmol/l [saline] vs. 7.1 ± 0.8 pmol/l [ghrelin], $P = 0.14$ at $t = 300$ min).

Resting energy expenditure and glucose and lipid metabolism. Data on resting energy expenditure and respiratory quotient (RQ) in study 2 are given in Table 1. Energy expenditure, RQ, or lipid oxidation were not significantly affected by ghrelin in the basal or in the clamp period. The increase in RQ ($RQ_{clamp} - RQ_{basal}$) during the clamp, however, was larger in the saline study (0.07 ± 0.01 vs. 0.03 ± 0.01 [ghrelin], $P = 0.03$).

FFAs. Ghrelin infusion induced an 80% increase in FFAs to 0.62 ± 0.03 mmol/l at $t = 120$ ($P < 0.05$), followed by a return to placebo levels during the clamp period (Fig. 2C).

Glucose. Ghrelin induced a rapid increase in plasma glucose levels with a peak value of 6.1 ± 0.2 mmol/l at $t = 120$ min ($P = 0.009$) (Fig. 2E). During the clamp, glucose levels gradually decreased toward postabsorptive levels on the ghrelin day, resulting in comparable glucose levels during the final 30 min of the clamp. The GIR was significantly decreased during ghrelin administration (Fig. 4A) ($P < 0.01$), and the corresponding M value was reduced by ~60% ($P < 0.001$). Ghrelin did not significantly impact glucose metabolism in the basal state (Table 1 and Fig. 4C) but reduced the rates of oxidative, nonoxidative, and total glucose disposal during the clamp period.

Regional substrate metabolism (microdialysis). Interstitial muscle glucose levels fluctuated in parallel with those in the circulation (Fig. 2F). By contrast, interstitial glucose in fat remained stable also during ghrelin infusion. Ghrelin did not significantly influence the levels of interstitial glycerol, lactate, or urea in either tissue (data not shown).

GH, insulin, and AMPK signaling. Densitometric quantitative bar graphs and representative Western blots from skeletal muscle biopsies are provided in Fig. 3. Adminis-

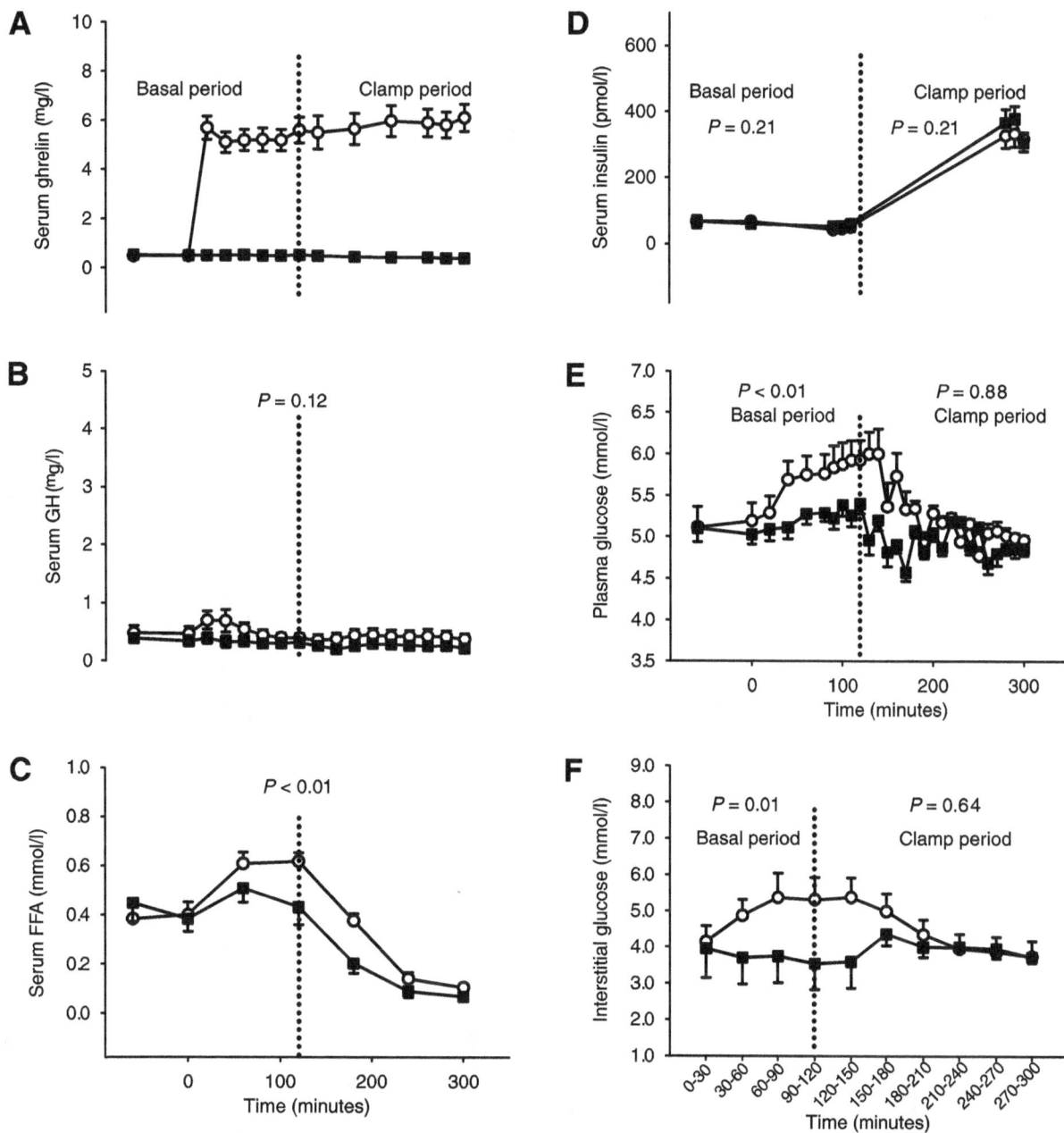

FIG. 2. Hormones and metabolites during saline and ghrelin administration in study 2. *A*: Serum levels of ghrelin increased in response to ghrelin infusion to a plateau of 5.33 ± 0.45 µg/l in the basal state and a higher plateau of 5.86 ± 0.50 µg/l during the clamp period (mean ghrelin levels basal period vs. clamp period *P* = 0.001). *B*: Serum levels of GH. *C*: Serum levels of FFA. *D*: Serum levels of insulin. Serum insulin was similar during both basal and clamp conditions. *E*: Plasma glucose levels. *F*: Interstitial skeletal muscle glucose levels. Printed *P* values refer to two-way ANOVA significance levels. ■, saline infusion; □, ghrelin infusion. All data are presented as means ± SE.

tration of ghrelin translated into STAT5 phosphorylation in the healthy subjects but not in the hypopituitary patients. Ghrelin exerted no effects on total protein levels, and no effects were recorded with regard to AMPK, ACC, STAT3, ERK-1 or -2, Akt, or AS160 phosphorylation in study 2. Insulin receptor substrate–associated PI3K activity was also not modified by ghrelin infusion (data not shown).

DISCUSSION

We document for the first time that ghrelin induces peripheral insulin resistance and stimulates lipolysis in the absence of GH and cortisol release. This investigation is also the first to document that ghrelin-induced endogenous GH release translates into Janus kinase/STAT signaling in skeletal muscle.

In some human studies, ghrelin administration increases plasma levels of glucose and FFAs (6–8,16) and reduces glucose disposal (5,8), indicating insulin resistance. These effects are, however, partly attributable to GH and/or cortisol secretion (5–8). There are both clinical and in vitro data to suggest that ghrelin directly suppresses glucose-induced insulin secretion from the β-cell (17), whereas administration of a ghrelin antagonist does the opposite (18). Moreover, ghrelin knockout mice display enhanced glucose-induced insulin release from isolated

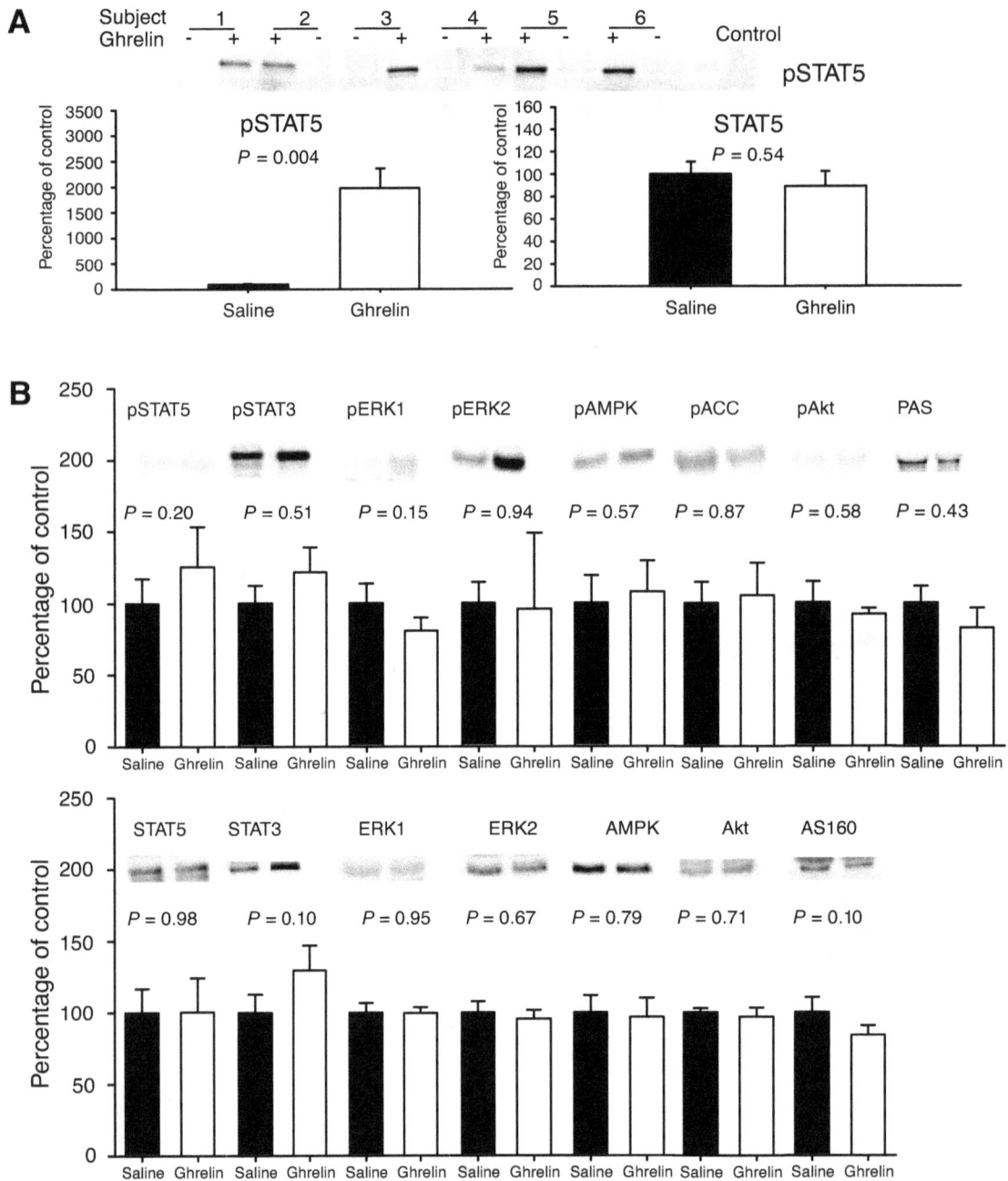

FIG. 3. *A*: Effects of ghrelin infusion on STAT5 phosphorylation and total STAT5 levels in skeletal muscle in healthy subjects (study 1). Values are means ± SE. *B*: Representative Western blots and quantitative bar-graphs regarding JAK/STAT, MAPK, AMPK, and insulin signaling pathways in skeletal muscle in hypopituitary patients (study 2) during ghrelin and saline infusion. PAS, pAkt substrate.

TABLE 1
Metabolic parameters during saline and ghrelin infusion in hypopituitary men (study 2)

	Basal period			Clamp period		
	Saline	Ghrelin	*P* value	Saline	Ghrelin	*P* value
RQ (ratio O_2/CO_2)	0.82 ± 0.02	0.83 ± 0.01	0.24	0.89 ± 0.01	0.86 ± 0.01	0.06
Energy expenditure (kcal/24 h)	1902 ± 58	1916 ± 61	0.80	1931 ± 49	1906 ± 66	0.72
Lipid oxidation ($mg \cdot kg^{-1} \cdot min^{-1}$)	0.74 ± 0.08	0.67 ± 0.05	0.37	0.34 ± 0.05	0.48 ± 0.08	0.19
Endogenous glucose production ($mg \cdot kg^{-1} \cdot min^{-1}$)	1.59 ± 0.18	1.63 ± 0.16	0.74	0.58 ± 0.19	0.57 ± 0.15	0.95

Data are means ± SE. Paired analysis of treatments.

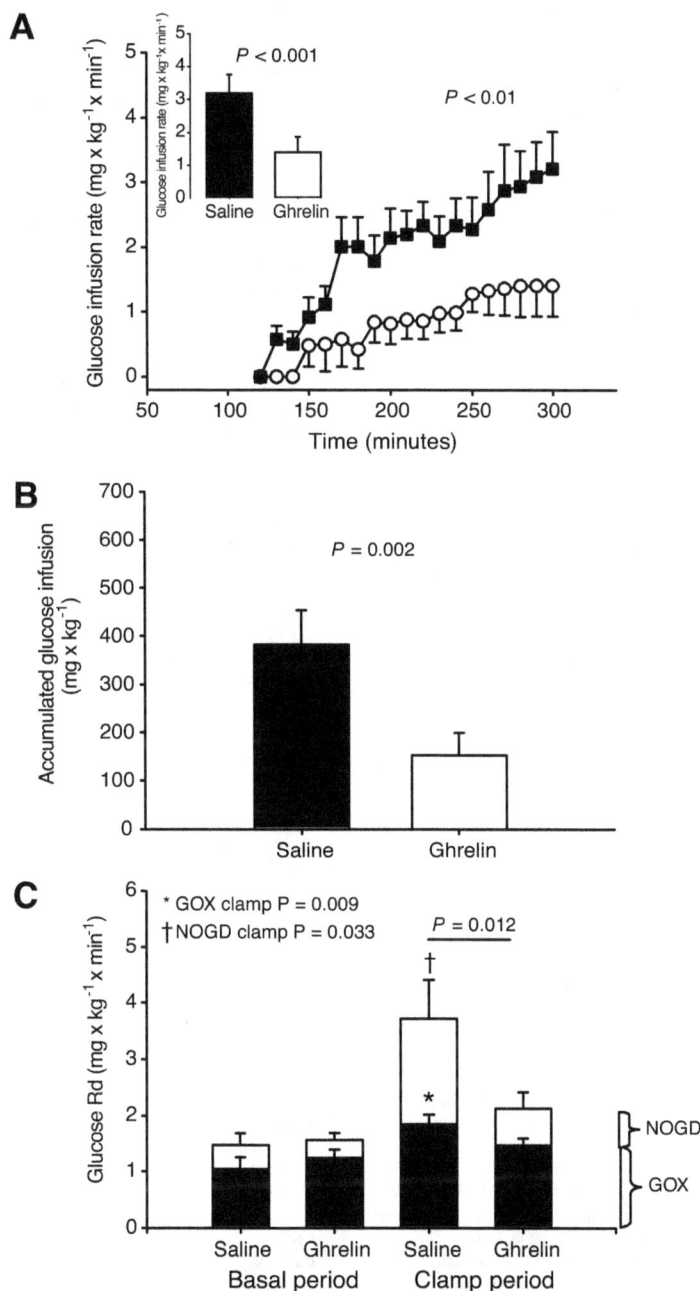

FIG. 4. *A*: Glucose metabolism during saline and ghrelin administration in study 2. Hyperinsulinemic clamp. Glucose infusion rates and *M* value during saline and ghrelin administration. ●, saline infusion; □, ghrelin infusion. *B*: Accumulative glucose infusion dosage during saline and ghrelin administration. The accumulative glucose dose was significantly decreased during the clamp period in the ghrelin study (*P* = 0.002). *C*: Glucose utilization during the terminal 30 min of basal and clamp periods in saline and ghrelin studies. Ghrelin did not significantly impact glucose metabolism in the basal period. During the clamp ghrelin infusion reduced the rates of oxidative, nonoxidative, and total glucose disposal (*P* = 0.009, *P* = 0.03, and *P* = 0.012, respectively). All data are presented as means ± SE.

islets (18,19) and exhibit increased peripheral insulin sensitivity (19). Ghrelin/GHS-R double knockout mice show lower glucose levels after a glucose tolerance test and a more rapid drop in plasma glucose levels after an insulin tolerance test (20).

Our study in hypopituitary men demonstrates that ghrelin in humans directly suppresses insulin-stimulated glucose disposal and stimulates FFA release. The observations at the whole-body level were corroborated by the demonstration of increased concentrations of glucose in skeletal muscle interstitial tissue. Previously, it has been demonstrated that in humans glucose disposal rates during hyperinsulinemic clamp conditions are predominantly determined by the rate of glucose uptake into skeletal muscle (21). By contrast, we observed no significant effect of ghrelin on hepatic insulin sensitivity. AMPK appears to be a key messenger in ghrelin signaling in several tissues (22–24), and AMPK is also a recognized cellular energy sensor (25). In our study, we did not record any significant effect of ghrelin on the activation of either AMPK or ACC in skeletal muscle. The biopsies, however, were only obtained in the basal period, which limits assessment of aberrations in insulin signaling pathways. The molecular mechanisms by which ghrelin causes insulin resistance in humans thus remain to be further ascertained and should be studied in both basal and insulin-stimulated conditions.

Serum FFA levels increased in response to ghrelin, which did not translate into increased lipid oxidation. It should be noted that hypopituitary adults are moderately obese, which is likely to influence any effect of ghrelin on FFA turnover. More importantly, infusion of ghrelin does not imitate the secretory pattern of endogenous ghrelin. Furthermore, this study was powered to detect effects of ghrelin on insulin sensitivity (8), and lack of significance with regard to lipid metabolism may be due to a β error.

In conclusion, we demonstrate for the first time in humans that ghrelin directly induces lipolysis and resistance to insulin-stimulated glucose disposal. We also demonstrate that ghrelin-induced GH release translates into GH signaling in skeletal muscle, emphasizing the significance of accounting for GH when evaluating any effects of ghrelin. The physiological significance of the direct metabolic effects of endogenous ghrelin remains unclear, but we propose that ghrelin in concert with GH partition substrate metabolism during conditions of energy shortage in such a way as to restrict glucose utilization to insulin-independent tissues such as the brain.

ACKNOWLEDGMENTS

This study was supported by an unrestricted grant from Novo Nordisk as well as grants from the Novo Nordisk Foundation, the A.P. Moller Foundation, the World Anti-Doping Agency, and the FOOD Study Group/Ministry of Food, Agriculture, and Fisheries and Ministry of Family and Consumer Affairs. Microdialysis catheters were kindly supplied by Roche.

The GCP unit of Aarhus University Hospital is acknowledged for monitoring that GCP guidelines were followed. S. Sorensen, M. Moller, E. Carstensen, and E. Hornemann are acknowledged for excellent technical assistance.

REFERENCES

1. Takaya K, Ariyasu H, Kanamoto N, Iwakura H, Yoshimoto A, Harada M, Mori K, Komatsu Y, Usui T, Shimatsu A, Ogawa Y, Hosoda K, Akamizu T, Kojima M, Kangawa K, Nakao K: Ghrelin strongly stimulates growth hormone release in humans. J Clin Endocrinol Metab 85:4908–4911, 2000
2. Wren AM, Seal LJ, Cohen MA, Brynes AE, Frost GS, Murphy KG, Dhillo WS, Ghatei MA, Bloom SR: Ghrelin enhances appetite and increases food intake in humans. J Clin Endocrinol Metab 86:5992–5995, 2001
3. Dornonville, dlC, Lindstrom E, Norlen P, Hakanson R: Ghrelin stimulates gastric emptying but is without effect on acid secretion and gastric endocrine cells. Regul. Pept. 120:23–32, 2004
4. Papotti M, Ghe C, Cassoni P, Catapano F, Deghenghi R, Ghigo E, Muccioli G: Growth hormone secretagogue binding sites in peripheral human tissues. J Clin Endocrinol Metab 85:3803–3807, 2000
5. Damjanovic SS, Lalic NM, Pesko PM, Petakov MS, Jotic A, Miljic D, Lalic KS, Lukic L, Djurovic M, Djukic VB: Acute Effects of Ghrelin on Insulin Secretion and Glucose Disposal Rate in Gastrectomized Patients. J Clin Endocrinol Metab 91:2574–2581, 2006
6. Vestergaard ET, Hansen TK, Gormsen LC, Jakobsen P, Moller N, Christiansen JS, Jorgensen JO: Constant intravenous ghrelin infusion in healthy young men: Clinical pharmacokinetics and metabolic effects. Am J Physiol Endocrinol Metab 292:E1829–E1836, 2007
7. Lucidi P, Murdolo G, Di Loreto C, Parlanti N, De Cicco A, Fatone C, Taglioni C, Fanelli C, Broglio F, Ghigo E, Bolli GB, Santeusanio F, De Feo P: Metabolic and endocrine effects of physiological increments in plasma ghrelin concentrations. Nutr. Metab Cardiovasc. Dis. 15:410–417, 2005
8. Vestergaard ET, Djurhuus CB, Gjedsted J, Nielsen S, Moller N, Holst JJ, Jorgensen JOL, Schmitz O: Acute Effects of Ghrelin Administration on Glucose and Lipid Metabolism. J Clin Endocrinol Metab 93:438–444, 2008
9. Steele R: Influences of glucose loading and of injected insulin on hepatic glucose output. Ann N Y Acad Sci 82:420–430, 1959
10. Ferrannini E: The theoretical bases of indirect calorimetry: a review. Metabolism 37:287–301, 1988
11. Gravholt CH, Schmitz O, Simonsen L, Bulow J, Christiansen JS, Moller N: Effects of a physiological GH pulse on interstitial glycerol in abdominal and femoral adipose tissue. Am J Physiol 277:E848–E854, 1999
12. Espelund U, Hansen TK, Hojlund K, Beck-Nielsen H, Clausen JT, Hansen BS, Orskov H, Jorgensen JO, Frystyk J: Fasting unmasks a strong inverse association between ghrelin and cortisol in serum: studies in obese and normal-weight subjects. J Clin Endocrinol Metab 90:741–746, 2005
13. Eriksson BM, Persson BA: Determination of catecholamines in rat heart tissue and plasma samples by liquid chromatography with electrochemical detection. J Chromatogr 228:143–154, 1982
14. Holst JJ: Molecular heterogeneity of glucagon in normal subjects and in patients with glucagon-producing tumours. Diabetologia 24:359–365, 1983
15. Wojtaszewski JF, Hansen BF, Urso B, Richter EA: Wortmannin inhibits both insulin- and contraction-stimulated glucose uptake and transport in rat skeletal muscle. J Appl. Physiol 81:1501–1509, 1996
16. Gauna C, Meyler FM, Janssen JA, Delhanty PJ, Abribat T, Van Koetsveld P, Hofland LJ, Broglio F, Ghigo E, Van der Lely AJ: Administration of acylated ghrelin reduces insulin sensitivity, whereas the combination of acylated plus unacylated ghrelin strongly improves insulin sensitivity. J Clin Endocrinol Metab 89:5035–5042, 2004
17. Kageyama H, Funahashi H, Hirayama M, Takenoya F, Kita T, Kato S, Sakurai J, Lee EY, Inoue S, Date Y, Nakazato M, Kangawa K, Shioda S: Morphological analysis of ghrelin and its receptor distribution in the rat pancreas. Regul. Pept. 126:67–71, 2005
18. Dezaki K, Sone H, Koizumi M, Nakata M, Kakei M, Nagai H, Hosoda H, Kangawa K, Yada T: Blockade of pancreatic islet-derived ghrelin enhances insulin secretion to prevent high-fat diet-induced glucose intolerance. Diabetes 55:3486–3493, 2006
19. Sun Y, Asnicar M, Saha PK, Chan L, Smith RG: Ablation of ghrelin improves the diabetic but not obese phenotype of ob/ob mice. Cell Metab 3:379–386, 2006
20. Pfluger PT, Kirchner H, Gunnel S, Schrott B, Perez-Tilve D, Fu S, Benoit SC, Horvath T, Joost HG, Wortley KE, Sleeman MW, Tschop MH: Simultaneous deletion of ghrelin and its receptor increases motor activity and energy expenditure. Am J Physiol Gastrointest. Liver Physiol 2007
21. DeFronzo RA, Jacot E, Jequier E, Maeder E, Wahren J, Felber JP: The effect of insulin on the disposal of intravenous glucose. Results from indirect calorimetry and hepatic and femoral venous catheterization. Diabetes 30:1000–1007, 1981
22. Andersson U, Filipsson K, Abbott CR, Woods A, Smith K, Bloom SR, Carling D, Small CJ: AMP-activated protein kinase plays a role in the control of food intake. J Biol. Chem. 279:12005–12008, 2004
23. Barazzoni R, Bosutti A, Stebel M, Cattin MR, Roder E, Visintin L, Cattin L, Biolo G, Zanetti M, Guarnieri G: Ghrelin regulates mitochondrial-lipid metabolism gene expression and tissue fat distribution in liver and skeletal muscle. Am J Physiol Endocrinol Metab 288:E228–E235, 2005
24. Kola B, Hubina E, Tucci SA, Kirkham TC, Garcia EA, Mitchell SE, Williams LM, Hawley SA, Hardie DG, Grossman AB, Korbonits M: Cannabinoids and ghrelin have both central and peripheral metabolic and cardiac effects via AMP-activated protein kinase. J Biol. Chem. 2005
25. Hardie DG, Carling D, Carlson M: The AMP-activated/SNF1 protein kinase subfamily: metabolic sensors of the eukaryotic cell? Annu Rev Biochem 67:821–855, 1998

Effects of a Protein Preload on Gastric Emptying, Glycemia, and Gut Hormones After a Carbohydrate Meal in Diet-Controlled Type 2 Diabetes

Jing Ma, mbbs[1,2]
Julie E. Stevens, bpharm, bsc[1,2]
Kimberly Cukier, mbbs[3]
Anne F. Maddox, ass dip rad tech[1,2]
Judith M. Wishart, bsc[1,2]

Karen L. Jones, phd[1,2]
Peter M. Clifton, mbbs, phd[3,4]
Michael Horowitz, mbbs, phd[1,2,3]
Christopher K. Rayner, mbbs, phd[1,2]

OBJECTIVE — We evaluated whether a whey preload could slow gastric emptying, stimulate incretin hormones, and attenuate postprandial glycemia in type 2 diabetes.

RESEARCH DESIGN AND METHODS — Eight type 2 diabetic patients ingested 350 ml beef soup 30 min before a potato meal; 55 g whey was added to either the soup (whey preload) or potato (whey in meal) or no whey was given.

RESULTS — Gastric emptying was slowest after the whey preload ($P < 0.0005$). The incremental area under the blood glucose curve was less after the whey preload and whey in meal than after no whey ($P < 0.005$). Plasma glucose-dependent insulinotropic polypeptide, insulin, and cholecystokinin concentrations were higher on both whey days than after no whey, whereas glucagon-like peptide 1 was greatest after the whey preload ($P < 0.05$).

CONCLUSIONS — Whey protein consumed before a carbohydrate meal can stimulate insulin and incretin hormone secretion and slow gastric emptying, leading to marked reduction in postprandial glycemia in type 2 diabetes.

Diabetes Care 32:1600–1602, 2009

The rate of gastric emptying and the incretin, glucagon-like peptide 1 (GLP-1) and glucose-dependent insulinotropic polypeptide (GIP), response to a meal are known to be major determinants of postprandial blood glucose excursions (1,2). One strategy to minimize postprandial glycemia could be to administer a small load of protein or fat before a meal, so that the presence of nutrients in the small intestine induces the release of peptides such as GLP-1, GIP, and cholecystokinin (CCK) to slow gastric emptying and stimulate insulin secretion in advance of the main nutrient load (3,4).

We hypothesized that a protein preload would reduce the postprandial glycemic excursion in type 2 diabetic patients by these mechanisms.

RESEARCH DESIGN AND METHODS — The protocol included eight diet-controlled type 2 diabetic patients (seven male, mean ± SE age 58 ± 3 years, BMI 28.6 ± 1.3 kg/m², duration of known diabetes 5.4 ± 1.1 years, and A1C 6.5 ± 0.2%) who attended the laboratory after an overnight fast (14 h for solids and 12 h for liquids) on three separate occasions. Each patient consumed beef-flavored soup (3.8 g noncaloric beef flavoring dissolved in 350 ml water) 30 min before a mashed potato meal containing 65 g powdered potato (Deb Instant Mashed Potato, Epping, Australia) with 20 g glucose (total: 59.1 g carbohydrate, 4.3 g fat, 5.2 g protein; 1,276.5 kJ), labeled with 20 MBq 99mTc-sulfur colloid (4). On one day, 55 g whey protein (876.7 kJ) was added to the soup. On another day, 55 g whey was mixed into the potato meal. On a third day, neither the preload nor the meal contained whey. Blood was sampled frequently for blood glucose and plasma hormone measurements.

Measurements
Gastric emptying was assessed by scintigraphy. Data were corrected for radionuclide decay, subject movement, and γ-ray attenuation, and the gastric half-emptying time (T50) was calculated (4).

Blood glucose concentrations were measured using a glucometer (Medisense Precision QID; Abbott Laboratories, Bedford, MA), which we have validated against the hexokinase technique (5). Plasma insulin was measured by enzyme-linked immunosorbent assay (ELISA; Diagnostic Systems Laboratories, Webster, TX). Total GLP-1 (GLPIT-36HK; Linco Research, St. Charles, MO), total GIP, and CCK-8 were measured by radioimmunoassay (6).

Cardiovascular autonomic function was assessed by the variation in R-R interval during deep breathing and the systolic blood pressure changes in response to standing (7).

Data were evaluated using repeated-measures ANOVA with treatment and time as factors (StatView 5.0; Abacus Concepts, Berkeley, CA). Data are shown as means ± SE; $P < 0.05$ was considered significant.

RESULTS — Two of the eight subjects had definite autonomic dysfunction. The study was well tolerated.

From the [1]Discipline of Medicine, University of Adelaide, Royal Adelaide Hospital, Adelaide, Australia; the [2]Centre of Clinical Research Excellence in Nutritional Physiology, Interventions and Outcomes, University of Adelaide, Adelaide, Australia; the [3]Endocrine & Metabolic Unit, Royal Adelaide Hospital, Adelaide, Australia; and the [4]Human Nutrition, Commonwealth Scientific and Industrial Research Organization, Adelaide, Australia.

Corresponding author: Christopher K. Rayner, chris.rayner@adelaide.edu.au.

Received 15 April 2009 and accepted 4 June 2009.

Published ahead of print at http://care.diabetesjournals.org on 18 June 2009. DOI: 10.2337/dc09-0723.

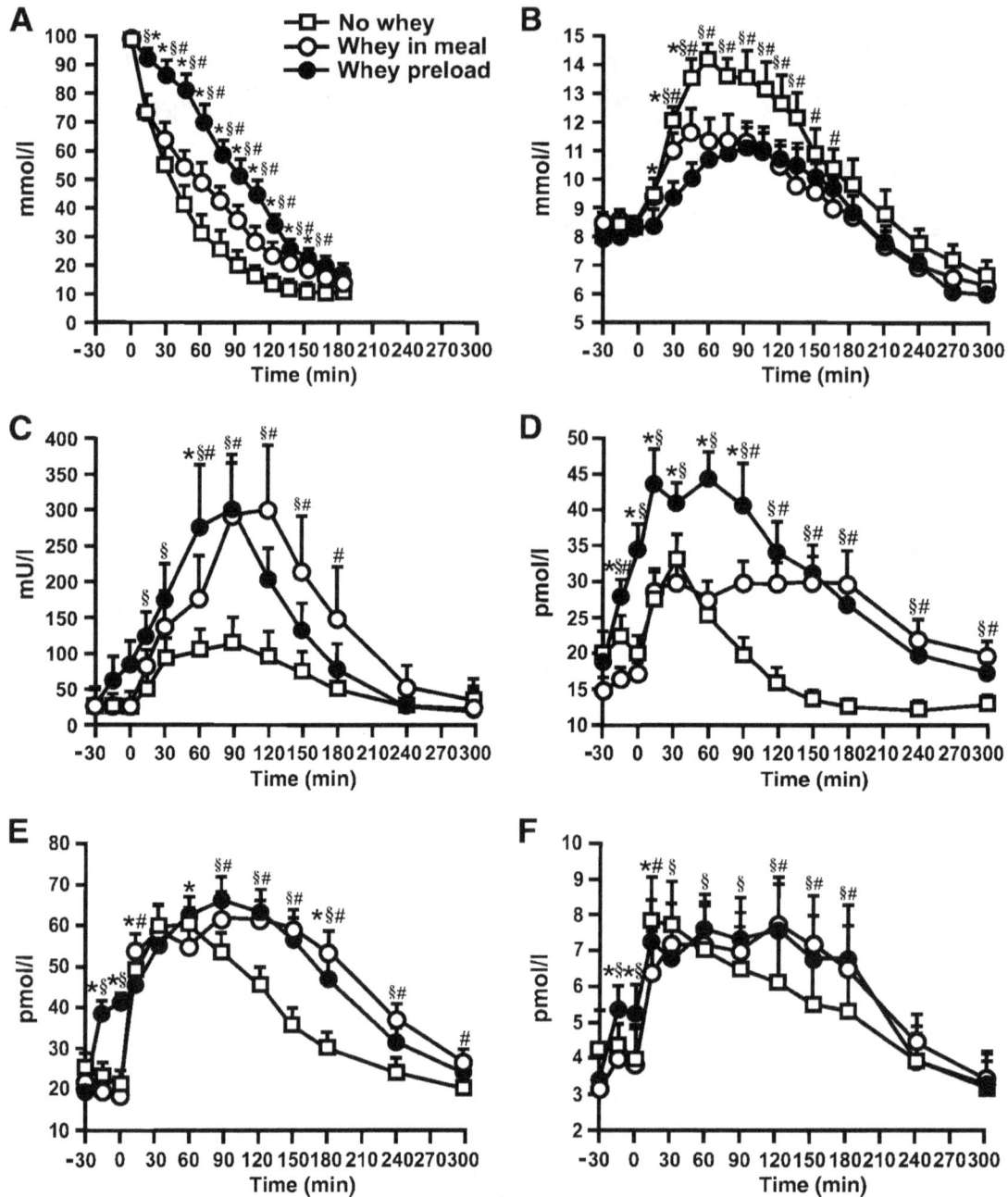

Figure 1—*Gastric emptying (A), concentrations of blood glucose (B), plasma insulin (C), plasma GLP-1 (D), plasma GIP (E), and plasma CCK (F) in response to a mashed potato meal in eight type 2 diabetic patients. On each study day, subjects ingested 350 ml beef-flavored soup 30 min before a radiolabeled mashed potato meal; 55 g whey protein was added either to the soup (whey preload) or to the potato (whey in meal) or no whey was given (no whey). Data are means ± SE. *P < 0.05, whey preload vs. whey in meal; #P < 0.05, whey in meal vs. no whey; §P < 0.05, whey preload vs. no whey.*

On the no whey and whey in meal days, emptying was rapid initially and subsequently slower, whereas emptying after the whey preload approximated a linear pattern. Gastric emptying was slowest on the whey preload day (T50: 87.3 ± 5.4 min; $P = 0.0001$) and was slower with whey in the meal (53.0 ± 8.3 min; $P < 0.01$) than with no whey (39.0 ± 6.2 min).

There were no differences in baseline blood glucose, plasma insulin, GLP-1, GIP, or CCK concentrations (Fig. 1). The incremental area under the curve (iAUC) for blood glucose was less after the whey preload (363.7 ± 64.5 mmol · min^{-1} · l^{-1}) and whey in meal (406.3 ± 85.9 mmol · min^{-1} · l^{-1}) compared with no whey (734.9 ± 98.9 mmol · min^{-1} · l^{-1}; $P < 0.005$ for both). The iAUCs for insulin, GLP-1, GIP, and CCK were greater when whey was given as a preload ($P < 0.05$ for all) or in the meal ($P < 0.005$ for all) compared with no whey. Despite an earlier response, the iAUC for insulin did not differ between whey preload and whey in meal ($P = 0.50$). GLP-1 was greater between -15 min and 90 min with the whey preload compared with whey in meal ($P = 0.0001$), but the overall iAUC did not differ significantly.

CONCLUSIONS— We demonstrated that whey protein, when given before or with a high-carbohydrate meal, resulted in a substantial reduction in postprandial glycemia in diet-controlled type 2 diabetic patients. Given that the magnitude of the reduction was comparable with what would be hoped for using pharmacological therapy, such as sulfonylureas, these data have considerable implications for nutritional strategies in the management of diabetes.

The pivotal role of the gastrointestinal tract in determining postprandial glycemia has often been overlooked, but it is assuming increasing prominence, partly because of the development of gut peptide–based therapies for diabetes, such as the GLP-1 analog exenatide (8) and the amylin analog pramlintide (9), which may act predominantly by slowing gastric emptying. Similar to what we reported after an oil preload (4), whey slowed gastric emptying substantially, in particular when given before the meal, and is associated with the stimulation of GLP-1 and CCK. However, in contrast to the delayed insulin response observed after oil, whey augmented insulin secretion markedly, possibly by a combination of the incretin effect and the direct stimulation of the β-cells by absorbed amino acids (10). It is likely that the stimulation of insulin by whey was responsible for the much greater reduction in glycemia after whey than after oil, given that the effects on gastric emptying were comparable.

Although our study involved a small number of subjects who had well-controlled, predominantly uncomplicated type 2 diabetes, the improvement in postprandial glycemia was marked and highly consistent. Further evaluation is

now required in poorly controlled patients and those taking oral hypoglycemic agents in order to determine whether the acute effects are sustained in the longer term. It would also be important to confirm whether the effects are evident with a smaller load of protein in order to minimize additional energy intake. Although concerns have been raised about hyperinsulinemia as a risk factor for vascular disease (11), it is more likely that it represents a marker for other risk factors (12), and in the UK Prospective Diabetes Study (UKPDS), stimulation of insulin by sulfonylureas was not associated with increased cardiovascular events (13).

The concept of using dietary manipulations to treat type 2 diabetes, based on our knowledge of the contribution of gastric emptying and gut peptides to postprandial glycemic responses, appears to hold much promise.

Acknowledgments— This work was supported by the National Health and Medical Research Council (NHMRC) of Australia. The salary of K.L.J. is also funded by the NHMRC.

No potential conflicts of interest relevant to this article were reported.

Parts of this study were presented in abstract form at Digestive Diseases Week, San Diego, California, 17–22 May 2008. Complete data have been submitted for presentation at the annual meeting of the European Association for the Study of Diabetes, Vienna, Austria, 29 September–2 October 2009

We thank Murray Goulburn for supply of the whey protein isolate and Jane Bowen for advice about formulating the preloads.

References
1. Chaikomin R, Rayner CK, Jones KL, Horowitz M. Upper gastrointestinal function and glycemic control in diabetes mellitus. World J Gastroenterol 2006;12: 5611–5621
2. Rayner CK, Samsom M, Jones KL, Horowitz M. Relationships of upper gastrointestinal motor and sensory function with glycemic control. Diabetes Care 2001;24: 371–381
3. Bowen J, Noakes M, Trenerry C, Clifton PM. Energy intake, ghrelin, and cholecys-
tokinin after different carbohydrate and protein preloads in overweight men. J Clin Endocrinol Metab 2006;91:1477–1483
4. Gentilcore D, Chaikomin R, Jones KL, Russo A, Feinle-Bisset C, Wishart JM, Rayner CK, Horowitz M. Effects of fat on gastric emptying of and the glycemic, insulin, and incretin responses to a carbohydrate meal in type 2 diabetes. J Clin Endocrinol Metab 2006;91:2062–2067
5. Horowitz M, Edelbroek MA, Wishart JM, Straathof JW. Relationship between oral glucose tolerance and gastric emptying in normal healthy subjects. Diabetologia 1993;36:857–862
6. Santangelo A, Peracchi M, Conte D, Fraquelli M, Porrini M. Physical state of meal affects gastric emptying, cholecystokinin release and satiety. Br J Nutr 1998; 80:521–527
7. Ewing DJ, Clarke BF. Diagnosis and management of diabetic autonomic neuropathy. Br Med J (Clin Res Ed) 1982;285: 916–918
8. Linnebjerg H, Park S, Kothare PA, Trautmann ME, Mace K, Fineman M, Wilding I, Nauck M, Horowitz M. Effect of exenatide on gastric emptying and relationship to postprandial glycemia in type 2 diabetes. Regul Pept 2008;151:123–129
9. Kong MF, King P, Macdonald IA, Stubbs TA, Perkins AC, Blackshaw PE, Moyses C, Tattersall RB. Infusion of pramlintide, a human amylin analogue, delays gastric emptying in men with IDDM. Diabetologia 1997;40:82–88
10. Fieseler P, Bridenbaugh S, Nustede R, Martell J, Orskov C, Holst JJ, Nauck MA. Physiological augmentation of amino acid-induced insulin secretion by GIP and GLP-I but not by CCK-8. Am J Physiol 1995;268:E949–E955
11. Reaven GM. Insulin resistance and compensatory hyperinsulinemia: role in hypertension, dyslipidemia, and coronary heart disease. Am Heart J 1991;121:1283–1288
12. Wingard DL, Barrett-Connor EL, Ferrara A. Is insulin really a heart disease risk factor? Diabetes Care 1995;18:1299–1304
13. UK Prospective Diabetes Study (UKPDS) Group. Intensive blood-glucose control with sulphonylureas or insulin compared with conventional treatment and risk of complications in patients with type 2 diabetes (UKPDS 33). Lancet 1998;352:837–853

Vasoactive Intestinal Peptide–Null Mice Demonstrate Enhanced Sweet Taste Preference, Dysglycemia, and Reduced Taste Bud Leptin Receptor Expression

Bronwen Martin,[1] Yu-Kyong Shin,[1] Caitlin M. White,[1] Sunggoan Ji,[1] Wook Kim,[1] Olga D. Carlson,[1] Joshua K. Napora,[1] Wayne Chadwick,[1] Megan Chapter,[1] James A. Waschek,[2] Mark P. Mattson,[1] Stuart Maudsley,[1] and Josephine M. Egan[1]

OBJECTIVE—It is becoming apparent that there is a strong link between taste perception and energy homeostasis. Recent evidence implicates gut-related hormones in taste perception, including glucagon-like peptide 1 and vasoactive intestinal peptide (VIP). We used VIP knockout mice to investigate VIP's specific role in taste perception and connection to energy regulation.

RESEARCH DESIGN AND METHODS—Body weight, food intake, and plasma levels of multiple energy-regulating hormones were measured and pancreatic morphology was determined. In addition, the immunocytochemical profile of taste cells and gustatory behavior were examined in wild-type and VIP knockout mice.

RESULTS—VIP knockout mice demonstrate elevated plasma glucose, insulin, and leptin levels, with no islet β-cell number/topography alteration. VIP and its receptors (VPAC1, VPAC2) were identified in type II taste cells of the taste bud, and VIP knockout mice exhibit enhanced taste preference to sweet tastants. VIP knockout mouse taste cells show a significant decrease in leptin receptor expression and elevated expression of glucagon-like peptide 1, which may explain sweet taste preference of VIP knockout mice.

CONCLUSIONS—This study suggests that the tongue can play a direct role in modulating energy intake to correct peripheral glycemic imbalances. In this way, we could view the tongue as a sensory mechanism that is bidirectionally regulated and thus forms a bridge between available foodstuffs and the intricate hormonal balance in the animal itself. *Diabetes* 59:1143–1152, 2010

Taste perception and its relationship to glucose homeostasis begins with stimulation of taste cells located in tongue taste buds. There are five basic taste modalities: bitter, sweet, umami, salty, and sour. Taste cells are clustered into taste buds in the tongue epithelium (1). Mammals have four different types of taste cells (types I, II, III, and IV), exhibiting different molecular phenotypes and functional roles (2–4). Type I cells are glial-like cells that maintain taste bud structure. Type II taste cells transduce sweet, bitter, or umami stimuli (5) and communicate information through G-protein–coupled transduction cascades (6,7). Type III cells synapse directly with afferent nerve fibers from three cranial nerves (8), and most release serotonin upon depolarization (9). Type IV "basal cells" are rapidly dividing progenitor cells that differentiate into type I, II, and III cells (10). Along with biogenic amine neurotransmitters, it is becoming evident that multiple peptide hormones including glucagon-like peptide-1 (GLP-1; [11]), cholecystokinin (12), and neuropeptide Y (13) as well as VIP (14) are located in taste cells, potentially acting as signaling modulators of multiple gustatory stimuli (15).

VIP is a 28–amino acid peptide expressed at multiple sites throughout the body. It was discovered by its potent muscle relaxant vasodilatory activity and as a stimulator of secretory activity (16). VIP exerts its effects through activation of two G-protein–coupled receptors (GPCRs): VPAC1 and VPAC2 (17). These receptors preferentially stimulate adenylate cyclase and increase intracellular cAMP. VIP activity at VPAC1/2 receptors in pancreatic islets is involved in insulin secretion (18). VIP expression has been identified in the taste cells of rat, hamster, carp, and human (12,14,19). In taste cells, VIP colocalizes with the taste transduction markers α-gustducin and T1R2 (20); any role, however, of VIP in gustation has not previously been established. Gustation is vital for locating food sources and determining which foodstuffs to ingest. Gustation is also involved in maintaining body weight and energy balance, that is, there is a strong link between peripheral somatic energy balance and "flavor perception." This link may be mediated by the coherent use of a cadre of neuropeptide hormones present in both the tongue and the periphery. We have previously shown that the gut incretin, GLP-1, in taste cells profoundly controls sweet and umami taste (11,21). Peripheral leptin (food intake regulator produced primarily in adipose tissue [22–24]), via activation of the leptin receptor (Ob-Rb) on taste cells, can inhibit responses to sweet tastants (25). Interestingly, such selective sweet taste inhibition by peripheral leptin is not present in leptin receptor–deficient *db/db* mice (26–28), suggesting that leptin, together with GLP-1, acts as a dual-functional sweet-sensation modulator involved in the regulation of food intake and somatic energy regulation.

In this study, we set out to uncover the role of VIP in gustation. We demonstrate, using VIP knockout mice, that VIP plays a specific role in modifying distinct taste modalities

From the [1]National Institutes of Health, National Institute on Aging, Baltimore, Maryland; and the [2]Department of Psychiatry and Behavioral Sciences, Mental Retardation Research Center, Semel Institute for Neuroscience and Human Behavior, University of California, Los Angeles, Los Angeles, California.

Corresponding author: Josephine Egan, eganj@mail.nih.gov.

Received 10 June 2009 and accepted 28 January 2010. Published ahead of print at http://diabetes.diabetesjournals.org on 11 February 2010. DOI: 10.2337/db09-0807.

B.M. and Y.-K.S. contributed equally to this study.

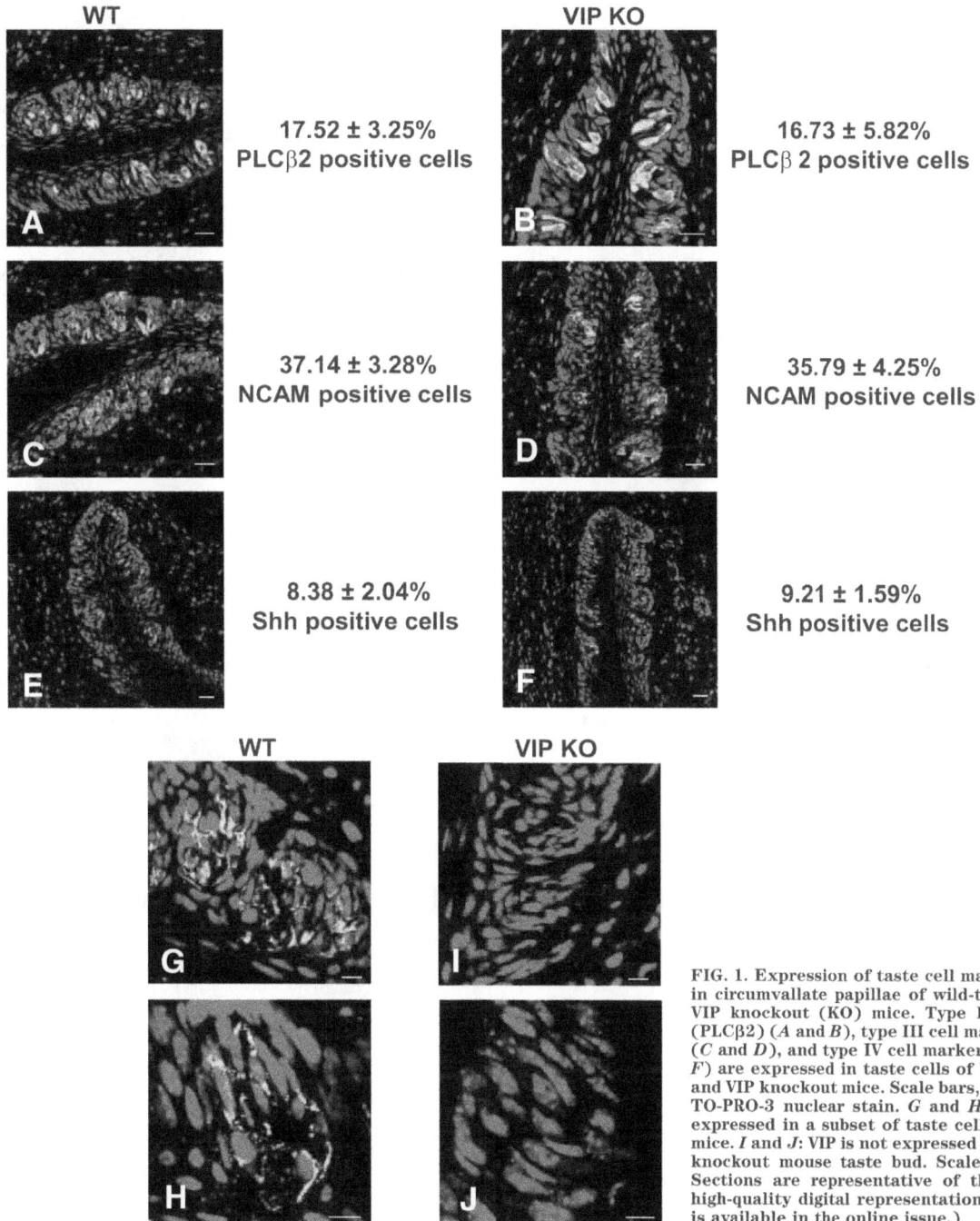

WT

17.52 ± 3.25%
PLCβ2 positive cells

VIP KO

16.73 ± 5.82%
PLCβ 2 positive cells

37.14 ± 3.28%
NCAM positive cells

35.79 ± 4.25%
NCAM positive cells

8.38 ± 2.04%
Shh positive cells

9.21 ± 1.59%
Shh positive cells

WT   VIP KO

FIG. 1. Expression of taste cell markers and VIP in circumvallate papillae of wild-type (WT) and VIP knockout (KO) mice. Type II cell marker (PLCβ2) (*A* and *B*), type III cell marker (NCAM) (*C* and *D*), and type IV cell marker (Shh) (*E* and *F*) are expressed in taste cells of both wild-type and VIP knockout mice. Scale bars, 20 μm. Blue is TO-PRO-3 nuclear stain. *G* and *H*: VIP (red) is expressed in a subset of taste cells of wild-type mice. *I* and *J*: VIP is not expressed within the VIP knockout mouse taste bud. Scale bars, 20 μm. Sections are representative of three mice. (A high-quality digital representation of this figure is available in the online issue.)

and that VIP knockout mice have significantly altered expression levels of other hormones and receptors that are involved in the control of taste modulation and energy balance.

RESEARCH DESIGN AND METHODS

Animal and tissue processing. Animal testing procedures were approved by the Animal Care and Use Committee of the National Institute on Aging. Methods are described in detail in the supplementary material, available in an online appendix at http://diabetes.diabetesjournals.org/cgi/content/full/db09-0807/DC1.

Immunohistochemistry. Methods are described in detail in the supplementary material. Serial sections (10-μm thickness) were cut from tissues containing circumvallate, foliate, and fungiform papillae, using a cryostat (Microm; Thermo Scientific). To obtain systematic samples without bias throughout the papillae, each papilla was sectioned and every tenth section was saved onto a slide. Taste buds are ~80–100 μm in length, therefore

sampling every tenth section ensures that no two sections will be from the same taste bud. Images were collected using a confocal microscope LSM-710 (Carl Zeiss). Approximately 100–120 taste buds per group were analyzed immunohistochemically as described previously (11,29). Only nuclear profile–positive cells were scored as immunoreactive. The total number of cells in the section was determined by counting the number of TO-PRO-3–stained nuclei present in each taste bud. The percentage of immunoreactive taste cells was calculated by: number of immunoreactive taste cells/total number of taste cells in each taste bud.

Immunoassay analyses of gut and appetite hormones in plasma. Plasma levels of gut and appetite hormones were measured using a mouse multiplex assay kit (Millipore) according to the manufacturer's instructions. Methods are described in detail in the supplementary material.

Pancreatic islet size quantification and Western blot analyses. Methods are described in detail in the supplementary material. Quantification of pancreatic immunohistochemistry images was performed in Matlab (Mathworks) as described previously (30). Hypothalamic protein levels of various factors involved in energy regulation were determined by Western blot analyses.

Taste behavioral tests. Taste behavioral testing was performed as previously described (11). VIP knockout and wild-type ($n = 8$) mice were habituated to the laboratory environment for 30 min each day prior to testing. The same animals were used for both the taste behavioral tests and analyses of physiological parameters (pancreatic function, gut/appetite plasma hormone analyses). Test stimuli consisted of various concentrations of sucrose (25, 75, 150, 300, and 600 mmol/l; Fisher Scientific), sodium chloride (NaCl: 100, 200, 400, 600, 800, and 1,000 mmol/l; Sigma), denatonium benzoate (0.001, 0.01, 0.1, 0.3, 1, 5, and 10 mmol/l; Sigma), and citric acid (0.01, 0.1, 1, 3, 5, 10, 30, and 100 mmol/l; Fisher Scientific). Brief-access taste testing took place in a Davis MS-160 gustometer (DiLog Instruments) as previously described (11,31–34). Brief-access procedures minimize postingestive effects that may confound other assays such as intake tests (33). To test salty, sour, and bitter stimuli responses, mice were water deprived prior to testing. For testing of the sweet stimulus, mice were both food and water restricted (2.5 ml of water, 1 g of food) prior to testing. All mice were tested with a single tastant at various concentrations per trial, to prevent the mice from being affected by prior experience. Data analysis is described in detail in the supplementary material.

RESULTS

VIP knockout mice possess normal taste bud morphology. Gross taste bud morphology and taste cell number were assessed in wild-type and VIP knockout mice using classical taste cell type–specific immunocytochemical markers (supplementary Tables 1 and 2). Compared with wild-type mice, VIP knockout mice showed no gross taste bud abnormalities and expressed similar distribution patterns of taste cell–specific markers (Fig. 1A–F, supplementary Table 2). VIP immunoreactivity was present in the taste cells of wild-type animals (Fig. 1G and H) but absent in the VIP knockout mice (Fig. 1I and J). The lack of VIP, therefore, did not significantly affect initial taste cell development and number.

VPAC1/2 receptors are expressed in taste cells. Both VPAC1/2 receptors were primarily expressed in phospholipase Cβ2 (PLCβ2)-positive taste cells (type II cells: Fig. 2; supplementary Figs. 2 and 3). The presence of VIP and its cognate receptors in type II taste cells suggests that VIP signaling is local to the taste bud and could likely affect tongue-localized gustation.

Reduced leptin receptor and increased GLP-1 expression in VIP knockout mice taste cells. VIP is coexpressed with the taste transduction marker α-gustducin and with the T1R2 GPCR (20). The majority of VIP-immunoreactive taste cells also coexpresses α-gustducin, although a subset also expresses T1R2. α-Gustducin and T1R2 are markers for type II cells, and based on this specific expression pattern, we hypothesized that VIP could be involved in the transduction of sweet and bitter stimuli. To investigate this, we first determined the expression patterns in the wild-type and VIP knockout mice of additional hormones and receptors known to play a functional role in sweet taste coding, that is, the T1R3 sweet stimulant receptor, GLP-1, and leptin receptor (Ob-Rb) (Fig. 3A–F). Both wild-type and VIP knockout mice showed similar expression patterns of T1R3 in the circumvallate papillae (Fig. 3A, B, and G). Interestingly, we found that GLP-1 expression was significantly increased in the taste cells of VIP knockout mice compared with wild type (Fig. 3C, D, and G, $P < 0.001$). Leptin receptor expression was markedly reduced in VIP knockout mice compared with wild type (Fig. 3E–G, $P < 0.001$). Peripheral leptin has been shown to suppress sweet taste preference through its action on the leptin receptors in the taste cells (26–28). Elevation in GLP-1 expression and the

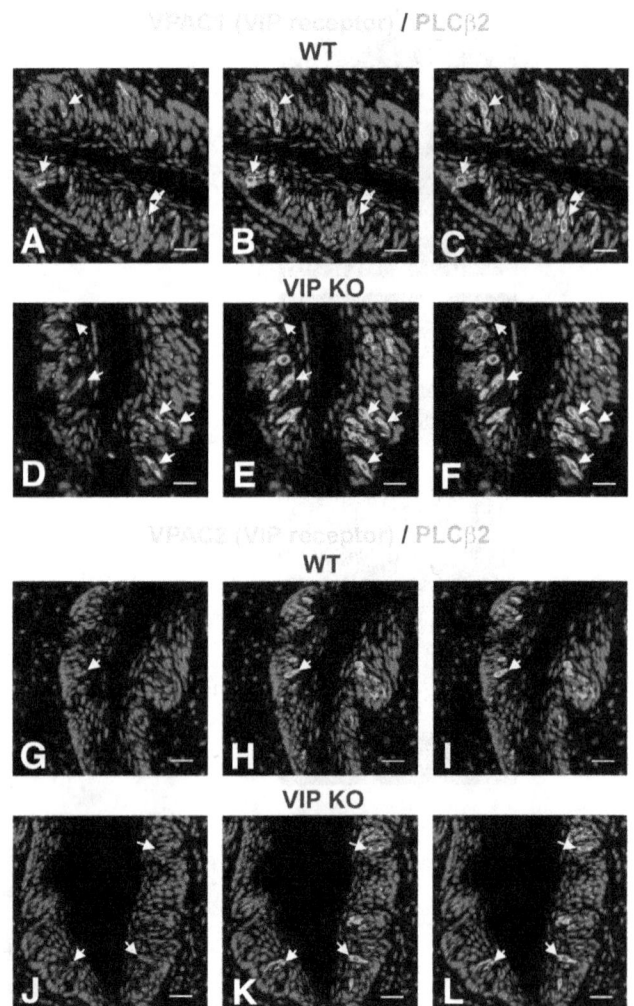

FIG. 2. Coexpression of VIP receptors (VPAC1/VPAC2) and PLCβ2 in circumvallate papillae of wild-type (WT) and VIP knockout (KO) mice. A–C: VPAC1 (red) and PLCβ2 (green) are colocalized in a subset of PLCβ2-positive cells (yellow cells) in wild-type mice. The arrows denote cells expressing both. D–F: VPAC1 (red) and PLCβ2 (green) are colocalized in a subset of PLCβ2-positive cells (yellow cells) in VIP knockout mice. G–I: VPAC2 (red) and PLCβ2 (green) are colocalized in a subset of PLCβ2-positive cells (yellow cells) in wild-type mice. The arrows denote cells expressing both. J–L: VPAC2 (red) and PLCβ2 (green) are colocalized in a subset of PLCβ2-positive cells (yellow cells) in VIP knockout mice. The arrows denote cells expressing both. Scale bars, 20 μm. Blue is TO-PRO-3 nuclear stain. (A high-quality digital representation of this figure is available in the online issue.)

reduction in leptin receptor expression strongly indicates that VIP could play a role in modulating sweet taste. Taken together, it is apparent that there are significant differences in the numbers of GLP-1– and Ob-Rb–immunopositive cells between wild-type and VIP knockout mice (Fig. 3G, supplementary Table 2). To enhance our understanding of these alterations in the taste cells of VIP knockout mice, we next determined whether other systemic alterations in appetite/energy-regulatory hormones occur in VIP knockout mice.

Elevation of plasma leptin and glucose in VIP knockout mice. As we detected reduced leptin receptor expression in VIP knockout mouse taste cells compared with wild type, we measured plasma leptin levels in these mice. Circulating leptin can bind to and activate the leptin receptor on taste cells, where it acts to specifically inhibit

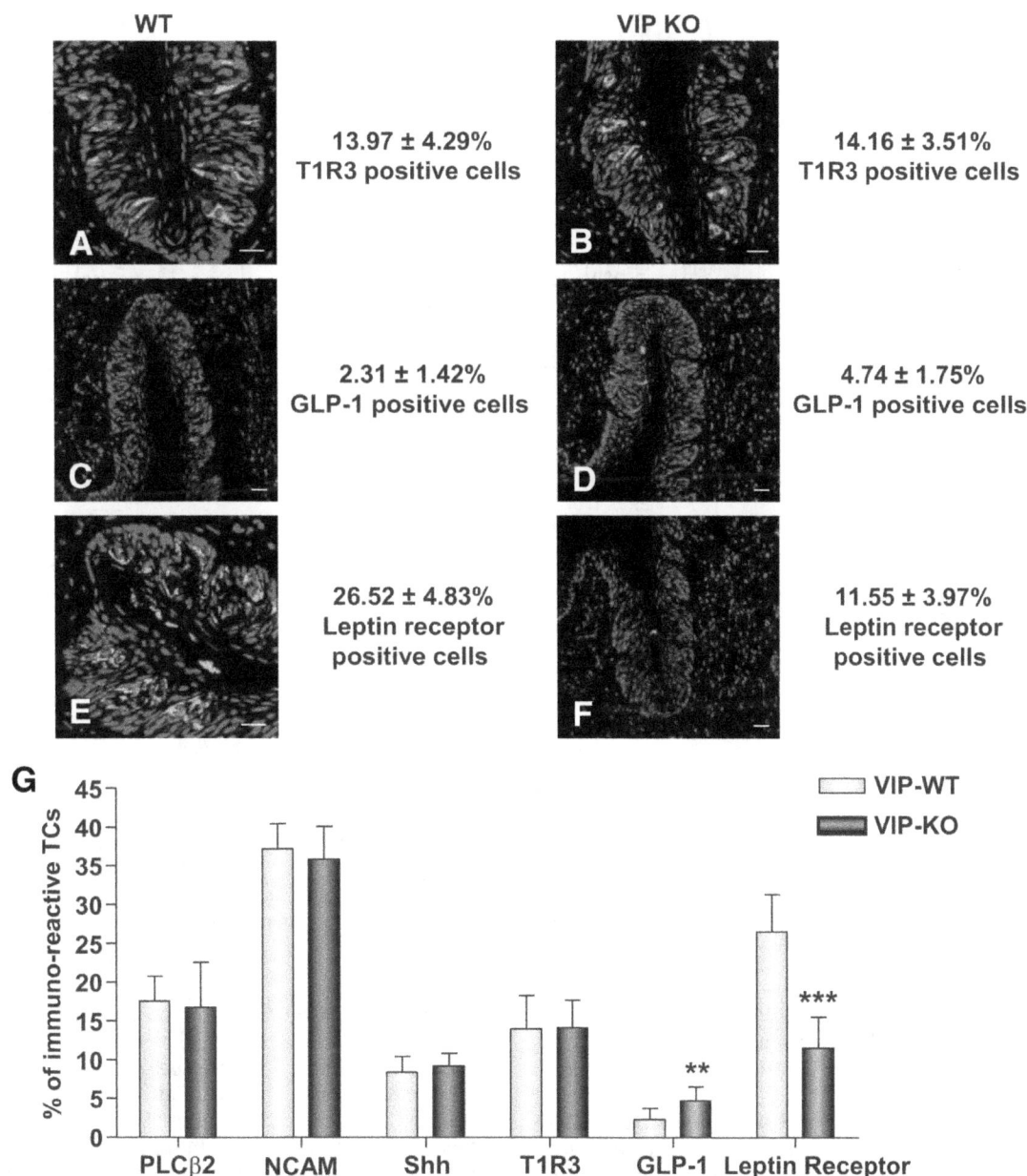

FIG. 3. Expression of taste-related proteins in circumvallate papillae of wild-type (WT) and VIP knockout (KO) mice. *A* and *B*: Sweet taste receptor (T1R3, green) is expressed in both wild-type and VIP knockout mice. *C* and *D*: GLP-1 (green) is expressed in wild-type and VIP knockout mice. *E* and *F*: Leptin receptor (green) is expressed in wild-type and VIP knockout mice. Scale bars, 20 μm. Blue is TO-PRO-3 nuclear stain. *G*: The percentage of immunopositive cells quantified in both wild-type and VIP knockout mice for the following markers: PLCβ2, NCAM, Shh, T1R3, GLP-1, and leptin receptor. Cells were scored as immunoreactive only if a nuclear profile was present within the cell. Values are the means ± SEM. **$P < 0.01$, ***$P < 0.001$. TCs, taste cells. (A high-quality digital representation of this figure is available in the online issue.)

gustatory responses to sweet substances, without affecting responses to sour, salty, and bitter substances in lean mice (26–28). In VIP knockout mice, both nonfasting and fasting glucose levels were elevated compared with wild type (Fig. 4*A* and *B*). In addition, we noted a significant elevation in fasting insulin in VIP knockout mice compared with wild type (Fig. 4*C*). We also found that plasma leptin levels were significantly elevated in VIP knockout mice compared with wild type (Fig. 4*D*). These data suggest that VIP knockout mice possess a diabetic-like pathology. Plasma levels of amylin (Fig. 4*E*) were not different between wild-type and VIP knockout mice, whereas VIP knockout mice possessed considerably

higher plasma gastrointestinal polypeptide (Fig. 4*F*), GLP-1 (Fig. 4*G*), and peptide tyrosine tyrosine (PYY) levels (Fig. 4*H*). Plasma pancreatic polypeptide (PP) levels between wild-type and VIP knockout mice were not significantly different despite a trend for lower PP levels in the VIP knockout mice (Fig. 4*I*).

VIP knockout mice have normal pancreatic islet cell morphology. As VIP knockout mice possessed significantly elevated plasma insulin levels compared with wild-type mice ($P < 0.01$), we next investigated pancreatic islet size and distribution of β-cells and α-cells. VIP knockout mice showed similar total β-cell area compared with wild-type (Fig. 5*A–C*). No signifi-

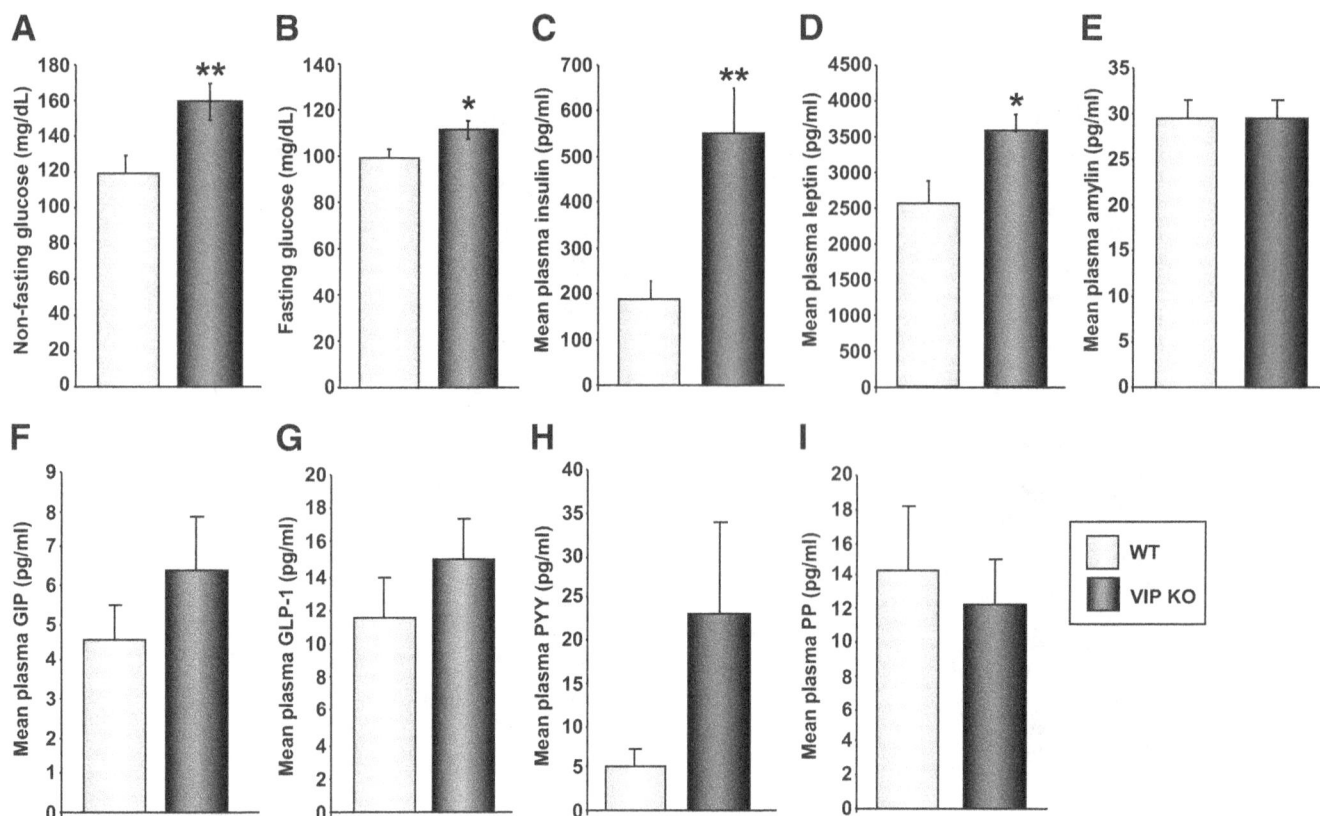

FIG. 4. VIP knockout (KO) mice possess alterations in multiple hormones controlling appetite and energy balance. Multiplex hormone analysis from plasma samples of wild-type (WT) and VIP knockout mice reveal multiple distinctions between the two animal groups. A and B: Significantly higher nonfasting and fasting glucose occurs in the VIP knockout mice. The VIP knockout mice also possessed significantly higher plasma insulin (C) and leptin (D) levels. No significant differences between wild-type and VIP knockout for amylin were noted (E). VIP knockout mice demonstrated higher levels of plasma gastrointestinal polypeptide (F), GLP-1 (G), and peptide tyrosine tyrosine (PYY) (H). No significant difference in the plasma levels of PP were noted between wild-type and VIP knockout mice (I). Each panel depicts means ± SEM from eight animals in each group. *$P < 0.05$, **$P < 0.01$.

cant difference in the total percentage of α- or β-cells in the islets (Fig. 5D) and the number of small-, middle-, and large-sized islets between wild-type and VIP knockout mice was observed (Fig. 5E).

VIP in taste cells regulates multiple taste modalities. As a considerable amount of our molecular/immunocytochemical data suggested a role for VIP in taste modulation, we next investigated VIP's role in taste perception. We tested the ability of wild-type and VIP knockout mice to detect prototypical taste stimuli, that is, sweet (sucrose), sour (citric acid), salty (sodium chloride), and bitter (denatonium benzoate). VIP knockout mice displayed significantly altered concentration-dependent licking for sucrose ($P = 0.0108$ between mean half-maximal effective concentration [EC_{50}] values) and denatonium benzoate ($P = 0.0003$ between mean EC_{50} values) compared with wild-type mice, demonstrated by their lower EC_{50} values compared with wild type (Fig. 6A and C, supplementary Fig. 1). VIP knockout mice also showed concentration-dependent changes in licking for citric acid ($P = 0.023$ between mean EC_{50} values) (Fig. 6B), but there was no significant alteration for sodium chloride in the VIP knockout mice compared with wild-type mice (Fig. 6D). Taken together, these results indicate that VIP plays a specific functional role in modulating taste perception of sweet, bitter, and sour stimuli.

VIP knockout mice attempt to ameliorate their dysglycemia. Our data indicate that there is an alteration in the biochemical, but not structural, nature of the tongue of VIP knockout mice, as well as complex alterations in circulating metabolic hormones. One paradoxical finding, however, was the reduction in leptin receptor levels in the tongue. VIP knockout mice demonstrate several features reminiscent of insulin resistance (e.g., high fasting glucose and insulin levels). In addition, VIP knockout animals possessed a heightened preference for appetitive sweet stimuli. Perhaps this change in taste preference—induced by increased tongue GLP-1 levels and reduced leptin receptor levels—could be a compensatory mechanism engendered to ameliorate their dysglycemia by attempting to reduce sugar intake. High circulating levels of leptin would be expected to reduce sweet taste preference (25), but with a significant ablation of the lingual Ob-Rb, this would be prevented. However, if this Ob-Rb ablation was universal, especially in the hypothalamus, then the animal would likely consume even more food and thus exacerbate its dysglycemic state. We, therefore, assessed the expression level of Ob-Rb in the hypothalami of wild-type and VIP knockout mice. In contrast to the tongue, no difference in Ob-Rb expression between wild-type and VIP knockout hypothalami was observed (Fig. 7A and B). In addition, we found no difference in insulin receptor substrate 2 (IRS2), T1R3 receptor, or GLP-1 expression in the

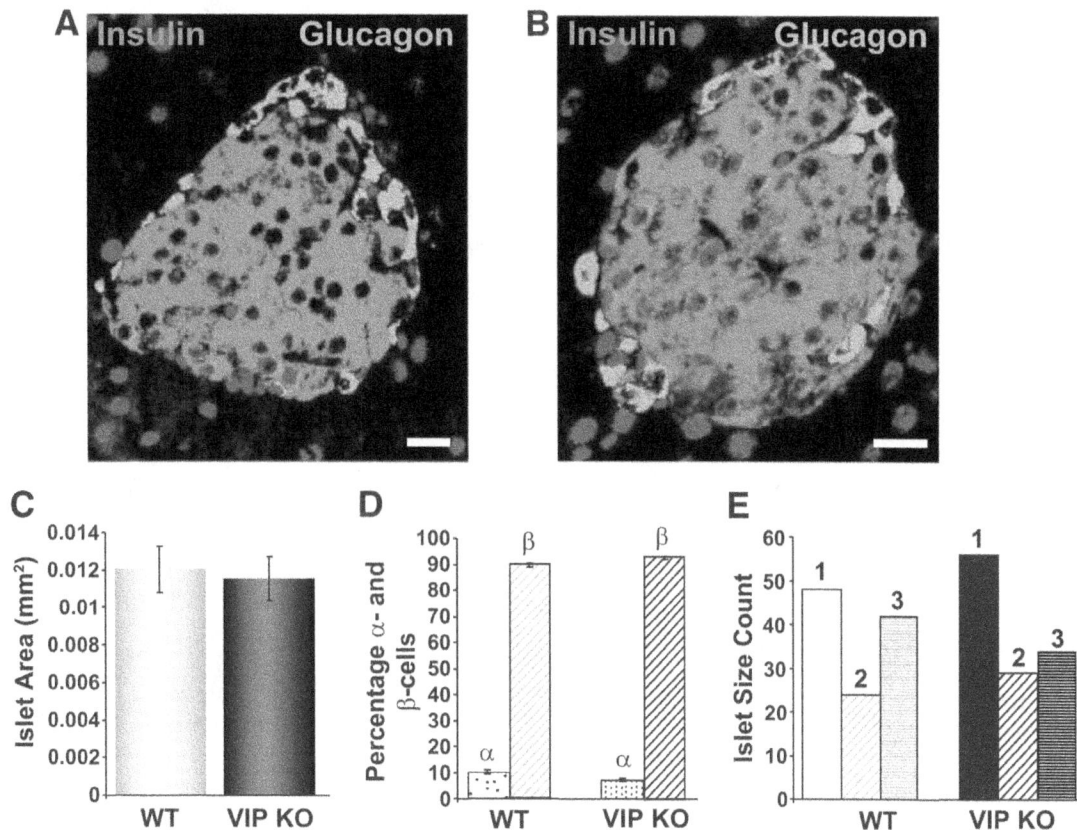

FIG. 5. Pancreatic islet sizing in VIP knockout (KO) and wild-type (WT) mice. Representative pancreatic islets from wild-type (A) or VIP knockout (B) mice demonstrate similar insulin (red fluorescence) and glucagon (green fluorescence) expression profiles. C: Mean islet area (mm²) measured in wild-type or VIP knockout pancreata. D: Similar mean α-cell (α) and β-cell (β) percentage in the islets of VIP knockout and wild-type mice. E: Relative distribution of the different islet sizes (1 = small; 2 = middle; 3 = large) for VIP knockout and wild-type mice. Values are expressed as the means ± SEM. (A high-quality digital representation of this figure is available in the online issue.)

hypothalami of wild-type or VIP knockout mice (Fig. 7A and C–E). VIP knockout mice showed a small reduction in food intake compared with wild-type mice (Fig. 7F) and there was no significant difference in body weight between VIP knockout and wild-type mice (Fig. 7G). Thus, it appears that the VIP knockout mice possess a complex physiological reaction to the imposed loss of VIP, one that may, in part, attempt to ameliorate their dysglycemia. VIP knockout mice show an increase in sweet taste preference and have elevated circulating leptin levels, which together could potentially be a mechanism to prevent additional excessive sugary food intake (summarized in Fig. 8). However, this mechanism would succeed only if there was localized lingual loss of the Ob-Rb, which was observed in the VIP-null mice.

DISCUSSION

We have demonstrated that VIP knockout mice possess alterations in their taste cells, circulating metabolic hormones, and taste preferences. Together, these factors appear to contribute to a unique dysglycemic pathophysiology. VIP and its cognate receptors are expressed in the type II taste cells of the circumvallate papillae. VIP knockout mice demonstrated normal gross taste bud morphology (Figs. 1 and 2). However, several key biochemical and pharmacologic alterations in their tongues were seen, that is, VIP knockout compared with wild-type mice exhibited significant increases and decreases in GLP-1 and leptin receptor, respectively, in taste cells (Fig. 3). In light of our

previous findings that GLP-1 in taste cells enhances sweet taste perception, this strongly indicated to us that taste cell VIP signaling may be involved in sweet taste perception. We demonstrated that VIP knockouts possess a greater preference for sweet compounds compared with wild-type mice (Fig. 6). VIP knockout mice also exhibited concentration-dependent changes in licking bitter stimuli and sour stimuli, but there was no change in salt perception compared with wild-type mice.

It is interesting to note that VPAC1/2 receptors were expressed on type II taste cells. Receptor systems responsive to bitter, sweet, and umami stimuli use similar signal transduction systems that themselves are narrowly tuned and achieve functional specificity by expression in non-overlapping subsets of type II cells. Interestingly, in this study, compared with our previous study (11), both VIP knockout and wild-type mice presented much higher sucrose/water lick ratios than GLP-1 receptor knockout (GLP-1R knockout) mice and their wild-type controls. It is unsurprising that distinct strains of mice possess different tastant responses, and this observation may be important for future experimental consideration of specific strains to facilitate efficient and sensitive detection of alterations in different taste modalities.

One unexpected finding in our VIP knockout mice was the significant reduction in leptin receptor (Ob-Rb) expression in the taste cells (Fig. 3F and G). Circulating leptin can activate leptin receptors on taste cells and specifically inhibit gustatory responses to sweet compounds (25).

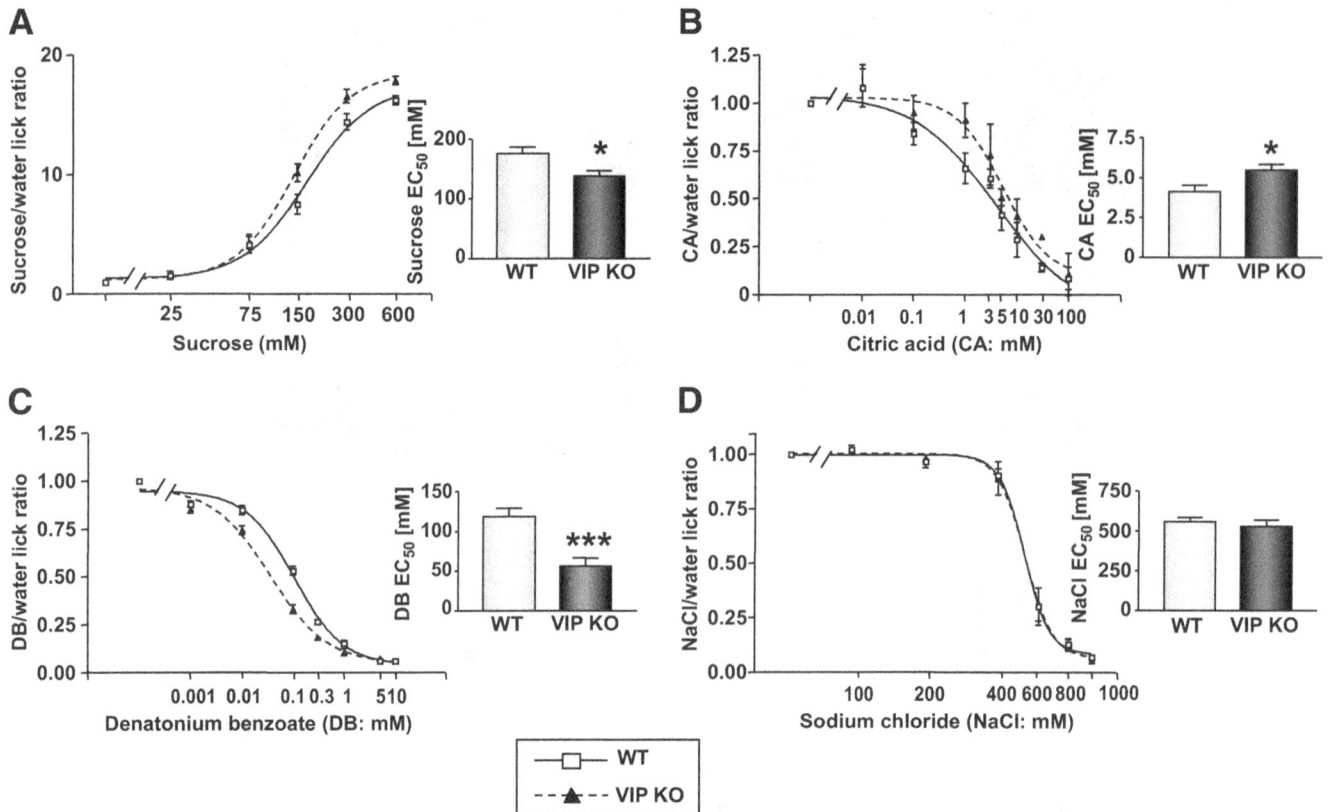

FIG. 6. Altered sweet, bitter, and sour taste responses of wild-type (WT) and VIP knockout (KO) mice in brief-access taste tests (*A–D*). Taste responses, expressed as tastant/water lick ratios and as a function of stimulus concentration, of VIP knockout (closed triangle, dotted line) and wild-type (open square, solid line) to sucrose (*A*), citric acid (CA; *B*), denatonium benzoate (DB; *C*), and sodium chloride (NaCl; *D*). Values are expressed as means ± SEM. Curves were fit as described in RESEARCH DESIGN AND METHODS. *$P < 0.05$, ***$P < 0.001$.

Hence, the significant reduction in taste cell leptin receptor expression in VIP knockout mice may, in part, account for their heightened preference for sweet tastants. Loss of the Ob-Rb would reduce any inhibitory action that circulating leptin would have upon sweet taste. This finding was interesting in light of our data showing that circulating levels of leptin in VIP knockout mice were considerably higher than those in wild type. Therefore, despite the presence of high concentrations of this sweet taste suppressor, the reduction of taste cell leptin receptor was able to facilitate enhanced sweet sensation by preventing inhibitory leptin signaling activity in the tongue. The elevated sweet preference of the VIP knockout mice may also stem from the elevated levels of taste cell GLP-1. We have previously shown that GLP-1's ability to activate the GLP-1R in the tongue strongly modulates sweet taste in mice (11). Increased levels of GLP-1 could, therefore, potentiate GLP-1R activity in the tongue, especially considering our previous findings that the enzyme that degrades GLP-1 in the peripheral circulation (dipeptidyl peptidase-4) is not present in taste cells of mice (11). The precise temporal nature of Ob-Rb loss, peripheral increase in leptin levels, or elevations in taste cell GLP-1 remains to be determined, but our data suggest that there is a strong connection between peripheral energy–regulatory hormones and lingual preference for foodstuffs. From our data, this physiological link may involve VIP. Because of the multiple sites and mechanisms of action of VIP in mammals, it is unsurprising that the metabolic phenotype of VIP knockout mice is complex. Hence, despite in-

creased leptin and PYY levels in VIP knockout mice there was no dramatic diminution of body weight or food intake. This may, in part, be due to removal of an inhibitory action of VIP upon food intake, demonstrated in multiple species including mice (35). Therefore, the resultant phenotype of the VIP knockout mice may be truly an intricate mixture of alterations of metabolic food desire and digestion.

In our study, several lines of evidence indicate a strong local taste cell action of VIP. First, VIP knockout mice demonstrated concentration-dependent changes in licking for sweet, bitter, and sour tastants, but not salt, indicating that there was not a generalized, widespread positive effect on all taste modalities. Second, VIP knockout and wild-type mice responded similarly to the salty taste stimulus; therefore, VIP knockout mice had no difficulty in learning and completing the taste test. Lastly, VIP and VIP receptors are specifically localized within sweet- and bitter-sensitive taste cells, consistent with the specific taste alterations we observed. Further reinforcing a selective local action of VIP, we found no VIP immunoreactivity in type I cells. It has been demonstrated that amiloride-sensitive Na^+ channels are expressed in type I cells of the fungiform papillae, suggesting that these taste cells could play a role in transducing salty taste stimuli (36). In line with this finding, we found that there was no difference in salt perception between VIP knockout and wild-type mice. Thus, it would be reasonable to propose that VIP signaling in the taste bud plays a local role in modulating sweet, bitter, and sour taste stimuli.

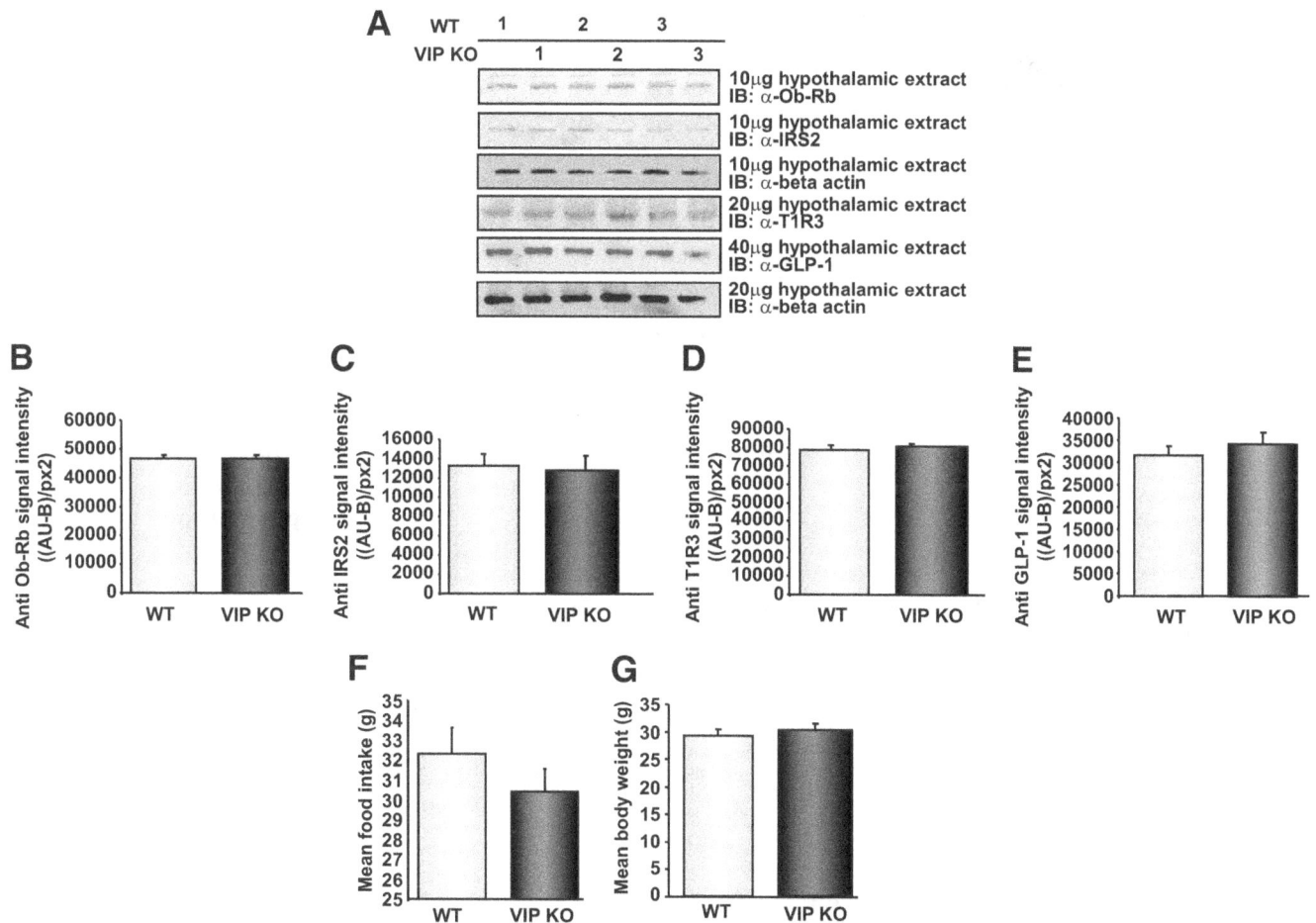

FIG. 7. Normal leptin receptor and IRS2 expression in the hypothalami of wild-type (WT) and VIP knockout (KO) mice. *A*: Representative Western blots of three wild-type (1–3) or VIP knockout (1–3) mice hypothalami. The tissue extracts were probed with specific antisera for the leptin receptor (Ob-Rb), IRS2, and β-actin as a loading control. For the Ob-Rb blot, a plasma membrane extract was used, whereas cytoplasmic tissue extracts were used for the IRS2 and actin blots. *B–E*: Mean ± SEM of the relative band intensities for the specific Western blots measured as relative absorbance units minus background absorbance per square pixel (AU-B/px2). *F*: Mean food intake (g) in wild-type and VIP knockout mice. *G*: Mean body weight of wild-type and VIP knockout mice. Values are expressed as means ± SEM.

There are numerous potential mechanisms by which VIP may affect both sweet and bitter stimuli. Sweet and bitter signal transduction is commonly mediated by PLCβ mechanisms involving taste receptor activation, as well as through adenylate cyclase–dependent mechanisms. VPAC1/2 receptors are coupled to multiple G-protein effectors to activate phospholipase D, PLCβ, and adenylate cyclase. VIP stimulation of VPAC receptors would therefore likely compete for availability of the PLCβ and adenylate cyclase signaling pathways, potentially diluting the functional signal transduction efficacy of the primary taste receptors. We have previously demonstrated that receptor stimulation of multiple related receptor systems can result in strong inhibitory effects that are profound and long-lasting (37). Genetic removal of the stimulating ligand will result in a diminution in the number of active VPAC1/2 receptors, reducing any diluting competitive actions upon the taste receptor's signaling capacity. Future experimentation upon the signaling efficiency of taste receptors in such an environment may shed light on this hypothesis.

The ability of VIP ablation to affect not only sweet and bitter taste perception, but also the response to a sour stimulus may be, in part, due to a role of VIP in controlling cell-cell signaling between taste cells and the type III ("presynaptic") cells possessing the putative sour receptor (PKD2L1). Recent data have shown that although presynaptic cells do not possess tastant-sensitive GPCRs (38), they still respond to tastant stimulation (5). Communication between taste cells and presynaptic cells is thought to involve ATP and serotonin secretion from the taste cells (39). In many areas of the gut, VIP is coreleased with both ATP and nitric oxide (NO) to exert relaxatory effects on smooth muscle (40). NO is commonly secreted from postsynaptic nervous tissue to act upon presynaptic neurons to control neurotransmitter release, and NO has also been associated with taste transduction (41). Therefore, it may be possible that in the tongue VIP may act in an analogous manner as in other parts of the digestive tract (i.e., in a concerted manner with NO and ATP). Therefore, genetic disruption of VIP may affect efficient taste cell–presynaptic cell communication, resulting in the reduction in sour taste we observed in VIP knockout mice.

We have demonstrated a complex physiological pattern of changes in VIP knockout mice that superficially may seem unconnected but together form a coherent and rational reactive mechanism to maintain energy homeostasis. VIP knockout animals demonstrate significantly ele-

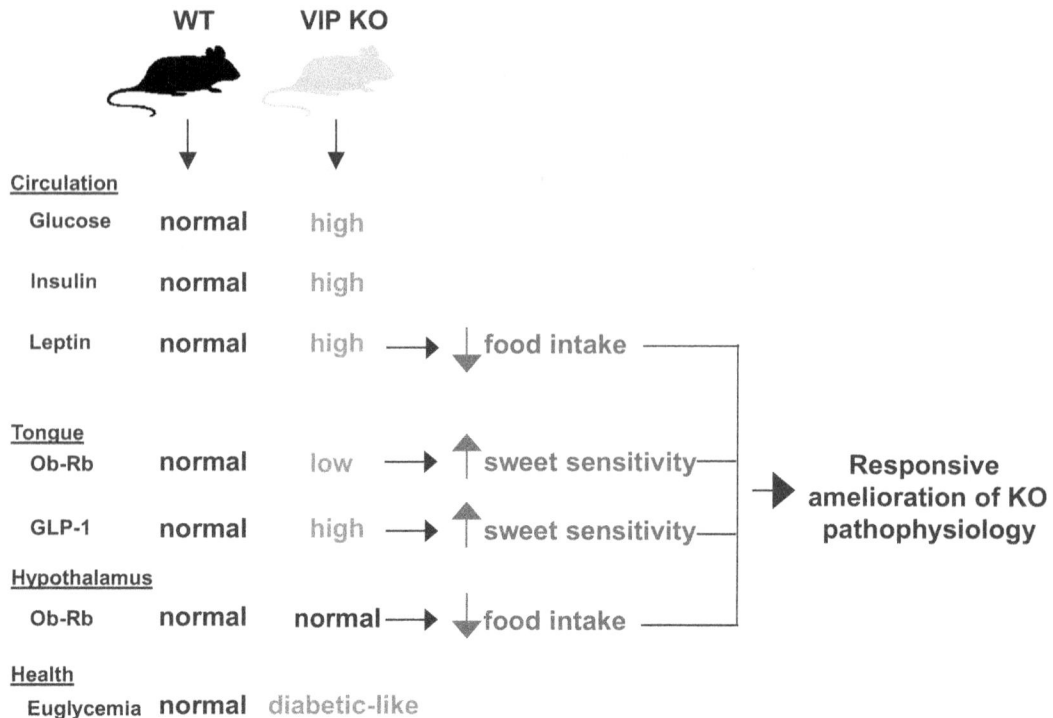

FIG. 8. A diagrammatic summary of the complex physiological parameters observed in the VIP knockout (KO) mice compared with the wild-type (WT) controls. The VIP knockout mice present with a diabetic-like state, and they actively attempt to ameliorate this condition with a series of physiological alterations (high circulating leptin, low tongue Ob-Rb expression, high tongue GLP-1 expression, normal hypothalamic Ob-Rb expression) that—in concert—could attenuate the animals' euglycemic disruption by enhancing their sweet taste and potentially reducing their desire to consume sweet foods.

vated blood glucose and insulin levels. They also possess significantly higher levels of circulating leptin but a striking reduction in Ob-Rb expression in the taste cells, while maintaining normal levels of Ob-Rb and other energy-regulatory factors (GLP-1, T1R3) in the hypothalamus. In addition, the animals demonstrate an altered preference for sweet tastants. The loss of VIP in our mice induces a dysglycemic state, that is, high resting glucose paired with a high insulin level. With knockout animals that survive birth, it is likely that they have physiologically adapted to counteract their deficits. For example, the lack of alteration of islet β-cell mass in the VIP knockout mice may be compensated for by the nonselective activity of structurally similar peptides, for example, pituitary adenylate cyclase activating polypeptide, which can activate VPAC2 receptors in the VIP knockout pancreata, substituting for VIP activity (18).

It would be interesting to speculate that reactive actions in VIP knockout mice have attempted to ameliorate their diabetic-like pathology by increasing their sweet preference (through reduced inhibitory leptin receptor activity and increased GLP-1 expression in the tongue) so as not to overconsume carbohydrates, while also trying to dampen their overall appetite (increased peripheral circulating leptin with normal hypothalamic Ob-Rb expression) (Fig. 8). Central nervous system VIP is antagonistic to dopamine and serotonin nervous activity (42,43). Both of these transmitters control food reward responses (44,45), and therefore VIP knockout mice may possess an elevated reward response, curtailing their intake and preventing weight increases. Human analogy of VIP knockout mice may be seen in "supertasters" (possessing increased sweet and bitter sensitivity) who tend to be more lean and

perhaps eat less than nonsupertasters (46). However, it is unclear whether the VIP knockout mice would not have gained weight if their chow was sweetened with sucrose, and more studies are needed to explore this further.

Thus, an interesting hypothesis would be that these multiple concerted responses in the VIP knockout mice suggest that the tongue could potentially act as a vessel for the animal to modulate its energy intake to correct any endogenous glycemic imbalances. In this way, we could potentially view the tongue as a sensory mechanism that is bidirectionally regulated, and thus forms a bridge between available foodstuffs and the intricate metabolic hormonal balance in the animal itself. Future studies would be needed to further explore this hypothesis.

To conclude, it is becoming apparent that there is a strong link between gustation and peripheral energy balance. Hormonal signaling within the taste buds of the tongue is likely to influence food intake and peripheral glucose homeostasis (15). For example, hormones such as GLP-1 and leptin, crucial to the control of peripheral somatic energy balance/appetite, are now thought to exert a strong local effect on the tongue with respect to food perception. This activity is mediated by their signaling roles in the gustatory system. Carbohydrates are among the most vital food stuffs for mammalian survival, and it would make evolutionary sense for mammals to have evolved multimodal carbohydrate sensing mechanisms. We feel that gaining a greater appreciation for which endocrine factors are present within taste cells and their putative roles in taste perception will shed much-needed light on how taste perception is linked to peripheral somatic energy balance. This knowledge will be invaluable for finding novel therapeutic targets and agents for the treatment of disorders such as metabolic syndrome and type 2 diabetes.

ACKNOWLEDGMENTS

This research was supported by the Intramural Research Program of the National Institutes of Health, National Institute on Aging.

No potential conflicts of interest relevant to this article were reported.

We thank Dr. Jacqueline Crawley, Dr. Joanna Hill, and Connor Stack (National Institute of Mental Health) for kindly providing us with VIP knockout mouse breeding pairs.

REFERENCES

1. Dulac C. The physiology of taste, vintage 2000. Cell 2000;100:607–610
2. Yoshie S, Wakasugi C, Teraki Y, Fujita T. Fine structure of the taste bud in guinea pigs: I, cell characterization and innervation patterns. Arch Histol Cytol 1990;53:103–119
3. Huang YJ, Lu KS. Unilateral innervation of guinea pig vallate taste buds as determined by glossopharyngeal neurectomy and HRP neural tracing. J Anat 1996;189:315–324
4. Yee CL, Yang R, Böttger B, Finger TE, Kinnamon JC. "Type III" cells of rat taste buds: immunohistochemical and ultrastructural studies of neuron-specific enolase, protein gene product 9.5, and serotonin. J Comp Neurol 2001;440:97–108
5. Tomchik SM, Berg S, Kim JW, Chaudhari N, Roper SD. Breadth of tuning and taste coding in mammalian taste buds. J Neurosci 2007;27:10840–10848
6. Chandrashekar J, Hoon MA, Ryba NJ, Zuker CS. The receptors and cells for mammalian taste. Nature 2006;444:288–294
7. Roper SD. Cell communication in taste buds. Cell Mol Life Sci 2006;63:1494–1500
8. Yang R, Stoick CL, Kinnamon JC. Synaptobrevin-2-like immunoreactivity is associated with vesicles at synapses in rat circumvallate taste buds. J Comp Neurol 2004;471:59–71
9. Huang YJ, Maruyama Y, Lu KS, Pereira E, Plonsky I, Baur JE, Wu D, Roper SD. Using biosensors to detect the release of serotonin from taste buds during taste stimulation. Arch Ital Biol 2005;143:87–96
10. Stone LM, Tan SS, Tam PP, Finger TE. Analysis of cell lineage relationships in taste buds. J Neurosci 2002;22:4522–4529
11. Shin YK, Martin B, Golden E, Dotson CD, Maudsley S, Kim W, Jang HJ, Mattson MP, Drucker DJ, Egan JM, Munger SD. Modulation of taste sensitivity by GLP-1 signaling. J Neurochem 2008;106:455–463
12. Kusakabe T, Matsuda H, Gono Y, Furukawa M, Hiruma H, Kawakami T, Tsukuda M, Takenaka T. Immunohistochemical localisation of regulatory neuropeptides in human circumvallate papillae. J Anat 1998;192:557–564
13. Zhao FL, Shen T, Kaya N, Lu SG, Cao Y, Herness S. Expression, physiological action, and coexpression patterns of neuropeptide Y in rat taste-bud cells. Proc Natl Acad Sci U S A 2005;102:11100–11105
14. Herness MS. Vasoactive intestinal peptide-like immunoreactivity in rodent taste cells. Neuroscience 1989;33:411–419
15. Martin B, Maudsley S, White CM, Egan JM. Hormones in the nasooropharynx: endocrine modulation of taste and smell. Trends Endocrinol Metab 2009;20:163–170
16. Dickson L, Finlayson K. VPAC and PAC receptors: from ligands to function. Pharmacol Ther 2009;121:294–316
17. Martin B, Lopez de Maturana R, Brenneman R, Walent T, Mattson MP, Maudsley S. Class II G protein-coupled receptors and their ligands in neuronal function and protection. Neuromolecular Med 2005;7:3–36
18. Winzell MS, Ahrén B. Role of VIP and PACAP in islet function. Peptides 2007;28:1805–1813
19. Witt M. Distribution of vasoactive intestinal peptide-like immunoreactivity in the taste organs of teleost fish and frog. Histochemical J 1995;27:161–165
20. Shen T, Kaya N, Zhao FL, Lu SG, Cao Y, Herness S. Co-expression patterns of the neuropeptides vasoactive intestinal peptide and cholecystokinin with the transduction molecules α-gustducin and T1R2 in rat taste receptor cells. Neuroscience 2005;130:229–238
21. Martin B, Dotson CD, Shin YK, Ji S, Drucker DJ, Maudsley S, Munger SD. Modulation of taste sensitivity by GLP-1 signaling in taste buds. Ann N Y Acad Sci 2009;1170:98–101
22. Zhang Y, Proenca R, Maffei M, Barone M, Leopold L, Friedman JM. Positional cloning of the mouse obese gene and its human homologue. Nature 1994;372:425–432
23. Lee GH, Proenca R, Montez JM, Carroll KM, Darvishzadeh JG, Lee JI, Friedman JM. Abnormal splicing of the leptin receptor in diabetic mice. Nature 1996;379:632–635
24. Chen H, Charlat O, Tartaglia LA, Woolf EA, Weng X, Ellis SJ, Lakey ND, Culpepper J, Moore KJ, Breitbart RE, Duyk GM, Tepper RI, Morgenstern JP. Evidence that the diabetes gene encodes the leptin receptor: identification of a mutation in the leptin receptor gene in db/db mice. Cell 1996;84:491–495
25. Nakamura Y, Sanematsu K, Ohta R, Shirosaki S, Koyano K, Nonaka K, Shigemura N, Ninomiya Y. Diurnal variation of human sweet taste recognition thresholds is correlated with plasma leptin levels. Diabetes 2008;57:2661–2665
26. Kawai K, Sugimoto K, Nakashima K, Miura H, Ninomiya Y. Leptin as a modulator of sweet taste sensitivities in mice. Proc Natl Acad Sci U S A 2000;97:11044–11049
27. Ninomiya Y, Sako N, Imai Y. Enhanced gustatory neural responses to sugars in the diabetic db/db mouse. Am J Physiol 1995;269:R930–R937
28. Shigemura N, Ohta R, Kusakabe Y, Miura H, Hino A, Koyano K, Nakashima K, Ninomiya Y. Leptin modulates behavioral responses to sweet substances by influencing peripheral taste structures. Endocrinology 2004;145:839–847
29. Ma H, Yang R, Thomas SM, Kinnamon JC. Qualitative and quantitative differences between taste buds of the rat and mouse. BMC Neurosci 2007;8:5
30. Martin B, Golden E, Carlson OD, Pistell P, Zhou J, Kim W, Frank BP, Thomas S, Chadwick WA, Greig NH, Bates GP, Sathasivam K, Bernier M, Maudsley S, Mattson MP, Egan JM. Exendin-4 improves glycemic control, ameliorates brain and pancreatic pathologies, and extends survival in a mouse model of Huntington's disease. Diabetes 2009;58:318–328
31. Boughter JD Jr, St John SJ, Noel DT, Ndubuizu O, Smith DV. A brief-access test for bitter taste in mice. Chem Senses 2002;27:133–142
32. Glendinning JI, Gresack J, Spector AC. A high-throughput screening procedure for identifying mice with aberrant taste and oromotor function. Chem Senses 2002;27:461–474
33. Nelson TM, Munger SD, Boughter JD Jr. Taste sensitivities to PROP and PTC vary independently in mice. Chem Senses 2003;28:695–704
34. Dotson CD, Spector AC. The relative affective potency of glycine, L-serine and sucrose as assessed by a brief-access taste test in inbred strains of mice. Chem Senses 2004;29:489–498
35. Morley JE, Horowitz M, Morley PM, Flood JF. Pituitary adenylate cyclase activating polypeptide (PACAP) reduces food intake in mice. Peptides 1992;13:1133–1135
36. Vandenbeuch A, Clapp TR, Kinnamon SC. Amiloride-sensitive channels in type I fungiform taste cells in mouse. BMC Neurosci 2008;9:1
37. Martin B, Brenneman R, Golden E, Walent T, Becker KG, Prabhu VV, Wood W 3rd, Ladenheim B, Cadet JL, Maudsley S. Growth factor signals in neural cells: coherent patterns of interaction control multiple levels of molecular and phenotypic responses. J Biol Chem 2009;284:2493–2511
38. DeFazio RA, Dvoryanchikov G, Maruyama Y, Kim JW, Pereira E, Roper SD, Chaudhari N. Separate populations of receptor cells and presynaptic cells in mouse taste buds. J Neurosci 2006;26:3971–3980
39. Huang YA, Dando R, Roper SD. Autocrine and paracrine roles for ATP and serotonin in mouse taste buds. J Neurosci 2009;29:13909–13918
40. Burnstock G. The journey to establish purinergic signaling in the gut. Neurogastroenterol Motil 2008;20:8–19
41. Nakamura T, Murata Y, Mashiko M, Okano K, Satoh H, Ozaki M, Amakawa T. The nitric oxide-cyclic GMP cascade in sugar receptor cells of the blowfly, Phormia regina. Chem Senses 2005;30:281–282
42. Gerhold LM, Sellix MT, Freeman ME. Antagonism of vasoactive intestinal peptide mRNA in the suprachiasmatic nucleus disrupts the rhythm of FRAs expression in neuroendocrine dopaminergic neurons. J Comp Neurol 2002;450:135–143
43. Karganov M, Romanova G, Braslawsky W, Tarshitz D, Telegdy G. Neuromodulator role of VIP in recovery of rat behavior and brain neurotransmitters level after frontal lobectomy. Ann N Y Acad Sci 1998;865:519–522
44. Wise RA. Role of brain dopamine in food reward and reinforcement. Philos Trans R Soc Lond B Biol Sci 2006;361:1149–1158
45. Ledonne A, Sebastianelli L, Federici M, Bernardi G, Mercuri NB. The anorexic agents, sibutramine and fenfluramine, depress GABA(B)-induced inhibitory postsynaptic potentials in rat mesencephalic dopaminergic cells. Br J Pharmacol 2009;156:962–969
46. Golding J, Steer C, Emmett P, Bartoshuk LM, Horwood J, Smith GD. Associations between the ability to detect a bitter taste, dietary behavior, and growth: a preliminary report. Ann N Y Acad Sci 2009;1170:553–557

Ghrelin Suppresses Glucose-Stimulated Insulin Secretion and Deteriorates Glucose Tolerance in Healthy Humans

Jenny Tong,[1] Ronald L. Prigeon,[2] Harold W. Davis,[1] Martin Bidlingmaier,[3] Steven E. Kahn,[4] David E. Cummings,[4] Matthias H. Tschöp,[1] and David D'Alessio[1,5]

OBJECTIVE—The orexigenic gut hormone ghrelin and its receptor are present in pancreatic islets. Although ghrelin reduces insulin secretion in rodents, its effect on insulin secretion in humans has not been established. The goal of this study was to test the hypothesis that circulating ghrelin suppresses glucose-stimulated insulin secretion in healthy subjects.

RESEARCH DESIGN AND METHODS—Ghrelin (0.3, 0.9 and 1.5 nmol/kg/h) or saline was infused for more than 65 min in 12 healthy patients (8 male/4 female) on 4 separate occasions in a counterbalanced fashion. An intravenous glucose tolerance test was performed during steady state plasma ghrelin levels. The acute insulin response to intravenous glucose (AIRg) was calculated from plasma insulin concentrations between 2 and 10 min after the glucose bolus. Intravenous glucose tolerance was measured as the glucose disappearance constant (Kg) from 10 to 30 min.

RESULTS—The three ghrelin infusions raised plasma total ghrelin concentrations to 4-, 15-, and 23-fold above the fasting level, respectively. Ghrelin infusion did not alter fasting plasma insulin or glucose, but compared with saline, the 0.3, 0.9, and 1.5 nmol/kg/h doses decreased AIRg (2,152 ± 448 vs. 1,478 ± 2,889, 1,419 ± 275, and 1,120 ± 174 pmol/l) and Kg (0.3 and 1.5 nmol/kg/h doses only) significantly ($P < 0.05$ for all). Ghrelin infusion raised plasma growth hormone and serum cortisol concentrations significantly ($P < 0.001$ for both), but had no effect on glucagon, epinephrine, or norepinephrine levels ($P = 0.44$, 0.74, and 0.48, respectively).

CONCLUSIONS—This is a robust proof-of-concept study showing that exogenous ghrelin reduces glucose-stimulated insulin secretion and glucose disappearance in healthy humans. Our findings raise the possibility that endogenous ghrelin has a role in physiologic insulin secretion, and that ghrelin antagonists could improve β-cell function. *Diabetes* **59:2145–2151, 2010**

From the [1]Department of Medicine, Division of Endocrinology, Diabetes and Metabolism, University of Cincinnati, Cincinnati, Ohio; the [2]School of Medicine, University of Maryland, Veterans Affairs Medical Center, Baltimore, Maryland; [3]Medizinische Klinik–Innenstadt, Ludwig-Maximilians-Universität, Munich, Germany; the [4]Division of Metabolism, Endocrinology and Nutrition, Department of Medicine, VA Puget Sound Health Care System and University of Washington, Seattle, Washington; and the [5]Cincinnati VA Medical Center, Cincinnati, Ohio.
Corresponding author: Jenny Tong, jenny.tong@uc.edu.

Received 15 April 2010 and accepted 15 June 2010. Published ahead of print at http://diabetes.diabetesjournals.org on 28 June 2010. DOI: 10.2337/db10-0504.

Ghrelin has gained considerable attention over the last decade for its unique role in regulating mealtime hunger and lipid metabolism, as well as short- and long-term energy homeostasis (1–3). It is the only known circulating factor that promotes food intake and increases fat mass. Ghrelin is secreted mainly from the stomach and proximal small bowel, and stimulates growth hormone (GH) secretion (4–6), in addition to its effect on energy balance. In healthy subjects, plasma ghrelin levels rise progressively before meals and fall to a nadir within 1 hour after eating, with changes in plasma levels during meals varying two- to threefold (7–8). Under pathologic conditions associated with severe malnutrition and weight loss, such as anorexia nervosa (9), cancer, or cardiac cachexia (10–11), plasma total ghrelin levels are increased up to threefold compared with healthy individuals. Besides its well known effects on feeding behavior, fat mass, and GH secretion, ghrelin has recently been implicated in the regulation of glucose homeostasis (12–13).

The GH secretagogue receptor (GHSR)-1a, also known as the ghrelin receptor, is widely distributed and has been localized to the hypothalamus, pituitary, liver, adipocyte, and pancreas (14–15). Both ghrelin and GHSR are expressed in human and rat pancreatic islets on both α- (16–17) and β-cells (18–19), and ghrelin is produced in a novel endocrine islet cell type that shares lineage with glucagon-secreting cells (20–21). Pancreatic ghrelin cells exist as the predominant cell type in fetal human islets, and expression in the pancreas during development significantly precedes its occurrence in the stomach (20). In animal mutant models, an early block in the differentiation of insulin-producing β cells leads to an enormous increase in ghrelin-producing ε cells, suggesting a developmental link between ghrelin and insulin (22). In vitro, ghrelin inhibits glucose-stimulated insulin secretion in a dose-dependent manner from cultured pancreata (23), isolated pancreatic islets (19,24), and immortalized β-cell lines (19,21), suggesting that it acts directly on β cells to achieve this effect. In experimental animals, both ghrelin released from pancreatic islets and exogenous ghrelin inhibit glucose-stimulated insulin secretion (16,24–26). Targeted gene deletion of ghrelin improves glucose tolerance and augments insulin secretion in *ob/ob* mice, suggesting a possible physiologic role which could be mediated by effects on islet function (27). Consistent with these findings, ghrelin gene deletion was shown to prevent glucose intolerance induced by a high-fat diet, an environmentally-induced model of hyperglycemia (26). Together, these findings indicate the potential of ghrelin blockade to prevent both genetically (*ob* gene)- and environmentally (high-fat diet)-induced glucose intolerance.

The effect of ghrelin on insulin secretion in humans is controversial. Intravenous injection of ghrelin decreases plasma insulin and increases blood glucose in some studies, suggesting inhibition of insulin secretion (12,28). However, this finding has not been universally observed (29), and it is unclear whether such effects occur at physiologic or only pharmacologic doses of ghrelin. Prior studies performed in humans primarily assessed the impact of ghrelin on β-cell function in the fasting state, and there is little information on the effect of the peptide on stimulated insulin release. Therefore, the role of ghrelin in the regulation of glucose homeostasis in humans remains poorly understood.

In this study, we determined the effect of ghrelin on glucose-stimulated insulin secretion and glucose tolerance. We infused acyl-ghrelin, the bioactive endogenous ligand of the GHSR-1a, at variable doses with the aim of raising plasma total ghrelin level to physiologic (less than twofold), supraphysiologic (two- to threefold) and pharmacologic (more than threefold) levels. An intravenous glucose tolerance test (IVGTT) was performed at steady state plasma ghrelin levels to determine the effect on glucose-stimulated insulin secretion and glucose tolerance in healthy, nonobese subjects.

RESEARCH DESIGN AND METHODS

Subjects. Healthy volunteers between the ages of 18 and 55 years with a BMI between 18 and 29 kg/m^2 were recruited from the greater Cincinnati area. Subjects with a history or clinical evidence of impaired fasting glucose or diabetes, recent myocardial infarction, congestive heart failure, active liver or kidney disease, growth hormone deficiency or excess, neuroendocrine tumor, anemia, or who were on medications known to alter insulin sensitivity were excluded.

All study procedures were conducted at the Cincinnati Veteran Affairs Medical Center General Clinical Research Center. All study participants gave informed consent for the study by signing a form approved by University of Cincinnati Institutional Review Board.

Experimental protocol. Subjects arrived at the Clinical Research Center between 0700 and 0730 after a 10–12 h fast for four separate experiments. intravenous catheters were placed in the veins of both forearms for blood sampling and infusion of test substances. The arm with the sampling catheter was heated to 55°C to arterialize venous blood.

Synthetic human acylated ghrelin was obtained from Bachem AG (Rubendorf, Switzerland). The authenticity of the peptide was verified by mass spectrometry, the purity was >95%, and reconstituted material was sterile and free of detectable pyrogens. On the morning of the 4 study days, either saline (as a control) or synthetic ghrelin dissolved in sterile saline solution was infused at doses of 0.3, 0.9, or 1.5 nmol/kg/h (equivalent to 1, 3, or 5 μg/kg/h) for a total of 65 min. The order of infusions was randomized, and study visits separated by at least 5 days. The use of synthetic human ghrelin was approved under the U.S. Food and Drug Administration Investigational New Drug 79,009.

After 55 min of ghrelin infusion, ∼6 plasma half-lives of acyl-ghrelin (28), subjects received an intravenous bolus of glucose (11.4 g/m^2 body surface area) over 60 s as the initiation of an IVGTT (time 0). Blood samples were removed at 2, 3, 4, 5, 6, 8, and 10 min after intravenous glucose bolus for the estimation of acute insulin response to glucose (AIRg) and acute C-peptide response to glucose (ACRg). Another seven blood samples were taken at 12, 14, 16, 20, 22, 25, and 30 min for the calculation of glucose disappearance and ghrelin pharmacokinetics. Blood was placed on ice and plasma separated by centrifugation within 1 hour, with the plasma stored at −80°C until used for assay. Blood pressure and heart rate were monitored every 15 min during the study procedure. A complete blood count, liver and kidney function tests, and an electrocardiogram were obtained as part of the safety monitoring of ghrelin use at the end of the last visit.

Assays. Blood glucose concentrations were determined by the glucose oxidase method using a glucose analyzer (YSI 2,300 STAT Plus; Yellow Springs Instruments, Yellow Springs, OH). Plasma immunoreactive insulin levels were measured using a double-antibody radioimmunoassay (RIA) as described previously (30). C-peptide levels were measured using a commercial RIA kit (Millipore). Total immunoreactive ghrelin was measured by RIA (Millipore, Billarica, MA). The lower and upper limits of detection were 27 and 1,765

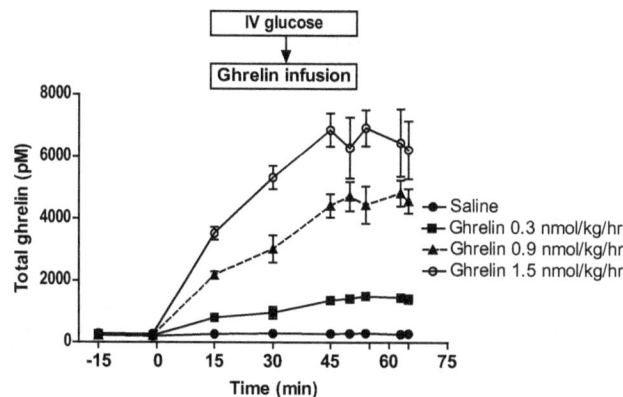

FIG. 1. Plasma total ghrelin levels during continuous intravenous infusions (minus 15 to 65 min) of saline, 0.3, 0.9, or 1.5 nmol/kg/h of acyl ghrelin in healthy men and women. A bolus intravenous dose of glucose (11.4 g/m^2 body surface area) was infused more than 1 min after plasma ghrelin had reached a steady state (55 min). The acyl ghrelin infusions resulted in a dose-dependent increase in plasma ghrelin.

pmol/l (93 and 6,000 pg/ml), respectively, and the intra-assay and interassay coefficients of variation (CV) were 6.4 and 16.3%, respectively. The ghrelin antibody used in the assay was directed toward the C-terminus of the molecule and binds both acyl- and desacyl-ghrelin, as well as truncated ghrelin species. Serum concentrations of human GH (hGH) were measured using the automated Immulite 2000 chemiluminescent assay system (Siemens, Bad Nauheim, Germany). This sandwich immunoassay uses a monoclonal mouse-anti-hGH capture- and a polyclonal rabbit-anti-hGH detection antibody. The intra-assay CV was 3%, and interassay variability ranged from 7%. Samples for glucagon were collected with benzamidine and heparin and were measured by RIA (Millipore, Billarica, MA). Cortisol levels were measured using the Corti-Cote RIA kit (MP Biomedicals, Orangeburg, NY). Plasma epinephrine and norepinephrine were measured using the CatCombi ELISA kit (IBL International; Hamburg, Germany). All samples were run in duplicate, and all specimens from a given participant were processed in the same assay.

Calculations. AIRg and ACRg were calculated as the average plasma insulin and C-peptide increment above baseline from 2–10 min after intravenous glucose administration, respectively. The glucose disappearance constant (31) was computed for each IVGTT as the slope of the natural logarithm of glucose from 10 to 30 min. The rate of ghrelin disappearance was calculated as the slope of the natural logarithm of ghrelin after cessation of the ghrelin infusion at 65 min (10 min after the glucose bolus was given).

Statistical analysis. The data were analyzed using ANOVA with 4 treatment levels (control, and ghrelin infusion rates of 0.3, 0.9, and 1.5 nmol/kg/h) and time of sampling being the repeated measure. Dependent variables included insulin, glucose, GH, cortisol, and glucagon concentrations. AIRg and ACRg for the 4 treatment levels were compared using a single-factor ANOVA. Post hoc analysis to compare control with each of the ghrelin infusion levels was performed using a Dunnett test. Data were analyzed using GraphPad Prism version 5.0 (GraphPad Software). All results are expressed as mean ± SEM unless otherwise noted.

RESULTS

Subject characteristics. Twelve healthy subjects (8 male and 4 female) age 26.0 ± 3.8 years with a BMI of 24.1 ± 1.4 kg/m^2 were enrolled in the study. No subject had a fasting blood glucose of >5.5 mmol/l. Mean fasting blood glucose for the group was 4.9 ± 0.2 mmol/l, and mean fasting plasma insulin was 37.8 ± 6.2 pmol/l.

Ghrelin pharmacokinetics. Steady-state levels were reached after ∼45 min for all 3 doses of acyl-ghrelin infusion. The average total ghrelin concentration during the time period between 45 and 54 min (10, 5, and 1 min before to intravenous glucose administration) for saline and the 3 acyl-ghrelin infusions were 304 ± 18, 1,429 ± 49, 4,629 ± 194, and 7,045 ± 295 pmol/l. The 0.3, 0.9 and 1.5 nmol/kg/h infusions raised the total ghrelin immunoreactivity 4.5 -, 15.4 -, and 22.6 - fold above an average basal level of 308 ± 30 pmol/l for the three infusions (Fig. 1;

TABLE 1
Basal plasma glucose and insulin levels during continuous intravenous infusions of saline, 0.3, 0.9, or 1.5 nmol/kg/h acyl ghrelin (0–54 min) before an IVGTT

Infusion rate	Plasma glucose (mg/dl)		Plasma insulin (pM)	
	Baseline	Ghrelin steady state (t = 45–54 min)	Baseline	Ghrelin steady state (t = 45–54 min)
Saline	83.8 ± 4.6	86.9 ± 1.0	34.1 ± 4.8	36.5 ± 5.8
Ghrelin (0.3 nmol/kg/h)	86.5 ± 2.4	96.7 ± 6.7	36.3 ± 4.8	30.4 ± 5.0
Ghrelin (0.9 nmol/kg/h)	91.4 ± 2.1	93.5 ± 2.7	42.0 ± 6.6	36.1 ± 6.9
Ghrelin (1.5 nmol/kg/h)	87.6 ± 1.6	91.5 ± 2.4	39.1 ± 5.8	25.6 ± 3.9

Data for baseline plasma glucose and insulin concentration were calculated as the average of the −15- and −1-min values. Data for plasma glucose and insulin at steady-state ghrelin concentration were calculated as the average of 45, 50, and 54 min values.

supplementary Table 1 is available in an online appendix at http://diabetes.diabetesjournals.org/cgi/content/full/db10 -0504/DC1). The intrasubject CV percentage for the saline, 0.3, 0.9, and 1.5 nmol/kg/h ghrelin infusions were 13.8, 7.7, 6.8, and 7.0%, respectively. The intersubject CV percentage for the steady-state total ghrelin measurement with different ghrelin infusion rates were 23.7, 20.1, 14.6, and 24.1%, respectively. After cessation of the ghrelin infusion at 65 min, total ghrelin levels declined after a first-order (exponential) decrease with an overall elimination rate constant (K_{el}) of 0.023 min^{-1}, corresponding to an elimination half-life of 30 min.

Effects of exogenous ghrelin on plasma insulin and glucose. The average fasting plasma glucose and insulin values at baseline and at times when ghrelin concentration reached a steady state (45 to 54 min) are shown in Table 1. Infusion of exogenous ghrelin did not alter fasting plasma concentrations of insulin and glucose from baseline ($P > 0.05$ for all comparisons).

Compared with saline, the doses of 0.3, 0.9, and 1.5 nmol/kg/h ghrelin each resulted in a significant reduction of AIRg (2,152 ± 448 to 1,478 ± 288, 1,419 ± 2,751 and 1,210 ± 188 pmol/l, $P < 0.05$, < 0.05, and < 0.01, respectively) during an IVGTT (Fig. 2A and B). The magnitude of suppression in AIRg increased with higher doses of ghrelin administration, suggesting a dose-dependent relationship between circulating ghrelin concentration and insulin secretion. Similar to AIRg, a significant suppression of C-peptide release in response to intravenous glucose was also seen with all three doses of ghrelin infusions (5.8 ± 0.9 to 4.1 ± 0.4, 4.2 ± 0.5, and 3.6 ± 0.6 nmol/l, $P < 0.05$, < 0.05, and < 0.01, respectively) (Fig. 2C). In addition, ghrelin infusion at the 0.3 and 1.5 nmol/kg/h doses also significantly decreased the rate of glucose disappearance ($P < 0.05$ for both comparisons; Fig. 3).

Effects of exogenous ghrelin on counterregulatory hormones. The three doses of ghrelin raised peak plasma GH levels by 12-, 114-, and 75-fold above baseline, respectively (Fig. 4). The 0.9 and 1.5 nmol/kg/h rates of ghrelin infusion also raised plasma cortisol levels significantly as compared with baseline at 30, 54, and 65 min ($P < 0.01$) (Fig. 5). Ghrelin infusion, regardless of dose, had no effect on glucagon secretion ($P = 0.44$) (supplementary Fig. 1). Plasma epinephrine and norepinephrine levels did not differ between baseline and 54 min when ghrelin in the circulation reached a steady state, regardless of the type of infusion the subjects received (supplementary Fig. 2).

Side effects. Ghrelin infusion was generally well tolerated. The most common complaints during infusion of ghrelin were hunger and "warm sensation." These symptoms were transient and resolved spontaneous after ces-

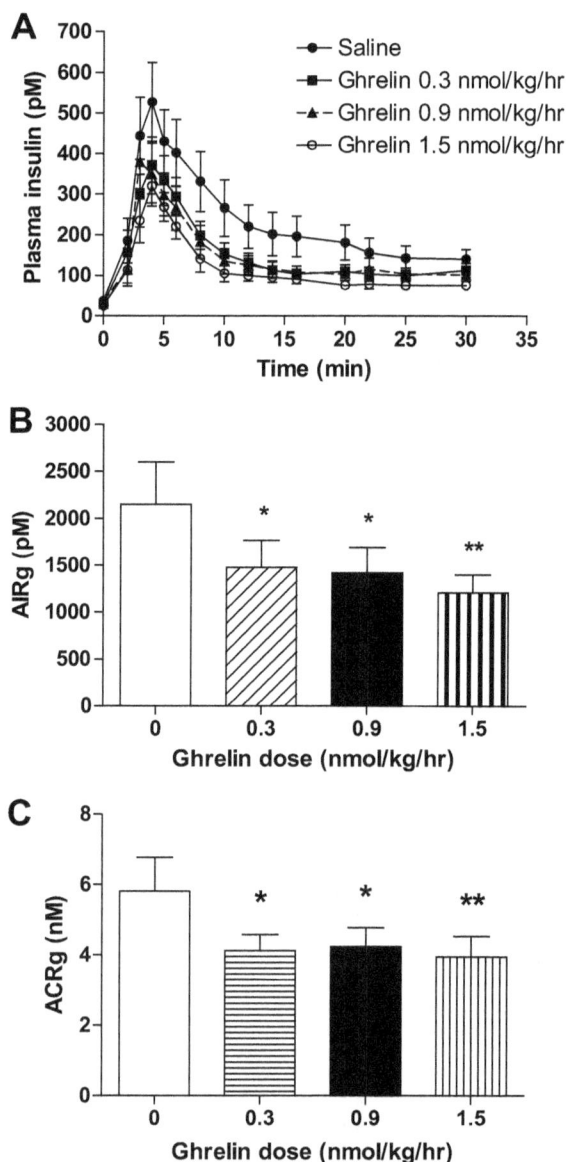

FIG. 2. A: Plasma insulin concentrations during an IVGTT after 55-min infusions of acyl ghrelin at 0.3, 0.9, or 1.5 nmol/kg/h, or saline. B: The acute insulin response to intravenous glucose (AIRg) determined during infusions of acyl ghrelin at 0.3, 0.9, or 1.5 nmol/kg/h dose, or saline. *$P < 0.05$, **$P < 0.01$. C: The acute C-peptide response to intravenous glucose (ACRg) determined during infusions of acyl ghrelin at 0.3, 0.9, or 1.5 nmol/kg/h dose, or saline. *$P < 0.05$, **$P < 0.01$.

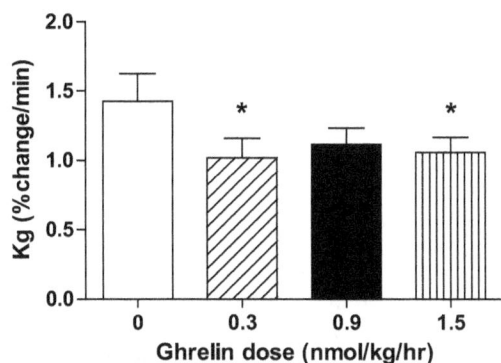

FIG. 3. Glucose disappearance constant (Kg) determined during infusions of acyl ghrelin at 0.3, 0.9, or 1.5 nmol/kg/h, or saline. *$P < 0.05$.

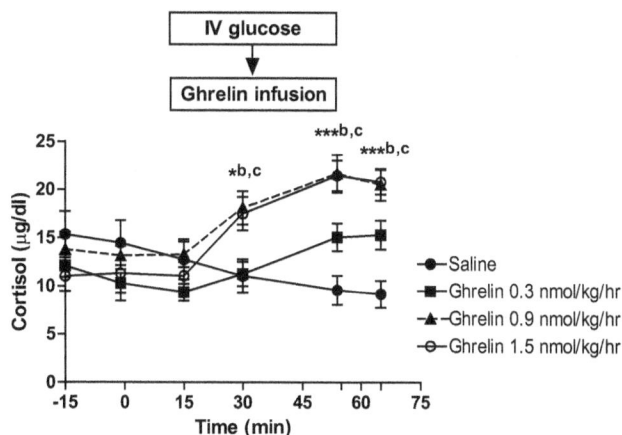

FIG. 5. Plasma cortisol concentrations during a 65-min infusion of acyl ghrelin at 0.3, 0.9, or 1.5 nmol/kg/h, or saline. Glucose was administered as an intravenous bolus after 55 min of the infusion. b and c are saline vs. 0.9 and 1.5 nmol/kg/h ghrelin, respectively; *$P < 0.05$, ***$P < 0.001$.

sation of the infusion. One subject, while receiving the 1.5 nmol/kg per hour ghrelin infusion, experienced a 23-mmHg decrease in mean arterial blood pressure without a significant change in heart rate. The subject was asymptomatic except for feeling "warm and hungry" during the event. The blood pressure returned to baseline within minutes after the ghrelin infusion was discontinued prematurely. This blood pressure change was not observed in any other subject or with any other dose.

DISCUSSION

Preclinical studies support a role for ghrelin to regulate glucose metabolism as well as energy balance and GH secretion. However, the effect of ghrelin on insulin secretion and glucose tolerance in humans has not been clearly established in the limited number of studies reported previously. In the present study, we examined the effect of a range of ghrelin doses on dynamic insulin secretion and glucose metabolism and demonstrated that acyl-ghrelin suppresses glucose-stimulated insulin secretion and worsens intravenous glucose tolerance in healthy humans. These effects appear to be present at concentrations of ghrelin above the usual physiologic range, and in a pattern consistent with dose-dependence. Our findings extend to humans the effects previously best demonstrated in mice, and suggest that ghrelin has a role in systemic glucose

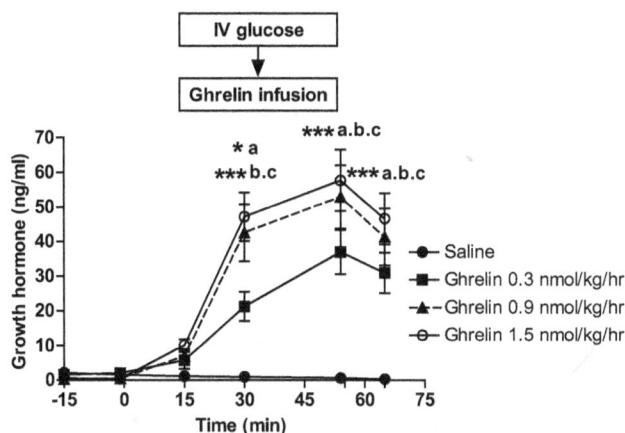

FIG. 4. Plasma growth hormone concentrations during a 65-min infusion of acyl ghrelin at 0.3, 0.9, or 1.5 nmol/kg/h, or saline. Glucose was administered as an intravenous bolus after 55 min of the infusion. a, b, and c are saline vs. 0.3, 0.9, or 1.5 nmol/kg/h of ghrelin, respectively; *$P < 0.05$, ***$P < 0.001$.

homeostasis. Moreover, our results raise possibilities for targeting the human ghrelin system as a means to improve disorders of glucose metabolism.

Several studies have examined the effect of ghrelin on insulin secretion in humans. In a study of healthy young males by Broglio et al. (12), an intravenous bolus injection of ghrelin (0.3 nmol/kg or 1.0 μg/kg) significantly increased fasting plasma glucose levels followed by a reduction in serum insulin levels beginning at 15 and 30 min after ghrelin administration, respectively, suggesting inhibition of insulin secretion. When the same dose of ghrelin was given as a continuous intravenous infusion to subjects who had undergone total gastrectomy, by necessity reducing the production of most endogenous ghrelin, C-peptide levels were suppressed when compared with saline infusion (32). In contrast, Lucidi et al. (29) infused acyl ghrelin at a rate of 7.5 or 15 pmol/kg/min for 2 hours in 8 healthy subjects and failed to observe a significant change in fasting plasma glucose and insulin levels. However, all previous studies in humans used fasting insulin as the marker of ghrelin effects on the β-cell, with no examination of stimulated insulin secretion. In the present study, we examined the effect of continuous infusions of low, medium, and high doses of acyl ghrelin on AIRg, a well established measure of insulin secretion that we think provides a more sensitive measure of β-cell function. The measure of C-peptide levels during the IVGTT confirms the changes in AIRg, and supports an effect of ghrelin on insulin secretion rather than insulin clearance. Moreover, the continuous infusion of ghrelin during the IVGTT also eliminated any potential bias in the β-cell response introduced by rapid changes in plasma ghrelin levels as occur with a bolus injection of the peptide. Based on these design advantages. we believe that ours is the most robust proof-of-concept study yet of the effect of ghrelin on insulin secretion in humans.

Similar to Lucidi et al. (29), we did not observe a significant change in fasting insulin or glucose levels with any of the 3 doses of ghrelin. On the other hand, we did find a clear suppressive effect of ghrelin on the first-phase insulin response in an apparent dose-dependent fashion, with the greatest effect seen with the highest dose ghrelin (Fig. 2). In addition, the decrease in intravenous glucose tolerance is consistent with a reduction of insulin secretion. Our observations are in keeping with several in vitro studies that have provided evidence that ghrelin has an inhibitory effect on stimulated insulin secretion from pancreatic β-cells (16,19,21,24–26) and in vivo studies that have shown a deteriorating effect on glucose tolerance (25,27). The mechanisms by which ghrelin could inhibit insulin secretion are unknown. Ghrelin may exert a direct effect on the β-cell or act indirectly by stimulating the secretion of counter-regulatory hormones that affect insulin secretion, or activating neural pathways that regulate islet function (33–38). The signaling mechanisms for insulinostatic ghrelin action in islet β-cells have been explored. Both endogenous and exogenous ghrelin has been shown to attenuate glucose-induced insulin release via $G\alpha_{i2}$-mediated activation of Kv channels, and suppression of action potential firing and $[Ca^{2+}]_i$ increases in β-cells (39). Furthermore, both ghrelin and its receptor are expressed in human and rat pancreatic islets (on α-, β-, and ε-cells) (16,18,20,40), and normal mouse pancreas contains a small population of ghrelin producing ε-cells which appear to be distinct from α- and β-cells (22,41). Ghrelin-immunoreactive cells are abundant in human islets during development, outnumbering those in the stomach, but few are present in adults (20). It is interesting to note that mice lacking the homeodomain protein Nkx2.2, which is essential for the differentiation of insulin-producing β-cells, have islets in which the β-cells are almost completely replaced by ε-cells (22). These findings raise the possibility of a shared common progenitor for both β- and ε-cells and suggest a role of ghrelin in the pancreatic islet, perhaps as a regulator of glucose homeostasis. Lastly, gut-brain crosstalk has been well described, and it is possible that ghrelin achieves its metabolic actions in the pancreas, muscle, adipose tissue, and liver via central ghrelin and insulin signaling (42–44).

As for possible indirect mechanisms of ghrelin action on the islet, previous studies in animals and humans have shown that both epinephrine and cortisol exhibit inhibitory effects on insulin secretion (33–36). We have shown here that cortisol levels were significantly elevated when higher doses of acyl ghrelin were given (0.9 and 1.5 nmol/kg/h). However, since steroid hormone action is thought to be mediated primarily by changes in gene transcription (45), it seems unlikely that the acute effect of ghrelin on AIRg can be explained by glucocorticoid activity. In contrast to a previous observation (46), we did not observe an increase in epinephrine levels with ghrelin administration. This could be caused by the difference in assay reproducibility (or perhaps sensitivity) or the method of ghrelin administration. As expected, GH levels were significantly elevated during ghrelin infusion (Fig. 5). Acutely, infusion of GH to levels within the physiologic range (27 ± 2 ng/ml) decrease insulin-mediated glucose uptake in the periphery within 2 to 12 h (37). In this study, the plasma insulin response to hyperglycemia was not altered by GH, and other investigators have noted increased plasma insulin concentration after 12-h infusion of GH to healthy volunteers (38). Therefore, we do not think the effects of ghrelin to reduce AIRg can be explained by changes in plasma GH.

Theoretically, the decrease in insulin secretion with ghrelin administration could be an adaptation to an increase in peripheral insulin sensitivity. However, previous studies in humans and animals seem to suggest that ghrelin consistently reduces, rather than improves, peripheral insulin sensitivity (12,28,32,47). The length of the IVGTT was limited by the total dose of ghrelin we could administer to each individual based on FDA requirements. For this reason, we do not have insulin sensitivity measures from IVGTT in this study. Overall, our data do not support indirect actions of counter-regulatory hormones or systemic insulin sensitivity to mediate the effects of ghrelin on insulin secretion.

Although in this study the effects of ghrelin on β-cell function occurred at supraphysiologic concentrations, it is important to consider that since ghrelin is produced in the islet ε cells (20–21), intraislet ghrelin concentrations may reach very high levels, raising the possibility that ghrelin could act locally on β cells via paracrine mechanisms (48–49), similarly to what has been demonstrated in adult rat islets (16). It is generally accepted that the level of hormone working in a paracrine/autocrine manner is higher than that working in an endocrine manner. Therefore, our observation of a suppressive effect of ghrelin on insulin secretion while the circulating level is in the supraphysiologic range does not exclude the possibility of a physiologic function of this hormone. Further studies will be necessary to delineate mechanisms by which endogenous ghrelin may affect islet function. Based on our results, endocrine, paracrine, and neural mechanisms are all plausible possibilities.

The role of ghrelin on α-cell function in humans has not been well established. Glucagon secretion is enhanced by ghrelin in vitro (25), but the effect of ghrelin on its release is less impressive in vivo, with levels largely unchanged or mildly increased after ghrelin administration (23,25,29,32). In our hands, no relevant change in glucagon level was seen with pharmacologic level ghrelin administration during fasting or IVGTT. Future studies that employ measurement of dynamic changes of glucagon level using more sensitive methods should be done to confirm this finding.

Conclusion. Our study demonstrates that exogenous ghrelin markedly reduces the first-phase insulin and C-peptide responses to intravenous glucose in healthy humans. These findings raise the possibility that endogenous ghrelin has a role in physiologic insulin secretion, and that ghrelin antagonists could improve β-cell function and serve as a novel drug target for the treatment of type 2 diabetes.

ACKNOWLEDGMENTS

Funding for this research was provided by NIH/NIDDK (5K23DK-80081 to J.T. and R0157900 to D.D.) and the Department of Veterans Affairs. M.H.T. is a scientific advisory board member and stockholder of Marcadia Biotech, Acylin Pharmaceutical, and Ambrx Inc.

No other potential conflicts of interest relevant to this article were reported.

J.T. researched data and wrote the manuscript. R.L.P. and H.W.D. researched data, contributed to discussion, and reviewed/edited the manuscript. M.B. researched data and reviewed/edited the manuscript. S.E.K. contributed to discussion and reviewed/edited the manuscript. D.E.C. reviewed/edited the manuscript. M.H.T. and D.D. contributed to discussion and reviewed/edited the manuscript.

The authors thank the General Clinical Research Center nursing staff, Kay Ellis, and Brianne Paxton for their excellent support for the study.

REFERENCES

1. Tschop M, Smiley DL, Heiman ML. Ghrelin induces adiposity in rodents. Nature 2000;407:908–913
2. Cummings DE. Ghrelin and the short- and long-term regulation of appetite and body weight. Physiol Behav 2006;89:71–84
3. Castaneda TR, Tong J, Datta R, Culler M, Tschop MH. Ghrelin in the regulation of body weight and metabolism. Front Neuroendocrinol 2010; 31:44–60
4. Bowers CY, Momany FA, Reynolds GA, Hong A. On the in vitro and in vivo activity of a new synthetic hexapeptide that acts on the pituitary to specifically release growth hormone. Endocrinology 1984;114:1537–1545
5. Kojima M, Hosoda H, Date Y, Nakazato M, Matsuo H, Kangawa K. Ghrelin is a growth-hormone-releasing acylated peptide from stomach. Nature 1999;402:656–660
6. Arvat E, Di Vito L, Broglio F, Papotti M, Muccioli G, Dieguez C, Casanueva FF, Deghenghi R, Camanni F, Ghigo E. Preliminary evidence that Ghrelin, the natural GH secretagogue (GHS)-receptor ligand, strongly stimulates GH secretion in humans. J Endocrinol Invest 2000;23:493–495
7. Tschop M, Wawarta R, Riepl RL, Friedrich S, Bidlingmaier M, Landgraf R, Folwaczny C. Post-prandial decrease of circulating human ghrelin levels. J Endocrinol Invest 2001;24:RC19–21
8. Cummings DE, Purnell JQ, Frayo RS, Schmidova K, Wisse BE, Weigle DS. A preprandial rise in plasma ghrelin levels suggests a role in meal initiation in humans. Diabetes 2001;50:1714–1719
9. Otto B, Cuntz U, Fruehauf E, Wawarta R, Folwaczny C, Riepl RL, Heiman ML, Lehnert P, Fichter M, Tschop M. Weight gain decreases elevated plasma ghrelin concentrations of patients with anorexia nervosa. Eur J Endocrinol 2001;145:669–673
10. Shimizu Y, Nagaya N, Isobe T, Imazu M, Okumura H, Hosoda H, Kojima M, Kangawa K, Kohno N. Increased plasma ghrelin level in lung cancer cachexia. Clin Cancer Res 2003;9:774–778
11. Nagaya N, Uematsu M, Kojima M, Date Y, Nakazato M, Okumura H, Hosoda H, Shimizu W, Yamagishi M, Oya H, Koh H, Yutani C, Kangawa K. Elevated circulating level of ghrelin in cachexia associated with chronic heart failure: relationships between ghrelin and anabolic/catabolic factors. Circulation 2001;104:2034–2038
12. Broglio F, Arvat E, Benso A, Gottero C, Muccioli G, Papotti M, van der Lely AJ, Deghenghi R, Ghigo E. Ghrelin, a natural GH secretagogue produced by the stomach, induces hyperglycemia and reduces insulin secretion in humans. J Clin Endocrinol Metab 2001;86:5083–5086
13. Sun Y, Asnicar M, Smith RG. Central and peripheral roles of ghrelin on glucose homeostasis. Neuroendocrinology 2007;86:215–228
14. Howard AD, Feighner SD, Cully DF, Arena JP, Liberator PA, Rosenblum CI, Hamelin M, Hreniuk DL, Palyha OC, Anderson J, Paress PS, Diaz C, Chou M, Liu KK, McKee KK, Pong SS, Chaung LY, Elbrecht A, Dashkevicz M, Heavens R, Rigby M, Sirinathsinghji DJ, Dean DC, Melillo DG, Patchett AA, Nargund R, Griffin PR, DeMartino JA, Gupta SK, Schaeffer JM, Smith RG, Van der Ploeg LH. A receptor in pituitary and hypothalamus that functions in growth hormone release. Science 1996;273:974–977
15. Guan XM, Yu H, Palyha OC, McKee KK, Feighner SD, Sirinathsinghji DJ, Smith RG, Van der Ploeg LH, Howard AD. Distribution of mRNA encoding the growth hormone secretagogue receptor in brain and peripheral tissues. Brain Res Mol Brain Res 1997;48:23–29
16. Dezaki K, Hosoda H, Kakei M, Hashiguchi S, Watanabe M, Kangawa K, Yada T. Endogenous ghrelin in pancreatic islets restricts insulin release by attenuating Ca2+ signaling in beta-cells: implication in the glycemic control in rodents. Diabetes 2004;53:3142–3151
17. Date Y, Nakazato M, Hashiguchi S, Dezaki K, Mondal MS, Hosoda H, Kojima M, Kangawa K, Arima T, Matsuo H, Yada T, Matsukura S. Ghrelin is present in pancreatic alpha-cells of humans and rats and stimulates insulin secretion. Diabetes 2002;51:124–129
18. Volante M, Allia E, Gugliotta P, Funaro A, Broglio F, Deghenghi R, Muccioli G, Ghigo E, Papotti M. Expression of ghrelin and of the GH secretagogue receptor by pancreatic islet cells and related endocrine tumors. J Clin Endocrinol Metab 2002;87:1300–1308
19. Colombo M, Gregersen S, Xiao J, Hermansen K. Effects of ghrelin and other neuropeptides (CART, MCH, orexin A and B, and GLP-1) on the release of insulin from isolated rat islets. Pancreas 2003;27:161–166
20. Wierup N, Svensson H, Mulder H, Sundler F. The ghrelin cell: a novel developmentally regulated islet cell in the human pancreas. Regul Pept 2002;107:63–69
21. Wierup N, Yang S, McEvilly RJ, Mulder H, Sundler F. Ghrelin is expressed in a novel endocrine cell type in developing rat islets and inhibits insulin secretion from INS-1 (832/13) cells. J Histochem Cytochem 2004;52:301–310
22. Prado CL, Pugh-Bernard AE, Elghazi L, Sosa-Pineda B, Sussel L. Ghrelin cells replace insulin-producing beta cells in two mouse models of pancreas development. Proc Natl Acad Sci U S A 2004;101:2924–2929
23. Egido EM, Rodriguez-Gallardo J, Silvestre RA, Marco J. Inhibitory effect of ghrelin on insulin and pancreatic somatostatin secretion. Eur J Endocrinol 2002;146:241–244
24. Reimer MK, Pacini G, Ahren B. Dose-dependent inhibition by ghrelin of insulin secretion in the mouse. Endocrinology 2003;144:916–921
25. Salehi A, Dornonville de la Cour C, Hakanson R, Lundquist I. Effects of ghrelin on insulin and glucagon secretion: a study of isolated pancreatic islets and intact mice. Regul Pept 2004;118:143–150
26. Dezaki K, Sone H, Koizumi M, Nakata M, Kakei M, Nagai H, Hosoda H, Kangawa K, Yada T. Blockade of pancreatic islet-derived ghrelin enhances insulin secretion to prevent high-fat diet-induced glucose intolerance. Diabetes 2006;55:3486–3493
27. Sun Y, Asnicar M, Saha PK, Chan L, Smith RG. Ablation of ghrelin improves the diabetic but not obese phenotype of ob/ob mice. Cell Metab 2006;3: 379–386
28. Akamizu T, Takaya K, Irako T, Hosoda H, Teramukai S, Matsuyama A, Tada H, Miura K, Shimizu A, Fukushima M, Yokode M, Tanaka K, Kangawa K. Pharmacokinetics, safety, and endocrine and appetite effects of ghrelin administration in young healthy subjects. Eur J Endocrinol 2004;150:447–455
29. Lucidi P, Murdolo G, Di Loreto C, Parlanti N, De Cicco A, Fatone C, Taglioni C, Fanelli C, Broglio F, Ghigo E, Bolli GB, Santeusanio F, De Feo P. Metabolic and endocrine effects of physiological increments in plasma ghrelin concentrations. Nutr Metab Cardiovasc Dis 2005;15:410–417
30. Elder DA, Prigeon RL, Wadwa RP, Dolan LM, D'Alessio DA. Beta-cell function, insulin sensitivity, and glucose tolerance in obese diabetic and nondiabetic adolescents and young adults. J Clin Endocrinol Metab 2006;91:185–191
31. Kahn SE, Montgomery B, Howell W, Ligueros-Saylan M, Hsu CH, Devineni D, McLeod JF, Horowitz A, Foley JE. Importance of early phase insulin secretion to intravenous glucose tolerance in subjects with type 2 diabetes mellitus. J Clin Endocrinol Metab 2001;86:5824–5829
32. Damjanovic SS, Lalic NM, Pesko PM, Petakov MS, Jotic A, Miljic D, Lalic KS, Lukic L, Djurovic M, Djukic VB. Acute effects of ghrelin on insulin secretion and glucose disposal rate in gastrectomized patients. J Clin Endocrinol Metab 2006;91:2574–2581
33. Tamagawa T, Henquin JC. Epinephrine modifications of insulin release and of 86Rb+ or 45Ca2+ fluxes in rat islets. Am J Physiol 1983;244:E245–E252
34. Sherwin RS, Sacca L. Effect of epinephrine on glucose metabolism in humans: contribution of the liver. Am J Physiol 1984;247:E157–E165
35. Barseghian G, Levine R. Effect of corticosterone on insulin and glucagon secretion by the isolated perfused rat pancreas. Endocrinology 1980;106: 547–552
36. Kalhan SC, Adam PA. Inhibitory effect of prednisone on insulin secretion in man: model for duplication of blood glucose concentration. J Clin Endocrinol Metab 1975;41:600–610
37. Bratusch-Marrain PR, Smith D, DeFronzo RA. The effect of growth hormone on glucose metabolism and insulin secretion in man. J Clin Endocrinol Metab 1982;55:973–982
38. Rizza RA, Mandarino LJ, Gerich JE. Effects of growth hormone on insulin action in man. Mechanisms of insulin resistance, impaired suppression of glucose production, and impaired stimulation of glucose utilization. Diabetes 1982;31:663–669
39. Dezaki K, Kakei M, Yada T. Ghrelin uses Galphai2 and activates voltage-dependent K+ channels to attenuate glucose-induced Ca2+ signaling and insulin release in islet β-cells: novel signal transduction of ghrelin. Diabetes 2007;56:2319–2327
40. Gnanapavan S, Kola B, Bustin SA, Morris DG, McGee P, Fairclough P, Bhattacharya S, Carpenter R, Grossman AB, Korbonits M. The tissue distribution of the mRNA of ghrelin and subtypes of its receptor, GHS-R, in humans. J Clin Endocrinol Metab 2002;87:2988
41. Andralojc KM, Mercalli A, Nowak KW, Albarello L, Calcagno R, Luzi L, Bonifacio E, Doglioni C, Piemonti L. Ghrelin-producing epsilon cells in the developing and adult human pancreas. Diabetologia 2009;52:486–493
42. Obici S, Zhang BB, Karkanias G, Rossetti L. Hypothalamic insulin signaling is required for inhibition of glucose production. Nat Med 2002;8:1376–1382
43. Obici S, Feng Z, Karkanias G, Baskin DG, Rossetti L. Decreasing hypothalamic insulin receptors causes hyperphagia and insulin resistance in rats. Nat Neurosci 2002;5:566–572
44. Pocai A, Morgan K, Buettner C, Gutierrez-Juarez R, Obici S, Rossetti L. Central leptin acutely reverses diet-induced hepatic insulin resistance. Diabetes 2005;54:3182–3189
45. Gronemeyer H. Control of transcription activation by steroid hormone receptors. FASEB J 1992;6:2524–2529

46. Nagaya N, Kojima M, Uematsu M, Yamagishi M, Hosoda H, Oya H, Hayashi Y, Kangawa K. Hemodynamic and hormonal effects of human ghrelin in healthy volunteers. Am J Physiol Regul Integr Comp Physiol 2001;280: R1483–R1487

47. Vestergaard ET, Gormsen LC, Jessen N, Lund S, Hansen TK, Moller N, Jorgensen JO. Ghrelin infusion in humans induces acute insulin resistance and lipolysis independent of growth hormone signaling. Diabetes 2008;57: 3205–3210

48. Ahima RS. Ghrelin–a new player in glucose homeostasis? Cell Metab 2006;3:301–302

49. van der Lely AJ. Ghrelin and new metabolic frontiers. Horm Res 71 Suppl 2009;1:129–133

NONALCOHOLIC FATTY LIVER DISEASE

Spectrum of Liver Disease in Type 2 Diabetes and Management of Patients With Diabetes and Liver Disease

KEITH G. TOLMAN, MD[1,2]
VIVIAN FONSECA, MD[3]

ANTHONY DALPIAZ, PHARMD[4]
MENG H. TAN, MD[5]

It is estimated that 20.8 million people, i.e., 7.0% of the U.S. population, have diabetes (1). Type 2 diabetes, with its core defects of insulin resistance and relative insulin deficiency, accounts for 90–95% of those with the disease. Another 5.2 million people are estimated to have undiagnosed type 2 diabetes. It is the sixth leading cause of death (1) in the U.S. and accounts for 17.2% of all deaths for those aged >25 years (2).

Liver disease is an important cause of death in type 2 diabetes. In the population-based Verona Diabetes Study (3), cirrhosis was the fourth leading cause of death and accounted for 4.4% of diabetes-related deaths. The standardized mortality ratio (SMR), i.e., the relative rate of an event compared with the background rate, for cirrhosis was 2.52 compared with 1.34 for cardiovascular disease (CVD). In another prospective cohort study (4), cirrhosis accounted for 12.5% of deaths in patients with diabetes.

Diabetes, by most estimates, is now the most common cause of liver disease in the U.S. Cryptogenic cirrhosis, of which diabetes is, by far, the most common cause, has become the third leading indication for liver transplantation in the U.S.

(5,6). Virtually the entire spectrum of liver disease is seen in patients with type 2 diabetes. This includes abnormal liver enzymes, nonalcoholic fatty liver disease (NAFLD), cirrhosis, hepatocellular carcinoma, and acute liver failure. In addition, there is an unexplained association of diabetes with hepatitis C. Finally, the prevalence of diabetes in cirrhosis is 12.3–57% (7). Thus, patients with diabetes have a high prevalence of liver disease and patients with liver disease have a high prevalence of diabetes.

The management of diabetes in patients with liver disease is theoretically complicated by liver-related alterations in drug metabolism, potential interactions between the drugs, and a low, albeit real, incidence of hepatotoxicity. In this article, we review the spectrum of liver disease found in patients with type 2 diabetes and the management of patients with concurrent diabetes and liver disease.

METHODS — A Medline search without limitations of date (as of October 2005), language, or humans was carried out by the authors. The following medical subject headings were used: "Diabetes Mellitus, type 2"; "Fatty Liver"; "Hepatitis,

Toxic"; "Sulfonylurea Compounds"; "Thiazolidinediones"; "Rosiglitazone"; "Pioglitazone"; "Troglitazone"; "Hydroxymethylglutaryl-CoA Reductase Inhibitors"; "Metformin"; "Acarbose"; and "Gemfibrozil" and free-text terms: "fatty liver", "steatohepatitis", "nonalcoholic steatohepatitis", "nonalcoholic fatty liver disease", "drug-induced hepatitis", each drug name and "hepat*", and each drug name. When full-text articles were not available in the English language, abstracts were included in the search. Abstracts from national meetings through October 2006 were included. The Food and Drug Administration (FDA) Web site was searched for hepatotoxicity reports using the free-text terms listed above.

SPECTRUM OF LIVER DISEASE IN TYPE 2 DIABETES

— The liver diseases seen in type 2 diabetes cover virtually the entire spectrum of liver disease.

Abnormal liver enzymes

Elevation of serum alanine aminotransferase (ALT), while uncommon (0.5%) in apparently normal subjects (7), is common in patients with type 2 diabetes. In four clinical trials involving 3,701 patients with type 2 diabetes, between 2 and 24% of screened patients had liver enzyme tests above the upper limit of normal (ULN) (8). In these studies, investigators noted that ~5% of the patients had concomitant liver disease at baseline. In another report involving 13 clinical trials and 5,003 patients with type 2 diabetes, in which patients with serum ALT, aspartate aminotransferase (AST), or alkaline phosphatase >2.5 times ULN were excluded, 5.6% had serum ALT values between 1 and 2.5 times ULN (9). Evaluation of asymptomatic individuals with mild elevations of ALT and AST reveals that 98% have liver disease—most commonly, fatty liver disease and chronic hepatitis (10). The most common cause of a mild elevation of serum ALT is NAFLD (11), the most prevalent liver disease in type 2 diabetes.

From the [1]Division of Gastroenterology, University of Utah School of Medicine, Salt Lake City, Utah; the [2]Department of Pharmacology, University of Utah School of Medicine, Salt Lake City, Utah; the [3]Division of Endocrinology, Tulane University, New Orleans, Louisiana; the [4]Department of Pharmacy, University Hospitals and Clinics, Salt Lake City, Utah; and [5]Lilly Research Laboratories, Eli Lilly and Company, Indianapolis, Indiana.

Address correspondence and reprint requests to Keith G. Tolman, MD, Department of Internal Medicine, University of Utah School of Medicine, 30 N. 1900 East, Salt Lake City, UT 84132. E-mail: keith.tolman@hsc.utah.edu.

Received for publication 21 July 2006 and accepted in revised form 20 November 2006.

K.G.T. is on the scientific advisory boards for TAP Pharmaceuticals, Takada, Santarus, Merck, Johnson & Johnson, and InterMune and is on the speakers bureau for TAP Pharmaceuticals, Takeda, Schering, Roche, Eli Lilly, Santarus, InterMune, and G.D. Searle. V.F. is a consultant for and on the speakers bureau for Eli Lilly, Novartis, Takeda, Pfizer, and Sanofi-Aventis and has received grants from GlaxoSmithKline, Novartis, Takeda, AstraZenca, Pfizer, Sanofi-Aventis, Eli Lilly, and the National Institutes of Health.

Abbreviations: ALT, alanine aminotransferase; AST, aspartate aminotransferase; CVD, cardiovascular disease; FDA, Food and Drug Administration; HCV, hepatitis C virus; NAFLD, nonalcoholic fatty liver disease; NASH, nonalcoholic steatohepatitis; SMR, standardized mortality ratio; TNF, tumor necrosis factor; TZD, thiazolidinedione; ULN, upper limit of normal.

A table elsewhere in this issue shows conventional and Système International (SI) units and conversion factors for many substances.

DOI: 10.2337/dc06-1539
© 2007 by the American Diabetes Association.

NAFLD

The most common chronic liver disease in the U.S. is NAFLD (5). It is defined as fatty liver disease in the absence of <20 g alcohol/day. NAFLD, which resembles alcoholic liver disease, consists of a spectrum of liver disease from steatosis (fatty infiltration of the liver) to nonalcoholic steatohepatitis (NASH), which consists of steatosis plus inflammation, necrosis, and fibrosis. The prevalence of NAFLD in diabetes is estimated at 34–74% (12–17) and, in diabetes with obesity, at virtually 100% (18). While once considered a benign process, NASH has been found to lead to cirrhosis and, in some cases, to hepatocellular carcinoma (13,19–21). Of patients with NAFLD, 50% have NASH and 19% have cirrhosis at the time of diagnosis (18,22,23) While these studies are subject to selection bias, the prevalence is undoubtedly very high.

The pathogenesis of NAFLD is only partially understood. Hepatic steatosis reflects an imbalance between the uptake and synthesis of fatty acids by the liver and their oxidation and export. Patients with type 2 diabetes have dyslipidemia, which is characterized by elevated plasma triglycerides, decreased HDL cholesterol, and predominance of small LDL, a pattern also seen in patients with NAFLD (24). A central abnormality in the pathogenesis of steatosis appears to be insulin resistance resulting in lipolysis, which increases circulating free fatty acids (25), which are then taken up by the liver as an energy source. The fatty acids overload the hepatic mitochondrial β-oxidation system, leading to accumulation of fatty acids in the liver (26). Indeed, some investigators suggest NAFLD to be the hepatic manifestation of the insulin resistance syndrome (22,27–29). NAFLD does not universally progress to NASH, and the precise pathogenesis of steatohepatitis is yet to be determined. However, dysregulation of peripheral lipid metabolism seems to be important.

Lipid metabolism is, in part, regulated by adipokines, including tumor necrosis factor (TNF)-α and adiponectin. TNF-α, which interferes with insulin signaling thereby favoring steatosis, is elevated in fatty liver disease albeit not specific to type 2 diabetes (30,31). TNF-α is also proinflammatory and, thus, may play a role in the pathogenesis of the inflammation in NASH (32,33). Adiponectin, in contrast to TNF-α, is antilipogenic and anti-inflammatory and, thus, may protect the liver from lipid accumulation

and inflammation. Adiponectin levels are decreased in conditions associated with NAFLD, including insulin resistance (34), obesity (35), type 2 diabetes (36,37), and NAFLD (36). Adiponectin and TNF-α therefore have opposing effects. The net effect of increased TNF-α and decreased adiponectin is prosteatotic and proinflammatory.

The mechanism of cell injury remains unclear. Fatty acids in the liver induce formation of free radicals (38), which cause lipid peroxidation and induce proinflammatory cytokines (39). The lipid peroxidation leads to the release of malondialdehyde and 4-hydroxynonenal, which in turn causes cell death and protein cross-linkage. This results in the formation of Mallory's hyaline in the hepatocyte (40) and activation of the stellate cells, which leads to collagen synthesis and fibrosis (41). The net effect of these processes is necrosis, formation of Mallory's hyaline, inflammation, and fibrosis—the characteristic histologic features of NASH.

The natural history of NAFLD is similar to that of alcoholic liver disease. The progression from steatosis to steatohepatitis to cirrhosis and, in some patients, to hepatocellular carcinoma over a period of many years is well established (13,42). The prognosis worsens with each stage of disease. Why some patients progress while most do not is not known. The only reliable way, to date, of determining this progression is liver biopsy, which may have significant economic implications (good or bad) for the management of patients with type 2 diabetes.

Cirrhosis in diabetes

Cirrhosis is an important cause of death in diabetes. An autopsy study in the U.S. has shown that patients with diabetes have an increased incidence of severe fibrosis (19). In the Verona study, the SMR for cirrhosis was 2.52, greater than the 1.34 for CVD. If the patient was being treated with insulin, the SMR increased to 6.84 (3). Cryptogenic cirrhosis, primarily diabetes 5, is the third leading indication for liver transplantation in this country (6).

The association of cirrhosis and diabetes is complicated by the fact that cirrhosis itself is associated with insulin resistance. Impaired glucose tolerance is seen in 60% and overt diabetes in 20% of patients with cirrhosis. Insulin-mediated glucose disposal has been shown to be reduced by ~50% in cirrhotic patients (43). However, the onset of type 2 diabe-

tes in cirrhotic patients is associated with decreased rather than increased insulin secretion (44). This interplay of associations has made it difficult to sort out the pathogenesis of cirrhosis in diabetes. Nevertheless, the association is incontrovertible and has implications for the treatment of diabetes in patients with cirrhosis.

Hepatocellular carcinoma in diabetes

Numerous studies have confirmed a fourfold increased prevalence of hepatocellular carcinoma in patients with diabetes as well as an increased prevalence of diabetes in patients with hepatocellular carcinoma (45–48). It is not known whether the increased prevalence of hepatocellular carcinoma is unique to diabetes or the increased prevalence of cirrhosis, the precursor lesion of hepatocellular carcinoma. The pathogenic sequence of events leading to hepatocellular carcinoma appears to be insulin resistance, increased lipolysis, lipid accumulation in the hepatocytes, oxidative stress, and cell damage followed by fibrosis and cell proliferation, which are procarcinogenic (49–52).

Acute liver failure

The incidence of acute liver failure appears to be increased in patients with diabetes: 2.31 per 10,000 person-years compared with 1.44 in the background population (53,54). It remains unclear whether it is diabetes, medications, or some other factor that accounts for the increased risk of acute liver failure. Troglitazone was factored out in these studies.

Hepatitis C in diabetes

The prevalence of hepatitis C virus (HCV) is higher in patients with diabetes than in the general population (55–63). Specifically, the prevalence of HCV antibodies is 4.2% in the diabetic population compared with 1.6% in the comparator group. The relative odds of HCV-infected patients developing diabetes is 2.1 (95% CI 1.12–3.90) (58). Patients with HCV are more likely to develop diabetes (21%) than patients with hepatitis B (10%), suggesting that HCV, rather than liver disease per se, predisposes patients to diabetes. Furthermore, patients who are transplanted for HCV (and universally become reinfected) are more likely to develop diabetes than those who are transplanted for other liver diseases (61). Taken together, these observations suggest that HCV may play a pathogenetic role in type

2 diabetes. Recent studies suggest that the core protein of HCV impairs insulin receptor substrate signaling, which plays an important role in the metabolic effects of insulin (64,65).

There are other peculiarities in the HCV-diabetes connection including HCV genotype specificity. There are six genotypes of HCV, with genotype 1 being the most prevalent in the U.S. The prevalence of fatty liver disease is disproportionately high in HCV genotype 3 (66), presumably secondary to insulin resistance (67,68). Patients with hepatitis C and fatty liver disease have elevated levels of TNF-α and reduced levels of adiponectin, which in combination are proinflammatory and prosteatotic (69,70), leading to oxidative stress in mitochondria (71) and steatosis in many genotype 3 patients (72–74). Finally, there is an association of diabetes with α-interferon treatment of HCV infection. Type 1 diabetes occurs more frequently in patients treated with interferon for HCV versus other conditions (75). The latency of diabetes ranges from 10 days to 4 years after starting treatment.

The interaction between HCV infection, diabetes, and interferon is the subject of intensive investigation. In the meantime, given the strong epidemiologic evidence for the increased prevalence of HCV in diabetes, it seems reasonable that all patients with type 2 diabetes and persistently elevated serum ALT should be screened for HCV.

TREATMENT OF PATIENTS WITH TYPE 2 DIABETES AND LIVER DISEASE — The severity of type 2 diabetes and the type and severity of liver disease influence the therapy. There are few clinical trials that specifically target patients with coexistent diabetes and liver disease, and all are limited by small numbers of patients. We will review the management of type 2 diabetes in patients with liver disease as well as the management of liver disease specifically associated with type 2 diabetes.

MANAGEMENT OF DIABETES IN PATIENTS WITH CONCOMITANT LIVER DISEASE

Lifestyle modification
Treatment of type 2 diabetes in patients with liver disease may be compromised by poor nutritional status and general health. More than 50% of patients with severe liver disease are malnourished. A number of uncontrolled studies indicate that weight loss decreases hepatic steatosis (76–78). The durability of weight loss on hepatic steatosis remains to be determined (79). Low-glycemic, low-calorie diets with a weight loss of 1–2 kg/week seem reasonable. Low-fat diets should be avoided (80,81). Some have suggested that a Mediterranean diet (i.e., high complex carbohydrates, high monounsaturated fats, moderate amounts of wine, and low amounts of red meat) is preferred in patients with type 2 diabetes and NAFLD (82,83). Exercise improves peripheral insulin sensitivity (84), albeit not specific to patients with diabetic liver disease. Alcohol should be avoided not only because of its toxic effects on the liver, but also because of its high caloric content and potential interaction with sulfonylureas (85,86).

Pharmacologic therapy
Pharmacologic therapy of type 2 diabetes in patients with liver diseases is, for the most part, the same as that without liver disease. While there are theoretical concerns about altered drug metabolism and hepatotoxicity, only patients with evidence of liver failure such as ascites, coagulopathy, or encephalopathy have altered drug metabolism. Furthermore, there is no evidence that patients with liver disease are predisposed to hepatotoxicity (87). Underlying liver disease, however, may compromise the diagnosis and increase the severity of drug-induced liver disease.

First-line therapy with metformin is appropriate in most patients but not recommended in patients with advanced hepatic disease because of a perceived increased risk of lactic acidosis. Recent trials have shown some benefit in patients with fatty liver and type 2 diabetes (88–91). Given that insulin resistance is the core defect in fatty liver disease, the case can be made for thiazolidinediones (TZDs) as front line therapy in these patients. Recent trials with pioglitazone and rosiglitazone have shown improvement in ALT and liver histology (92–97). Weight gain is a concern with TZDs, and cost is prohibitive for many patients. If metformin or TZDs are contraindicated, pharmacotherapy can begin with a secretagogue such as a sulfonylurea with rapid advancement to insulin if glycemic control is not achieved.

Insulin secretagogues. Sulfonylureas are generally safe in patients with liver disease but may not overcome the insulin resistance and defects in insulin secretion seen in patients with coexistent alcoholic liver disease and pancreatic damage (84). Sulfonylureas with a short half-life such as glipizide or glyburide are preferred in these patients. Patients with decompensated cirrhosis, i.e., encephalopathy, ascites, or coagulopathy, may have a reduced ability to counteract hypoglycemia, and thus, the response to therapy should be monitored closely. Historically, chlorpropamide (84,98–100) was associated with hepatitis and jaundice.

Clinical trials assessing the efficacy of meglitinides in the treatment of patients with liver disease have not been reported. The pharmacokinetics and tolerability of nateglinide in patients with cirrhosis is not significantly different than in control subjects (101). Repaglinide and nateglinide have not been associated with hepatotoxicity.

Biguanides. Metformin may be particularly useful in obese patients in whom it may cause mild weight loss (102). It is relatively contraindicated in patients with advanced liver disease or in binge drinkers because it may predispose to lactic acidosis. It is unclear whether the liver disease or alcohol is the predisposing factor. Metformin has not been reported to cause hepatotoxicity and has shown some benefit in patients with NAFLD (88–91).

α-Glucosidase inhibitors. The α-glucosidase inhibitors may be particularly useful in patients with liver disease because they act directly on the gastrointestinal tract to decrease carbohydrate digestion and thus glucose absorption, thereby decreasing postprandial hyperglycemia

A randomized double-blind trial evaluated the use of acarbose for the control of postprandial hyperglycemia in 100 patients with compensated liver cirrhosis and type 2 diabetes treated with insulin (103). Glycemic control improved significantly in both the fasting and postprandial state. In a recent placebo-controlled cross-over trial in patients with hepatic encephalopathy, acarbose significantly decreased fasting and postprandial glucose as well as A1C (104). There was also a reduction in blood ammonia levels, which paralleled an increase in bowel movement frequency. It was speculated that the increased bowel frequency favored the proliferation of saccharolytic bacteria while reducing the proliferation of proteolytic bacteria, resulting in a reduction in intestinal ammonia production.

Acarbose frequently causes mild transient elevations of ALT and, on rare occasions, severe liver disease (105–107).

While the labeling of acarbose has a warning for patients with liver disease, it appears to be safe and effective in patients with hepatic encephalopathy and type 2 diabetes. Miglitol, another α-glucosidase inhibitor, has not been associated with hepatotoxicity.

TZDs. TZDs may be especially useful because they enhance insulin sensitivity, the underlying defect in NAFLD. There has been concern about their potential hepatotoxicity because of the experience with troglitazone (since withdrawn from the U.S. market). However, in pre-approval clinical trials of rosiglitazone and pioglitazone, threefold elevations of ALT were seen with the same frequency for rosiglitazone (0.26%), pioglitazone (0.2%), and placebo (0.2 and 0.25%) (Physicians' Desk Reference 2005, Avandia Tablets and Actos Tablets). Lebovitz et al. (9) have reported that there was no difference in the incidence of liver abnormalities in patients treated with rosiglitazone, placebo, metformin, or a sulfonylurea in trials involving >5,000 patients. Rosiglitazone, in fact, decreased serum ALT by a mean of 5 units/l (9), as did pioglitazone in another trial (8). Furthermore, in the latter trial (8), serum ALT three times ULN occurred less frequently in the pioglitazone group (0.9%) than in the metformin (1.9%) or gliclazide (1.9%) groups.

The risk of acute liver failure with rosiglitazone and pioglitazone is much less than that with troglitazone (108,109). At the time of that review (109), 68 cases of "hepatitis" or "acute liver failure" due to rosiglitazone and 37 cases due to pioglitazone had been reported to the Food and Drug Administration (110–116). However, attestation as to cause was not provided, and many cases were confounded by concomitant medications and cardiovascular events (fluid retention and heart failure).

It is currently recommended that serum ALT levels be evaluated before the initiation of rosiglitzone and pioglitazone therapy and that therapy not be initiated if there is evidence of active liver disease or if the serum ALT level exceeds 2.5 times ULN (product labeling, 2005). Monitoring is recommended periodically thereafter as clinically indicated rather than every 2 months as previously recommended. Paradoxically, TZDs are emerging as the treatment of choice for NASH (92–97).

Insulin. Insulin treatment is frequently required in patients with diabetes and liver disease. Insulin requirements, however, may vary. For example, in patients

with decompensated liver disease, the requirement may be decreased due to reduced capacity for gluconeogenesis and reduced hepatic breakdown of insulin. However, patients with impaired hepatic function may have an increased need for insulin due to insulin resistance (43). Thus, careful glucose monitoring and frequent dose adjustments of insulin may be necessary.

In patients with hepatic encephalopathy who require high-carbohydrate diets, resulting in postprandial hyperglycemia, rapid-acting insulin analogs such as insulin lispro, aspart, or glulisine may be particularly useful.

Other drugs used in the management of disorders associated with type 2 diabetes

Statins are frequently used in patients with type 2 diabetes to treat hyperlipidemia and prevent cardiovascular events. Statin therapy, like all cholesterol-lowering therapy including bariatric surgery (117,118), causes minor but transient elevations in liver enzymes (119). However, the liver adapts with continuing therapy, and there are no long-term consequences of these abnormalities. Severe liver damage and liver failure are very rare (119). Paradoxically, statins are currently used to treat NAFLD (120,121), and recent studies suggest that statins are hepatoprotective in patients with HCV (122).

All of the ACE inhibitors have been implicated in hepatic injury including fulminant hepatic failure (123–126). The reactions are mostly hepatocellular, but cholestatic reactions have also been reported. Although losartan has been associated with hepatotoxicity (127) it has also been used to treat fatty liver disease (128). There are no current recommendations for hepatic monitoring of these idiosyncratic events.

Even aspirin is potentially hepatotoxic albeit at very high doses. Hepatotoxicity has not been described at doses used for cardioprotection.

MANAGEMENT OF LIVER DISEASE IN PATIENTS WITH CONCOMITANT TYPE 2 DIABETES AND LIVER DISEASE

Abnormal liver function tests
Given the fact that at least 50% of patients with type 2 diabetes have NAFLD, all patients with type 2 diabetes should have an

ALT and AST test done as part of their initial evaluation. At least 95% of patients with a confirmed minor elevation of ALT or AST have chronic liver disease independent of the degree of elevation. Thus, it is always necessary to obtain a specific diagnosis (10). The most likely etiologies of minor elevations of ALT/AST are NAFLD, hepatitis C, hepatitis B, and alcohol. Moderate social drinking, i.e., <20 g/day, does not cause an elevation of liver enzymes. The initial workup should include testing for hepatitis C (anti-HCV or HCV PCR), hepatitis B (HBV surface antigen), hemochromatosis (iron and iron saturation), and an abdominal ultrasound. Patients with hepatitis C, hepatitis B, and increased iron saturation need referral for further workup and treatment. Ultrasound has a positive predictive value of 96% for detecting NAFLD in the absence of other liver diseases (129). Unfortunately the negative predictive value is only 19%; thus, patients with a negative ultrasound will also need referral. The impact of this approach on cost of care and manpower is not known, and the cost-effectiveness of screening ALT has not been established, although the American Association for the Study of Liver Disease is now recommending yearly ALT screening for everyone.

Fatty liver disease
The diagnosis of NAFLD or NASH should be suspected in any patient with type 2 diabetes, especially if there are abnormal liver function tests. It should be specifically looked for in all obese patients with type 2 diabetes. ALT is typically elevated two- to threefold above ULN but is often normal. Mild elevations of serum alkaline phosphatase and glutamyl transferase may be present. Serum ferritin levels are frequently elevated, while iron and iron-binding capacity are normal (42,130).

Ultrasound studies may reveal a diffuse increase in echogenicity, so-called "bright" liver. The sensitivity of ultrasound in patients with elevated ALT is 89% with a specificity of 93% for detecting steatosis (131). If the ultrasound reveals fatty liver, it is appropriate to look for etiologies other than diabetes such as dyslipidemia. There are shortcomings to this approach. The sensitivity of ultrasound decreases greatly as hepatic steatosis decreases to 30% or less (132). Most patients with NAFLD found incidentally or by screening ultrasound have a normal ALT. These observations suggest that the sensitivity of ultrasound overall is really not very high. In patients with abnormal ALTs and other diseases ruled out, the positive predictive value of ultrasound is 96% but the negative predictive value only 19% (129). Magnetic resonance spectroscopy is capable of quantitative assessment of steatosis (133) but is not indicated for routine clinical practice. Thus, the gold standard for diagnosis of NAFLD remains the liver biopsy. Furthermore, the diagnosis of progressive liver disease (i.e., NASH), the precursor of cirrhosis, can only be made by liver biopsy. However, certain patients including those with reversed ALT-to-AST ratio, hypertriglyceridemia, and thrombocytopenia are at high risk for progressive disease (134,135).

Treatment of NAFLD

Most patients do not need to be treated. Only patients with biopsy-proved NASH or the risk factors listed above should be treated. Whether or not all patients need a liver biopsy is controversial in that the sensitivity of the risk factors for progressive disease is not known. It is also not known whether treatment, other than bariatric surgery, affects the ultimate prognosis. The treatment consists of measures to lose weight as well as pharmacologic intervention. There are no FDA-approved treatments and, in fact, no FDA guidelines for approving drugs for NAFLD.

Exercise and weight reduction. The initial treatment of NASH consists of weight loss and exercise, which enhance insulin sensitivity and result in reduction of steatosis (136–141). Rapid weight reduction, however, may increase necrosis, inflammation, and fibrosis (117,118,142). This paradoxical effect is thought to be due to an increase in circulating free fatty acids due to increased lipolysis seen with fasting. The ideal rate of weight loss is not known, but 1.5 kg/week has been recommended (143). The ideal content of the diet is not known. However, saturated fatty acids increase insulin resistance, and for that reason a Mediterranean diet, i.e., a diet enriched with monounsaturated fatty acids and low-glycemic carbohydrates, seems reasonable (82,83). Recent studies have demonstrated that bariatric surgery either improves or completely reverses steatosis in patients with obesity with or without diabetes (141,144).

Pharmacologic therapy. Pharmacologic therapy of NAFLD is evolving. While many studies have shown improvement in steatosis, there are neither long-term

studies to determine whether they alter the natural history of the disease nor studies to indicate whether relapse occurs after treatment withdrawal. Gemfibrozil (145), vitamin E (146), metformin (88–91), betaine (147), pioglitazone (92–96), rosiglitazone (97), atorvastatin (120, 121), losartan (128), orlistat (148), and pentoxifylline (149) have all been tried and have all been shown in small trials to improve liver enzymes. Modest histologic improvement over 6–12 months is seen with some of the agents. Long-term outcome trials with the various treatment modalities are yet to be completed.

Given that insulin resistance is central to the pathogenesis of NAFLD, insulin-sensitizing agents should have utility (even in the absence of diabetes), and there is increasing evidence that they do (80–90,92–97). Five studies using pioglitazone from 16 to 48 weeks have been published, and a large multicenter placebo-controlled trial is near completion (94). All have shown improvement in serum ALT and most in histology (92–96). One study showed an increase in adiponectin, a decrease in A1C, enhanced insulin sensitivity, and improved hepatic histology including steatosis, inflammation, and fibrosis (150). There have been three trials including a placebo-controlled trial with rosiglitazone (97,151,152). A 24-week study with rosiglitazone showed histologic improvement (97). In another study of 30 patients treated with rosiglitazone 8 mg/day for 48 weeks, there was significant improvement in ALT, AST, γ-glutamyl transferase, and insulin sensitivity. Of the 22 patients who had histologic evaluation, steatosis improved in 13, and fibrosis improved in 8 (152). This study was confounded by the use of statins. Interestingly, in the recently presented French multicenter trial known as FLIRT (French Multicenter Trail), ~50% of the patients had ALT and/or histologic improvement, but nondiabetic patients were more likely than diabetic patients to respond (153).

Metformin has shown mixed results in human trials (88–91) with some improvement in ALT but not in histology. Two long-term trials initiated by the National Institutes of Health are underway. At this time, treatment with metformin is not recommended outside of clinical trials. In the meantime, it seems reasonable to treat patients with NASH and type 2 diabetes with TZDs, recognizing that the patients may gain weight. In the absence of a histologic diagnosis of NASH, only

those with risk factors for progressive disease as mentioned above should be treated. TZDs, despite shortcomings, are emerging as the treatment of choice even in the absence of diabetes.

Three prospective controlled studies using ursodeoxycholic acid, which reduces apoptosis and has cytoprotective properties, have been conducted. The results have been mixed (121,154,155). There is increasing interest in this agent because of its antiapoptotic effect as nonspecific or add-on therapy.

Statins may reduce hepatic fat content in patients with hyperlipidemia and NASH (120,121). Atorvastatin and ursodeoxycholic acid were evaluated in a small comparative trial of 44 obese adults with NASH, including 10 patients with diabetes. Normolipidemic patients received ursodeoxycholic acid, 13–15 mg · kg^{-1} · day^{-1}, and hyperlipidemic patients received atorvastatin, 10 mg daily for 6 months. Liver chemistries improved in both groups; however, an increase in liver density, suggesting a decrease in fat content, occurred only in the atorvastatin group.

Oxidative stress has been shown to be important in the pathogenesis of NASH. It seems reasonable, therefore, to try therapy with antioxidants. Pilot studies with vitamin E have been conducted (146,156–158) with promising results, but a meta-analysis of high-dose vitamin E revealed an increase in overall mortality (159).

TNF-α is proinflammatory and increased in NASH. Pentoxifylline is a methylxanthine compound that inhibits TNF-α. It is used in the treatment of alcoholic hepatitis. A pilot study (149) has shown improvement in liver enzymes in patients with NASH. However, the high incidence of side effects led to early withdrawal in many patients, and it seems unlikely that it will find a place in the treatment of NASH.

In summary, the ideal therapy for NAFLD is yet to be identified, and no evidence-based recommendations can be made. Outside of clinical trials, therapy should be directed toward the underlying etiology.

Hepatitis C. The most effective treatment of HCV is a combination of pegylated α-interferon and ribavirin (160). Interferon, however, affects insulin sensitivity and glucose tolerance. Studies in nondiabetic patients report that interferon impairs glucose tolerance (161–163). A recent trial, however, failed to detect a difference in insulin sensitivity and glucose tolerance after 6 months of interferon treatment (164), while another study reported that fasting plasma glucose and fasting immunoreactive insulin decreased during interferon treatment (72). The practical implications of the observed changes in glucose homeostasis in patients being treated with interferon are not known. Given the unpredictable effect of interferon in diabetes, it is reasonable to monitor diabetes carefully when using interferon.

SUMMARY — Type 2 diabetes is associated with a large number of liver disorders including elevated liver enzymes, fatty liver disease, cirrhosis, hepatocellular carcinoma, and acute liver failure. In addition, there is an unexplained association with HCV. The SMR for cirrhosis is higher than that for CVD in type 2 diabetes. Many consider NAFLD to be part of the insulin resistance syndrome. However, the presence of liver disease (unless decompensated) has little implication for the specific treatment of diabetes, and the presence of diabetes has little implication for the specific treatment of liver disease. Patients with decompensated liver disease are more susceptible to hypoglycemia and require careful monitoring. There continues to be a need for long-term placebo-controlled trials for the treatment of NAFLD and for the treatment of diabetes in patients with liver disease.

References

1. http://diabetes.niddk.nih.gov/dm/pubs/statistics. Accessed 30 July 2005
2. Geiss LS, Herman WH, Smith PJ: Mortality in non-insulin dependent diabetes. In *Diabetes in America*. 2nd Edition, 1995 p. 233–252 (NIH publ. no. 95-1468)
3. de Marco R, Locatelli F, Zoppini G, Verlato G, Bonora E, Muggeo M: Cause-specific mortality in type 2 diabetes: The Verona Diabetes Study. *Diabetes Care* 22:756–761, 1999
4. Balkau B, Eschwege E, Ducimetiere P, Richard JL, Warnet JM: The high risk of death by alcohol related diseases in subjects diagnosed as diabetic and impaired glucose tolerant: the Paris Prospective Study after 15 years of follow-up. *J Clin Epidemiol* 44:465–474, 1991
5. Caldwell SH, Oelsner DH, Iezzoni JC, Hespenheide EE, Battle EH, Driscoll CJ: Cryptogenic cirrhosis: clinical characterization and risk factors for underlying disease. *Hepatology* 29:664–669, 1999
6. The U.S. Organ Procurement and Transplantation Network and the Scientific Registry of Transplant Recipients: OPTN/SRTR annual report: table 9.4a: transplant recipient characteristics, 1995 to 2004: recipients of deceased donor livers [Internet], 2 May 2005. Available from http://www.optn.org/AR2005/904a_rec-dgn_li.htm. Ann Arbor, MI. Accessed on 1 September 2006
7. Trombetta M, Spiazzi G, Zoppini G, Muggeo M: Review article: type 2 diabetes and chronic liver disease in the Verona diabetes study. *Aliment Pharmacol Ther* 22 (Suppl. 2):24–27, 2005
8. Belcher G, Schernthaner G: Changes in liver tests during 1-year treatment of patients with type 2 diabetes with pioglitazone, metformin or gliclazide. *Diabet Med* 22:973–979, 2005
9. Lebovitz HE, Kreider M, Freed MI: Evaluation of liver function in type 2 diabetic patients during clinical trials: evidence that rosiglitazone does not cause hepatic dysfunction. *Diabetes Care* 25:815–821, 2002
10. Hultcrantz R, Glaumann H, Lindberg G, Nilsson LH: Liver investigation in 149 asymptomatic patients with moderately elevated activities of serum aminotransferases. *Scand J Gastroenterol* 21:109–113, 1986
11. Harris MI, Flegal KM, Cowie CC, Eberhardt MS, Goldstein DE, Little RR, Wiedmeyer HM, Byrd-Holt DD: Prevalence of diabetes, impaired fasting glucose, and impaired glucose tolerance in U.S. adults: the Third National Health and Nutrition Examination Survey, 1988–1994. *Diabetes Care* 21:518–524, 1998
12. Ludwig J, Viggiano TR, McGill DB, Oh BJ: Nonalcoholic steatohepatitis: Mayo Clinic experiences with a hitherto unnamed disease. *Mayo Clin Proc* 55:434–438, 1980
13. Powell EE, Cooksley WG, Hanson R, Searle J, Halliday JW, Powell LW: The natural history of nonalcoholic steatohepatitis: a follow-up study of forty-two patients for up to 21 years. *Hepatology* 11:74–80, 1990
14. Lee RG: Nonalcoholic steatohepatitis: a study of 49 patients. *Hum Pathol* 20:594–598, 1989
15. Itoh S, Yougel T, Kawagoe K: Comparison between nonalcoholic steatohepatitis and alcoholic hepatitis. *Am J Gastroenterol* 82:650–654, 1987
16. Diehl AM, Goodman Z, Ishak KG: Alcohol-like liver disease in nonalcoholics: a clinical and histologic comparison with alcohol-induced liver injury. *Gastroenterology* 95:1056–1062, 1988
17. Pinto HC, Baptista A, Camilo ME, Valente A, Saragoca A, de Moura MC: Nonalcoholic steatohepatitis: clinicopathological comparison with alcoholic hepatitis in ambulatory and hospitalized patients. *Dig Dis Sci* 41:172–179, 1996
18. Silverman JF, O'Brien KF, Long S, Leggett N, Khazanie PG, Pories WJ, Norris HT, Caro JF: Liver pathology in morbidly obese patients with and without diabetes. *Am J Gastroenterol* 85:1349–1355, 1990
19. Wanless IR, Lentz JS: Fatty liver hepatitis (steatohepatitis) and obesity: an autopsy study with analysis of risk factors. *Hepatology* 12:1106–1110, 1990
20. Teli MR, James OF, Burt AD, Bennett MK, Day CP: The natural history of nonalcoholic fatty liver: a follow-up study. *Hepatology* 22:1714–1719, 1995
21. Matteoni CA, Younossi ZM, Gramlich T, Boparai N, Liu YC, McCullough AJ: Nonalcoholic fatty liver disease: a spectrum of clinical and pathological severity. *Gastroenterology* 116:1413–1419, 1999
22. Marchesini G, Bugianesi E, Forlani G, Cerrelli F, Lenzi M, Manini R, Natale S, Vanni E, Villanova N, Melchionda N, Rizzetto M: Nonalcoholic fatty liver, steatohepatitis, and the metabolic syndrome. *Hepatology* 37:917–923, 2003
23. Silverman JF, O'Brien KF, Long S, Leggett N, Khazanie PG, Pories WJ, Norris HT, Caro JF: Liver pathology in morbidly obese patients with and without diabetes. *Am J Gastroenterol* 85:1349–1355, 1990
24. Cassader M, Gambino R, Musso G, Depetris N, Mecca F, Cavallo-Perin P, Pacini G, Rizzetto M, Pagano G: Postprandial triglyceride-rich lipoprotein metabolism and insulin sensitivity in nonalcoholic steatohepatitis patients. *Lipids* 36:1117–1124, 2001
25. Marchesini G, Brizi M, Morselli-Labate AM, Bianchi G, Bugianesi E, McCullough AJ, Forlani G, Melchionda N: Association of nonalcoholic fatty liver disease with insulin resistance. *Am J Med* 107:450–455, 1999
26. Angulo P: Nonalcoholic fatty liver disease. *N Engl J Med* 346:1221–1231, 2002
27. Chitturi S, Abeygunasekera S, Farrell GC, Holmes-Walker J, Hui JM, Fung C, Karim R, Lin R, Samarasinghe D, Liddle C, Weltman M, George J: NASH and insulin resistance: insulin hypersecretion and specific association with the insulin resistance syndrome. *Hepatology* 35:373–379, 2002
28. Crespo J, Cayon A, Fernandez-Gil P, Hernandez-Guerra M, Mayorga M, Dominguez-Diez A, Fernandez-Escalante JC, Pons-Romero F: Gene expression of tumor necrosis factor alpha and TNF-receptors, p55 and p75, in nonalcoholic steatohepatitis patients. *Hepatology* 34:1158–1163, 2001
29. Hui JM, Farrell GC: Clear messages from sonographic shadows?: links between metabolic disorders and liver disease, and what to do about them. *J Gastroenterol Hepatol* 18:1115–1117, 2003

30. Kugelmas M, Hill DB, Vivian B, Marsano L, McClain CJ: Cytokines and NASH: a pilot study of the effects of lifestyle modification and vitamin E. *Hepatology* 38:413–419, 2003

31. Wigg AJ, Roberts-Thomson IC, Dymock RB, McCarthy PJ, Grose RH, Cummins AG: The role of small intestinal bacterial overgrowth, intestinal permeability, endotoxaemia, and tumour necrosis factor alpha in the pathogenesis of non-alcoholic steatohepatitis. *Gut* 48:206–211, 2001

32. Hui JM, Hodge A, Farrell GC, Kench JG, Kriketos A, George J: Beyond insulin resistance in NASH: TNF-alpha or adiponectin? *Hepatology* 40:46–54, 2004

33. Crespo J, Cayon A, Fernandez-Gil P, Hernandez-Guerra M, Mayorga M, Dominguez-Diez A, Fernandez-Escalante JC, Pons-Romero F: Gene expression of tumor necrosis factor alpha and TNF-receptors, p55 and p75, in nonalcoholic steatohepatitis patients. *Hepatology* 34:1158–1163, 2001

34. Weyer C, Funahashi T, Tanaka S, Hotta K, Matsuzawa Y, Pratley RE, Tataranni PA: Hypoadiponectinemia in obesity and type 2 diabetes: close association with insulin resistance and hyperinsulinemia. *J Clin Endocrinol Metab* 86:1930–1935, 2001

35. Arita Y, Kihara S, Ouchi N, Takahashi M, Maeda K, Miyagawa J, Hotta K, Shimomura I, Nakamura T, Miyaoka K, Kuriyama H, Nishida M, Yamashita S, Okubo K, Matsubara K, Muraguchi M, Ohmoto Y, Funahashi T, Matsuzawa Y: Paradoxical decrease of an adipose-specific protein, adiponectin, in obesity. *Biochem Biophys Res Commun* 257:79–83, 1999

36. Hotta K, Funahashi T, Arita Y, Takahashi M, Matsuda M, Okamoto Y, Iwahashi H, Kuriyama H, Ouchi N, Maeda K, Nishida M, Kihara S, Sakai N, Nakajima T, Hasegawa K, Muraguchi M, Ohmoto Y, Nakamura T, Yamashita S, Hanafusa T, Matsuzawa Y: Plasma concentrations of a novel, adipose-specific protein, adiponectin, in type 2 diabetic patients. *Arterioscler Thromb Vasc Biol* 20:1595–1599, 2000

37. Hotta K, Funahashi T, Bodkin NL, Ortmeyer HK, Arita Y, Hansen BC, Matsuzawa Y: Circulating concentrations of the adipocyte protein adiponectin are decreased in parallel with reduced insulin sensitivity during the progression to type 2 diabetes in rhesus monkeys. *Diabetes* 50:1126–1133, 2001

38. Weltman MD, Farrell GC, Hall P, Ingelman-Sundberg M, Liddle C: Hepatic cytochrome P450 2E1 is increased in patients with nonalcoholic steatohepatitis. *Hepatology* 27:128–133, 1998

39. Esterbauer H, Schaur RJ, Zollner H: Chemistry and biochemistry of 4-hydroxynonenal, malonaldehyde and related aldehydes. *Free Radic Biol Med* 11:81–128, 1991

40. Zatloukal K, Bock G, Rainer I, Denk H, Weber K: High molecular weight components are main constituents of Mallory bodies isolated with a fluorescence activated cell sorter. *Lab Invest* 64:200–206, 1991

41. Leonarduzzi G, Scavazza A, Biasi F, Chiarpotto E, Camandola S, Vogel S, Dargel R, Poli G: The lipid peroxidation end product 4-hydroxy-2,3-nonenal upregulates transforming growth factor beta1 expression in the macrophage lineage: a link between oxidative injury and fibrosclerosis. *Faseb J* 11:851–857, 1997

42. Bacon BR, Farahvash MJ, Janney CG, Neuschwander-Tetri BA: Nonalcoholic steatohepatitis: an expanded clinical entity. *Gastroenterology* 107:1103–1109, 1994

43. Petrides AS: Liver disease and diabetes mellitus. *Diabet Rev* 2:2–18, 1994

44. Baig NA, Herrine SK, Rubin R: Liver disease and diabetes mellitus. *Clin Lab Med* 21:193–207, 2001

45. Adami HO, Chow WH, Nyren O, Berne C, Linet MS, Ekbom A, Wolk A, McLaughlin JK, Fraumeni JF Jr: Excess risk of primary liver cancer in patients with diabetes mellitus. *J Natl Cancer Inst* 88:1472–1477, 1996

46. Wideroff L, Gridley G, Mellemkjaer L, Chow WH, Linet M, Keehn S, Borch-Johnsen K, Olsen JH: Cancer incidence in a population-based cohort of patients hospitalized with diabetes mellitus in Denmark. *J Natl Cancer Inst* 89:1360–1365, 1997

47. Fujino Y, Mizoue T, Tokui N, Yoshimura T: Prospective study of diabetes mellitus and liver cancer in Japan. *Diabetes Metab Res Rev* 17:374–379, 2001

48. El-Serag HB, Tran T, Everhart JE, Kaserer K, Fiedler R, Steindl P, Muller CH, Wrba F, Ferenci P, Rubbia-Brandt L, Leandro G, Spahr L, Giostra E, Quadri R, Male PJ, Negro F, Hui JM, Kench J, Farrell GC, Lin R, Samarasinghe D, Liddle C, Byth K, George J, Castera L, Hezode C, Roudot-Thoraval F, Lonjon I, Zafrani ES, Pawlotsky JM, Dhumeaux D, Lonardo A, Adinolfi LE, Loria P, Carulli N, Ruggiero G, Day CP: Diabetes increases the risk of chronic liver disease and hepatocellular carcinoma. *Gastroenterology* 126:460–468, 2004

49. Kazachkov Y, Yoffe B, Khaoustov VI, Solomon H, Klintmalm GB, Tabor E: Microsatellite instability in human hepatocellular carcinoma: relationship to p53 abnormalities. *Liver* 18:156–161, 1998

50. Macdonald GA, Greenson JK, Saito K, Cherian SP, Appelman HD, Boland CR: Microsatellite instability and loss of heterozygosity at DNA mismatch repair gene loci occurs during hepatic carcinogenesis. *Hepatology* 28:90–97, 1998

51. Morgan DO, Edman JC, Standring DN, Fried VA, Smith MC, Roth RA, Rutter WJ: Insulin-like growth factor II receptor as a multifunctional binding protein. *Nature* 329:301–307, 1987

52. Kishimoto Y, Shiota G, Wada K, Kitano M, Nakamoto K, Kamisaki Y, Suou T, Itoh T, Kawasaki H: Frequent loss in chromosome 8p loci in liver cirrhosis accompanying hepatocellular carcinoma. *J Cancer Res Clin Oncol* 122:585–589, 1996

53. El-Serag HB, Everhart JE: Diabetes increases the risk of acute hepatic failure. *Gastroenterology* 122:1822–1828, 2002

54. Chan KA, Truman A, Gurwitz JH, Hurley JS, Martinson B, Platt R, Everhart JE, Moseley RH, Terrault N, Ackerson L, Selby JV: A cohort study of the incidence of serious acute liver injury in diabetic patients treated with hypoglycemic agents. *Arch Intern Med* 163:728–734, 2003

55. Gray H, Wreghitt T, Stratton IM, Alexander GJ, Turner RC, O'Rahilly S: High prevalence of hepatitis C infection in Afro-Caribbean patients with type 2 diabetes and abnormal liver function tests. *Diabet Med* 12:244–249, 1995

56. Simo R, Hernandez C, Genesca J, Jardi R, Mesa J: High prevalence of hepatitis C virus infection in diabetic patients. *Diabetes Care* 19:998–1000, 1996

57. Allison ME, Wreghitt T, Palmer CR, Alexander GJ: Evidence for a link between hepatitis C virus infection and diabetes mellitus in a cirrhotic population. *J Hepatol* 21:1135–1139, 1994

58. Ozyilkan E, Arslan M: Increased prevalence of diabetes mellitus in patients with chronic hepatitis C virus infection. *Am J Gastroenterol* 91:1480–1481, 1996

59. Lonardo A, Adinolfi LE, Loria P, Carulli N, Ruggiero G, Day CP: Steatosis and hepatitis C virus: mechanisms and significance for hepatic and extrahepatic disease. *Gastroenterology* 126:586–597, 2004

60. Mason AL, Lau JY, Hoang N, Qian K, Alexander GJ, Xu L, Guo L, Jacob S, Regenstein FG, Zimmerman R, Everhart JE, Wasserfall C, Maclaren NK, Perrillo RP: Association of diabetes mellitus and chronic hepatitis C virus infection. *Hepatology* 29:328–333, 1999

61. Knobler H, Stagnaro-Green A, Wallenstein S, Schwartz M, Roman SH: Higher incidence of diabetes in liver transplant recipients with hepatitis C. *J Clin Gastroenterol* 26:30–33, 1998

62. Mehta SH, Brancati FL, Sulkowski MS, Strathdee SA, Szklo M, Thomas DL: Prevalence of type 2 diabetes mellitus among persons with hepatitis C virus infection in the United States. *Ann Intern Med* 133:592–599, 2000

63. Mehta SH, Brancati FL, Strathdee SA, Pankow JS, Netski D, Coresh J, Szklo M, Thomas DL: Hepatitis C virus infection and incident type 2 diabetes. *Hepatology* 38:50–56, 2003

64. Cantley LC: The phosphoinositide 3-kinase pathway. *Science* 296:1655–1657, 2002

65. Kawaguchi T, Yoshida T, Harada M, Hisamoto T, Nagao Y, Ide T, Taniguchi E, Kumemura H, Hanada S, Maeyama M, Baba S, Koga H, Kumashiro R, Ueno T, Ogata H, Yoshimura A, Sata M: Hepatitis C virus down-regulates insulin receptor substrates 1 and 2 through upregulation of suppressor of cytokine signaling 3. *Am J Pathol* 165:1499–1508, 2004

66. Rubbia-Brandt L, Leandro G, Spahr L, Giostra E, Quadri R, Male PJ, Negro F: Liver steatosis in chronic hepatitis C: a morphological sign suggesting infection with HCV genotype 3. *Histopathology* 39:119–124, 2001

67. Hui JM, Kench J, Farrell GC, Lin R, Samarasinghe D, Liddle C, Byth K, George J: Genotype-specific mechanisms for hepatic steatosis in chronic hepatitis C infection. *J Gastroenterol Hepatol* 17:873–881, 2002

68. Di Fiore F, Charbonnier F, Martin C, Frerot S, Olschwang S, Wang Q, Boisson C, Buisine MP, Nilbert M, Lindblom A, Frebourg T: Screening for genomic rearrangements of the MMR genes must be included in the routine diagnosis of HNPCC. *J Med Genet* 41:18–20, 2004

69. Durante-Mangoni E, Zampino R, Marrone A, Tripodi MF, Rinaldi L, Restivo L, Cioffi M, Ruggiero G, Adinolfi LE: Hepatic steatosis and insulin resistance are associated with serum imbalance of adiponectin/tumour necrosis factor-alpha in chronic hepatitis C patients. *Aliment Pharmacol Ther* 24:1349–1357, 2006

70. Sabile A, Perlemuter G, Bono F, Kohara K, Demaugre F, Kohara M, Matsuura Y, Miyamura T, Brechot C, Barba G: Hepatitis C virus core protein binds to apolipoprotein AII and its secretion is modulated by fibrates. *Hepatology* 30:1064–1076, 1999

71. Okuda M, Li K, Beard MR, Showalter LA, Scholle F, Lemon SM, Weinman SA: Mitochondrial injury, oxidative stress, and antioxidant gene expression are induced by hepatitis C virus core protein. *Gastroenterology* 122:366–375, 2002

72. Tanaka H, Shiota G, Kawasaki H: Changes in glucose tolerance after interferon-alpha therapy in patients with chronic hepatitis C. *J Med* 28:335–346, 1997

73. Konrad T, Zeuzem S, Vicini P, Toffolo G, Briem D, Lormann J, Herrmann G, Berger A, Kusterer K, Teuber G, Cobelli C, Usadel KH: Evaluation of factors controlling glucose tolerance in patients with HCV infection before and after 4 months therapy with interferon-alpha. *Eur J Clin Invest* 30:111–121, 2000

74. Castera L, Hezode C, Roudot-Thoraval F, Lonjon I, Zafrani ES, Pawlotsky JM, Dhumeaux D: Effect of antiviral treatment on evolution of liver steatosis in patients with chronic hepatitis C: indirect evidence of a role of hepatitis C virus genotype 3 in steatosis. *Gut* 53:420–424, 2004

75. Fabris P, Floreani A, Tositti G, Vergani D, De Lalla F, Betterle C: Type 1 diabetes mellitus in patients with chronic hepatitis C before and after interferon therapy. *Aliment Pharmacol Ther* 18:549–558, 2003

76. Huang MA, Greenson JK, Chao C, Anderson L, Peterman D, Jacobson J, Emick D, Lok AS, Conjeevaram HS: One-year intense nutritional counseling results in histological improvement in patients with non-alcoholic steatohepatitis: a pilot study. *Am J Gastroenterol* 100:1072–1081, 2005

77. Suzuki A, Lindor K, St Saver J, Lymp J, Mendes F, Muto A, Okada T, Angulo P: Effect of changes on body weight and lifestyle in nonalcoholic fatty liver disease. *J Hepatol* 43:1060–1066, 2005

78. Petersen KF, Dufour S, Befroy D, Lehrke M, Hendler RE, Shulman GI: Reversal of nonalcoholic hepatic steatosis, hepatic insulin resistance, and hyperglycemia by moderate weight reduction in patients with type 2 diabetes. *Diabetes* 54:603–608, 2005

79. Douketis JD, Feightner JW, Attia J, Feldman WF: Periodic health examination, 1999 update. I. Detection, prevention and treatment of obesity: Canadian Task Force on Preventive Health Care. *Cmaj* 160:513–525, 1999

80. Kang H, Greenson JK, Omo JT, Chao C, Peterman D, Anderson L, Foess-Wood L, Sherbondy MA, Conjeevaram HS: Metabolic syndrome is associated with greater histologic severity, higher carbohydrate, and lower fat diet in patients with NAFLD. *Am J Gastroenterol* 101:2247–2253, 2006

81. Solga S, Alkhuraishe AR, Clark JM, Torbenson M, Greenwald A, Diehl AM, Magnuson T: Dietary composition and nonalcoholic fatty liver disease. *Dig Dis Sci* 49:1578–1583, 2004

82. Esposito K, Marfella R, Ciotola M, Di Palo C, Giugliano F, Giugliano G, D'Armiento M, D'Andrea F, Giugliano D: Effect of a Mediterranean-style diet on endothelial dysfunction and markers of vascular inflammation in the metabolic syndrome: a randomized trial. *JAMA* 292:1440–1446, 2004

83. Musso G, Gambino R, De Michieli F, Cassader M, Rizzetto M, Durazzo M, Faga E, Silli B, Pagano G: Dietary habits and their relations to insulin resistance and postprandial lipemia in nonalcoholic steatohepatitis. *Hepatology* 37:909–916, 2003

84. Petrides AS, Vogt C, Schulze-Berge D, Matthews D, Strohmeyer G: Pathogenesis of glucose intolerance and diabetes mellitus in cirrhosis. *Hepatology* 19:616–627, 1994

85. Marks V, Teale JD: Drug-induced hypoglycemia. *Endocrinol Metab Clin North Am* 28:555–577, 1999

86. Burge MR, Zeise TM, Sobhy TA, Rassam AG, Schade DS: Low-dose ethanol predisposes elderly fasted patients with type 2 diabetes to sulfonylurea-induced low blood glucose. *Diabetes Care* 22:2037–2043, 1999

87. Zimmerman HJ: Drug-induced liver disease. In *Hepatotoxicity: The Adverse Effects of Drugs and Other Chemicals on the Liver*. 2nd ed. Philadelphia, Lippincott Williams and Williams, 1991, p. 430

88. Nair S, Diehl AM, Wiseman M, Farr GH, Jr., Perrillo RP: Metformin in the treatment of non-alcoholic steatohepatitis: a pilot open label trial. *Aliment Pharmacol Ther* 20:23–28, 2004

89. Marchesini G, Brizi M, Bianchi G, Tomassetti S, Zoli M, Melchionda N: Metformin in non-alcoholic steatohepatitis. *Lancet* 358:893–894, 2001

90. Uygun A, Kadayifci A, Isik AT, Ozgurtas T, Deveci S, Tuzun A, Yesilova Z, Gulsen M, Dagalp K: Metformin in the treatment of patients with non-alcoholic steatohepatitis. *Aliment Pharmacol Ther* 19:537–544, 2004

91. Nair S, Diehl AM, Perille R: Metformin in non-alchoholic steatohepatitis: efficacy and safety: a preliminary report (Abstract). *Gastroenterology* 122 (Suppl. 2) 2002

92. Bajaj M, Suraamornkul S, Pratipanawatr T, Hardies LJ, Pratipanawatr W, Glass L, Cersosimo E, Miyazaki Y, DeFronzo RA: Pioglitazone reduces hepatic fat content and augments splanchnic glucose uptake in patients with type 2 diabetes. *Diabetes* 52:1364–1370, 2003

93. Freedman R, Uwaifo G, Lutchman G, Kittichaipromrat., Park Y, Kleiner D, Yanovski J, Hoofnagle J: Changes in insulin sensitivity and improvements in liver histology in patients with nonalcoholic steatohepatitis (NASH) treated with pioglitazone (PIO) (Abstract). *Diabetes* 52 (Suppl. 1):A76, 2003

94. Harrison S, Belfort R, Brown K, Darland C, Finch J, Fincke C, Havranek R, Hardies J, Dwivedi S, Berria R, Tio F, Schenker S, Cusi K: A double-blind, placebo-controlled trial of pioglitazone in the treatment of non-alcoholic steatohepatitis (NASH) (Abstract). *Gastroenterology* 128 (Suppl 2):A681, 2005

95. Acosta R, Molina E, O'Brien C, Cobo M, Amaro R, Neff G, Schiff E: The use of pioglitazone in non-alcoholic steato-

hepatitis (Abstract). *Gastroenterology* 120 (Suppl. 1):A-546, 2001

96. Promrat K, Lutchman G, Uwaifo GI, Freedman RJ, Soza A, Heller T, Doo E, Ghany M, Premkumar A, Park Y, Liang TJ, Yanovski JA, Kleiner DE, Hoofnagle JH: A pilot study of pioglitazone treatment for nonalcoholic steatohepatitis. *Hepatology* 39:188–196, 2004

97. Neuschwander-Tetri BA, Brunt EM, Wehmeier KR, Sponseller CA, Hampton K, Bacon BR: Interim results of a pilot study demonstrating the early effects of the PPAR-gamma ligand rosiglitazone on insulin sensitivity, aminotransferases, hepatic steatosis and body weight in patients with non-alcoholic steatohepatitis. *J Hepatol* 38:434–440, 2003

98. Frier BM, Stewart WK: Cholestatic jaundice following chlorpropamide self-poisoning. *Clin Toxicol* 11:13–17, 1977

99. Gupta R, Sachar DB: Chlorpropamide-induced cholestatic jaundice and pseudomembranous colitis. *Am J Gastroenterol* 80:381–383, 1985

100. Reichel J, Goldberg S, Ellenberg M, Schaffner F: Intrahepatic cholestasis following administration of chlorpropamide: report of a case with electron microscope observations. *Am J Med* 28:654, 1960

101. Choudhury S, Hirschberg Y, Filipek R, Lasseter K, McLeod JF: Single-dose pharmacokinetics of nateglinide in subjects with hepatic cirrhosis. *J Clin Pharmacol* 40:634–640, 2000

102. Bailey CJ, Turner RC: Metformin. *N Engl J Med* 334:574–579, 1996

103. Gentile S, Turco S, Guarino G, Oliviero B, Annunziata S, Cozzolino D, Sasso FC, Turco A, Salvatore T, Torella R: Effect of treatment with acarbose and insulin in patients with non-insulin-dependent diabetes mellitus associated with non-alcoholic liver cirrhosis. *Diabetes Obes Metab* 3:33–40, 2001

104. Gentile S, Guarino G, Romano M, Alagia IA, Fierro M, Annunziata S, Magliano PL, Gravina AG, Torella R: A randomized controlled trial of acarbose in hepatic encephalopathy. *Clin Gastroenterol Hepatol* 3:184–191, 2005

105. Andrade RJ, Lucena MI, Rodriguez-Mendizabal M: Hepatic injury caused by acarbose. *Ann Intern Med* 124:931, 1996

106. Carrascosa M, Pascual F, Aresti S: Acarbose-induced acute severe hepatotoxicity (Letter). *Lancet* 349:698, 1998

107. Diaz-Gutierrez FL, Ladero JM, Diaz-Rubio M: Acarbose-induced acute hepatitis. *Am J Gastroenterol* 93:481, 1998

108. Zawadski J, Green L, Graham B: Troglitazone-associated 15-month post-marketing hepatotoxicity: FDA science forum [article online]. Available from http://www.cfsan.fda.gov~frf/forum 02/a 187 ab4.htm. Accessed 5 February 5 2002

109. Tolman KG, Fonseca V, Tan MH, Dalpiaz A: Narrative review: hepatobiliary disease in type 2 diabetes mellitus. *Ann Intern Med* 141:946–956, 2004

110. Bonkovsky HL, Azar R, Bird S, Szabo G, Banner B: Severe cholestatic hepatitis caused by thiazolidinediones: risks associated with substituting rosiglitazone for troglitazone. *Dig Dis Sci* 47:1632–1637, 2002

111. Al-Jalman J, Arjomand H, Kemp DG, Mittal M: Hepatocellular injury in a patient receiving rosiglitazone: a case report. *Ann Intern Med* 132:121–124, 2000

112. Forman LM, Simmons DA, Diamond RH: Hepatic failure in a patient taking rosiglitazone. *Ann Intern Med* 132:118–121, 2000

113. Gouda HE, Khan A, Schwartz J, Cohen RI: Liver failure in a patient treated with long-term rosiglitazone therapy. *Am J Med* 111:584–585, 2001

114. Chase MP, Yarze JC: Pioglitazone-associated fulminant hepatic failure. *Am J Gastroenterol* 97:502–503, 2002

115. Maeda K: Hepatocellular injury in a patient receiving pioglitazone. *Ann Intern Med* 135:306, 2001

116. May LD, Lefkowitch JH, Kram MT, Rubin DE: Mixed hepatocellular-cholestatic liver injury after pioglitazone therapy. *Ann Intern Med* 136:449–452, 2002

117. Andersen T, Gluud C, Franzmann MB, Christoffersen P: Hepatic effects of dietary weight loss in morbidly obese subjects. *J Hepatol* 12:224–229, 1991

118. Drenick EJ, Simmons F, Murphy JF: Effect on hepatic morphology of treatment of obesity by fasting, reducing diets and small-bowel bypass. *N Engl J Med* 282:829–834, 1970

119. Tolman KG: The liver and lovastatin. *Am J Cardiol* 89:1374–1380, 2002

120. Horlander J, Kwo P, Cummings O: Atorvastatin for the treatment of NASH (Abstract). *Gastroenterology* 5:A-544 , 2001

121. Kiyici M, Gulten M, Gurel S, Nak SG, Dolar E, Savci G, Adim SB, Yerci O, Memik F: Ursodeoxycholic acid and atorvastatin in the treatment of nonalcoholic steatohepatitis. *Can J Gastroenterol* 17:713–718, 2003

122. Chalasani N, Aljadhey H, Kesterson J, Murray MD, Hall SD: Patients with elevated liver enzymes are not at higher risk for statin hepatotoxicity. *Gastroenterology* 126:1287–1292, 2004

123. Putterman C, Livshitz T: Captopril-induced liver dysfunction. *Harefuah* 121:92–93, 1991 [article in Hebrew]

124. Shionoiri H, Nomura S, Oda H,: Hepatitis associated with captopril and enalapril but not with delapril in a patient with congestive heart failure receiving chronic hemodialysis. *Curr Ther Res* 42:1171–1176, 1986

125. Rosellini SR, Costa PL, Gaudio M, Saragoni A, Miglio F: Hepatic injury related to enalapril (Letter). *Gastroenterology* 97:810, 1989

126. Larrey D, Babany G, Bernuau J, Andrieux J, Degott C, Pessayre D, Benhamou JP: Fulminant hepatitis after lisinopril administration. *Gastroenterology* 99:1832–1833, 1990

127. Tabak F, Mert A, Ozaras R, Biyikli M, Ozturk R, Ozbay G, Senturk H, Aktuglu Y: Losartan-induced hepatic injury. *J Clin Gastroenterol* 34:585–586, 2002

128. Yokohama S, Yoneda M, Haneda M, Okamoto S, Okada M, Aso K, Hasegawa T, Tokusashi Y, Miyokawa N, Nakamura K: Therapeutic efficacy of an angiotensin II receptor antagonist in patients with nonalcoholic steatohepatitis. *Hepatology* 40:1222–1225, 2004

129. Lavine JE, Schwimmer JB: Nonalcoholic fatty liver disease in the pediatric population. *Clin Liver Dis* 8:549–558, viii–ix, 2004

130. Angulo P, Keach JC, Batts KP, Lindor KD: Independent predictors of liver fibrosis in patients with nonalcoholic steatohepatitis. *Hepatology* 30:1356–1362, 1999

131. Joseph AE, Saverymuttu SH, al-Sam S, Cook MG, Maxwell JD: Comparison of liver histology with ultrasonography in assessing diffuse parenchymal liver disease. *Clin Radiol* 43:26–31, 1991

132. Saadeh S, Younossi ZM, Remer EM, Gramlich T, Ong JP, Hurley M, Mullen KD, Cooper JN, Sheridan MJ: The utility of radiological imaging in nonalcoholic fatty liver disease. *Gastroenterology* 123:745–750, 2002

133. Longo R, Pollesello P, Ricci C, Masutti F, Kvam BJ, Bercich L, Croce LS, Grigolato P, Paoletti S, de Bernard B, et al.: Proton MR spectroscopy in quantitative in vivo determination of fat content in human liver steatosis. *J Magn Reson Imaging* 5:281–285, 1995

134. Dixon JB, Bhathal PS, O'Brien PE: Nonalcoholic fatty liver disease: predictors of nonalcoholic steatohepatitis and liver fibrosis in the severely obese. *Gastroenterology* 121:91–100, 2001

135. Goessling W, Friedman LS: Increased liver chemistry in an asymptomatic patient. *Clin Gastroenterol Hepatol* 3:852–858, 2005

136. Luyckx FH, Desaive C, Thiry A, Dewe W, Scheen AJ, Gielen JE, Lefebvre PJ: Liver abnormalities in severely obese subjects: effect of drastic weight loss after gastroplasty. *Int J Obes Relat Metab Disord* 22:222–226, 1998

137. Palmer M, Schaffner F: Effect of weight reduction on hepatic abnormalities in overweight patients. *Gastroenterology* 99:1408–1413, 1990

138. Eriksson S, Eriksson KF, Bondesson L: Nonalcoholic steatohepatitis in obesity: a reversible condition. *Acta Med Scand*

220:83–88, 1986

139. Ueno T, Sugawara H, Sujaku K, Hashimoto O, Tsuji R, Tamaki S, Torimura T, Inuzuka S, Sata M, Tanikawa K: Therapeutic effects of restricted diet and exercise in obese patients with fatty liver. *J Hepatol* 27:103–107, 1997

140. Hickman IJ, Jonsson JR, Prins JB, Ash S, Purdie DM, Clouston AD, Powell EE: Modest weight loss and physical activity in overweight patients with chronic liver disease results in sustained improvements in alanine aminotransferase, fasting insulin, and quality of life. *Gut* 53: 413–419, 2004

141. Dixon JB, Bhathal PS, Hughes NR, O'Brien PE: Nonalcoholic fatty liver disease: improvement in liver histological analysis with weight loss. *Hepatology* 39: 1647–1654, 2004

142. Rozental P, Biava C, Spencer H, Zimmerman HJ: Liver morphology and function tests in obesity and during total starvation. *Am J Dig Dis* 12:198–208, 1967

143. Comar KM, Sterling RK: Review article: Drug therapy for non-alcoholic fatty liver disease. *Aliment Pharmacol Ther* 23: 207–215, 2006

144. Clark JM, Alkhuraishi AR, Solga SF, Alli P, Diehl AM, Magnuson TH: Roux-en-Y gastric bypass improves liver histology in patients with non-alcoholic fatty liver disease. *Obes Res* 13:1180–1186, 2005

145. Basaranoglu M, Acbay O, Sonsuz A: A controlled trial of gemfibrozil in the treatment of patients with nonalcoholic steatohepatitis (Letter). *J Hepatol* 31:384, 1999

146. Lavine JE: Vitamin E treatment of nonalcoholic steatohepatitis in children: a pilot study. *J Pediatr* 136:734–738, 2000

147. Abdelmalek MF, Angulo P, Jorgensen RA, Sylvestre PB, Lindor KD: Betaine, a promising new agent for patients with nonalcoholic steatohepatitis: results of a pilot study. *Am J Gastroenterol* 96:2711–2717, 2001

148. Harrison SA, Fincke C, Helinski D, Torgerson S, Hayashi P: A pilot study of orlistat treatment in obese, non-alcoholic steatohepatitis patients. *Aliment Pharmacol Ther* 20:623–628, 2004

149. Adams LA, Zein CO, Angulo P, Lindor KD: A pilot trial of pentoxifylline in non-alcoholic steatohepatitis. *Am J Gastroenterol* 99:2365–2368, 2004

150. Lutchman G, Promrat K, Kleiner DE, Heller T, Ghany MG, Yanovski JA, Liang TJ, Hoofnagle JH: Changes in serum adipokine levels during pioglitazone treatment for nonalcoholic steatohepatitis: relationship to histological improvement. *Clin Gastroenterol Hepatol* 4: 1048–1052, 2006

151. Tiikkainen M, Hakkinen AM, Korsheninnikova E, Nyman T, Makimattila S, Yki-Jarvinen H: Effects of rosiglitazone and metformin on liver fat content, hepatic insulin resistance, insulin clearance, and gene expression in adipose tissue in patients with type 2 diabetes. *Diabetes* 53:2169–2176, 2004

152. Neuschwander-Tetri BA, Brunt EM, Wehmeier KR, Oliver D, Bacon BR: Improved nonalcoholic steatohepatitis after 48 weeks of treatment with the PPAR-gamma ligand rosiglitazone. *Hepatology* 38:1008–1017, 2003

153. Ratziu V, Charlotte F, Jacqueminet S, Podevin P, Serfaty L, Bruckert E, Grimaldi A, Poynard T: A one year randomized, placebo-controlled, double-blind trial of rosiglitazone in non alcoholic steatohepatitis: results of the FLIRT pilot trial (Abstract). *Hepatology* 44 (Suppl. 1):201A, 2006

154. Holoman J, Glasa J, Kasar J et al: Serum markers of liver fibrosis in patients with non-alcoholic steatohepatitis (NASH): correlation to liver morphology and effect of therapy (Abstract). *J Hepatol* 32 (Suppl. 2):210, 2000

155. Lindor K: Ursodeoxycholic acid for treatment of nonalcoholic steatohepatitis: results of a randomized, placebo-controlled study (Abstract). *Gastroenterology* 124 (Suppl.1):A336, 2003

156. Hasegawa T, Yoneda M, Nakamura K, Makino I, Terano A: Plasma transforming growth factor-beta1 level and efficacy of alpha-tocopherol in patients with non-alcoholic steatohepatitis: a pilot study. *Aliment Pharmacol Ther* 15: 1667–1672, 2001

157. Harrison SA, Torgerson S, Hayashi P, Ward J, Schenker S: Vitamin E and vitamin C treatment improves fibrosis in patients with nonalcoholic steatohepatitis. *Am J Gastroenterol* 98:2485–2490, 2003

158. Sanyal AJ, Mofrad PS, Contos MJ, Sargeant C, Luketic VA, Sterling RK, Stravitz RT, Shiffman ML, Clore J, Mills AS: A pilot study of vitamin E versus vitamin E and pioglitazone for the treatment of nonalcoholic steatohepatitis. *Clin Gastroenterol Hepatol* 2:1107–1115, 2004

159. Miller ER, 3rd, Pastor-Barriuso R, Dalal D, Riemersma RA, Appel LJ, Guallar E: Meta-analysis: high-dosage vitamin E supplementation may increase all-cause mortality. *Ann Intern Med* 142:37–46, 2005

160. Strader DB, Wright T, Thomas DL, Seeff LB: Diagnosis, management, and treatment of hepatitis C. *Hepatology* 39: 1147–1171, 2004

161. Koivisto VA, Pelkonen R, Cantell K: Effect of interferon on glucose tolerance and insulin sensitivity. *Diabetes* 38:641–647, 1989

162. Imano E, Kanda T, Ishigami Y, Kubota M, Ikeda M, Matsuhisa M, Kawamori R, Yamasaki Y: Interferon induces insulin resistance in patients with chronic active hepatitis C. *J Hepatol* 28:189–193, 1998

163. Ishigami Y, Kanda T, Wada M, Shimizu Y: Glucose intolerance during interferon therapy in patients with chronic hepatitis type C. *Nippon Rinsho* 52:1901–1904, 1994 [article in Japanese]

164. Ito Y, Takeda N, Ishimori M, Akai A, Miura K, Yasuda K: Effects of long-term interferon-alpha treatment on glucose tolerance in patients with chronic hepatitis C. *J Hepatol* 31:215–220, 1999

Habitual Physical Activity Is Associated With Intrahepatic Fat Content in Humans

Gianluca Perseghin, MD[1,2,3]
Guido Lattuada, PhD[1]
Francesco De Cobelli, MD[2,4]
Francesca Ragogna, PhD[1]
Georgia Ntali, MD[1]
Antonio Esposito, MD[4]

Elena Belloni, MD[4]
Tamara Canu[4]
Ileana Terruzzi, PhD[1]
Paola Scifo, PhD[5]
Alessandro Del Maschio, MD[2,4,6]
Livio Luzi, MD[1,2,3]

OBJECTIVE — Fatty liver may be involved in the pathogenesis of type 2 diabetes. Physical exercise is a tool to improve insulin sensitivity, but little is known about its effect on intrahepatic fat (IHF) content. The purpose of this study was to examine the association of habitual physical activity, insulin resistance, and adiponectin with IHF content.

RESEARCH DESIGN AND METHODS — Participants were 191 (77 female and 114 male) apparently healthy, nonalcoholic individuals (aged 19–62 years; BMI 17.0–35.5 kg/m^2). IHF content was assessed in a quantitative fashion and noninvasively as a continuous variable by means of ^{1}H magnetic resonance spectroscopy (MRS), and habitual physical activity was assessed by means of a questionnaire. Fatty liver was defined as IHF content of >5% wet weight, and insulin sensitivity was estimated using the computer homeostasis model assessment (HOMA)-2 indexes.

RESULTS — A reduced prevalence of fatty liver in the quartile of the most physically active individuals (25, 11, 25, and 2% in quartile 1, 2, 3, and 4, respectively; $\chi^2 = 15.63$; $P = 0.001$) was found along with an inverse correlation between the physical activity index and the IHF content when plotted as continuous variables (Pearson's $r = -0.27$; $P < 0.000$). This association was not attenuated when adjusted for age, sex, BMI, HOMA-2, and adiponectin (partial correlation $r = -0.25$; $P < 0.001$).

CONCLUSIONS — This study demonstrated that a higher level of habitual physical activity is associated with a lower IHF content and suggested that this relationship may be due to the effect of exercise per se.

Diabetes Care 30:683–688, 2007

A lanine aminotransferase and γ-glutamyltransferase are associated with type 2 diabetes risk (1–3), and it is thought that the link is represented by the intrahepatic fat (IHF) content. Ectopic fat accumulation within the liver, in fact, has been reported in association with impairment of insulin-stimulated glucose metabolism, of suppression of endogenous glucose production, and of whole-body lipolysis in nondiabetic individuals with nonalcoholic fatty liver disease (NAFLD) (4,5). Additional results also demonstrated that decreased levels of circulating adiponectin in NAFLD are related to hepatic insulin sensitivity and to the IHF content, suggesting that hypoadiponectinemia may be involved in excessive hepatic fat accumulation (6).

Physical exercise was found to be associated with a reduced risk of development of type 2 diabetes (7,8) and is a well-recognized tool to improve insulin sensitivity at the level of the skeletal muscle (9). However, whether physical exercise may affect insulin sensitivity and diabetes risk via an effect on the IHF content and adiponectin remains unknown.

The IHF content may be assessed as a continuous variable by means of ^{1}H magnetic resonance spectroscopy (MRS) (10), and recently this technique was found to be a sensitive, quantitative, and noninvasive method also when applied to a large population (11) without the need for the use of a more invasive approach such as liver biopsy. The purpose of this study was, therefore, to examine the association of habitual physical activity, insulin resistance, and plasma adiponectin concentration with the IHF content in a population of 191 nonalcoholic, healthy individuals using a cross-sectional approach.

RESEARCH DESIGN AND METHODS — One-hundred and ninety-one individuals were recruited via a survey performed to assess the prevalence of fatty liver among the employees of the San Raffaele Scientific Institute. These individuals were recruited in the outpatient service of the Center of Nutrition/Metabolism of the San Raffaele Scientific Institute. Their body weight had to be stable for at least 6 months for inclusion; exclusion criteria included a history of hepatic disease, substance abuse, or daily consumption of >1 alcohol drink (<20 g/day) or the equivalent in beer and wine. Normal or higher than normal IHF content was set at 5% wet weight as suggested by the American Association for the Study of Liver Diseases (AASLD) (12). The anthropometric characteristics of the subjects are summarized in Table 1. Subjects were in good health as assessed by medical history, physical examination, hematological analysis, and urinalysis. Recruited subjects gave their informed written consent after explanation of the

From [1]Internal Medicine, Section of Nutrition/Metabolism, San Raffaele Scientific Institute, Milan, Italy; the [2]Unit of Clinical Spectroscopy, San Raffaele Scientific Institute, Milan, Italy; the [3]Center "Physical Exercise for Health and Wellness," Faculty of Exercise Sciences, Università degli Studi di Milano, Milan, Italy; [4]Diagnostic Radiology, San Raffaele Scientific Institute, Milan, Italy; [5]Nuclear Medicine, San Raffaele Scientific Institute, Milan, Italy; and the [6]Università Vita e Salute San Raffaele, Milan, Italy.

Address correspondence and reprint requests to Gianluca Perseghin, MD, Faculty of Exercise Sciences, Università degli Studi di Milano and San Raffaele Scientific Institute, Internal Medicine, via Olgettina 60, 20132, Milan, Italy. E-mail: perseghin.gianluca@hsr.it.

Received for publication 2 October 2006 and accepted in revised form 30 November 2006.

Abbreviations: FFA, free fatty acid; HOMA, homeostasis model assessment; HOMA2-%B, HOMA2-derived index of β-cell insulin sensitivity; HOMA2-%S, HOMA2-derived index of insulin sensitivity; IHF, intrahepatic fat; MRS, magnetic resonance spectroscopy; NAFLD, nonalcoholic fatty liver disease; TSH, thyroid-stimulating hormone.

A table elsewhere in this issue shows conventional and Système International (SI) units and conversion factors for many substances.

DOI: 10.2337/dc06-2032

Table 1—*Anthropometric and laboratory features of individuals with fatty liver (IHF content >5% wet weight) and normal subjects (IHF content <5% wet weight)*

	Individuals with fatty liver	Normal subjects	P value
Sex (female/male)	31 (4/27)	160 (73/87)	0.001*
Age (years)	36 ± 8	34 ± 9	0.52
Height (cm)	173 ± 7	170 ± 16	0.35
Weight (kg)	82 ± 15	70 ± 14	0.0001
BMI (kg/m²)	27.4 ± 3.8	23.7 ± 3.6	0.0001
Systolic blood pressure (mmHg)	128 ± 10	117 ± 10	0.0001
Diastolic blood pressure (mmHg)	83 ± 8	77 ± 8	0.0001
Total cholesterol (mmol/l)	5.25 ± 1.24	4.65 ± 0.80	0.002
HDL cholesterol (mmol/l)	1.22 ± 0.31	1.53 ± 0.39	0.0001
Triglycerides (mmol/l)	1.66 ± 0.92	0.86 ± 0.36	0.0001
FFAs (mmol/l)	0.62 ± 0.16	0.57 ± 0.23	0.22
Creatinine (μmol/l)	74 ± 17	74 ± 15	0.86
TSH (mU/l)	1.26 ± 0.97	1.18 ± 0.91	0.77
Fasting glucose (mmol/l)	5.11 ± 0.61	4.72 ± 0.50	0.0001
Fasting insulin (pmol/l)	97 ± 37	70 ± 32	0.0001
HOMA2-%B	153 ± 43	142 ± 58	0.15
HOMA2-%S	56 ± 24	83 ± 38	0.0001
Adiponectin (μg/ml)	5.3 ± 2.0	8.2 ± 3.7	0.0001
PAI work	2.60 ± 0.50	2.59 ± 0.53	0.92
PAI sport	2.06 ± 0.69	2.61 ± 1.06	0.006
PAI leisure time	3.03 ± 0.65	3.10 ± 0.60	0.58
PAI total	7.69 ± 1.23	8.30 ± 1.41	0.02

Data are means ± SD. Independent-samples t test (two tailed). The range of possible scores for the total physical activity index (PAI) is 3–15; the lowest value corresponds to the level of physical activity of a clerical worker who plays a light sport (energy expended is <0.76 MJ/h; e.g., bowling) and who participates in sedentary activities during leisure time. The highest value corresponds to the level of physical activity of a person who is very physically active at work (e.g., a construction worker), who plays heavy sports (energy expended is at least 1.76 MJ/h; e.g., boxing, basketball, football, or rugby), and who is very physically active during leisure time (e.g., walking >1 h/day or biking >45 min/day). *Pearson χ^2 test.

purpose, nature, and potential risks of the study.

Subjects were instructed by a registered dietitian to consume an isocaloric diet containing at least 250 g of carbohydrates and 70–90 g of protein/day and to abstain from exercise activity for 3 days before the study. They were studied after an 8- to 10-h overnight fast by means of ¹H-MRS for the assessment of IHF content. Blood samples were collected for measurement of serum insulin, plasma glucose, free fatty acids (FFAs), the lipid profile, and biochemical parameters.

Experimental protocol
Assessment of habitual physical activity. Habitual physical activity was assessed using a validated questionnaire that had been developed for the various socioeconomic classes in the general population (13). Briefly, three meaningful factors can be distinguished within habitual physical activity: 1) occupational physical activity (precoded according to three levels of physical activity at work);

2) sport during leisure time subdivided in three levels and a sport score calculated from a combination of the intensity of the sport (low level, 0.76 MJ/h: sailing, bowling, billiards, and golf; middle level, 1.26 MJ/h: cycling, dancing, swimming, and tennis; and high level, 1.76 MJ/h: basketball, football, and rowing), the amount of time per week (from 0.5 to >4 h), and the proportion of the year (from <1 to >9 months) during which the sport was played regularly; and 3) other physical activity during leisure time (this specifically relates to watching television, walking, and cycling during leisure time). The test-retest reliability of this questionnaire, validated in a Dutch population, was tested for Italian individuals in our laboratory in previous studies; the questionnaire was administered twice 2 weeks apart and the coefficients of variation (CVs) of the work, sport, and leisure time indexes were 2, 3, and 8%, respectively.

¹H-MRS. Hepatic ¹H-MRS was performed at rest and with patients in the supine position with the use of a 1.5-T

whole-body scanner (Gyroscan Intera Master 1.5 MR System; Philips Medical Systems, Best, Netherlands) using a conventional circular superficial coil as described previously (14). First, coronal and transverse images of the liver were obtained for all patients. Next, T1 in-phase and out-of-phase sequences were obtained to look for a potential loss of signal on out-of-phase images, indicating the presence of IHF accumulation. Then an 8-cm³ spectroscopic volume of interest was positioned within the right lobe, avoiding major blood vessels, intrahepatic bile ducts, and the lateral margin of the liver. The voxel shimming was executed to optimize the homogeneity of the magnetic field within the specific volume of interest. Two ¹H spectra were collected from the hepatic parenchyma with the same prescanning conditions using a PRESS pulse sequence (interpulse delay TR = 3,000 ms, spin-echo time TE = 25 ms, 1,024 data points over a 1,000-Hz spectral width and 64 acquisitions) with and without suppression of the water signal, respectively. Area of resonances from protons of water (4.8 ppm) and methylene groups in fatty acid chains of the hepatic triglycerides (1.4 ppm) were obtained with a time-domain nonlinear fitting routine using commercial software (VARPRO-MRUI; http://www.mrui.uab.es). The percent IHF was calculated by dividing the integral of the methylene groups in fatty acid chains of the hepatic triglycerides (obtained from the water-suppressed spectrum) by the sum of methylene groups and water (obtained from the nonwater-suppressed spectrum) × 100. The CV of the IHF content assessed using the above-described setting in our laboratory is 4.7% in individuals with <5% wet weight and 3.1% in individuals with an IHF content >5% wet weight, and the CV was calculated using the row data obtained from two consecutive acquisitions performed using the same volume of interest and the same prescanning procedures.

Analytical determinations
Glucose (Beckman Coulter, Fullerton, CA), FFAs, triglycerides, total cholesterol, HDL cholesterol, and serum creatinine were measured as described previously (14). Plasma levels of insulin (sensitivity 2 μU/ml; intra- and interassay CVs of <3.1 and 6%, respectively) were measured with a radioimmunoassay (Linco Research, St. Charles, MO). Serum adiponectin was measured, as described

Table 2—*Characteristics of study subjects by quartiles of physical activity index (PAI)*

	Quartile 1 (4.63–7.25)	Quartile 2 (7.26–8.00)	Quartile 3 (8.01–9.08)	Quartile 4 (9.09–13.06)	P value
Sex (female/male)	23/29	20/24	18/30	16/31	0.63*
Age (years)	34 ± 7	35 ± 7	35 ± 9	35 ± 11	0.82
BMI (kg/m²)	24.9 ± 4.3	24.2 ± 4.6	25.1 ± 3.4	23.1 ± 2.8	0.036
Systolic blood pressure (mmHg)	119 ± 13	119 ± 11	121 ± 11	118 ± 8	0.35
Diastolic blood pressure (mmHg)	77 ± 9	79 ± 7	80 ± 9	76 ± 7	0.15
Total cholesterol (mmol/l)	4.76 ± 0.80	4.68 ± 0.70	5.02 ± 1.14	4.58 ± 0.88	0.09
HDL cholesterol (mmol/l)	1.42 ± 0.39	1.45 ± 0.41	1.50 ± 0.44	1.55 ± 0.36	0.37
Triglycerides (mmol/l)	1.13 ± 0.79	1.05 ± 0.90	1.01 ± 0.45	0.76 ± 0.30	0.06
Fasting glucose (mmol/l)	4.77 ± 0.56	4.77 ± 0.56	4.83 ± 0.55	4.72 ± 0.56	0.85
Fasting insulin (pmol/l)	85 ± 37	67 ± 27	73 ± 34	66 ± 32†	0.03
HOMA2-%B	157 ± 58	131 ± 35	137 ± 39	139 ± 68	0.11
HOMA2-%S	69 ± 24	81 ± 22	80 ± 30	88 ± 29‡	0.01
Adiponectin (μg/ml)	6.8 ± 2.8	7.2 ± 4.1	8.4 ± 3.7	8.4 ± 3.6	0.08
IHF content (% wet weight)	5.1 ± 6.5	2.8 ± 3.6	4.9 ± 7.1	1.5 ± 1.0§	0.0001
Fatty liver	13/52 (25)	5/44 (11)	12/48 (25)	1/46 (2)	0.001*
PAI work	2.2 ± 0.4‖	2.6 ± 0.5§	2.8 ± 0.4	2.8 ± 0.6	0.000
PAI sport	1.7 ± 0.4‖	2.2 ± 0.5	2.4 ± 0.7	3.8 ± 1.1‖	0.000
PAI leisure time	2.7 ± 0.5¶	2.9 ± 0.5¶	3.3 ± 0.5	3.5 ± 0.5	0.000

Data are means ± SD or n (%). *Pearson χ^2 test. †$P < 0.05$ vs. quartile 1; ‡$P < 0.05$ vs. quartile 1 and quartile 2; §$P < 0.02$ vs. quartile 1 and quartile 3; ‖$P < 0.001$ vs. all; ¶$P < 0.001$ vs. quartiles 3 and 4, Bonferroni post hoc analysis.

previously (15), with an enzyme-linked immunosorbent kit (B-Bridge International, Sunnyvale, CA) with a sensitivity of 25 pg/ml. The intra- and interassay CVs were <3.7 and <6%, respectively. Thyroid-stimulating hormone (TSH) was measured by an immunofluorometric method as described previously (16).

Calculations

Insulin resistance was determined by updated computer homeostasis model assessment (HOMA)-2 indexes (17) available from http://www.OCDEM.ox. ac.uk. The percent IHF was calculated by dividing the integral of the methylene groups in fatty acid chains of the hepatic triglycerides by the sum of methylene groups and water × 100. Signal decay due to spin-spin relaxation was calculated using mean T2 relaxation times for water and fat of 50 and 60 ms, respectively, and the exponential relaxation equation $I_m = I_0 \exp(-Te/T2)$, where I_m is the measured signal intensity obtained at the selected echo-time Te, I_0 is the signal intensity immediately after the 90° pulse, and T2 is the spin-spin relaxation time. Average T2 relaxation times were used for these calculations (10,18) as previously performed (11). These values represent a relative quantity of water and hepatic triglyceride fatty acid chain protons in the volume of interest. To convert these values to absolute concentrations expressed

as percent fat by weight of volume, we used equations validated by Longo et al. (10). A liver fat content >50 mg/g (5% by wet weight and equivalent to 6.5% of the ratio of methylene to methylene + water × 100 in our setting) is diagnostic of hepatic steatosis (12), and study subjects could be segregated into a group of individuals with normal (<5% wet weight) or higher than normal IHF content (>5% wet weight).

Statistical analysis

Data in text and tables are means ± SD. Analyses were performed using the SPSS software (version 10.0; SPSS, Chicago, IL). Variables with skewed distribution assessed using the Kolmogorov-Smirnov test of normality (IHF content, HDL cholesterol, triglycerides, systolic and diastolic blood pressure, insulin, TSH, HOMA2-derived index of insulin sensitivity [HOMA2-%S], and HOMA2-derived index of β-cell insulin sensitivity [HOMA2-%B]) were log transformed before the analysis. One-way ANOVA or a Kruskal-Wallis nonparametric test was used when appropriate to compare variables between subjects with and subjects without fatty liver (Table 1) or among quartiles of the physical activity index (Table 2). The Bonferroni post hoc test was used. $P < 0.05$ was considered to be significant. The relationship between IHF content and the physical activity index

was examined by a two-tailed Pearson's correlation. Partial correlation was used to examine these relationships independently of age, sex, BMI, adiponectin, and HOMA2-%S.

RESULTS

Anthropometric and laboratory features of study subjects with or without fatty liver

A higher than normal IHF content (>5% wet weight) was found in 31 individuals (16%) with a higher prevalence in men than in women (Table 1). These individuals were characterized by a higher BMI, systolic and diastolic blood pressure, total cholesterol, and triglycerides along with a reduced HDL cholesterol (Table 1). Plasma FFAs, serum creatinine, and TSH were not different between individuals with or without fatty liver. Two volunteers had impaired fasting glucose (one man with 6.1 mmol/l and fatty liver and one woman with 6.3 mmol/l and normal IHF content) and were included in the study. Fasting plasma glucose and insulin concentrations were increased in individuals with fatty liver compared with normal subjects (Table 1) ($P < 0.0001$); in association, the HOMA2-%S was reduced in subjects with than in those without fatty liver ($P < 0.0001$), whereas the HOMA2-%B was not different (Table 1). The serum adiponectin concentration was reduced in individuals with fatty liver more than in the normal subjects ($P <$ 0.0001). The score for the total physical activity index was reduced in individuals with fatty liver more than in the normal subjects (Table 1) ($P < 0.02$), and this difference was due exclusively to physical exercise during sport activities ($P <$ 0.006), whereas scores for physical activity during work ($P = 0.92$) and leisure time ($P = 0.58$) were not different.

Characteristics of study subjects by quartiles of the physical activity index

To assess in a cross-sectional fashion the impact of habitual physical activity, study subjects were segregated in subgroups of quartiles of the score of total physical activity index (cutoffs 7.25, 8.00, and 9.08) as summarized in Table 2. The subgroups were not different per sex and age; for BMI, one-way ANOVA showed that it was different even if the Bonferroni post hoc analysis did not reveal a significant difference among quartiles. Blood pressure, total cholesterol ($P = 0.09$), HDL cholesterol, triglycerides ($P = 0.06$), and fasting plasma glucose were not different. In contrast, fasting plasma insulin was lower in the most physically active (quartile 4) compared with the least active (quartile 1) individuals. β-Cell insulin sensitivity was not different among quartiles, whereas HOMA2-%S (Table 2) was higher in quartile 4 compared with quartiles 1 and 2. The fasting serum adiponectin concentration was not different among quartiles ($P = 0.08$) (Table 2). Finally, IHF content was lower in the quartile of the most physically active (quartile 4) individuals compared with those in quartiles 1 and 3 ($P < 0.02$) (Table 2 and Fig. 1A), and this finding was confirmed by analyzing the prevalence of fatty liver, which was the lowest (2%) in the quartile of the most physically active individuals (Pearson χ^2 test: $P < 0.001$).

Correlative analysis

Based on the working hypothesis, we tested whether the IHF content correlated with the total score of the physical activity index ($r = -0.27$; $P < 0.000$), with the sport index ($r = -0.26$; $P < 0.000$), and with the leisure time physical activity index ($r = -0.17$; $P < 0.02$) but not with the work physical activity index ($r = 0.08$; $P = 0.92$) in the entire population. The same findings were reproducible when the correlative analysis was performed separately in individuals with or

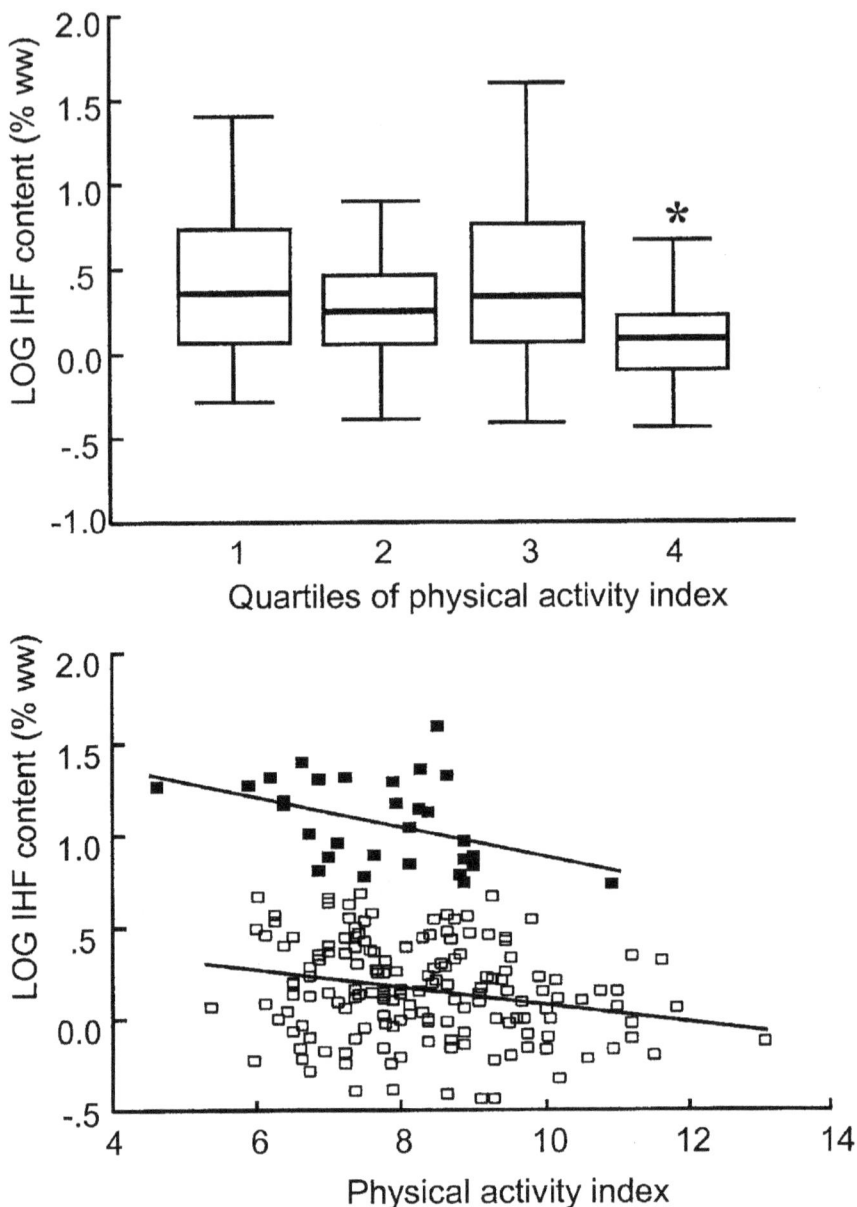

Figure 1—A: *IHF content by quartiles of physical activity index. Box plot of the log IHF content in individuals within quartiles of physical activity index showing that the higher level of habitual physical activity (quartile 4) is associated with lower IHF content. *P < 0.02 versus quartiles 1 and 3, one-way ANOVA and Bonferroni post hoc analysis. B: Correlation between the IHF content and physical activity index. Scatter plot of the log IHF content and the score of total physical activity.* ■, *individuals with fatty liver (>5% wet weight);* □, *individuals with normal IHF content (<5% wet weight). Pearson's correlation analysis showed that the variables were significantly associated in the entire population (r = -0.27; P < 0.000, regression line not shown) and also in the two subgroups of individuals separately (r = -0.21, P < 0.008 in the 160 subjects with normal IHF content and r = -0.39, P < 0.03 in the 31 subjects with fatty liver).*

without fatty liver. In particular, the total score of the physical activity index was significantly associated with individuals with normal IHF content and with fatty liver (Fig. 1B). The IHF content correlated strongly also with the BMI ($r = 0.54$; $P < 0.000$), HOMA2-%S ($r = -0.31$; $P <$ 0.000), and adiponectin ($r = -0.45$; $P <$ 0.000). We therefore performed a correlative analysis between the IHF content and the total score of the physical activity index, controlling for age, sex, BMI, HOMA2-%S, and adiponectin, and found that it was not attenuated (partial correlation $r = -0.25$; $P < 0.001$). The adjusted correlative analysis remained unaffected also when it was performed separately in the two subgroups: partial correlation factor from -0.21 to -0.29 ($P < 0.001$) in the subgroup of individuals with normal IHF content and from -0.39 to -0.33 ($P < 0.05$) in the subgroup of individuals with fatty liver.

CONCLUSIONS — The present study is based on the hypothesis that part of the well-known beneficial impact of physical exercise on the prevention and treatment of insulin resistance and type 2 diabetes might be mediated by a depleting effect on ectopic fat accumulation within the liver. In support of this hypothesis we demonstrated in this study, using a cross-sectional approach, that a higher level of habitual physical activity is associated with lower IHF content in humans; in addition, the results suggested that this association is detectable regardless of other key factors involved in the pathogenesis of type 2 diabetes: age, sex, obesity, insulin resistance, and circulating adiponectin levels.

In support of this conclusion, we found in a population of 191 nonalcoholic, apparently healthy individuals, in which the prevalence of fatty liver was found to be 16%, that 1) those segregated in the quartile of the highest score of physical activity were characterized by the lowest IHF content when analyzed as a continuous variable (Fig. 1A), 2) they were characterized by the lowest prevalence of fatty liver (Table 2) when analyzed as a categorical variable (IHF content >5% wet weight), and 3) the physical activity index was inversely associated with the IHF content within the entire population and within each subgroup of individuals with or without fatty liver (Fig. 1B). These results are in agreement with previous cross-sectional studies showing an association of physical activity with indirect markers of fatty liver: Lawlor et al. (19) showed an independent association of the level of physical activity with alanine aminotransferase and γ-glutamyltransferase, whereas Church et al. (20) showed an association between physical fitness and the prevalence of NAFLD. An additional study reported a significant correlation between cardiorespiratory fitness and a semiquantitative, computed tomography–derived value obtained as a ratio of the liver-to-spleen attenuation signal in men (21). With respect to these studies, the impor-

tance of our own report was 1) to provide for the first time a direct and absolute quantification of the IHF content using a reliable, highly sensitive and specific in vivo technique and 2) to obtain the determination of additional variables strongly involved in the pathogenesis of type 2 diabetes and in the development of ectopic fat accumulation. Studies have pointed to insulin resistance as pathogenic factors in NAFLD and fatty liver (22,23). On the basis of the measurement of fasting plasma glucose and insulin concentration, we estimated insulin sensitivity using the computer HOMA2 indexes and showed that, not surprisingly, the individuals segregated in the quartile of highest score of physical activity were characterized by higher insulin sensitivity (Table 2) and the IHF content and HOMA2-%S were strongly correlated. Similarly, it was suggested that adiponectin was independently associated with fatty liver (6), and also in our own population the IHF content strongly correlated with adiponectin. Because exercise training may influence both insulin sensitivity and circulating levels of adiponectin, it might be that the association between lower IHF content and higher habitual physical activity was due to an effect mediated by the fitness status on insulin sensitivity and adiponectin rather than being a direct effect on liver storage. Against the hypothesis of an indirect effect of physical activity mediated by the modulation of insulin sensitivity or adiponectin, as well as age, sex, and obesity, the correlation analysis adjusted for all these variables revealed that the association between IHF content and the physical activity score was not lessened, suggesting that the relationship between the two variables was an independent one. Taking into account the fact that excessive fatty liver accumulation appeared to be peculiarly associated with hepatic insulin resistance (5) and that reduction of the IHF content due to a moderate weight reduction was associated with improvement of hepatic insulin sensitivity (24), the potential beneficial effect of physical exercise would represent an additional tool to improve the metabolic profile of patients type 2 diabetes. The precise mechanisms by which physical exercise may reduce hepatic steatosis remains unknown and needs to be extensively explored, even if it was suggested that it would stimulate lipid oxidation and inhibit lipid synthesis in liver through the activation of the AMP-activated protein kinase pathway (25).

The score of habitual physical activity was based on three factors: occupational physical activity, sport activity, and physical activity during leisure time. The study population was rather homogeneous in terms of occupational physical activity because these individuals were employees in our institute and were similarly involved in mild occupational activity. Consequently, it was not surprising that the occupational physical activity was not different between groups (Table 1). Also physical activity during leisure time was not apparently different between the individuals with or without fatty liver despite the observation that when plotted as a continuous variable, it correlated with IHF content even if in a weaker fashion than the sport physical activity. Therefore, we should emphasize that among the three components of the physical activity index, the habit of playing a sport regularly was the most relevant in the correlation with IHF content (Table 1).

The strength of this work is based on the highly sensitive and specific absolute quantification of IHF content using a noninvasive technique, controlling for anthropometric, metabolic, and endocrine variables; on the other hand, some major limitations need to be stated. One limitation is the cross-sectional nature of the study; unfortunately, we are not aware of any study in which the effect of acute exercise or of an exercise training program on IHF content was assessed. Only data in animal models are available, and they showed that physical exercise performed for 8 weeks in rats during the administration of a high-fat diet (26) or introduced midway through a 16-week period (27) largely reduced fat accumulation. Therefore, studies aimed to assess longitudinally the effect of physical exercise are warranted and need to be performed in the near future. In addition, diet habits may affect IHF content (28), but we did not have valuable dietary data for this population to assess its potential influence and interplay with habitual physical activity. These limitations are not trivial issues; in fact we can say that, in general, there exists a consensus that lifestyle changes and increasing physical activity through exercise are cornerstones to therapy of insulin-resistant states and fatty liver, and these sorts of interventions are typically part of initial recommendations. However, the efficacy of this common sense approach remains to be established, and the relative merits of different levels of diet and exercise on IHF metabolism remain to be defined. This is confirmed by the fact that on the basis of the results of the present work, the impact of habitual physical activity, even if significant, explained only 8% of the variance of the IHF content, suggesting that the amount of IHF is mainly regulated by a factor other than habitual physical activity.

Thus, it may be concluded that by using a cross-sectional approach in the present work, we provided evidence that habitual physical activity is associated with a lower IHF content in humans. However, it is possible that physical exercise may only modulate the severity of the degree of hepatic fat accumulation.

Acknowledgments— This study was supported by grants from the Italian Minister of Health (RF01.1831). G.N. was the recipient of the Marie Curie Host Fellowship of the European Community (Contract HPMT-CT-2001-00329); she is currently a clinical fellow in endocrinology, Polikliniki Hospital, Athens, Greece, and a PhD candidate in Nutrition and Dietetics, Harokopio University, Athens, Greece.

References

1. Vozarova B, Stefan N, Lindsay RS, Saremi A, Pratley RE, Bogardus C, Tataranni PA: High alanine aminotransferase is associated with decreased hepatic insulin sensitivity and predicts the development of type 2 diabetes. *Diabetes* 51:1889–1895, 2002
2. Sattar N, Scherbakova O, Ford I, O'Reilly DS, Stanley A, Forrest E, Macfarlane PW, Packard CJ, Cobbe SM, Shepherd J; West of Scotland Coronary Prevention Study: Elevated alanine aminotransferase predicts new-onset type 2 diabetes independently of classical risk factors, metabolic syndrome, and C-reactive protein in the west of Scotland coronary prevention study. *Diabetes* 53:2855–2860, 2004
3. Perry IJ, Wannamethee SG, Shaper AG: Prospective study of serum γ-glutamyltransferase and risk of NIDDM. *Diabetes Care* 21:732–737, 1998
4. Marchesini G, Brizi M, Bianchi G, Tomassetti S, Bugianesi E, Lenzi M, McCullough AJ, Natale S, Forlani G, Melchionda N: Nonalcoholic fatty liver disease: a feature of the metabolic syndrome. *Diabetes* 50:1844–1850, 2001
5. Seppala-Lindroos A, Vehkavaara S, Hakkinen AM, Goto T, Westerbacka J, Sovijarvi A, Halavaara J, Yki-Jarvinen H: Fat accumulation in the liver is associated with defects in insulin suppression of glucose production and serum free fatty acids independent of obesity at a normal men. *J Clin Endocrinol Metab* 87:3023–3028, 2002
6. Bugianesi E, Pagotto U, Manini R, Vanni E, Gastaldelli A, de Iasio R, Gentilcore E, Natale S, Cassader M, Rizzetto M, Pasquali R, Marchesini G: Plasma adiponectin in nonalcoholic fatty liver is related to hepatic insulin resistance and hepatic fat content, not to liver disease severity. *J Clin Endocrinol Metab* 90:3498–3504, 2005
7. Hu FB, Manson JE, Stampfer MJ, Colditz G, Liu S, Solomon CG, Willett WC: Diet, lifestyle, and the risk of type 2 diabetes mellitus in women. *N Engl J Med* 345:790–797, 2001
8. Hu G, Qiao Q, Silventoinen K, Eriksson JG, Jousilahti P, Lindstrom J, Valle TT, Nissinen A, Tuomilehto J: Occupational, commuting, and leisure-time physical activity in relation to risk for type 2 diabetes in middle-aged Finnish men and women. *Diabetologia* 46:322–329, 2003
9. Perseghin G, Price TB, Petersen KF, Roden M, Cline GW, Gerow K, Rothman DL, Shulman GI: Increased glucose transport/phosphorylation and muscle glycogen synthesis after exercise training in insulin resistant subjects. *N Engl J Med* 335:1357–1362, 1996
10. Longo R, Ricci C, Masutti F, Vidimari R, Croce LS, Bercich L, Tiribelli C, Dalla Palma L: Fatty infiltration of the liver quantification by ^{1}H localized magnetic resonance spectroscopy and comparison with computed tomography. *Invest Radiol* 28:297–302, 1993
11. Szczepaniak LS, Nurenberg P, Leonard D, Browning JD, Reingold JS, Grundy S, Hobbs HH, Dobbins RL: Magnetic resonance spectroscopy to measure hepatic triglyceride content: prevalence of hepatic steatosis in the general population. *Am J Physiol Endocrinol Metab* 288:E462–E468, 2004
12. Neuschwander-Tetri BA, Caldwell SH: Nonalcoholic steatohepatitis: summary of an AASLD single topic conference. *Hepatology* 37:1202–1219, 2003
13. Baecke JAH, Burema J, Frijters JER: A short questionnaire for the measurement of habitual physical activity in epidemiological studies. *Am J Clin Nutr* 36:936–942, 1982
14. Perseghin G, Lattuada G, De Cobelli F, Esposito A, Costantino F, Canu T, Ragogna F, Scifo P, De Taddeo F, Maffi P, Secchi A, Del Maschio A, Luzi L: Reduced intra-hepatic fat content is associated with increased whole body lipid oxidation in patients with type 1 diabetes. *Diabetologia* 48:2615–2621, 2005
15. Perseghin G, Lattuada G, De Cobelli F, Ntali G, Esposito A, Burska A, Belloni E, Canu T, Ragogna F, Scifo P, Del Maschio A, Luzi L Serum resistin and intra-hepatic fat content in non-diabetic individuals. *J Clin Endocrinol Metab* 81:5122–5125, 2006
16. Perseghin G, Bonfanti R, Magni S, Lattuada G, De Cobelli F, Canu T, Esposito A, Scifo P, Ntali G, Costantino F, Bosio L, Ragogna F, Del Maschio A, Chiumello G, Luzi L: Insulin resistance and whole body energy homeostasis in obese adolescents with fatty liver disease. *Am J Physiol* 291:E697–E703, 2006
17. Wallace TM, Levy JC, Matthews DR: Use and abuse of HOMA modeling. *Diabetes Care* 27:1487–1495, 2004
18. Thomsen C, Becker U, Winkler K, Christoffersen P, Jensen M, Henriksen O: Quantification of liver fat by using magnetic resonance spectroscopy. *Magn Reson Imaging* 12:487–495, 1994
19. Lawlor DA, Sattar N, Smith GD, Ebrahim S: The associations of physical activity and adiposity with alanine aminotransferase and gamma-glutamyltransferase. *Am J Epidemiol* 161:1081–1088, 2005
20. Church TS, Kuk JL, Ross R, Priest EL, Biltoff E, Blair SN: Association of cardiorespiratory fitness, body mass index, and waist circumference to nonalcoholic fatty liver disease. *Gastroenterology* 130:2023–2030, 2006
21. Nguyen-Duy TB, Nichaman MZ, Church TS, Blair SN, Ross R: Visceral fat and liver fat are independent predictors of metabolic risk factors in men. *Am J Physiol* 284:E1065–E1071, 2003
22. Marchesini G, Brizi M, Morselli Labate AM, Bianchi G, Bugianesi G, McCullough AJ, Forlani G, Melchionda N: Association of non-alcoholic fatty liver disease to insulin resistance. *Am J Med* 107:450–455, 1999
23. Lewis GF, Carpentier A, Adeli K, Giacca A: Disordered fat storage and mobilization in the pathogenesis of insulin resistance and type 2 diabetes. *Endocr Rev* 23:201–229, 2002
24. Petersen KF, Dufour S, Befroy D, Lehrke M, Hendler RE, Shulman GI: Reversal of nonalcoholic hepatic steatosis, hepatic insulin resistance, and hyperglycemia by moderate weight reduction in patients with type 2 diabetes. *Diabetes* 54:603–608, 2005
25. Lavoie JM, Gauthier MS: Regulation of fat metabolism in the liver: link to non-alcoholic hepatic steatosis and impact of physical exercise. *Cell Mol Life Sci* 63:1393–1409, 2006
26. Gauthier MS, Couturier K, Latour JG, Lavoie JM: Concurrent exercise prevents high-fat-diet-induced macrovesicular hepatic steatosis. *J Appl Physiol* 94:2127–2134, 2003
27. Gauthier MS, Couturier K, Charbonneau A, Lavoie JM: Effects of introducing physical training in the course of a 16-week high-fat diet regimen on hepatic steatosis, adipose tissue fat accumulation, and plasma lipid profile. *Int J Obes Relat Metab Disord* 28:1064–1071, 2004
28. Westerbacka J, Lammi K, Hakkinen A-M, Rissanen A, Salminen I, Aro A, Yki-Jarvinen H: Dietary fat content modifies liver fat in overweight nondiabetic subjects. *J Clin Endocrinol Metab* 90:2804–2809, 2005

Prevalence of Nonalcoholic Fatty Liver Disease and Its Association With Cardiovascular Disease Among Type 2 Diabetic Patients

Giovanni Targher, MD[1,2]
Lorenzo Bertolini, MD[1]
Roberto Padovani, MD[1]
Stefano Rodella, MD[3]

Roberto Tessari, MD[1]
Luciano Zenari, MD[1]
Christopher Day, MD[4]
Guido Arcaro, MD[1]

OBJECTIVE — To determine the prevalence of nonalcoholic fatty liver disease (NAFLD) in type 2 diabetic population and to compare the prevalence of cardiovascular disease (CVD) and its risk factors between people with and without NAFLD.

RESEARCH DESIGN AND METHODS — The entire sample of type 2 diabetic outpatients ($n = 2,839$) who regularly attended our clinic was screened. Main outcome measures were NAFLD (by patient history and liver ultrasound) and manifest CVD (by patient history, review of patient records, electrocardiogram, and echo-Doppler scanning of carotid and lower limb arteries).

RESULTS — The unadjusted prevalence of NAFLD was 69.5% among participants, and NAFLD was the most common cause (81.5%) of hepatic steatosis on ultrasound examination. The prevalence of NAFLD increased with age (65.4% among participants aged 40–59 years and 74.6% among those aged ≥60 years; $P < 0.001$) and the age-adjusted prevalence of NAFLD was 71.1% in men and 68% in women. NAFLD patients had remarkably ($P < 0.001$) higher age and sex-adjusted prevalences of coronary (26.6 vs. 18.3%), cerebrovascular (20.0 vs. 13.3%), and peripheral (15.4 vs. 10.0%) vascular disease than their counterparts without NAFLD. In logistic regression analysis, NAFLD was associated with prevalent CVD independent of classical risk factors, glycemic control, medications, and metabolic syndrome features.

CONCLUSIONS — NAFLD is extremely common in people with type 2 diabetes and is associated with a higher prevalence of CVD. Follow-up studies are needed to determine whether NAFLD predicts the development and progression of CVD.

Diabetes Care 30:1212–1218, 2007

Nonalcoholic fatty liver disease (NAFLD) is the most common cause of abnormal liver function tests among adults in Western countries (1–4). The spectrum of NAFLD ranges from simple steatosis to nonalcoholic ste- atohepatitis (NASH), which can progress to end-stage liver disease. NAFLD is commonly associated with obesity, type 2 diabetes, dyslipidemia, and insulin resistance, all of which are components of the metabolic syndrome, strongly sup- porting the notion that NAFLD is the hepatic manifestation of the syndrome (1–4). The prevalence of NAFLD has been reported to be in the 15–30% range in the general population in various countries (5–7) and is almost certainly increasing. Accordingly, a huge number of individuals are at risk of developing advanced liver disease.

Compared with nondiabetic subjects, people with type 2 diabetes appear to have an increased risk of developing NAFLD and certainly have a higher risk of developing fibrosis and cirrhosis (1–4). It has been estimated that ~70–75% of type 2 diabetic patients may have some form of NAFLD (8); however, the "pre- cise" prevalence of NAFLD in type 2 dia- betes is unknown. The few available studies have been small and performed in highly selected populations or have esti- mated only the prevalence of abnormal aminotransferase levels (9–12), which are a poor proxy measure of NAFLD (1–3).

Recent data suggest that the presence of NAFLD in type 2 diabetes may also be linked to increased cardiovascular disease (CVD) risk independently of components of the metabolic syndrome (13,14), al- though this hypothesis needs verification in larger studies. However, if correct, these data suggest that the identification of NAFLD in type 2 diabetes may help in CVD risk prediction with important man- agement implications. Identifying people with NAFLD would also highlight a sub- group of diabetic patients who should be targeted with more intensive therapy to decrease their risk of future CVD events. The main purpose of this study was to determine the prevalence of NAFLD, as diagnosed by patient history and liver ul- trasound, which is the most widely used imaging test for detecting hepatic steato- sis, and to establish whether there is an association between NAFLD and CVD in a large cohort of type 2 diabetic adults.

RESEARCH DESIGN AND METHODS

All of the outpatients ($n = 3,166$) with type 2 diabetes who reg- ularly attended our clinic during the pe-

From the ¹Department of Internal Medicine, "Sacro Cuore" Hospital, Negrar, Italy; the ²Section of Endocri- nology, Department of Biomedical and Surgical Sciences, University Hospital of Verona, Verona, Italy; the ³Department of Radiology, "Sacro Cuore" Hospital, Negrar, Italy; and the ⁴Institute of Cellular Medicine, Newcastle University, Newcastle upon Tyne, U.K.

Address correspondence and reprint requests to Giovanni Targher, MD, Division of Internal Medicine and Diabetes Unit, Ospedale "Sacro Cuore–don Calabria," Via A. Semprebони, 5, 37024 Negrar (VR), Italy. E-mail: targher@sacrocuore.it.

Received for publication 2 November 2006 and accepted in revised form 16 January 2007.

Published ahead of print at http://care.diabetesjournals.org on 2 February 2007. DOI: 10.2337/dc06- 2247.

Abbreviations: ALT, alanine aminotransferase; ATP III, Adult Treatment Panel III; CVD, cardiovascular disease; NAFLD, nonalcoholic fatty liver disease; NASH, nonalcoholic steatohepatitis.

A table elsewhere in this issue shows conventional and Système International (SI) units and conversion factors for many substances.

riod between 1 January 2005 and 1 January 2006 were screened. Excluding those for whom a liver ultrasound examination was not available ($n = 327$, 10.3%), 2,839 type 2 diabetic outpatients were studied; 800 of them were previously included in a study (14). The local ethics committee approved the study. All participants provided written informed consent.

BMI was calculated by dividing weight in kilograms by the square of height in meters. Waist circumference was measured in a standing position at the level of the umbilicus. Blood pressure was measured with a standard mercury manometer. Information on daily alcohol consumption, smoking status, and use of medications (including also hepatotoxic drugs such as glucocorticoids, amiodarone, methotrexate, or antineoplastic drugs) was obtained from all participants by a questionnaire (13). Most participants were abstainers ($n = 2,169$, 76.4%) or drank minimally (alcohol consumption <20 g/day; $n = 312$, 11%); only 12.6% of participants drank >20 g/day of alcohol.

Venous blood was drawn in the morning after an overnight fast. Plasma liver tests and other biochemical blood measurements were determined by standard laboratory procedures. Normal ranges for serum aminotransferase levels, in our laboratory, were 10–35 units/l for women and 10–50 units/l for men, respectively. In this study, a single measurement of liver enzymes that was obtained within ~1 month of liver ultrasonography was used in statistical analyses. However, as all participants attended our clinic regularly, repeated aminotransferase measurements were available for each participant (>2 per year); none of those without NAFLD had raised serum aminotransferase levels at any time. Serology for viral hepatitis B and C was assessed in all participants. LDL cholesterol was calculated by the Friedewald equation. A1C was measured by a high-performance liquid chromatography analyzer (HA-8140; Menarini Diagnostics, Florence, Italy); the upper limit of normal for the laboratory was 5.9%.

Metabolic syndrome was diagnosed by the Adult Treatment Panel III (ATP III) definition. In accordance with this definition (15), a person with type 2 diabetes was classified as having the syndrome if he or she had at least two of the following four components: 1) waist circumference >102 cm in men or >88 cm in women, 2) triglycerides ≥1.7 mmol/l, 3) HDL

<1.0 mmol/l in men and <1.29 mmol/l in women or receiving treatment, and 4) blood pressure ≥130/85 mmHg or receiving treatment.

Hepatic ultrasonography scanning was performed in all participants by a single experienced radiologist, who was blinded to subjects' details. The diagnosis of hepatic steatosis was made on the basis of characteristic sonographic features (1–3). It is known that ultrasonography has a sensitivity of ~90% and a specificity of ~95% in detection of moderate and severe hepatic steatosis (1,2), although ultrasonography is not totally sensitive, particularly when hepatic fat infiltration on liver biopsy is <30% (16). Semiquantitative sonographic scoring for the degree of hepatic steatosis was not available. Repeated measurements that were done on a random subgroup of 150 of the same subjects gave coefficients of variation within 3% (13,14).

The presence of CVD was assessed as follows. A detailed medical history was collected by a questionnaire (14) administered by a trained physician to record previous or current coronary (myocardial infarction, angina, or revascularization procedures), cerebrovascular (ischemic stroke, recurrent transient ischemic attacks, carotid endarterectomy, or carotid stenosis ≥70% as diagnosed by echo-Doppler scanning), and peripheral (intermittent claudication, rest pain, as confirmed by echo-Doppler scanning, lower extremity amputation, or revascularization procedures) vascular disease. The presence of CVD was confirmed by reviewing hospital medical records of all patients and by a thorough physical examination by one of the investigators that also included vascular laboratory studies (electrocardiogram and echo-Doppler scanning of carotid and lower limb arteries, which were performed for all participants). Data on CVD were collected only for those with and without NAFLD but not for those with other causes of chronic liver disease.

Statistical analysis
Data are means ± SD or proportions. Skewed variables (triglycerides and liver enzymes) were logarithmically transformed to improve normality before analysis. Statistical analyses included the unpaired t test and the χ^2 test with Yates' correction for continuity (for categorical variables). The independence of the associations of variables with prevalent CVD, included as the dependent variable, was

assessed by multivariable logistic regression analysis and expressed as odds ratios (ORs). In this analysis, men and women were combined and first-order interaction terms for sex-by-NAFLD interactions on risk for CVD were examined. Because the interactions were not statistically significant, sex-pooled multivariable logistic regression analysis was used to assess the independence of the association of NAFLD with CVD. In that analysis, CVD was considered as the composite end point inclusive of those patients with coronary, cerebrovascular, or peripheral vascular disease (as defined above). In the fully adjusted regression models, NAFLD, sex, age, BMI, smoking status, diabetes duration, A1C, LDL cholesterol, use of medications (hypoglycemic, antihypertensive, lipid-lowering, or antiplatelet drugs), and presence of ATP III–defined metabolic syndrome were also included as covariates. Separate models were also tested with the four individual components of the metabolic syndrome included as categorical or continuous measures. $P < 0.05$ was considered statistically significant.

RESULTS — As shown in Fig. 1, 3,166 type 2 diabetic outpatients, who regularly attended our clinic, were initially screened. Excluding those ($n = 327$) who did not have a liver ultrasound examination left 2,839 participants, aged 40–86 years, who were included in analyses. There were no significant differences in main study variables between those who did and those who did not have a liver ultrasound examination. Of the 2,839 participants, 2,421 had hepatic steatosis on ultrasound, whereas 418 had negative liver ultrasound tests as well as normal liver tests and the absence of viral hepatitis or excessive alcohol consumption. Among those with hepatic steatosis, 358 participants admitted alcohol abuse or drank >20 g/day and 89 had other causes of chronic liver disease (viral hepatitis or medications), whereas the remaining 1,974 participants met the criteria for diagnosis of NAFLD, i.e., hepatic steatosis among individuals without excessive alcohol consumption or other causes of chronic liver disease. Thus, the unadjusted prevalence of NAFLD was 69.5% (95% CI 68.5–70.5), and NAFLD represented the most common cause (81.5%) of hepatic steatosis on ultrasound. The prevalence of NAFLD increased with increasing age (65.4% among participants aged 40–59 years and 74.6% among

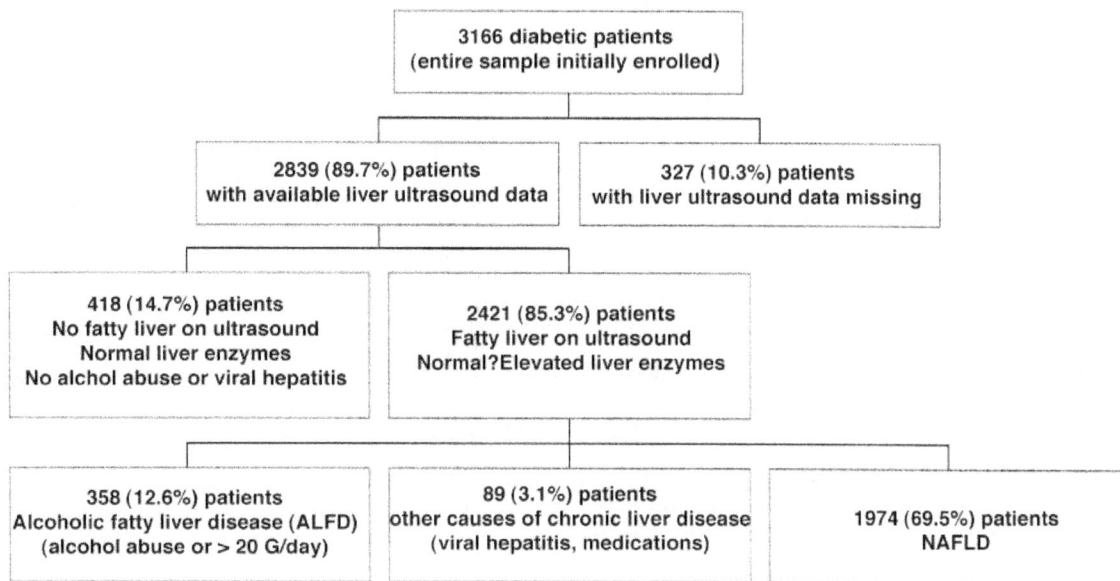

```
                    ┌─────────────────────────────────┐
                    │      3166 diabetic patients       │
                    │ (entire sample initially enrolled) │
                    └─────────────────────────────────┘
```

Figure 1—*Details of the study design.*

those aged ≥60 years; $P < 0.001$), and the age-adjusted prevalence of NAFLD was 71.1% in men and 68.0% in women ($P = 0.20$).

The baseline characteristics of the study participants, grouped according to NAFLD status, after exclusion of those with other known causes of chronic liver disease ($n = 447$), are presented in Table 1. Individuals with NAFLD were older, more likely to be male, and had longer diabetes duration than those without NAFLD. They also had higher values of A1C and liver enzymes, although the vast majority of patients with NAFLD (86%) had normal serum alanine aminotransferase (ALT) levels. Metabolic syndrome and its individual components occurred more frequently among patients with NAFLD. Smoking history, plasma LDL cholesterol, and creatinine concentrations were not significantly different between the groups. The proportion using insulin or antihypertensive or antiplatelet drugs was higher among patients with NAFLD, whereas the proportion using lipid-lowering drugs was similar in both groups.

Overall, 1,074 (44.4% [95% CI 43.4–45.4]) of 2,421 participants with and without NAFLD were coded positive for CVD (as composite end point). Of these, 546 patients (22.6% [21.6–23.6]) had coronary heart disease (398 with myocardial infarction and 148 subjects with angina or revascularization procedures), 398 patients (16.4% [15.4–17.4])

had cerebrovascular disease (298 with ischemic stroke, recurrent transient ischemic attack, or carotid endarterectomy and 100 with carotid stenosis ≥70% as ascertained by echo-Doppler scanning),

and 307 patients (12.7% [11.7–13.7]) had peripheral vascular disease (182 of them with rest pain or claudication as confirmed by echo-Doppler scanning and 125 subjects with prior lower extremity

Table 1—*Baseline characteristics of the study participants, grouped according to NAFLD status*

Variables	Without fatty liver	With NAFLD	P value
n	418	1,974	
Sex (% men)	54	57	<0.001
Age (years)	60 ± 4	65 ± 6	<0.001
BMI (kg/m^2)	26.5 ± 3	28.3 ± 4	<0.001
Diabetes duration (years)	7 ± 2	12 ± 3	<0.001
Oral hypoglycemic users (%)	67	66	0.80
Insulin users (%)	17	25	<0.001
Antihypertensive drug users (%)	60	73	<0.001
Aspirin users (%)	48	57	<0.001
Lipid-lowering drug users (%)	41	43	0.60
Current smokers (%)	25	27	0.60
Systolic blood pressure (mmHg)	135 ± 10	139 ± 12	<0.001
Diastolic blood pressure (mmHg)	83 ± 7	85 ± 10	<0.001
A1C (%)	6.7 ± 0.6	7.3 ± 1.1	<0.001
Triglycerides (mmol/l)	1.40 ± 0.6	1.68 ± 1.0	<0.001
HDL cholesterol (mmol/l)	1.41 ± 0.3	1.34 ± 0.4	<0.001
LDL cholesterol (mmol/l)	3.40 ± 0.4	3.37 ± 0.4	0.40
Creatinine (μmol/l)	90 ± 12	92 ± 14	0.40
Aspartate aminotransferase (units/l)	23 ± 3	28 ± 10	<0.001
ALT (units/l)	25 ± 3	33 ± 12	<0.001
Elevated ALT (men >50 units/l; women >35 units/l) (%)	0	14	<0.001
ATP III–defined metabolic syndrome (%)	70	86	<0.001

Data are means ± SD or proportions. $n = 2,392$.

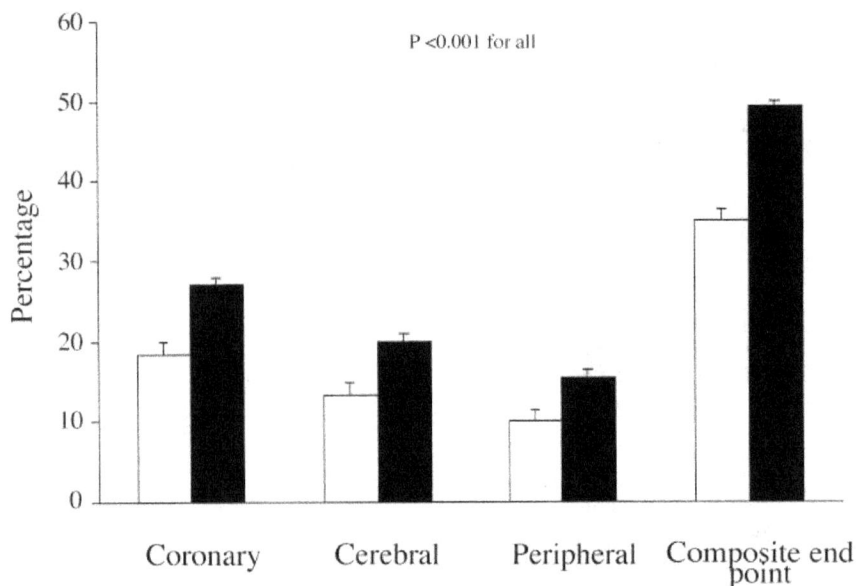

Figure 2—*Age- and sex-adjusted prevalence of CVD in type 2 diabetic adults with (■) and without (□) NAFLD. Data are expressed as percentages ± SE. P < 0.001 for differences between the groups.*

amputation or revascularization procedures); many subjects had CVD in multiple sites. Interestingly, compared with previous reports, in which comparable diagnostic noninvasive measures were used, the prevalence of CVD in this study was similar to that described in other populations with comparable age, diabetes duration, glycemic control, and smoking status (17–20). As shown in Fig. 2, the age- and sex-adjusted prevalences of coronary, cerebrovascular, and peripheral vascular disease were remarkably higher in patients with NAFLD than in those without NAFLD.

In univariate logistic regression analysis, together with NAFLD (Fig. 3, *top bar*), age, male sex, BMI, smoking, diabetes duration, A1C, LDL cholesterol, presence of ATP III–defined metabolic syndrome, and use of medications (particularly the aspirin use) were significantly associated with CVD (not shown). The relationship between NAFLD and CVD was little affected by adjustment for age, sex, BMI, smoking, diabetes duration, A1C, LDL cholesterol, and medications (Fig. 3, *second* and *third bars*); additional adjustment for the metabolic syndrome did not appreciably change this relationship (Fig. 3, *bottom bar*). In this fully adjusted regression model, together with NAFLD, male sex (OR 1.5 [95% CI 1.2–1.9]), older age (1.08 [1.06–1.1]), smoking (1.4 [1.1–1.8]), and the metabolic syndrome (1.6 [1.3–2.6]) were also

independently (*P* < 0.001) associated with CVD.

Almost identical results were obtained in models that also adjusted for the individual components of the metabolic syndrome (not shown). Exclusion of participants who have asymptomatic CVD

(carotid stenosis ≥70%) or who were light-to-moderate drinkers (alcohol consumption <20 g/day) did not alter the observed associations between NAFLD and CVD (OR 1.49 [95% CI 1.1–2.0], *P* = 0.032).

CONCLUSIONS — There is a pressing unmet need to determine the prevalence of NAFLD in the type 2 diabetic population and to evaluate its association with CVD. It has only recently been recognized that NAFLD represents an important burden of disease for patients with type 2 diabetes (1–4,21), but the magnitude of the problem of NAFLD in patients with type 2 diabetes is currently unknown. It is also becoming evident that NAFLD is related to CVD in people with type 2 diabetes (13,14), but further research in this area is required to ascertain whether NAFLD is a (independent) CVD risk factor. Indeed, the impact of NAFLD on CVD risk deserves particular attention in view of the implications for screening/surveillance strategies in the growing number of patients with NAFLD.

To our knowledge, this is the largest cross-sectional study with the specific aims of establishing the prevalence of NAFLD in a large cohort of type 2 diabetic patients and assessing the association of NAFLD with CVD. A major finding of this

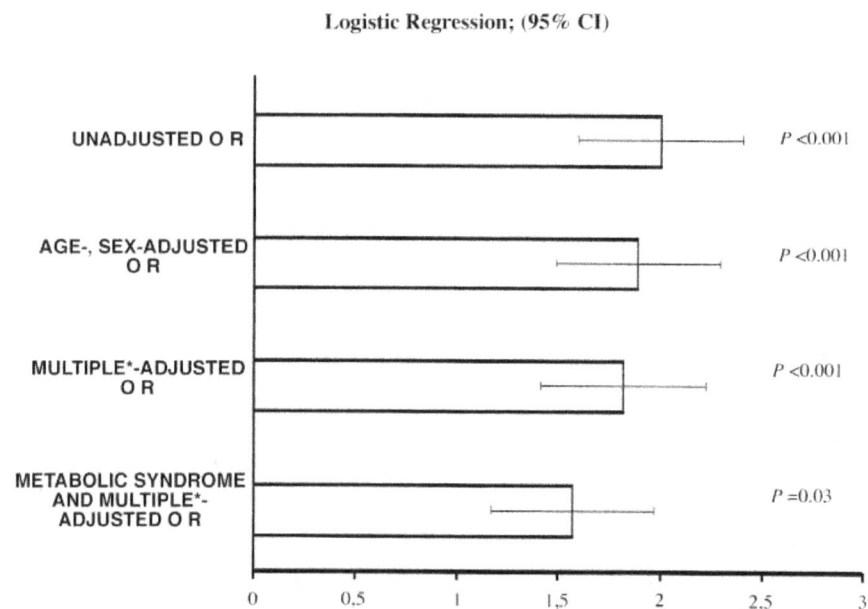

Figure 3—*Association between NAFLD and prevalent CVD in type 2 diabetic adults with and without NAFLD (n = 2,392). Data are expressed as ORs ± 95% CI. *The multiple adjustment reported in the third and fourth bars was as follows: age, sex, BMI, smoking status, diabetes duration, A1C, LDL cholesterol, and current use of medications (hypoglycemic, antihypertensive, lipid-lowering, or antiplatelet drugs).*

study is that the prevalence of NAFLD, as diagnosed by patient history and characteristic sonographic features, in the type 2 diabetic population is very high. Indeed, NAFLD is present in ~70% of our population and represents the most common explanation (81.5%) for any form of hepatic steatosis on ultrasound examination.

Interestingly, this study provides further evidence that a normal serum ALT level provides little diagnostic or prognostic value when assessing patients for NAFLD, because more than four-fifths (86%) of our patients with NAFLD had normal ALT levels. Even when more stringent criteria were used (i.e., ALT >30 units/l in men and >19 units/l in women) (22), most patients with NAFLD (63%) had normal ALT levels. Therefore, serum ALT levels appear to be insensitive markers for NAFLD. Indeed, it is known that the full histological spectrum of NAFLD may be present among patients with normal liver enzymes (23), which therefore cannot be reliably used to exclude the presence of more advanced stages of NAFLD (1–4).

Another major finding of this study is that NAFLD is associated with a higher prevalence of CVD in multiple sites (coronary, cerebrovascular, and peripheral vascular disease). Importantly, this association remains statistically significant after adjustment for a broad spectrum of prognostic factors, including the metabolic syndrome, a chronic inflammatory cardiovascular condition that is closely associated with NAFLD (as also confirmed by our results).

Given our study design, we are unable to draw conclusions about causality in the relation between NAFLD and CVD and to determine whether the higher CVD prevalence among patients with NAFLD affects long-term mortality. The most likely explanation for our findings could be that the relationship between NAFLD and CVD mainly reflects the overall, adverse, impact of the metabolic syndrome phenotype, principally insulin resistance. Although our results have been adjusted for the metabolic syndrome, a condition that is closely associated with insulin resistance, we did not directly measure insulin resistance (by glucose clamp) in our diabetic population, so we cannot be certain that identical results could be obtained after additional adjustment for this CVD risk factor. However, the glucose clamp would be impossible to perform routinely in a large epidemiological study.

On the other hand, the homeostasis model assessment score is not a reliable method for determining insulin resistance in diabetic patients treated with antidiabetes agents, particularly in those receiving insulin treatment (24).

A significant association between NAFLD and increased CVD prevalence in type 2 diabetic individuals has been previously shown in our smaller study (14). In that study, however, the association between NAFLD and CVD was no longer apparent after adjustment for the metabolic syndrome. These apparently discrepant results can be principally explained by the larger sample size of this study, which provided a greater statistical power and permitted more complete adjustment for potential confounders. Moreover, our findings are validated by a follow-up study demonstrating that NAFLD is associated with increased CVD incidence in type 2 diabetic patients independent of traditional risk factors and the presence of the metabolic syndrome (13). Others have cross-sectionally shown that individuals with modestly elevated serum ALT levels, as surrogate measures of NAFLD, have an increased CVD risk (as calculated by the Framingham risk score) (25). Currently, it is not known whether improving NAFLD will ultimately prevent the development of CVD. However, it is notable that interventions that are known to be effective in preventing CVD in type 2 diabetic people, including weight reduction and treatment with insulin-sensitizing antidiabetes agents (26–32), may possibly improve NAFLD.

Overall, these findings might have possible clinical and public health implications. Our results indicate that the majority of patients with type 2 diabetes have NAFLD, and previous studies showing that type 2 diabetes is an independent predictor of advanced liver disease in NAFLD suggest that consideration should be given to referring patients to a hepatologist for further evaluation. This will be particularly important once an effective treatment for NASH has been established, and better noninvasive methods for assessing disease severity are validated. Additionally, our findings complement recent observations that the severity of NAFLD histology is associated with greater carotid intima-media thickness and plaques (33) and lower endothelial flow-mediated vasodilation (34) independent of underlying metabolic abnormalities and that NAFLD is associated with higher all-cause death (35–37) and pre-

dicts the risk of future CVD events (13,37). There is therefore now growing evidence that NAFLD is not simply a marker of CVD but may also be, directly or indirectly, involved in its pathogenesis. The possible molecular mediators linking NAFLD and CVD have been extensively reviewed elsewhere but include the release of proatherogenic mediators from the liver including C-reactive protein, interleukin-6, and plasminogen activator inhibitor-1 (38).

The present study has some limitations that should be noted. The cross-sectional design of our study precludes the establishment of causal or temporal relations among NAFLD, metabolic syndrome, and CVD. Another limitation of this study is that the diagnosis of NAFLD was based on ultrasound imaging and exclusion of other causes of chronic liver disease but was not confirmed by liver biopsy. It is known that none of the radiological features can distinguish between NASH and other forms of NAFLD and that only liver biopsy can assess the severity of damage and the prognosis (1–3). However, liver biopsy would be impossible to perform routinely in a large epidemiological study. Conversely, ultrasonography is by far the most common way of diagnosing NAFLD in clinical practice and has good sensitivity and specificity in detecting moderate and severe steatosis (1,2). Indeed, it has been reported that the presence of >30% fat on liver biopsy is optimal for ultrasound detection of steatosis, whereas ultrasonography is not totally sensitive, particularly when hepatic fat infiltration is <30% (16). Thus, although some nondifferential misclassification of NAFLD on the basis of ultrasonography is likely (i.e., some of the diabetic control subjects could have underlying NAFLD despite normal liver enzymes and negative ultrasonography examination), this limitation would serve to attenuate the magnitude of our effect measures toward the null; thus, our results can probably be considered as conservative estimates of the relationship between NAFLD and CVD.

In conclusion, our results suggest that NAFLD is extremely common in people with type 2 diabetes and is associated with a higher prevalence of CVD. The association between NAFLD and CVD appears to be independent of classical risk factors, glycemic control, medications, and presence of the metabolic syndrome. Thus, these results further confirm the hypothesis that the identification of NAFLD in type 2 diabetes may help in CVD prediction. Future experimental and follow-up studies are needed to elucidate the possible molecular mechanisms linking NAFLD and CVD and to determine whether NAFLD predicts the development and progression of CVD.

References

1. Angulo P: Nonalcoholic fatty liver disease. *N Engl J Med* 346:1221–1231, 2002
2. Day CP: Non-alcoholic fatty liver disease: current concepts and management strategies. *Clin Med* 6:19–25, 2006
3. McCullough AJ: Pathophysiology of nonalcoholic steatohepatitis. *J Clin Gastroenterol* 40 (Suppl. 1):S17–29, 2006
4. Marchesini G, Marzocchi R, Agostini F, Bugianesi E: Nonalcoholic fatty liver disease and the metabolic syndrome. *Curr Opin Lipidol* 16:421–427, 2005
5. Clark JM, Brancati FL, Diehl AM: The prevalence and aetiology of elevated aminotransferase levels in the United States. *Am J Gastroenterol* 98:960–967, 2003
6. Bedogni G, Miglioli L, Masutti F, Tiribelli C, Marchesini G, Bellentani S: Prevalence of and risk factors for nonalcoholic fatty liver disease: the Dionysos Nutrition and Liver Study. *Hepatology* 42:44–52, 2005
7. Browning JD, Szczepaniak LS, Dobbins R, Nuremberg P, Horton JD, Cohen JC, Grundy SM, Hobbs HH: Prevalence of hepatic steatosis in an urban population in the United States: impact of ethnicity. *Hepatology* 40:1387–1395, 2004
8. Medina J, Fernandez-Salazar LI, Garcia-Buey L, Moreno-Otero R: Approach to the pathogenesis and treatment of nonalcoholic steatohepatitis. *Diabetes Care* 27:2057–2066, 2004
9. Jick SS, Stender M, Myers MW: Frequency of liver disease in type 2 diabetic patients treated with oral antidiabetic agents. *Diabetes Care* 22:2067–2071, 1999
10. Erbey JR, Silberman C, Lydick E: Prevalence of abnormal serum alanine aminotransferase levels in obese patients and patients with type 2 diabetes. *Am J Med* 109:588–590, 2000
11. Younossi ZM, Gramlich T, Matteoni CA, Boparai N, McCullough AJ: Nonalcoholic fatty liver disease in patients with type 2 diabetes. *Clin Gastroenterol Hepatol* 2:262–265, 2004
12. Jimba S, Nakagami T, Takahashi M, Wakamatsu T, Hirota Y, Iwamoto Y, Wasada T: Prevalence of nonalcoholic fatty liver disease and its association with impaired glucose metabolism in Japanese adults. *Diabet Med* 22:1141–1145, 2005
13. Targher G, Bertolini L, Poli F, Rodella S, Scala L, Tessari R, Zenari L, Falezza G: Nonalcoholic fatty liver disease and risk of future cardiovascular events among type 2 diabetic patients. *Diabetes* 54:3541–3546, 2005
14. Targher G, Bertolini L, Padovani R, Poli F, Scala L, Tessari R, Zenari L, Falezza G: Increased prevalence of cardiovascular disease among type 2 diabetic patients with non-alcoholic fatty liver disease. *Diabet Med* 23:403–409, 2006
15. National Cholesterol Education Program: Executive summary of the Third Report of the National Cholesterol Education Program (NCEP) Expert Panel on Detection, Evaluation, and Treatment of High Blood Cholesterol in Adults (Adult Treatment Panel III). *JAMA* 285:2486–2497, 2001
16. Saadeh S, Younossi ZM, Remer EM, Gramlich T, Ong JP, Hurley M, Mullen KD, Cooper JN, Sheridan MJ: The utility of radiological imaging in nonalcoholic fatty liver disease. *Gastroenterology* 123:745–750, 2002
17. DAI Study Group: The prevalence of coronary heart disease in type 2 diabetic patients in Italy: the DAI study. *Diabet Med* 21:738–745, 2004
18. Meijer WT, Hoes AW, Rutgers D, Bots ML, Hofman A, Grobbee DE: Peripheral arterial disease in the elderly: the Rotterdam Study. *Arterioscler Thromb Vasc Biol* 18:185–192, 1998
19. Arteagoitia JM, Larranaga MI, Rodriguez JL, Fernandez I, Pinies JA: Incidence, prevalence and coronary heart disease risk level in known type 2 diabetes: a sentinel practice network study in the Basque Country, Spain. *Diabetologia* 46:899–909, 2003
20. Bonora E, Formentini G, Calcaterra F, Lombardi S, Marini F, Zenari L, Saggiani F, Poli M, Perbellini S, Raffaelli A, Cacciatori V, Santi L, Targher G, Bonadonna RC, Muggeo M: HOMA-estimated insulin resistance is an independent predictor of cardiovascular disease in type 2 diabetic subjects: prospective data from the Verona Diabetes Complications Study. *Diabetes Care* 25:1135–1141, 2002
21. Harrison SA: Liver disease in patients with diabetes mellitus. *J Clin Gastroenterol* 40:68–76, 2006
22. Prati D, Taioli E, Zanella A, Della Torre E, Buttelli S, Del Vecchio E, Vianello L, Zanuso F, Mozzi F, Milani S, Conte D, Colombo M, Sirchia G: Updated definitions of healthy ranges for serum alanine aminotransferase levels. *Ann Intern Med* 137:1–10, 2002
23. Mofrad P, Contos MJ, Haque M, Sargeant C, Fisher RA, Luketic VA, Sterling RK, Shiffman ML, Stravitz RT, Sanyal AJ: Clinical and histological spectrum of nonalcoholic fatty liver disease associated with normal ALT values. *Hepatology* 37:1286–1292, 2003
24. Bonora E, Targher G, Alberiche M, Bonadonna RC, Saggiani F, Zenere MB, Monauni T, Muggeo M: Homeostasis model assessment closely mirrors the glucose clamp technique in the assessment of insulin sensitivity: studies in subjects with various degrees of glucose tolerance and insulin sensitivity. *Diabetes Care* 23:57–63, 2000
25. Ioannou GN, Weiss NS, Boyko EJ, Mozaffarian D, Lee SP: Elevated serum alanine aminotrasferase activity and calculated risk of coronary heart disease in the United States. *Hepatology* 43:1145–1151, 2006
26. Ueno T, Sugawara H, Sujaku K, Hashimoto O, Tsuji R, Tamaki S, Torimura T, Inuzuka S, Sata M, Tanikawa K: Therapeutic effects of restricted diet and exercise in obese patients with fatty liver. *J Hepatol* 27:103–107, 1997
27. Petersen KF, Dufour S, Befroy D, Lehrke M, Hendler RE, Shulman GI: Reversal of nonalcoholic hepatic steatosis, hepatic insulin resistance, and hyperglycemia by moderate weight reduction in patients with type 2 diabetes. *Diabetes* 54:603–608, 2005
28. Uygun A, Kadayifci A, Isik A, Ozgurtas T, Deveci S, Tuzun A, Yesilova Z, Gulsen M, Dagalp K: Metformin in the treatment of patients with non-alcoholic steatohepatitis. *Aliment Pharmacol Ther* 19:537–544, 2004
29. Bugianesi E, Gentilcore E, Manini R, Natale S, Vanni E, Villanova N, David E, Rizzetto M, Marchesini G: A randomized controlled trial of metformin versus vitamin E or prescriptive diet in non-alcoholic fatty liver disease. *Am J Gastroenterol* 100:1082–1090, 2005
30. Neuschwander-Tetri BA, Brunt E, Wehmeier K, Oliver D, Bacon B: Improved nonalcoholic steatohepatitis after 48 weeks of treatment with the PPAR-gamma ligand rosiglitazone. *Hepatology* 38:1008–1017, 2003
31. Promrat K, Lutchman G, Uwaifo G, Freedman R, Soza A, Heller T, Doo E, Ghany M, Premkumar A, Park Y, Liang TJ, Yanovski JA, Kleiner DE, Hoofnagle JH: A pilot study of pioglitazone treatment for nonalcoholic steatohepatitis. *Hepatology* 39:188–196, 2004
32. Tiikkainen M, Hakkinen AM, Korsheninnikova E, Nyman T, Makimattila S, Yki-Jarvinen H: Effects of rosiglitazone and metformin on liver fat content, hepatic insulin resistance, insulin clearance, and gene expression in adipose tissue in patients with type 2 diabetes. *Diabetes* 53:2169–2176, 2004
33. Targher G, Bertolini L, Padovani R, Rodella S, Zoppini G, Zenari L, Cigolini M, Falezza G, Arcaro G: Relations between carotid artery wall thickness and liver histology in subjects with nonalcoholic fatty liver disease. *Diabetes Care* 29:1325–1330, 2006
34. Villanova N, Moscatiello S, Ramilli S, Bugianesi E, Magalotti D, Vanni E, Zoli M,

Marchesini G: Endothelial dysfunction and cardiovascular risk profile in nonalcoholic fatty liver disease. *Hepatology* 42: 473–478, 2005

35. Matteoni CA, Younossi ZM, Gramlich T, Boparai N, Liu LC, McCullough AJ: Nonalcoholic fatty liver disease: a spectrum of clinical and pathological severity. *Gastro-* *enterology* 116:1413–1419, 1999

36. Adams LA, Lymp JF, St Sauver J, Sanderson SO, Lindor KD, Feldstein A, Angulo P: The natural history of nonalcoholic fatty liver disease: a population-based cohort study. *Gastroenterology* 129:113–121, 2005

37. Ekstedt M, Franzen LE, Mathiesen UL, Thorelius L, Holmqvist M, Bodemar G, Kechagias S: Long-term follow-up of patients with NAFLD and elevated liver enzymes. *Hepatology* 44:865–873, 2006

38. Targher G, Arcaro G: Review: Nonalcoholic fatty liver disease and increased risk of cardiovascular disease. *Atherosclerosis* 2006, doi:10.1016/j.atherosclerosis.2006.08.021

Serum Alanine Aminotransferase Levels Decrease Further With Carbohydrate Than Fat Restriction in Insulin-Resistant Adults

Marno Celeste Ryan, MD[1]
Fahim Abbasi, MD[1]
Cindy Lamendola, MSN[2]

Susan Carter, MS, RD[2]
Tracey Lynn McLaughlin, MD, MS[2]

OBJECTIVE — Although weight loss interventions have been shown to reduce steatosis in nonalcoholic fatty liver disease (NAFLD), the impact of dietary macronutrient composition is unknown. We assessed the effect on serum alanine aminotransferase (ALT) concentrations of two hypocaloric diets varying in amounts of carbohydrate and fat in obese insulin-resistant individuals, a population at high risk for NAFLD.

RESEARCH DESIGN AND METHODS — Post hoc analysis of ALT concentrations was performed in 52 obese subjects with normal baseline values and insulin resistance, as quantified by the steady-state plasma glucose (SSPG) test, who were randomized to hypocaloric diets containing either 60% carbohydrate/25% fat or 40% carbohydrate/45% fat (15% protein) for 16 weeks. The primary end point was change in ALT, which was evaluated according to diet, weight loss, SSPG, and daylong insulin concentrations.

RESULTS — Although both diets resulted in significant decreases in weight and SSPG, daylong insulin, and serum ALT concentrations, the 40% carbohydrate diet resulted in greater decreases in SSPG ($P < 0.04$), circulating insulin ($P < 0.01$), and ALT (9.5 ± 9.4 vs. 4.2 ± 8.3 units/l; $P < 0.04$) concentrations. ALT changes correlated with improvement in insulin sensitivity ($P = 0.04$) and daylong insulin ($P < 0.01$). Individuals with ALT concentrations above the proposed upper limits experienced significant declines in ALT, unlike those with lower ALT levels.

CONCLUSIONS — In a population at high risk for NAFLD, a hypocaloric diet moderately lower in carbohydrate decreased serum ALT concentrations to a greater degree than a higher-carbohydrate/low-fat diet, despite equal weight loss. This may result from a relatively greater decline in daylong insulin concentrations. Further research with histological end points is needed to further explore this finding.

Diabetes Care 30:1075–1080, 2007

N onalcoholic fatty liver disease (NAFLD) is a clinicopathologic syndrome that encompasses a spectrum of conditions ranging from simple hepatic fat (steatosis) to nonalcoholic steatohepatitis (NASH), fibrosis, and end-stage liver disease (1–3). NAFLD affects up to 74% of obese individuals (4,5) and is almost always associated with both hepatic and peripheral insulin resistance (6–9).

There has been recent interest in the optimal diet to reduce the cardiometabolic complications of obesity-associated insulin resistance. As the same population also is at risk of NAFLD, it is of interest to identify the optimal dietary approach to prevent steatosis, the initial lesion, in this group. Furthermore, the development of steatosis per se, even in the absence of fibrosis, may stimulate inflammatory pathways that adversely affect metabolism (10–12), possibly contributing to systemic insulin resistance and risk for cardiovascular disease and diabetes.

Current therapeutic guidelines for NAFLD advocate weight loss as a first-line treatment (13). Although a number of studies (14–17) have demonstrated a reduction in steatosis with weight loss, there are no published studies comparing the relative benefits for NAFLD of a hypocaloric diet that is restricted in fat versus carbohydrate. In this regard, it seems intuitive that a low-fat diet would be preferable to a high-fat diet in preventing or reversing established steatosis. Indeed, the American Heart Association, the American Diabetes Association, and the National Heart, Lung, and Blood Institute all recommend for weight loss a diet with <30% of total calories derived from fat. However, we and others have previously shown that diets enriched in carbohydrate lead to increased circulating insulin concentrations (18,19), which contribute to elevated fasting and daylong triacylglycerol concentrations and lower HDL cholesterol concentrations under isocaloric conditions. Even under weight loss conditions, diets that are lower in carbohydrate and higher in fat have relatively greater benefits on insulin, triacylglycerol, and HDL cholesterol concentrations than similarly hypocaloric, low-fat diets (20–22). We hypothesized that a lower-carbohydrate diet, via greater reductions in daylong insulin concentrations, also may be relatively more effective in reducing intrahepatic fat in the insulin-resistant obese population. This hypothesis is based on the observation that de novo lipogenesis in the liver is increased fourfold in insulin-resistant individuals (23), possibly as a result of insulin stimulation of the transcription factor sterol regulatory binding protein-1c, which regulates expression of lipogenic genes in the liver (24). Thus, we sought to determine, in an obese insulin-resistant population without established liver disease, whether restriction in dietary carbohydrate or fat

From the [1]Division of Cardiovascular Medicine, Falk Cardiovascular Research Center, Stanford University School of Medicine, Stanford University, Stanford, California; and the [2]Division of Endocrinology, Stanford University School of Medicine, Stanford University, Stanford, California.

Address correspondence and reprint requests to Marno C. Ryan, MD, Falk Cardiovascular Research Center, 300 Pasteur Dr., Stanford University, Stanford, CA 94305-5406. E-mail: mryan@cvmed.stanford.edu.

Received for publication 20 October 2006 and accepted in revised form 31 January 2007.

Published ahead of print at http://care.diabetesjournals.org on 10 March 2007. DOI: 10.2337/dc06-2169.

Abbreviations: ALT, alanine aminotransferase; AUC, area under the curve; NAFLD, nonalcoholic fatty liver disease; SSPG, steady-state plasma glucose.

A table elsewhere in this issue shows conventional and Système International (SI) units and conversion factors for many substances.

would yield relatively greater reduction in serum alanine aminotransferase (ALT) concentrations during dietary weight loss.

It has been suggested that the upper limits of normal for serum ALT concentrations set in the 1980s may have been falsely elevated by undiagnosed NAFLD in the reference population (25). A secondary goal of this study was to determine whether ALT values within the current normal limits decrease with weight loss, presumably to truly "normal" concentrations. Insulin-sensitizing thiazolidenedione treatment has been demonstrated to cause a decrease in ALT concentrations in the normal range (26), and we hypothesized that a similar decrease would be seen with weight loss. Thus, we compared change in ALT in those above and below the newly proposed upper limit for the normal range (30 units/l for men and 19 units/l for women) (25).

RESEARCH DESIGN AND METHODS
— The study population consisted of 52 apparently healthy, obese, and insulin-resistant individuals, selected on the basis of baseline ALT concentrations in the normal range at our institution (<60 units/l), from a larger group of subjects ($n = 57$) who participated in a weight loss study (20). All participants gave written informed consent, and the protocol was approved by the Stanford University Human Subjects Committee. To determine eligibility, blood frozen at $-80°C$ was sent to the clinical laboratory at Stanford Medical Center for measurement of baseline serum ALT.

Inclusion criteria included BMI 30.0–36.0 kg/m^2, fasting plasma glucose <126 mg/dl, stable body weight, and no preexisting heart disease, anemia, or kidney disease. Subjects with positive viral serology, previously abnormal serum hepatic transaminases, or alcohol use of more than two standard alcoholic drinks per day were excluded.

Insulin-mediated glucose uptake was quantified by a modification (27) of the insulin suppression test, as originally described and validated (28,29). This approach to the quantification of insulin-mediated glucose uptake has been used for >30 years, and the results are highly correlated with the euglycemic-hyperinsulinemic clamp technique (29). Briefly, after a 12-h overnight fast, an intravenous catheter is placed into each of the patient's arms. A 180-min infusion of somatostatin (0.27 μg/m^2 per min), insulin (32 mU/m^2

per min), and glucose (267 mg/m^2 per min) is administered into one arm. Blood is drawn from the other arm at 30-min intervals, increasing to 10-min intervals for the last 30 min of the study, to determine steady-state plasma glucose (SSPG) and insulin concentrations. As steady-state insulin concentrations are similar for all subjects, the SSPG directly measures the subject's ability to dispose of the glucose load. All subjects entering the dietary intervention phase were required to be insulin resistant on the basis of an SSPG concentration ≥180 mg/dl. This level corresponds to the most insulin-resistant third of 490 apparently healthy individuals (30), a cut point that predicts the development of a variety of adverse clinical outcomes (31,32).

Daylong plasma glucose and insulin concentrations were determined, as described previously (33), at hourly intervals before and after two standardized meals given at 8:00 A.M. and noon. Both meals contained (as percentages of total calories) 15% protein, 43% carbohydrate, and 42% fat (<10% saturated fat), with breakfast comprising 20% and lunch comprising 40% of estimated daily caloric requirements. Insulin was measured in a stepwise sandwich enzyme-linked immunosorbent assay procedure on an ES 300 (Boehringer Mannheim Diagnostics).

Glucose was measured using the hexokinase method on the Hitachi 747 (Boehringer Mannheim Diagnostics).

Following baseline testing, subjects were randomized to follow a hypocaloric diet containing either 60% carbohydrate/25% fat or 40% carbohydrate/45% fat. Both diets contained 15% protein and 7% saturated fat. American Diabetes Association–modified diabetes exchange lists were used. Choices included complex carbohydrates with high fiber content, lean protein, and low saturated fat. All subjects were encouraged to attempt to consume 25 g of fiber. No glycemic index targets were set. Following 2 h of individualized dietary instruction, meals were prepared at home according to weekly diet plans from the study dietitians. Calorie deficit for both diets was -750 kcal/day, as estimated by the Harris Benedict equation (34) and an activity factor for each subject. Subjects were required to keep a daily food diary, which was reviewed weekly with study dietitians to monitor weight and enhance compliance. Actual macronutrient intake was estimated by FOOD PROCESSOR software (version 8.0; ESHA, Salem, OR) analysis of food diaries. Adjustments in intake were recommended as needed to enhance compliance with assigned diets. Sixteen weeks of a hypocaloric diet was followed

Table 1—*Baseline characteristics and reported macronutrient composition consumed by subjects assigned to a 60 vs. 40% carbohydrate diet*

	60% carbohydrate diet	40% carbohydrate diet	P
n	26	26	
Age (years)	54 ± 10	49 ± 11	0.08
Sex (male/female)	14/12	12/14	0.48
Postmenopausal women [n (%)]	9 (35)	7 (27)	0.56
Ethnicity (% Caucasian)	92	93	0.89
BMI (kg/m^2)	33.0 ± 2.4	32.3 ± 1.8	0.20
Weight (kg)	95.1 ± 13.0	94.2 ± 12.3	0.80
SSPG (mg/dl)*	227 ± 26	247 ± 47	0.77
AUC glucose (mg · dl^{-1} · 8 h^{-1})*	869 ± 88	852 ± 98	0.53
AUC insulin (μU · ml^{-1} · 8 h^{-1})*	435 ± 439	459 ± 256	0.82
Serum ALT (units/l)	27.0 ± 10.4	29.0 ± 9.5	0.49
Carbohydrate (%)	58 ± 4	42 ± 5	**<0.01**
Protein (%)	18 ± 2	18 ± 2	0.69
Total fat (%)	23 ± 4	39 ± 5	**<0.01**
Saturated fat (%)	8 ± 2	9 ± 2	0.14
Monounsaturated fat (%)	8 ± 2	13 ± 2	**<0.01**
Polyunsaturated fat (%)	4 ± 1	7 ± 2	**0.01**
Fiber (g)	26 ± 6	23 ± 8	0.27
kcal/day	1,699 ± 334	1,595 ± 262	0.24

Data are means ± SD unless otherwise indicated. P values were calculated using Student's unpaired t tests. Two women in each dietary group were taking hormone replacement therapy. *P values for variables that are not normally distributed refer to analyses performed with logarithmically transformed data. Data in bold face are statistically significant.

by 2 weeks of weight maintenance, with calorie requirements for each subject recalculated according to their current weight. Following the weight maintenance phase, baseline measurements were repeated.

To test our theory that the current normal range of serum ALT included undiagnosed NAFLD, a secondary analysis was performed. Subjects were divided into two groups, regardless of diet, based on whether their baseline ALT was above ("abnormal") or below ("normal") the cut points suggested by Prati et al. (25). We then compared the decline in ALT in the two groups, with the hypothesis that those with the abnormal ALT at baseline, suggestive of NAFLD, would have a greater decline in serum ALT with the hypocaloric diet.

Results are expressed as means ± SD, unless otherwise stated. Between-group differences in experimental variables were assessed with Student's unpaired t tests, whereas within-group changes resulting from the diets were assessed with Student's paired t tests. Differences in categorical variables were tested with χ^2 analysis. SSPG, glucose, and insulin area under the curve (AUC) values were log transformed for normality. All other variables were normally distributed. For clarity of presentation, actual values of variables are presented. P values were done with log-transformed values as per above. Because of the relatively great number of potential confounders for our sample size, stepwise multiple linear regression models were used for the magnitude of change in each dependent variable (weight and ALT, insulin, glucose, and SSPG concentrations) to assess the independent effect of the dietary group (between-group difference). Potential confounders entered into each model included age, sex, baseline concentration of the dependent variable, and amount of weight lost. In all cases, P values <0.05 were considered statistically significant. Analyses were performed using SAS 9.2 and SPPS (version 12).

RESULTS — Twenty-six subjects from each dietary group were eligible for the current analysis. As shown in Table 1, demographic characteristics did not differ significantly between the two groups. Among women, postmenopausal status was not significantly different, and only two women in each group used hormone replacement therapy. There also were no significant differences between the base-

line metabolic variables of weight; BMI; and SSPG, plasma insulin, glucose, and ALT concentrations for the two diet groups. Table 1 also details the estimated actual macronutrient composition of meals consumed. Amounts of carbohydrate and total, mono-, and polyunsaturated fats differ significantly between groups.

Both groups experienced a significant decrease in weight (7.0 ± 3.8 kg [$P < 0.001$] vs. 5.7 ± 4.1 kg [$P < 0.001$]) as a result of the dietary intervention (Table 2), but the amount of weight loss did not differ significantly between the two groups. Serum ALT concentrations decreased twice as much in the group assigned to the 40% carbohydrate compared with the 60% carbohydrate diet group (−9.5 ± 9.4 vs. −4.2 ± 8.3; $P < 0.01$). This difference remained statistically significant ($P < 0.02$) after adjusting for baseline ALT concentration, sex, age, and weight loss.

Insulin resistance, as quantified by SSPG, declined significantly in both groups (Table 2). The magnitude of decline was greater in the 40% carbohydrate group, but after adjustment for age, sex, baseline SSPG, and weight loss this difference was not statistically significant. Daylong insulin concentrations declined significantly only in the 40% carbohydrate diet group, and this decline was significantly greater than the decline in the 60% carbohydrate group, even after adjustment for baseline insulin concentration, age, sex, and weight loss. Daylong glucose concentrations did not change significantly in either group.

Based on the proposal that the upper limits of normal for ALT concentrations should be adjusted to be 30 units/l for men and 19 units/l for women (25), we divided our study subjects into those who had baseline ALT concentrations above (abnormal) or below (normal) these proposed alternative cut points. There were no significant differences between the abnormal versus normal ALT groups in terms of age (51 ± 11 vs. 52 ± 10; $P = 0.83$), number of women (64 vs. 42%; $P = 0.14$), postmenopausal status (27 vs. 37%; $P = 0.56$), BMI (32.5 ± 2.6 vs. 32.5 ± 1.9; $P = 0.97$), SSPG (237 ± 38 vs. 234 ± 41; $P = 0.83$), glucose AUC (859 ± 90 vs. 864 ± 98; $P = 0.85$), or insulin AUC (391 ± 164 vs. 534 ± 539; $P = 0.18$), and the mean baseline ALT concentrations for two groups were significantly different (19.5 ± 5.5 vs. 32.9 ± 8.6 units/l; $P < 0.01$). Comparison of the

Table 2—Change in metabolic variables as a result of hypocaloric dietary intervention in individuals assigned to the 40 vs. 60% carbohydrate diet

	60% carbohydrate diet (n = 26)				40% carbohydrate diet (n = 26)					
	Prediet	Postdiet	Δ	P*	Prediet	Postdiet	Δ	P*	P†	P‡
Weight (kg)	95.1 ± 13.0	89.4 ± 13.0	−5.7 ± 4.1	<0.01	94.2 ± 12.3	87.1 ± 11.3	−7.0 ± 3.8	0.20	0.20	0.23
ALT units/l	27.0 ± 10.4	22.9 ± 7.7	−4.2 ± 8.3	0.02	29.0 ± 9.5	19.5 ± 4.7	−9.5 ± 9.4	<0.01	<0.01	0.02
SSPG (mg/dl)	226.5 ± 26.4	194.1 ± 42.9	−32.4 ± 40.7	<0.01	246.6 ± 47.2	185.4 ± 67.9	−61.3 ± 52.3	<0.02	<0.01	0.06
AUC insulin (μU · ml^{-1} · 8 h^{-1})	435 ± 439	400 ± 383	−35 ± 115	0.14	459 ± 256	295 ± 180	−164 ± 151	0.03	0.03	0.04
AUC glucose (mg · dl^{-1} · 8 h^{-1})	869 ± 88	873 ± 87	−4 ± 68	0.75	852 ± 98	826 ± 92	26 ± 76	0.12	0.16	0.74

Data are means ± SD unless otherwise indicated. *Within-group comparison for each diet (paired Student's t test). †Unadjusted between-group comparison (unpaired Student's t test) of the change in dependent variable. ‡Adjusted for age, sex, baseline concentration of variable, and weight loss (stepwise multiple linear regression analysis).

Diabetes Care • May 2007 • 30:1075–1080

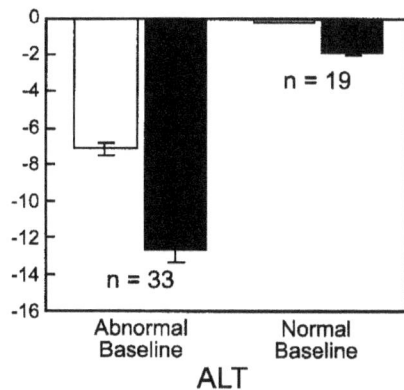

Figure 1—*The change in ALT is shown in the two diet groups divided into those with an abnormal and a normal baseline ALT based on proposed upper limits of 19 units/l for women and 30 units/l for men (24). P < 0.01 for the decrease in ALT in those with abnormal versus normal ALT at baseline (both dietary groups combined, n = 52). In the abnormal ALT group (n = 33), P < 0.01 for the between-diet comparison of the decrease in ALT after adjustment for age, sex, baseline ALT, and weight loss by stepwise multiple linear regression. P = 0.97 for the between-diet comparison of the decrease in ALT in the normal baseline group (n = 19). Carbohydrate diet: □, 60%; ■, 40%.*

ALT responses of those with abnormal or normal baseline ALT concentrations to the 40 and 60% carbohydrate diets is shown in Fig. 1. Irrespective of dietary macronutrient content, the decline (mean ± SD) in ALT concentrations with weight loss in the 33 subjects with baseline abnormal ALT concentrations was 10-fold greater than in the 19 with normal baseline values (-10.2 ± 9.3 vs. -1.0 ± 5.4 units/l; $P < 0.01$). In addition, in the abnormal baseline ALT group, concentrations fell to a greater degree in those assigned to the 40% carbohydrate diet ($n = 18$) compared with those on the 60% carbohydrate diet ($n = 15$) (-12.8 ± 8.8 vs. -7.2 ± 9.1 unit/l; $P < 0.01$ after adjustment for age, sex, baseline ALT, and weight loss). Among those with normal baseline ALT concentrations ($n = 19$), ALT decreases were -2.0 ± 1.4 vs. -0.8 ± 0.6 units/l ($P = 0.97$) on the 40 and 60% carbohydrate diets, respectively.

CONCLUSIONS — The main finding of this study is that among obese, otherwise-healthy, insulin-resistant individuals, a hypocaloric diet moderately restricted in carbohydrate (40%) and enriched in fat (45%), compared with a traditional low-fat hypocaloric diet (25% fat and 60% carbohydrate), lowers serum ALT concentrations to a significantly greater degree, even after

adjustment for amount of weight loss and other potential confounders, including baseline concentration of ALT. Of note, the subjects in our study were selected to have no prior diagnosis of liver disease and baseline ALT concentrations that did not exceed the current upper limit of the normal range. Thus, it is important to consider that even in apparently healthy obese, insulin-resistant individuals, weight loss can reduce ALT concentrations, suggesting that steatosis was present. Furthermore, our study adds to the accumulating data suggesting that among this population at particularly high risk for obesity-related morbidities, hypocaloric diets that differ in macronutrient composition yield different weight loss–related benefits. For example, we and others (20–22,35,36) have previously shown that hypocaloric diets lower in carbohydrate are more effective in reducing triglyceride and increasing HDL cholesterol concentrations, which may be related to relatively greater reductions in insulin concentrations (18,20,21,35,36) as a result of lower dietary carbohydrate intake. Indeed, it is plausible that relatively greater reductions in ambient insulin concentrations in the current study also contributed to the lowering of serum ALT, given that significantly greater reductions were seen on the 40% compared with the 60% carbohydrate diet.

There are several lines of evidence supporting a biological link between insulin concentrations and hepatic steatosis. First, strong correlations have been observed between the degree of hyperinsulinemia and the extent of hepatic steatosis (9,37). Also, in NAFLD, the area of the lobule containing the highest number of steatotic hepatocytes is zone 3, the area closest to portal drainage with the highest concentration of insulin (38). The more insulin resistant an individual, and the higher the daylong insulin and free fatty acid concentrations, the greater is hepatic VLDL-triacylglycerol synthesis and secretion (39–42). Furthermore, ex vivo hepatic perfusion studies have shown that the higher the ambient in vivo insulin concentration, the greater the stimulatory effect of a given increment in perfusate free fatty acid concentrations on hepatic triglyceride synthesis and secretion (43). In regard to ALT, links between glucose-mediated insulin sensitivity and serum ALT have been demonstrated previously (37,44,45). On a molecular level, sterol regulatory binding protein 1, the peroxisome proliferator–activated receptor system, and Fas genes are key transcriptional

factors regulated by insulin. In situations of insulin and free fatty acid abundance, such as obesity, insulin binding increases the expression of sterol regulatory binding protein-1c, leading to increased expression of lipogenic genes and a consequent increase in de novo lipogenesis (46). All of these observations support the biologic plausibility of our observation that those assigned to the 40% carbohydrate diet experienced a greater decline in ALT concentrations as a result of greater reductions in ambient insulin concentrations.

Alternatively, there is a growing body of evidence that intrahepatic fat accumulation potentiates insulin resistance via stimulation of inflammatory pathways regulated by nuclear factor-κB (10–12). In this regard, prevention/reduction of early intrahepatic fat accumulation may not only prevent the development of NASH and subsequent cirrhosis in a minority of affected patients but may potentiate improvement in insulin sensitivity and other metabolic parameters.

Baseline ALT concentrations for our subjects did not exceed the upper limit of the normal range (60 units/l), but 63% of subjects had a baseline ALT above that of new, more conservative limits (<19 units/l for women and <30 units/l for men) (25). Our results further support these limits, as individuals with ALT levels above these limits decreased with dietary weight loss, while those below the new upper limits did not. Furthermore, even in this smaller subgroup, the impact of dietary macronutrient composition was statistically significant, with greater reductions in ALT observed in the 40% carbohydrate diet group. Although ALT is not a precise marker of NAFLD, these results suggest that the majority of our subjects did indeed have some degree of steatosis.

Our findings are limited to the obese, insulin-resistant population who *1*) have compensatory hyperinsulinemia and may be more sensitive to variations in dietary macronutrient composition with regard to insulin concentrations and *2*) have a high likelihood of steatosis (5,6,9). Furthermore, our subjects were engaged in dietary weight loss, and, thus, we cannot extrapolate the results of our study to eucaloric diets. We also did not quantify variability in micronutrients consumed, including relative proportions of refined and unrefined carbohydrates, types of carbohydrate, or n-6/n-3 polyunsaturated fats and thus cannot rule out the possibility that these factors and/or glycemic index or differences in fiber intake in our two study diets had an impact on our results. Finally, we did not quantify hepatic steatosis radiologically or histologically, but given the current findings, it would be reasonable to use more costly and/or invasive studies in this subject pool as well as in those with established steatohepatitis to evaluate the potential benefits of moderate reductions in dietary carbohydrate.

In summary, it appears that a hypocaloric diet moderately restricted in carbohydrate may be beneficial in reducing hepatic steatosis in obese, insulin-resistant adults. Given the ongoing debate as to which macronutrient composition is optimal for reducing health risks associated with obesity, our results demonstrate yet another benefit of a carbohydrate-restricted diet moderately enriched in fat compared with the currently recommended higher carbohydrate diets typically prescribed for weight loss in this population (47–49). Further research is needed to identify the mechanism by which lowering carbohydrate lowers ALT concentrations in patients with steatosis and the relative benefit to those with more advanced NASH.

Acknowledgments— This research was supported by the National Institutes of Health (grants RR2HLL406 and RR000070) and the Stanford University Deans' Fellowship (to M.C.R.).

References
1. Ludwig J, Viggiano TR, McGill DB, Ott BJ: Nonalcoholic steatohepatitis: Mayo Clinic experience with a hitherto unnamed disease. *Mayo Clin Proc* 55:434–438, 1980
2. Angulo P, Lindor KD: Nonalcoholic liver disease. *N Engl J Med* 346:1221–1231, 2002
3. Clark JM: The epidemiology of nonalcoholic fatty liver disease in adults. *J Clin Gastroenterol* 40 (Suppl. 1):S5–S10, 2006
4. Luyckx FH, Desaive C, Thiry A, Dewe W, Scheen AJ, Gielen JE, Lefebvre PJ: Liver abnormalities in severely obese subjects: effect of drastic weight loss after gastroplasty. *Int J Obes Relat Metab Disord* 22:222–226, 1998
5. Wanless IR, Lentz JS: Fatty liver hepatitis and obesity: an autopsy study with analysis of risk factors. *Hepatology* 12:1106–1110, 1990
6. Chalasani N, Deeg MA, Persohn S, Crabb DW: Metabolic and anthropometric evaluation of insulin resistance in nondiabetic patients with nonalcoholic steatohepatitis. *Am J Gastroenterol* 98:1849–1855, 2003
7. Seppala-Lindroos A, Vehkavaara S, Hakkinen AM, Goto T, Westerbacka J, Sovijarvi A, Halavaara J, Yki-Jarvinen H: Fat accumulation in the liver is associated with defects in insulin suppression of glucose production and serum free fatty acids independent of obesity in normal men. *J Clin Endocrinol Metab* 87:3023–3028, 2002
8. Tiikkainen M, Tamminen M, Hakkinen AM, Bergholm R, Vehkavaara S, Halavaara J, Teramo K, Rissanen A, Yki-Jarvinen H: Liver-fat accumulation and insulin resistance in obese women with previous gestational diabetes. *Obes Res Sep* 10:859–867, 2002
9. Bugianesi E, Gastaldelli A, Vanni E, Gambino R, Cassader M, Baldi S, Ponti V, Pagano G, Ferrannini E, Rizzetto M: Insulin resistance in non-diabetic patients with non-alcoholic fatty liver disease: sites and mechanisms. *Diabetologia* 48:634–642, 2005
10. Shoelson SE, Lee J, Goldfine AB: Inflammation and insulin resistance. *J Clin Invest* 116:1793–1801, 2006
11. Arkan MC, Havener AL, Greten FR, Maeda S, Li ZW, Long JM, Wynshaw-Boris A, Poli G, Olefsky J, Karin M: IKK-beta links inflammation to obesity-induced insulin resistance. *Nat Med* 11:191–198, 2005
12. Boden G, She P, Mozzoli M, Cheung P, Gumireddy K, Reddy P, Xiang X, Luo Z, Ruderman N: Free fatty acids produce insulin resistance and activate the proinflammatory nuclear factor-kB pathway in rat liver. *Diabetes* 54:3458–3465, 2005
13. American Gastroenterological Association: Medical position statement: nonalcoholic fatty liver disease. *Gastroenterology* 123:1702–1704, 2002
14. Park HS, Kim MW, Shin ES: Effect of weight control on hepatic abnormalities in obese patients with fatty liver. *J Korean Med Sci* 10:414–421, 1995
15. Palmer M, Schaffner F: Effect of weight reduction on hepatic abnormalities in overweight patients. *Gastroenterology* 99:1408–1413, 1990
16. Huang MA, Greenson JK, Chao C, Anderson L, Peterman D, Jacobson J, Emick D, Lok AS, Conjeevaram HS: One-year intense nutritional counseling results in histological improvement in patients with non-alcoholic steatohepatitis: a pilot study. *Am J Gastroenterol* 100:1072–1081, 2005
17. Ueno T, Sugawara H, Sujaku K, Hashimoto O, Tsuji R, Tamaki S, Torimura T, Inuzuka S, Sata M, Tanikawa K: Therapeutic effects of restricted diet and exercise in obese patients with fatty liver. *J Hepatol* 27:103–107, 1997
18. Garg A, Bantle JP, Henry RR, Coulston AM, Griver KA, Raatz SK, Brinkley L, Chen YD, Grundy SM, Huet BA, Reaven GM: Effects of varying carbohydrate content of diet in patients with non-insulin-dependent diabetes mellitus. *JAMA* 271:1421–1428, 1994
19. McLaughlin T, Abbasi F, Lamendola C, Yeni-Komshian H, Reaven GM: Carbohydrate-induced hypertriglyceridemia: an insight into the link between plasma insulin and triglyceride concentrations. *J Clin Endocrinol Metab* 85:3085–3088, 2000
20. McLaughlin TL, Carter S, Lamendola C, Abbasi F, Yee G, Schaaf P, Basina M, Reaven GM: Effects of moderate variations in macronutrient composition on weight loss and cardiovascular risk reduction in obese, insulin resistant adults. *Am J Clin Nutr* 84:813–821, 2006
21. Foster GD, Wyatt HR, Hill JO, McGuckin BG, Brill C, Mohammed BS, Szapary PO, Rader DJ, Edman JS, Klein SA: randomized trial of a low-carbohydrate diet for obesity. *N Engl J Med* 348:2082–2090, 2003
22. Cornier MA, Donahoo WT, Pereira R, Gurevich I, Westergren R, Enerback S, Eckel PJ, Goalstone ML, Hill JO, Eckel RH, Draznin B: Insulin sensitivity determines the effectiveness of dietary macronutrient composition on weight loss in obese women. *Obes Res* 13:703–709, 2005
23. Diraison F, Dusserre E, Vidal H, Sothier M, Beylot M: Increased hepatic lipogenesis but decreased expression of lipogenic gene in adipose tissue in human obesity. *Am J Physiol Endocrinol Metab* 282:E46–E51, 2002
24. Girard J, Perdereau D, Foufelle F, Prip-Buus C, Ferre P: Regulation of lipogenic enzyme gene expression by nutrients and hormones. *FASEB J* 8:36–42, 1994
25. Prati D, Taioli E, Zanella A, Della Torre E, Butelli S, Del Vecchio E, Vianello L, Zanuso F, Mozzi F, Milani S, Conte D, Colombo M, Sirchia G: Updated definitions of healthy ranges for serum alanine aminotransferase levels. *Ann Intern Med* 137:1–10, 2002
26. Cataldo NA, Abbasi F, McLaughlin TL, Basina M, Fechner PY, Giudice LC, Reaven GM: Metabolic and ovarian effects of rosiglitazone treatment for 12 weeks in insulin-resistant women with polycystic ovary syndrome. *Hum Reprod* 21:109–120, 2006
27. Pei D, Jones CN, Bhargava R, Chen YD, Reaven GM: Evaluation of octreotide to assess insulin-mediated glucose disposal by the insulin suppression test. *Diabetologia* 37:843–845, 1994
28. Shen SW, Reaven GM, Farquhar JW: Comparison of impedance to insulin-mediated glucose uptake in normal subjects and in subjects with latent diabetes. *J Clin Invest* 49:2151–2160, 1970
29. Greenfield MS, Doberne L, Kraemer F,

Tobey T, Reaven G: Assessment of insulin resistance with the insulin suppression test and the euglycaemic clamp. *Diabetes* 30:387–392, 1981

30. Yeni-Komshian H, Carantoni M, Abbasi F, Reaven GM: Relationship between several surrogate estimates of insulin resistance and quantification of insulin-mediated glucose disposal in 490 healthy nondiabetic volunteers. *Diabetes Care* 23: 171–175, 2000

31. Yip J, Facchini FS, Reaven GM: Resistance to insulin-mediated glucose disposal as a predictor of cardiovascular disease. *J Clin Endocrinol Metab* 83:2773–2776, 1998

32. McLaughlin T, Abbasi F, Cheal K, Chu J, Lamendola C, Reaven G: Use of metabolic markers to identify overweight individuals who are insulin resistant. *Ann Intern Med* 139:802–809, 2003

33. McLaughlin T, Stuhlinger M, Lamendola C, Abbasi F, Bialek J, Reaven GM, Tsao P: Plasma asymmetric dimethylarginine concentrations are elevated in obese, insulin-resistant women and fall with weight loss. *J Clin Endocrin Metab* 91: 1896–1900, 2006

34. Harris JA, Benedict FG: *A Biometric Study of Basal Metabolism in Man.* Washington DC, Carnegie Institute of Washington, 1919 (publ. no. 279)

35. Boden G, Sargrad K, Homko C, Mozzoli M, Stein P: Effect of a low carbohydrate diet on appetite, blood glucose levels and insulin resistance in obese patients with type 2 diabetes. *Ann Intern Med* 142:403–411, 2005

36. Pelkman CL, Fishell VK, Maddox DH, Pearson TA, Mauger DT, Kris-Etherton PM: Effects of moderate-fat (from monounsaturated fat) and low-fat weight-loss diets on the serum lipid profile in overweight and obese men and women. *Am J Clin Nutr* 79:204–212, 2004

37. Ardigo D, Numeroso F, Valtuena S, Franzini L, Piatti PM, Monti L, Delsignore R, Reaven GM, Zavaroni I: Hyperinsulinemia predicts hepatic fat content in healthy individuals with normal transaminase concentrations. *Metabolism* 54:1566–1570, 2005

38. MacDonald GA, Bridle KR, Ward PJ, Walker NI, Houglum K, George DK, Smith JL, Powell LW, Crawford DH, Ramm GA: Lipid peroxidation in hepatic steatosis in humans is associated with hepatic fibrosis and occurs predominately in acinar zone 3. *J Gastroenterol Hepatol* 16: 599–606, 2001

39. Reaven GM: Compensatory hyperinsulinemia and the development of an atherogenic lipoprotein profile: the price paid to maintain glucose homeostasis in insulin-resistant individuals. *Endocrinol Metab Clin North Am* 34:49–62, 2005

40. Reaven GM, Lerner RL, Stern MP, Farquhar JW: Role of insulin in endogenous hypertriglyceridemia. *J Clin Invest* 46: 1756–1767, 1967

41. Olefsky JM, Farquhar JW, Reaven GM: Reappraisal of the role of insulin in hypertriglyceridemia. *Am J Med* 57:551–560, 1974

42. Jeng C-Y, Fuh MM-T, Sheu WH-H, Chen Y-DI, Reaven GM: Hormone and substrate modulation of plasma triglyceride concentration in primary hypertriglyceridemia. *Endocrinol Metab* 1:15–21, 1994

43. Reaven GM, Mondon CE: Effect of in vivo plasma insulin levels on the relationship between perfusate free fatty acid concentration and triglyceride secretion by perfused rat livers. *Horm Metabol Res* 16: 230–232, 1984

44. Wang CH, Leung CH, Liu SC, Chung CH: Safety and effectiveness of rosiglitazone in type 2 diabetes patients with nonalcoholic fatty liver disease. *J Formos Med Assoc* 105: 743–752, 2006

45. Burgert TS, Taksali SE, Dziura J, Goodman TR, Yeckel CW, Papademetris X, Constable RT, Weiss R, Tamborlane WV, Savoye M, Seyal AA, Caprio S: Alanine aminotransferase levels and fatty liver in childhood obesity: associations with insulin resistance, adiponectin and visceral fat. *J Clin Endocrinol Metab* 91:4287–4294, 2006

46. Foufelle F, Ferre P: New perspectives in the regulation of hepatic glycolytic and lipogenic genes by insulin and glucose: a role for the transcription factor sterol regulatory element binding protein-1c 4. *Biochem J* 366:377–391, 2002

47. American Diabetes Association: Nutrition principles and recommendations in diabetes. *Diabetes Care* 27 (Suppl. 1):S36–S46, 2004

48. American Heart Association: Dietary guidelines, revision 2000. *Circulation* 102: 2284–2299, 2000

49. National Institutes of Health, National Heart, Lung, and Blood Institute: Clinical guidelines on the identification, evaluation, and treatment of overweight and obesity in adults: the evidence report. *Obes Res* 6 (Suppl. 2):51S–209S, 1998

Relationships Between Estimates of Adiposity, Insulin Resistance, and Nonalcoholic Fatty Liver Disease in a Large Group of Nondiabetic Korean Adults

Ki Chul Sung, md[1,2]
Marno C. Ryan, md[2]
Bum Soo Kim, md[1]
Yong Kyun Cho, md[1]
Byung Ik Kim, md[1]
Gerald M. Reaven, md[2]

OBJECTIVE — Nonalcoholic fatty liver disease (NAFLD) is emerging as a major health problem in parallel with an increasing prevalence of obesity. Insulin resistance and abdominal and overall adiposity are closely associated with NAFLD; however, the interplay between them in the relationship with NAFLD is unclear, especially in nondiabetic individuals.

RESEARCH DESIGN AND METHODS — Abdominal ultrasound, hepatitis serology, and measurements of fasting plasma insulin (FPI), lipid concentrations, overall obesity (BMI), and abdominal obesity (waist circumference) were performed in 56,249 Korean subjects.

RESULTS — After rigorous exclusion criteria, 36,654 nondiabetic subjects (54% male) were enrolled. Subjects were divided into control (no fatty liver on ultrasound, serum alanine aminotransferase [ALT] <30 units/l [men] or <19 units/l [women]), fatty liver with normal ALT (FL-NALT), and fatty liver with a high ALT (FL-HALT) groups. After adjusting for age, BMI, and waist circumference, FPI and ratio of triglycerides to HDL cholesterol (TG/HDL-C ratio) were significantly higher in the FL-NALT than in the control group and even higher in the FL-HALT group. Odds ratios for the presence of FL-HALT with increasing quartiles of FPI and TG/HDL-C ratio were increased five- to sevenfold over those of the control group, independent of age, BMI, and waist circumference.

CONCLUSIONS — In this large population of individuals of Korean ancestry, results indicate that while overall (BMI) and abdominal (waist circumference) overweight/obesity are associated with features of NAFLD, surrogate estimates of insulin resistance, FPI concentration, and TG/HDL-C ratio predict NAFLD independently of age, BMI, and waist circumference.

Diabetes Care 30:2113–2118, 2007

N onalcoholic fatty liver disease (NAFLD) represents a spectrum of disease, ranging from simple fatty liver or steatosis, a generally benign accumulation of triglyceride in hepatocytes, to nonalcoholic steatohepatitis, which can progress to chronic liver disease, cirrhosis, and hepatocellular carcinoma (1,2). Along with the "obesity epidemic," the worldwide prevalence of NAFLD is increasing rapidly and is generally assumed to be a consequence of obesity-induced insulin resistance (1–3). On the other hand, not all obese individuals are insulin resistant, nor are all insulin-resistant individuals obese

(4–6). Furthermore, many reports of the relationship between obesity, insulin resistance, and NAFLD have included relatively few individuals, often predominantly overweight and/or with some degree of glucose intolerance (7–9).

The current study was initiated to address some of these issues by taking advantage of a database of a large group of apparently healthy, nondiabetic, middle-aged subjects that included measurements of hepatic ultrasonography and serum hepatic transaminases. The primary goal of our analysis was to evaluate the relationship between NAFLD and two surrogate markers of insulin resistance taking into consideration the potentially confounding impact of differences in overall and abdominal obesity. The two surrogate markers of insulin resistance chosen for this purpose were fasting plasma insulin (FPI) concentration and plasma concentration ratio of triglycerides to HDL cholesterol (TG/HDL-C ratio). Both of these variables have been shown to be significantly correlated with a specific measure of insulin-mediated glucose uptake (10), with r values of ~0.6.

RESEARCH DESIGN AND METHODS — The initial study population consisted of 56,249 subjects (33,546 men and 22,703 women) who volunteered for a health status evaluation in between 1 January and 30 September 2005 at Kangbuk Samsung Hospital, College of Medicine, Sungkyunkwan University. Data were obtained from a retrospective medical record review, and the study protocol was approved by the Kangbuk Samsung Hospital Ethics Committee. In addition to a complete medical history, physical examination, and chemical screening battery, all 56,249 subjects underwent an abdominal ultrasound and had blood drawn for serum levels of viral markers. To avoid confounding factors, the results of these preliminary observations resulted in the exclusion of a significant number from this analysis, based on: *1*) a past history of diabetes or a fasting

From the [1]Division of Medicine, Kangbuk Samsung Hospital, Sungkyunkwan University School of Medicine, Seoul, South Korea; and the [2]Division of Medicine, Stanford University Medical Center, Stanford, California.

Address correspondence and reprint requests to Ki Chul Sung, MD, Kangbuk Samsung Hospital, Sungkyunkwan University, Pyung Dong, Jongro-Ku, Seoul, Korea 110-746. E-mail: kcmd.sung@samsung.com.

Received for publication 14 March 2007 and accepted in revised form 26 April 2007.

Published ahead of print at http://care.diabetesjournals.org on 7 May 2007. DOI: 10.2337/dc07-0512.

K.C.S. and M.C.R. contributed equally to this article.

Abbreviations: ALT, alanine aminotransferase; FL-HALT, fatty liver with a high ALT; FL-NALT, fatty liver with normal ALT; FPI, fasting plasma insulin; NAFLD, nonalcoholic fatty liver disease; TG/HDL-C ratio, ratio of triglycerides to HDL cholesterol.

A table elsewhere in this issue shows conventional and Système International (SI) units and conversion factors for many substances.

Table 1—Clinical characteristics of the control group and the two fatty liver groups divided by grade of fatty liver and sex

Men (n = 17,616)

	Control	FL-NALT Grade 1	FL-NALT Grade 2/3	FL-NALT P*	FL-HALT Grade 1	FL-HALT Grade 2/3	FL-HALT P*	P overall
n	10,461	2,815	128		3,334	878		
(years)	40 ± 8	42 ± 8	40 ± 9	0.08	40 ± 7	39 ± 7	<0.01	<0.01
kg/m²	22.9 ± 2.4	25.2 ± 2.2	26.9 ± 2.5	<0.01	26.1 ± 2.3	27.5 ± 2.6	<0.01	<0.01
circumference (cm)	79 ± 7	86 ± 6	90 ± 8	<0.01	88 ± 6	92 ± 7	<0.01	<0.01
mmol/l	45 ± 15	56 ± 18	65 ± 22	<0.01	65 ± 23	77 ± 39	<0.01	<0.01
rides (mmol/l)	1.3 ± 0.7	1.9 ± 1.0	2.2 ± 1.2	<0.01	2.1 ± 1.1	2.4 ± 1.3	<0.01	<0.01
cholesterol (mmol/l)	1.3 ± 0.3	1.2 ± 0.2	1.1 ± 0.2	<0.01	1.2 ± 0.2	1.1 ± 1.8	<0.01	<0.01
DL-C ratio (mmol/l)	1.0 ± 0.5	1.6 ± 0.4	2.0 ± 0.8	<0.01	1.8 ± 0.6	2.2 ± 1.4	<0.01	<0.01

Women (n = 13,624)

	Control	FL-NALT Grade 1	FL-NALT Grade 2/3	FL-NALT P*	FL-HALT Grade 1	FL-HALT Grade 2/3	FL-HALT P*	P overall
n	11,757	695	21		988	163		
(years)	39 ± 8	45 ± 10	46 ± 12	0.85	49 ± 11	47 ± 11	0.14	<0.01
kg/m²	21.6 ± 2.4	25.0 ± 2.8	28.6 ± 5.2	<0.05	25.6 ± 2.8	28.3 ± 3.3	<0.01	<0.01
circumference (cm)	71 ± 7	80 ± 7	96 ± 14	<0.01	82 ± 7	88 ± 8	<0.01	<0.01
mmol/l	47 ± 17	62 ± 22	77 ± 25	<0.02	70 ± 25	73 ± 26	0.03	<0.01
rides (mmol/l)	1.0 ± 0.5	1.6 ± 1.0	2.3 ± 1.5	<0.01	1.8 ± 1.0	2.1 ± 1.3	<0.01	<0.01
cholesterol (mmol/l)	1.5 ± 0.3	1.3 ± 0.3	1.2 ± 0.3	0.02	1.3 ± 0.3	1.3 ± 0.2	<0.01	<0.01
DL-C ratio (mmol/l)	0.7 ± 0.4	1.2 ± 0.5	1.9 ± 0.7	0.02	1.4 ± 0.5	1.6 ± 0.6	<0.01	<0.01

Data are means ± SD. *Comparison between grades 1 and 2 fatty liver (unpaired student's t test); P overall = ANOVA including the FL-NALT, FL-HALT (without dividing by grade of fatty liver), and control groups. ALT: steatosis detected on ultrasound with ALT <30 units/l (men) or <19 units/l (women); FL-HALT: steatosis detected on ultrasound with ALT >30 units/l (men) or >19 units/l (women).

plasma glucose concentration >125 mg/dl (n = 2,630), 2) a history of malignancy (n = 293), 3) consumption of alcohol in amounts in excess of 70 g/week for women (n = 986) and 140 g/week for men (n = 8,688), or 4) hepatitis C antibody (HCV Ab) positivity (n = 107), hepatitis B surface antigen (HBsAg) positivity (n = 2,408), or solitary hepatitis B core antibody (HBcAb) positivity (n = 2,679). Also excluded from this analysis were subjects who took a variety of drugs reported to affect liver function (n = 376) and individuals with abnormal abdominal sonography results (evidence of malignancy, cirrhosis, or gall bladder disease) (n = 3,060). Thus, as some individuals met more than one exclusion criteria, the final number of subjects available for study was 36,654 (19,618 men and 17,036 women).

All subjects were seen after an overnight fast. Height and weight were determined, and BMI was expressed as weight (in kilograms) divided by the square of the height (in meters). Waist circumference was measured at the midlevel between the lowest rib and the iliac crest with the subject standing and breathing normally. Blood samples were collected, plasma separated, and alanine aminotransferase (ALT) measured by ultraviolet without P5P method (Advia 1650 Autoanalyzer; Byer Diagnostics, Leverkusen, Germany). HBsAg and HBsAb were measured by chemiluminescent microparticle immunoassay (Architect i2000 SR; Abbott, Abbott Park, IL). HBcAb immunoglobulin G was measured by radioimmunoassay (Titertek, AL). HCV Ab was measured by polymerase chain reaction (Cobas Amplicor; Roche, Basel, Switzerland). Insulin concentrations were determined by immunoradiometric assay (Biosource, Nivelles, Belgium), with intra- and interassay CVs of 2.1–4.5 and 4.7–12.2%, respectively. An enzymatic colorimetric test was used to measure total cholesterol and triglyceride concentrations (Hitachi 912 analyzer; Roche Diagnostics). The selective inhibition method was used to measure the level of HDL cholesterol, and a ho-

LDL cholesterol (Advia 1650 Autoanalyzer; Byer Diagnostics).

Abdominal ultrasonography (Aspen, Acuson, PA) was performed to detect the presence of fatty infiltration in the liver by a core laboratory of experienced radiologists, all of whom used standard criteria in evaluating the images for hepatic fat (11). The severity of the fatty liver was classified into three groups, grades 1–3, according to the Mittelstaedt classification (11). Subjects with both fatty liver and an ALT of <30 units/l for men and <19 units/l for women, as described by Prati et al. (12), were classified as having fatty liver with a normal ALT (FL-NALT). Patients with fatty liver and a serum ALT >30 units/l for men and >19 units/l for women were classified as having fatty liver with a high ALT (FL-HALT). These ALT cut points were determined after a review of previous work both in Koreans (13,14) and non-Koreans (12,15) in an effort to use sex-specific cut points that accurately detected abnormal values. Finally, subjects without fatty liver on ultrasound but an ALT >30 units/l for men or >19 units/l for women (n = 5,414 subjects) were not included in this analysis, but the mean FPI and TG/HDL-C ratio concentrations for this group were compared with the other groups and are presented.

Since specific measures of insulin-mediated glucose uptake had not been performed, the two following surrogate estimates of insulin sensitivity were used to assess the relationship between insulin resistance/hyperinsulinemia and fatty liver. FPI concentrations are significantly correlated with direct measures of insulin resistance (10,16). The plasma concentration of TG/HDL-C ratio is as closely related to direct measures of insulin resistance as FPI concentration (10) but has been shown to be superior to both triglycerides and HDL cholesterol alone (17).

Statistics

Statistical analysis of the data were performed using SPSS version 14.0 (SPSS, Point Richmond, CA), and the continuous variable data are presented as means ± SD. Student's unpaired t test was used to compare the means of grade 1 fatty liver versus grades 2 and 3 combined. ANOVA was used to evaluate the overall differences in means. ANCOVA was used to assess the effect of weight (BMI and waist circumference) on the re-

Table 2—*Mean ± SD values for FPI and TG/HDL-C ratio concentrations adjusted for differences in age, BMI, and waist circumference in the three groups (control, FL-NALT, and FL-HALT) divided by sex (ANCOVA)*

	Control	FL-NALT	FL-HALT	Multiple comparison
Men (N = 17,616)				
n	10,461	2,943	4,212	
FPI (pmol/l)	49 ± 16	55 ± 18	62 ± 27	1≠2, 1≠3, 2≠3
TG/HDL-C ratio (mmol/l)	1.2 ± 0.7	1.6 ± 1.1	1.8 ± 2.2	1≠2, 1≠3, 2≠3
Women (N = 16,483)				
n	11,757	716	1,151	
FPI (pmol/l)	50 ± 17	60 ± 22	68 ± 25	1≠2, 1≠3, 2≠3
TG/HDL-C ratio (mmol/l)	0.7 ± 0.5	1.1 ± 0.9	1.2 ± 0.9	1≠2, 1≠3, 2≠3

FL-NALT: steatosis detected on ultrasound with ALT <30 units/l (men) or <19 units/l (women); FL-HALT: steatosis detected on ultrasound with ALT >30 units/l (men) or >19 units/l (women). ≠, two groups are different.

For the comparison of nominal variables, the χ^2 method was used for cross-tabulation analysis. Multiple logistic regression analysis was used to analyze relationships between age, BMI, waist circumference, and insulin and the TG/HDL-C ratio and the presence of FL-NALT and FL-HALT. P values <0.05 were considered to be statistically significant.

RESULTS — Overall, the 36,654 subjects were relatively young (mean ± SD age 41 ± 9 years [men 41 ± 8, women 41 ± 9]) and nonobese (BMI 23.0 ± 3.0 kg/m² [men 24.3 ± 2.8, women 22.2 ± 2.9] and waist circumference 78 ± 9 cm [men 83 ± 8, women 72 ± 8]). Hepatic ultrasonography indicated that 27,632 subjects were without evidence of fatty liver (75.4%), while the remaining subjects had grade 1 (21.4%, 6,149 men, 1,683 women), grade 2 (3.2%, 977 men, 181 women), or grade 3 (0.09%, 29 men, 3 women) fatty liver. In Table 1, the subjects are separated by fatty liver grade and sex. Subjects with grades 2 and 3 were combined into one category due to the

very small numbers in grade 3. For the remainder of the presented analyses the fatty liver grades are not separated, and the data are presented for two groups: FL-NALT and FL-HALT.

The presence of fatty liver and elevation of ALT increased with the degree of both overall and abdominal obesity
The relevant clinical characteristics of the 36,654 subjects, divided into the three experimental groups (control, FL-NALT, and FL-HALT) are shown in Table 1, with the two fatty liver groups also divided into fatty liver grades. In general, the fatty liver groups had a higher overall (BMI) and abdominal (waist circumference) obesity than the control group, and the FL-HALT group was significantly more obese by both measures than the FL-NALT group. These data also show a significant trend of worsening metabolic variables (FPI, triglyceride, and HDL cholesterol concentrations and TG/HDL-C ratio) across the groups from the control to the FL-

NALT and FL-HALT groups. After division of the two fatty liver groups into grades of fatty liver, the same can be said of men with grade 2 fatty liver in comparison with those with grade 1 fatty liver, within both the FL-NALT and the FL-HALT groups. Thus, in men, the degree of steatosis was positively associated with worsening metabolic variables. For women, although the division into grades of fatty liver also demonstrated an association between worsening metabolic variables and a higher grade of fatty liver, women with grade 2/3 fatty liver in the two fatty liver/ALT groups had equivalent mean values for variables.

Table 2 presents the mean values for FPI concentration and the TG/HDL-C ratio of the three experimental groups this time adjusted for differences in age, BMI, and waist circumference. These results indicate that the estimates of insulin resistance increased in magnitude in parallel with presence of fatty liver and increased ALT level, with each group being significantly different from the other two groups.

Odds ratios for features of NAFLD increased with increasing insulin resistance, independently of obesity
To quantify the adverse impact of obesity on the degree of liver disease, odds ratios (ORs) were calculated between age, BMI, and waist circumference and the presence of FL-NALT or FL-HALT (Table 3). For men, in this relatively young population, being older did not seem to have an adverse effect on the presence of NAFLD. However, in women, the two fatty liver groups were significantly older than the control subjects. In terms of adiposity, the larger the BMI or waist circumference, the greater the OR of having either FL-NALT

Table 3—*Age, BMI, and waist circumference ORs and 95% CIs for risk of sonographic liver fat and elevated ALT level in men and women*

	FL-NALT			FL-HALT		
	OR	95% CI	P	OR	95% CI	P
Men						
Age	1.02	1.01–1.02	0.001	0.97	0.96–0.98	<0.001
BMI	1.12	1.08–1.16	<0.001	1.26	1.22–1.31	<0.001
Waist circumference	1.03	1.01–1.04	<0.001	1.11	1.09–1.12	<0.001
Women						
Age	1.02	1.00–1.03	0.007	1.05	1.04–1.09	<0.001
BMI	1.20	1.11–1.24	<0.001	1.29	1.23–1.36	<0.001
Waist circumference	1.06	1.03–1.08	<0.001	1.06	1.04–1.09	<0.001

FL-NALT: steatosis detected on ultrasound with ALT <30 units/l (men) or <19 units/l (women); FL-HALT: steatosis detected on ultrasound with ALT >30 units/l (men) or >19 units/l (women).

Table 4—*ORs and 95% CIs for risk of sonographic liver fat with and without an elevated serum ALT, with increasing FPI and TG/HDL-C ratio concentration quartiles, independent of age, BMI, and waist circumference for men and women*

	FL-NALT			FL-HALT		
	OR	95% CI	*P*	OR	95% CI	*P*
Men						
FPI quartiles (mmol/l)						
I (12.6~37.2)	1			1		
II (37.3~48.6)	1.70	1.41–2.04	<0.001	1.89	1.51–2.36	<0.001
III (48.7~62.4)	2.84	1.97–3.82	<0.001	2.80	2.26–3.47	<0.001
IV (62.58~804.0)	1.79	1.48–2.16	<0.001	6.25	5.07–7.70	<0.001
TG/HDL-C ratio quartiles (mmol/l)						
I (0.19~0.77)	1			1		
II (1.77~1.14)	1.92	1.59–2.32	<0.001	2.06	1.63–2.52	<0.001
III (1.15~1.73)	2.36	1.97–2.84	<0.001	3.27	2.66–4.02	<0.001
IV (1.74~13.3)	2.73	2.27–3.29	<0.001	5.88	4.80–7.21	<0.001
Women						
FPI quartiles (mmol/l)						
I (12.0~37.8)	1			1		
II (37.9~47.4)	1.78	1.16–2.73	0.008	1.24	0.80–1.91	0.339
III (47.5~60.6)	2.29	1.53–3.43	<0.001	2.23	1.53–3.36	<0.001
IV (60.7~495.6)	2.89	1.95–4.28	<0.001	6.40	4.42–9.25	<0.001
TG/HDL-C ratio quartiles (mmol/l)						
I (0.12~0.44)	1			1		
II (0.45~0.63)	2.68	1.54–4.66	<0.001	1.36	0.85–2.19	0.205
IIII (0.64~0.95)	5.13	3.05–8.61	<0.001	2.62	1.71–4.01	<0.001
IV (0.96~23.5)	7.66	4.59–12.77	<0.001	6.65	4.43–9.98	<0.001

FL-NALT: steatosis detected on ultrasound with ALT <30 units/l (men) or <19 units/l (women); FL-HALT: steatosis detected on ultrasound with ALT >30 units/l (men) or >19 units/l (women).

or FL-HALT. The increase in ORs ranged from 10 to 30%, with the values for BMI and waist circumference of seemingly comparable magnitude.

As shown in Table 4, the impact of insulin resistance was assessed with the calculation of ORs between FPI and TG/HDL-C ratio concentrations and the presence of FL-NALT or FL-HALT. For this purpose, the experimental population was divided into quartiles on the basis of their FPI concentration or their TG/HDL-C ratio. Age, BMI, and waist circumference were included in the regression model for both the FPI and TG/HDL-C ratio analyses, so that the increasing quartiles of the two markers of insulin resistance are independent of these three variables. In terms of FPI concentration, when comparing each of the three highest insulin quartiles with the lowest, ORs for the presence of FL-HALT increased significantly in both men and women, with the OR increasing five- to sixfold in the quartile with the highest FPI concentration. Similar results are seen for TG/HDL-C ratio. When examining the ORs

for FPI and TG/HDL-C ratio concentrations in predicting the presence of FL-NALT, the results are similar for women, albeit of smaller magnitude. However, for men, the OR for FL-NALT decreased with the highest FPI quartile, indicating a decrease in risk with this degree of hyperinsulinemia. This is difficult to explain but could indicate that in men an increasing FPI concentration is less associated with steatosis alone and more associated with steatohepatitis. This is with the caveat that ALT is only a moderately accurate marker of inflammatory activity. Thus, apart from this one exception, the higher the FPI and TG/HDL-C ratio concentrations, the significantly greater the OR of having either FL-NALT or FL-HALT.

Secondary analyses

A total of 5,414 subjects (3,412 women, 2,002 men) with an isolated elevated ALT (>30 units/l for men and >19 units/l for women), i.e., no fatty liver on ultrasound, were excluded from the above analyses. We compared the mean FPI and TG/HDL-C ratio concentrations

for this group with those of our other groups and found that for both of these measures the mean values for the isolated ALT group were significantly lower than those in either the FL-NALT or the FL-HALT groups after adjusting for age, BMI, and waist circumference (data not shown).

CONCLUSIONS — Both obesity and insulin resistance have been identified as factors associated with deposition of fat in the liver, although it is unclear whether they are a cause of hepatic fat (18–21) or a result of hepatic fat (22–25). Because obesity and insulin resistance are themselves significantly correlated (26,27), it is difficult to clarify which of these two variables is most closely related to increased hepatic fat content. The problem is further confounded by questions as to the relative adverse impact of overall obesity as compared with abdominal obesity. This study is, to the best of our knowledge, the largest that has been performed in analyzing associations between measures of overall and abdominal obesity, insulin resistance, hepatic transaminases, and fatty liver, using a comprehensive evaluation including ultrasound, hepatic enzymes, and serum viral markers, in a nondiabetic apparently healthy population.

Based on the results in Tables 1 and 2, it appears that both surrogate estimates of insulin resistance used in this study (FPI and TG/HDL-C ratio concentrations) are independently associated with severity of liver disease. Thus, although the results in Table 1 indicate that both estimates of obesity (BMI and waist circumference) and the two surrogate estimates of insulin resistance all increased significantly as a function of the presence of steatosis and a raised ALT, it can be seen from Table 2 that FPI and TG/HDL-C ratio concentrations continued to be statistically associated with these features of liver disease when adjusted for differences in age, BMI, and waist circumference. Furthermore, when the subjects were divided into quartiles based on magnitude of surrogate estimates of insulin resistance, the OR of having evidence of FL-HALT increased significantly with each successively higher quartile (Table 4). As in the results in Table 2, these findings were independent of differences in age, BMI, and waist circumference and, with the exception of relatively minor quantitative differences, were true of both sexes. Thus, in answer to the question we posed, the evidence strongly supports the notion that although both overall and abdominal obesity are associated with fatty liver, the specific relationship between insulin resistance and fatty liver is independent of either overall or abdominal obesity.

It is of interest that the relationships between either index of obesity and hepatic fat content were quite comparable, so that neither waist circumference nor BMI was more predictive of hepatic fat than the other. However, the population under study was a very specific population of East Asian ancestry, with a lower mean BMI and waist circumference than seen in Caucasians, and these findings may not be applicable to other ethnic groups. Further, it should be emphasized that the specific cut points that performed the best in this analysis may only be applicable to individuals of Korean ethnicity.

Although the results of this study seem relatively straight forward, certain weaknesses should be acknowledged. First, subjects with sonographic evidence of cirrhosis were excluded, and in doing so some NAFLD chronic liver disease or cirrhosis may have also been excluded, explaining why we found such small numbers with grade 3 fatty liver. Second, NAFLD cirrhosis, where the hepatic fat tends to be greatly diminished, can be mistaken sonographically for normal nonfatty liver (28). Third, and most importantly, our conclusions are based on the combined use of hepatic ultrasonography and ALT measurements as markers of NAFLD, without morphological examination of hepatic tissue. We used "FL-HALT" to attempt to measure prevalence of inflammatory activity in the liver, to distinguish this from benign fatty liver. We acknowledge that serum ALT levels have been shown to be at best a moderate predictor of hepatic necroinflammatory damage or steatohepatitis (29–31); however, we would argue that the large number of apparently healthy individuals studied precludes the possibility of obtaining histology.

In summary, we demonstrate that although both adiposity and surrogate estimates of insulin resistance (FPI and TG/HDL-C ratio concentrations) are associated with the estimates of NAFLD in this healthy nondiabetic Korean population, these measures of insulin resistance predict NAFLD independently of both overall and abdominal overweight/obesity.

Acknowledgments— We acknowledge the efforts of the health screening group at Kangbuk Samsung Hospital, Seoul, South Korea.

References

1. Angulo P: Nonalcoholic fatty liver disease. *N Engl J Med* 346: 1221–1231, 2002
2. Clark JM, Brancati FL, Diehl AM: Nonalcoholic fatty liver disease. *Gastroenterology* 122:1649–1657, 2002
3. McCullough AJ: Pathophysiology of nonalcoholic steatohepatitis (Review). *J Clin Gastroenterol* 40 (Suppl. 1):S17–S29, 2006
4. Ferrannini E, Natali A, Bell P, Cavallo-Perin P, Lalic N, Mingrone G: Insulin resistance and hypersecretion in obesity: European Group for the Study of Insulin Resistance (EGIR). *J Clin Invest* 100: 1166–1173, 1997
5. Abbasi F, Brown BW Jr, Lamendola C, McLaughlin T, Reaven GM: Relationship between obesity, insulin resistance, and coronary heart disease risk. *J Am Coll Cardiol* 40:937–943, 2002
6. Jones CN, Abbasi F, Carantoni M, Polonsky KS, Reaven GM: Roles of insulin resistance and obesity in regulation of plasma insulin concentrations. *Am J Physiol Endocrinol Metab* 278:E501—E508, 2000
7. Marchesini G, Brizi M, Morselli-Labate AM, Bianchi G, Bugianesi E, McCullough AJ, Forlani G, Melchionda N: Association of nonalcoholic fatty liver disease with insulin resistance. *Am J Med* 107:450–455, 1999
8. Chitturi S, Abeygunasekera S, Farrell GC, Holmes-Walker J, Hui JM, Fung C, Karim R, Lin R, Samarasinghe D, Liddle C, Weltman M, George J: NASH and insulin resistance: insulin hypersecretion and specific association with the insulin resistance syndrome. *Hepatology* 35:373–379, 2002
9. Tiikkainen M, Tamminen M, Häkkinen AM, Bergholm R, Vehkavaara S, Halavaara J, Teramo K, Rissanen A, Yki-Järvinen H: Liver fat accumulation and insulin resistance in obese women with previous GDM. *Obes Res* 10:859–867, 2002
10. McLaughlin T, Abbasi F, Cheal K, Chu J, Lamendola C, Reaven GM: Use of metabolic markers to identify individuals who are insulin resistant. *Ann Intern Med* 139: 802–809, 2003
11. Mittelstaedt CA, Vincent LM: *Abdominal Ultrasound*. New York, Churchill Livingston, 1987
12. Prati D, Taioli E, Zanella A, Della Torre E, Butelli S, Del Vecchio E, Vianello L, Zanuso F, Mozzi F, Milani S, Conte D, Colombo M, Sirchia G: Updated definitions of healthy ranges for serum alanine aminotransferase levels. *Ann Intern Med* 137:

1–10, 2002
13. Kim HC, Choi KS, Jang YH, Shin HW, Kim DJ: Normal serum aminotransferase levels and the metabolic syndrome: Korean National Health and Nutrition Examination Surveys. *Yonsei Med J* 47:542–550, 2006
14. Park HS, Han JH, Choi KM, Kim SM: Relation between elevated serum alanine aminotransferase and metabolic syndrome in Korean adolescents. *Am J Clin Nutr* 82:1046–1051, 2005
15. Clark JM, Diehl AM: Defining nonalcoholic fatty liver disease: implications for epidemiologic studies. *Gastroenterology* 124:248–250, 2003
16. Lee S, Choi S, Kim HJ, Chung YS, Lee KW, Lee HC, Huh KB, Kim DJ: Cutoff values of surrogate measures of insulin resistance for metabolic syndrome in Korean non-diabetic adults. *J Korean Med Sci* 21:695–700, 2006
17. McLaughlin T, Reaven G, Abbasi F, Lamendola C, Saad M, Waters D, Simon J, Krauss RM: Is there a simple way to identify insulin-resistant individuals at increased risk of cardiovascular disease? *Am J Cardiol* 96:399–404, 2005
18. Marchesini G, Bugianesi E, Forlani G, Cerrelli F, Lenzi M, Manini R, Natale S, Vanni E, Villanova N, Melchionda N, Rizzetto M: Nonalcoholic fatty liver, steatohepatitis, and the metabolic syndrome. *Hepatology* 37:917–923, 2003
19. Marchesini G, Brizi M, Bianchi G, Tomassetti S, Bugianesi E, Lenzi M, McCullough AJ, Natale S, Forlani G, Melchionda N: Nonalcoholic fatty liver disease: a feature of the metabolic syndrome. *Diabetes* 50: 1844–1850, 2001
20. Haukeland JW, Konopski Z, Linnestad P, Azimy S, Marit Løberg E, Haaland T, Birkeland K, Bjøro K: Abnormal glucose tolerance is a predictor of steatohepatitis and fibrosis in patients with nonalcoholic fatty liver disease. *Scand J Gastroenterol* 40: 1469–1477, 2005
21. Marceau P, Biron S, Hould FS, Marceau S, Simard S, Thung SN, Kral JG: Liver pathology and the metabolic syndrome X in severe obesity. *J Clin Endocrinol Metab* 84: 1513–1517, 1999
22. Seppälä-Lindroos A, Vehkavaara S, Häkkinen AM, Goto T, Westerbacka J, Sovijärvi A, Halavaara J, Yki-Järvinen H: Fat accumulation in the liver is associated with defects in insulin suppression of glucose production and serum free fatty acids independent of obesity in normal men. *J Clin Endocrinol Metab* 87:3023–3028, 2002
23. Shoelson SE, Lee J, Goldfine AB: Inflammation and insulin resistance. *J Clin Invest* 116:1793–1801, 2006
24. Arkan MC, Havener AL, Greten FR, Maeda S, Li ZW, Long JM, Wynshaw-Boris A, Poli G, Olefsky J, Karin M: IKK-beta links inflammation to obesity-induced insulin re-

sistance. *Nat Med* 11:191–198, 2005

25. Boden G, She P, Mozzoli M, Cheung P, Gumireddy K, Reddy P, Xiang X, Luo Z, Ruderman N: Free fatty acids produce insulin resistance and activate the proinflammatory nuclear factor-kB pathway in rat liver. *Diabetes* 54:3458–3465, 2005

26. Kim SH, Abbasi F, Reaven GM: Impact of degree of obesity on surrogate estimates of insulin resistance. *Diabetes Care* 27:1998–2002, 2004

27. Farin HM, Abbasi F, Reaven GM: Body mass index and waist circumference both contribute to differences in insulin-mediated glucose disposal in nondiabetic adults. *Am J Clin Nutr* 83:47–51, 2006

28. Saadeh S, Younossi ZM, Remer EM, Gramlich T, Ong JP, Hurley M, Mullen KD, Cooper JN, Sheridan MJ: The utility of radiological imaging in nonalcoholic fatty liver disease. *Gastroenterology* 123:745–750, 2002

29. Dixon JB, Bhathal PS, O'Brien PE: Nonalcoholic fatty liver disease: predictors of nonalcoholic steatohepatitis and liver fibrosis in the severely obese. *Gastroenterology* 121:91–100, 2001

30. Amarapurka DN, Amarapurkar AD, Patel ND, Agal S, Baigal R, Gupte P, Pramanik S: Nonalcoholic steatohepatitis (NASH) with diabetes: predictors of liver fibrosis. *Ann Hepatol* 5:30–33, 2006

31. Palekar NA, Naus R, Larson SP, Ward J, Harrison SA: Clinical model for distinguishing nonalcoholic steatohepatitis from simple steatosis in patients with nonalcoholic fatty liver disease. *Liver Int* 26:151–156, 2006

Nonalcoholic Fatty Liver Disease Is Independently Associated With an Increased Incidence of Cardiovascular Events in Type 2 Diabetic Patients

Giovanni Targher, MD[1,2]
Lorenzo Bertolini, MD[1]
Stefano Rodella, MD[3]
Roberto Tessari, MD[1]

Luciano Zenari, MD[1]
Giuseppe Lippi, MD[4]
Guido Arcaro, MD[1]

Recent data suggest that the presence of nonalcoholic fatty liver disease (NAFLD) in type 2 diabetes may be linked to increased cardiovascular disease (CVD) independent of components of the metabolic syndrome (1–3), although this hypothesis needs verification in larger studies. We assessed whether NAFLD, as diagnosed by ultrasound, predicts the risk of incident CVD events in a large cohort of type 2 diabetic adults.

RESEARCH DESIGN AND METHODS

Study subjects were participants in the Valpolicella Heart Diabetes Study (1). Briefly, we enrolled all of the type 2 diabetic outpatients ($n =$ 2,103) who regularly attended our clinic in the period January–December 2000 after excluding those who had manifest CVD and/or secondary causes of chronic liver disease (alcohol abuse, viral infection, or medications). The local ethics committee approved the study. All participants provided written informed consent.

During 6.5 years of follow-up (through December 2006; follow-up range: 5–84 months), 384 participants subsequently developed CVD events (myocardial infarction, ischemic stroke, coronary revascularization, or cardiovascular death), whereas 1,719 patients re-mained free of diagnosed CVD. These events were ascertained by patient history, chart review, autopsy reports, and family contact (1).

Plasma liver enzymes, A1C, and other biochemical blood measurements were determined by standard procedures. At baseline, most participants (~86%) had normal liver enzymes (reference ranges for aminotransferases were 10–35 and 10–50 units/l for female and male subjects, respectively) and were abstainers (77%) or drank minimally (13%); only 10% of participants drank >20 g/day of alcohol. No participants had seropositivity for viral hepatitis.

Hepatic ultrasonography scanning was performed in all participants by an experienced radiologist who was blind to subjects' details. Hepatic steatosis was diagnosed by characteristic sonographic features (4,5). Metabolic syndrome was diagnosed by a recently modified Adult Treatment Panel III definition (6).

Statistical analyses included unpaired t test, χ^2 test, and multivariate Cox proportional hazards analysis. In this latter analysis, CVD was considered a composite end point inclusive of nonfatal coronary heart disease, ischemic stroke, and cardiovascular death.

RESULTS

During follow-up, we documented 384 CVD events: 219 cases of nonfatal coronary heart disease (151 myocardial infarction and 68 revascularization procedures), 44 cases of nonfatal ischemic stroke, and 121 cardiovascular deaths.

As shown in Table 1, subjects who developed CVD events during follow-up were older, had higher liver enzymes and A1C, and had greater prevalence of metabolic syndrome than those who did not develop CVD events. Sex, smoking, LDL cholesterol, diabetes duration, and treatment did not differ between the groups. The frequency of NAFLD was markedly higher in those who developed CVD events than in those who did not, without significant sex differences (not shown).

In univariate regression analysis, NAFLD (hazard ratio [HR] 2.01 [95% CI 1.4–2.9]), metabolic syndrome (1.74 [1.3–3]), age (1.11 [1.05–1.2]), male sex (1.52 [1.3–1.8]), smoking (1.48 [1.2–2.2]), A1C (1.44 [1.4–2.9]), LDL cholesterol (1.37 [1.1–1.8]), alanine aminotransferase (1.47 [1.2–1.9]), and other liver enzymes were significantly ($P < 0.01$) associated with incident CVD, whereas diabetes duration and medications were not. In multivariate regression analysis, the significant association between NAFLD and incident CVD was little affected (1.96 [1.4–2.7], $P < 0.001$) by adjustment for sex, age, smoking, diabetes duration, A1C, LDL cholesterol, and medications (hypoglycemic, antihypertensive, lipid-lowering, or antiplatelet drugs); further adjustment for the metabolic syndrome did not appreciably change the association (1.87 [1.2–2.6], $P < 0.001$).

Almost identical results were obtained in models that also adjusted for individual components of the metabolic syndrome and/or liver enzymes. No liver enzymes were independently associated with incident CVD after controlling for the metabolic syndrome and/or ultrasound-diagnosed NAFLD. Exclusion of participants who were light/moderate drinkers did not alter the association be-

From the [1]Unit of Internal Medicine and Diabetes, "Sacro Cuore" Hospital of Negrar, Negrar, Italy; the [2]Section of Endocrinology, Biomedical and Surgical Sciences, University Hospital of Verona, Verona, Italy; the [3]Department of Radiology, "Sacro Cuore" Hospital of Negrar, Negrar, Italy; and the [4]Section of Clinical Chemistry, Biomedical and Morphological Sciences, University Hospital of Verona, Verona, Italy.

Address correspondence and reprint requests to Dr. Giovanni Targher, Endocrinology and Metabolic Diseases, Ospedale Civile Magglore, Piazzale Stefani, 1, 37126 Verona, Italy. E-mail: giovanni.targher@univr.it.

Received for publication 21 February 2007 and accepted in revised form 13 May 2007.

Published ahead of print at http://care.diabetesjournals.org on 22 May 2007. DOI: 10.2337/dc07-0349.

Abbreviations: CVD, cardiovascular disease; NAFLD, nonalcoholic fatty liver disease.

A table elsewhere in this issue shows conventional and Système International (SI) units and conversion factors for many substances.

Table 1—*Baseline characteristics of the diabetic cohort (n = 2,103) by CVD status*

Variables	Control subjects	Case subjects	P
n	1,719	384	
Sex (% men)	62%	63%	0.80
Age (years)	59 ± 3	61 ± 4	0.001
BMI (kg/m^2)	26 ± 3	28 ± 4	0.001
Waist circumference (cm)	93 ± 11	99 ± 13	0.001
Duration of diabetes (years)	14 ± 3	16 ± 3	0.60
Diabetes treatment			
Diet only	21	15	0.20
Oral hypoglycemic drugs	62	65	0.30
Insulin only	17	20	0.20
Antihypertensive users	60	73	0.001
Aspirin users	49	48	0.80
Lipid-lowering users	34	36	0.60
Current smokers	22	23	0.70
Systolic blood pressure (mmHg)	127 ± 12	131 ± 16	0.001
Diastolic blood pressure (mmHg)	80 ± 12	83 ± 14	0.001
A1C (%)	6.9 ± 0.8	7.3 ± 1.0	0.001
Triglycerides (mmol/l)	1.32 ± 0.6	1.62 ± 1.0	0.001
HDL cholesterol (mmol/l)	1.40 ± 0.3	1.32 ± 0.4	0.001
LDL cholesterol (mmol/l)	3.35 ± 0.4	3.32 ± 0.5	0.80
AST (units/l)	20 ± 6	26 ± 12	0.001
ALT (units/l)	24 ± 6	32 ± 13	0.001
GGT (units/l)	23 ± 10	34 ± 14	0.001
Metabolic syndrome	59	75	0.001
NAFLD	61	96	0.001

Data are means ± SD or percentages unless otherwise indicated. Differences are assessed by the unpaired *t* test (for normally distributed variables) and by the χ^2 test (for categorical variables). ALT, alanine aminotransferase; AST, aspartate aminotransferase; GGT, γ-glutamyl transferase.

tween NAFLD and CVD risk (HR 1.80 [95% CI 1.2–2.7], *P* < 0.005).

CONCLUSIONS — The major finding of this study is that NAFLD, as diagnosed by ultrasound, is associated with an increased incidence of CVD in a large cohort of type 2 diabetic adults. Notably, this association appears to be independent of a broad spectrum of risk factors, thus suggesting that NAFLD might confer an excess of CVD risk over and above what would be expected because of increased prevalence of the underlying metabolic risk factors. Moreover, this study provides further evidence that normal liver enzymes provide little diagnostic or prognostic value when assessing patients for NAFLD (3–5,7) because more than four-fifths (~86%) of our NAFLD patients had liver enzymes within the normal range.

Our findings complement recent observations that the severity of NAFLD histology is associated with greater carotid intima-media thickness (8) and lower endothelial flow-mediated vasodilation (9), independent of underlying metabolic abnormalities, and that NAFLD is associated

with higher all-cause death (10,11) and higher prevalence (2,3,12–15) and incidence (1,11) of CVD in nondiabetic and type 2 diabetic individuals. Others have shown that individuals with slightly elevated liver enzymes, as surrogate markers of NAFLD, have an increased CVD risk (16–19).

There is therefore now growing evidence suggesting that NAFLD is not merely a marker of CVD but may also be involved in its pathogenesis. The possible molecular mediators linking NAFLD and CVD have been extensively reviewed elsewhere (20) but include the release of proatherogenic mediators from the liver, including C-reactive protein, fibrinogen, and plasminogen activator inhibitor-1.

This study has some limitations. First, we did not directly measure abdominal visceral fat (by computed tomography) or insulin resistance (by euglycemic clamp), so we cannot be certain that these data completely exclude an independent contribution of insulin resistance and visceral fat to accelerated CVD in NAFLD. Second, NAFLD diagnosis was based on ultrasonography but was not confirmed by biopsy. It is known that ultrasonography

has a good sensitivity/specificity in detecting moderate and severe liver steatosis, but its sensitivity is reduced when hepatic fat infiltration on biopsy is <33% (5). Thus, although some nondifferential misclassification of NAFLD on the basis of ultrasonography is likely (some of the diabetic control subjects could have underlying NAFLD despite normal liver enzymes and negative ultrasonography), this limitation would serve to attenuate the magnitude of our effect measures toward the null; thus, our results can probably be considered conservative estimates of the relationship between NAFLD and CVD risk.

In conclusion, our findings suggest that NAFLD is associated with an increased incidence of CVD in type 2 diabetic patients, independent of traditional CVD risk factors and metabolic syndrome components. These findings support the hypothesis that the identification of NAFLD in type 2 diabetes may help in CVD risk prediction, with important management implications. Further studies are needed to extend these findings to NAFLD patients without type 2 diabetes.

References
1. Targher G, Bertolini L, Poli F, Rodella S, Scala L, Tessari R, Zenari L, Falezza G: Nonalcoholic fatty liver disease and risk of future cardiovascular events among type 2 diabetic patients. *Diabetes* 54:3541–3546, 2005
2. Targher G, Bertolini L, Padovani R, Poli F, Scala L, Tessari R, Zenari L, Falezza G: Increased prevalence of cardiovascular disease among type 2 diabetic patients with non-alcoholic fatty liver disease. *Diabet Med* 23:403–409, 2006
3. Targher G, Bertolini L, Padovani R, Rodella S, Tessari R, Zenari L, Day C, Arcaro G: Prevalence of nonalcoholic fatty liver disease and its association with cardiovascular disease among type 2 diabetic patients. *Diabetes Care* 30:1212–1218, 2007
4. Angulo P: Nonalcoholic fatty liver disease. *N Engl J Med* 346:1221–1231, 2002
5. Saadeh S, Younossi ZM, Remer EM, Gramlich T, Ong JP, Hurley M, Mullen KD, Cooper JN, Sheridan MJ: The utility of radiological imaging in nonalcoholic fatty liver disease. *Gastroenterology* 123:745–750, 2002
6. Grundy SM, Cleeman JI, Daniels SR, Donato KA, Eckel RH, Franklin BA, Gordon DJ, Krauss RM, Savage PJ, Smith SC Jr, Spertus JA, Costa F; American Heart Association; National Heart, Lung, and Blood Institute: Diagnosis and management of the metabolic syndrome: an

American Heart Association/National Heart, Lung, and Blood Institute scientific statement. *Circulation* 112:2735–2752, 2005

7. Day CP: Nonalcoholic fatty liver disease: current concepts and management strategies. *Clin Med* 6:19–25, 2006
8. Targher G, Bertolini L, Padovani R, Rodella S, Zoppini G, Zenari L, Cigolini M, Falezza G, Arcaro G: Relations between carotid artery wall thickness and liver histology in subjects with nonalcoholic fatty liver disease. *Diabetes Care* 29:1325–1330, 2006
9. Villanova N, Moscatiello S, Ramilli S, Bugianesi E, Magalotti D, Vanni E, Zoli M, Marchesini G: Endothelial dysfunction and cardiovascular risk profile in nonalcoholic fatty liver disease. *Hepatology* 42:473–478, 2005
10. Adams LA, Lymp JF, St Sauver J, Sanderson SO, Lindor KD, Feldstein A, Angulo P: The natural history of nonalcoholic fatty liver disease: a population-based cohort study. *Gastroenterology* 129:113–121, 2005
11. Ekstedt M, Franzen LE, Mathiesen UL, Thorelius L, Holmqvist M, Bodemar G, Kechagias S: Long-term follow-up of patients with NAFLD and elevated liver enzymes. *Hepatology* 44:865–873, 2006
12. Lin YC, Lo HM, Chen JD: Sonographic fatty liver, overweight and ischaemic heart disease. *World J Gastroenterol* 11:4838–4842, 2005
13. Kessler A, Levy Y, Roth A, Zelber-Sagi S, Leshno M, Blendis L, Halpern Z, Oren R: Increased prevalence of NAFLD in patients with acute myocardial infarction independent of BMI (Abstract). *Hepatology* 42:623A, 2005
14. Volzke H, Robinson DM, Kleine V, Deutscher R, Hoffmann W, Ludemann J, Schminke U, Kessler C, John U: Hepatic steatosis is associated with an increased risk of carotid atherosclerosis. *World J Gastronterol* 11:1848–1853, 2005
15. Targher G, Bertolini L, Padovani R, Zenari L, Zoppini G, Falezza G: Relation of nonalcoholic hepatic steatosis to early carotid atherosclerosis in healthy men: role of visceral fat accumulation. *Diabetes Care* 27:1498–1500, 2004
16. Wannamethee G, Ebrahim S, Shaper AG: Gamma-glutamyltransferase: determinants and association with mortality from ischaemic heart disease and all causes. *Am J Epidemiol* 142:699–708, 1995
17. Ruttmann E, Brant LJ, Concin H, Diem G, Rapp K, Ulmer H: Gamma-glutamyltransferase as a risk factor for cardiovascular disease mortality: an epidemiological investigation in a cohort of 163,944 Austrian adults. *Circulation* 112:2130–2137, 2005
18. Schindhelm RK, Dekker JM, Nijpels G, Bouter LM, Stehouwer CD, Heine RJ, Diamant M: Alanine aminotransferase predicts coronary heart disease events: a 10-year follow-up of the Hoorn Study. *Atherosclerosis* 191:391–396, 2007
19. Ioannou GN, Weiss NS, Boyko EJ, Mozaffarian D, Lee SP: Elevated serum alanine aminotrasferase activity and calculated risk of coronary heart disease in the United States. *Hepatology* 43:1145–1151, 2006
20. Targher G, Arcaro G: Non-alcoholic fatty liver disease and increased risk of cardiovascular disease. *Atherosclerosis* 191:235–240, 2007

Intrauterine Growth Retardation, Insulin Resistance, and Nonalcoholic Fatty Liver Disease in Children

Valerio Nobili, md[1]
Matilde Marcellini, md[1]
Giulio Marchesini, md[2]
Ester Vanni, md[3]

Melania Manco, md[1]
Alberto Villani, md[4]
Elisabetta Bugianesi, md[3]

Intrauterine growth retardation is associated with the development of abnormalities in glucose tolerance in adulthood (1,2). Studies in adults and children born small for gestational age (SGA) (3–7) indicate that insulin resistance is the earliest component associated with low birth weight, irrespective of confounding factors, including obesity (8) and a family history of type 2 diabetes.

In SGA children, the typical central fat accumulation may actively contribute to insulin resistance (9). Visceral fat and fatty liver represent special depots of ectopic fat, independently associated with insulin resistance (10–12). In the liver, hepatic triglyceride accumulation characterizes nonalcoholic fatty liver disease (NAFLD), a highly prevalent and potentially progressive condition in adults, now considered the hepatic expression of the metabolic syndrome (13). In the pediatric population, the prevalence of NAFLD is only 2–3% but increases to 53% in the presence of obesity (14,15).

We studied the association of low birth weight with histologically assessed pediatric NAFLD to test the hypothesis that intrauterine growth retardation might be an additional factor responsible for metabolic liver disease in children via insulin resistance.

RESEARCH DESIGN AND METHODS — We studied 90 children with NAFLD, consecutively observed in the Liver Unit, Bambino Gesù Children's Hospital, Rome, Italy, from June 2001 to April 2003. Part of this cohort group was reported elsewhere (16). All had a complete anthropometric and laboratory investigation, including a 2-h oral glucose tolerance test, within 2 months of a liver biopsy confirming the diagnosis of NAFLD. To compare BMI across different ages and sexes, we calculated the BMI Z score (17). Obesity was defined as BMI above the 97th percentile and overweight as BMI from the 85th to 97th percentile. The control group consisted of 90 children pair matched by age and sex, with normal liver scanning and liver function tests, selected among 200 consecutive subjects observed in the general pediatric department.

All children were born at term ($\geq$37 weeks). They were defined SGA or appropriate for gestational age when their weight at birth was, respectively, $\leq$10th and >10th percentile, corrected for gestational age, sex, and the local standard growth curve (18). The study was approved by the ethics committee of the Bambino Gesù Children's Hospital.

RESULTS — Of 90 NAFLD children, 35 (38.9%) were classified as SGA, compared with 6.7% of control subjects ($P <$ 0.0001). The prevalence of SGA in NAFLD was also approximately fourfold higher compared with the average SGA prevalence of children admitted to our pediatric department in the last decade (10%). Obesity and altered glucose regulation (American Diabetes Association criteria [19]) were more common in NAFLD patients (Table 1). Insulin resistance (20), assessed by homeostasis model assessment of insulin resistance (21) and by the insulin sensitivity index derived from the oral glucose tolerance test (22), was very common in children with NAFLD, independent of obesity. SGA children with NAFLD had higher basal glucose and insulin levels and were more insulin resistant. The family history of metabolic diseases was not systematically different between groups, with the notable exception of type 2 diabetes in second-degree relatives.

In multivariate regression, SGA was independently associated with NAFLD (odds ratio [OR] 7.94 [95% CI 2.71–23.24]) after correction for age, sex, BMI Z score, and glucose regulation. Among children with NAFLD, SGA was significantly associated with both homeostasis model assessment of insulin resistance (1.75 [1.17–2.62]) and insulin sensitivity index (0.73 [0.56–0.95] after correction for age, sex, and BMI Z score, and the association was maintained after exclusion of type 2 diabetes cases.

The main histological features of NALFD (steatosis, necro-inflammation, and fibrosis) were scored according to the Non-Alcoholic Steatohepatitis (NASH) Clinical Research Network proposal (23) and combined into the NAFLD activity score (NAS) (NAS $\geq$5, "NASH"; NAS $\leq$2, "non-NASH"; and NAS 3–4, "borderline"). Thirty-six patients (40%) met the criteria for NASH. After correction for age, sex, BMI, insulin resistance (both basal and postload), and the presence of pre-diabetes/diabetes, the risk of NAS >5 associated with SGA was highly significant (OR 3.45 [95% CI 1.20–9.91]). Fibrosis was present in 56 cases (62%), but its presence (1.28 [0.53–3.09]) and severity (stage 3: 1.61 [0.22–11.96]) was not associated with SGA.

CONCLUSIONS — The major finding of the study is the association of pediatric NAFLD with intrauterine growth

From the [1]Liver Unit, Bambino Gesù Children's Hospital, Rome, Italy; the [2]Unit of Clinical Dietetics, University of Bologna, Bologna, Italy; [3]Gastroenterology, University of Turin, Turin, Italy; and [4]Pediatrics, Bambino Gesù Children's Hospital, Rome, Italy.

Address correspondence and reprint requests to Valerio Nobili, MD, Liver Unit, Research Institute, Bambino Gesù Children's Hospital, Piazza S. Onofrio 4, 00165 Rome, Italy. E-mail: nobili66@yahoo.it.

Received for publication 10 February 2007 and accepted in revised form 22 May 2007.

Published ahead of print at http://care.diabetesjournals.org on 29 May 2007. DOI: 10.2337/dc07-0281.

Abbreviations: NAFLD, nonalcoholic fatty liver disease; NAS, NAFLD activity score; NASH, nonalcoholic steatohepatitis; SGA, small for gestational age.

A table elsewhere in this issue shows conventional and Système International (SI) units and conversion factors for many substances.

Table 1—*Anthropometric, clinical, and biochemical characteristics of children with NAFLD, subgrouped according to weight at birth, and of control subjects, matched for age and sex*

Variables	Control subjects	NAFLD	AGA NAFLD	SGA NAFLD
n	90	90	55	35
Age (years)	11.3 ± 3.8	11.7 ± 3.2	11.3 ± 3.3	12.3 ± 3.0
Sex (male/female)	63/27	63/27	37/18	26/9
Birth weight (kg)	3.38 ± 0.42	3.12 ± 0.66*	3.57 ± 0.36	2.41 ± 0.29†
Gestational age (weeks)	39.3 ± 1.0	39.3 ± 1.1	39.1 ± 1.2	39.6 ± 0.7
BMI (kg/m^2)	19.7 ± 2.7	26.3 ± 3.6‡	26.5 ± 3.6	26.0 ± 3.5
BMI Z score	1.14 ± 0.38	1.78 ± 0.72‡	1.82 ± 0.85	1.73 ± 0.43
Obesity	6 (2–13)	44 (34–54)‡	44 (31–56)	46 (29–60)
NGT/IFG-IGT/diabetes (%)	99/1/0	84/9/7‡	89/9/2	78/19/3
Family history of diabetes				
First degree (%)	NA	8 (3–15)	10 (4–20)	3 (1–14)
Second degree (%)	NA	21 (13–30)	29 (18–41)	9 (2–20)§
AST (IU/l)	28 ± 7	48 ± 25‡	49 ± 26	47 ± 23
ALT (IU/l)	28 ± 5	74 ± 61‡	77 ± 60	71 ± 63
gGT (IU/l)	22 ± 6	26 ± 21	26 ± 22	26 ± 18
Cholesterol (mg/dl)	138 ± 28	154 ± 34*	148 ± 34	164 ± 34§
Triglycerides (mg/dl)	79 ± 22	95 ± 53*	93 ± 36	99 ± 73
Fasting glucose (mg/dl)	81 ± 6	82 ± 10	81 ± 9	85 ± 11§
Fasting insulin (μU/l)	6.7 ± 2.3	11.4 ± 6.0‡	10.5 ± 5.1	13.5 ± 6.7†
HOMA-IR	1.34 ± 0.46	2.32 ± 1.25‡	1.99 ± 0.98	2.85 ± 1.46†
ISI	NA	4.42 ± 1.98	4.86 ± 1.87	3.73 ± 1.98†
HOMA-IR >2.6¶	11 (6–19)	48 (37–54)‡	38 (25–50)	63 (45–76)§
ISI <6.0¶	NA	73 (63–81)	65 (51–76)	86 (69–93)§
Liver histology				
NAS index	NA	4.41 ± 2.06	4.29 ± 2.11	4.60 ± 1.99
Fibrosis stage	NA	0.74 ± 0.73	0.73 ± 0.73	0.77 ± 0.73

Data are means ± SD and percent cases (95% CI) unless otherwise indicated. *P vs. control subjects <0.01; †P vs. NAFLD appropriate for gestational age (AGA) <0.01; ‡P vs. control subjects <0.001; §P vs. NAFLD AGA <0.05. ¶These cutoffs, representing the upper (homeostasis model assessment of insulin resistance [HOMA-IR]) and lower (insulin sensitivity index derived from oral glucose load [ISI]) quartiles of a control population, respectively (ref. 20), identify subjects considered insulin resistant. ALT, alanine aminotransferase; AST, aspartate aminotransferase; IFG, impaired fasting glucose; IGT, impaired glucose tolerance; NGT, normal glucose tolerance; γGT, γ-glutamyl transpeptidase.

retardation independent of and in addition to insulin resistance. SGA children with NAFLD represent a subset with a higher prevalence of both metabolic abnormalities and NASH, the most severe form of liver damage, independently of age, sex, BMI, and genetic inheritance.

Intrauterine growth has a strong independent effect on insulin resistance. The relative risk of metabolic syndrome in adulthood increases by 1.72 times for each tertile decrease in birth weight (24). Insulin resistance probably appears early in the postnatal period, during the catch-up growth period, but the metabolic derangements are initially moderate (25–27).

At an average age of 11 years, most of our study's subjects (80%) were insulin resistant, despite normal BMI and a very low prevalence of metabolic abnormalities. Insulin resistance in adipose tissue develops early during fetal growth restriction (5) and is maintained during the neo-natal period and adulthood. NAFLD has been proposed as part of a generalized abnormality of the adipose tissue (28) known as lipotoxicity, leading to fat accumulation in ectopic sites, including muscle and liver, and to an altered pattern of circulating and intracellular adipokines (29). This defect might stem from a combination of acquired and genetic factors. Notably, the family history of type 2 diabetes was less common in SGA NAFLD, suggesting that genetic factors have lower relevance in the onset of NAFLD in this cohort, counterbalanced by an adverse in utero environment favoring the future development of abnormal adipose tissue.

SGA was also associated with more severe disease activity at histology independently of age, sex, and insulin resistance. This confirms that factors known to affect insulin sensitivity may also independently contribute to liver disease progression (30). Insulin-resistant states are characterized by chronic subclinical inflammation, and an imbalance in cytokine activity produced by dysfunctional fat cells may be the link between metabolic and liver disorders. In conclusion, intrauterine growth retardation is an important risk factor for pediatric NAFLD; careful monitoring of SGA children may be considered.

References
1. Hales CN, Barker DJ, Clark PM, Cox LJ, Fall C, Osmond C, Winter PD: Fetal and infant growth and impaired glucose tolerance at age 64. *BMJ* 303:1019–1022, 1991
2. Lithell HO, McKeigue PM, Berglund L, Mohsen R, Lithell UB, Leon DA: Relation of size at birth to non-insulin dependent diabetes and insulin concentrations in men aged 50–60 years. *BMJ* 312:406–410, 1996
3. Flanagan DE, Moore VM, Godsland IF, Cockington RA, Robinson JS, Phillips DI: Fetal growth and the physiological control of glucose tolerance in adults: a min-

imal model analysis. *Am J Physiol Endocrinol Metab* 278:E700–E706, 2000

4. Hofman PL, Cutfield WS, Robinson EM, Bergman RN, Menon RK, Sperling MA, Gluckman PD: Insulin resistance in short children with intrauterine growth retardation. *J Clin Endocrinol Metab* 82:402–406, 1997

5. Jaquet D, Gaboriau A, Czernichow P, Levy-Marchal C: Insulin resistance early in adulthood in subjects born with intrauterine growth retardation. *J Clin Endocrinol Metab* 85:1401–1406, 2000

6. Phillips DI, Barker DJ, Hales CN, Hirst S, Osmond C: Thinness at birth and insulin resistance in adult life. *Diabetologia* 37:150–154, 1994

7. Veening MA, Van Weissenbruch MM, Delemarre-Van De Waal HA: Glucose tolerance, insulin sensitivity, and insulin secretion in children born small for gestational age. *J Clin Endocrinol Metab* 87:4657–4661, 2002

8. Hovi P, Andersson S, Eriksson JG, Jarvenpaa A-L, Strang-Karlsson S, Makitie O, Kajantie E: Glucose regulation in young adults with very low birth weight. *N Engl J Med* 356:2053–2063, 2007

9. Rasmussen EL, Malis C, Jensen CB, Jensen JE, Storgaard H, Poulsen P, Pilgaard K, Schou JH, Madsbad S, Astrup A, Vaag A: Altered fat tissue distribution in young adult men who had low birth weight. *Diabetes Care* 28:151–153, 2005

10. Marchesini G, Brizi M, Bianchi G, Tomassetti S, Bugianesi E, Lenzi M, McCullough AJ, Natale S, Forlani G, Melchionda N: Nonalcoholic fatty liver disease: a feature of the metabolic syndrome. *Diabetes* 50:1844–1850, 2001

11. Gastaldelli A, Miyazaki Y, Pettiti M, Matsuda M, Mahankali S, Santini E, DeFronzo RA, Ferrannini E: Metabolic effects of visceral fat accumulation in type 2 diabetes. *J Clin Endocrinol Metab* 87:5098–5103, 2002

12. Medina J, Fernandez-Salazar LI, Garcia-Buey L, Moreno-Otero R: Approach to the pathogenesis and treatment of nonalcoholic steatohepatitis. *Diabetes Care* 27:

2057–2066, 2004

13. Eckel RH, Grundy SM, Zimmet PZ: The metabolic syndrome. *Lancet* 365:1415–1428, 2005

14. Franzese A, Vajro P, Argenziano A, Puzziello A, Iannucci MP, Saviano MC, Brunetti F, Rubino A: Liver involvement in obese children: ultrasonography and liver enzyme levels at diagnosis and during follow-up in an Italian population. *Dig Dis Sci* 42:1428–1432, 1997

15. Tominaga K, Kurata JH, Chen YK, Fujimoto E, Miyagawa S, Abe I, Kusano Y: Prevalence of fatty liver in Japanese children and relationship to obesity: an epidemiological ultrasonographic survey. *Dig Dis Sci* 40:2002–2009, 1995

16. Nobili V, Marcellini M, Devito R, Ciampalini P, Piemonte F, Comparcola D, Sartorelli MR, Angulo P: NAFLD in children: a prospective clinical-pathological study and effect of lifestyle advice. *Hepatology* 44:458–465, 2006

17. Cole TJ, Bellizzi MC, Flegal KM, Dietz WH: Establishing a standard definition for child overweight and obesity worldwide: international survey. *BMJ* 320:1240–1243, 2000

18. Gairdner D, Pearson J: A growth chart for premature and other infants. *Arch Dis Child* 46:783–787, 1971

19. The Expert Committee on the Diagnosis and Classification of Diabetes Mellitus: Follow-up report on the diagnosis of diabetes mellitus. *Diabetes Care* 26:3160–3167, 2003

20. Bugianesi E, Pagotto U, Manini R, Vanni E, Gastaldelli A, De Iasio R, Gentilcore E, Natale S, Rizzetto M, Pasquali R, Marchesini G: Plasma adiponectin in nonalcoholic fatty liver is related to hepatic insulin resistance and hepatic fat content, not to liver disease severity. *J Clin Endocrinol Metab* 90:3498–3504, 2005

21. Matthews DR, Hosker JP, Rudenski AS, Naylor BA, Treacher DF, Turner RC: Homeostasis model assessment: insulin resistance and beta-cell function from plasma fasting glucose and insulin concentrations in man. *Diabetologia* 28:412–419, 1985

22. Matsuda M, DeFronzo RA: Insulin sensitivity indices obtained from oral glucose tolerance testing: comparison with the euglycemic insulin clamp. *Diabetes Care* 22:1462–1470, 1999

23. Kleiner DE, Brunt EM, Van Natta M, Behling C, Contos MJ, Cummings OW, Ferrell LD, Liu YC, Torbenson MS, Unalp-Arida A, Yeh M, McCullough AJ, Sanyal AJ: Design and validation of a histological scoring system for nonalcoholic fatty liver disease. *Hepatology* 41:1313–1321, 2005

24. Valdez R, Athens MA, Thompson GH, Bradshaw BS, Stern MP: Birthweight and adult health outcomes in a biethnic population in the USA. *Diabetologia* 37:624–631, 1994

25. Soto N, Bazaes RA, Pena V, Salazar T, Avila A, Iniguez G, Ong KK, Dunger DB, Mericq MV: Insulin sensitivity and secretion are related to catch-up growth in small-for-gestational-age infants at age 1 year: results from a prospective cohort. *J Clin Endocrinol Metab* 88:3645–3650, 2003

26. Yajnik CS, Fall CH, Vaidya U, Pandit AN, Bavdekar A, Bhat DS, Osmond C, Hales CN, Barker DJ: Fetal growth and glucose and insulin metabolism in four-year-old Indian children. *Diabet Med* 12:330–336, 1995

27. Bo S, Bertino E, Bagna R, Trapani A, Gambino R, Martano C, Mombro M, Pagano G: Insulin resistance in pre-school very-low-birth weight pre-term children. *Diabet Metab* 32:151–158, 2006

28. Unger RH: Lipotoxic diseases. *Annu Rev Med* 53:319–336, 2002

29. Bugianesi E, McCullough AJ, Marchesini G: Insulin resistance: a metabolic pathway to chronic liver disease. *Hepatology* 42:987–1000, 2005

30. Marchesini G, Bugianesi E, Forlani G, Cerrelli F, Lenzi M, Manini R, Natale S, Vanni E, Villanova N, Melchionda N, Rizzetto M: Nonalcoholic fatty liver, steatohepatitis, and the metabolic syndrome. *Hepatology* 37:917–923, 2003

Relationship of Liver Enzymes to Insulin Sensitivity and Intra-Abdominal Fat

Tara M. Wallace, md[1]
Kristina M. Utzschneider, md[1]
Jenny Tong, md[1]
Darcy B. Carr, md[2]

Sakeneh Zraika, phd[1]
Daniel D. Bankson, md[3]
Robert H. Knopp, md[4]
Steven E. Kahn, mb, chb[1]

OBJECTIVE — The purpose of this study was to determine the relationship between plasma liver enzyme concentrations, insulin sensitivity, and intra-abdominal fat (IAF) distribution.

RESEARCH DESIGN AND METHODS — Plasma γ-glutamyl transferase (GGT), aspartate transaminase (AST), alanine transaminase (ALT) levels, insulin sensitivity (insulin sensitivity index [S_I]), IAF area, and subcutaneous fat (SCF) area were measured in 177 nondiabetic subjects (75 men and 102 women, aged 31–75 years) with no history of liver disease. On the basis of BMI (< or $\geq$27.5 kg/m^2) and S_I (< or $\geq 7.0 \times 10^{-5}$ min/pmol) subjects were divided into lean insulin sensitive (LIS, $n = 53$), lean insulin resistant (LIR, $n = 60$), and obese insulin resistant (OIR, $n = 56$) groups.

RESULTS — Levels of all three liver enzymes were higher in men than in women ($P < 0.0001$ for each). In men, GGT levels were higher in insulin-resistant than in insulin-sensitive subjects ($P < 0.01$). In women, GGT levels were higher in the OIR than in the LIS group ($P < 0.01$) but no different in the LIR group. There was no difference in ALT and AST levels among the LIS, LIR, and OIR groups. GGT was associated with S_I ($r = -0.26$, $P < 0.0001$), IAF area ($r = 0.22$, $P < 0.01$), waist-to-hip ratio (WHR) ($r = 0.25$, $P = 0.001$), BMI ($r = 0.17$, $P < 0.05$), and SCF area ($r = 0.16$, $P < 0.05$) after adjustments for age and sex. In men, only S_I ($r = -0.29$, $P < 0.05$) remained independently correlated with GGT in multiple regression analysis. In women, IAF area ($r = 0.29$, $P < 0.01$) and WHR ($r = 0.29$, $P < 0.01$) were independently associated with GGT, but S_I was not.

CONCLUSIONS — In nondiabetic men GGT but not AST or ALT levels, are inversely related to insulin sensitivity independent of IAF area. However in women, GGT is related to measures of central body fat rather than to insulin sensitivity.

Diabetes Care 30:2673–2678, 2007

R elatively recently, the liver has been recognized as a major target of injury in patients with insulin resistance or the metabolic syndrome. Non-alcoholic fatty liver disease (NAFLD) is characterized by accumulation of hepatic fat in the absence of significant alcohol intake. In a proportion of patients, NAFLD may progress to nonalcoholic steatohepatitis (NASH), characterized by the presence of hepatic inflammation and hepatocellular damage, which may eventually progress to cirrhosis (1). The prevalence of NAFLD is about 20% and that of NASH is 2–3% in adults (2,3).

NAFLD is strongly associated with insulin resistance, dyslipidemia, obesity, and hypertension (4) and is probably the most common cause of abnormal liver function tests in diabetes (5). In nondiabetic subjects, elevated plasma liver enzyme levels are risk factors for the development of type 2 diabetes; however, γ-glutamyl transferase (GGT) may be a stronger predictor than aspartate transaminase (AST) or alanine transaminase (ALT) (6–8). Although GGT has been widely used as a marker of alcohol consumption, it has recently been found to be associated with an increased risk of development of type 2 diabetes independent of alcohol intake (9) as well as an increased risk of hypertension and cardiovascular mortality (10,11).

Because diabetes, dyslipidemia, hypertension, cardiovascular disease, and NAFLD have all been shown to be associated with central adiposity and insulin resistance (12), we hypothesized that differences in liver enzyme levels in healthy subjects are related in part to differences in fat distribution and insulin sensitivity. To test this hypothesis, we analyzed the relationship between liver enzymes, insulin sensitivity, and body fat distribution in a large cohort of apparently healthy normal subjects.

RESEARCH DESIGN AND METHODS — The data presented are baseline measurements from 177 subjects (75 men and 102 women) from a study population of 234 subjects in whom data on insulin sensitivity, body fat distribution, and plasma liver enzyme concentrations were available. There were no significant differences in subject characteristics between all 234 subjects and the 177 who form the basis of the current analysis. The subjects, who had been recruited by advertisement to participate in a study of the effect of egg consumption on plasma lipids in people with various degrees of insulin sensitivity, were aged 31–75 years and were apparently healthy, had no history of diabetes, dyslipidemia, or uncontrolled hypertension, and had no known liver disease (13). Specific testing

From the [1]Department of Medicine, VA Puget Sound Health Care System, and University of Washington, Seattle, Washington; the [2]Department of Obstetrics and Gynecology, University of Washington, Seattle, Washington; the [3]Department of Pathology and Laboratory Medicine, VA Puget Sound Health Care System, and University of Washington, Seattle, Washington; and [4]Harborview Medical Center, University of Washington, Seattle, Washington.

Address correspondence and reprint requests to Steven E. Kahn, MB, ChB, VA Puget Sound Health Care System (151), 1660 S. Columbian Way, Seattle, WA 98108. E-mail: skahn@u.washington.edu.

Received for publication 18 August 2006 and accepted in revised form 29 June 2007.

Published ahead of print at http://care.diabetesjournals.org on 31 July 2007. DOI: 10.2337/dc06-1758.

T.M.W., K.M.U., and J.T. contributed equally to this work.

Abbreviations: ALT, alanine aminotransferase; AST, aspartate aminotransferase; FSIGT, frequently sampled intravenous glucose tolerance test; GGT, γ-glutamyl transferase; IAF, intra-abdominal fat; IQR, interquartile range; LIR, lean insulin resistant; LIS, lean insulin sensitive; NAFLD, nonalcoholic fatty liver disease; NASH, nonalcoholic steatohepatitis; OIR, obese insulin resistant; SCF, subcutaneous fat; S_I, insulin sensitivity index; WHR, waist-to-hip ratio.

A table elsewhere in this issue shows conventional and Système International (SI) units and conversion factors for many substances.

for liver disease was not performed at the time of the study. Subjects with fasting plasma glucose ≥6.4 mmol/l (≥115 mg/dl), biochemical evidence of renal disease, uncontrolled thyroid disease, coronary or other vascular disease, or anemia were excluded, but formal oral glucose tolerance tests were not performed. The subjects were predominantly Caucasian: Caucasian ($n = 161$), Asian ($n = 5$), African American ($n = 7$), Native American ($n = 2$), and Hispanic ($n = 2$). The study was approved by the Human Subjects Review Committee of the University of Washington, and subjects provided written informed consent.

Subjects were divided a priori into three groups on the basis of BMI and insulin sensitivity index (S_I) to analyze the relationship between liver enzyme concentrations, obesity, and insulin sensitivity. These three groups were lean insulin sensitive (LIS) (BMI <27.5 kg/m² and S_I ≥7.0 ×10⁻⁵ min/[pmol/l]), lean insulin resistant (LIR) (BMI <27.5 kg/m² and S_I <7.0 ×10⁻⁵ min/[pmol/l]), and obese insulin resistant (OIR) (BMI ≥27.5 kg/m² and S_I <7.0 ×10⁻⁵ min/[pmol/l]). The cutoff of 27.5 kg/m² was based on the criteria in place before the more recent definition of the criteria for overweight and obesity. The cutoff of 7.0 ×10⁻⁵ min/(pmol/l) for S_I represents the highest value for this parameter among a group of apparently healthy obese subjects studied in Seattle (14). Obese insulin-sensitive subjects were excluded from this analysis because of their small number ($n = 8$).

Measures of anthropometry and body fat distribution
The averages of two weight and height measurements were used to calculate BMI as weight in kilograms divided by the square of height in meters. Waist and hip circumferences were calculated as the average of two measurements. Waist circumference was measured at the smallest circumference of the waist, and hip circumference was measured at the widest level of the buttocks, using a previously described protocol (*National Health and Nutrition Examination Survey III Anthropometric Measurements*. Videotape, National Center for Health Statistics).

A computed tomography scan of the abdomen was performed at the level of the umbilicus to quantify subcutaneous fat (SCF) area and intra-abdominal fat (IAF) area as described previously (15). Fat area was computed as the area with an attenuation range of −250 to −50

Hounsfield units. IAF and SCF areas were quantified by delineating the border of the peritoneal cavity. These measurements were performed by a single observer using standard GE 8800 computer software. The variability of these measures made by a single observer was 1.5% (15).

Fasting plasma and insulin sensitivity measurements
Subjects underwent a tolbutamide-modified, frequently sampled intravenous glucose tolerance test (FSIGT) to quantify insulin sensitivity as the S_I using Bergman's minimal model of glucose kinetics (16). Three basal blood samples were drawn at 15, 5, and 1 min before the intravenous administration of glucose at time 0. Glucose (11.4 g/m² body surface area) was infused over 1 min, and tolbutamide (125 mg/m² body surface area) was injected intravenously over 30 s at time 20 min. Blood samples were taken at 32 time points over 240 min after commencement of the glucose injection. Fasting glucose and insulin concentrations were calculated as the average of the three basal samples. Liver function tests were performed on the 3-min sample obtained during the FSIGT.

Alcohol intake
Alcohol intake was assessed using a standardized questionnaire and quantified as self-reported number of drinks per week.

Assays
Glucose was measured in duplicate using the glucose oxidase method. Immunoreactive insulin was measured in duplicate by radioimmunoassay using a modification of the double antibody technique. Samples for liver enzymes were assayed between 5 and 7 years after sampling. GGT was measured using an enzymatic colorimetric method (Modular P; Roche Diagnostics, Indianapolis, IN). AST and ALT were measured using the standardized kinetic method (Modular P). Samples were stored at −70°C before assay.

Calculations and statistics
Statistical analyses were performed using SPSS 12.0 (SPSS, Chicago, IL). For regression analysis, dependent variables were logarithmically transformed where appropriate to satisfy the statistical assumptions of linear regression. Multiple regression analysis was used to determine whether associations between the dependent (liver transaminase levels) and independent variables of interest remained

significant after adjustments for other potentially confounding independent variables. Model 1 contained S_I, IAF area, BMI, and age for each sex. Model 2 contained S_I, WHR, BMI, and age for each sex. Comparisons between groups were assessed by ANOVA with Tukey post hoc analysis, Kruskal-Wallis test, t test, or Mann-Whitney U test as appropriate. Data are presented as means ± SD unless specified. Non-normally distributed data with kurtosis were log transformed before parametric statistical tests were applied. $P < 0.05$ was considered significant.

RESULTS

Demographic, anthropometric, and metabolic characteristics
Characteristics for all subjects are shown in Table 1 ($n = 177$) and subdivided into LIS ($n = 53$), LIR ($n = 60$), and OIR ($n = 56$) subjects and into men ($n = 75$) and women ($n = 102$). In this apparently healthy group of nondiabetic subjects, 66% were insulin resistant (defined as S_I <7.0 ×10⁻⁵ min/[pmol/l]) and 32% were obese (defined as BMI >27.5 kg/m²). In accordance with the a priori classification, the BMI of the obese group was significantly higher than that of both of the lean groups ($P < 0.0001$) (Table 1). S_I values were 2.3- and 2.8-fold higher in the LIS group than in the LIR and OIR groups, respectively ($P ≤ 0.0001$). The mean age of the LIS subjects was slightly lower than that of the insulin-resistant subjects.

LIR subjects were more centrally obese than LIS subjects, as evidenced by higher WHR ($P = 0.009$) and IAF area ($P < 0.0001$), despite a similar BMI in the two groups. LIR subjects were significantly less centrally obese (WHR $P = 0.0005$; IAF area $P < 0.0001$) and more insulin sensitive ($P = 0.0001$) than OIR subjects.

As listed in Table 1, fasting glycemia increased with increasing obesity and insulin resistance (LIS vs. LIR and LIR vs. OIR, $P < 0.03$; LIS vs. OIR, $P < 0.0001$), and a similar pattern was seen for triglycerides (LIS vs. LIR $P < 0.006$; LIR vs. OIR, $P < 0.05$; LIS vs. OIR, $P < 0.0001$). Systolic blood pressure was significantly higher in OIR subjects than in LIR and LIS subjects. There was no significant difference in alcohol intake, reported as median number of drinks per week (interquartile range [IQR]) between groups.

Table 1—*Demographics and clinical variables in all subjects, LIS, LIR, OIR, men, and women*

	All	LIS	LIR	OIR	Men	Women
n	177	53	60	56	75	102
Age (years)	52.3 ± 9.9	49.6 ± 8.0	53.8 ± 11.4*	53.2 ±9.6	52.6 ± 10.2	52.0 ± 9.8
Sex (male/female)	75/102	18/35	27/33	25/31	—	—
BMI (kg/m²)	26.4 ± 4.3	23.4 ± 2.3	24.3 ± 1.8	31.0 ± 3.4*†	26.8 ± 3.5	26.2 ± 4.8
Waist circumference (cm)	87.2 ± 13.2	77.9 ± 8.5	83.7 ± 9.2*	99.3 ± 11.1*†	94.9 ± 10.6‡	81.9 ± 12.2
WHR	0.84 ± 0.09	0.80 ± 0.08	0.83 ± 0.09*	0.89 ± 0.08*†	0.92 ± 0.06‡	0.78 ± 0.06
SCF area (cm²)	195.8 (135.6)	125.7 (102.7)	179.6 (114.1)*	299.1 (164.1)*†	166.9 (117.3)§	225.9 (162.9)
IAF area (cm²)	88.4 (84.9)	43.3 (36.4)	76.8 (69.3)*	140.6 (57.9)*†	113.8 (86.9)‡	71.9 (79.1)
Systolic blood pressure (mmHg)	118 ± 12	114 ± 10	117 ± 10	123 ± 12*†	120 ± 11¶	117 ± 12
S_I (×10^{-5} min^{-1}/[pmol/l])	5.65 (4.61)	9.35 (3.94)	5.04 (2.54)*	3.59 (2.10)*†	4.93 (4.88)	6.03 (4.18)
Fasting plasma glucose (mmol/l)	5.4 ± 0.4	5.3 ± 0.4	5.4 ± 0.4*	5.6 ± 0.5*†	5.6 ± 0.4‡	5.3 ± 0.4
Triglycerides (mmol/l)	1.4 (0.79)	0.99 (0.72)	1.4 (0.5)*	1.6 (0.75)*†	1.4 (0.82)	1.3 (0.75)
HDL cholesterol (mmol/l)	1.4 ± 0.4	1.5 ± 0.4	1.3 ± 0.4*	1.2 ± 0.4*	1.2 ± 0.3‡	1.5 ± 0.4
Alcohol intake (drinks/week)	1.0 (3.0)	1.0 (2.0)	1.0 (4.0)	1.5 (4.0)	2.0 (7.0)#	1.0 (2.0)

Data are means ± SD or median (IQR). Normal ranges: GGT <51 IU/l, ALT <40 IU/l, and AST <38 IU/l. LIS vs. LIR vs. OIR: ANOVA *P < 0.05 vs. LIS; †P < 0.05 vs. LIR (eight OIR subjects were excluded from this analysis because of the small number). Men vs. women: t test ‡P < 0.0001, §P < 0.005, ¶P < 0.05; Mann Whitney U test #P < 0.05.

Effect of sex on liver enzymes

There was no sex-based difference in age or BMI (Table 1). As expected, men had higher WHR ($P < 0.0001$) and IAF area ($P < 0.001$) than women, whereas women had more SCF area ($P < 0.005$) than men (Table 1). Fasting glucose was higher in men ($P < 0.001$), but S_I did not differ between men and women ($P = 0.1$) (Table 1). All liver transferase levels, reported as median (IQR) were significantly higher in men compared with women: GGT 17 (14) vs. 10 (6) IU/l, ALT 16 (10) vs. 11 (6) IU/l, and AST 21 (7) vs. 17.5 (5) IU/l ($P < 0.0001$ for each).

Effect of obesity and insulin sensitivity on liver enzymes

Because transaminase levels were significantly higher in men than in women, the effect of obesity and insulin sensitivity on transaminase levels was analyzed separately for each sex. In men, GGT levels were significantly higher in insulin-resistant subjects (LIR and OIR) compared with LIS subjects (Fig. 1A). GGT levels did not differ between LIR and OIR subjects ($P = 0.6$). In women, GGT levels were also significantly higher in the OIR group than in the LIS group and tended to be higher in the LIR than in the LIS group ($P = 0.09$) (Fig. 1A). ALT and AST levels did not differ significantly among the LIS, LIR, and OIR groups in either men or women (Figs. 1B and C).

Relationship between liver enzymes, body anthropometrics, insulin sensitivity, and sex

GGT was negatively associated with S_I and positively associated with IAF area, SCF area, WHR, and BMI (Table 2) after adjustment for age and sex. Waist circumference and alcohol consumption were not associated with GGT levels. ALT and AST were not associated with any of the variables and were thus not included in the multiple regression models.

Multiple linear regression analyses stratified by sex were performed with GGT as the dependent variable. In men, only S_I remained significantly associated with GGT levels independent of IAF area and WHR (models 1 and 2 in Table 3), age, and BMI. In contrast, in women, IAF area and WHR (models 1 and 2 in table 3) were significantly associated with GGT levels, but S_I was not.

CONCLUSIONS — We examined the relationship between body fat distribution, insulin sensitivity, and liver enzymes in a cohort of 177 nondiabetic subjects of whom >97% had GGT levels within the normal range. It is well recognized that body fat distribution and insulin sensitivity are associated (17,18), and in this cohort of apparently healthy individuals, we found that GGT was negatively associated with insulin sensitivity in men, whereas in women GGT was associated with central obesity. In common with other studies (19), we found that men had higher GGT levels and increased central adiposity than women, and these differences may explain the different results in men and women. ALT and AST were not associated with insulin sensitivity or body fat measures in our study.

The association between elevated liver transaminase levels and insulin resistance in the context of NAFLD is well established (20). In the Tübingen Family Study, GGT was associated with insulin sensitivity and glucose tolerance in both men and women. In addition, in this same study GGT was positively correlated with hepatic lipid content measured by magnetic resonance spectroscopy (21). ALT has previously been shown to be inversely related to insulin sensitivity, determined by the euglycemic clamp, and it has also been shown to have this same relationship with endothelial function in subjects with type 2 diabetes (22). Recently, the role of liver transaminases in predicting the development of type 2 diabetes has been examined in two large studies. In a study of 906 subjects, Hanley et al. (6) found that ALT and, to a lesser extent, AST were associated with the development of diabetes; however, they did not examine whether GGT predicted the development of hyperglycemia. In another study of 5,974 nondiabetic subjects, Sattar et al. (23) found that ALT levels within the normal range predicted incident diabetes. In the Mexico City Diabetes Study, GGT was shown to be an independent risk factor for the development of impaired glucose tolerance and diabetes (24), whereas Vozarova et al. (25) found that only ALT predicted progression to diabetes in Pima Indians.

Although GGT has been widely used as a marker of alcohol consumption, Lee et al. (9) have shown that GGT levels are also associated with an increased risk of development of type 2 diabetes independent of alcohol intake. In another study of >4,000 subjects, although an association

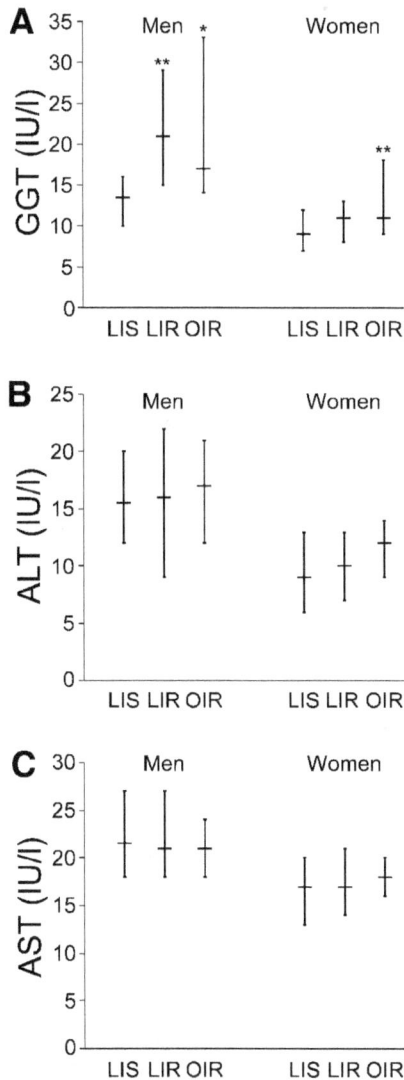

Figure 1—GGT (A), ALT (B), and AST (C) levels in men (left) (LIS, n = 18; LIR, n = 27; and OIR, n = 25) and women (right) (LIS, n = 35; LIR, n = 33; and OIR, n = 31). Data are median (IQR). *P < 0.05 vs. LIS; **P < 0.01 vs. LIS.

Table 2—Linear regression analyses for liver transferases adjusted for age and sex

	GGT		ALT		AST	
	r	P	r	P	r	P
S_I	−0.26	<0.0001	−0.07	0.326	0.02	0.754
IAF area	0.22	0.003	0.12	0.127	0.02	0.844
WHR	0.25	0.001	0.15	0.054	0.08	0.292
BMI	0.17	0.027	0.14	0.066	0.02	0.766
SCF area	0.16	0.036	0.10	0.192	0.01	0.916
Waist circumference	0.04	0.569	0.07	0.403	0.05	0.501
Alcohol consumption	0.09	0.220	−0.03	0.688	-0.12	0.118

Data in bold are significant.

ity we found here. The basis of the proposed link between GGT and oxidative stress is that glutathione is a major intracellular defense against free radicals and peroxides. However, as intact glutathione cannot be taken up by cells, the intracellular synthesis of glutathione depends on the metabolism of extracellular glutathione by GGT to release cysteine, which is then transported into the cell and used as a substrate for the de novo intracellular synthesis of glutathione (28). In vitro studies have demonstrated a protective effect of GGT against oxidative stress and cell death (29). Thus, increased GGT expression may initially represent an adaptive protective response to persistent oxidative stress. This would be consistent with the recent in vivo finding of a positive association between GGT and C-reactive protein levels (30). GGT levels have also been shown to predict future levels of inflammatory markers including C-reactive protein, fibrinogen, and F2-isoprostanes (a biomarker of lipid peroxidation) (10).

Yki-Jarvinen's group has shown that fatty liver is associated with fasting insulin as a surrogate measure of insulin sensitivity independently of IAF and SCF areas. In their study ALT was more strongly correlated with liver fat than GGT (31). We found that in men, GGT but not ALT or AST was associated with insulin sensitivity independently of body fat measures. As we quantified insulin sensitivity directly, we believe that our data raise the possibility that GGT may be a more sensitive marker of the liver's response to insulin sensitivity than ALT and AST. The finding that, even across the normal range, GGT levels are related to insulin sensitivity is of clinical relevance in the light of the emerging possible therapeutic role of the peroxisome proliferator–activated receptor-γ agonists in the treatment of NASH. Promrat et al. (32)

demonstrated an improvement in transaminases and amelioration of insulin resistance in subjects with NASH after 48 weeks of treatment with pioglitazone. Lifestyle changes with weight loss and increased exercise have also been shown to improve liver enzymes and histological findings in subjects with NAFLD (4). Our data raise the possibility that increasing GGT levels (even within the normal range) in the context of insulin resistance may be an indication for lifestyle changes with the aim of weight loss or treatment with peroxisome proliferator–activated receptor-γ agonists.

The advantages of our analysis are that we examined a large number of subjects in whom insulin sensitivity had been determined by the FSIGT, and all of whom had fat distribution measured using computed tomography scans. However, the lack of any direct measure of hepatic fat is a drawback. Another potential limitation is that because alcohol intake was assessed by self-reported questionnaire, consumption may have been underestimated. Although liver en-

Table 3—Multiple regression models with GGT as the dependent variable

	Men		Women	
	Partial		Partial	
	r	P	r	P
Model 1				
S_I	−0.29	0.014	−0.08	0.449
IAF area	−0.15	0.206	0.29	0.004
BMI	0.15	0.210	−0.15	0.137
Age	0.01	0.921	−0.01	0.955
Model 2				
S_I	−0.32	0.010	−0.15	0.162
WHR	0.06	0.647	0.29	0.005
BMI	−0.06	0.660	−0.13	0.198
Age	−0.02	0.896	0.02	0.821

Data in bold are significant.

between the incidence of diabetes and ALT levels was found, this was most strongly observed in the abnormal range of ALT and was weaker than the association with GGT levels (26). Others have found a strong, independent, and graded association between GGT levels and type 2 diabetes but not ALT or AST levels (7,8,27). However, to our knowledge, no previous study has examined the relationship between GGT, IAF area, and insulin sensitivity in nondiabetic subjects.

The recent emergence of the potential protective role of GGT against oxidative stress may explain the inverse association between GGT levels and insulin sensitiv-

zyme measurements were made on a sample taken just after glucose administration, we doubt this affected our findings, as nutrient intake has been shown not to affect liver enzyme levels (33). The transferase levels were uniformly lower than would be expected in a normal population, which may be due to the fact that transaminase levels tend to decrease slightly (about 8%) with time, even when stored at −80°C (34,35). However, all samples were handled in the same manner. Although the absolute levels may have been affected, all samples should have been affected to the same degree, and therefore it is likely that although the absolute values may be lower, relative differences would have been robust and maintained.

In summary, GGT but not ALT or AST levels are inversely related to insulin sensitivity independently of central obesity in nondiabetic men. In contrast, in women GGT levels were positively associated with IAF area and WHR but were not associated with insulin sensitivity. If GGT is a marker of hepatic fat accumulation, this sex difference suggests that body fat distribution may be a more important player in the development of hepatic steatosis in women than in men. This finding suggests that GGT is a more sensitive marker of insulin resistance, at least in men, but whether this liver enzyme will prove useful to guide treatment decisions related to insulin resistance awaits further research.

Acknowledgments— This work was supported by the Medical Research Service of the Veterans Affairs; the American Egg Board; National Institutes of Health Grants DK-02654, DK-17047, DK-35747, DK-35816, HL-30086, HL-07028, RR-37, and RR-16066; the U.S. Department of Agriculture; the McMillen Family Trust; and an American Diabetes Association Distinguished Clinical Scientist Award to S.E.K.

We thank the subjects, Diane Collins, and the nursing staff of the General Clinical Research Center at University of Washington.

References
1. Browning JD, Horton JD: Molecular mediators of hepatic steatosis and liver injury. *J Clin Invest* 114:147–152, 2004
2. Hilden M, Christoffersen P, Juhl E, Dalgaard JB: Liver histology in a 'normal' population—examinations of 503 consecutive fatal traffic casualties. *Scand J Gastroenterol* 12:593–597, 1977
3. Browning JD, Szczepaniak LS, Dobbins R, Nuremberg P, Horton JD, Cohen JC, Grundy SM, Hobbs HH: Prevalence of hepatic steatosis in an urban population in the United States: impact of ethnicity. *Hepatology* 40:1387–1395, 2004
4. Utzschneider KM, Kahn SE: Review: The role of insulin resistance in nonalcoholic fatty liver disease. *J Clin Endocrinol Metab* 91:4753–4761, 2006
5. Daniel S, Ben-Menachem T, Vasudevan G, Ma CK, Blumenkehl M: Prospective evaluation of unexplained chronic liver transaminase abnormalities in asymptomatic and symptomatic patients. *Am J Gastroenterol* 94:3010–3014, 1999
6. Hanley AJ, Williams K, Festa A, Wagenknecht LE, D'Agostino RB Jr, Kempf J, Zinman B, Haffner SM: Elevations in markers of liver injury and risk of type 2 diabetes: the Insulin Resistance Atherosclerosis Study. *Diabetes* 53:2623–2632, 2004
7. Perry IJ, Wannamethee SG, Shaper AG: Prospective study of serum γ-glutamyltransferase and risk of NIDDM. *Diabetes Care* 21:732–737, 1998
8. Nakanishi N, Nishina K, Li W, Sato M, Suzuki K, Tatara K: Serum γ-glutamyltransferase and development of impaired fasting glucose or type 2 diabetes in middle-aged Japanese men. *J Intern Med* 254:287–295, 2003
9. Lee DH, Silventoinen K, Jacobs DR Jr, Jousilahti P, Tuomileto J: γ-Glutamyltransferase, obesity, and the risk of type 2 diabetes: observational cohort study among 20,158 middle-aged men and women. *J Clin Endocrinol Metab* 89:5410–5414, 2004
10. Lee DH, Jacobs DR Jr, Gross M, Kiefe CI, Roseman J, Lewis CE, Steffes M: γ-Glutamyltransferase is a predictor of incident diabetes and hypertension: the Coronary Artery Risk Development in Young Adults (CARDIA) Study. *Clin Chem* 49:1358–1366, 2003
11. Wannamethee G, Ebrahim S, Shaper AG: γ-Glutamyltransferase: determinants and association with mortality from ischemic heart disease and all causes. *Am J Epidemiol* 142:699–708, 1995
12. Kissebah AH: Intra-abdominal fat: is it a major factor in developing diabetes and coronary artery disease? *Diabetes Res Clin Pract* 30:25–30, 1996
13. Knopp RH, Retzlaff B, Fish B, Walden C, Wallick S, Anderson M, Aikawa K, Kahn SE: Effects of insulin resistance and obesity on lipoproteins and sensitivity to egg feeding. *Arterioscler Thromb Vasc Biol* 23:1437–1443, 2003
14. Kahn SE, Prigeon RL, McCulloch DK, Boyko EJ, Bergman RN, Schwartz MW, Neifing JL, Ward WK, Beard JC, Palmer JP, Porte D Jr: Quantification of the relationship between insulin sensitivity and β-cell function in human subjects: evidence for a hyperbolic function. *Diabetes* 42:1663–1672, 1993
15. Shuman WP, Morris LL, Leonetti DL, Wahl PW, Moceri VM, Moss AA, Fujimoto WY: Abnormal body fat distribution detected by computed tomography in diabetic men. *Invest Radiol* 21:483–487, 1986
16. Bergman R, Ider Y, Bowden C, Cobelli C: Quantitative estimation of insulin sensitivity. *Am J Physiol* 236:E667–E677, 1979
17. Cnop M, Landchild MJ, Vidal J, Havel PJ, Knowles NG, Carr DR, Wang F, Hull RL, Boyko EJ, Retzlaff BM, Walden CE, Knopp RH, Kahn SE: The concurrent accumulation of intra-abdominal and subcutaneous fat explains the association between insulin resistance and plasma leptin concentrations : distinct metabolic effects of two fat compartments. *Diabetes* 51:1005–1015, 2002
18. Despres JP, Lemieux I: Abdominal obesity and metabolic syndrome. *Nature* 444:881–887, 2006
19. Nilssen O, Forde OH, Brenn T: The Tromso Study: distribution and population determinants of γ-glutamyltransferase. *Am J Epidemiol* 132:318–326, 1990
20. Machado M, Cortez-Pinto H: Non-alcoholic fatty liver disease and insulin resistance. *Eur J Gastroenterol Hepatol* 17:823–826, 2005
21. Thamer C, Tschritter O, Haap M, Shirkavand F, Machann J, Fritsche A, Schick F, Haring H, Stumvoll M: Elevated serum GGT concentrations predict reduced insulin sensitivity and increased intrahepatic lipids. *Horm Metab Res* 37:246–251, 2005
22. Schindhelm RK, Diamant M, Bakker SJ, van Dijk RA, Scheffer PG, Teerlink T, Kostense PJ, Heine RJ: Liver alanine aminotransferase, insulin resistance and endothelial dysfunction in normotriglyceridaemic subjects with type 2 diabetes mellitus. *Eur J Clin Invest* 35:369–374, 2005
23. Sattar N, Scherbakova O, Ford I, O'Reilly DS, Stanley A, Forrest E, Macfarlane PW, Packard CJ, Cobbe SM, Shepherd J: Elevated alanine aminotransferase predicts new-onset type 2 diabetes independently of classical risk factors, metabolic syndrome, and C-reactive protein in the West of Scotland Coronary Prevention Study. *Diabetes* 53:2855–2860, 2004
24. Nannipieri M, Gonzales C, Baldi S, Posadas R, Williams K, Haffner SM, Stern MP, Ferrannini E: Liver enzymes, the metabolic syndrome, and incident diabetes: the Mexico City Diabetes Study. *Diabetes Care* 28:1757–1762, 2005
25. Vozarova B, Stefan N, Lindsay RS, Saremi A, Pratley RE, Bogardus C, Tataranni PA: High alanine aminotransferase is associated with decreased hepatic insulin sensitivity and predicts the development of type 2 diabetes. *Diabetes* 51:1889–1895, 2002

26. Lee DH, Ha MH, Kim JH, Christiani DC, Gross MD, Steffes M, Blomhoff R, Jacobs DR Jr: γ-Glutamyltransferase and diabetes—a 4 year follow-up study. *Diabetologia* 46:359–364, 2003

27. Andre P, Balkau B, Born C, Royer B, Wilpart E, Charles MA, Eschwege E: Hepatic markers and development of type 2 diabetes in middle aged men and women: a three-year follow-up study: the D.E.S.I.R. Study (Data from an Epidemiological Study on the Insulin Resistance Syndrome). *Diabetes Metab* 31:542–550, 2005

28. Pastore A, Federici G, Bertini E, Piemonte F: Analysis of glutathione: implication in redox and detoxification. *Clin Chim Acta* 333:19–39, 2003

29. Karp DR, Shimooku K, Lipsky PE: Expression of γ-glutamyl transpeptidase protects Ramos B cells from oxidation-induced cell death. *J Biol Chem* 276:3798–3804, 2001

30. Lee DH, Jacobs DR Jr: Association between serum γ-glutamyltransferase and C-reactive protein. *Atherosclerosis* 178:327–330, 2005

31. Westerbacka J, Corner A, Tiikkainen M, Tamminen M, Vehkavaara S, Hakkinen AM, Fredriksson J, Yki-Jarvinen H: Women and men have similar amounts of liver and intra-abdominal fat, despite more subcutaneous fat in women: implications for sex differences in markers of cardiovascular risk. *Diabetologia* 47:1360–1369, 2004

32. Promrat K, Lutchman G, Uwaifo GI, Freedman RJ, Soza A, Heller T, Doo E, Ghany M, Premkumar A, Park Y, Liang TJ, Yanovski JA, Kleiner DE, Hoofnagle JH: A pilot study of pioglitazone treatment for nonalcoholic steatohepatitis. *Hepatology* 39:188–196, 2004

33. Siest G, Schiele F, Galteau MM, Panek E, Steinmetz J, Fagnani F, Gueguen R: Aspartate aminotransferase and alanine aminotransferase activities in plasma: statistical distributions, individual variations, and reference values. *Clin Chem* 21:1077–1087, 1975

34. Williams KM, Williams AE, Kline LM, Dodd RY: Stability of serum alanine aminotransferase activity. *Transfusion* 27:431–433, 1987

35. Clark JM, Brancati FL, Diehl AM: The prevalence and etiology of elevated aminotransferase levels in the United States. *Am J Gastroenterol* 98:960–967, 2003

FGFR4 Prevents Hyperlipidemia and Insulin Resistance but Underlies High-Fat Diet–Induced Fatty Liver

Xinqiang Huang, Chaofeng Yang, Yongde Luo, Chengliu Jin, Fen Wang, and Wallace L. McKeehan

OBJECTIVE—Fibroblast growth factor (FGF) family signaling largely controls cellular homeostasis through short-range intercell paracrine communication. Recently FGF15/19, 21, and 23 have been implicated in endocrine control of metabolic homeostasis. The identity and location of the FGF receptor isotypes that mediate these effects are unclear. The objective was to determine the role of FGFR4, an isotype that has been proposed to mediate an ileal FGF15/19 to hepatocyte FGFR4 axis in cholesterol homeostasis, in metabolic homeostasis in vivo.

RESEARCH DESIGN AND METHODS—FGFR4$^{-/-}$ mice—mice overexpressing constitutively active hepatic FGFR4—and FGFR4$^{-/-}$ with constitutively active hepatic FGFR4 restored in the liver were subjected to a normal and a chronic high-fat diet sufficient to result in obesity. Systemic and liver-specific metabolic phenotypes were then characterized.

RESULTS—FGFR4-deficient mice on a normal diet exhibited features of metabolic syndrome that include increased mass of white adipose tissue, hyperlipidemia, glucose intolerance, and insulin resistance, in addition to hypercholesterolemia. Surprisingly, the FGFR4 deficiency alleviated high-fat diet–induced fatty liver in obese mice, which is also a correlate of metabolic syndrome. Restoration of FGFR4, specifically in hepatocytes of FGFR4-deficient mice, decreased plasma lipid levels and restored the high-fat diet–induced fatty liver but failed to restore glucose tolerance and sensitivity to insulin.

CONCLUSIONS—FGFR4 plays essential roles in systemic lipid and glucose homeostasis. FGFR4 activity in hepatocytes that normally serves to prevent systemic hyperlipidemia paradoxically underlies the fatty liver disease associated with chronic high-fat intake and obesity. *Diabetes* 56:2501–2510, 2007

Metabolic syndrome (also known as insulin resistance syndrome or syndrome X) is a multicomponent disorder characterized by central body obesity, dyslipidemia, insulin resistance, glucose intolerance, and hypertension, which are risk factors for numerous diseases including type 2 diabetes, cardiovascular diseases, neurodegenerative diseases, liver disease, and cancer (1,2). The hepatic manifestation of the metabolic syndrome is nonalcoholic fatty liver disease (NAFLD), which is evident from triglyceride accumulation in macroscopic fat droplets (3–5). NAFLD is the most common liver disease in developed countries. NAFLD may be an indicator of metabolic syndrome and risk for its associated diseases equal to body mass and shape, insulin resistance, blood triglycerides, and HDL/LDL cholesterol (6,7). The mechanisms underlying NAFLD and its relationship to the other components of metabolic syndrome are largely unknown.

The fibroblast growth factor (FGF) signaling system is a ubiquitous microenvironmental regulator of cell-to-cell communication in development and adult homeostasis (8–12). Recent developments indicate that specific members of the family may regulate metabolic homeostasis by endocrine mechanisms where FGF originates in one tissue and acts distally on FGFR in another. Administration of FGF19 (13,14) and FGF21 (15) or their expression in the liver of transgenic animals impacts metabolic rate and multiple parameters associated with metabolic syndrome. Circulating FGF23 that resides in the same FGF subgroup as FGF15/19 and FGF21 based on sequence homology and affinity for heparan sulfate (16) regulates vitamin D and phosphate homeostasis (17,18). The regulation of expression and the tissue and cellular origin of FGF15/19, FGF21, and FGF23, as well as the isotype and location of the FGFR isotype underlying the metabolic effects of the three factors, is not well resolved.

An ileal origin of FGF15/19 under control of the bile acid–activated farnesoid X receptor (FXR) (NR1H4) that activates hepatocyte FGFR4 has been proposed to regulate cholesterol–to–bile acid metabolism (19). Hepatocyte FGFR4 regulates cholesterol–to–bile acid synthesis in the liver by transcriptional downregulation of cholesterol 7α-hydroxylase (CYP7A1), the rate-limiting enzyme for classical bile acid synthesis (20,21). A gut-to-liver FGF15/19-to-FGFR4 axis explains why only intestinal, compared with portal or intravenous, administration of bile acids represses hepatic *cyp7a1* expression and bile acid synthesis (19). In contrast to FGF15/19, which is not expressed in liver (19), low-level FGF21 expression that increases on liver perturbation is relatively restricted to hepatocytes (22). When expressed in the hepatocyte, FGF21 improved glucose clearance and insulin sensitivity similar to systemic treatment of animals with FGF21 (15). We have shown that targeted expression of FGF21 in hepatocytes delays the appearance of diethyluitrosamine-induced liver adenoma. However, it has no effect on hepatocellular carcinoma incidence and burden. Although hepatocytes are a candidate for the autocrine action of FGF21, the most dramatic effects are on adipose tissue where neither FGF21 nor FGFR4 are significantly expressed (15,23). In adipocytes in vitro, FGF21 synergizes with the peroxisome proliferator–activated receptor (PPAR)γ ligand and an-

From the Center for Cancer and Stem Cell Biology, Institute of Biosciences and Technology, Texas A&M Health Science Center, Houston, Texas.

Address correspondence and reprint requests to Wallace L. McKeehan, PhD, Center for Cancer and Stem Cell Biology, Institute of Biosciences and Technology, Texas A&M Health Science Center, 2121 W. Holcombe Blvd., Houston, TX 77030. E-mail: wmckeehan@ibt.tamhsc.edu.

Received for publication 14 May 2007 and accepted in revised form 18 July 2007.

Published ahead of print at http://diabetes.diabetesjournals.org on 30 July 2007. DOI: 10.2337/db07-0648.

Additional information for this article can be found in an online appendix at http://dx.doi.org/10.2337/db07-0648.

FGF, fibroblast growth factor; FXR, farnesoid X receptor; G6Pase, glucose-6-phosphatase; NAFLD, nonalcoholic fatty liver disease; PPAR, peroxisome proliferator–activated receptor; SCD, stearoyl-CoA desaturase.

tidiabetes agent rogsiglitazone to increase insulin-independent glucose uptake (23).

Because of the strong evidence that hepatocyte FGFR4 controls cholesterol–to–bile acid metabolism, which occurs primarily in the liver, it is a strong candidate for the mediator either directly or indirectly of some of the effects of FGF15/19 on general metabolic homeostasis. In this report, we evaluated the consequences of a general ablation of FGFR4 and hepatocyte-specific FGFR4 restoration on features associated with metabolic syndrome. We show that FGFR4 plays a general role in the maintenance of both lipid and glucose metabolism under normal dietary conditions in addition to its established role in cholesterol metabolism. Hepatocyte FGFR4 appears to exert a primary control on lipid metabolism. Effects on glucose metabolism could not be explained by activity of hepatocyte FGFR4 alone, suggesting an additional role of FGFR4 at other organ sites. Ironically, hepatocyte FGFR4, which normally protects against hyperlipidemia and hypercholesterolemia, underlies the fatty liver induced by high-fat intake and obesity.

RESEARCH DESIGN AND METHODS

Animals and diets. Mice lacking FGFR4 (FGFR4$^{-/-}$) and expressing constitutively activated human FGFR4 (Alb-caFGFR4), specifically in hepatocytes, have been previously described (20,21). The FGFR4$^{-/-}$ mice were a mixed 129Sv-C57BL/6 background, and Alb-caFGFR4 mice were an FVB background. FGFR4$^{-/-}$ and wild-type mice were produced from an FGFR4$^{+/-}$ mating. Alb-caFGFR4 and wild-type FVB mice were produced by mating heterozygous Alb-caFGFR4 transgenic males with wild-type FVB females. FGFR4$^{-/-}$ mice were crossed with Alb-caFGFR4 transgenic mice to obtain hybrids from the two strain backgrounds expressing caFGFR4 in the hepatocytes. Mice were maintained in 12-h light/dark cycles with free access to food and water. Except where indicated, experimental animals were male.

The normal diet (Prolab Isopro RMH 3000; PMI Nutrition International, Brentwood, MO) contained 3.46 kcal/g, of which 60 and 14% of the kilocalories were from carbohydrate and fat, respectively. Animals on a normal diet were analyzed at 6 months of age. Where indicated, mice were presented with a high-fat diet beginning at weaning over a period of 4 months to induce obesity. The high-fat diet (D12451; Research Diets, New Brunswick, NJ) presented 4.73 kcal/g, of which 35 and 45% of kilocalories were from carbohydrate and fat, respectively. Animals were killed and weighed, body fat depots were examined, and tissue was excised, weighed, and then subjected to analysis. All animal work was performed in accordance with the institutional animal care and use committee at the Institute of Biosciences and Technology, Texas A&M Health Science Center.

Histochemistry. Tissues were fixed with Histochoice Tissue Fixative MB (Amresco, Solon, OH), and paraffin-embedded serial sections were prepared and archived; then, sections were stained for general pathological examination with hematoxylin and eosin. Lipid droplets were revealed by staining with Oil Red O. Livers were frozen in Neg-50 frozen section medium (Richard-Allan Scientific, Kalamazoo, MI). Frozen sections (10 μm) were prepared on glass slides, which were then incubated with Oil Red O for 8 min at 60°C. After washing with 85% isopropanol, tissue was counterstained with hematoxylin.

Analysis of blood chemistries and tissue lipids. Blood was collected by retro-orbital puncture after anesthetization with 2,2,2-Tribromoethanol (avertin) (Sigma, St. Louis, MO). Serum was prepared by centrifugation of the clotted blood at 2,000g for 10 min, frozen in aliquots, and stored at −70°C for future analysis. Lipids were extracted from ~50 mg tissue after homogenization in 1 ml PBS and incubation with 1 ml chloroform/methanol (2:1) overnight at room temperature. After centrifugation of the homogenate at 12,000g for 15 min, the lower organic phase–containing lipid was collected and evaporated under a vacuum in a rotary evaporator. The lipid pellet was dissolved in 200 μl PBS containing 1% Triton X-100. Triglyceride, free fatty acids, and cholesterol were measured enzymatically (Wako Pure Chemicals, Richmond, VA). Serum glucose was determined with the Glucometer Elite system (Bayer, Elkhart, IN). Serum insulin, leptin, and adiponectin levels were measured by enzyme-linked immunosorbent assay (Linco Research, St. Charles, MO).

Glucose tolerance and insulin responsiveness. Conventional glucose and insulin tolerance tests were performed on mice fasted for 12 and 4 h, respectively. Mice were injected intraperitoneally with either 1 g glucose/kg body wt or 0.4 or 0.6 units recombinant human insulin/kg body wt (Eli Lilly,

Indianapolis, IN). Blood was collected from the tail immediately before and 30, 60, 90, and 120 min after injection. Plasma glucose was measured as described above.

Analysis of gene expression. Steady-state mRNA levels were quantified by real-time PCR analysis. Total RNA was prepared from tissues using the Ultraspec RNA isolation system (Biotecx Laboratories, Houston, TX). Equal amounts of RNA from four to five mice were pooled and subjected to reverse transcription with Superscript II (Life Technologies, Grand Island, NY) and random primers according to protocols provided by the manufacturer. Oligonucleotide primer sequences are shown in supplemental Table 1 (available in an online appendix at http://dx.doi.org/10.2337/db07-0648). Real-time PCR was performed using the Stratagene Mx 3000P QPCR system and SYBR Green JumpStart Taq Ready Mix (Sigma). All reactions were done in triplicate, and relative amounts of mRNA were calculated using the comparative threshold (C_t) cycle method. Mouse β-actin was used as the internal control.

Fatty acid β-oxidation activity. Fatty acid oxidation activity was measured as previously described (24). Briefly, fresh livers were homogenized in four volumes of 0.25 mol/l sucrose containing 1 mmol/l EDTA. About 1 mg homogenate was incubated in 0.2 ml assay medium (150 mmol/l KCl, 10 mmol/l HEPES [pH 7.2], 0.1 mmol/l EDTA, 1 mmol/l potassium phosphate buffer [pH 7.2], 5 mmol/l malonate, 10 mmol/l MgCl$_2$, 1 mmol/l carnitine, 0.5% BSA, 5 mmol/l ATP, and palmitic acid containing [9,10 (n)-^{3}H]palmitic acid). The reaction was run for 30 min at 25°C and stopped by the addition of 0.2 ml of 0.6 N perchloric acid. The mixture was centrifuged at 2,000g for 10 min, and the unreacted fatty acid in the supernatant was removed with three extractions with 2 ml n-hexane. Radioactive degradation products in the water phase were counted.

Liver triglyceride secretion. Liver triglyceride secretion rate was measured as previously described (25). Mice were fasted 4 h before intraperitoneal injection with 1 mg/g body wt Poloxamer 407. Blood samples were collected retro-orbitally immediately before injection and at 1, 2, and 4 h following injection. The triglyceride accumulation was linear during this time period. Hepatic triglyceride secretion rate was calculated from the slope of the curve and assuming a value of 0.071 ml plasma vol/g body wt (26).

Statistical analysis. Metabolic parameters were expressed as means ± SD from the numbers of replicates described in the text. Statistical significance was determined by Student's t test, and $P < 0.05$ was considered significant.

RESULTS

FGFR4$^{-/-}$ mice exhibit increased white adipose tissue and hyperlipidemia. FGFR4$^{-/-}$ mice appeared normal with respect to feeding behavior and physical activity. The impact of ablation of FGFR4 on body, liver, and adipose tissue mass in mice of both sexes that were fed normal diets was examined over a 6-month period (Table 1). No significant changes in body mass between wild-type and FGFR4$^{-/-}$ males or females were noted. Liver mass was slightly higher in FGFR4$^{-/-}$ females and significantly higher in FGFR4$^{-/-}$ males. Despite a similar body weight, the absence of FGFR4 caused a 1.5- and 2-fold increase, respectively, in mass of reproductive white adipose tissue in males and females (Table 1 and Fig. 1A). The weight of subcutaneous and perirenal fat pads was also higher in the FGFR4$^{-/-}$ mice but less notable (data not shown). The mass of brown adipose tissue was similar between the two genotypes (Table 1). A histological analysis of the reproductive white adipose tissue showed that the increase in mass was associated with an increase in size of adipocytes in the FGFR4$^{-/-}$ mice (Fig. 1B–E) and confirmed that there was no difference in brown adipose cell or tissue morphology (Fig. 1F–I). Although plasma leptin and adiponectin did not differ between FGFR4$^{-/-}$ and wild-type mice, triglycerides, free fatty acids, and cholesterol were 30–40% higher in FGFR4$^{-/-}$ mice under normal dietary conditions (Fig. 2).

Both FGFR4$^{-/-}$ and wild-type mice exhibited the expected increases in body and white adipose tissue mass when presented with only a high-fat diet over a 4-month period after weaning. No significant differences in the two parameters were noted between the two genotypes (Table 1 and Fig. 1). Wild-type mice on the high-fat diet exhibited

TABLE 1
Body and tissue mass in wild-type and FGFR4$^{-/-}$ mice

Parameters	Male: normal diet		Female: normal diet		Male: high-fat diet	
	Wild type	FGFR4$^{-/-}$	Wild type	FGFR4$^{-/-}$	Wild type	FGFR4$^{-/-}$
Body mass (g)	27.90 ± 3.30	29.68 ± 4.41	24.22 ± 1.91	24.25 ± 1.30	38.33 ± 6.15	40.97 ± 5.77
Liver mass (g)	1.25 ± 0.19	1.44 ± 0.19*	1.13 ± 0.15	1.21 ± 0.20	1.41 ± 0.55	1.54 ± 0.44
Liver mass/body mass (%)	3.89 ± 0.32	4.48 ± 0.75*	4.19 ± 0.55	4.31 ± 0.57	3.00 ± 0.53	3.12 ± 0.44
Reproductive WAT (g)	0.65 ± 0.15	0.96 ± 0.24*	0.86 ± 0.19	1.57 ± 0.39*	4.42 ± 1.19	4.71 ± 1.40
Reproductive WAT/body mass (%)	2.25 ± 0.54	3.14 ± 0.45*	3.07 ± 0.52	6.10 ± 1.29†	9.62 ± 1.51	9.69 ± 1.05
BAT (g)	0.16 ± 0.05	0.15 ± 0.04	0.11 ± 0.01	0.13 ± 0.02	0.53 ± 0.20	0.56 ± 0.14

Data are means ± SD (n = 9–25 mice). Wild-type and FGFR4$^{-/-}$ mice on a normal diet were examined at 6 months of age, and mice on a high-fat diet were examined after 4 months of exposure to the diet since weaning. *$P < 0.05$, †$P < 0.01$. BAT, brown adipose tissue; WAT, white adipose tissue.

elevated levels of free fatty acids ($P < 0.05$), cholesterol ($P < 0.001$), and leptin ($P < 0.001$), while plasma triglycerides and adiponectin remained constant (Fig. 2). Plasma leptin, adiponectin, and free fatty acids did not differ between the two groups, but triglycerides and cholesterol were elevated by 1.4- ($P < 0.05$) and 1.25- ($P < 0.001$) fold, respectively, over wild-type levels in the FGFR4$^{-/-}$ mice. These results indicate that FGFR4 plays a key role in maintenance of systemic lipid homeostasis.

Hyperglycemia, glucose intolerance, and insulin resistance in FGFR4$^{-/-}$ mice. To determine whether glucose metabolism was altered along with lipid metabolism and fat deposition in the FGFR4$^{-/-}$ mice, we examined fasting plasma glucose and insulin levels. Although insulin levels were similar, plasma glucose in fasting FGFR4$^{-/-}$ mice was about 1.3 times ($P < 0.05$) that observed in wild-type mice (Fig. 3A and B). When subjected to the glucose tolerance test by administration of 1 g glucose/kg body wt, FGFR4$^{-/-}$ mice exhibited elevated levels of glucose over wild-type mice at all times (183 ± 26 vs. 243 ± 33 mg/dl, wild-type vs. FGFR4$^{-/-}$, respectively, $P < 0.001$) 30 min after the infusion, and levels were still elevated at 2 h when levels had almost returned to normal (121 ± 15 vs. 180 ± 42 mg/dl, wild-type vs. FGFR4$^{-/-}$, respectively, $P < 0.01$) in wild-type mice (Fig. 3C). Administration of 0.4 units insulin/kg caused plasma glucose

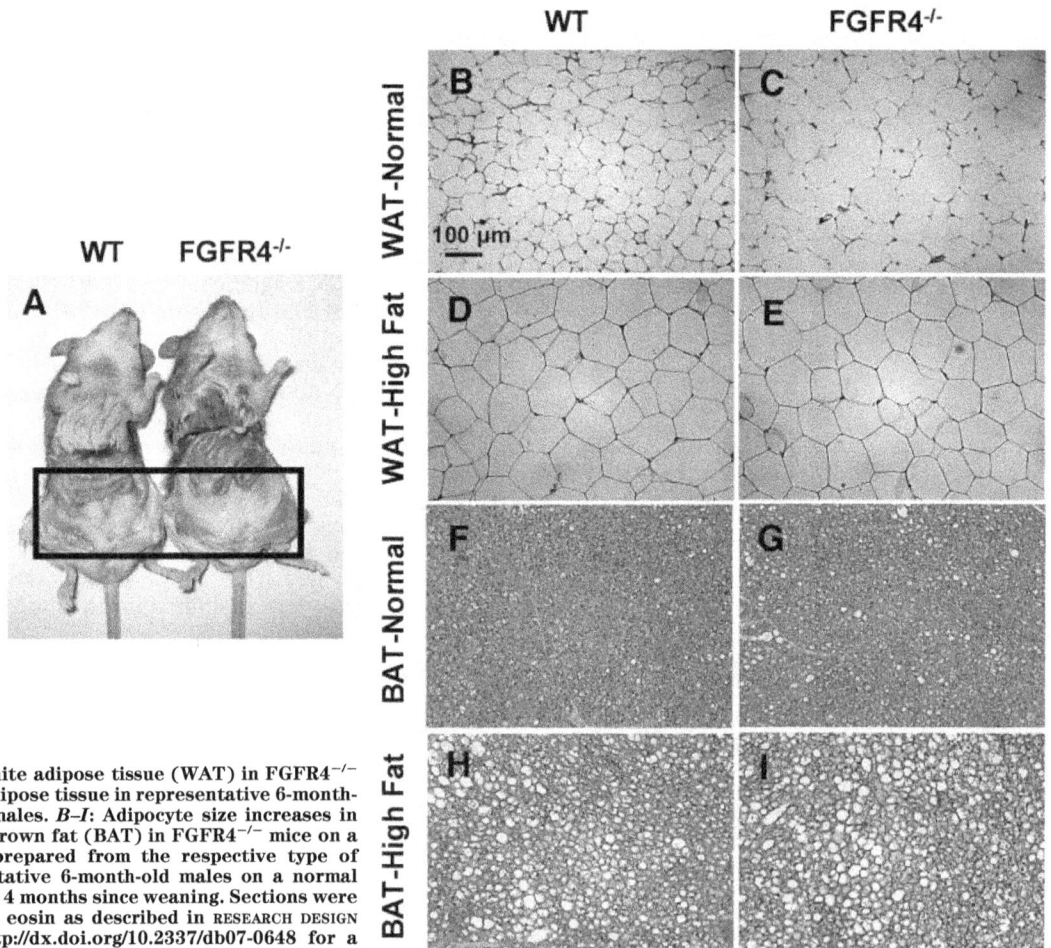

FIG. 1. Increase in mass of white adipose tissue (WAT) in FGFR4$^{-/-}$ mice. A: Reproductive white adipose tissue in representative 6-month-old wild-type and FGFR4$^{-/-}$ males. B–I: Adipocyte size increases in white adipose tissue but not brown fat (BAT) in FGFR4$^{-/-}$ mice on a normal diet. Sections were prepared from the respective type of adipose tissue from representative 6-month-old males on a normal diet or males on a high-fat diet 4 months since weaning. Sections were stained with hematoxylin and eosin as described in RESEARCH DESIGN AND METHODS. (Please see http://dx.doi.org/10.2337/db07-0648 for a high-quality digital representation of this figure.)

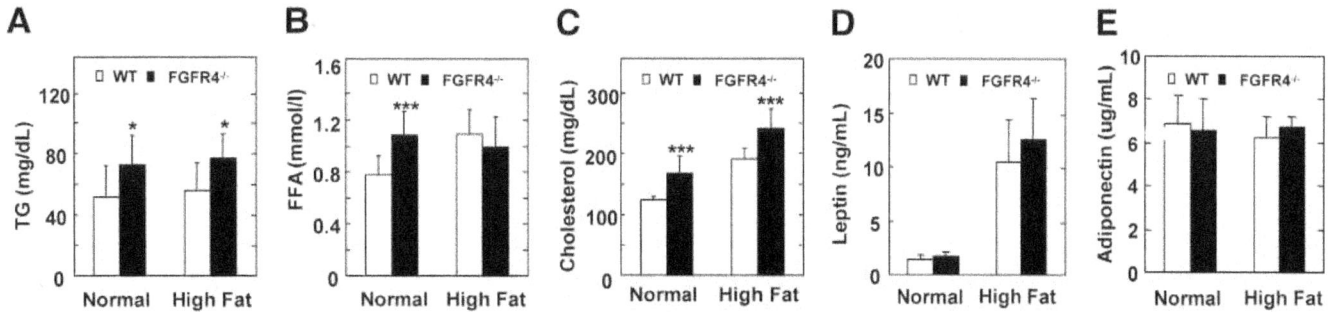

FIG. 2. Increased fasting plasma lipid levels in FGFR4$^{-/-}$ mice. Fasting plasma triglycerides (TG) (*A*), free fatty acids (FFA) (*B*), cholesterol (*C*), leptin (*D*), and adiponectin (*E*) levels of wild-type and FGFR4$^{-/-}$ mice on normal and high-fat diets were measured. Data are means ± SD (*n* = 8–18 mice). *$P < 0.05$; ***$P < 0.001$.

levels to drop to only 60% of normal in FGFR4$^{-/-}$ mice compared with 45% ($P = 0.06$) observed in wild-type mice after 1 h (Fig. 3*D*). At 90 and 120 min, glucose levels were at 87 and 113% of normal, respectively, in the FGFR4$^{-/-}$ mice, whereas they remained depressed at 51 and 57% of normal in wild-type mice ($P < 0.01$ and $P < 0.001$, respectively). These results show that FGFR4$^{-/-}$ mice exhibited reduced glucose tolerance concurrent with increased insulin resistance.

Wild-type mice subjected to chronic high-fat diet exhibited hyperinsulinemia (Fig. 3*A*) that was apparently sufficient to maintain similar fasting plasma glucose levels in animals on a normal diet in this strain of mouse (Fig. 3*B*). However, the high-fat diet caused a reduced glucose tolerance and increased insulin resistance, similar to the

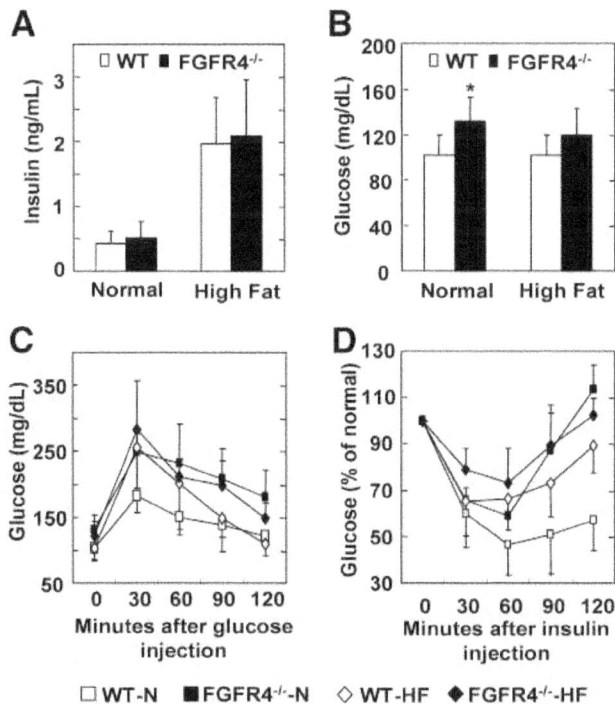

FIG. 3. Glucose intolerance and insulin resistance in FGFR4$^{-/-}$ mice. *A* and *B*: Fasting plasma insulin and glucose levels were assessed in mice with the indicated genotype on a normal (N) and high-fat (HF) diet. *C*: Plasma glucose levels were measured at the indicated times after intraperitoneal administration of 1 g glucose/kg body wt to fasting mice. *D*: Plasma glucose levels were measured at the indicated times following administration of 0.4 units insulin/kg body wt. Data are means ± SD (*n* = 8–10 mice). *$P < 0.05$. WT, wild type.

mice deficient in FGFR4 on the normal diet (Fig. 3*C* and *D*). No significant differences between wild-type and FGFR4$^{-/-}$ mice subjected to chronic high-fat diet were detected. This suggests that FGFR4 deficiency or high-fat diet causes glucose intolerance and insulin resistance. Any additional effects of the FGFR4 deficiency are overridden or masked by the high-fat diet.

The FGFR4 deficiency reduces high-fat diet–induced fatty liver. Livers of FGFR4$^{-/-}$ mice on a normal diet exhibited no notable morphological differences coincident with the observed hyperlipidemia and insulin resistance. As expected, the chronic high-fat diet induced severe fatty liver in wild-type males and, to a lesser extent, in wild-type females (Fig. 4*A* and *C*). Surprisingly, fatty liver was dramatically reduced in FGFR4$^{-/-}$ males and undetectable in females (Fig. 4*B* and *D*). Oil Red O staining confirmed the reduction of lipid droplets caused by the absence of FGFR4 in livers of mice on the high-fat diet (Fig. 4*E–H*). A direct analysis further confirmed the effect of the FGFR4 deficiency on the elevated hepatic lipid content under the high-fat dietary load (Fig. 4*I–K*). No difference was observed between wild-type and FGFR4$^{-/-}$ mice on a normal diet. The 71% reduction ($P < 0.001$) in triglyceride content in FGFR4$^{-/-}$ mice was most dramatic (Fig. 4*I*). Cholesterol levels were also reduced by 36% ($P < 0.01$) (Fig. 4*J*), whereas a reduction in free fatty acids was less significant (18.4 ± 4.2 vs. 14.9 ± 1.5 μmol/g, $P = 0.06$) (Fig. 4*K*). Despite the reduction in lipid accumulation in the liver, no significant reduction of total liver weight was observed in the FGFR4$^{-/-}$ mice (Table 1) since lipid mass accounts for less than 10% of total mass (Fig. 4). Thus, while FGFR4 maintains systemic glucose homeostasis and prevents plasma hyperlipidemia and fat accumulation in the white adipose tissue under normal dietary conditions, it underlies hepatic accumulation of lipid and the fatty liver that results from a chronic high-fat dietary load.

The FGFR4 deficiency alters liver lipid metabolism but not glucose metabolism. Liver plays a key role in metabolic homeostasis of organisms by hormone and metabolite-responsive transcriptional level regulation of rate-limiting enzymes in both synthetic and catabolic pathways in lipid and glucose metabolism (27,28). Therefore, steady-state levels of mRNA coding for key factors involved in hepatic lipid and glucose metabolism were examined in wild-type and FGFR4$^{-/-}$ mice subjected to normal and high-fat diets (Fig. 5*A*). No change in expression of sterol regulatory element–binding protein 1C, a major regulator of lipogenesis (29,30), was observed. However, expression of lipogenic transcription factor

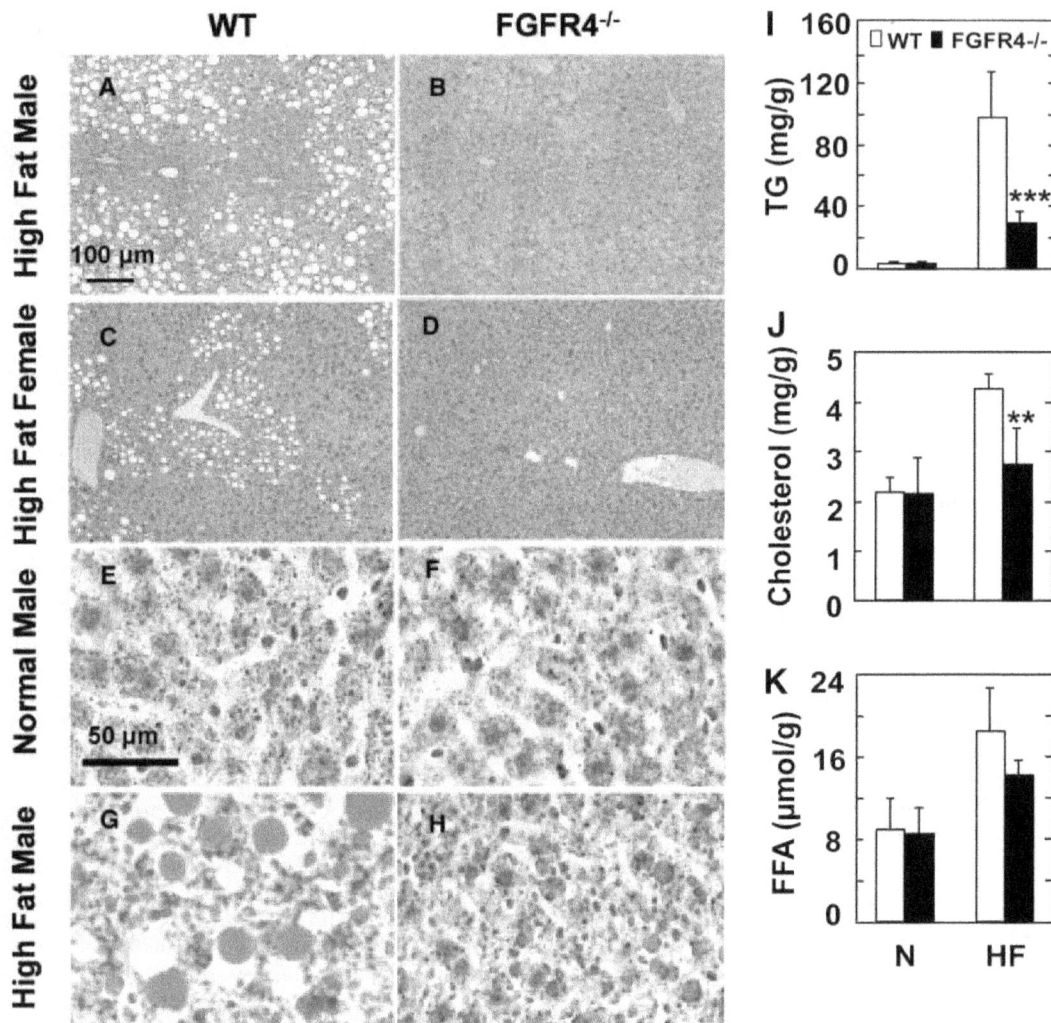

FIG. 4. FGFR4 deficiency alleviates high-fat diet–induced fatty liver. *A–D*: Sections from livers of representative wild-type (WT) and FGFR4$^{-/-}$ mice of the indicated sex on the high-fat diet were prepared and fixed and stained with hematoxylin and eosin. *E–H*: Lipid in sections of livers from representative male wild-type and FGFR4$^{-/-}$ mice on a normal or high-fat diet was stained with Oil Red O. Intense red indicates lipid droplets. *I–K*: Triglycerides (TG), cholesterol, and free fatty acids (FFA) were measured in lipid extracts of livers of wild-type and FGFR4$^{-/-}$ males on the indicated diet (HF, high fat; N, normal). Data are means ± SD ($n = 7$–12 mice). **$P < 0.01$; ***$P < 0.001$. (Please see http://dx.doi.org/10.2337/db07-0648 for a high-quality digital representation of this figure.)

PPARγ (31,32) was elevated by 2.3- ($P < 0.01$) and 1.7- ($P < 0.05$) fold above wild-type levels in FGFR4$^{-/-}$ mice under normal and high-fat dietary conditions, respectively. Under normal dietary conditions, expression of lipogenic genes involved in fatty acid synthesis and uptake was generally higher in the FGFR4$^{-/-}$ livers compared with wild type. Most significant was the 2.5-fold increase ($P < 0.05$) in stearoyl-CoA desaturase (SCD)1 that converts saturated to monounsaturated fatty acids and a 2.6-fold increase ($P < 0.01$) in fatty acid translocase (CD36/FAT). Expression levels of fatty acid synthase, SCD1, and CD36, but not acetyl-CoA carboxylase (ACC1), increased 2- to 3.5-fold ($P < 0.01$) after administration of the high-fat diet in wild-type mice. However, no additional changes in the elevated levels were observed in the FGFR4$^{-/-}$ mice except a 2.6-fold increase of fatty acid synthase ($P < 0.01$). The increase in PPARγ, SCD1, and CD36 in the FGFR4$^{-/-}$ mice may contribute to the hyperlipidemia observed under normal dietary conditions.

In contrast to lipogenic transcripts PPARγ, SCD1, and CD36, expression of liver PPARα and its downstream targets, medium-chain acyl-CoA dehydrogenase that stimulates fatty acid oxidation (33) and microsomal triglyceride transfer protein that is required for the assembly and secretion of apoB-containing lipoproteins (34), were unaffected by FGFR4 deficiency or the high-fat dietary load (Fig. 5A). However levels of these genes were elevated by ~40–60% ($P < 0.05$) in FGFR4$^{-/-}$ mice on the high-fat diet. As we previously reported (20), hepatic FGFR4 is a negative regulator of expression of CYP7A, the rate-limiting enzyme for the canonical pathway of cholesterol–to–bile acid synthesis, under normal dietary conditions. Figure 5A shows that the threefold elevation of CYP7A expression in FGFR4$^{-/-}$ mice relative to wild type was also apparent in the obese mice under the high-fat dietary load. Thus, the reduction in liver cholesterol may also contribute to the alleviation of fatty liver in mice devoid of FGFR4.

We then determined rates of liver fatty acid oxidation and triglyceride secretion. Fatty acid oxidation was 1.43 ($P < 0.05$) times higher in FGFR4$^{-/-}$ livers in mice on a high-fat diet, although they were similar to wild type under

A

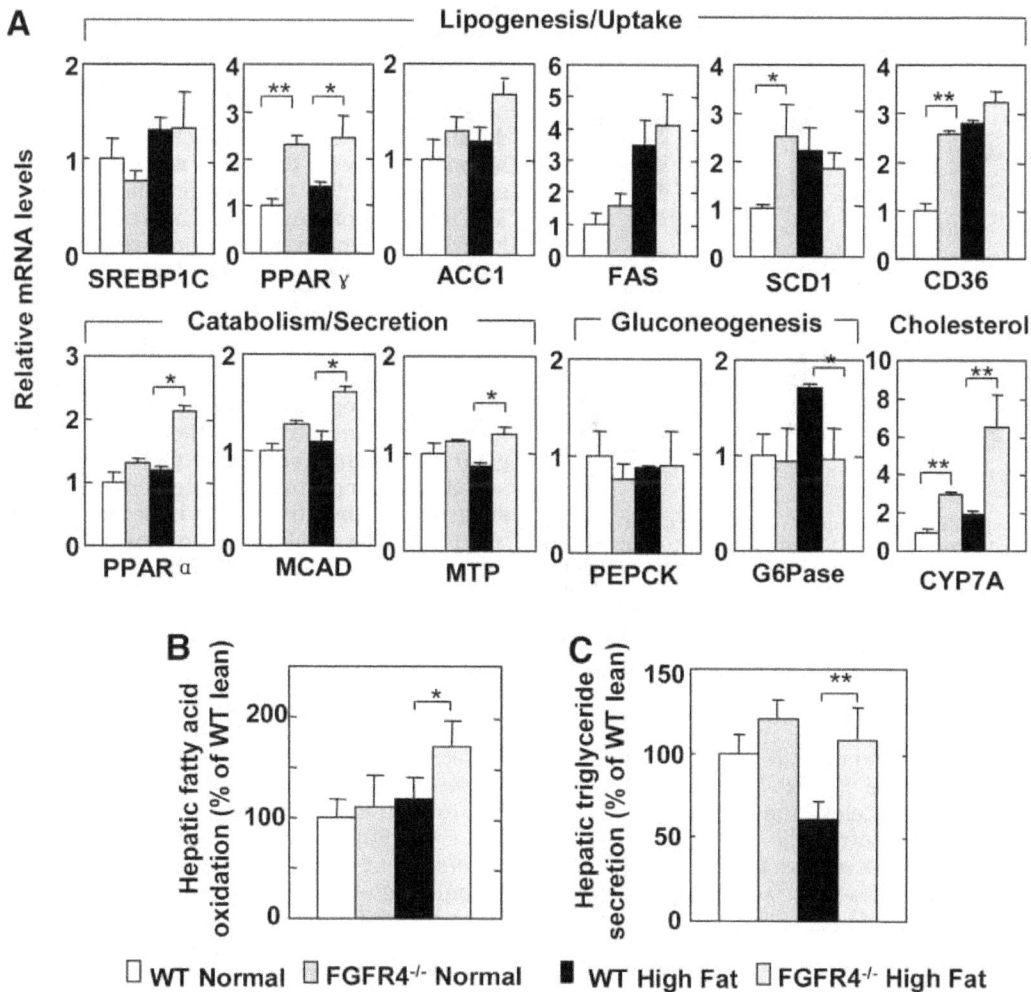

FIG. 5. FGFR4 deficiency alters liver lipid but not glucose metabolism. *A*: Expression of hepatic genes involved in lipid and glucose metabolism. Expression levels were determined in the indicated mice on the indicated diet by quantitative real-time PCR analysis of steady-state mRNA levels and normalized to β-actin expression. Values in wild-type (WT) mice on a normal diet were set to 1. Data are means ± SD of three independent experiments for each gene with four to five mice of each genotype on each dietary regimen. *B*: Hepatic fatty acid oxidation. *C*: Hepatic triglyceride secretion. Values are expressed relative to wild-type mice on a normal diet. Data are means ± SD ($n = 6$–9 mice). *$P < 0.05$; **$P < 0.01$ relative to the corresponding wild-type mice. ACC1, acetyl-CoA carboxylase; CYP7A, cholesterol 7α-hydroxylase; FAS, fatty acid synthase; MCAD, medium-chain acyl-CoA dehydrogenase; MTP, microsomal triglyceride transfer protein; SREBP1, sterol regulatory element-binding protein 1.

normal dietary conditions (Fig. 5*B*). FGFR4$^{-/-}$ mice on a normal diet exhibited an insignificant 20% ($P = 0.08$) increase in rate of hepatic triglyceride secretion. Similar to observations in obese *ob/ob* mice (35), the rate of secretion was reduced in the wild-type obese mice on the chronic high-fat diet. The absence of FGFR4 abolished the resultant reduction in obese mice (Fig. 5*C*). Obese FGFR4$^{-/-}$ mice exhibited an 82% ($P < 0.01$) increase in hepatic triglyceride secretion compared with wild-type littermates.

Lastly, we examined the effect of FGFR4 deficiency on expression of the two key transcriptionally regulated regulators of hepatic gluconeogenesis, PEPCK and glucose-6-phosphatase (G6Pase). The FGFR4 deficiency had no effect on expression of either PEPCK or G6Pase under normal dietary conditions. The high-fat dietary load caused an ~1.8-fold increase in G6Pase mRNA ($P < 0.05$) that was reduced to normal levels in the FGFR4$^{-/-}$ mice (Fig. 5*A*). We then determined whether insulin responsiveness was altered in livers of the FGFR4-deficient mice. Although insulin-stimulated phosphorylation of the insulin

receptor and Akt were significantly decreased in obese compared with normal animals, no significant difference was observed between livers of wild-type and FGFR4$^{-/-}$ mice under either condition (supplemental Fig. 1). This indicated normal insulin signaling in the FGFR4$^{-/-}$ mouse livers upstream through Akt. Together, these results suggest that lipid but not glucose metabolism in the liver is impaired by the absence of germline FGFR4.

Hepatocyte FGFR4 is the determinant of plasma lipid levels and fatty liver. To determine the contribution of hepatocyte FGFR4 to lipid and glucose metabolism, we examined the impact of overexpression of FGFR4 in hepatocytes driven by the albumin promoter in FVB mice (21). A constitutively active FGFR4 (caFGFR4) mutant was used to ensure a sustained signal and to bypass the need for an activating ligand. No significant changes relative to the wild-type control in body, liver, or white or brown adipose tissue weight were observed in the Alb-caFGFR4 mice expressing hyperactive FGFR4 in hepatocytes (data not shown). Basal fasting levels of plasma triglycerides, free fatty acids, and cholesterol were higher

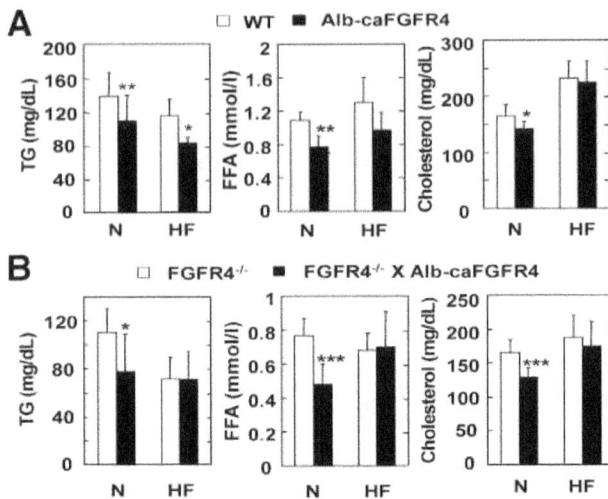

FIG. 6. **Hepatocyte-specific expression of activated FGFR4 reduces plasma lipid levels.** *A*: Fasting plasma triglycerides (TG), free fatty acids (FFA), and cholesterol were determined in mice overexpressing constitutively active FGFR4 in hepatocytes (Alb-caFGFR4) and compared with the wild-type (WT) FVB strain on a normal (N) or high fat (HF) diet. *B*: Fasting plasma lipid levels were determined in the FGFR4$^{-/-}$ × Alb-caFGFR4 hybrid and compared with the FGFR4$^{-/-}$ littermates. Data are means ± SD ($n = 8$–11 mice). *$P < 0.05$; **$P < 0.01$; ***$P < 0.001$.

in the wild-type FVB mice relative to the wild-type littermate control strain for the FGFR4$^{-/-}$ mice (Fig. 6*A*). However, in contrast to the elevation in FGFR4$^{-/-}$ mice relative to their wild-type control, the three parameters in Alb-caFGFR4 mice were decreased to about 80% ($P < 0.01$), 70% ($P < 0.01$), and 85% ($P < 0.05$), respectively, of the wild-type control (Fig. 6*A*).

To determine whether restoration of FGFR4 to the hepatocytes could rescue the metabolic phenotype of the FGFR4$^{-/-}$ mice, the two strains were crossed to produce a FGFR4$^{-/-}$/Alb-caFGFR4 hybrid. Littermates from the cross were compared to minimize strain differences. The FGFR4$^{-/-}$/Alb-caFGFR4 mice exhibited normal liver morphology, although their weight was reduced compared with FGFR4$^{-/-}$ littermates (1.51 ± 0.22 vs. 1.27 ± 0.18 g, $P < 0.05$). The hybrid mice exhibited a less significant 15% reduction in reproductive white adipose tissue. Plasma levels of triglyceride, free fatty acids, and cholesterol were also significantly reduced in the FGFR4$^{-/-}$/Alb-caFGFR4 mice relative to their FGFR4$^{-/-}$ littermates (Fig. 6*B*). Except for a 30% reduction ($P < 0.05$) in blood triglyceride levels in Alb-caFGFR4 mice, no differences in other parameters measured were observed when the mice were administrated a high-fat diet (Fig. 6). This suggests an inability of FGFR4 activity to compensate for the increase in plasma lipids levels caused by the high-fat diet.

We then determined whether restoration of FGFR4 to hepatocytes of the germline FGFR4-deficient mice, which are resistant to high-fat diet–induced fatty liver (Fig. 4), would restore the fatty liver condition. A fatty liver similar to wild-type mice on the chronic high-fat dietary load was apparent in the FGFR4$^{-/-}$/Alb-caFGFR4 hybrids (Fig. 7*A*–*D*). Quantification revealed that restored hepatocyte FGFR4 expression increased liver triglyceride levels (35.9 ± 8.69 vs. 108.6 ± 33.8 mg/g, $P < 0.01$). Analysis of gene expression revealed that restoration of hepatic FGFR4 largely reversed the altered gene expression related to lipid metabolism caused by FGFR4 deficiency but

as expected had no impact on genes related to glucose metabolism (supplemental Fig. 2). These results show that specifically hepatocyte FGFR4 plays a major role in lipid metabolism in the liver. Its activity directly impacts plasma lipid homeostasis and underlies the fatty liver disease that results from a chronic high-fat diet.

Hepatocyte FGFR4 does not directly affect glucose metabolism. We then determined whether hyperactive FGFR4 in hepatocytes or the restoration of hepatocyte FGFR4 to deficient livers would restore defects in glucose metabolism induced by the global absence of FGFR4 (Fig. 3). In contrast to FGFR4$^{-/-}$ mice that exhibited hyperglycemia and hyperinsulinemia, neither Alb-caFGFR4 nor FGFR4$^{-/-}$/Alb-caFGFR4 hybrids exhibited changes in these parameters relative to their appropriate wild-type or FGFR4$^{-/-}$ littermate controls (Fig. 8*A* and *B*). Glucose and insulin tolerance tests further confirmed that the transgenic mice exhibited similar glucose tolerance and insulin sensitivity as controls (supplemental Fig. 3). These results suggest that the absence of hepatocyte FGFR4 activity is insufficient to explain the abnormalities in glucose homeostasis observed in FGFR4$^{-/-}$ mice. They suggest a potential role of FGFR4 on glucose homeostasis at another organ site.

DISCUSSION

In this study, we showed that FGFR4$^{-/-}$ mice displayed multiple elements of metabolic syndrome that included increased white adipose tissue, hyperlipidemia, and insulin resistance. However, despite the beneficial effects of FGFR4 activity on plasma lipid and glucose homeostasis under normal dietary conditions, FGFR4 underlies the development of fatty liver with obesity that is caused by a chronic high-fat diet. The alleviation of fatty liver induced by the high-fat dietary load by ablation of FGFR4 was associated with elevated plasma triglycerides without effect on an increase in body mass, adiposity, glucose intolerance, and insulin resistance. In other words, the normal protection against hyperlipidemia mediated by hepatocyte FGFR4 is to the detriment of the liver under conditions of chronic high-fat diet and obesity. Our observations revealed the physiological importance of FGFR4 signaling in normal lipid and glucose homeostasis in addition to cholesterol and bile acid metabolism. Hyperlipidemia and fatty liver are clinically associated with hyperglycemia and insulin resistance—all of which are part of metabolic syndrome. Type 2 diabetic patients with fatty liver are substantially more insulin resistant and have higher levels of plasma free fatty acids than those without (6). Thus, reduced fatty liver in FGFR4$^{-/-}$ mice may explain the similar extent of insulin resistance of these mice under a high-fat diet, although FGFR4$^{-/-}$ mice on a normal diet were more insulin resistant.

Our findings that hepatocyte FGFR4 activity maintains systemic lipid homeostasis under normal dietary conditions but underlies fatty liver in obese mice on a high-fat diet indicate dramatically different roles of FGFR4 that are dependent on nutritional status. At the molecular level under normal dietary conditions, FGFR4 deficiency is associated with elevation of liver lipogenic genes PPARγ, SCD1, and CD36, with no change in catabolic factors, which is consistent with the hyperlipidemia observed in FGFR4$^{-/-}$ mice. In contrast, on a high-fat diet, FGFR4 deficiency caused a net increase in PPARα and its downstream target genes medium-chain acyl-CoA dehydrogenase and microsomal triglyceride transfer protein, which

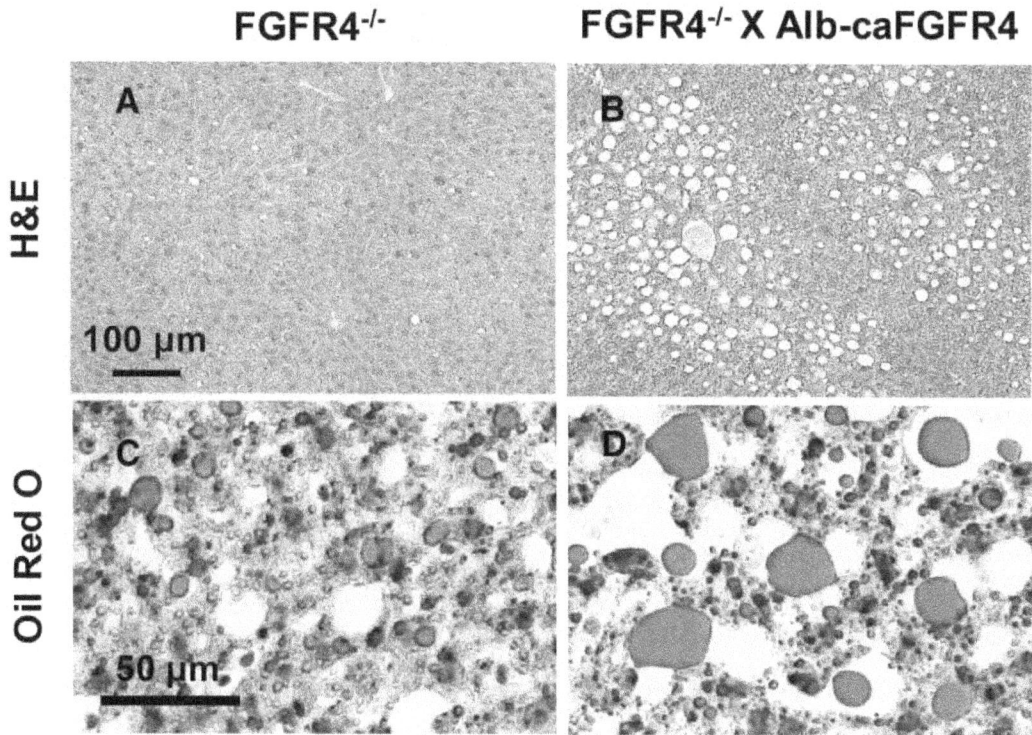

FIG. 7. Hepatocyte-specific restoration of FGFR4 in FGFR4$^{-/-}$ mice restores high-fat diet–induced fatty liver. *A* and *B*: Representative livers from FGFR4$^{-/-}$ and hybrid FGFR4$^{-/-}$/Alb-caFGFR4 mice on a high-fat diet were processed and stained with hematoxylin and eosin (H&E) as described in Fig. 4*C* and *D*. Sections from the same livers were stained with Oil Red O. (Please see http://dx.doi.org/10.2337/db07-0648 for a high-quality digital representation of this figure.)

is accompanied by elevated levels of fatty acid oxidation and hepatic triglyceride secretion. How high-fat dietary overload causes the FGFR4 deficiency to increase gene expression associated with fatty acid oxidation and he-

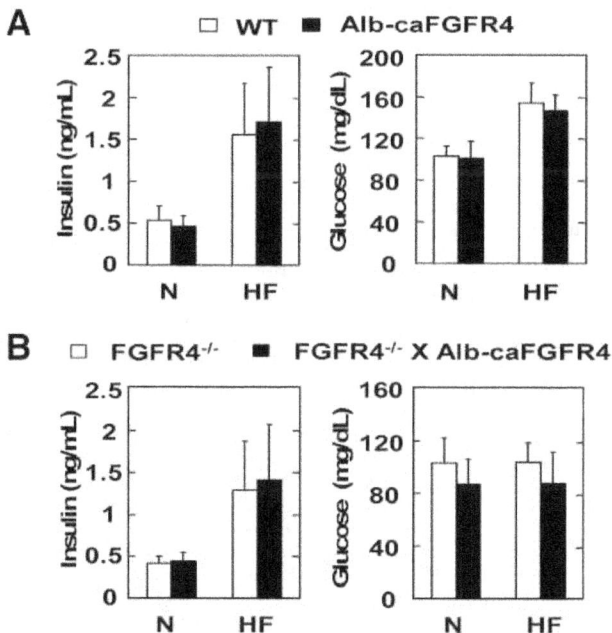

FIG. 8. Hepatocyte FGFR4 does not affect glucose metabolism. *A* and *B*: Fasting plasma insulin and glucose levels were determined in the caFGFR4 and FGFR4$^{-/-}$/Alb-caFGFR4 hybrids as described in RESEARCH DESIGN AND METHODS. Data are means ± SD ($n = 8$–11 mice). HF, high-fat diet; N, normal diet.

patic triglyceride secretion remains to be determined. Such dual and seemingly opposing effects dependent on nutritional status are not without precedent. When overexpressed in hepatocytes, transcriptional regulator liver X receptor α, which directly senses diverse lipid metabolites as ligands (38), elevates mouse serum lipid profiles on a normal diet but improves high blood lipid profiles and protects from atherosclerosis in mice on a Western diet (39). It should also be noted that bile acids reduce high-fat diet–induced hyperglycemia and triglyceride accumulation in liver (36). FGFR4$^{-/-}$ mice display increased bile acid levels (20).

An unresolved issue from our study is the contribution of other organs or tissues where FGFR4 is expressed other than liver for metabolic abnormalities in the FGFR4-deficient mice. We have shown that both overexpression and restoration of FGFR4 to, specifically, hepatocytes decreased plasma lipid levels but failed to improve glucose tolerance and insulin sensitivity. Consistent with this, FGFR4 deficiency neither affects liver gluconeogenic enzymes nor hepatic insulin signaling. This indicates that hepatocyte FGFR4 plays a major role in control of hyperlipidemia (but not hyperglycemia), glucose intolerance, and insulin resistance caused by the general deficiency of FGFR4. Cholesterol synthesis and conversion to bile acids are limited to mature liver hepatocytes where FGFR4 is the only FGFR isotype (40). In contrast, lipid and glucose homeostasis is a partnership between liver and peripheral organs, most significant of which are skeletal muscle and adipose tissue. This suggests that peripheral sites other than liver or the complex interaction of multiple sites are the determinant of hyperglycemia and insulin resistance in FGFR4-deficient mice. FGFR4 is not expressed in adipose tissue (13,15) but is functional in skeletal muscle and has been implicated in its cellular homeostasis during embryogenesis and regeneration (41,42). Compared with other obese mouse models that have a significantly increased body weight, FGFR4$^{-/-}$ mice displayed an increase in the mass of reproductive white adipose tissue without a change in overall body weight and levels of two major adipokines, leptin and adiponectin. Apparently neither an increase in caloric intake nor obesity is the primary factor in determining the basal FGFR4$^{-/-}$ metabolic phenotype. One candidate for the obesity-independent upset in both systemic lipid and glucose metabolism due to FGFR4 deficiency is FXR, which has been implicated in both systemic lipid and glucose metabolism (43–45). An enterohepatic FXR-FGF15-FGFR4 axis has been suggested for regulation of hepatic cholesterol–to–bile acid metabolism, and this may also extend to hepatic lipid metabolism. Since hepatocyte FGFR4 does not play a major role in glucose metabolism and FGFR4 is not at play in adipose tissue (13,15), an FXR-regulated FGF15–to–muscle FGFR4 axis that contributes to glucose metabolism is conceivable. Results not shown here indicated that skeletal muscle in FGFR4$^{-/-}$ mice exhibited elevated levels of lipid compared with wild-type mice. Elevation of skeletal muscle lipids is associated with metabolic syndrome and insulin resistance (46,47). Additional experiments using mice with muscle-specific alterations in FGFR4 should clarify the relative contributions of muscle FGFR4 to aberrant lipid and glucose metabolism.

The opposite phenotypes between FGFR4-deficient mice on a normal diet and those caused by systemic administration or overexpression of FGF19, the human ortholog of mouse FGF15 (13,14), further suggest FGF15/19 as a candidate activator of FGFR4. However, both systemic administration or overexpression of FGF19 (13,14) and the FGFR4 deficiency reduced triglyceride content in the liver in obese mice. It has also been reported that mice with an FGFR4 gene deletion are still metabolically responsive to systemic FGF19 (13). Although it has been argued that FGF19 may be a specific FGF ligand for FGFR4 (48,49), this specificity has yet to be confirmed, particularly in tissues where FGFR4 has impact. Another candidate FGF ligand for FGFR4 particularly in hepatocytes is FGF21. Systemic administration or forced expression of FGF21 in hepatocytes results in reduced adiposity, improved glucose clearance, and insulin sensitivity (15). FGF21 is expressed at low levels in hepatocytes and increases dramatically with liver perturbation (22,50). We have shown that constitutive expression of FGF21 in hepatocytes delays development of chemically induced early hepatic adenomas in mice (22). The FGF21-dependent delay of adenoma development may suggest an internal autocrine activation of hepatocyte FGFR4 since resident hepatocyte FGFR4 exerts a suppressive effect on chemically induced hepatomas (22, X.H., W.L.K., unpublished observations). However, the autocrine action of hepatocyte FGF21 on hepatocyte FGFR4 alone cannot explain the effects of systemic administration of FGF21 on systemic glucose metabolism. Hepatic glucose metabolism is insensitive to hepatic FGFR4 activity. From cell culture studies, Kharitonenkov and colleagues (15,23) have shown that FGF21 stimulates PPARγ agonist-enhanced glucose uptake and metabolism in adipocytes that express other isotypes of FGFR kinase isotypes than FGFR4. An endocrine activity of hepatocyte FGF21 on adipose tissue under control of FXR-FGF15/19–activated hepatocyte FGFR4 is an attractive adjunct to FGF signal-mediated four-way communication among ileum, liver, skeletal muscle, and adipose tissue in control of lipid and glucose homeostasis.

In summary, we have shown that in addition to cholesterol and bile acid homeostasis, FGFR4 plays an important role in systemic lipid and glucose homeostasis. Similar to bile acid metabolism, hepatocyte FGFR4 exerts a major impact on lipid metabolism, but it appears that FGFR4 at other organ sites affects glucose homeostasis. Ironically, hepatocyte FGFR4 is also responsible for the fatty liver associated with obesity induced by chronic high-fat intake. General agonists of FGFR4 may be beneficial in alleviation of elements and consequences of metabolic syndrome related to hyperglycemia and hyperlipidemia. However, in the obese, under conditions of high-caloric intake, the benefits may be at the expense of aggravating fatty liver. General antagonists of FGFR4 may relieve fatty liver in the obese but aggravate the other consequences of metabolic syndrome. A complete knowledge of FGF ligand and tissue context specificity of FGFR4 signaling will be essential to designing tissue-specific agonists and antagonists to alleviate all elements of metabolic syndrome in the obese.

ACKNOWLEDGMENTS

This work was supported by Public Health Service grants R01DK35310 and R01CA59971 (to W.L.M.).

We thank Dr. Wemin He (Institute of Biosciences and Technology, Texas A&M Health Science Center) for helpful advice and sharing reagents.

REFERENCES

1. Eckel RH, Grundy SM, Zimmet PZ: The metabolic syndrome. *Lancet* 365:1415–1428, 2005
2. Biddinger SB, Kahn CR: From mice to man: insights into the insulin resistance syndromes. *Annu Rev Physiol* 68:123–158, 2006
3. Mach T: Fatty liver–current look at the old disease. *Med Sci Monit* 6:209–216, 2000
4. Angulo P: Nonalcoholic fatty liver disease. *N Engl J Med* 346:1221–1231, 2002
5. McClain CJ, Mokshagundam SP, Barve SS, Song Z, Hill DB, Chen T, Deaciuc I: Mechanisms of non-alcoholic steatohepatitis. *Alcohol* 34:67–79, 2004
6. Kelley DE, McKolanis TM, Hegazi RA, Kuller LH, Kalhan SC: Fatty liver in type 2 diabetes mellitus: relation to regional adiposity, fatty acids, and insulin resistance. *Am J Physiol Endocrinol Metab* 285:E906–E916, 2003
7. Schwimmer JB, Deutsch R, Behling C, Lavine JE: Fatty liver as a determinant of atherosclerosis (Abstract). *Hepatology* 42:610A, 2005
8. McKeehan WL, Wang F, Kan M: The heparan sulfate-fibroblast growth factor family: diversity of structure and function. *Prog Nucleic Acid Res Mol Biol* 59:135–176, 1998
9. Wang F, McKeehan WL: The fibroblast growth factor (FGF) signaling complex. In *Handbook of Cell Signaling*. Bradshaw R, Dennis E, Eds. New York, Elsevier, 2003, p. 265–270
10. Powers CJ, McLeskey SW, Wellstein A: Fibroblast growth factors, their receptors and signaling. *Endocr Relat Cancer* 7:165–197, 2000
11. Klint P, Claesson-Welsh L: Signal transduction by fibroblast growth factor receptors. *Front Biosci* 4:D165–D177, 1999
12. Ornitz DM, Itoh N: Fibroblast growth factors. *Genome Biol* 2:REVIEWS3005, 2001
13. Fu L, John LM, Adams SH, Yu XX, Tomlinson E, Renz M, Williams PM, Soriano R, Corpuz R, Moffat B, Vandlen R, Simmons L, Foster J, Stephan JP, Tsai SP, Stewart TA: Fibroblast growth factor 19 increases metabolic rate and reverses dietary and leptin-deficient diabetes. *Endocrinology* 145:2594–2603, 2004
14. Tomlinson E, Fu L, John L, Hultgren B, Huang X, Renz M, Stephan JP, Tsai SP, Powell-Braxton L, French D, Stewart TA: Transgenic mice expressing human fibroblast growth factor-19 display increased metabolic rate and decreased adiposity. *Endocrinology* 143:1741–1747, 2002
15. Kharitonenkov A, Shiyanova TL, Koester A, Ford AM, Micanovic R, Galbreath EJ, Sandusky GE, Hammond LJ, Moyers JS, Owens RA, Gromada J, Brozinick JT, Hawkins ED, Wroblewski VJ, Li DS, Mehrbod F, Jaskunas SR, Shanafelt AB: FGF-21 as a novel metabolic regulator. *J Clin Invest* 115:1627–1635, 2005

16. Zhang X, Ibrahimi OA, Olsen SK, Umemori H, Mohammadi M, Ornitz DM: Receptor specificity of the fibroblast growth factor family: the complete mammalian FGF family. *J Biol Chem* 281:15694–15700, 2006

17. Yu X, White KE: FGF23 and disorders of phosphate homeostasis. *Cytokine Growth Factor Rev* 16:221–232, 2005

18. Schiavi SC: Fibroblast growth factor 23: the making of a hormone. *Kidney Int* 69:425–427, 2006

19. Inagaki T, Choi M, Moschetta A, Peng L, Cummins CL, McDonald JG, Luo G, Jones SA, Goodwin B, Richardson JA, Gerard RD, Repa JJ, Mangelsdorf DJ, Kliewer SA: Fibroblast growth factor 15 functions as an enterohepatic signal to regulate bile acid homeostasis. *Cell Metab* 2:217–225, 2005

20. Yu C, Wang F, Kan M, Jin C, Jones RB, Weinstein M, Deng CX, McKeehan WL: Elevated cholesterol metabolism and bile acid synthesis in mice lacking membrane tyrosine kinase receptor FGFR4. *J Biol Chem* 275: 15482–15489, 2000

21. Yu C, Wang F, Jin C, Huang X, McKeehan WL: Independent repression of bile acid synthesis and activation of c-Jun N-terminal kinase (JNK) by activated hepatocyte fibroblast growth factor receptor 4 (FGFR4) and bile acids. *J Biol Chem* 280:17707–17714, 2005

22. Huang X, Yu C, Jin C, Yang C, Xie R, Cao D, Wang F, McKeehan WL: Forced expression of hepatocyte-specific fibroblast growth factor 21 delays initiation of chemically induced hepatocarcinogenesis. *Mol Carcinog* 45:934–942, 2006

23. Moyers JS, Shiyanova TL, Mehrbod F, Dunbar JD, Noblitt TW, Otto KA, Reifel-Miller A, Kharitonenkov A: Molecular determinants of FGF-21 activity-synergy and cross-talk with PPARγ signaling. *J Cell Physiol* 210:1–6, 2007

24. Linden D, William-Olsson L, Ahnmark A, Ekroos K, Hallberg C, Sjogren HP, Becker B, Svensson L, Clapham JC, Oscarsson J, Schreyer S: Liver-directed overexpression of mitochondrial glycerol-3-phosphate acyltransferase results in hepatic steatosis, increased triacylglycerol secretion and reduced fatty acid oxidation. *FASEB J* 20:434–443, 2006

25. Millar JS, Cromley DA, McCoy MG, Rader DJ, Billheimer JT: Determining hepatic triglyceride production in mice: comparison of poloxamer 407 with Triton WR-1339. *J Lipid Res* 46:2023–2028, 2005

26. Ishikawa T, Fidge N: Changes in the concentration of plasma lipoproteins and apoproteins following the administration of Triton WR 1339 to rats. *J Lipid Res* 20:254–264, 1979

27. Postic C, Dentin R, Girard J: Role of the liver in the control of carbohydrate and lipid homeostasis. *Diabetes Metab* 30:398–408, 2004

28. Roden M, Bernroider E: Hepatic glucose metabolism in humans: its role in health and disease. *Best Pract Res Clin Endocrinol Metab* 17:365–383, 2003

29. Shimano H: Sterol regulatory element-binding protein-1 as a dominant transcription factor for gene regulation of lipogenic enzymes in the liver. *Trends Cardiovasc Med* 10:275–278, 2000

30. Horton JD, Goldstein JL, Brown MS: SREBPs: activators of the complete program of cholesterol and fatty acid synthesis in the liver. *J Clin Invest* 109:1125–1131, 2002

31. Bocher V, Pineda-Torra I, Fruchart JC, Staels B: PPARs: transcription factors controlling lipid and lipoprotein metabolism. *Ann N Y Acad Sci* 967:7–18, 2002

32. Lehrke M, Lazar MA: The many faces of PPARgamma. *Cell* 123:993–999, 2005

33. Gulick T, Cresci S, Caira T, Moore DD, Kelly DP: The peroxisome proliferator-activated receptor regulates mitochondrial fatty acid oxidative enzyme gene expression. *Proc Natl Acad Sci U S A* 91:11012–11016, 1994

34. Ameen C, Edvardsson U, Ljungberg A, Asp L, Akerblad P, Tuneld A, Olofsson SO, Linden D, Oscarsson J: Activation of peroxisome proliferator-activated receptor alpha increases the expression and activity of microsomal triglyceride transfer protein in the liver. *J Biol Chem* 280:1224–1229, 2005

35. Li X, Grundy SM, Patel SB: Obesity in db and ob animals leads to impaired hepatic very low density lipoprotein secretion and differential secretion of apolipoprotein B-48 and B-100. *J Lipid Res* 38:1277–1288, 1997

36. Ikemoto S, Takahashi M, Tsunoda N, Maruyama K, Itakura H, Kawanaka K, Tabata I, Higuchi M, Tange T, Yamamoto TT, Ezaki O: Cholate inhibits high-fat diet-induced hyperglycemia and obesity with acyl-CoA synthetase mRNA decrease. *Am J Physiol* 273:E37–E45, 1997

37. Miyake JH, Doung XD, Strauss W, Moore GL, Castellani LW, Curtiss LK, Taylor JM, Davis RA: Increased production of apolipoprotein B-containing lipoproteins in the absence of hyperlipidemia in transgenic mice expressing cholesterol 7alpha-hydroxylase. *J Biol Chem* 276:23304–23311, 2001

38. Kalaany NY, Mangelsdorf DJ: LXRS and FXR: the yin and yang of cholesterol and fat metabolism. *Annu Rev Physiol* 68:159–191, 2006

39. Lehrke M, Lebherz C, Millington SC, Guan HP, Millar J, Rader DJ, Wilson JM, Lazar MA: Diet-dependent cardiovascular lipid metabolism controlled by hepatic LXRalpha. *Cell Metab* 1:297–308, 2005

40. Kan M, Wu X, Wang F, McKeehan WL: Specificity for fibroblast growth factors determined by heparan sulfate in a binary complex with the receptor kinase. *J Biol Chem* 274:15947–15952, 1999

41. Marics I, Padilla F, Guillemot JF, Scaal M, Marcelle C: FGFR4 signaling is a necessary step in limb muscle differentiation. *Development* 129:4559–4569, 2002

42. Zhao P, Caretti G, Mitchell S, McKeehan WL, Boskey AL, Pachman LM, Sartorelli V, Hoffman EP: Fgfr4 is required for effective muscle regeneration in vivo. Delineation of a MyoD-Tead2-Fgfr4 transcriptional pathway. *J Biol Chem* 281:429–438, 2006

43. Ma K, Saha PK, Chan L, Moore DD: Farnesoid X receptor is essential for normal glucose homeostasis. *J Clin Invest* 116:1102–1109, 2006

44. Cariou B, van Harmelen K, Duran-Sandoval D, van Dijk TH, Grefhorst A, Abdelkarim M, Caron S, Torpier G, Fruchart JC, Gonzalez FJ, Kuipers F, Staels B: The farnesoid X receptor modulates adiposity and peripheral insulin sensitivity in mice. *J Biol Chem* 281:11039–11049, 2006

45. Sinal CJ, Tohkin M, Miyata M, Ward JM, Lambert G, Gonzalez FJ: Targeted disruption of the nuclear receptor FXR/BAR impairs bile acid and lipid homeostasis. *Cell* 102:731–744, 2000

46. Perseghin G: Muscle lipid metabolism in the metabolic syndrome. *Curr Opin Lipidol* 16:416–420, 2005

47. Goodpaster BH, Wolf D: Skeletal muscle lipid accumulation in obesity, insulin resistance, and type 2 diabetes. *Pediatr Diabetes* 5:219–226, 2004

48. Xie MH, Holcomb I, Deuel B, Dowd P, Huang A, Vagts A, Foster J, Liang J, Brush J, Gu Q, Hillan K, Goddard A, Gurney AL: FGF-19, a novel fibroblast growth factor with unique specificity for FGFR4. *Cytokine* 11:729–735, 1999

49. Harmer NJ, Pellegrini L, Chirgadze D, Fernandez-Recio J, Blundell TL: The crystal structure of fibroblast growth factor (FGF) 19 reveals novel features of the FGF family and offers a structural basis for its unusual receptor affinity. *Biochemistry* 43:629–640, 2004

50. Nishimura T, Nakatake Y, Konishi M, Itoh N: Identification of a novel FGF, FGF-21, preferentially expressed in the liver. *Biochim Biophys Acta* 1492:203–206, 2000

Genes Involved in Fatty Acid Partitioning and Binding, Lipolysis, Monocyte/Macrophage Recruitment, and Inflammation Are Overexpressed in the Human Fatty Liver of Insulin-Resistant Subjects

Jukka Westerbacka,[1] Maria Kolak,[2] Tuula Kiviluoto,[3] Perttu Arkkila,[4] Jukka Sirén,[3] Anders Hamsten,[2] Rachel M. Fisher,[2] and Hannele Yki-Järvinen[1,5]

OBJECTIVE—The objective of this study is to quantitate expression of genes possibly contributing to insulin resistance and fat deposition in the human liver.

RESEARCH DESIGN AND METHODS—A total of 24 subjects who had varying amounts of histologically determined fat in the liver ranging from normal ($n = 8$) to steatosis due to a nonalcoholic fatty liver (NAFL) ($n = 16$) were studied. The mRNA concentrations of 21 candidate genes associated with fatty acid metabolism, inflammation, and insulin sensitivity were quantitated in liver biopsies using real-time PCR. In addition, the subjects were characterized with respect to body composition and circulating markers of insulin sensitivity.

RESULTS—The following genes were significantly upregulated in NAFL: peroxisome proliferator–activated receptor (PPAR)γ2 (2.8-fold), the monocyte-attracting chemokine CCL2 (monocyte chemoattractant protein [MCP]-1, 1.8-fold), and four genes associated with fatty acid metabolism (acyl-CoA synthetase long-chain family member 4 [ACSL4] [2.8-fold], fatty acid binding protein [FABP]4 [3.9-fold], FABP5 [2.5-fold], and lipoprotein lipase [LPL] [3.6-fold]). PPARγ coactivator 1 (PGC1) was significantly lower in subjects with NAFL than in those without. Genes significantly associated with obesity included nine genes: plasminogen activator inhibitor 1, PPARγ, PPARδ, MCP-1, CCL3 (macrophage inflammatory protein [MIP]-1α), PPARγ2, carnitine palmitoyltransferase (CPT1A), FABP4, and FABP5. The following parameters were associated with liver fat independent of obesity: serum adiponectin, insulin, C-peptide, and HDL cholesterol concentrations and the mRNA concentrations of MCP-1, MIP-1α, ACSL4, FABP4, FABP5, and LPL.

CONCLUSIONS—Genes involved in fatty acid partitioning and binding, lipolysis, and monocyte/macrophage recruitment and inflammation are overexpressed in the human fatty liver.
Diabetes 56:2759–2765, 2007

E xcess fat accumulation in the liver characterizes insulin-resistant subjects with both too much and too little subcutaneous fat (1). Obesity and insulin resistance are the most common associates of nonalcoholic fatty liver disease (NAFLD), a condition characterized by >10% fat (by histology) in the liver in the absence of other causes of steatosis (2). NAFLD covers a spectrum from simple steatosis (nonalcoholic fatty liver [NAFL]) to nonalcoholic steatohepatitis (NASH), including NASH with cirrhosis, and predicts type 2 diabetes, cardiovascular disease, and liver failure (1). The mechanisms underlying fat accumulation in the human liver and those linking fat to insulin resistance are poorly understood.

Insulin resistance is frequently accompanied by low-grade inflammation. Circulating markers of inflammation include elevated serum levels of C-reactive protein (3) and cytokines and chemokines attracting monocytes/macrophages, such as monocyte chemoattractant protein (MCP)-1 (4). An absence of the C-C motif chemokine receptor-2 (CCR2) regulating monocyte/macrophage recruitment protects the liver against fat accumulation in diet-induced obesity in mice (5). MCP-1 is overexpressed in insulin-resistant human adipose tissue (6,7). Adipose tissue of obese subjects is also characterized by increased accumulation of macrophages as determined by immunohistochemistry (6,8) and expression of macrophage-specific markers, such as CD68 (6–8). The fatty liver of obese mice overexpresses plasminogen activator inhibitor 1 (PAI-1) (9). We have previously demonstrated circulating PAI-1 concentrations to be closely correlated with liver fat content in patients with lipoatrophy (10), but it is unknown whether the human fatty liver of insulin-resistant subjects overexpresses MCP-1, macrophage inflammatory protein (MIP)-1α, CD68, or PAI-1.

In human NAFL, the main source of free fatty acid (FFA) in triglycerides in hepatocytes is peripheral lipolysis from subcutaneous sources (11). In addition, postprandially, de novo lipogenesis contributes significantly to hepatic fat accumulation (11). Fatty acid transport proteins (FATPs) and fatty acid binding proteins (FABPs) regulate fatty acid fluxes. FATP5 is exclusively expressed in the liver, and its overexpression in cell cultures increases FFA uptake (12). Conversely, FFA uptake is reduced in hepatocytes isolated

From the [1]Department of Medicine, Division of Diabetes, University of Helsinki, Helsinki, Finland; the [2]Atherosclerosis Research Unit, King Gustaf V Research Institute, Karolinska Institutet, Stockholm, Sweden; the [3]Department of Surgery, University of Helsinki, Helsinki, Finland; the [4]Department of Medicine, Division of Gastroenterology, University of Helsinki, Helsinki, Finland; and [5]Minerva Foundation Institute for Medical Research, Helsinki, Finland.

Address correspondence and reprint requests to Jukka Westerbacka, MD, PhD, Department of Medicine, Division of Diabetes, University of Helsinki, P.O. Box 700, Room C418b, FIN-00029 HUCH, Helsinki, Finland. E-mail: jukka.westerbacka@helsinki.fi.

Received for publication 18 March 2007 and accepted in revised form 10 August 2007.

Published ahead of print at http://diabetes.diabetesjournals.org on 17 August 2007. DOI: 10.2337/db07-0156.

ADIPOR, adiponectin receptor; CCR2, C-C motif chemokine receptor-2; FATP, fatty acid transport protein; FABP, fatty acid binding protein; FFA, free fatty acid; LPL, lipoprotein lipase; MCP, monocyte chemoattractant protein; MIP, macrophage inflammatory protein; NAFL, nonalcoholic fatty liver; NAFLD, NAFL disease; NASH, nonalcoholic steatohepatitis; PAI-1, plasminogen activator inhibitor 1; PGC1, PPARγ coactivator 1; PPAR, peroxisome proliferator–activated receptor. RPLP0, ribosomal protein, large P0; TBP, TATA-binding protein.

from FATP5 knockout animals (12). FABP4- and FABP5-deficient mice are protected against diet-induced obesity, insulin resistance, type 2 diabetes, and a fatty liver (13,14). There are no data on expression of FATPs or FABPs or other genes, such as acyl-CoA synthetase long-chain family member 4 (ACSL4) and FAS, in the human fatty liver. Peroxisome proliferator–activated receptor (PPAR)γ has two major isoforms, -γ1 and -γ2. Both isoforms activate several adipogenic and lipogenic genes regulating adipocyte maturation, lipid accumulation, and insulin sensitivity. In mice, PPARγ2 is overexpressed in the fatty liver (15), but data regarding PPARγ, -α, and -δ expression in the human fatty liver are lacking.

In the present study, we quantified, by real-time PCR, expression of genes related to inflammation (CD68, MCP-1, MIP-1α, and PAI-1), lipolysis (lipoprotein lipase [LPL]), FFA binding (FABP4 and FABP5), transport (FATP5 and CPT1), and synthesis (ACSL4, SCD1 [stearoyl-coenzyme A desaturase 1], and acetyl-coenzyme A carboxylase-α [ACACA]) in the liver of subjects with varying amounts of liver fat ranging from normal to NAFL ($>$10% fat as determined by histology [2]). In addition, expression of PPARα, -γ, -δ, PPARγ coactivator 1 (PGC1), and adiponectin receptors 1 and 2 were measured. Data were also analyzed after dividing the subjects into groups based on the presence and absence of NAFL.

RESEARCH DESIGN AND METHODS

A total of 30 Caucasian subjects were recruited from patients undergoing a laparoscopic gastric bypass operation or among those referred to the gastroenterologist because of elevated liver function tests. Inclusion criteria were as follows: 1) age of 18–60 years; 2) alcohol consumption less than two drinks, i.e., 20 g ethanol/day; and 3) no histological evidence of NASH. The following causes of liver diseases were excluded: chronic hepatitis B or C, thyroid dysfunction, autoimmune hepatitis (smooth muscle and anti-nuclear antibodies), primary biliary cirrhosis (anti-mitochondrial antibodies), primary sclerosing cholangitis, use of hepatotoxic medications or herbal products, or use of medications known to be associated with steatohepatitis. None of the subjects used antidiabetic or lipid-lowering medications, including PPARα or -γ agonists. The liver biopsy was taken if considered clinically indicated. The subjects were divided into groups with (NAFL+) or without (NAFL−) NAFL (2). Of the 30 patients, 6 were excluded because of NASH ($n = 2$), undefined hepatitis ($n = 1$), cirrhosis ($n = 1$), or insufficient sample for RNA isolation ($n = 2$), resulting in the patient sample of 24 patients for final analysis.

The nature and potential risks of the study were explained to all subjects before obtaining their written informed consent. The study was carried out in accordance with the principles of the Declaration of Helsinki. The protocol was approved by the ethics committee of the Helsinki University Central Hospital.

Liver biopsy and total RNA cDNA preparation. Needle or wedge biopsies (10–400 mg) were taken after an overnight fast. Approximately one-half of the sample was sent to the pathologist for routine histopathological assessment, while the rest was immediately frozen and stored in liquid nitrogen. Frozen tissue samples (2–30 mg) were homogenized in 1 ml QIAzol Lysis Reagent (Qiagen, Valencia, CA), and total RNA was isolated as previously described (16). RNA was stored at −80°C until quantification of target mRNAs. A total of 0.1 μg RNA was transcribed into cDNA using Moloney murine leukemia virus reverse transcriptase (Life Technologies, Paisley, U.K.) and oligo (dT)$_{12-18}$ primers (16).

PCR analyses. The mRNA concentrations were quantified by real-time PCR using the ABI 7000 Sequence Detection System instrument and software (Applied Biosystems). cDNA synthesized from 10 ng total RNA was mixed with TaqMan Universal PCR Master Mix (Applied Biosystems) and a gene-specific primer and probe mixture (predeveloped TaqMan Gene Expression Assays; Applied Biosystems) in a final volume of 25 μl. The assays used were as follows: Hs00167155_m1 for PAI-1, Hs00234592_m1 for PPARγ, Hs00602622_m1 for PPARδ, Hs00360422_m1 for adiponectin receptor (ADIPOR)1, Hs00154355_m1 for CD68, Hs00231882_m1 for PPARα, Hs00748952_s1 for SCD, Hs00234140_m1 for MCP-1, Hs00234142_m1 for MIP-1α, Hs00226105_m1 for ADIPOR2, Hs00173304_m1 for PGC1α, Hs01115510_m1 for

TABLE 1
Characteristics of the study subjects

	All subjects	NAFL−	NAFL+
n	24	8	16
Histological liver fat (%)	38.5 ± 6.8	2.6 ± 1.2	56.4 ± 6.5*
Women/men	14/10	4/4	10/6
Age (years)	44 ± 2	47 ± 4	42 ± 3
Body weight (kg)	105 ± 6	85 ± 9	116 ± 8†
BMI (kg/m^2)	37.1 ± 2.4	29.9 ± 3.8	40.8 ± 2.6†
Components of the MetS			
Waist circumference (cm)	113 ± 4	85 ± 9	116 ± 8
Systolic blood pressure (mmHg)	133 ± 2	130 ± 5	134 ± 3
Diastolic blood pressure (mmHg)	83 ± 2	78 ± 3	86 ± 2†
fS triglycerides (mmol/l)	1.7 ± 0.2	1.1 ± 0.2	1.9 ± 0.2†
fS HDL cholesterol (mmol/l)	1.5 ± 0.1	2 ± 0.3	1.3 ± 0.1†
fP glucose (mmol/l)	5.9 ± 0.2	5.3 ± 0.2	6.1 ± 0.3
Other parameters			
fS insulin (mU/l)	12 ± 2	6 ± 1	15 ± 3†
fS C-peptide (nmol/l)	0.9 ± 0.1	0.6 ± 0.1	1.1 ± 0.1‡
fS FFA (μmol/l)	588 ± 45	509 ± 90	628 ± 49
fS adiponectin (μg/ml)	9.7 ± 1	12.3 ± 2.1	8.4 ± 1§
fP PAI-1 (ng/ml)	31 ± 3	24 ± 6	35 ± 3
fS LDL cholesterol (mmol/l)	2.7 ± 0.2	2.7 ± 0.3	2.7 ± 0.2
fS ALT (units/l)	87 ± 13	97 ± 21	82 ± 17
fS AST (units/l)	53 ± 6	55 ± 9	53 ± 8
MCV (fl)	90 ± 1	90 ± 1	90 ± 1
Daily alcohol dose	0.5 ± 0.2	0.4 ± 0.2	0.5 ± 0.2

Data are means ± SE. *$P < 0.001$, †$P < 0.05$, ‡$P < 0.01$, §$0.1 > P > 0.05$, for subjects without (NAFL−) versus with (NAFL+) NAFLD. ALT, alanine aminotransferase; ASP, aspartate aminotransferase; fP, fasting plasma, fS, fasting serum; MCV, mean corpuscular volume; MetS, metabolic syndrome; NA, not applicable.

PPARγ2, Hs00244871_m1 for ACSL4, Hs00157079_m1 for carnitine palmitoyltransferase 1A (CPT1A), Hs00236877_m1 and Hs00426285_m1 for IGFBP1 (insulin-like growth factor binding protein-1), Hs00167385_m1 for ACACA, Hs00202073_m1 for FATP5, Hs00609791_m1 for FABP4, Hs02339439_g1 for FABP5, Hs00173425_m1 for LPL, Hs00194145_m1 for HMGCS2, Hs99999910_m1 for TATA-binding protein (TBP), and Hs99999902_m1 for ribosomal protein, large P0 (RPLP0). All samples were run in duplicate. Relative expression levels were determined using a 7-point serially diluted standard curve, generated from cDNA of human liver. The mRNA concentrations of specific genes were expressed in arbitrary units and normalized to the mean of the mRNA concentrations of RPLP0 and TBP to correct for differences in cDNA loading.

Other measurements. Blood samples were taken after an overnight fast for measurement of plasma glucose, serum insulin, C-peptide, serum triglycerides, and total and HDL cholesterol concentrations as described previously (7). Serum adiponectin concentrations were measured using an enzyme-linked immunosorbent assay kit from B-Bridge International (San Jose, CA). Serum FFA were measured by an enzymatic colorimetric method using a kit from Wako Chemicals (Neuss, Germany) and PAI-1 antigen using an enzyme-linked immunosorbent assay kit from Trinity Biotech (Wicklow, Ireland).

Statistical analyses. Comparisons between NAFL+ and NAFL− groups were performed using nonparametric methods, and correlations coefficients were calculated using Spearman's rank correlation coefficient. Nonparametric statistics were used because of relatively small sample size, although all gene expression data passed the normality test. Adjustment of liver fat for BMI was performed using analysis of covariance after logarithmic transformation of the variables if necessary. A P value of <0.05 was considered statistically significant. The calculations were performed using SPSS 11.0 for Windows (SPSS, Chicago, IL). All data are shown as means ± SE.

RESULTS

The NAFL+ group had significantly higher concentrations of fasting serum insulin, C-peptide, and triglycerides and

TABLE 2
Nonparametric correlations (Spearman's r) between hepatic gene expression (as expressed relative to housekeeping gene mRNA expression) and the amount of liver fat and liver fat adjusted for BMI

Gene	Liver fat	Liver fat adjusted for BMI	NAFL−	NAFL+	Fold difference
PAI1	0.32	0.05	2.12 ± 0.9	1.85 ± 0.28	0.9
PPARγ	0.39	0.22	0.13 ± 0.01	0.17 ± 0.01	1.3
PPARγ2	0.64*	0.34	0.05 ± 0.01	0.15 ± 0.02†	2.8
PGC1	−0.19	−0.19	5.6 ± 1.37	3.29 ± 0.56‡	0.6
PPARα	0.06	−0.05	4.58 ± 0.97	4.31 ± 0.52	0.9
PPARδ	0.29	0.1	0.18 ± 0.03	0.24 ± 0.03	1.3
ADIPOR1	−0.08	−0.14	1.23 ± 0.1	1.29 ± 0.13	1.1
ADIPOR2	0.05	0.03	3.01 ± 0.53	3.03 ± 0.46	1.0
HMGCS2	−0.07	−0.17	6.36 ± 0.71	5.96 ± 0.44	0.9
IGFBP1	−0.11	−0.28	4.88 ± 1.38	6.76 ± 2.5	1.4
CD68	0.14	0.17	0.17 ± 0.03	0.2 ± 0.02	1.1
MCP-1	0.61§	0.45†	0.32 ± 0.05	0.57 ± 0.05§	1.8
MIP-1α	0.42†	0.36	0.03 ± 0.01	0.04 ± 0.01	1.6
SCD	0.18	0.22	0.44 ± 0.13	0.48 ± 0.09	1.1
ACSL4	0.53§	0.43†	0.11 ± 0.05	0.31 ± 0.07‡	2.8
CPT1A	0.24	0.11	2.69 ± 0.53	3.39 ± 0.44	1.3
ACACA	0.27	0.2	1.39 ± 0.31	1.89 ± 0.18	1.4
FATP5	−0.16	−0.22	8.57 ± 0.87	7.81 ± 0.7	0.9
FABP4	0.83¶	0.76¶	0.002 ± 0.001	0.009 ± 0.001§	3.9
FABP5	0.74*	0.62§	0.016 ± 0.003	0.039 ± 0.008†	2.5
LPL	0.73*	0.66*	0.002 ± 0.001	0.006 ± 0.002	3.6

Data are means ± SE. mRNA concentration of selected genes in the liver in control subjects and subjects with NAFL. *$P < 0.001$, †$P < 0.05$, ‡$0.1 > P > 0.05$, §$P < 0.01$, ¶$P < 0.0001$ for correlation or control versus NAFL.

lower concentrations of HDL cholesterol than the NAFL+ group (Table 1). Five of the eight NAFL− patients had slightly elevated serum alanine aminotransferases and/or aspartate aminotransferases without any known cause.

Liver fat and markers of insulin resistance. In all subjects, liver fat correlated with BMI (Spearman's rank correlation coefficient $r = 0.46$, $P < 0.05$). Liver fat was positively correlated with fasting serum insulin ($r = 0.59$, $P < 0.01$), C-peptide ($r = 0.83$, $P < 0.0001$), and serum triglycerides ($r = 0.53$, $P < 0.01$) and negatively with serum HDL cholesterol ($r = -0.59$, $P < 0.01$). After adjusting for BMI, liver fat was significantly correlated with fasting serum insulin ($r = 0.45$, $P < 0.05$), C-peptide ($0.63, P < 0.01$), and HDL cholesterol ($r = -0.41, P < 0.05$) concentrations. Serum adiponectin did not correlate with BMI but was inversely related with liver fat (unadjusted for BMI, $r = -0.49, P < 0.05$; adjusted for BMI, $r = -0.44$,

$P < 0.05$). Serum PAI-1 concentrations were also correlated with liver fat ($r = 0.41$, $P < 0.04$) but not with BMI ($r = 0.19$, NS).

Liver fat and hepatic gene expression. The correlation coefficients between liver fat and gene expression are shown in Table 2. Liver fat was significantly associated with increased expression of PPARγ2, MCP-1, and MIP-1α (Table 2; Figs. 1 and 2) and ACSL4, FABP4, FABP5, and LPL (Table 2; Figs. 2 and 3). When adjusted for BMI, the relationships between liver fat and MCP-1, ACSL4, FABP4, FABP5, and LPL expression remained statistically significant.

NAFL and hepatic gene expression. Data on gene expression in the subjects divided into groups based on NAFL are shown in Table 2. The NAFL+ group had significantly increased hepatic expression of PPARγ2, MCP-1, FABP4, FABP5, and LPL compared with the NAFL− group.

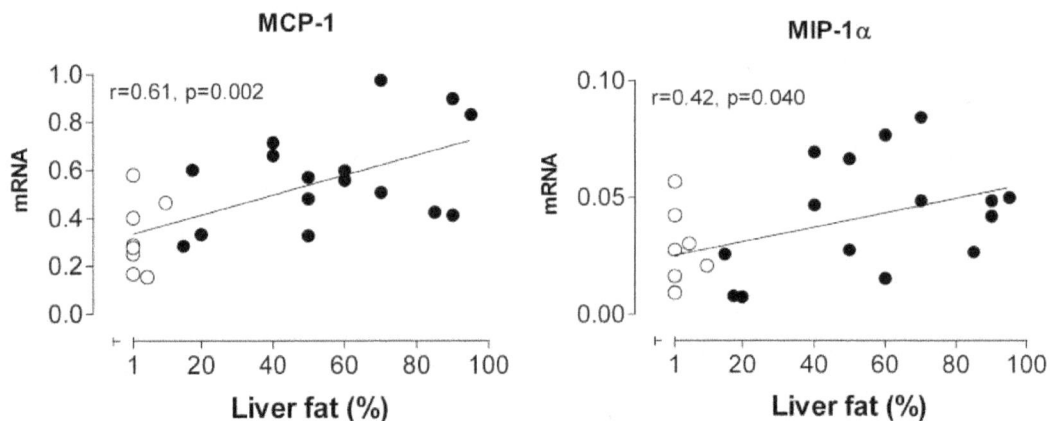

FIG. 1. The relationship between liver fat and hepatic mRNA concentrations of MCP-1 and MIP-1α expressed relative to the mean of housekeeping genes (RPLP0 and TBP) and the percentage of liver fat in the entire study group. ○, without NAFLD; ●, with NAFLD.

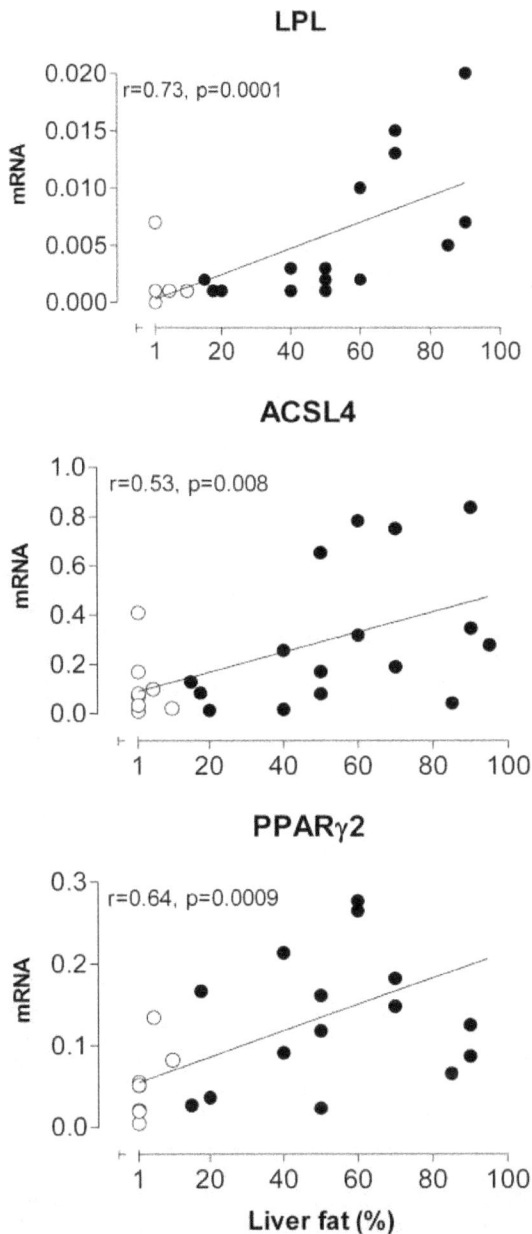

FIG. 2. The relationship between liver fat and hepatic mRNA concentrations of LPL, ACSL4, and PPARγ2 expressed relative to the mean of housekeeping genes (RPLP0 and TBP) and the percentage of liver fat in the entire study group. ○, without NAFLD; ●, with NAFLD.

DISCUSSION

We quantified expression of genes thought to be important in fatty acid trafficking, synthesis and storage, and inflammation in human liver samples with varying amounts of fat. We found the expression of PPARγ2, of two monocyte-attracting chemokines (MCP-1 and MIP-1α) and of four genes associated with fatty acid metabolism (ACSL4, FABP4, FABP5, and LPL) to be increased in proportion to liver fat content. Interestingly, of these genes, PPARγ2, FABP4, and LPL are normally expressed, especially in adipose tissue. The relationships between liver fat and MCP-1, ACSL4, FABP4, FABP5, and LPL expression remained significant even when adjusted for BMI, although statistical adjustment for the impact of obesity is inferior

to study of weight-matched groups with and without NAFL. When the subjects were divided into those with NAFL using the cutoff point of 10% liver fat, those with NAFL had higher expression of PPARγ2, MCP-1, FABP4, and FABP5.

Studies examining gene expression in human NAFL are very limited. Younossi et al. (17) compared gene expression using microarray between 12 steatosis patients and 7 obese controls. Ten of the 5,220 genes examined were differentially expressed in the liver. None was related to inflammation, insulin action, or fatty acid transport or synthesis (17). The steatosis (NAFL) subjects did not, however, differ with respect to serum insulin concentrations or the homeostasis model assessment insulin resistance index from the nonsteatosis control subjects. Younossi et al. (18) also reported results of microarray analysis comprising 5,220 genes in 29 patients with NASH, 14 subjects with steatosis alone, and 7 obese and 6 nonobese control subjects. A total of 34 genes were differentially expressed between obese patients with NASH and nonobese subjects. Altered expression of four of these genes was verified using real-time PCR. Results regarding differences between subjects with and without steatosis were not reported. Chiappini et al. (19) recently reported microarray data comparing hepatic gene expression between obese steatotic ($n = 9$) and significantly leaner subjects. Features of insulin resistance or degree of alcohol consumption were not reported. Of 110 differentially expressed genes, expression of one mitochondrial (mtDNA) and three inflammatory genes (SIGIRR, TOLLIP, and STIPEC) were verified using real-time PCR in a larger group of 40 liver donors, but characteristics of these subjects were not reported.

The chemokines MCP-1 and MIP-1α are low–molecular weight proteins secreted by several tissues. These chemokines primarily stimulate leukocyte recruitment. Haukeland et al. (20) reported, using immunohistochemistry, that MCP-1 was expressed in normal human livers and in livers from patients with simple steatosis and NASH. Positive staining was found in bile duct epithelial cells, endothelial cells, leukocytes, and hepatocytes (20). Our data support these observations by showing a significant positive correlation between liver fat and MCP-1 gene expression.

CD68 is a transmembrane glycoprotein that is highly expressed by human monocytes and tissue macrophages. In the present study, expression of CD68 was not associated with liver fat and did not differ between those with and without NAFL. Although this was somewhat unexpected, it is noteworthy that the subjects did not have histological signs of inflammation as determined by histopathological examination. Possibly, expression of macrophage markers could be increased in more advanced forms of NAFLD.

FABPs are members of the superfamily of lipid-binding proteins with tissue-specific distribution (21). They regulate fatty acid uptake and are involved in intracellular trafficking of long-chain fatty acids for oxidation and storage. In the present study, expression of both FABP4 and FABP5 were closely positively correlated with liver fat content. FABP4 is considered to be adipocyte specific (22), although it is expressed also in stimulated human monocytes and macrophages (23). FABP5 (epidermal FABP) is expressed in many tissues, such as brain, kidney, adipose tissue, and liver (24). In livers of *ob/ob* mice, FABP expression has been found to be increased twofold com-

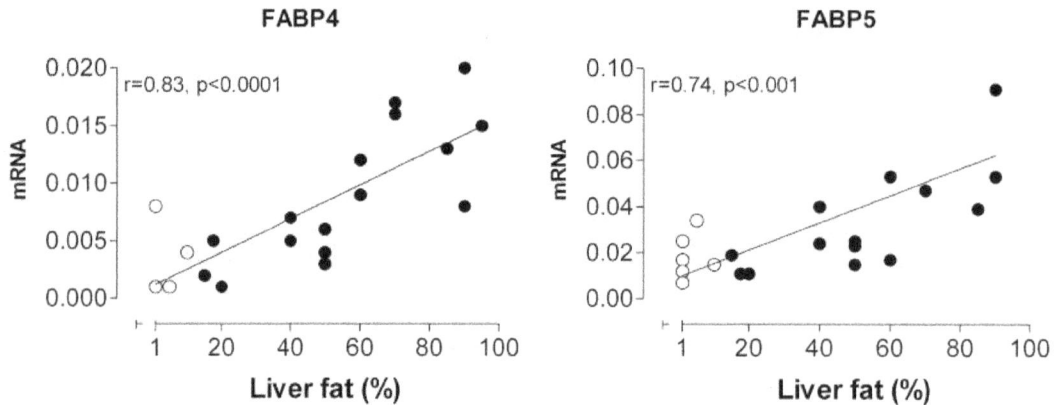

FIG. 3. The relationship between liver fat and hepatic mRNA concentrations of FABP4 and FABP5 expressed relative to the mean of housekeeping genes (RPLP0 and TBP) and the percentage of liver fat in the entire study group. ○, without NAFLD; ●, with NAFLD.

pared with that in lean control mice (25), in keeping with the present data in humans. In these mice, FATP has been reported to be unchanged, as in the present study (25). Mice lacking both FABP4 and FABP5 are protected from diet-induced obesity and accumulation of fat in the liver (13), implying that these proteins may play a role in regulating liver fat.

LPL is a rate-limiting enzyme for intravascular hydrolysis of lipoprotein-rich triglyceride particles, which is expressed at high levels in adipose tissue, heart and skeletal muscle, kidney, and the mammary gland and at lower levels in the liver, adrenal gland, and brain (26). In the liver, LPL has been shown to be upregulated by liver X receptor (LXR) agonists (27). In addition, LPL expression is induced in the liver by tumor necrosis factor-α (28). A study performed in rats suggested LPL activity in the liver and in peripheral tissues to be reciprocally regulated (29). Liver-specific overexpression of LPL in mice causes hepatic steatosis and insulin resistance (30). In humans, LPL activity in adipose tissue is high in obese, insulin-resistant subjects (31). It is thus possible that LPL is reciprocally regulated even in humans, a combination that would favor fat accumulation in the liver.

Acyl-CoA synthetases catalyze the initial step of acyl-CoA formation from long-chain fatty acids. These enzymes have been classified by their preferences for short, medium, long, and very long chain fatty acids, although there is considerable overlap (32). Isoforms 1, 3, 4, and 5 are abundant in the liver (33). Overexpression of ACSL isoforms has been shown to increase fatty acid uptake (34). Rat ACSL4 is a membrane-associated long-chain acyl-CoA synthetase that can activate both saturated and unsaturated fatty acids from 14 to 26 carbons (35). Increased ACSL4 expression in the liver could thus promote fatty acid uptake, although the exact function of this isoform in the liver is unexplored.

Studies using animal models, such as lipoatrophic A-ZIP/F-1 mice with PPARγ ablation (15), leptin-deficient mice with liver-specific disruption of PPARγ (36), and mice with hepatic overexpression of either PPARγ1 (37) or PPARγ2 (38), have established that increased PPARγ activity can cause hepatic steatosis. In mice, PPARγ and a fatty liver can be induced by synthetic and natural ligands, such as those generated by a high-fat diet (39). The 2.8-fold increase in PPARγ2 expression in the NAFL patients is consistent with these data. We have previously found in two cross-sectional studies that liver fat content is posi-

tively correlated with the percentage of calories originating from fat and especially saturated fat (40,41). A high-fat diet compared with a eucaloric low-fat diet increases liver fat content in humans (42). The possibility that high relative fat intake contributed to the increased PPARγ2 expression in the NAFL group remains to be tested. In mice, saturated fats also appear to increase hepatic steatosis and obesity via activation of SREBP1 and SCD (43–45). Disruption of SCD alone is sufficient to protect against steatosis and obesity (43). Although SREBP1c expression was not measured, expression of two of its target lipogenic mRNAs, ACACA and SCD, was not increased in the NAFL+ compared with the control group (43). No measurement of fatty acid oxidation was performed, but the mRNA concentration of CPT1A, the rate-limiting enzyme for mitochondrial β-oxidation, was unchanged.

PPARγ activation changes the transcription of hundreds of genes in vitro in cell lines, such as 3T3-L1 adipocytes. However, in a recent study examining the effect of chronic rosiglitazone treatment in type 2 diabetic patients on gene expression, only 13 of 50 genes, which have been most frequently reported to be regulated by PPARγ agonism in animal studies, were altered. Nevertheless, some of the genes in which expression was studied in the present study could represent PPARγ targets. These include the adiponectin receptors in addition to LPL, FABP4, and FABP5, which were discussed above. Whereas FABP4 is a classic PPARγ-regulated gene in adipose tissue (46), FABP5 has also been shown to be overexpressed in the liver in response to adenovirus-induced overexpression of PPARγ in PPARα$^{-/-}$ mice (37). Such treatment induced profound adipogenic transformation of the gene expression pattern in hepatocytes. Rosiglitazone has been shown to increase the mRNA and protein levels of ADIPOR2 in HepG2 cells (47), but expression of both ADIPOR1 and ADIPOR2 were unchanged in the present study. It may seem paradoxical that PPARγ agonists markedly lower liver fat content in humans (48), although PPARγ2 is overexpressed in the human fatty liver. The reason for this paradox is poorly understood, but possibly, the decrease in FFA flux and increase in serum adiponectin via PPARγ agonism in adipose tissue could be more important regulators of liver fat than direct effect of these drugs in the liver.

In conclusion, the human steatotic liver due to NAFL overexpresses PPARγ2 and genes normally found abundantly in adipose tissue, such as FABP4 and LPL, the chemokine genes MCP-1 and CCL3, and two other genes facilitating fatty acid transport and synthesis, FATP5 and ACSL4. These changes in the human fatty liver bear some resemblance to the adipogenic transformation described in the PPARα$^{-/-}$ overexpressing PPARγ in the liver. This conclusion awaits verification of the now described alterations in gene expression functionally and at the level of protein expression.

ACKNOWLEDGMENTS

J.W. has received support from the Academy of Finland, the EVO Foundation, and Biovitrum. A.H. has received support from the Karolinska Institute, the Swedish Heart-Lung Foundation, and Biovitrum. R.M.F. has received support from the Swedish Research Council (project 15352), the Novo Nordisk Foundation, and Biovitrum. H.Y.-J. has received support from the Academy of Finland, the Sigrid Juselius and EVO Foundations, the Novo Nordisk Foundation, and Biovitrum. This work is part of the project "Hepatic and Adipose Tissue and Functions in the Metabolic Syndrome" (www.hepadip.org), which is supported by the European Commission as an Integrated Project under the 6th Framework Programme (contract LSHM-CT-2005-018734).

We gratefully acknowledge Dr. Päivi Kärkkäinen for histological analysis of the liver samples and Katja Tuominen and Mia Urjansson for excellent technical assistance.

REFERENCES

1. Yki-Jarvinen H, Westerbacka J: The fatty liver and insulin resistance. *Curr Mol Med* 5:287–295, 2005
2. Neuschwander-Tetri BA, Caldwell SH: Nonalcoholic steatohepatitis: summary of an AASLD Single Topic Conference. *Hepatology* 37:1202–1219, 2003
3. Festa A, D'Agostino R Jr, Howard G, et al.: Chronic subclinical inflammation as part of the insulin resistance syndrome: the Insulin Resistance Atherosclerosis Study (IRAS). *Circulation* 102:42–47, 2000
4. Sartipy P, Loskutoff DJ: Monocyte chemoattractant protein 1 in obesity and insulin resistance. *Proc Natl Acad Sci U S A* 100:7265–7270, 2003
5. Weisberg SP, Hunter D, Huber R, Lemieux J, Slaymaker S, Vaddi K, Charo I, Leibel RL, Ferrante AW: CCR2 modulates inflammatory and metabolic effects of high-fat feeding. *J Clin Invest* 116:115–124, 2006
6. Weisberg SP, McCann D, Desai M, et al.: Obesity is associated with macrophage accumulation in adipose tissue. *J Clin Invest* 112:1796–1808, 2003
7. Westerbacka J, Corner A, Kannisto K, et al.: Acute in vivo effects of insulin on gene expression in adipose tissue in insulin-resistant and insulin-sensitive subjects. *Diabetologia* 49:132–140, 2006
8. Xu H, Barnes GT, Yang Q, et al.: Chronic inflammation in fat plays a crucial role in the development of obesity-related insulin resistance. *J Clin Invest* 112:1821–1830, 2003
9. Alessi MC, Bastelica D, Mavri A, et al.: Plasma PAI-1 levels are more strongly related to liver steatosis than to adipose tissue accumulation. *Arterioscler Thromb Vasc Biol* 23:1262–1268, 2003
10. Yki-Jarvinen H, Sutinen J, Silveira A, et al.: Regulation of plasma PAI-1 concentrations in HAART-associated lipodystrophy during rosiglitazone therapy. *Arterioscler Thromb Vasc Biol* 23:688–694, 2003
11. Donnelly KL, Smith CI, Schwarzenberg SJ, et al.: Sources of fatty acids stored in liver and secreted via lipoproteins in patients with nonalcoholic fatty liver disease. *J Clin Invest* 115:1343–1351, 2005
12. Doege H, Baillie RA, Ortegon AM, et al.: Targeted deletion of FATP5 reveals multiple functions in liver metabolism: alterations in hepatic lipid homeostasis. *Gastroenterology* 130:1245–1258, 2006
13. Maeda K, Cao H, Kono K, et al.: Adipocyte/macrophage fatty acid binding proteins control integrated metabolic responses in obesity and diabetes. *Cell Metab* 1:107–119, 2005
14. Newberry EP, Xie Y, Kennedy SM, et al.: Protection against Western diet-induced obesity and hepatic steatosis in liver fatty acid-binding protein knockout mice. *Hepatology* 44:1191–1205, 2006
15. Gavrilova O, Haluzik M, Matsusue K, et al.: Liver peroxisome proliferator-activated receptor gamma contributes to hepatic steatosis, triglyceride clearance, and regulation of body fat mass. *J Biol Chem* 278:34268–34276, 2003
16. Sutinen J, Kannisto K, Korsheninnikova E, et al.: Effects of rosiglitazone on gene expression in subcutaneous adipose tissue in highly active antiretroviral therapy-associated lipodystrophy. *Am J Physiol Endocrinol Metab* 286:E941–E949, 2004
17. Younossi ZM, Baranova A, Ziegler K, et al.: A genomic and proteomic study of the spectrum of nonalcoholic fatty liver disease. *Hepatology* 42:665–674, 2005
18. Younossi ZM, Gorreta F, Ong JP, et al.: Hepatic gene expression in patients with obesity-related non-alcoholic steatohepatitis. *Liver Int* 25:760–771, 2005
19. Chiappini F, Barrier A, Saffroy R, et al.: Exploration of global gene expression in human liver steatosis by high-density oligonucleotide microarray. *Lab Invest* 86:154–165, 2006
20. Haukeland JW, Damas JK, Konopski Z, et al.: Systemic inflammation in nonalcoholic fatty liver disease is characterized by elevated levels of CCL2. *J Hepatol* 44:1167–1174, 2006
21. Chmurzynska A: The multigene family of fatty acid-binding proteins (FABPs): function, structure and polymorphism. *J Appl Genet* 47:39–48, 2006
22. Amri EZ, Bertrand B, Ailhaud G: Regulation of adipose cell differentiation. I. Fatty acids are inducers of the aP2 gene expression. *J Lipid Res* 32:1449–1456, 1991
23. Makowski L, Boord JB, Maeda K, et al.: Lack of macrophage fatty-acid-binding protein aP2 protects mice deficient in apolipoprotein E against atherosclerosis. *Nat Med* 7:699–705, 2001
24. Krieg P, Feil S, Furstenberger G, et al.: Tumor-specific overexpression of a novel keratinocyte lipid-binding protein: identification and characterization of a cloned sequence activated during multistage carcinogenesis in mouse skin. *J Biol Chem* 268:17362–17369, 1993
25. Memon RA, Fuller J, Moser AH, et al.: Regulation of putative fatty acid transporters and Acyl-CoA synthetase in liver and adipose tissue in *ob/ob* mice. *Diabetes* 48:121–127, 1999
26. Kirchgessner TG, Svenson KL, Lusis AJ, et al.: The sequence of cDNA encoding lipoprotein lipase: a member of a lipase gene family. *J Biol Chem* 262:8463–8466, 1987
27. Zhang Y, Repa JJ, Gauthier K, et al.: Regulation of lipoprotein lipase by the oxysterol receptors, LXRalpha and LXRbeta. *J Biol Chem* 276:43018–43024, 2001
28. Enerback S, Semb H, Tavernier J, et al.: Tissue-specific regulation of guinea pig lipoprotein lipase: effects of nutritional state and of tumor necrosis factor on mRNA levels in adipose tissue, heart, and liver. *Gene* 64:97–106, 1988
29. Chajek T, Stein O, Stein Y: Pre- and post-natal development of lipoprotein lipase and hepatic triglyceride hydrolase activity in rat tissues. *Atherosclerosis* 26:549–561, 1977
30. Kim JK, Fillmore JJ, Chen Y, et al.: Tissue-specific overexpression of lipoprotein lipase causes tissue-specific insulin resistance. *Proc Natl Acad Sci U S A* 98:7522–7527, 2001
31. Ong JM, Kern PA: Effect of feeding and obesity on lipoprotein lipase activity, immunoreactive protein, and messenger RNA levels in human adipose tissue. *J Clin Invest* 84:305–311, 1989
32. Coleman RA, Lewin TM, Van Horn CG, et al.: Do long-chain acyl-CoA synthetases regulate fatty acid entry into synthetic versus degradative pathways? *J Nutr* 132:2123–2126, 2002
33. Mashek DG, Li LO, Coleman RA: Rat long-chain acyl-CoA synthetase mRNA, protein, and activity vary in tissue distribution and in response to diet. *J Lipid Res* 47:2004–2010, 2006
34. Mashek DG, McKenzie MA, Van Horn CG, et al.: Rat long chain acyl-CoA synthetase 5 increases fatty acid uptake and partitioning to cellular triacylglycerol in McArdle-RH7777 cells. *J Biol Chem* 281:945–950, 2006
35. Kang MJ, Fujino T, Sasano H, et al.: A novel arachidonate-preferring acyl-CoA synthetase is present in steroidogenic cells of the rat adrenal, ovary, and testis. *Proc Natl Acad Sci U S A* 94:2880–2884, 1997
36. Matsusue K, Haluzik M, Lambert G, et al.: Liver-specific disruption of PPARgamma in leptin-deficient mice improves fatty liver but aggravates diabetic phenotypes. *J Clin Invest* 111:737–747, 2003
37. Yu S, Matsusue K, Kashireddy P, et al.: Adipocyte-specific gene expression and adipogenic steatosis in the mouse liver due to peroxisome proliferator-activated receptor gamma1 (PPARgamma1) overexpression. *J Biol Chem* 278:498–505, 2003
38. Schadinger SE, Bucher NL, Schreiber BM, et al.: PPARgamma2 regulates lipogenesis and lipid accumulation in steatotic hepatocytes. *Am J Physiol Endocrinol Metab* 288:E1195–E1205, 2005

39. Ferre P: The biology of peroxisome proliferator-activated receptors: relationship with lipid metabolism and insulin sensitivity. *Diabetes* 53 (Suppl. 1):S43–S50, 2004

40. Tiikkainen M, Bergholm R, Vehkavaara S, et al.: Effects of identical weight loss on body composition and features of insulin resistance in obese women with high and low liver fat content. *Diabetes* 52:701–707, 2003

41. Pietilainen KH, Rissanen A, Kaprio J, et al.: Acquired obesity is associated with increased liver fat, intra-abdominal fat, and insulin resistance in young adult monozygotic twins. *Am J Physiol Endocrinol Metab* 288: E768–E774, 2005

42. Westerbacka J, Lammi K, Hakkinen AM, et al.: Dietary fat content modifies liver fat in overweight nondiabetic subjects. *J Clin Endocrinol Metab* 90:2804–2809, 2005

43. Sampath H, Miyazaki M, Dobrzyn A, et al.: Stearoyl CoA desaturase-1 mediates the pro-lipogenic effects of dietary saturated fat. *J Biol Chem* 282:2483–2493, 2007

44. Lin J, Yang R, Tarr PT, et al.: Hyperlipidemic effects of dietary saturated fats mediated through PGC-1beta coactivation of SREBP. *Cell* 120:261–273, 2005

45. Miyazaki M, Kim YC, Gray-Keller MP, et al.: The biosynthesis of hepatic cholesterol esters and triglycerides is impaired in mice with a disruption of the gene for stearoyl-CoA desaturase 1. *J Biol Chem* 275:30132–30138, 2000

46. Rosen ED, Spiegelman BM: PPARgamma: a nuclear regulator of metabolism, differentiation, and cell growth. *J Biol Chem* 276:37731–37734, 2001

47. Sun X, Han R, Wang Z, et al.: Regulation of adiponectin receptors in hepatocytes by the peroxisome proliferator-activated receptor-gamma agonist rosiglitazone. *Diabetologia* 49:1303–1310, 2006

48. Yki-Jarvinen H: Thiazolidinediones. *N Engl J Med* 351:1106–1118, 2004

Should Nonalcoholic Fatty Liver Disease Be Included in the Definition of Metabolic Syndrome?

A cross-sectional comparison with Adult Treatment Panel III criteria in nonobese nondiabetic subjects

Giovanni Musso, md[1]
Roberto Gambino, md[2]
Simona Bo, md[2]
Barbara Uberti, md[2]

Giampaolo Biroli, md[2]
Gianfranco Pagano, md[2]
Maurizio Cassader, md[2]

OBJECTIVE — The ability of the Adult Treatment Panel III (ATP III) criteria of metabolic syndrome to identify insulin-resistant subjects at increased cardiovascular risk is suboptimal, especially in the absence of obesity and diabetes. Nonalcoholic fatty liver disease (NAFLD) is associated with insulin resistance and is emerging as an independent cardiovascular risk factor. We compared the strength of the associations of ATP III criteria and of NAFLD to insulin resistance, oxidative stress, and endothelial dysfunction in nonobese nondiabetic subjects.

RESEARCH DESIGN AND METHODS — Homeostasis model assessment of insulin resistance (HOMA-IR) >2, oxidative stress (nitrotyrosine), soluble adhesion molecules (intracellular adhesion molecule-1, vascular cell adhesion molecule-1, and E-selectin), and circulating adipokines (tumor necrosis factor-α, leptin, adiponectin, and resistin) were cross-sectionally correlated to ATP III criteria and to NAFLD in 197 unselected nonobese nondiabetic subjects.

RESULTS — NAFLD more accurately predicted insulin resistance than ATP III criteria: sensitivity 73 vs. 38% ($P = 0.0001$); positive predictive value: 81 vs. 62% ($P = 0.035$); negative predictive value 87 vs. 74% ($P = 0.012$); positive likelihood ratio 4.39 vs. 1.64 ($P = 0.0001$); and negative likelihood ratio 0.14 vs. 0.35 ($P = 0.0001$). Adding NAFLD to ATP III criteria significantly improved their diagnostic accuracy for insulin resistance. Furthermore, NAFLD independently predicted HOMA-IR, nitrotyrosine, and soluble adhesion molecules on logistic regression analysis; the presence of NAFLD entailed more severe oxidative stress and endothelial dysfunction, independent of adiposity or any feature of the metabolic syndrome in insulin-resistant subjects.

CONCLUSIONS — NAFLD is more tightly associated with insulin resistance and with markers of oxidative stress and endothelial dysfunction than with ATP III criteria in nonobese nondiabetic subjects and may help identify individuals with increased cardiometabolic risk in this population.

Diabetes Care 31:562–568, 2008

From the [1]Gradenigo Hospital, Turin, Italy; and the [2]Department of Internal Medicine, University of Turin, Turin, Italy.

Address correspondence and reprint requests to Giovanni Musso, Gradenigo Hospital, Corso R. Margherita 8, 10132 Turin, Italy. E-mail: giovanni_musso@yahoo.it.

Received for publication 3 August 2007 and accepted in revised form 19 November 2007.

Published ahead of print at http://care.diabetesjournals.org on 4 December 2007. DOI: 10.2337/dc07-1526.

Additional information for this article can be found in an online appendix at http://dx.doi.org/10.2337/dc07-1526.

Abbreviations: ALT, alanine aminotransferase; ATP III, Adult Treatment Panel III; HOMA-IR, homeostasis model assessment of insulin resistance; ICAM-1, intercellular adhesion molecule-1; NAFLD, nonalcoholic fatty liver disease; OGTT, oral glucose tolerance test; TNF-α, tumor necrosis factor-α; VCAM-1, vascular cell adhesion molecule-1.

Metabolic syndrome is a cluster of metabolic and cardiovascular risk factors that sharing the hallmark of insulin resistance; its prevalence according to Adult Treatment Panel III (ATP III) criteria is 20% among Western adults (1). Insulin resistance is an independent predictor of cardiovascular disease and type 2 diabetes and should be identified and treated early (2–5).

Nonalcoholic fatty liver disease (NAFLD) is the most common chronic liver disease in Western countries (1). NAFLD predicts incident diabetes independent of classic risk factors and C-reactive protein in large prospective cohort studies and may therefore be an early marker of mechanisms predisposing to future metabolic events (1,6). In a parallel way, NAFLD is emerging as a marker of early atherosclerosis: liver enzymes predicted incident cardiovascular disease independent of traditional risk factors, C-reactive protein and metabolic syndrome, and liver histology correlated with early carotid atherosclerosis in NAFLD, suggesting that the vessels and the liver share common inflammatory mediators (7–9).

Despite the number of studies connecting fatty liver to insulin resistance, it is still unclear whether a diagnosis of NAFLD can help identify apparently healthy individuals with an increased cardiometabolic risk more accurately than current diagnostic criteria. ATP III criteria for metabolic syndrome correlate fairly well with insulin resistance (sensitivity of 46% and specificity of 76% for insulin resistance, respectively) in the general population, and this association is weaker in the absence of obesity and diabetes (10–13).

By directly comparing subjects with NAFLD with insulin-resistant subjects without fatty liver, we tested the hypotheses that 1) NAFLD might be more tightly associated with insulin resistance than current ATP III criteria in nonobese nondiabetic subjects and 2) fatty liver per se conveys a higher cardiovascular risk in otherwise healthy insulin-resistant subjects, independent of insulin resistance, metabolic syndrome, and circulating adipokines.

RESEARCH DESIGN AND METHODS

A total of 197 Caucasians (87 women, age range 24–63 years, BMI range 19.9–29.9 kg/m²) were selected from a population-based cohort participating in previous institutional studies over the past 5 years (14). All were nondiabetic and nonobese, in good general health, and with normal findings on medical history, physical examination, blood count, and chemical screening battery. Insulin resistance was defined by a homeostasis model assessment of insulin resistance (HOMA-IR) index >2. The HOMA-IR index closely correlated with clamp measures in nondiabetic Northern Italian subjects (15) and with oral glucose tolerance test (OGTT)-derived indexes of insulin sensitivity in our subjects with NAFLD (G.M., unpublished data); furthermore, a cutoff value >2 predicted insulin resistance and increased cardiovascular risk in the general population independent of traditional risk factors (2–4,14,15).

NAFLD was diagnosed by persistently (>6 months) elevated aminotransferases (defined by alanine aminotransferase [ALT] ≥30 units/l in men and ≥20 units/l in women, based on recently proposed cutoff values, which increase the sensitivity for detection of NAFLD) (16,17) and ultrasonographic bright liver with no other liver disease; histological confirmation was available for 66% of the subjects. Exclusion criteria were a history of alcohol consumption >70 g/week (assessed by a detailed inquiry of patients and relatives and a validated questionnaire filled in daily for 1 week by the patients); diabetes (fasting plasma glucose ≥126 mg/dl or ≥200 mg/dl at +2 h with a standard oral glucose load on an OGTT); obesity (BMI ≥30 kg/m²); positive serum markers of viral disease; and exposure to occupational hepatotoxins or to drugs known to be steatogenic or to affect glucose metabolism.

Modified ATP III criteria for the diagnosis of metabolic syndrome were the following: hypertension (systolic/diastolic blood pressure ≥130/85 mmHg or receiving antihypertensive therapy); hypertriglyceridemia (fasting plasma triglycerides ≥150 mg/dl [1.7 mmol/l] or

Table 1—*Main characteristics of study subjects according to HOMA-IR index*

	Insulin sensitive: HOMA-IR ≤2	Insulin resistant: HOMA-IR >2	P value
n	129	68	
Age (years)	47 ± 12	44 ± 10	0.083
Sex (male/female)	72/57	38/30	0.928
BMI (kg/m²)	25.0 ± 2.0	25.8 ± 2.2	0.030
Overweight (% subjects)	39	71	0.000
% Smokers	40	38	0.931
Waist (cm)	88 ± 8	92 ± 8	0.005
Systolic BP (mmHg)	130 ± 14	131 ± 16	0.700
Diastolic BP (mmHg)	81 ± 8	87 ± 9	0.009
Triglycerides (mmol/l)	1.32 ± 0.59	1.47 ± 0.75	0.198
Total cholesterol (mmol/l)	5.53 ± 0.96	5.69 ± 1.06	0.126
HDL cholesterol (mmol/l)	1.53 ± 0.28	1.29 ± 0.28	0.0002
Triglyceride-to-HDL ratio	2.2 ± 1.2	2.7 ± 1.6	0.037
LDL cholesterol (mmol/l)	3.39 ± 0.85	3.52 ± 0.93	0.406
Glucose (mmol/l)	4.83 ± 0.68	5.08 ± 0.62	0.032
Insulin (pmol/l)	32.2 ± 12.0	116.7 ± 55.2	0.0002
HOMA-IR	0.90 ± 0.67	3.74 ± 2.01	0.0001
AST (units/l)	17 ± 9	29 ± 16	0.0001
ALT (units/l)	24 ± 11	61 ± 16	0.0001
GGT (units/l)	27 ± 31	76 ± 63	0.0001
Resistin (ng/ml)	3.35 ± 0.22	3.62 ± 0.24	0.729
Adiponectin (ng/ml)	9851 ± 639	5401 ± 349	0.0002
Leptin (pg/ml)	7988 ± 1289	8247 ± 1502	0.863
TNF-α (pg/ml)	1.35 ± 0.18	1.49 ± 0.24	0.546
C-reactive protein (mg/l)	1.11 ± 1.01	2.96 ± 1.86	0.002
Nitrotyrosine (mmol/ml)	5.1 ± 6.0	19.9 ± 17.6	0.00001
E-selectin (mg/ml)	22.7 ± 11.5	36.1 ± 10.9	0.0001
ICAM-1 (mg/ml)	203.6 ± 46.4	241.8 ± 28.9	0.0002
VCAM-1 (mg/ml)	448.6 ± 155.4	486.7 ± 138.6	0.043
Metabolic syndrome (ATP III) (% subjects)	11	38	0.0003
NAFLD (% subjects)	8	73	0.0001

Data are means ± SD unless indicated otherwise. AST, aspartate aminotransferase; BP, blood pressure; GGT, γ-glutamyl transferase.

receiving lipid-lowering therapy; low plasma HDL cholesterol (<40 mg/dl [1.03 mmol/l] in men and <50 mg/dl [1.29 mmol/l]) in women]); impaired glucose regulation (impaired fasting glycemia, i.e., fasting plasma glucose ≥100 but <126 mg/dl [5.6–7.0 mmol/l] or impaired glucose tolerance, i.e., plasma glucose ≥140 mg/dl [7.8 mmol/l] at +2 h on an OGTT]; or abdominal obesity, modified according to ethnic-specific cutoff values to increase sensitivity for "metabolically obese" lean subjects (for Europeans, cutoff ranges were a waist circumference >94 cm [37 inches] in men and >80 cm [31 inches] in women) (12). A diagnosis of metabolic syndrome required fulfillment of at least three criteria.

Oxidative stress
Nitrosative stress is believed to be involved in diabetic endothelial dysfunc-

tion and cardiovascular complications (1) and in liver oxidative injury in NAFLD (18,19). Fasting plasma nitrotyrosine, as a marker of nitrosative stress, was determined by a commercial ELISA kit product by HyCult Biotechnology (Pantec, Turin, Italy).

Endothelial dysfunction
Soluble adhesion molecules E-selectin, vascular cell adhesion molecule-1 (VCAM-1), and intercellular adhesion molecule 1 (ICAM-1) have been associated with endothelial dysfunction and early cardiovascular disease (20,21). Serum E-selectin, VCAM-1, and ICAM-1 levels were measured by a solid-phase ELISA (R&D Systems, Minneapolis, MN). Minimal detectable doses and intra- and interassay coefficients of variation (CVs) were, respectively, <0.1 ng/ml, 4.7–5.0%, and 7.4–8.8%, 0.17–1.26 pg/ml,

Table 2—Comparison of the ability of the individual components of the metabolic syndrome, of metabolic syndrome overall, and of NAFLD to identify insulin-resistant subjects

	No. of case subjects			Sensitivity × IR	Specificity × IR	PPV × IR	NPV × IR	LR+ × IR	LR− × IR
	Total	IR	IS						
Obesity	77	35	42	0.54 (0.40–0.68)	0.68 (0.59–0.77)	0.46 (0.33–0.59)	0.75 (0.66–0.84)	0.84 (0.71–0.97)	0.33 (0.29–0.49)
IGR	76	35	41	0.54 (0.40–0.68)	0.69 (0.59–0.78)	0.46 (0.33–0.59)	0.75 (0.66–0.84)	0.87 (0.66–0.84)	0.33 (0.26–0.40)
Triglycerides	46	22	24	0.33 (0.20–0.47)	0.82 (0.75–0.90)	0.48 (0.31–0.66)	0.71 (0.63–0.80)	0.94 (0.73–1.15)	0.40 (0.32–0.48)
HDL	16	13	3	0.21 (0.09–0.32)	0.98 (0.96–1.00)	0.83 (0.67–0.99)	0.71 (0.64–0.79)	5.00 (4.00–6.00)	0.40 (0.33–0.47)
Hypertension	103	47	57	0.73 (0.60–0.85)	0.57 (0.47–0.67)	0.45 (0.34–0.57)	0.81 (0.72–0.90)	0.83 (0.70–0.95)	0.23 (0.19–0.27)
Overall cases of MS:									
ATP III	40	26	14	0.38 (0.24–0.51)	0.89 (0.82–0.95)	0.62 (0.44–0.80)	0.74 (0.66–0.82)	1.64 (1.16–2.12)	0.35 (0.30–0.40)
NAFLD	59	49	10	0.73 (0.60–0.85)*	0.92 (0.86–0.97)	0.81 (0.70–0.93)†	0.87 (0.81–0.94)†	4.90 (4.01–5.79)*	0.14 (0.12–0.16)*
Overall cases of MS: ATP III + NAFLD	64	47	17	0.69 (0.58–0.84)*	0.87 (0.80–0.93)	0.72 (0.59–0.85)	0.85 (0.78–0.92)†	2.53 (2.07–2.99)†	0.18 (0.16–0.20)*

95% CIs are reported in parentheses. *$P < 0.001$ vs. ATP III criteria. †$P < 0.01$ vs. ATP III criteria. ‡$P < 0.05$ vs. ATP III criteria. IGR, impaired glucose regulation; IR, insulin resistance; IS, insulin sensitive; LR+, positive likelihood ratio; LR−, negative likelihood ratio; MS, metabolic syndrome; NPV, negative predictive value; PPV, positive predictive value.

2.3–3.6%, and 5.5–7.8%, and <0.1 ng/ml, 4.7–5.0%, and 7.4–8.8%.

Adipokines

Serum tumor necrosis factor-α (TNF-α), leptin, and adiponectin were measured by a sandwich ELISA (R&D Systems Europe, Abingdon, UK). For TNF-α the kit has a sensitivity of 0.12 pg/ml in a 200-μl sample size and a range of 0.5 to 32 pg/ml. Intra- and interassay CVs were 5.9 and 12.6%, respectively. For adiponectin, the kit has a sensitivity of 0.25 pg/ml in a 50-μl sample size and a range of 3.9 to 250 ng/ml. The intra- and interassay CVs were 3.4 and 5.8%, respectively. Resistin was measured by a biotin-labeled antibody-based sandwich enzyme immunoassay (BioVendor Laboratory Medicine, Brno, Czech Republic).

Statistics

Data are expressed as means ± SD. Differences between groups were analyzed by ANOVA when variables were normally distributed; otherwise (for triglycerides, insulin, HOMA-IR, adipokines, nitrotyrosine, and adhesion molecules), the Mann-Whitney test was used. A χ^2 test was used to compare categorical variables. Normality was evaluated by the Shapiro-Wilk test. For multiple comparisons, ANOVA and the Kruskal-Wallis test, followed by the Bonferroni correction or a Dunn test, were used, as appropriate. Spearman correlation coefficients were used to estimate the relationship between variables. Logistic regression analysis was applied when multiple associations were detected on univariate analysis. Differences were considered statistically significant if $P < 0.05$.

Sensitivity, specificity, positive and negative predictive value, and likelihood ratios of different criteria for the presence of insulin resistance were calculated. The positive likelihood ratio is the true-positive rate divided by the false-positive rate; the negative likelihood ratio is the inverse of the true-negative rate divided by the false-negative rate. For each parameter 95% CIs were provided.

RESULTS — Of the subjects, 50% were overweight (39% of insulin-sensitive and 71% of insulin-resistant subjects) (Table 1). The prevalence of NAFLD was 30% (8% in insulin-sensitive and 73% in insulin-resistant subjects). Insulin-resistant subjects also had higher circulating markers of oxidative stress and

Table 3—*Main characteristics of insulin-resistant subjects grouped according to the presence of NAFLD*

	IR, NAFLD	IR, no NAFLD	P value
n			
Age (years)	45 ± 10	48 ± 7	0.313
Sex (male/female)	29/5	10/6	0.277
BMI (kg/m^2)	25.6 ± 2.1	26.3 ± 2.5	0.350
Overweight (% subjects)	61	74	0.786
Smokers (%)	35	42	0.921
Waist (cm)	92 ± 7	94 ± 8	0.112
Systolic BP (mmHg)	130 ± 14	128 ± 14	0.468
Diastolic BP (mmHg)	87 ± 8	87 ± 12	0.920
Triglycerides (mmol/l)	1.34 ± 0.69	1.78 ± 0.83	0.091
Total cholesterol (mmol/l)	6.39 ± 1.24	5.64 ± 0.98	0.282
HDL cholesterol (mmol/l)	1.27 ± 0.21	1.42 ± 0.39	0.173
Triglyceride-to-HDL ratio	2.5 ± 1.4	3.2 ± 2.3	0.252
LDL cholesterol (mmol/l)	3.69 ± 0.72	3.36 ± 0.98	0.195
Glucose (mmol/l)	5.14 ± 0.61	4.89 ± 0.83	0.189
Insulin (pmol/l)	125.6 ± 68.9	105.7 ± 59.1	0.279
HOMA-IR	3.78 ± 2.27	2.88 ± 2.06	0.178
AST (units/l)	35 ± 12	15 ± 5	0.0001
ALT (units/l)	78 ± 21	17 ± 9	0.0001
GGT (units/l)	97 ± 89	21 ± 12	0.0003
C-reactive protein (mg/l)	2.91 ± 1.25	2.02 ± 1.12	0.391
Nitrotyrosine(mmol/ml)	27.1 ± 18.9	9.9 ± 7.6	0.002
E-selectin (mg/ml)	51.3 ± 17.1	32.7 ± 16.6	0.004
ICAM-1(mg/ml)	261.2 ± 38.5	225.6 ± 24.0	0.002
VCAM-1(mg/ml)	512.5 ± 141.5	474.2 ± 113.9	0.191
Abdominal obesity (% subjects)	50	64	0.559
Impaired glucose regulation (% subjects)	78	44	0.115
Hypertension (% subjects)	74	71	0.835
Hypertriglyceridemia (% subjects)	29	43	0.217
Low HDL cholesterol (% subjects)	24	14	0.745
Metabolic syndrome (ATP III) (% subjects)	32	50	0.412

Data are means ± SD unless indicated otherwise. AST, aspartate aminotransferase; GGT, γ-glutamyl transferase; IR, insulin resistance.

endothelial dysfunction and lower adiponectin levels.

The prevalence of different features of the metabolic syndrome and of NAFLD were higher in insulin-resistant subjects. Seventy-three percent of insulin-resistant versus 43% of insulin-sensitive subjects were hypertensive (P = 0.001), 54% of insulin-resistant versus 32% of insulin-sensitive subjects had abdominal obesity (P = 0.017), 33% of insulin-resistant versus 18% of insulin-sensitive subjects were hypertriglyceridemic (P = 0.054), 21% of insulin-resistant versus 2% of insulin-sensitive subjects had low HDL cholesterol, and 54% of insulin-resistant versus 31% of insulin-sensitive control subjects had impaired glucose regulation (P = 0.012). The prevalence of metabolic syndrome was 20% according to ATP III criteria (12).

Relationship of ATP III criteria and NAFLD to insulin resistance

Table 2 shows the relationship of different ATP III criteria and of NAFLD to insulin resistance. Hypertension and NAFLD were the most sensitive (73% for both) and had the highest negative predictive value (81 and 87%, respectively) for insulin resistance. The negative likelihood ratio (i.e., the extent to which the odds of insulin resistance decrease if the test result is negative) was greatest with hypertension (0.23) and NAFLD (0.14). HDL cholesterol and NAFLD were most specific for insulin resistance (98 and 92%, respectively) and had the highest positive predictive value (83 and 81%, respectively) and positive likelihood ratio (i.e., the odds of insulin resistance if the test result is positive: 5.00 and 4.39, respectively).

ATP III criteria had a positive predictive value of 62% for the presence of insulin resistance; the addition of NAFLD to ATP criteria yielded a prevalence of metabolic syndrome of 32%, with a positive predictive value for insulin resistance of 72%. The sensitivity of ATP III criteria for insulin resistance was 38%, but rose to 69% with the inclusion of NAFLD as a criterion (P = 0.002). The specificity of ATP III criteria for insulin resistance was 89% without NAFLD and 87% with NAFLD (P = 0.002). The positive likelihood ratio for insulin resistance increased from 1.64 to 2.53 when NAFLD was included (P = 0.010), whereas the negative likelihood ratio, i.e., the odds of insulin resistance in the absence of a certain condition, decreased from 35 to 18% with the inclusion of NAFLD in the diagnostic criteria of metabolic syndrome (P = 0.0002).

Insulin resistance with NAFLD versus insulin resistance without fatty liver

With subgrouping of insulin-resistant subjects according to the presence of NAFLD, patients with NAFLD had higher levels of nitrotyrosine and of soluble adhesion molecules than subjects without fatty liver (Table 3).

Correlative analysis

The main Spearman correlation coefficients are presented in Table 1 of the online appendix (available at http://dx.doi.org/10.2337/dc07-1526). HOMA-IR correlated with age, ALT (Fig. 1 of the online appendix), HDL cholesterol, triglyceride-to-HDL cholesterol ratio, C-reactive protein, adiponectin, nitrotyrosine, waist, adhesion molecules, and the number of ATP criteria.

On logistic regression analysis, HOMA-IR >2 was independently predicted by NAFLD, adiponectin, and nitrotyrosine (Table 4). Nitrotyrosine was independently predicted by NAFLD and C-reactive protein, NAFLD (β = 0.36; P = 0.008) and HOMA-IR independently predicted E-selectin, ICAM-1 was independently predicted by ALT and adiponectin, and adiponectin predicted VCAM-1 (Table 4).

CONCLUSIONS — By directly comparing NAFLD with ATP III criteria for metabolic syndrome in nonobese nondiabetic subjects, we found that 1) fatty liver, as diagnosed by ALT levels and ul-

Table 4—*Logistic regression analysis for factors associated with insulin resistance (HOMA-IR >2), plasma nitrotyrosine, and soluble adhesion molecule levels in study subjects*

Factor	Odds ratio	95% CI	P value
Insulin resistance (HOMA-IR >2)			
Age (quartiles)	1.4	0.5–2.5	0.791
NAFLD (present vs. absent)	2.8	1.9–4.3	0.007
HDL cholesterol (quartiles)	1.7	0.6–6.2	0.100
Triglyceride-to-HDL cholesterol ratio (quartiles)	1.5	0.6–3.9	0.231
C-reactive protein (quartiles)	1.6	0.7–2.8	0.072
Adiponectin (quartiles)	1.8	1.0–3.4	0.045
Nitrotyrosine (quartiles)	2.1	1.6–3.1	0.021
Waist (quartiles)	1.1	0.5–2.2	0.692
No. ATP III criteria	1.5	0.4–2.9	0.571
Nitrotyrosine (upper quartile)			
Age (quartiles)	1.2	0.8–3.1	0.680
NAFLD (present vs. absent)	3.2	2.0–4.8	0.002
HOMA-IR (quartiles)	1.5	1.2–2.8	0.112
No. ATP III criteria	1.7	1.0–2.9	0.213
HDL cholesterol (quartiles)	1.4	0.6–3.2	0.427
C-reactive protein (quartiles)	2.0	1.5–3.9	0.038
E-selectin (upper quartile)			
NAFLD (present vs. absent)	1.9	1.5–2.6	0.009
BMI (quartiles)	1.3	0.6–2.3	0.238
TNF-α (quartiles)	1.1	0.4–2.1	0.85
Triglyceride-to-HDL cholesterol ratio (quartiles)	1.0	0.6–1.5	0.871
No. ATP III criteria	1.3	0.8–2.1	0.276
HOMA-IR (quartiles)	1.7	1.4–2.3	0.01
C-reactive protein (quartiles)	1.4	0.9–1.9	0.457
ICAM-1 (upper quartile)			
NAFLD (present vs. absent)	1.8	1.4–2.5	0.010
BMI (quartiles)	0.9	0.4–1.8	0.348
Adiponectin (quartiles)	1.7	1.3–2.1	0.015
HOMA-IR (quartiles)	1.5	1.2–2.4	0.079
No. ATP III metabolic syndrome criteria	1.2	0.9–2.9	0.575
VCAM-1 (upper quartile)			
NAFLD (present vs. absent)	1.7	1.3–2.9	0.069
Adiponectin (quartiles)	1.9	1.5–2.7	0.008
HOMA-IR (quartiles)	1.5	0.9–3.2	0.134
C-reactive protein (quartiles)	1.6	1.2–3.5	0.397

n = 197.

trasonography, is more closely associated to insulin resistance than to ATP III criteria and 2) the presence of NAFLD in insulin-resistant subjects implies more severe systemic oxidative stress and endothelial dysfunction, independently of metabolic syndrome, adiposity, and adipokines.

The aim of the ATP III criteria is to identify individuals at increased risk for cardiovascular disease and diabetes to allow early treatment. Current ATP III criteria were selected because they tend to cluster together, share insulin resistance as their common denominator, and have individually been associated with an increased cardiovascular risk. However, they correlate weakly with the presence of

insulin resistance, having a sensitivity and positive predictive value of 46 and 76%, respectively, in the general population (10). Because of their low sensitivity, many cases of insulin resistance remain undiagnosed, particularly in nonobese nondiabetic subjects, in whom the diagnosis of metabolic syndrome is less assisted by obesity and glucose criteria (10–13).

ATP III criteria consistently identified only 39% of insulin-resistant subjects in our population, with a positive predictive value of 62% and a positive likelihood ratio of 1.64. The presence of NAFLD alone doubled the sensitivity and significantly elevated positive predictive value and positive likelihood ratio, keeping the

same specificity for insulin resistance (92% vs. 89%). The addition of NAFLD to the ATP III criteria improved their sensitivity by 72%, from 39 to 69%, with only a slight decrease in specificity, from 89 to 87%. Pathogenetically, these findings suggest that in nonobese nondiabetic subjects hepatic fat accumulation is more tightly related to insulin resistance than visceral adiposity, as estimated by waist circumference or any other feature of the metabolic syndrome, as defined by ATP III criteria.

The mechanism(s) underlying the association between NAFLD and insulin resistance are under investigation, but impaired hepatic lipid and lipoprotein handling and increased oxidative stress may enhance liver fat accumulation and lead to insulin resistance by nuclear factor-κB pathway activation (22–26). Increased nitrosative stress, in particular, seems to be operating in NAFLD even in the absence of insulin resistance (27).

The second intriguing finding relates to the additive information that NAFLD carries in the setting of insulin resistance. Patients with NAFLD displayed more severe oxidative stress and endothelial dysfunction than nonsteatotic insulin-resistant subjects, despite similar HOMA-IR and adiposity, and NAFLD independently entailed more severe oxidative stress and endothelial dysfunction.

Nitrotyrosine is an index of peroxynitrite formation, which is believed to play a key role in diabetic endothelial dysfunction and in liver oxidative injury in NAFLD (18,19). Mechanisms underlying increased oxidative stress in NAFLD cannot be elucidated in our study, but impaired mitochondrial β-oxidation, dietary saturated fat excess, and reduced antioxidant intake have been proposed (22,23,26). Increased oxidative stress can induce not only steatosis but also necroinflammation and fibrosis in NAFLD: high oxidative stress experimentally impaired VLDL secretion, leading to hepatocyte triglyceride accumulation (24,28); oxidation end products trigger the inflammatory cascade and extracellular matrix deposition, paralleling the severity of liver fibrosis in NAFLD (23).

Soluble adhesion molecule levels were higher in NAFLD than in insulin resistance without fatty liver, and fatty liver predicted increased E-selectin and ICAM-1 levels independently of HOMA-IR, adipokines, and visceral fat accumulation. Plasma concentrations of these molecules were consistently related to incident cardiovascular disease in apparently healthy individuals in large prospective studies (20,21). Our findings therefore suggest that NAFLD may be an early marker of endothelial dysfunction, independently of insulin resistance and traditional risk factors (7). Mechanism(s) linking NALFD to endothelial dysfunction are unclear, but impaired lipoprotein metabolism and oxidized LDL accumulation are potential candidates (22,23,26, 27).

In nonobese, nondiabetic insulin-resistant subjects, the presence of NAFLD may therefore indicate a host of unsuspected derangements in oxidative balance and endothelial function, not routinely assessed, that contribute to increased cardiovascular disease risk: in day-to-day clinical practice, a diagnosis of NAFLD would simply require chronically elevated liver enzyme levels, an ultrasonographic bright liver, and exclusion of viral infection and of exposure to hepatotoxins (including alcohol) by interview of patient and relatives. Early identification of such patients at higher cardiometabolic risk may trigger earlier lifestyle and pharmacological interventions. Consistently, therapeutic measures in NAFLD also ameliorate insulin sensitivity and cardiovascular risk profile, the ultimate goal of a diagnosis of metabolic syndrome (29–31).

Further studies are required to test the validity of this proposal and to overcome the limitations of our study: its cross-sectional nature, which prevents any causal inference, and the absence of obese and diabetic subjects. However, the prevalence of NAFLD and insulin resistance is even higher in obesity and diabetes, so the association between NAFLD and insulin resistance could be further strengthened. Consistent with previous findings, lower sex-specific ALT cutoff levels identified insulin-resistant subjects more accurately (16,17). However, because liver fat content was not directly measured, some control subjects might have fatty liver despite normal ultrasound and liver enzyme levels; even so, this definition of NAFLD proved to be useful in clinical practice. Furthermore, misclassification of NAFLD would attenuate the magnitude of the difference in oxidative stress and endothelial dysfunction observed toward the null hypothesis, making our results a conservative estimate of the relationship between NAFLD, oxidative stress, and endothelial dysfunction.

References

1. Bloomgarden ZT: Second World Congress on the Insulin Resistance Syndrome: insulin resistance syndrome and nonalcoholic fatty liver disease. *Diabetes Care* 28:1518–1523, 2005
2. Saely CH, Aczel S, Marte T, Langer P, Hoefle G, Drexel H: The metabolic syndrome, insulin resistance, and cardiovascular risk in diabetic and nondiabetic patients. *J Clin Endocrinol Metab* 90:698–703, 2005
3. Resnick HE, Jones K, Ruotolo G, Jain AK, Henderson J, Lu W, Howard BV: Strong Heart Study: insulin resistance, the metabolic syndrome, and risk of incident cardiovascular disease in nondiabetic American Indians: the Strong Heart Study. *Diabetes Care* 26:861–867, 2003
4. Bonora E, Kiechl S, Willeit J, Oberhollenzer F, Egger G, Meigs JB, Bonadonna RC, Muggeo M: Insulin resistance as estimated by homeostasis model assessment predicts incident symptomatic cardiovascular disease in Caucasian subjects from the general population: the Bruneck study. *Diabetes Care* 30:318–324, 2007
5. Yokoyama H, Emoto M, Fujiwara S, Motoyama K, Morioka T, Komatsu M, Tahara H, Shoji T, Okuno Y, Nishizawa Y: Quantitative insulin sensitivity check index and the reciprocal index of homeostasis model assessment in normal range weight and moderately obese type 2 diabetic patients. *Diabetes Care* 26:2426–2432, 2003
6. Sattar N, Scherbakova O, Ford I, O'Reilly DSJ, Stanley A, Forrest E, Macfarlane PW, Packard CJ, Cobbe SM, Shepherd J: Elevated alanine aminotransferase predicts new-onset type 2 diabetes independently of classical risk factors, metabolic syndrome, and C-reactive protein in the West of Scotland Coronary Prevention Study. *Diabetes* 53:2855–2860, 2004
7. Schindhelm RK, Dekker JM, Nijpels G, Bouter LM, Stehouwer CD, Heine RJ, Diamant M: Alanine aminotransferase predicts coronary heart disease events: a 10-year follow-up of the Hoorn Study. *Atherosclerosis* 191:391–396, 2007
8. Targher G, Bertolini L, Poli F, Rodella S, Scala L, Tessari R, Zenari L, Falezza G: Nonalcoholic fatty liver disease and risk of future cardiovascular events among type 2 diabetic patients. *Diabetes* 54:3541–3546, 2005
9. Targher G, Bertolini L, Padovani R, Rodella S, Zoppini G, Zenari L, Cigolini M, Falezza G, Arcaro G: Relations between carotid artery wall thickness and liver histology in subjects with nonalcoholic fatty liver disease. *Diabetes Care* 29:1325–1330, 2006
10. St-Onge MP, Janssen L, Heymsfield SB: Metabolic syndrome in normal-weight Americans. *Diabetes Care* 27:2222–2228, 2004
11. Cheal KL, Abbasi F, Lamendola C, McLaughlin T, Reaven GM, Ford ES: Relationship to insulin resistance of the adult treatment panel III diagnostic criteria for identification of the metabolic syndrome. *Diabetes* 53:1195–1200, 2004
12. Grundy SM, Cleeman JI, Daniels SR, Donato KA, Eckel RH, Franklin BA, Gordon DJ, Krauss RM, Savage PJ, Smith SC Jr, Spertus JA, Costa F, American Heart Association, National Heart, Lung, and Blood Institute: Diagnosis and management of. the metabolic syndrome: an AHA/NHLBI Scientific Statement. *Circulation* 112:2735–2752, 2005
13. Hu G, Qiao Q, Tuomilehto J, Balkau B, Borch-Johnsen K, Pyorala K: Prevalence of the metabolic syndrome and its relation to all-cause and cardiovascular mortality in nondiabetic European men and women. *Arch Intern Med* 164:1066–1076, 2004
14. Bo S, Gambino R, Uberti B, Mangiameli MP, Colosso G, Repetti E, Gentile L, Cassader M, Pagano GF: Does C-reactive protein identify a subclinical metabolic disease in healthy subjects? *Eur J Clin Invest* 35:265–270, 2005
15. Bonora E, Targher G, Alberiche M, Bonadonna RC, Saggiani F, Zenere MB, Monauni T, Muggeo M: Homeostasis model assessment closely mirrors the glucose clamp technique in the assessment of insulin sensitivity: studies in subjects with various degrees of glucose tolerance and insulin sensitivity. *Diabetes Care* 23:57–63, 2000
16. Prati D, Taioli E, Zanella A, Della Torre E, Butelli S, Del Vecchio E, Vianello L, Zanuso F, Mozzi F, Milani S, Conte D, Colombo M, Sirchia G: Updated definitions ranges for serum alanine aminotransferase levels. *Ann Intern Med* 137:1–9, 2002
17. Chang Y, Ryu S, Sung E, Jang Y: Higher concentrations of alanine aminotransferase within the reference interval predict nonalcoholic fatty liver disease. *Clin Chem* 53:686–692, 2007
18. Pacher P, Szabo C: Role of peroxynitrite in the pathogenesis of cardiovascular complications of diabetes. *Curr Opin Pharmacol* 6:136–141, 2006
19. Sanyal AJ, Campbell-Sargent C, Mirshahi F, Rizzo WB, Contos MJ, Sterling RK, Luketic VA, Shiffman ML, Clore JN: Nonalcoholic steatohepatitis: association of insulin resistance and mitochondrial abnormalities. *Gastroenterology* 120:1183–1192, 2001
20. Hwang SJ, Ballantyne CM, Sharrett AR, Smith LC, Davis CE, Gotto AM Jr, Boerwinkle E: Circulating adhesion molecules VCAM-1, ICAM-1, and E-selectin in carotid atherosclerosis and incident coronary heart disease cases. *Circulation* 96:4219–4225, 1997
21. Ridker PM, Hennekens CH, Roitman-

Johnson B, Stampfer MJ, Allen J: Plasma concentration of soluble intercellular adhesion molecule 1 and risks of future myocardial infarction in apparently healthy men. *Lancet* 351:88–92, 1998

22. Musso G, Gambino R, Durazzo M, Biroli G, Carello M, Faga E, Pacini G, De Michieli F, Rabbione L, Premoli A, Cassader M, Pagano G: Adipokines in NASH: postprandial lipid metabolism as a link between adiponectin and liver disease. *Hepatology* 42:1175–1183, 2005

23. Musso G, Cassader M, Gambino R, Durazzo M, Pagano G: Association between postprandial LDL conjugated dienes and the severity of liver fibrosis in NASH. *Hepatology* 43:1169–1170, 2006

24. Pan M, Cederbaum AI, Zhang YL, Ginsberg HW, Williams KJ, Fisher FA: Lipid peroxidation and oxidant stress regulate hepatic apolipoprotein B degradation and VLDL production. *J Clin Invest* 113:1277–1287, 2004

25. Gambino R, Cassader M, Pagano G, Durazzo M, Musso G: Polymorphism in microsomal triglyceride transfer protein: a link between liver disease and athero-genic postprandial lipid profile in NASH? *Hepatology* 45:1097–1107, 2007

26. Musso G, Gambino R, De Michieli F, Cassader M, Rizzetto M, Durazzo M, Fagà E, Silli B, Pagano G: Dietary habits and their relations to insulin resistance and postprandial lipemia in non-alcoholic steatohepatitis. *Hepatology* 37:909–916, 2003

27. Musso G, Gambino R, De Michieli F, Biroli G, Premoli A, Pagano G, Bo S, Durazzo M, Cassader M: Nitrosative stress predicts the presence and severity of non-alcoholic fatty liver at different stages of the development of insulin resistance and metabolic syndrome: possible role of vitamin A intake. *Am J Clin Nutr* 86:661–671, 2007

28. Botham KM, Zheng X, Napoletano M, Avella M, Cavallai C, Rivabene R, Bravo E: The effects of dietary n-3 polyunsaturated fatty acids delivered in chylomicron remnants on the transcription of genes regulating synthesis and secretion of very-low-density lipoprotein by the liver: modulation by cellular oxidative state. *Exp Biol Med (Maywood)* 228:143–151, 2003

29. Athyros VG, Mikhailidis DP, Didangelos TP, Giouleme OI, Liberopoulos EN, Karagiannis A, Kakafika AI, Tziomalos K, Burroughs AK, Elisaf MS: Effect of multifactorial treatment on non-alcoholic fatty liver disease in metabolic syndrome: a randomized study. *Curr Med Res Opin* 22:873–883, 2006

30. DREAM (Diabetes REduction Assessment with ramipril and rosiglitazone Medication) Trial Investigators, Gerstein HC, Yusuf S, Bosch J, Pogue J, Sheridan P, Dinccag N, Hanefeld M, Hoogwerf B, Laakso M, Mohan V, Shaw J, Zinman B, Holman RR: Effect of rosiglitazone on the frequency of diabetes in patients with impaired glucose tolerance or impaired fasting glucose: a randomised controlled trial. *Lancet* 368:1096–1105, 2006

31. Huang MA, Greenson JK, Chao C, Anderson L, Peterman D, Jacobson J, Emick D, Lok AS, Conjeevaram HS: One-year intense nutritional counseling results in histological improvement in patients with non-alcoholic steatohepatitis: a pilot study. *Am J Gastroenterol* 100:1072–1081, 2005

Serum Adipocyte Fatty Acid–Binding Protein Levels Are Associated With Nonalcoholic Fatty Liver Disease in Type 2 Diabetic Patients

Jang Hyun Koh, md[1]
Young Goo Shin, md, phd[2]
Soo Min Nam, md[2]

Mi Young Lee, md[2]
Choon Hee Chung, md, phd[2]
Jang Yel Shin, md[2]

OBJECTIVE — Adipocyte fatty acid–binding protein (A-FABP) is a major cytoplasmic protein in adipocytes and macrophages and is closely associated with metabolic syndrome, type 2 diabetes, and atherosclerosis. Here, we investigated whether A-FABP was associated with nonalcoholic fatty liver disease (NAFLD) in type 2 diabetes.

RESEARCH DESIGN AND METHODS — We enrolled 181 type 2 diabetic patients. Clinical and biochemical metabolic parameters were measured. The severity of NAFLD was measured by ultrasound. A-FABP, adiponectin, and retinol-binding protein-4 (RBP-4) were determined by enzyme-linked immunosorbent assay.

RESULTS — A-FABP levels, defined as more than a moderate degree of fatty liver compared with men, those without metabolic syndrome, and those without NAFLD, were higher in women, patients with metabolic syndrome, and patients with overt NAFLD, respectively. Adiponectin was decreased according to the severity of NAFLD, but RBP-4 showed no difference. Age- and sex-adjusted A-FABP showed positive correlations with BMI, waist-to-hip ratio, waist circumference, triglycerides, γ-glutamyltransferase, fasting insulin, homeostasis model assessment of insulin resistance (HOMA-IR), A1C, and C-reactive protein (CRP) but showed negative correlation with HDL cholesterol. The odds ratio (OR) for the risk of overt NAFLD with increasing levels of sex-specific A-FABP was significantly increased (OR 2.90 [95% CI 1.15–7.29] vs. 7.87 [3.20–19.38]). The OR in the highest tertile of A-FABP remained significant after adjustments for BMI, waist circumference, A1C, HDL cholesterol, triglycerides, HOMA-IR, CRP, and hepatic enzymes.

CONCLUSIONS — Our study demonstrates that serum A-FABP is significantly associated with NAFLD in type 2 diabetes, independent of BMI, waist circumference, HOMA-IR, A1C, triglycerides, HDL cholesterol, and CRP.

Diabetes Care 32:147–152, 2009

Nonalcoholic fatty liver disease (NAFLD) is one of the most common causes of chronic elevation of hepatic enzymes in the general population without known liver disease. NAFLD is observed in 20–30% of the total population (1) and in 75% of type 2 diabetic patients (2,3) in developed countries. NAFLD is characterized by hepatic insulin resistance. In epidemiologic studies, NAFLD has been reported to be closely associated with obesity, dyslipidemia, and diabetes (4–6). In prospective studies, NAFLD was a risk factor for type 2 diabetes and cardiovascular disease independent of the classic risk factors (7,8). Hence, NAFLD is considered a hepatic manifestation of metabolic syndrome.

Adipocyte fatty acid–binding protein (A-FABP; also known as FABP-4 or aP2)

is a major cytoplasmic protein and is involved in the regulation of lipid metabolism. A-FABP is expressed abundantly in mature adipocytes and activated macrophages. A-FABP binds fatty acid ligands with high affinity and functions in intracellular fatty acid trafficking, regulation of lipid metabolism, and modulation of gene expression (9,10). In obese mice lacking A-FABP, dyslipidemia and peripheral insulin resistance are improved and β-cell function is preserved (11). Boord et al. (12) reported that combined adipocyte-macrophage fatty acid–binding protein deficiency improves glucose and lipid metabolism, reduces atherosclerosis, and improves survival in apoE[-/-] mice. In cross-sectional studies, A-FABP was closely associated with obesity and metabolic syndrome (13,14). In prospective studies, A-FABP levels predicted the development of metabolic syndrome and type 2 diabetes (15,16). Furthermore, Yeung et al. (17) reported that A-FABP levels were independently associated with carotid atherosclerosis. Tuncman et al. (18) reported that individuals with an aP2 variant had lower triglycerides and a reduced risk of coronary heart disease and obesity-induced type 2 diabetes. These findings suggested that A-FABP is closely associated with insulin resistance and plays a central role in the development of metabolic syndrome, type 2 diabetes, and atherosclerosis. Maeda et al. (19) demonstrated protection against fatty liver disease in mice lacking aP2 and mal1 on high-fat diet. However, a relationship between A-FABP and NAFLD, a hepatic manifestation of metabolic syndrome, has not yet been established in a human study.

We hypothesized that patients with NAFLD might have higher A-FABP levels and that A-FABP might show a positive correlation with the severity of NAFLD on ultrasound. To test this hypothesis, we investigated the relationship between serum A-FABP levels and NAFLD in type 2 diabetic patients.

From the [1]Health Promotion Center, Samsung Seoul Hospital, Sungkyunkwan University School of Medicine, Seoul, Korea; and the [2]Department of Internal Medicine, Yonsei University, Wonju College of Medicine, Wonju, Korea.
Corresponding author: Jang Yel Shin, sjy3290@yonsei.ac.kr.
Received 25 July 2008 and accepted 18 September 2008.
Published ahead of print at http://care.diabetesjournals.org on 3 October 2008. DOI: 10.2337/dc08-1379.

RESEARCH DESIGN AND METHODS

— We enrolled 181 type 2 diabetic subjects using the following inclusion criteria: *1*) ages >35 and <75 years, *2*) serum creatinine levels less than 1.4 mg/dl and albumin excretion rate less than 300 mg/day, *3*) hepatic enzymes levels less than three times upper normal, and *4*) alcohol consumption less than 20 g/day. Patients with known hepatic disease, cardiovascular disease, acute or chronic inflammation, and malignancy were excluded. The mean age of the subjects was 54.3 ± 10.4 years, and 55.2% of the total subjects were male. The protocol was approved by the ethics committee of Yonsei University Wonju College of Medicine. All of the subjects gave written informed consent, and all of the reported investigations were carried out according to the principles of the Declaration of Helsinki (the year 2000 revision).

Alcohol intake, smoking habits, medication history, and medical history were assessed using a standardized questionnaire. Anthropometric data including weight, height, waist and hip circumference, and blood pressure were assessed. BMI was calculated as weight in kilograms divided by the square of height in meters (kg/m^2). All blood samples were obtained after overnight fasting. Fasting plasma glucose, insulin, A1C, urine albumin excretion rate, hepatic enzyme levels, high-sensitivity C-reactive protein (CRP), and lipid profiles were measured.

All of the abdominal ultrasounds were performed by the same specialist. The severity of NAFLD on ultrasound was graded as follows: mild (grade 1), defined as a slight diffuse increase in liver echogenicity in the hepatic parenchyma with normal visualization of the diaphragm and the portal veins; moderate (grade 2), defined as a moderately diffuse increase in liver echogenicity with a slightly impaired visualization of the diaphragm and the portal veins; and severe (grade 3), defined as a marked increase in liver echogenicity with poor or no visualization of the diaphragm and the portal veins. We defined overt NAFLD in this study as more than a moderate degree of fatty liver.

Adiponectin and retinol-binding protein-4 (RBP-4) levels were determined by ELISA (Adipogen, Seoul, Korea). A-FABP levels were also assessed by ELISA (Bio vendor Laboratory Medicine, Modrice, Czech Republic). Insulin resistance was measured by the homeostasis model of assessment for insulin resistance (HOMA-IR). The HOMA-IR index was calculated

using the following formula: fasting plasma glucose (mg/dl) × fasting insulin /405 (μU/ml).

Statistical analyses

Statistical analysis was performed using SPSS (version 13.0; SPSS, Chicago, IL). Data are presented as means ± SD and as a number (in percentages) for categorical measures. Data that were not normally distributed were logarithmically transformed before analysis. For continuous variables, the differences between groups were compared using either an unpaired Student's *t* test or one-way ANOVA. The χ^2 test was used to compare categorical variables between groups. Correlations of A-FABP with various metabolic parame-

Table 1—*Characteristics of the subjects according to the severity of fatty liver*

	Normal	Mild	Moderate	P
n	42	78	61	
Age (years)	53.4 ± 10.5	54.0 ± 9.3	55.2 ± 11.8	0.7
Sex (male %)	64.3	57.7	45.9	0.2
Hypertension (%)	52.4	34.6	44.1	0.2
Current smoker (%)	26.2	23.1	11.5	0.1
PPARγ agonists use (%)	9.5	5.1	8.2	0.6
Insulin use (%)	7.1	5.1	1.6	0.4
ARB and ACEi use (%)	40.5	21.8	23.0	0.06
Statins use (%)	21.4	12.8	19.7	0.4
Diabetes duration (years)	6.7 ± 6.0	4.6 ± 4.7	4.6 ± 6.3	0.1
Systolic BP (mmHg)	129.6 ± 21.1	131.5 ± 13.7	134.8 ± 17.2	0.3
Diastolic BP (mmHg)	75.4 ± 15.0	77.1 ± 8.2	78.7 ± 11.6	0.4
BMI (kg/m^2)	24.0 ± 2.3	25.3 ± 3.3*	27.1 ± 3.4‡	<0.001
Waist circumference (cm)	84.8 ± 8.0	88.1 ± 7.5*	91.2 ± 8.7‡	<0.001
Male	85.8 ± 7.1	88.6 ± 6.7	92.7 ± 6.7†	0.001
Female	83.1 ± 9.4	87.4 ± 8.5	91.8 ± 10.1†	0.01
WHR	0.91 ± 0.06	0.93 ± 0.05*	0.94 ± 0.05†	0.003
Total cholesterol (mg/dl)	180.3 ± 34.4	193.4 ± 39.5	190.3 ± 39.1	0.2
Triglycerides (mg/dl)	149.4 ± 101.8	182.0 ± 115.1	186.7 ± 83.4	0.2
HDL cholesterol (mg/dl)	50.0 ± 13.1	48.0 ± 12.1	47.8 ± 8.8	0.6
Male	48.8 ± 9.4	46.6 ± 10.2	48.1 ± 8.7	0.6
Female	52.1 ± 18.3	49.4 ± 14.4	47.5 ± 8.9	0.5
LDL cholesterol (mg/dl)	104.9 ± 30.8	112.4 ± 36.6	111.5 ± 33.7	0.5
AST (units/l)	20.5 ± 6.5	24.9 ± 10.2	33.8 ± 19.2‡	<0.001
ALT (units/l)	23.5 ± 10.2	32.6 ± 22.6*	42.6 ± 24.7‡	<0.001
GGT (units/l)	27.8 ± 18.5	42.0 ± 35.9*	52.1 ± 41.9†	0.003
A-FABP total (μg/l)	13.9 ± 10.1	15.9 ± 10.1	24.7 ± 17.9‡	<0.001
Male	12.3 ± 9.0	13.6 ± 10.2	15.9 ± 6.6	0.3
Female	16.7 ± 11.6	19.1 ± 9.3	32.2 ± 20.9†	0.001
RBP-4 total (μg/ml)	72.7 ± 28.7	74.1 ± 32.6	72.1 ± 26.1	0.9
Male	76.2 ± 23.3	83.3 ± 38.1	77.8 ± 23.6	0.6
Female	66.3 ± 36.5	61.6 ± 17.0	67.3 ± 27.5	0.7
Adiponectin total (μg/ml)	5.0 ± 2.2	4.1 ± 2.6*	3.8 ± 2.3†	0.03
Male	5.1 ± 2.2	3.5 ± 2.0†	2.7 ± 1.2‡	<0.001
Female	5.0 ± 2.3	4.9 ± 3.2	4.7 ± 2.5	0.9
CRP (mg/l)	1.50 ± 2.50	2.39 ± 4.46	3.60 ± 4.66*	0.04
FPG (mg/dl)	207.9 ± 142.5	180.0 ± 68.8	174.5 ± 58.5	0.2
Fasting insulin (μU/ml)	6.4 ± 6.7	7.5 ± 6.1	11.1 ± 8.2†	0.001
HOMA-IR	3.1 ± 3.5	3.1 ± 2.3	4.6 ± 3.6*	0.01
A1C (%)	8.9 ± 2.7	8.2 ± 2.2	8.8 ± 2.0	0.2
24-h albumin (mg/day)	40.3 ± 45.1	31.4 ± 38.6	30.3 ± 40.6	0.5
Serum creatinine (mg/dl)	0.87 ± 0.28	0.78 ± 0.17*	0.80 ± 0.18	0.07
Metabolic syndrome (n [%])	17 (41.5)	55 (71.4)	47 (77.0)	<0.001

Data are means ± SD, unless indicated otherwise. P value: the difference among three groups using ANOVA test. *$P < 0.05$ compared with normal. †$P < 0.01$ compared with normal. ‡$P < 0.001$ compared with normal. ACEi, angiotensin converting enzyme inhibitors; ARB, angiotensin II receptor blockers; ALT, alanine aminotransferase; AST, aspartate aminotransferase; BP, blood pressure; FPG, fasting plasma glucose; GGT, γ-glutamyltransferase.

ters were analyzed using Pearson correlation and multiple regression analysis after adjustments for age and sex. Logistic regression analysis was performed to assess the odds ratio (OR) of the metabolic parameters for the presence of overt NAFLD after adjustments for age and sex. A-FABP levels were grouped into tertiles in a sex-specific manner. Multiple logistic regression analysis was used to assess the OR for the presence of overt NAFLD in subjects with the higher A-FABP tertiles compared with those with the lowest tertile. Two-sided values of $P < 0.05$ were considered significant.

RESULTS

Baseline characteristics of the subjects

Duration of diabetes and mean A1C levels for all of the subjects were 5.1 years and 8.6%, respectively. Of the 181 type 2 diabetic patients, the users of peroxisome proliferator–activated receptor-γ (PPAR-γ) agonists, insulin, statins, and angiotensin-converting enzyme inhibitors and/or angiotensin II receptor blockers were 7.2, 4.4, 17.1, and 26.5%, respectively. The percentage of patients with metabolic syndrome and NAFLD were 66.5 and 76.8%, respectively. As shown in Table 1, all subjects were divided into three subgroups according to the severity of their fatty liver disease: normal, mild degree, and more-than-moderate degree. The proportions of each group were 23.2, 43.1, and 33.7%, respectively. Patients with overt NAFLD had higher BMI, waist circumference, waist-to-hip ratio (WHR), hepatic enzymes, CRP, A-FABP, and HOMA-IR ($P < 0.05$) and had lower adiponectin levels ($P < 0.05$) compared with those without NAFLD. Also, patients with overt NAFLD were more likely to have metabolic syndrome than those without. Serum A-FABP levels were significantly higher in women than men (24.0 ± 16.7 vs. 13.9 ± 9.0 μg/l; $P < 0.001$). Also, A-FABP levels in patients with overt NAFLD and metabolic syndrome were significantly higher than in those without NAFLD (24.7 ± 17.9 vs. 15.3 ± 10.2 μg/l; $P < 0.001$) and those without metabolic syndrome (20.6 ± 14.4 vs. 14.2 ± 12.2 μg/l; $P = 0.004$). A-FABP levels in users of PPAR-γ agonists were slightly higher compared with nonusers, but this difference was not significant.

Table 2—Correlation between A-FABP levels and various metabolic parameters

| | A-FABP* | | | |
| | Model 1 | | Model 2 | |
	r	P	β	P
Male sex	−0.43	<0.001	—	—
PPARγ agonists use	0.09	0.2	—	—
ACEi or ARB use	0.05	0.3	—	—
BMI	0.22	0.003	0.22	0.004
WHR	0.33	<0.001	0.35	<0.001
Waist circumference	0.28	<0.001	0.32	<0.001
Current smoking	−0.22	0.003	−0.03	0.7
Triglycerides*	0.15	0.03	0.20	0.003
HDL cholesterol	−0.18	0.01	−0.17	0.03
GGT*	0.12	0.06	0.22	0.001
Fasting insulin	0.18	0.01	0.17	0.03
HOMA-IR*	0.22	0.003	0.22	0.004
A1C	0.19	0.008	0.23	0.003
Metabolic syndrome	0.31	<0.001	0.25	0.001
CRP*	0.32	<0.001	0.30	<0.001
Adiponectin*	0.09	0.1	—	—

Model 1: Pearson correlation coefficient. Model 2: Regression coefficient adjusted for age and sex. *Log transformed data before analysis. ACEi, angiotensin converting enzyme inhibitors; ARB, angiotensin II receptor blockers; GGT, γ-glutamyltransferase.

Correlations between serum A-FABP levels and various metabolic parameters

As shown in Table 2, age- and sex-adjusted A-FABP showed significant positive correlations with BMI, WHR, waist circumference, triglycerides, γ-glutamyltransferase, fasting insulin, HOMA-IR, A1C, and CRP. However, A-FABP was negatively correlated with HDL cholesterol ($P < 0.05$). However, there were no significant correlations between age- and sex-adjusted A-FABP and adiponectin, RBP-4, and the use of PPAR-γ agonists, statins, or antihypertensive drugs (data not shown).

OR of the metabolic parameters for the presence of overt NAFLD

In multivariate linear regression analysis after adjustment for age and sex, A-FABP was significantly associated with overt NAFLD independent of BMI, waist circumference, HOMA-IR, and A1C ($P < 0.01$) (data not shown). In multiple logistic regression analysis after adjustment for age and sex, high A-FABP was associated with overt NAFLD (OR 2.87 [95% CI 1.47–5.61]; $P = 0.002$). Also, waist circumference, BMI, WHR, HOMA-IR, CRP, triglycerides, aspartate aminotransferase, alanine aminotransferase, and γ-glutamyltransferase were significantly associ-

Table 3—OR of metabolic parameters for the presence of overt fatty liver after adjustment for age and sex

	OR	95% CI	P
BMI	1.24	1.11–1.38	<0.001
Waist circumference	1.07	1.02–1.13	0.003
WHR	2.20	1.18–4.11	0.01
HOMA-IR*	1.46	1.07–1.98	0.02
A-FABP*	2.87	1.47–5.61	0.002
CRP*	2.40	1.36–4.23	0.002
Triglycerides*	1.99	1.07–3.68	0.03
ALT*	3.97	2.10–7.49	<0.001
AST*	7.16	2.93–17.45	<0.001
GGT*	2.55	1.53–4.23	<0.001

Data are OR (95% CI) unless otherwise indicated. *Log transformed data before analysis. ALT, alanine aminotransferase; AST, aspartate aminotransferase; GGT, γ-glutamyltransferase.

Table 4—*Characteristics according to A-FABP tertile levels*

	A-FABP tertile			
	1 (<8.6 μg/l [men], <150 μg/l [women])	2 (8.6–14.3 μg/l [men], 15.0–24.1 μg/l [women])	3 (>14.3 μg/l [men], >24.1 μg/l [women])	P
Age (years)	53.1 ± 8.1	55.3 ± 11.4	54.4 ± 11.4	0.5
BMI (kg/m²)	24.6 ± 3.2	25.8 ± 3.1	26.3 ± 3.5†	0.02
Waist circumference (cm)	85.0 ± 7.0	89.3 ± 7.7†	91.6 ± 9.2‡	<0.001
WHR	0.91 ± 0.05	0.93 ± 0.05*	0.95 ± 0.06‡	0.001
Triglycerides (mg/dl)	148.9 ± 94.1	190.1 ± 124.3*	187.3 ± 82.1*	0.05
HDL cholesterol (mg/dl)	52.6 ± 11.6	45.7 ± 9.3†	46.7 ± 11.9†	0.001
A-FABP (μg/l)	9.0 ± 2.9	14.6 ± 4.2†	31.1 ± 16.9‡	<0.001
RBP-4 (μg/ml)	67.1 ± 19.6	78.6 ± 34.4	73.4 ± 31.5	0.1
Adiponectin (μg/ml)	4.3 ± 2.0	3.9 ± 2.2	4.4 ± 3.0	0.5
CRP (mg/l)	1.70 ± 3.55	2.57 ± 4.14	3.39 ± 4.69*	0.1
FPG (mg/dl)	172.5 ± 69.2	188.2 ± 119.3	192.5 ± 70.4	0.4
Fasting insulin (μU/ml)	7.7 ± 7.6	7.3 ± 6.2	10.1 ± 7.5	0.07
HOMA-IR	3.2 ± 3.3	3.3 ± 3.2	4.3 ± 2.8	0.08
A1C (%)	8.1 ± 2.0	8.6 ± 2.3	9.1 ± 2.4*	0.04
24-h albumin (mg/day)	29.3 ± 38.2	29.0 ± 26.3	40.4 ± 52.6	0.2
Serum creatinine (mg/dl)	0.76 ± 0.16	0.82 ± 0.24	0.84 ± 0.21*	0.1
Estimated GFR (ml/min/1.73 m²)	103.8 ± 19.6	96.5 ± 26.7	94.5 ± 23.4*	0.08
Metabolic syndrome (n [%])	25 (43.1)	46 (76.7)‡	48 (78.7)‡	<0.001

Data are means ± SD unless indicated otherwise. P = the difference among three groups using ANOVA test. * P < 0.05 compared with tertile 1. †P < 0.01 compared with tertile 1. ‡P < 0.001 compared with tertile 1. FPG, fasting plasma glucose.

ated with the presence of overt NAFLD (Table 3). As shown in Table 4, the patients in the highest tertile of sex-specific A-FABP had significantly higher BMI, waist circumference, WHR, triglycerides, A1C, and serum creatinine but had lower HDL cholesterol and estimated glomerular filtration rate (GFR) compared with those in the lowest tertile (P < 0.05). Patients in the higher tertiles of sex-specific A-FABP had higher OR for the presence of overt NAFLD compared with those in the lowest tertile (2.90 [1.15–7.29] vs. 7.87 [3.20–19.38]). The OR in the highest tertile of sex-specific A-FABP remained significant after adjustment for BMI, waist circumference, A1C, HDL cholesterol, HOMA-IR, CRP, triglycerides, and hepatic enzymes (8.53 [2.63–27.65]) (Table 5).

CONCLUSIONS — In the present study, we demonstrate that serum A-

FABP levels in type 2 diabetic patients are closely associated with NAFLD independent of BMI, waist circumference, HOMA-IR, A1C, triglycerides, HDL cholesterol, and CRP levels. Patients in the highest tertile of A-FABP were eight times more likely to have overt NAFLD compared with those in the lowest tertile. In animal studies, there was no protection against fatty liver disease in aP2-deficient mice because of compensation through increased expression of mal1 (20). However, a profound protection against fatty liver disease was shown in aP2-mal1 combined–deficient mice on high-fat diet (19). Also, Cao et al. (21) demonstrated that there was striking protection from liver fatty infiltration in *ob/ob*-aP2-mal1–deficient mice with strong suppression of liver stearoyl-CoA desaturase-1. Furthermore, Furuhashi et al. (22) reported that fatty infiltration of the liver was attenuated and total liver triglyceride content

was reduced in aP2-inhibitor–treated *ob/ob* mice. However, the relationship between A-FABP and fatty liver disease has not yet been established in a human study. This study is the first to demonstrate an association between A-FABP and NAFLD in type 2 diabetic patients. Taken together, these findings suggest that chemical inhibition of A-FABP might show beneficial effects against fatty liver disease.

Like previous studies, serum A-FABP levels in our type 2 diabetic patients were associated with markers of obesity, dyslipidemia, hyperglycemia, insulin resistance, and inflammation. However, there are discrepancies in the correlation between A-FABP and adiponectin. Xu et al. (13) reported that A-FABP in nondiabetic subjects was positively correlated with HOMA-IR but was negatively correlated with adiponectin. On the contrary, Cabre et al. (23) reported that A-FABP in type 2 diabetes was positively correlated with adiponectin but was not correlated with HOMA-IR. In our type 2 diabetic patients, A-FABP was not correlated with adiponectin but was positively correlated with HOMA-IR. Differences in the adiposity of the populations and sex difference of A-FABP and adiponectin levels might partly explain this discrepancy. Recently, Cabre et al. (24) reported that high A-FABP plasma concentrations were as-

Table 5—*OR for the presence of overt fatty liver according to the tertile of sex-specific A-FABP levels*

	OR (95% CI)		
	Tertile 1	Tertile 2	Tertile 3
Model 1	1	2.90 (1.15–7.29)	7.87 (3.20–19.38)
Model 2	1	3.14 (0.99–9.99)	8.53 (2.63–27.65)

Data are OR (95% CI). Model 1: unadjusted. Model 2: model 1 + adjustments for BMI, waist circumference, triglycerides, HDL cholesterol, A1C, HOMA-IR, CRP, alanine aminotransferase, aspartate aminotransferase, and γ-glutamyltransferase.

sociated with high plasma creatinine and low GFR in type 2 diabetic patients. In our study, patients with estimated GFR <60 ml/min per $1.73 m^2$ were only 2.8% of the total subjects. In multiple regression analysis, A-FABP was associated with serum creatinine after adjustments for age, sex, and BMI but was not associated with estimated GFR (data not shown).

Similar to previous studies (15,23), sex difference in A-FABP was observed in our study. A-FABP was significantly higher in women than in men. The sex difference is explained partly by the higher fat and subcutaneous fat percentages in women compared with men because adipose tissue is a major source of circulating A-FABP and A-FABP expression is higher in subcutaneous fat than in visceral fat. In our data, patients with NAFLD had higher A-FABP levels than those without NAFLD. In women, A-FABP levels in patients with overt NAFLD were significantly higher than in those without overt NAFLD. However, it was not significant in men. These findings suggest that A-FABP is a more specific marker of NAFLD in women than in men.

This study has several limitations. One limitation of the present study is that it is cross-sectional. We could not prove a causal link between serum A-FABP levels and the development of NAFLD. Second, we could not analyze our data stratified by sex because of the small sample size. Nevertheless, we assessed the OR for the presence of NAFLD according to the sex-specific tertiles of A-FABP. Third, the severity of NAFLD was assessed by ultrasound in this study but was not confirmed pathologically. Although liver biopsy is the gold standard to assess pathologic grading of NAFLD, it is difficult to perform liver biopsies for the assessment of NAFLD in clinical practice. It has been reported that the sensitivity and specificity of ultrasound in the diagnosis of fatty liver, as assessed on liver biopsy, were 60–94 and 84–95%, respectively (25).

In conclusion, we demonstrated that serum A-FABP was closely associated with NAFLD in type 2 diabetic patients. Our data suggest that A-FABP may be an independent marker of NAFLD in type 2 diabetes, independent of BMI, waist circumference, HOMA-IR, A1C, triglycerides, HDL cholesterol, and CRP levels. Large population-based prospective studies are warranted to confirm whether A-FABP is an independent predictor of NAFLD and whether it plays a causative role in the pathogenesis of NAFLD.

Acknowledgments— No potential conflicts of interest relevant to this article were reported.

References

1. Tilg H, Kaser A: Treatment strategies in nonalcoholic fatty liver disease. *Nat Clin Pract Gastroenterol Hepatol* 2:148–155, 2005
2. Gupte P, Amarapurkar D, Agal S, Baijal R, Kulshrestha P, Pramanik S, Patel N, Madan A, Amarapurkar A, Hafeezunnisa: Non-alcoholic steatohepatitis in type 2 diabetes mellitus. *J Gastroenterol Hepatol* 19: 854–858, 2004
3. Leite NC, Salles GF, Araujo AL, Villela-Nogueira CA, Cardoso CR: Prevalence and associated factors of non-alcoholic fatty liver disease in patients with type-2 diabetes mellitus. *Liver Int* in press, 2008
4. Wanless IR, Lentz JS: Fatty liver hepatitis (steatohepatitis) and obesity: an autopsy study with analysis of risk factors. *Hepatology* 12:1106–1110, 1990
5. Angelico F, Del Ben M, Conti R, Francioso S, Feole K, Fiorello S, Cavallo G, Zalunardo B, Lirussi F, Alessandri C, Violi F: Insulin resistance, the metabolic syndrome, and nonalcoholic fatty liver disease. *J Clin Endocrinol Metab* 90:1578–1582, 2005
6. Kotronen A, Yki-Jarvinen H: Fatty liver: a novel component of the metabolic syndrome. *Arterioscler Thromb Vasc Biol* 28: 27–38, 2008
7. Shibata M, Kihara Y, Taguchi M, Tashiro M, Otsuki M: Nonalcoholic fatty liver disease is a risk factor for type 2 diabetes in middle-aged Japanese men. *Diabetes Care* 30:2940–2944, 2007
8. Brea A, Mosquera D, Martin E, Arizti A, Cordero JL, Ros E: Nonalcoholic fatty liver disease is associated with carotid atherosclerosis: a case-control study. *Arterioscler Thromb Vasc Biol* 25:1045–1050, 2005
9. Coe NR, Bernlohr DA: Physiological properties and functions of intracellular fatty acid binding proteins. *Biochim Biophys Acta* 1391:287–306, 1998
10. Hertzel AV, Bernlohr DA: The mammalian fatty acid-binding protein multigene family: molecular and genetic insights into function. *Trends Endocrinol Metab* 11: 175–180, 2000
11. Uysal KT, Scheja L, Wiesbrock SM, Bonner-Weir S, Hotamisligil GS: Improved glucose and lipid metabolism in genetically obese mice lacking aP2. *Endocrinology* 141:3388–3396, 2000
12. Boord JB, Maeda K, Makowski L, Babaev VR, Fazio S, Linton MF, Hotamisligil GS: Combined adipocyte-macrophage fatty acid-binding protein deficiency improves metabolism, atherosclerosis, and survival in apolipoprotein E-deficient mice. *Circu-*

lation 110:1492–1498, 2004
13. Xu A, Wang Y, Xu JY, Stejskal D, Tam S, Zhang J, Wat NM, Wong WK, Lam KS: Adipocyte fatty acid-binding protein is a plasma biomarker closely associated with obesity and metabolic syndrome. *Clin Chem* 25:405–413, 2006
14. Stejskal D, Karpisek M: Adipocyte fatty acid binding protein in a Caucasian population: a new marker of metabolic syndrome? *Eur J Clin Invest* 36:621–625, 2006
15. Xu A, Tso AW, Cheung BM, Wang Y, Wat NM, Fong CH, Yeung DC, Janus ED, Sham PC, Lam KS: Circulating adipocyte-fatty acid binding protein levels predict the development of the metabolic syndrome: a 5-year prospective study. *Circulation* 115:1537–1543, 2007
16. Tso AW, Xu A, Sham PC, Wat NM, Wang Y, Fong CH, Cheung BM, Janus ED, Lam KS: Serum adipocyte fatty acid binding protein as a new biomarker predicting the development of type 2 diabetes: a 10-year prospective study in a Chinese cohort. *Diabetes Care* 30:2667–2672, 2007
17. Yeung DC, Xu A, Cheung CW, Wat NM, Yau MH, Fong CH, Chau MT, Lam KS: Serum adipocyte fatty acid-binding protein levels were independently associated with carotid atherosclerosis. *Arterioscler Thromb Vasc Biol* 27:1796–1802, 2007
18. Tuncman G, Erbay E, Hom X, De Vivo I, Campos H, Rimm EB, Hotamisligil GS: A genetic variant at the fatty acid-binding protein aP2 locus reduces the risk for hypertriglyceridemia, type 2 diabetes, and cardiovascular disease. *Proc Natl Acad Sci U S A* 103:6970–6975, 2006
19. Maeda K, Cao H, Kono K, Gorgun CZ, Furuhashi M, Uysal KT, Cao Q, Atsumi G, Malone H, Krishnan B, Minokoshi Y, Kahn BB, Parker RA, Hotamisligil GS: Adipocyte/macrophage fatty acid binding proteins control integrated metabolic responses in obesity and diabetes. *Cell Metab* 1:107–119, 2005
20. Hotamisligil GS, Johnson RS, Distel RJ, Ellis R, Papaioannou VE, Spiegelman BM: Uncoupling of obesity from insulin resistance through a targeted mutation in aP2, the adipocyte fatty acid binding protein. *Science* 274:1377–1379, 1996
21. Cao H, Maeda K, Gorgun CZ, Kim HJ, Park SY, Shulman GI, Kim JK, Hotamisligil GS: Regulation of metabolic responses by adipocyte/macrophage fatty acid–binding proteins in leptin-deficient mice. *Diabetes* 55:1915–1922, 2006
22. Furuhashi M, Tuncman G, Gorgun CZ, Makowski L, Atsumi G, Vaillancourt E, Kono K, Babaev VR, Fazio S, Linton MF, Sulsky R, Robl JA, Parker RA, Hotamisligil GS: Treatment of diabetes and atherosclerosis by inhibiting fatty-acid-binding protein aP2. *Nature* 447:959–965
23. Cabre A, Lazaro I, Girona J, Manzanares

JM, Marimon F, Plana N, Heras M, Masana L: Fatty acid binding protein 4 is increased in metabolic syndrome and with thiazolidinedione treatment in diabetic patients. *Atherosclerosis* 195:e150–

e158, 2007
24. Cabre A, Lazaro I, Girona J, Manzanares JM, Marimon F, Plana N, Heras M, Masana L: Plasma fatty acid-binding protein 4 increases with renal dysfunction in type 2 di-

abetic patients without microalbuminuria. *Clin Chem* 54:181–187, 2008
25. Joy D, Thava VR, Scott BB: Diagnosis of fatty liver disease: is biopsy necessary? *Eur J Gastroenterol Hepatol* 15:539–543, 2003

Histological Course of Nonalcoholic Fatty Liver Disease in Japanese Patients

Tight glycemic control, rather than weight reduction, ameliorates liver fibrosis

ERIKA HAMAGUCHI, MD, PHD[1]
TOSHINARI TAKAMURA, MD, PHD[1]
MASARU SAKURAI, MD, PHD[2]
EISHIRO MIZUKOSHI, MD, PHD[3]
YOH ZEN, MD, PHD[4]
YUMIE TAKESHITA, MD, PHD[1]

SEIICHIRO KURITA, MD, PHD[1]
KUNIAKI ARAI, MD, PHD[3]
TATSUYA YAMASHITA, MD, PHD[3]
MOTOKO SASAKI, MD, PHD[5]
YASUNI NAKANUMA, MD, PHD[5]
SHUICHI KANEKO, MD, PHD[3]

OBJECTIVE — The goal of this study was to examine whether metabolic abnormalities are responsible for the histological changes observed in Japanese patients with nonalcoholic fatty liver disease (NAFLD) who have undergone serial liver biopsies.

RESEARCH DESIGN AND METHODS — In total, 39 patients had undergone consecutive liver biopsies. Changes in their clinical data were analyzed, and biopsy specimens were scored histologically for stage.

RESULTS — The median follow-up time was 2.4 years (range 1.0–8.5). Liver fibrosis had improved in 12 patients (30.7%), progressed in 11 patients (28.2%), and remained unchanged in 16 patients (41%). In a Cox proportional hazard model, decrease in A1C and use of insulin were associated with improvement of liver fibrosis independent of age, sex, and BMI. However, ΔA1C was more strongly associated with the improvement of liver fibrosis than use of insulin after adjustment for each other (χ^2; 7.97 vs. 4.58, respectively).

CONCLUSIONS — Tight glycemic control may prevent histological progression in Japanese patients with NAFLD.

Diabetes Care 33:284–286, 2010

A
ccumulating trans-sectional evidence suggests that the presence of multiple metabolic disorders, including obesity, diabetes, dyslipidemia, hypertension, and ultimately metabolic syndrome, are associated with nonalcoholic fatty liver disease (NAFLD) (1). However, it remains unclear which metabolic abnormalities are responsible for the pathological progression of NAFLD, especially in Japanese patients, who generally are not severely obese compared with Western patients.

We retrospectively compared clinical features with the histological changes in the livers of Japanese patients with NAFLD who had undergone serial liver biopsies.

RESEARCH DESIGN AND METHODS

— We recruited 195 patients with clinically suspected NAFLD who had undergone liver biopsies at Kanazawa University Hospital from 1997 through 2008. For details about the study subjects and the exclusion criteria, see supplementary Fig. 1 in the online appendix, available at http://care.diabetesjournals.org/cgi/content/full/dc09-0148/DC1. Of 178 patients diagnosed histologically as having NAFLD, 39 had undergone serial liver biopsies.

Data collection

Clinical information, including age, sex, body measurements, and prevalence of metabolic abnormalities, was obtained for each patient. Venous blood samples drawn for laboratory testing before the liver biopsies were obtained. All subjects had been administered a 75-g oral glucose tolerance test at baseline and at follow-up.

Liver biopsies

Biopsies were obtained after a thorough clinical evaluation and receipt of signed informed consent from each patient. All biopsies were analyzed twice and at separate times randomly by a single pathologist who was blinded to the clinical information and the order in which the biopsies were obtained. The biopsied tissues were scored for steatosis, stage, and grade as described (2), according to the standard criteria for grading and staging of nonalcoholic steatohepatitis proposed by Brunt et al. (3).

For additional details on subjects, data collection methods, liver pathology, and statistical analyses, see supplementary Methods in the online appendix.

RESULTS — The basal clinical and biochemical data from 39 patients with NAFLD are described in supplementary Table 1. Prevalence of type 2 diabetes, hypertension, and dyslipidemia were 77, 36, and 64%, respectively. The median follow-up period was 2.4 years (range 1.0–8.5). Medications for diabetes and medication changes during the follow-up period are described in supplementary Table 2. Seventeen patients treated with oral diabetic agents were switched to insulin therapy after the initial biopsy. No patients initiated pioglitazone during follow-up.

From the [1]Department of Disease Control and Homeostasis, Kanazawa University Graduate School of Medical Science, Ishikawa, Japan; the [2]Department of Epidemiology and Public Health, Kanazawa Medical University, Ishikawa, Japan; the [3]Department of Gastroenterology, Kanazawa University Hospital, Ishikawa, Japan; the [4]Division of Pathology, Kanazawa University Hospital, Ishikawa, Japan; and the [5]Department of Human Pathology, Kanazawa University Graduate School of Medical Science, Ishikawa, Japan.

Corresponding author: Toshinari Takamura, ttakamura@m-kanazawa.jp.

Received 8 February 2009 and accepted 20 October 2009. Published ahead of print at http://care.diabetesjournals.org on 30 October 2009. DOI: 10.2337/dc09-0148.

Table 1—*Baseline and follow-up clinical features and gradients of laboratory markers associated with changes in liver fibrosis in 39 patients with NAFLD*

	Baseline				Follow-up			
	Improved	Stable	Progressed	P	Improved	Stable	Progressed	P
n	12	16	11		12	16	11	—
Simple fatty liver:nonalcoholic steatohepatitis (n)	3:9	9:7	10:1		10:2	9:7	6:5	
Age (years)	51.5 (29–66)	48.5 (20–79)	51.5 (29–66)	0.97				
Sex (M:F)	5:7	12:4	5:7	0.17				
BMI (kg/m^2)	27.5 (23.2–34.1)	27.7 (22.5–44.4)	30.9 (23.4–37.7)	0.74	26.9 (22.8–31.2)	29.1 (24.3–44.8)	30.7 (24.1–36.3)	0.13
Aspartate transaminase (IU/l)	70 (11–106)	29 (14–86)	32 (13–83)	0.05	23 (11–28)	26 (15–71)	24 (14–164)	0.20
Alanine transaminase (IU/l)	71 (10–209)	48 (23–81)	40 (11–162)	0.13	21 (11–53)	36 (21–66)	31 (12–202)	0.10
Fasting plasma glucose (mg/dl)	133 (96–207)	143 (87–414)	111 (76–167)	0.20	103 (93–220)	121 (83–198)	116 (88–199)	0.51
A1C (%)	8.2 (4.7–11.6)	8.0 (4.9–13.6)	6.2 (5.1–9.5)	0.27	6.0 (5.0–9.0)	6.2 (5.0–10.0)	7.0 (6.0–11.0)	0.10
HOMA-IR	3.9 (0.7–5.5)	3.4 (1.9–7.7)	3.9 (1.6–11.1)	0.91	3.1 (1.5–8.5)	3.4 (1.9–7.7)	3.9 (1.6–11.1)	0.76
QUICKI	0.32 (0.29–0.40)	0.31 (0.27–0.34)	0.31 (0.29–0.35)	0.32	0.33 (0.28–0.37)	0.32 (0.30–0.35)	0.31 (0.29–0.34)	0.82
Muscle insulin resistance	2.1 (1.5–4.0)	1.7 (0.3–3.3)	3.0 (2.1–4.4)	0.20	2.0 (1.3–5.9)	2.4 (1.6–4.5)	1.9 (1.3–4.5)	0.80
Hepatic insulin resistance (×10^6)	5.3 (2.3–10.2)	5.0 (2.3–10.0)	3.7 (1.4–10.6)	0.66	3.9 (1.4–9.8)	4.3 (1.9–15.9)	4.5 (2.3–8.8)	0.75
Total cholesterol (mg/dl)	191 (128–276)	187 (129–252)	206 (163–244)	0.57	192 (114–224)	195 (136–273)	194 (162–234)	0.74
Triglycerides (mg/dl)	111 (28–224)	114 (36–204)	96 (36–521)	0.87	104 (22–241)	115 (57–241)	131 (36–173)	0.68
HDL cholesterol (mg/dl)	47 (35–82)	51 (31–73)	48 (20–74)	0.68	53 (40–71)	52 (39–64)	52 (36–79)	0.92
Platelets (×10^4/μl)	21.1 (9.4–30.8)	23.0 (7.0–38.2)	24.3 (20.2–41.2)	0.29	23.3 (14.5–27.6)	21.5 (6.3–31.8)	24.0 (15.2–32.6)	0.60
Ferritin (μg/dl)	185 (13–452)	397 (190–604)	46 (10–347)	0.14	74 (16–211)	162 (110–614)	62 (10–171)	0.05
hs-CRP	0.40 (0.08–7.53)	0.14 (0.02–0.61)	0.06 (0.00–0.30)	0.23	0.09 (0.04–0.23)	0.10 (0.00–0.24)	0.09 (0.00–0.89)	0.89
Type IV collagen 7S (ng/dl)	5.1 (2.7–10.0)	4.1 (3.1–7.2)	3.7 (3.3–4.5)	0.27	3.5 (2.3–3.9)	8.3 (3.2–14.0)	4.0 (3.2–5.0)	0.21
HA (ng/dl)	20.6 (0.0–144.7)	25.5 (11.5–299)	30.4 (0.0–61.7)	0.66	32.8 (0.0–117.2)	24.5 (0.0–570)	24.3 (0.0–140.3)	0.63
P-III-P (U/ml)	0.6 (0.5–1.2)	0.6 (0.4–45.0)	0.5 (0.4–0.6)	0.07	0.6 (0.3–0.8)	0.5 (0.5–233.0)	0.6 (0.4–1.0)	0.96
Diabetes (%)	82	69	64	0.59	82	75	64	0.56
Dyslipidemia (%)	73	63	73	0.95	73	63	73	0.86
Hypertension (%)	64	18	36	0.03	64	18	36	0.10
Metabolic syndrome (%)	73	38	27	0.18	67	50	45	0.43
ΔA1C					−1.9 (−6.0 to 0.4)	−1.2 (−6.1 to 4.4)	0.3 (−1.8 to 7.1)	0.02
ΔBody weight					−4.7 (−10.6 to 10.2)	2.2 (−9.4 to 13.4)	−0.9 (−12.7 to 9.6)	0.04
ΔHOMA-IR					−1.3 (−4.4 to 1.2)	−0.3 (−4.3 to 3.3)	−0.7 (−6.1 to 1.8)	0.81

Data are medians (range) or %. A Kruskal-Wallis test and a χ^2 test were used to compare the continuous and categorical variables among three groups. HA, hyaluronic acid; hs-CRP, high-sensitivity C-reactive protein; P-III-P, procollagen III peptide.

Liver fibrosis improved in 12 patients (30.7%), progressed in 11 patients (28.2%), and remained unchanged in 16 patients (41%). As shown in Table 1, fasting plasma glucose, A1C, insulin resistance indicators, and prevalence of metabolic disorders were not significantly different among the three liver fibrosis groups. In the Cox proportional hazard model (supplementary Table 3), although some of the confidence intervals were very wide because of the small sample size, improvement of liver fibrosis was significantly associated with changes in A1C between the initial and final liver biopsies (ΔA1C) ($P = 0.005$) and use of insulin for the treatment of diabetes ($P = 0.019$). Both ΔA1C and use of insulin were independently associated with the improvement of liver fibrosis after adjusted for each other. However, ΔA1C was more strongly associated with the improvement of liver fibrosis than use of insulin (χ^2; 7.97 vs. 4.58, respectively; supplementary Table 3).

CONCLUSIONS — In the present study, we showed that a change in glycemic control (ΔA1C), but not changes in insulin resistance indicators, was an independent predictor of the progression of liver fibrosis in Japanese patients with NAFLD. This is the first report identifying a change in A1C as a predictor of the histological course in the liver of patients with NAFLD. Two of five previous longitudinal studies have identified obesity, higher BMI, and homeostasis model assessment of insulin resistance (HOMA-IR) as predictors of liver fibrosis progression in Western populations (4,5). The difference between those results and the results of the present study may be due in part to differences in the assessed severity of obesity and insulin resistance between the populations. We previously demonstrated that diabetes is an independent risk factor for the progression of liver fibrosis in hepatitis C (6) and that diabetes accelerates the pathology of nonalcoholic steatohepatitis in the type 2 diabetic rat model OLETF (7).

Liver fibrosis is closely associated with two regulators of fibrosis: transforming growth factor (TGF)-β (8,9) and plasminogen activator inhibitor type 1 (PAI-1) (8,10). High glucose levels induce the expression of TGF-β (11) and PAI-1 (12). We previously reported that the expression of TGF family member genes, PAI-1, and genes involved in fibrogenesis are upregulated in the livers of patients with type 2 diabetes (13,14), suggesting that a diabetic state increases the risk for liver fibrosis.

In the present study, only ΔA1C was associated with the progression of liver fibrosis, but not liver inflammation (data not shown). We speculate that the reduction of A1C inhibits the expression of master genes such as *TGF-β* and *PAI-1* that are involved in the regulation of fibrogenesis, rather than genes involved in liver inflammation, and thereby improves liver fibrosis in NAFLD.

The major limitation of this study was small population size. We could not evaluate the changes of liver histology according to the difference in detail characteristics such as treatment of diabetes. Lower statistical power of this study should be consider when we evaluate the results.

In conclusion, our study suggested that ΔA1C could predict liver fibrosis progression in Japanese patients with NAFLD, and tight glycemic control may ameliorate liver fibrosis. Future large-scale prospective studies are needed to confirm our results.

Acknowledgments — This study was supported in part by a grant-in-aid from the Ministry of Education, Culture, Sports, Science and Technology, Japan.

No potential conflicts of interest relevant to this article were reported.

We thank Dr. Akiko Shimizu, Dr. Tsuguhito Ota, and Dr. Hirofumi Misu for recruiting the patients.

References
1. Duvnjak M, Lerotic I, Barsic N, Tomasic V, Virovic Jukic L, Velagic V. Pathogenesis and management issues for non-alcoholic fatty liver disease. World J Gastroenterol 2007;13:4539–4550
2. Sakurai M, Takamura T, Ota T, Ando H, Akahori H, Kaji K, Sasaki M, Nakanuma Y, Miura K, Kaneko S. Liver steatosis, but not fibrosis, is associated with insulin resistance in nonalcoholic fatty liver disease. J Gastroenterol 2007;42:312–317
3. Brunt EM, Janney CG, Di Bisceglie AM, Neuschwander-Tetri BA, Bacon BR. Nonalcoholic steatohepatitis: a proposal for grading and staging the histological lesions. Am J Gastroenterol 1999;94:2467–2474
4. Ekstedt M, Franzen LE, Mathiesen UL, Thorelius L, Holmqvist M, Bodemar G, Kechagias S. Long-term follow-up of patients with NAFLD and elevated liver enzymes. Hepatology 2006;44:865–873
5. Fassio E, Alvarez E, Dominguez N, Landeira G, Longo C. Natural history of nonalcoholic steatohepatitis: a longitudinal study of repeat liver biopsies. Hepatology 2004;40:820–826
6. Kita Y, Mizukoshi E, Takamura T, Sakurai M, Takata Y, Arai K, Yamashita T, Nakamoto Y, Kaneko S. Impact of diabetes mellitus on prognosis of patients infected with hepatitis C virus. Metabolism 2007;56:1682–1688
7. Ota T, Takamura T, Kurita S, Matsuzawa N, Kita Y, Uno M, Akahori H, Misu H, Sakurai M, Zen Y, Nakanuma Y, Kaneko S. Insulin resistance accelerates a dietary rat model of nonalcoholic steatohepatitis. Gastroenterology 2007;132:282–293
8. Matsuzawa N, Takamura T, Kurita S, Misu H, Ota T, Ando H, Yokoyama M, Honda M, Zen Y, Nakanuma Y, Miyamoto K, Kaneko S. Lipid-induced oxidative stress causes steatohepatitis in mice fed an atherogenic diet. Hepatology 2007;46:1392–1403
9. Uno M, Kurita S, Misu H, Ando H, Ota T, Matsuzawa-Nagata N, Kita Y, Nabemoto S, Akahori H, Zen Y, Nakanuma Y, Kaneko S, Takamura T. Tranilast, an antifibrogenic agent, ameliorates a dietary rat model of nonalcoholic steatohepatitis. Hepatology 2008;48:109–118
10. Bergheim I, Guo L, Davis MA, Lambert JC, Beier JI, Duveau I, Luyendyk JP, Roth RA, Arteel GE. Metformin prevents alcohol-induced liver injury in the mouse: critical role of plasminogen activator inhibitor-1. Gastroenterology 2006;130:2099–2112
11. Sugimoto R, Enjoji M, Kohjima M, Tsuruta S, Fukushima M, Iwao M, Sonta T, Kotoh K, Inoguchi T, Nakamuta M. High glucose stimulates hepatic stellate cells to proliferate and to produce collagen through free radical production and activation of mitogen-activated protein kinase. Liver Int 2005;25:1018–1026
12. Suzuki M, Akimoto K, Hattori Y. Glucose upregulates plasminogen activator inhibitor-1 gene expression in vascular smooth muscle cells. Life Sci 2002;72:59–66
13. Takamura T, Sakurai M, Ota T, Ando H, Honda M, Kaneko S. Genes for systemic vascular complications are differentially expressed in the livers of type 2 diabetic patients. Diabetologia 2004;47:638–647
14. Takeshita Y, Takamura T, Hamaguchi E, Shimizu A, Ota T, Sakurai M, Kaneko S. Tumor necrosis factor-alpha-induced production of plasminogen activator inhibitor 1 and its regulation by pioglitazone and cerivastatin in a nonmalignant human hepatocyte cell line. Metabolism 2006;55:1464–1472

Effect of a 12-Month Intensive Lifestyle Intervention on Hepatic Steatosis in Adults With Type 2 Diabetes

Mariana Lazo, md, scm[1]
Steven F. Solga, md[2]
Alena Horska, phd[3]
Susanne Bonekamp, dvm[2]
Anna Mae Diehl, md[4]
Frederick L. Brancati, md, mhs[1,2]

Lynne E. Wagenknecht, drph[5]
F. Xavier Pi-Sunyer, md, mph[6]
Steven E. Kahn, mb, chb[7]
Jeanne M. Clark, md, mph[1,2]
for the Fatty Liver Subgroup of the
Look AHEAD Research Group

OBJECTIVE — Weight loss through lifestyle changes is recommended for nonalcoholic fatty liver disease (NAFLD). However, its efficacy in patients with type 2 diabetes is unproven.

RESEARCH DESIGN AND METHODS — Look AHEAD (Action for Health in Diabetes) is a 16-center clinical trial with 5,145 overweight or obese adults with type 2 diabetes, who were randomly assigned to an intensive lifestyle intervention (ILI) to induce a minimum weight loss of 7% or a control group who received diabetes support and education (DSE). In the Fatty Liver Ancillary Study, 96 participants completed proton magnetic resonance spectroscopy to quantify hepatic steatosis and tests to exclude other causes of liver disease at baseline and 12 months. We defined steatosis >5.5% as NAFLD.

RESULTS — Participants were 49% women and 68% white. The mean age was 61 years, mean BMI was 35 kg/m^2, mean steatosis was 8.0%, and mean aspartate aminotransferase (AST) and alanine aminotransferase (ALT) were 20.5 and 24.2 units/l, respectively. After 12 months, participants assigned to ILI ($n = 46$) lost more weight (-8.5 vs. -0.05%; $P < 0.01$) than those assigned to DSE and had a greater decline in steatosis (-50.8 vs. -22.8%; $P = 0.04$) and in A1C (-0.7 vs. -0.2%; $P = 0.04$). There were no significant 12-month changes in AST or ALT levels. At 12 months, 26% of DSE participants and 3% (1 of 31) of ILI participants without NAFLD at baseline developed NAFLD ($P < 0.05$).

CONCLUSIONS — A 12-month intensive lifestyle intervention in patients with type 2 diabetes reduces steatosis and incident NAFLD.

Diabetes Care 33:2156–2163, 2010

N onalcoholic fatty liver disease (NAFLD) is one of the most common chronic liver diseases in the general population with up to 20–30% of adults having hepatic steatosis. Furthermore, NAFLD is known to lead to serious liver-related complications and cardiovascular disease, especially in individuals with type 2 diabetes (1,2). Obesity, diabetes, and insulin resistance are the main risk factors for more advanced forms of the disease; up to 70–80% of individuals with NAFLD have insulin resistance or metabolic syndrome (3). Currently, there is no approved therapy, and identifying an effective treatment remains a priority area for research. In their last Medical Position Statement in 2002, the American Gastroenterology Association and American Association for the Study of Liver Diseases stated that "Weight loss should be considered in overweight patients with NAFLD" (4). However, both organizations acknowledged that this recommendation was based on clinical impressions rather than on objective evidence.

Although a number of clinical studies have been conducted since 1990 to assess the effect of lifestyle change and/or weight loss on hepatic steatosis, these studies have differed in treatment intensity and have been limited by small study size, short duration, and the presence of confounding by other factors related to weight changes and NAFLD. In addition, most studies have relied on nonspecific (liver enzymes) or semiquantitative (ultrasound) outcomes to assess changes in hepatic steatosis. Finally, large controlled trials focused on patients with type 2 diabetes are lacking.

To fill this gap, we conducted an ancillary study within the Look AHEAD (Action for Health in Diabetes) trial, a National Institutes of Health–funded, randomized controlled trial investigating the long-term health impact of an intensive lifestyle intervention (ILI) in overweight or obese adults with type 2 diabetes. We hypothesized that the ILI would reduce hepatic steatosis and incident NAFLD compared with those of individuals in the comparison group who received diabetes support and education (DSE).

RESEARCH DESIGN AND METHODS

— This study was conducted at one of the 16 Look AHEAD clinical sites (https://www.lookaheadtrial.org/public/home.cfm). The design of the Look AHEAD trial has been published previously (5). In brief, participants were eligible for the study if they were aged between 45 and 76 years, had type 2 diabetes, had a BMI of at least 25 kg/m^2, and were able to complete a maximal exercise test. For the main Look AHEAD study, participants were excluded if they had known chronic liver disease, cirrhosis, or inflammatory bowel disease requiring

From the [1]Johns Hopkins Bloomberg School of Public Health, Department of Epidemiology, Welch Center for Prevention, Epidemiology and Clinical Research, Baltimore, Maryland; the [2]Johns Hopkins Medicine, Baltimore, Maryland; the [3]Department of Radiology and Radiological Science, Johns Hopkins University School of Medicine, Baltimore, Maryland; the [4]Duke University Medical Center, Durham, North Carolina, the [5]Division of Public Health Sciences, Wake Forest University, Winston-Salem, North Carolina; the [6]Division of Endocrinology, Diabetes and Nutrition, St. Luke's-Roosevelt Hospital Center, Columbia University College of Physicians and Surgeons, New York, New York; and the [7]Division of Metabolism, Endocrinology and Nutrition, Department of Medicine, VA Puget Sound Health Care System and University of Washington, Seattle, Washington.

Corresponding author: Mariana Lazo, mlazo@jhsph.edu.

Received 5 May 2010 and accepted 14 July 2010. Published ahead of print at http://care.diabetesjournals.org on 27 July 2010. DOI: 10.2337/dc10-0856. Clinical trial registry no. NCT00017953, clinicaltrials.gov.

treatment in the past year, consumed >14 alcoholic drinks per week, had prior bariatric surgery, were currently using weight loss medications (e.g., sibutramine, phentermine, and orlistat), or had uncontrolled medical conditions (e.g., A1C >11% or blood pressure ≥160/100 mmHg), chronic use of systemic corticosteroids, or known conditions that would limit their adherence to the study protocol (e.g., inability to engage in moderate exercise) or their life span (e.g., cancer). All participants were required to have a regular source of medical care outside the study.

After random assignment, all 318 participants at The Johns Hopkins University site were invited to participate in the Fatty Liver Ancillary Study; 244 participants in the ILI ($n = 124$) and DSE ($n = 120$) groups agreed. A representative sample of them ($n = 185$) also agreed to undergo proton magnetic resonance spectroscopy (^{1}H MRS) and, of these, 151 had successful ^{1}H MRS at baseline. Of the 151 participants who completed a baseline ^{1}H MRS, 102 successfully underwent a 12-month ^{1}H MRS and were eligible for the current analyses. After exclusion for alcohol consumption (>1 drink/day for women and >2 drinks/day for men) or other potential causes of liver disease (see below) (total $n = 6$), a total of 96 participants were included in the current analyses (Fig. S1, available in an online appendix at http://care. diabetesjournals.org/cgi/content/full/ dc09-0856/DC1).

The study was reviewed and approved by local institutional review board. All participants gave written informed consent.

Measurements

As a part of both the parent Look AHEAD trial and our ancillary study, participants underwent extensive data collection at baseline and 12 months after the intervention. Age, sex, race/ethnicity, and medication use were obtained by questionnaire. Lifetime alcohol use was estimated using the Skinner Lifetime Drinking History (6). Weight, height, and waist circumference were directly measured by trained data collectors using standardized techniques. Blood samples were obtained from all patients after an overnight fast; analyses included serum aminotransferases, A1C (NGSP-certified autoanalyzer [G7 Tosoh] with interassay coefficients of variation [CVs]) of 0.9 and 0.6% for the low- and high-quality con-

trol samples, respectively), creatinine, and lipid levels.

For those who completed the ^{1}H MRS, blood samples were also tested for hepatitis B surface antigen, hepatitis C antibody, α-1-antitrypsin phenotype, iron, transferrin saturation, iron-binding capacity, antinuclear antibodies, antimitochondrial antibodies, and anti–smooth muscle antibodies. After centrifugation, serum for insulin, adipokines, cytokines, and inflammatory markers were frozen at −70°F and subsequently hand transported on dry ice to the Core Laboratory at The Johns Hopkins General Clinical Research Center. After a single thaw, the following assays were performed: interleukin IL-8 (R&D Systems) (interassay CV 10.32% and intra-assay CV 2.33%), IL-10 (R&D Systems) (10.17% and 3.38%), tumor necrosis factor-α (TNF-α) (R&D Systems) (8.79% and 7.0%), insulin (Linco) (8.77% and 5.78%), ghrelin (Linco) (5.72% and 5.17%), resistin (ALPCO Diagnostics) (3.16% and 2.11%), and adiponectin (Linco) (3.5% and 3.6%).

^{1}H MRS was performed on a 1.5-T whole-body scanner (Philips Gyroscan ACS-NT; Philips Medical Systems, Best, the Netherlands). Percent hepatic steatosis was calculated as fat/fat + water as determined from proton magnetic resonance spectra by integration of the respective signals. In our center, the reproducibility of steatosis measurement by ^{1}H MRS was excellent with intra- and interrater intraclass correlation coefficients of 0.99.

Hepatic steatosis was defined as ≥5.5% hepatic fat by ^{1}H-MRS and NAFLD as hepatic steatosis plus alcohol consumption <1 drink/day for women or <2 drinks/day for men and negative serology for hepatitis B and hepatitis C.

To estimate intra-abdominal fat volume, eight axial magnetic resonance T_1-weighted spin echo images were also acquired at vertebral bodies L2–L3 during a single breath-hold and estimated using "NIH Image" (http://rsb.info.nih.gov/nih-image/Default.html). These measurements were also highly reliable (intraclass correlation coefficients 0.96–0.99) (7).

Look AHEAD interventions

A description of the Look AHEAD intervention has been published previously (8). In brief, participants assigned to the ILI were encouraged to lose at least 10% of initial weight at 12 months through a combination of moderate caloric restric-

tion (1,200–1,500 kcal/day for those individuals weighing <114 kg and 1,500–1,800 kcal/day for those weighing >114 kg, with <30% calories from fat and <10% from saturated fat) and increased physical activity with a goal of 175 min of moderate intensity physical activity per week. During the first 6 months, participants attended weekly meetings, including one individual and three group sessions per month. During months 7–12, participants attended monthly individual session and the group sessions.

Participants assigned to the DSE group attended three group sessions per year, which provided general information on nutrition, physical activity, and social support. DSE participants were given no individual goals, were not weighed during the sessions, and received no counseling in behavioral strategies for changing diet and physical activity.

Statistical analysis

Twelve-month changes in measures of adiposity, biochemical and metabolic parameters, adipokines and cytokines, and medication use by group were assessed using ANCOVA. Despite the randomized design of the parent study, our study groups were not comparable in all respects. To address these imbalances, we adjusted all of our analyses by differences in sex, baseline weight, and baseline hepatic steatosis.

We analyzed changes in steatosis using two approaches: first as the absolute difference between 12 months and baseline (change steatosis = steatosis [percent]) at 12 months minus steatosis [percent] at baseline) and then as relative difference (percent change steatosis = [(steatosis [percent] at 12 months minus steatosis [percent] at baseline)/steatosis [percent] at baseline] × 100). Because the distribution of percent change in steatosis was skewed, we used quintile regression methods to model the median percent change steatosis from baseline to 12 months in hepatic steatosis in the ILI compared with the DSE group, adjusting for other covariates.

We used multivariate regression analyses to assess the influence of potential mediators of the intervention including changes in weight and other measures of adiposity, metabolic parameters, and adipokines and cytokines. First, we assessed the role of changes in other adiposity deposits. Second, we evaluated changes in metabolic parameters and, third, we determined changes in adipokines and cytokines. All

Table 1—*Baseline and 1-year characteristics of Look AHEAD participants*

Variable	ILI (intervention)			
	Baseline	1 year	Absolute change	Relative change
n			46	
Measures of adiposity				
Hepatic fat	4.2 (2.3−7.2)*	2.9 (1.3−3.9)	−2.3 (−4.3 to −0.4)	−50.8 (−66.9 to −27.8)
0−1 (%)	7 (15.2)	8 (17.4)		
1.1−5.49 (%)	24 (52.2)	29 (63.0)		
5.5−10 (%)	5 (10.9)	5 (10.9)		
10.1−20 (%)	8 (17.4)	3 (6.5)		
>20 (%)	2 (4.4)	1 (2.2)		
BMI	34.7 ± 5.4	32.1 ± 5.2	−2.6 ± 2.6	−7.3 ± 6.8
25−29.9 kg/m^2	8 (17.4)	15 (68.2)		
30−34.9 kg/m^2	21 (44.7)	20 (43.5)		
35−39.9 kg/m^2	12 (26.1)	9 (19.6)		
≥40 kg/m^2	5 (10.9)	2 (4.4)		
Weight (kg)	98.1 ± 16.6*	90.6 ± 14.9	−8.5 ± 8.3	−8.3 ± 6.9
Waist circumference (cm)	112.0 ± 11.7*	102.4 ± 11.7	−9.9 ± 11.1	−8.4 ± 8.9
Total fat (per 10 cm^2)	51.3 ± 15.4	46.4 ± 14.8	−5.3 ± 11.0	−8.8 ± 17.2
Subcutaneous (per 10 cm^2)	28.8 ± 13.2	26.6 ± 11.8	−2.9 ± 7.2	−6.7 ± 19.2
Intraperitoneal (per 10 cm^2)	15.5 ± 6.6	13.0 ± 5.5	−2.5 ± 4.4	−12.7 ± 28.5
Retroperitoneal (per 10 cm^2)	5.8 ± 2.7	5.9 ± 3.1	0.2 ± 1.6	5.3 ± 27.4
Biochemical and metabolic parameters				
ALT (units/l)	17.5 (14−28)	20 (16−27)	1 (−3 to 7)	
AST (units/l)	18 (15−24)	21 (18−25)	3 (−2 to 5)	
ALT−to−AST ratio	1 (0.8−1.1)	1 (0.8−1.2)	0.1 (−0.2 to 0.2)	
GGT (units/l)	24 (18−36)	22 (17.5−32.0)	−3 (−6 to 1)	
A1C (%)	7.1 ± 1.0	6.5 ± 0.9	−0.7 ± 1.1	
HDL cholesterol (mg/dl)	47.9 ± 11.7	52.7 ± 12.0	4.1 ± 7.0	
Triglycerides (mg/dl)	111.5 (88−169)	107 (66−139)	−5 (−46 to 18)	
LDL cholesterol (mg/dl)	118.0 ± 34.5	107.3 ± 30.7	−9.3 ± 23.3	
HDL−to−triglyceride ratio	2.3 (1.6−3.9)	2.1 (1.31−3.1)	−0.2 (−1.1 to 0.3)	
Adipokines and cytokines				
IL−8 (pg/ml)	31.7 (24.3−38.2)	23.0 (17.0−29.6)	−9.3 (−17.3 to 5.9)	
IL−10 (pg/ml)	5.5 (4.8−5.9)	6.8 (5.5−7.8)	0.9 (−0.2 to 3.0)	
TNF−α (pg/ml)	1.7 (1.2−2.6)	1.7 (1.4−2.2)	0.2 (−0.7 to 0.6)	
Adiponectin (μg/ml)	5.9 (4.5−7.2)	11.5 (7.67−21.21)	6.7 (2.4 to 10.8)	
Ghrelin (ng/ml)	1.2 (0.9−2.0)	1.4 (0.9−1.8)	−0.03 (−0.9 to 0.7)	
Resistin (ng/ml)	4.1 (2.9−6.6)	6.8 (4.7−8.8)	1.9 (0.5 to 2.6)	
Medications				
No. of diabetes medications	1.3 ± 0.8	1.2 ± 0.9	−0.1 ± 0.5	
0−1	29 (63.0)	30 (65.2)		
2	12 (26.1)	11 (23.9)		
3	5 (10.9)	5 (10.9)		
Use of insulin (%)	13	11	−2	
Use of metformin (%)	52.20	45.70	−6.5	
Use of thiazolidinedione (%)	28.30	23.90	−4.4	
Use of lipid-lowering drug (%)	41.3*	45.70	4.4	

Data are means ± SEM, median (interquartile range), or frequency (%). *ILI vs. DSE baseline difference $P > 0.05$, adjusted for sex and baseline weight.

models were also adjusted for sex, baseline weight, and baseline steatosis.

To assess the correlations between hepatic steatosis and other parameters we used partial Spearman rank coefficients to account for the nonnormal distribution of liver fat while adjusting for treatment group and sex. The odds of incident NAFLD was assessed using logistic regression and included only individuals with baseline steatosis <5.5%.

RESULTS

Baseline characteristics

We included 96 participants randomly assigned to ILI ($n = 46$) and DSE ($n = 50$). The sample had a mean ± SD age of 61.6 ± 6.7 years and BMI of 34.9 ± 5.0 kg/m^2; 60% were white, 32% were African American, 5% were other, and 2% were Hispanic. Overall 49% were women, with slightly more women in the ILI group than in the DSE group (59 vs. 40% $P = 0.06$). A1C was 7.2 ± 1.0%, and 87% of participants were using any diabetes medication, including 12% taking insulin and 50% taking met-

Table 1—*Continued*

	DSE (control)			P value deltas
Baseline	1 year	Absolute change	Relative change	(ILI vs. DSE) 1 year
		50		
6.3 (2.7−12.7)	4.9 (1.9−8.6)	−1.1 (−3.1 to 1.2)	−22.8 (−51.2 to 32.2)	0.04
5 (10.0)	6 (12.2)			
18 (36.0)	20 (40.8)			
9 (18.0)	13 (26.5)			
14 (28.0)	6 (12.2)			
4 (8.0)	4 (8.2)			
35.3 ± 4.7	35.3 ± 4.8	−0.02 ± 2.0	0.03 ± 5.7	<0.001
3 (6.0)	7 (14.0)			
26 (52.0)	19 (38.0)			
14 (28.0)	15 (30.0)			
7 (14.0)	9 (18.0)			
104.8 ± 16.7	104.7 ± 16.9	−0.05 ± 5.7	−0.02 ± 5.2	<0.001
115.0 ± 11.8	113.5 ± 12.4	−1.8 ± 6.5	−1.4 ± 5.5	<0.001
56.0 ± 14.5	56.0 ± 15.6	−0.03 ± 7.8	0.5 ± 14.1	0.002
29.1 ± 10.3	28.4 ± 10.7	−0.8 ± 4.16	−1.9 ± 16.8	0.02
18.7 ± 7.7	18.2 ± 7.3	−0.4 ± 4.4	1.8 ± 24.4	0.02
7.1 ± 3.2	8.2 ± 4.1	1.1 ± 2.0	15.4 ± 26.6	0.05
20 (17−26)	19 (14−24)	−2 (−6 to 1)		0.31
19 (15−24)	17 (15−22)	0 (−3 to 2)		0.45
0.8 (0.7−1)	0.9 (0.8−1.1)	0.1 (−0.04 to 0.2)		0.19
25 (22−45)	23 (18−35)	−4 (−11 to 2)		0.27
7.3 ± 1.0	7.1 ± 1.0	−0.2 ± 0.8		0.04
42.9 ± 12.0	44.2 ± 11.4	2 ± 6.5		0.11
122.5 (91−194)	121 (87−190)	−5 (−31 to 20)		0.23
109.8 ± 29.9	98.1 ± 27.7	−12.3 ± 25.0		0.53
3.2 (2.1−5.4)	2.6 (1.9−4.7)	−0.2 (−0.9 to 0.4)		0.4
31.9 (21.1−41.7)	21.0 (15.9−26.3)	−9.3 (−21.1 to −0.1)		0.65
5.3 (4.8−6.4)	7.1 (5.9−8.7)	1.4 (0.04−3.4)		0.08
1.8 (1.4−2.8)	1.9 (1.6−2.5)	0.03 (−0.7 to 0.7)		0.82
5.4 (4.3−6.3)	9.3 (6.8−15.2)	3.8 (1.7 to 8.9)		0.1
1.2 (0.9−2.1)	0.9 (0.8−1.2)	−0.3 (−1.1 to 0.2)		0.35
4.5 (3.5−5.9)	6.2 (4.8−8.2)	1.5 (0.1 to 3.0)		0.84
1.4 ± 0.8	1.5 ± 0.8	0.1 ± 0.6		0.06
27 (44.0)	22 (44.0)			
19 (38.0)	23 (46.0)			
4 (8.0)	5 (10.0)			
10	8	−2		0.94
48	54.20	6.2		0.38
34	30.00	−4		0.95
70	70.80	0.8		0.82

formin. Although this study was nested in the main Look AHEAD trial, the final sample included a subset of the randomly assigned participants, and there were significant differences in baseline weight, steatosis, waist circumference, and use of lipid-lowering medications between the groups (Table 1). Hepatic steatosis (≥5.5%) was present in 44% including 15 (36%) in the ILI group and 27 (64%) in the DSE group (P = 0.04). All analyses were adjusted for these baseline differences.

Baseline levels of alanine aminotransferase (ALT), aspartate aminotransferase (AST), and γ-glutamyl transferase (GGT) were 23.9, 20.4, and 45.1 units/l, respectively, and did not differ by group (all P ≥ 0.05). Overall, 6 participants (6%) had elevated ALT levels (≥40 units/l) and 43 (45%) had an AST-to-ALT ratio ≥1.

12-Month changes in steatosis, adiposity, and other metabolic parameters
As shown in Table 1, the ILI was effective and resulted in significant decreases in BMI (−2.6 vs. 0.03 kg/m^2; P < 0.001), weight (−8.5 vs. −0.05 kg; P < 0.001), percent weight (−8.3 vs. −0.03%; P < 0.001), waist circumference (−9.5 vs. −1.8 cm; P < 0.001), percent total fat

(−8.8 vs. 0.53%; $P = 0.001$), percent subcutaneous fat (−6.7 vs. −1.9%; $P = 0.02$), and percent intraperitoneal fat (−12.7 vs. 1.8%; $P = 0.02$) compared with the DSE. These findings are similar to the 1-year results of the main Look AHEAD trial (9).

After adjustment for sex, baseline weight, and baseline steatosis, the 12-month median absolute change in steatosis in the ILI group was more than double that in the DSE group (−2.3 vs. −1.1; $P = 0.04$). The median percent decrease in steatosis was −50.8% in the ILI group and −22.8% in the DSE group ($P = 0.04$).

Participants in the ILI group also had significant decreases in A1C (−0.7 vs. −0.2%; $P = 0.04$). This difference in glucose control occurred despite the fact that the proportion of individuals using any diabetes medicine decreased from baseline in the ILI group compared with that in the DSE group. No statistically significant differences were observed in liver enzymes or lipids at 12 months.

Variables associated with changes in hepatic steatosis

As shown in Table 2, after adjustment for intervention group and sex, absolute changes in steatosis were significantly correlated with changes in weight ($r = 0.231$, $P = 0.03$), A1C ($r = 0.311$, $P = 0.004$), glucose ($r = 0.291$, $P = 0.007$), and ALT, AST, and GGT ($r = 0.294$, $r = 0.348$ and $r = 0.277$, all $P \leq 0.001$). No significant correlations were found between absolute changes in steatosis and changes in any measured cytokine or adipokine. On a relative scale, the percent change in liver fat showed significant and strong correlation coefficients with changes in all of the above parameters. In addition, percent change in steatosis was significantly correlated with changes in BMI ($r = 0.259$, $P = 0.02$), insulin levels ($r = −0.302$, $P = 0.02$), triglycerides ($r = 0.336$, $P = 0.002$), and the HDL-to-triglyceride ratio ($r = 0.276$, $P = 0.011$).

Greater weight loss was associated with the largest decreases in steatosis. Compared with those with little weight change (±1%), those with the largest weight loss (≥10%) had a significantly higher median percent reduction in steatosis of −79.5 vs. −13.7% (Fig. 1). We used multivariate models to assess whether these correlations were independently associated with changes in steatosis. After adjustment for any of the following: changes in weight, changes in BMI, changes in retroperitoneal fat,

Table 2—*Correlation of changes in liver fat with changes in other parameters, adjusted for sex and intervention group*

	Absolute Δ liver fat	P value	Percent Δ liver fat	P value
Measures of adiposity				
Δ weight	0.231	0.030	0.349	0.001
Δ waist	0.022	0.835	0.116	0.281
Δ BMI	0.194	0.070	0.259	0.015
Δ total fat	0.095	0.378	0.097	0.367
Δ subcutaneous fat	0.135	0.209	0.111	0.304
Δ intraperitoneal fat	0.056	0.604	0.045	0.676
Δ retroperitoneal fat	0.080	0.456	0.145	0.179
Metabolic parameters				
Δ A1C	0.311	0.004	0.419	<0.0001
Δ glucose	0.291	0.007	0.373	0.001
Δ insulin*	−0.186	0.137	−0.302	0.015
Δ total cholesterol	0.050	0.654	0.042	0.701
Δ HDL	0.072	0.517	0.005	0.964
Δ triglycerides	0.187	0.089	0.336	0.002
Δ LDL	−0.084	0.447	−0.105	0.342
Δ HDL-to-triglyceride ratio	0.128	0.246	0.276	0.011
Liver tests				
Δ ALT	0.294	0.005	0.211	0.047
Δ AST	0.348	0.001	0.280	0.008
Δ GGT	0.277	0.009	0.287	0.006
Δ AST-to-ALT ratio	−0.030	0.781	−0.033	0.762
Inflammatory markers				
Δ IL-8	0.014	0.904	−0.085	0.466
Δ IL-10	0.136	0.245	−0.010	0.934
Δ TNF-α	−0.024	0.840	−0.002	0.986
Δ adiponectin	0.062	0.600	−0.124	0.290
Δ ghrelin	0.195	0.094	0.214	0.065
Δ resistin	−0.122	0.297	−0.079	0.498

*Among non–insulin users.

changes in A1C, changes in triglycerides, and changes in the HDL-to-triglyceride ratio as well as sex, treatment group, and baseline weight and hepatic fat, the effect of the intervention was no longer significant. Changes in adipokines or cytokines did not attenuate the effect of the intervention.

NAFLD incidence

Finally, during the 12-months of follow-up, 6 of 23 (26%) DSE participants and 1 of 31 (3%) ILI participants without NAFLD at baseline developed NAFLD at 12 months (odds ratio 0.07 [95% CI 0.007–0.71]).

CONCLUSIONS — Among adults with type 2 diabetes, 12 months of an intensive lifestyle intervention leading to 8% loss of body weight was successful in both reducing hepatic steatosis and decreasing the risk of incident NAFLD, compared with those in a control group. Furthermore, a dose-response relation-

ship was observed with weight loss, with the greatest reduction observed in those with the greatest weight loss (≥10%). Our findings therefore support the current recommendation for weight loss using lifestyle modification as the first step in the management of patients with NAFLD, including patients with type 2 diabetes and for those at risk for NAFLD.

We found that the decrease in steatosis was nearly double in the ILI group compared with that in the DSE group. In addition, as in the main Look AHEAD 1-year results (9), the use of overall and specific medications such as thiazolidinedione and metformin tended to decrease more among the intervention arm. We would anticipate that these differences would then favor the control arm, leading to a more conservative estimate. These findings are important because NAFLD not only disproportionately affects individuals with type 2 diabetes but also because once NAFLD is present, the risk of developing more advanced forms

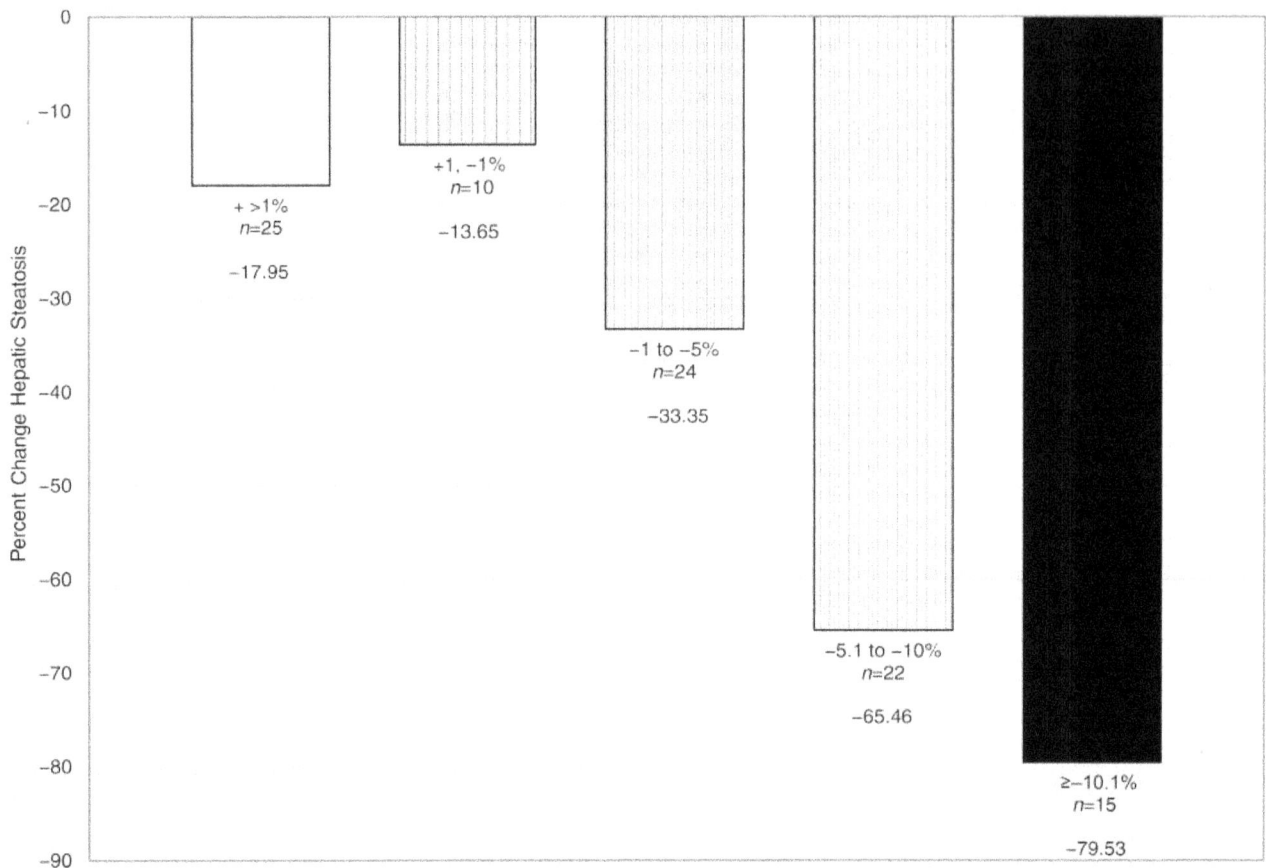

Figure 1—*Median percent change in hepatic steatosis by percent weight change.*

of NAFLD, such as nonalcoholic steato-hepatitis and hepatocellular carcinoma is higher in this group than in the general population (3,10–13).

Our results are consistent and extend previous trials of weight loss for patients with NAFLD, suggesting improvement in hepatic steatosis. To our knowledge there have been a total of nine clinical studies of lifestyle intervention on hepatic steatosis measured by ^{1}H MRS (14–22), and, of these, only two have been conducted among individuals with type 2 diabetes (17,18). Petersen et al. (17) treated eight individuals with obesity and diabetes with a 1,200-calorie liquid diet for 3–12 weeks to achieve 8% weight loss. Steatosis decreased on average 81% (from 12 to 2.2%). Tamura et al. (17) randomly assigned 14 subjects to a controlled diet only (25–30 kcal/kg ideal body weight) or exercise and diet (same diet plus two or three 30-min sessions of walking 5–6 days/week) for 2 weeks. In this inpatient study, the mean decreases in hepatic steatosis were 25 and 28% for the diet only and diet plus exercise group, respectively (18). Our study extends these findings in patients with type 2 diabetes by including a larger and diverse sample and a longer intervention.

Because most participants had normal liver enzymes at baseline, it is understandable that there was no significant change with weight loss and decrease in steatosis. However, consistent with other studies, our data show that normal liver test results are not good indicators of the presence or absence of hepatic steatosis.

Cytokines and adipokines have been posited to play an important role as mediators of improved hepatic insulin sensitivity with weight loss. In our study, changes in steatosis and adiposity were not associated with changes in IL-8, IL-10, TNF-α, adiponectin, ghrelin, or resistin. These results are consistent with two other previous studies (16,17) and suggest that among individuals with type 2 diabetes these may not play a major role in changing insulin sensitivity in the liver.

Although a clinically meaningful change in steatosis remains to be defined, our results suggest that among patients with type 2 diabetes, reduction in hepatic steatosis is significantly associated with levels of A1C and triglycerides, both of which are important markers of disease risk and control (23). Longer studies are needed to identify meaningful changes in liver fat, with respect to liver outcomes.

Our study has some limitations. First, we had no histopathological data to assess the effect of the intervention. Although ^{1}H MRS is an excellent method to quantify changes in steatosis because it is noninvasive and reliable, it cannot assess inflammation or fibrosis. Recently, Promrat et al. (24) reported the results of an smaller trial of lifestyle intervention for 31 overweight patients with biopsy-proven nonalcoholic steatohepatitis, and their results are in agreement with our findings. In addition, our study included older individuals with type 2 diabetes and mostly with normal liver enzyme levels, probably reflecting a different spectrum of the disease. Second, even though this trial is by far is the largest of its kind, the study sample was not large enough to study participant subgroups (i.e., sex and race or to assess sex-treatment or race-treatment interactions). Third, we studied participants in a large randomized clinical trial who are likely to represent a very motivated group; however, although limiting generalizability, this setting is ideal to assess the efficacy of this intervention. Future studies will be needed to assess the effectiveness of this approach. Fourth, even though the parent study had a randomized design, our study groups were not comparable in all respects, probably because enrollment into this ancillary study occurred after randomization and by random chance. To address these imbalances we adjusted all our analyses by these baseline differences. Finally, because obesity hinders the successful acquisition of ^{1}H MRS, the results may be conservative.

In summary, in patients with type 2 diabetes, an intensive lifestyle intervention that produced 8% weight loss resulted in a significant, 25% greater reduction in hepatic steatosis and a substantially lower incidence of NAFLD compared with that of a comparison group after 12 months of the intervention. The long-term efficacy as well as the effectiveness of an intensive lifestyle intervention needs to be further established.

Acknowledgments— The study was supported by the National Institutes of Health National Institute of Diabetes and Digestive and Kidney Diseases (grants R01-DK-060427 and U01-DK-57149), The Johns Hopkins University School of Medicine General Clinical Research Center (grant M01-RR-00052), and the Department of Veterans Affairs.

No potential conflicts of interest relevant to this article were reported.

M.L. analyzed and interpreted data, performed statistical analysis, wrote the manuscript, and reviewed/edited the manuscript. S.F.S., A.M.D., and F.L.B. provided the study concept and design, analyzed and interpreted data, and reviewed/edited the manuscript. A.H. and S.B., acquired data and reviewed/edited the manuscript. L.E.W., F.X.P.-S., and S.E.K. analyzed and interpreted data and reviewed/edited the manuscript. J.M.C. provided the study concept and design, analyzed and interpreted data, wrote the manuscript, and reviewed/edited the manuscript.

Parts of this study were presented in abstract form at the Liver Meeting 2008, San Francisco, California, 31 October–4 November 2008.

References

1. Targher G, Bertolini L, Padovani R, Rodella S, Tessari R, Zenari L, Day C, Arcaro G. Prevalence of nonalcoholic fatty liver disease and its association with cardiovascular disease among type 2 diabetic patients. Diabetes Care 2007;30:1212–1218
2. Neuschwander-Tetri BA, Caldwell SH. Nonalcoholic steatohepatitis: summary of an AASLD Single Topic Conference. Hepatology 2003;37:1202–1219
3. Marchesini G, Bugianesi E, Forlani G, Cerrelli F, Lenzi M, Manini R, Natale S, Vanni E, Villanova N, Melchionda N, Rizzetto M. Nonalcoholic fatty liver, steatohepatitis, and the metabolic syndrome. Hepatology 2003;37:917–923
4. American Gastroenterological Association Medical Position Statement: nonalcoholic fatty liver disease. Gastroenterology 2002;123:1702–1704
5. Ryan DH, Espeland MA, Foster GD, Haffner SM, Hubbard VS, Johnson KC, Kahn SE, Knowler WC, Yanovski SZ. Look AHEAD (Action for Health in Diabetes): design and methods for a clinical trial of weight loss for the prevention of cardiovascular disease in type 2 diabetes. Control Clin Trials 2003;24:610–628
6. Skinner HA, Sheu WJ. Reliability of alcohol use indices. The Lifetime Drinking History and the MAST. J Stud Alcohol 1982;43:1157–1170
7. Bonekamp S, Ghosh P, Crawford S, Solga SF, Horska A, Brancati FL, Diehl AM, Smith S, Clark JM. Quantitative comparison and evaluation of software packages for assessment of abdominal adipose tissue distribution by magnetic resonance imaging. Int J Obes (Lond) 2008;32:100–111
8. Wadden TA, West DS, Delahanty L, Jakicic J, Rejeski J, Williamson D, Berkowitz RI, Kelley DE, Tomchee C, Hill JO, Kumanyika S. The Look AHEAD study: a description of the lifestyle intervention and the evidence supporting it. Obesity (Silver Spring) 2006;14:737–752
9. Pi-Sunyer X, Blackburn G, Brancati FL, Bray GA, Bright R, Clark JM, Curtis JM, Espeland MA, Foreyt JP, Graves K, Haffner SM, Harrison B, Hill JO, Horton ES, Jakicic J, Jeffery RW, Johnson KC, Kahn S, Kelley DE, Kitabchi AE, Knowler WC, Lewis CE, Maschak-Carey BJ, Montgomery B, Nathan DM, Patricio J, Peters A, Redmon JB, Reeves RS, Ryan DH, Safford M, Van Dorsten B, Wadden TA, Wagenknecht L, Wesche-Thobaben J, Wing RR, Yanovski SZ. Reduction in weight and cardiovascular disease risk factors in individuals with type 2 diabetes: one-year results of the look AHEAD trial. Diabetes Care 2007;30:1374–1383
10. Adams LA, Lymp JF, St Sauver J, Sanderson SO, Lindor KD, Feldstein A, Angulo P. The natural history of nonalcoholic fatty liver disease: a population-based cohort study. Gastroenterology 2005;129:113–121
11. Adams LA, Sanderson S, Lindor KD, Angulo P. The histological course of nonalcoholic fatty liver disease: a longitudinal study of 103 patients with sequential liver biopsies. J Hepatol 2005;42:132–138
12. Bugianesi E, Leone N, Vanni E, Marchesini G, Brunello F, Carucci P, Musso A, De Paolis P, Capussotti L, Salizzoni M, Rizzetto M. Expanding the natural history of nonalcoholic steatohepatitis: from cryptogenic cirrhosis to hepatocellular carcinoma. Gastroenterology 2002;123:134–140
13. Caldwell SH, Oelsner DH, Iezzoni JC, Hespenheide EE, Battle EH, Driscoll CJ. Cryptogenic cirrhosis: clinical characterization and risk factors for underlying disease. Hepatology 1999;29:664–669
14. Cowin GJ, Jonsson JR, Bauer JD, Ash S, Ali A, Osland EJ, Purdie DM, Clouston AD, Powell EE, Galloway GJ. Magnetic resonance imaging and spectroscopy for monitoring liver steatosis. J Magn Reson Imaging 2008;28:937–945
15. Larson-Meyer DE, Heilbronn LK, Redman LM, Newcomer BR, Frisard MI, Anton S, Smith SR, Alfonso A, Ravussin E. Effect of calorie restriction with or without exercise on insulin sensitivity, β-cell function, fat cell size, and ectopic lipid in overweight subjects. Diabetes Care 2006;29:1337–1344
16. Larson-Meyer DE, Newcomer BR, Heilbronn LK, Volaufova J, Smith SR, Alfonso AJ, Lefevre M, Rood JC, Williamson DA, Ravussin E. Effect of 6-month calorie restriction and exercise on serum and liver lipids and markers of liver function. Obesity 2008;16:1355–1362
17. Petersen KF, Dufour S, Befroy D, Lehrke M, Hendler RE, Shulman GI. Reversal of nonalcoholic hepatic steatosis, hepatic insulin resistance, and hyperglycemia by moderate weight reduction in patients with type 2 diabetes. Diabetes 2005;54:603–608
18. Tamura Y, Tanaka Y, Sato F, Choi JB, Watada H, Niwa M, Kinoshita J, Ooka A, Kumashiro N, Igarashi Y, Kyogoku S, Maehara T, Kawasumi M, Hirose T, Kawamori R. Effects of diet and exercise on muscle and liver intracellular lipid contents and insulin sensitivity in type 2 diabetic patients. J Clin Endocrinol Metab 2005;90:3191–3196
19. Thamer C, Machann J, Stefan N, Haap M, Schafer S, Brenner S, Kantartzis K, Claussen C, Schick F, Haring H, Fritsche A. High visceral fat mass and high liver fat are associated with resistance to lifestyle intervention. Obesity (Silver Spring) 2007;15:531–538
20. Thomas EL, Brynes AE, Hamilton G, Patel N, Spong A, Goldin RD, Frost G, Bell JD, Taylor-Robinson SD. Effect of nutritional counselling on hepatic, muscle and adipose tissue fat content and distribution in non-alcoholic fatty liver disease. World J Gastroenterol 2006;12:5813–5819
21. Tiikkainen M, Bergholm R, Vehkavaara S, Rissanen A, Häkkinen AM, Tamminen M, Teramo K, Yki-Järvinen H. Effects of identical weight loss on body composition and features of insulin resistance in obese women with high and

low liver fat content. Diabetes 2003;52: 701–707

22. Viljanen AP, Iozzo P, Borra R, Kankaanpää M, Karmi A, Lautamäki R, Järvisalo M, Parkkola R, Rönnemaa T, Guiducci L, Lehtimäki T, Raitakari OT, Mari A, Nuutila P. Effect of weight loss on liver free fatty acid uptake and hepatic insulin resistance. J Clin Endocrinol Metab 2009;94:50–55

23. Standards of medical care in diabetes—2010. Diabetes Care 2010;33(Suppl. 1): S11–S61

24. Promrat K, Kleiner DE, Niemeier HM, Jackvony E, Kearns M, Wands JR, Fava JL, Wing RR. Randomized controlled trial testing the effects of weight loss on non-alcoholic steatohepatitis. Hepatology 2010;51:121–129

Adipose Tissue Dysfunction Signals Progression of Hepatic Steatosis Towards Nonalcoholic Steatohepatitis in C57Bl/6 Mice

Caroline Duval,[1,2] Uwe Thissen,[2,3] Shohreh Keshtkar,[1,2] Bertrand Accart,[1,2] Rinke Stienstra,[1,2] Mark V. Boekschoten,[1,2] Tania Roskams,[4] Sander Kersten,[1,2] and Michael Müller[1,2]

OBJECTIVE—Nonalcoholic fatty liver disease (NAFLD) is linked to obesity and diabetes, suggesting an important role of adipose tissue in the pathogenesis of NAFLD. Here, we aimed to investigate the interaction between adipose tissue and liver in NAFLD and identify potential early plasma markers that predict nonalcoholic steatohepatitis (NASH).

RESEARCH DESIGN AND METHODS—C57Bl/6 mice were chronically fed a high-fat diet to induce NAFLD and compared with mice fed a low-fat diet. Extensive histological and phenotypical analyses coupled with a time course study of plasma proteins using multiplex assay were performed.

RESULTS—Mice exhibited pronounced heterogeneity in liver histological scoring, leading to classification into four subgroups: low-fat low (LFL) responders displaying normal liver morphology, low-fat high (LFH) responders showing benign hepatic steatosis, high-fat low (HFL) responders displaying pre-NASH with macrovesicular lipid droplets, and high fat high (HFH) responders exhibiting overt NASH characterized by ballooning of hepatocytes, presence of Mallory bodies, and activated inflammatory cells. Compared with HFL responders, HFH mice gained weight more rapidly and exhibited adipose tissue dysfunction characterized by decreased final fat mass, enhanced macrophage infiltration and inflammation, and adipose tissue remodeling. Plasma haptoglobin, IL-1β, TIMP-1, adiponectin, and leptin were significantly changed in HFH mice. Multivariate analysis indicated that in addition to leptin, plasma CRP, haptoglobin, eotaxin, and MIP-1α early in the intervention were positively associated with liver triglycerides. Intermediate prognostic markers of liver triglycerides included IL-18, IL-1β, MIP-1γ, and MIP-2, whereas insulin, TIMP-1, granulocyte chemotactic protein 2, and myeloperoxidase emerged as late markers.

CONCLUSIONS—Our data support the existence of a tight relationship between adipose tissue dysfunction and NASH pathogenesis and point to several novel potential predictive biomarkers for NASH. *Diabetes* 59:3181–3191, 2010

From the [1]Nutrition, Metabolism and Genomics Group, Division of Human Nutrition, Wageningen University, Wageningen, the Netherlands; the [2]Nutrigenomics Consortium, Top Institute Food & Nutrition, Wageningen, the Netherlands; [3]TNO Quality of Life, Zeist, the Netherlands; the [4]Liver Research Unit, Department of Morphology and Molecular Pathology, University of Leuven, Leuven, Belgium.

Corresponding author: Sander Kersten, sander.kersten@wur.nl.

Received 13 February 2010 and accepted 12 September 2010. Published ahead of print at http://diabetes.diabetesjournals.org on 21 September 2010. DOI: 10.2337/db10-0224.

Obesity is associated with a number of metabolic perturbations that increase risk for type 2 diabetes, coronary heart disease, and liver dysfunction. These metabolic perturbations, collectively referred to as the metabolic syndrome, include hypertension, dyslipidemia, and insulin resistance. Additionally, metabolic syndrome is often characterized by nonalcoholic fatty liver disease (NAFLD) (1).

It is evident that obesity represents a state of chronic low-grade inflammation that likely originates in the adipose tissue. Upon fat expansion, macrophages and other leukocytes infiltrate the adipose tissue and account for secretion of various cytokines and adipokines (2,3). Because many of these cytokines reduce insulin sensitivity, the elevated inflammatory status may provide a mechanistic explanation for the well-established link between obesity and insulin resistance (4). Alternatively, the complications of obesity may be traced to aberrant storage of lipids in nonadipose tissues, which can profoundly disturb organ function (5).

Excess storage of fat in liver is the hallmark of NAFLD, which refers to a wide histological spectrum of liver diseases ranging from hepatic steatosis to pathological nonalcoholic steatohepatitis (NASH) and fibrotic complications (6). Steatosis alone is considered relatively innocuous, but prognosis is much more grim for NASH, which might progress to cirrhosis and liver cancer (7). Several theories have been proposed to explain why steatosis occasionally progresses to NASH. One popular model is the two-hit hypothesis, in which the first hit is the accumulation of fat in the hepatocytes that renders the liver more susceptible to second hits comprised of inflammatory insults or oxidative stress (7). Alternatively, progression of steatosis to NASH may be stimulated by cellular lipotoxicity mediated by lipotoxic fatty acids, cholesterol, and/or ceramides (8).

Since NAFLD is strongly linked to obesity, an important role of adipose tissue in the pathogenesis of NAFLD is suspected. Indeed, growing evidence indicates that proteins secreted from adipose tissue may be implicated in NAFLD (9). To gain insight into the nature of the interaction between adipose tissue and liver in the context of obesity-related NAFLD and to identify potential early plasma markers that predict steatosis and/or NASH, we subjected C57Bl/6 mice to a chronic high-fat diet to induce NAFLD and coupled extensive histological and phenotypical analyses with a time course study of plasma proteins using multiplex assay. The results indicate a tight relationship between adipose tissue dysfunction and NASH pathogenesis and point to several novel potential predictive biomarkers for NASH.

RESEARCH DESIGN AND METHODS

Twenty male C57BL/6JOlaHsd (C57Bl/6) mice at 8 weeks of age were purchased from Harlan (Horst, the Netherlands) and housed individually. Detailed information about the mouse strain is available at the following Web site: http://www.harlan.com/research_models_and_services/research_models_by_product_type/inbred_mice/c57bl6j_inbred_mice.hl. After 3 weeks on a low-fat diet (LFD), mice were divided into two weight-matched groups. One group continued on the LFD while the other group switched to a high fat diet (HFD) containing 10 or 45% energy as triglycerides, respectively (D12450B and D12451; Research Diets) for 21 weeks. Lard in these diets was replaced by palm oil. Palm oil is devoid of cholesterol, which may have proinflammatory properties. Food intake was measured by weighing the pellets once per week. Mice were housed individually, allowing for assessment of food consumption of individual mice. Food intake was averaged over the 20-week intervention and multiplied by the caloric value of the feed to determine energy intake in kcal · mouse^{-1} · day^{-1}. Numbers were subsequently averaged per group. At weeks 0, 2, 4, 8, 12, 16, and 20, tail vein plasma samples were collected after a 6-h fast. Two mice within the HFD group died before the end of the experiment for reasons unrelated to the dietary intervention. After 21 weeks, ad libitum–fed mice were anesthetized using isofluorane. Blood was collected by orbital puncture, followed by sacrifice via cervical dislocation. Liver and epididymal white adipose tissues were removed, weighed, and immediately frozen in liquid nitrogen. For histology, liver was frozen with OCT compound, and adipose tissue samples were fixed in 10% formalin and processed for paraffin embedding. Animal experiments were approved by the local animal ethics committee at Wageningen University.

Hepatic triglyceride content determination, RNA extraction, real-time PCR, and Affymetrix Microarrays. Liver triglycerides were determined enzymatically as previously described (10). Other techniques were employed as previously described (11). Microarray data were analyzed as previously described (12). Genes with a P value <0.05 were considered significantly regulated. Array data have been submitted to the Gene Expression Omnibus (accession no. GSE24031). Gene set enrichment analysis was used to identify significantly regulated pathways (13). Gene sets with a false discovery rate <0.25 were considered significant.

Plasma measurements. Plasma concentrations of multiple chemokines were measured with multiplex technologies (Rodent Map 2.0; Rules Based Medicine, Austin, TX). Plasma free fatty acids and alanine aminotransferase were measured with commercially available kits from Instruchemie (Delfzijl, the Netherlands). Plasma leptin and insulin levels were measured using kits from Linco (St. Louis, MO).

Liver immunohistochemistry. For oil red O staining, 5 μm frozen liver sections were air-dried for 30 min, followed by fixation in formal calcium (4% formaldehyde and 1% CaCl$_2$). Oil red O staining was performed using standard protocols. Hematoxylin-eosin (H-E) staining of frozen liver sections was carried out as described at http://www.ihcworld.com/histology.htm. Collagen was stained using fast green FCF/sirius red F3B.

For immunohistochemistry, 5 μm frozen liver sections were cut, dried overnight, fixed in acetone for 10 min, and washed in PBS prior to use. For visualization of hepatic stellate cell activation, rabbit anti–glial fibrillary acidic protein (GFAP) polyclonal antibody was used (Dako, Glostrup, Denmark). For detection of macrophages/monocytes, a rat polyclonal anti-Cd68 antibody (Serotec, Oxford, U.K.) was used. Sections were incubated for 30 min at room temperature with GFAP (1:1,000 dilution) or Cd68 (1:100 dilution) primary antibodies, followed by incubation for 30 min at room temperature with anti-rabbit peroxidase-conjugated En Vision (GFAP; Dako) or 1:20 diluted anti-rat IgG peroxidase-conjugated secondary antibodies (Cd68; Serotec). Visualization of the complex was done using 3-amino-9-ethylcarbazole chromogen for 15 min, followed by staining with H-E. Negative controls were performed by omitting the primary antibody.

Immunohistochemistry of adipose tissue. 5-μm-thick paraffin-embedded sections were cut, dried for 30 min at 37°C, and washed in PBS prior to use. Staining of adipose tissue macrophages was carried out using an antibody against Cd68 as described above. H-E staining of sections was done using standard protocols. Collagen was stained using fast green FCF/sirius red F3B.

Multivariate Rules-Based Medicine data analysis. The data obtained from the commercial Rules-Based Medicine multiplex analysis (70 proteins measured in 126 plasma samples) contained a number of technically unreliable entries for specific samples and proteins that were: 1) lower than the least detectable dose (LDD): replaced by 0.5 × LDD, 2) not detectable (i.e., not measured on the standard curve): replaced by 0.1 × LDD, or 3) not measurable (i.e., not sufficient sample material available): replaced by 0.1 × LDD. Proteins were removed if they did not contain more than 50% reliable

entries for two or more groups of the totally available 14 groups (7 time points × 2 diets). This approach assures that potentially relevant group differences are retained in the data. Of the 70 proteins screened, 19 were excluded, 18 contained more than 50% reliable entries for at least two groups, and 33 proteins contained 100% reliable entries for all groups. One mouse was removed from the dataset for multivariate analysis on the basis that some plasma proteins display atypical outlying values.

Multiway partial least squares (PLS) (MPLS) is a multivariate statistical technique that is an extension of standard PLS analysis able to analyze data across different time points (14–16). Both methods are able to analyze large numbers of variables in small sample sizes by reducing the dimensionality of the data. In contrast to standard two-dimensional data (matrix), multiway data can be represented as a collection of matrices (a cube) where each matrix contains data from one specific time point. For MPLS, the data were centered across the samples (i.e., zero mean) to remove offsets followed by autoscaling for the variables (i.e., a mean ± SD of 0 ± 1 to remove arbitrary differences in measurement scales [16]).

Validation of the MPLS models using a double cross-validation strategy and the selection of most important proteins from the models have been performed as previously described (17). Because (double) cross-validation relies on a random subdivision of data, the complete validation procedure was repeated five times on the basis of different random subdivisions of the data during cross-validation. A model was considered to be reliable if at least four (out of five) models could be calculated with an $R^2 > 0.7$.

Statistical analyses. Statistically significant differences were calculated using Student's T test. The cutoff for statistical significance was set at $P < 0.05$. MPLS was performed using the N-way toolbox (http://www.models.life.ku.dk/nwaytoolbox) in combination with Matlab, version 7.1.0, release 14 (The Mathworks, Natick, MA) and homemade software.

RESULTS

Development of NASH in a subpopulation of C57Bl/6 mice fed a HFD.
To study the effect of chronic high-fat feeding on liver metabolic functions, C57Bl/6 mice were fed an LFD or HFD for 21 weeks. Mice fed the HFD gained more weight compared with mice fed the LFD (Fig. 1A), which was already evident after 2 weeks. Enhanced weight gain in mice fed a HFD may be related to increased energy intake (Fig. 1B). After 21 weeks, weight of the epididymal fat pad, which was assumed to reflect overall adiposity of the animals, was markedly higher in mice fed an HFD (Fig. 1C).

To characterize the effect of an HFD on hepatic steatosis, liver sections were stained with H-E (Fig. 1D) and oil red O (Fig. 1E). Remarkably, a marked heterogeneity in fat accumulation and histology was observed within each group. Scoring of the sections by a pathologist (T.R.) indicated different stages of NAFLD and led to classification of mice into four subgroups, which surprisingly but not deliberately ended up being of approximately equal size. These subgroups were low-fat low (LFL) responders (n = 4), which display normal liver morphology; low-fat high (LFH) responders (n = 6), which develop benign hepatic steatosis; high-fat low (HFL) responders (n = 4), which show a pre-NASH phenotype of macrovesicular lipid droplets; and high-fat high (HFH) responders (n = 4), which develop overt NASH characterized by ballooning of hepatocytes, presence of Mallory bodies, and activated inflammatory cells (Fig. 1D).

Quantitation of hepatic triglycerides confirmed the heterogeneity between the subgroups, with HFH mice accumulating the highest amount of triglycerides (Fig. 1F). Consequently, liver–to–body weight ratio was increased specifically in HFH mice, indicating hepatomegaly (Fig. 1G). Finally, plasma alanine aminotransferase activity was highest in the HFH subgroup, reflecting increased liver damage (Fig. 1H).

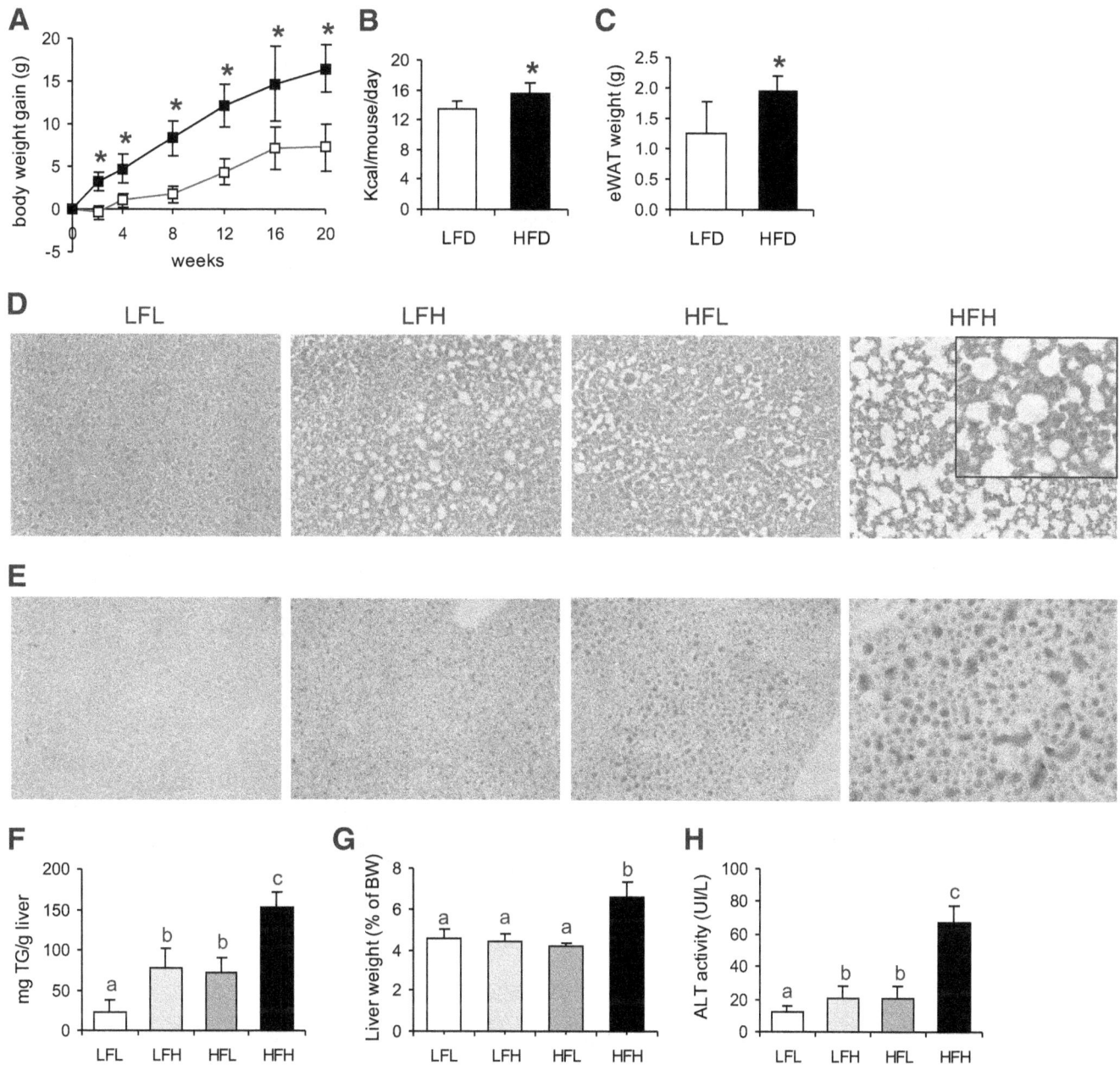

FIG. 1. A subpopulation of mice fed an HFD develops NASH. *A*: Changes in body weight in C57Bl/6 mice fed an LFD (□; n = 10) or HFD (■; n = 8). *B*: Mean energy intake of mice fed an LFD or HFD during 21 weeks of dietary intervention. *C*: Weight of epididymal fat pad after 21 weeks of dietary intervention. Error bars reflect SD. *Significantly different from mice fed an LFD according to Student's *t* test (P < 0.05). H-E staining (*D*) and oil red O staining (*E*) of representative liver sections of the four subgroups (LFL, LFH, HFL, and HFH). *F*: liver triglyceride concentration. *G*: Liver weight (expressed as percentage of total body weight [BW]). *H*: Activity of alanine aminotransferase (ALT) (glutamate pyruvate transaminase) in plasma. Error bars reflect SD. Bars with different letters are statistically different (P < 0.05 according to Student's *t* test). *n* = 4 mice per group for LFL, HFL, and HFH, and *n* = 6 mice per group for LFH. (A high-quality digital representation of this figure is available in the online issue.)

NASH-related metabolic pathways are exclusively impaired in HFH Responders. To correlate changes in liver functions with gene expression, expression profiling was performed on individual mouse livers. Microarray data were processed according to subgroups, with LFL mice serving as the reference group for calculation of fold change and *P* values. The most dramatic effects were observed in HFH responders as shown by changes in expression of >3,000 genes (Fig. 2*A*). To identify genes regulated exclusively in HFH responders, we selected genes that were statistically significantly regu-

lated in HFH versus all subgroups but unchanged in other comparisons. This HFH responder gene expression signature comprised 388 upregulated and 319 downregulated genes. One dominant pathway within the HFH expression signature was lipid metabolism, illustrated by the marked induction of *Cidec* and *Mogat1* (Fig. 2*B*). Other lipid metabolism genes such as *Cd36* and *Pparγ* increased gradually from LFL to HFH, correlating with hepatic triglycerides (Fig. 1*F* and Fig. 2*B*). Another pathway well represented within the HFH expression signature was inflammation, as shown by

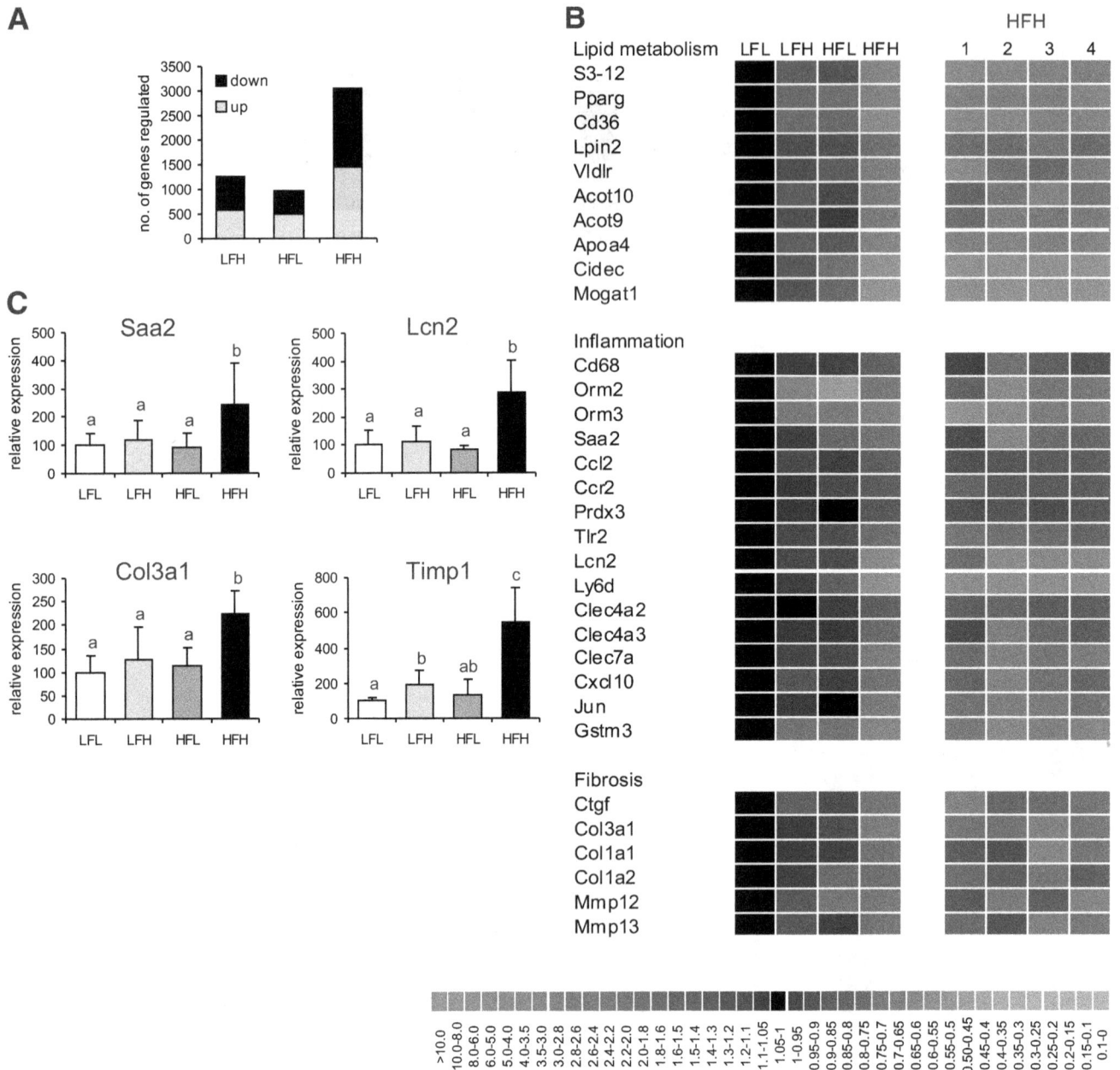

FIG. 2. Upregulation of inflammatory and fibrotic gene expression in HFH responder mice. *A*: Number of genes up- or downregulated in the various subgroups in comparison with the LFL mice as determined by Affymetrix GeneChip analysis. Genes with a *P* value <0.05 were considered significantly regulated. *B*: Heat map showing changes in expression of selected genes involved in lipid metabolism, inflammation, and fibrosis in liver. Mean expression in LFL mice was set at 1. Gene expression changes in individual mice within the HFH group are shown on the right. *C*: Changes in gene expression of selected genes as determined by real-time quantitative PCR. Mean expression in LFL mice was set at 100%. Error bars reflect SD. Bars with different letters are statistically different (*P* < 0.05 according to Student's *t* test). Number of mice per group: *n* = 4 for the LFL, HFL, and HFH groups and *n* = 6 for the LFH group.

marked and specific induction of acute phase genes encoding orosomucoid, serum amyloid-A, and lipocalin-2 in the HFH subgroup (Fig. 2*B*), and confirmed by quantitative PCR (Fig. 2*C*). Finally, many genes in the HFH expression signature were related to fibrosis, including *Ctgf*, collagens, metalloproteases, and *Timp1* (Fig. 2*B* and *C*). Expression analysis of individual mice within the HFH group showed uniform induction of genes involved in the above-mentioned pathways (Fig. 2*B*). Gene set enrichment analysis indicated that while pathways related to lipid metabolism were upregulated in all subgroups when compared with LFL mice, with most

prominent effects observed in HFH mice, numerous pathways of inflammation, cell cycle, and oxidative stress were specifically induced in HFH mice (supplemental Table 1, available in an online appendix [available at http://diabetes.diabetesjournals.org/cgi/content/full/db10-0224/DC1]). The complete microarray dataset is available at http://humannutrition2.wur.nl/duval2010.

The elevated inflammatory status in HFH livers was corroborated by immunostaining for macrophage marker Cd68 (Fig. 3*A*). Early fibrosis was detected in one HFH mouse (Fig. 3*B*). Finally, hepatic stellate activation was demonstrated in HFH mice by GFAP

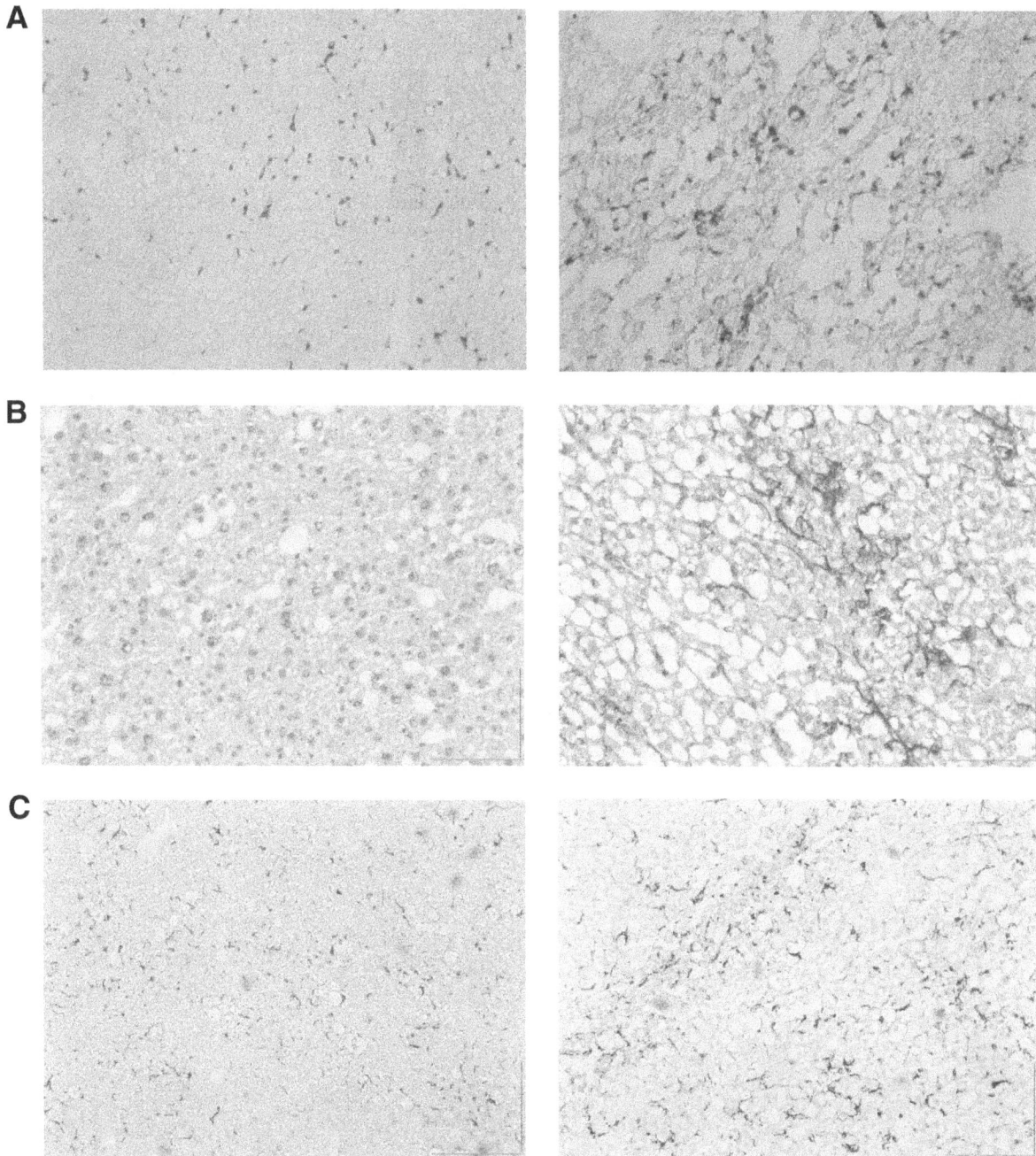

FIG. 3. (Immuno)histochemical staining confirms enhanced inflammation and early fibrosis in HFH mice. *A*: Immunohistochemical staining of macrophage activation in representative liver sections of HFL (*left panel*) and HFH (*right panel*) mice using antibody against the specific macrophage marker Cd68. *B*: Collagen staining using fast green FCF/sirius red F3B. *C*: Staining of stellate cell activation using antibody against GFAP. (A high-quality digital representation of this figure is available in the online issue.)

immunostaining (Fig. 3*C*). Overall, these analyses support induction of inflammation and fibrosis in HFH responders, indicating NASH.

HFH responder mice exhibit adipose tissue dysfunction. Mice classified as high responders also gained the most body weight (Fig. 4*A*), likely related to increased food intake (Fig. 4*B*). Indeed, a positive correlation was found between final body weight and hepatic triglycerides (Fig. 4*C*). Remarkably, despite increased weight gain, weight of the epididymal fat pad at sacrifice was markedly lower in HFH compared with that in HFL mice (Fig. 4*D*). As expected, leptin expression in adipose tissue mirrored

adiposity (Fig. 4*E*), which was also true for the plasma free fatty acids (Fig. 4*F*). Evaluation of the morphology of the epididymal fat pad in HFH mice after H-E staining revealed atrophied adipocytes surrounded by inflammatory cells, which were hardly observed in HFL responders (Fig. 4*G*). Cd68 immunostaining indicated increased presence of macrophages in HFH mice (Fig. 4*H*), which was supported by gene expression of *F4/80* and *Cd68* (Fig. 5). In contrast, expression of the anti-inflammatory adipokine adiponectin was markedly reduced in HFH mice, as was resistin (Fig. 5). Interestingly, expression of adipogenic (*Pparγ* and *Fabp4*) and lipogenic (*Dgat2*, *Srebp-1*, and fatty acid

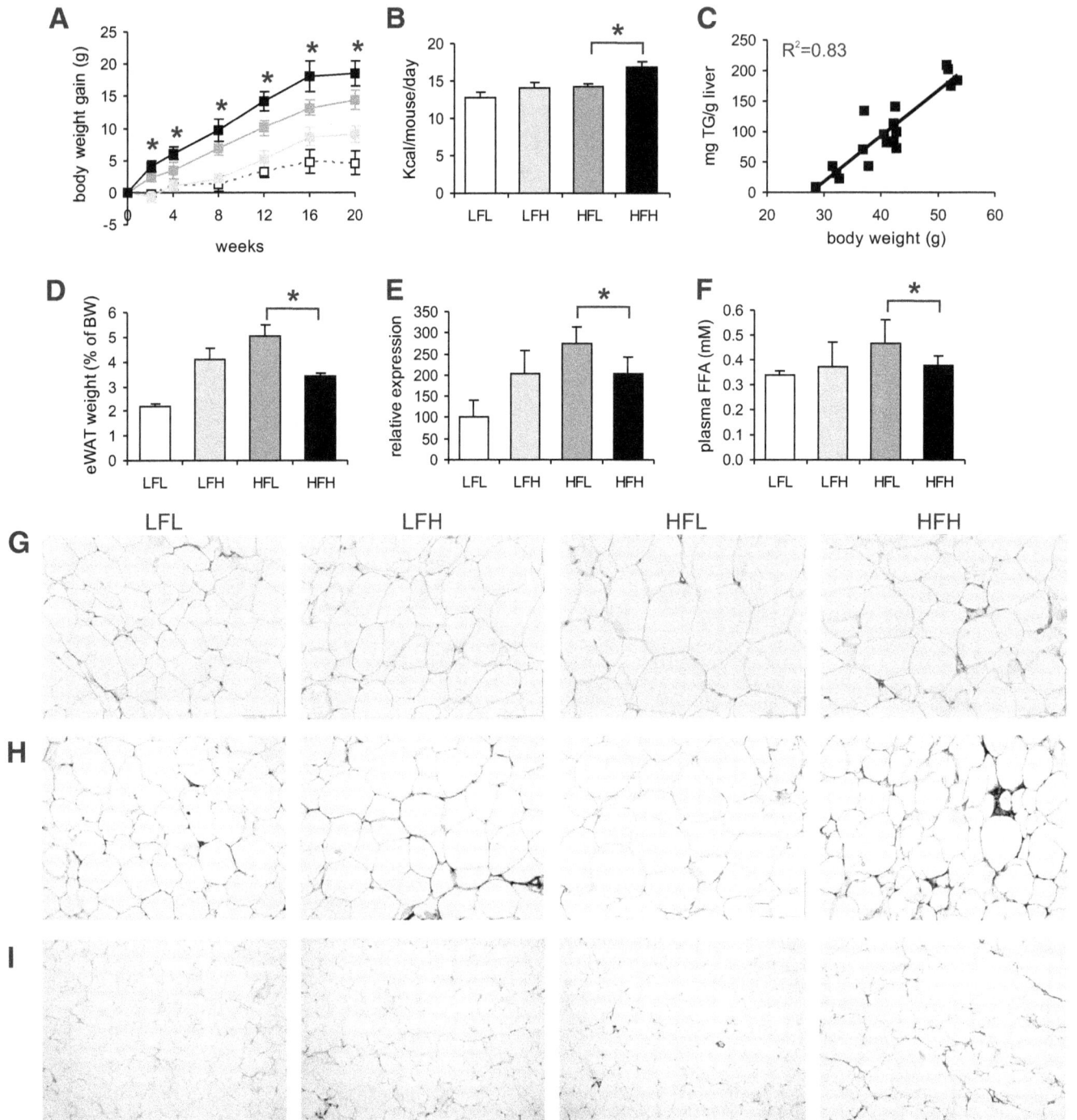

FIG. 4. Adipose dysfunction in HFH mice. *A*: Body weight changes in the four subgroups during the 21-week dietary intervention. White squares, LFL; light-gray squares, LFH; dark-gray squares, HFL; black squares, HFH. *B*: Mean daily energy intake. *C*: Positive correlation between final body weight and liver triglyceride concentration ($P < 0.05$). *D*: Weight of epididymal fat depot. *E*: Adipose tissue leptin mRNA expression as determined by quantitative PCR. Mean expression in LFL mice was set at 100%. *F*: Plasma free fatty acid levels. Error bars reflect SD. *Significantly different from HFL mice according to Student's *t* test ($P < 0.05$). Number of mice per group: $n = 4$ for LFL, HFL, and HFH and $n = 6$ for LFH. *G*: H-E staining of representative adipose tissue sections. *H*: Immunohistochemical staining of macrophages using antibody against Cd68. *I*: Collagen staining using fast green FCF/sirius red F3B. (A high-quality digital representation of this figure is available in the online issue.)

synthase, *Fasn*) marker genes was significantly downregulated in HFH mice compared with HFL mice, suggesting adipose tissue dysfunction. Finally, collagen staining revealed fibrotic adipose tissue in HFH mice (Fig. 4*I*), which was supported by increased expression of tissue inhibitor of matrix metalloproteinases (*Timp-1*) (Fig. 5). These data suggest that HFH responders, classification of which is

entirely determined by liver histology, exhibit adipose tissue dysfunction characterized by decreased fat mass, enhanced macrophage infiltration, inflammation, and adipose tissue remodelling.

Plasma biomarkers are significantly associated with liver triglycerides. To find early biomarkers that may predict NASH in C57Bl/6 mice and that may serve as

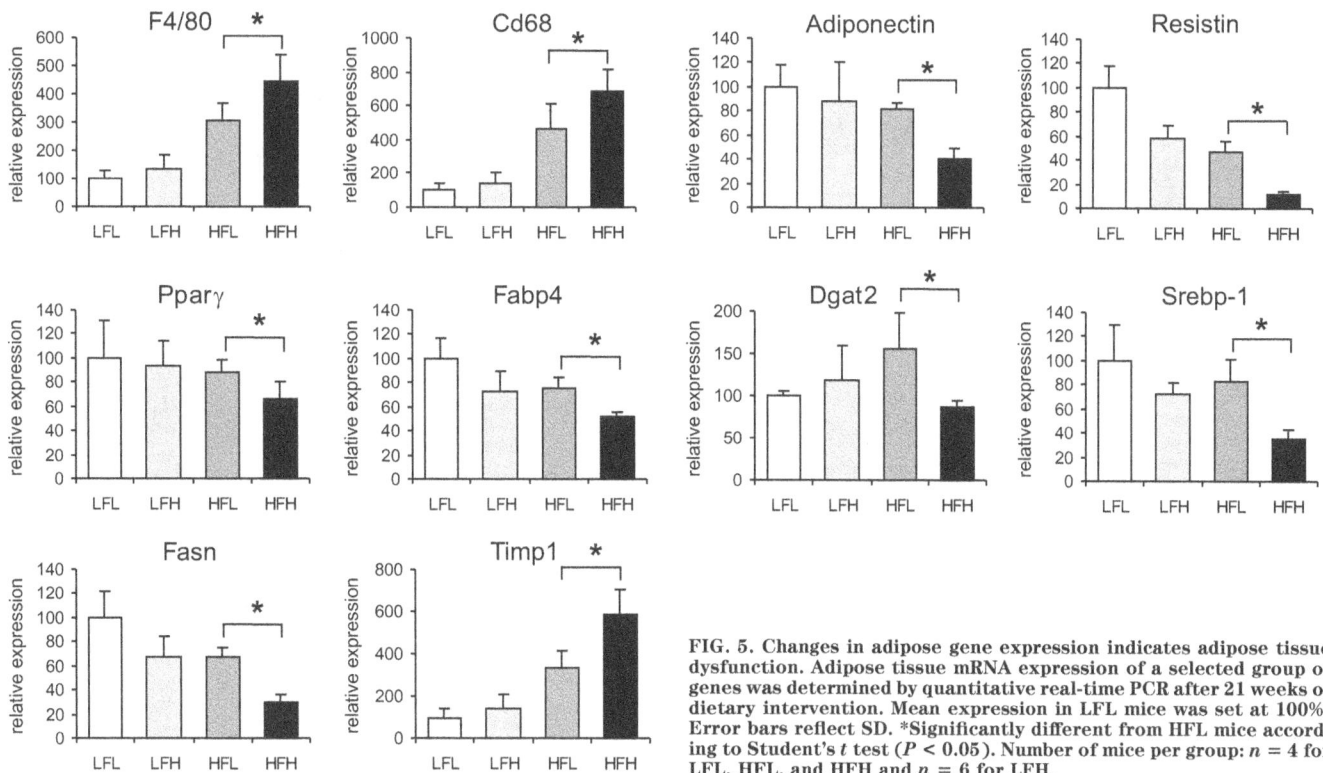

FIG. 5. Changes in adipose gene expression indicates adipose tissue dysfunction. Adipose tissue mRNA expression of a selected group of genes was determined by quantitative real-time PCR after 21 weeks of dietary intervention. Mean expression in LFL mice was set at 100%. Error bars reflect SD. *Significantly different from HFL mice according to Student's t test ($P < 0.05$). Number of mice per group: $n = 4$ for LFL, HFL, and HFH and $n = 6$ for LFH.

potential mediators between adipose tissue dysfunction and NASH, plasma was collected at different time points of diet intervention and assayed for 70 plasma proteins using multiplex analysis. Levels of most plasma proteins were not consistently different between the subgroups. One exception was the acute phase protein haptoglobin, which was elevated in HFH mice after 12 weeks of diet intervention (Fig. 6A). Similarly, plasma levels of the fibrosis marker TIMP-1 started to deviate at week 12 and further increased until the end. Remarkably, interleukin (IL)-1β and leptin levels were already elevated in HFH after 2 weeks and this pattern was maintained throughout the intervention. Finally, plasma insulin levels indicated that HFH mice became hyperinsulinemic from week 12, suggesting development of insulin resistance.

To systematically screen for plasma biomarkers that predict liver triglycerides, multivariate analysis was performed using MPLS. The results of multivariate analysis between plasma proteins at different time points and liver triglycerides are depicted in Fig. 6B and supplemental Table 2. In addition to leptin, plasma levels of C-reactive protein (CRP), eotaxin, haptoglobin, and macrophage inflammatory protein (MIP)-1α early in the intervention were positively associated with liver triglycerides at 20 weeks. Intermediate prognostic markers of liver triglycerides included IL-18, IL-1β, MIP-1γ, and MIP-2, whereas insulin, TIMP-1, GCP-2, and MPO emerged as late markers. Throughout the diet intervention, highest regression coefficients were obtained for CRP, haptoglobin, leptin, and IL-1β (supplemental Table 2). Adiponectin was not significantly associated with liver triglycerides. The complete multivariate dataset is available at http://humannutrition2.wur.nl/duval2010. Besides potentially serving as predictive biomarkers of liver triglycerides, these proteins may provide a functional link between adipose tissue dysfunction and NAFLD.

DISCUSSION

C57Bl/6 mice fed a HFD represent a popular animal model for human obesity and insulin resistance. Despite development of hepatic steatosis and other features of patients with NAFLD (18), except for a recent report the model has not been extensively used to study NAFLD (19). As expected, high-fat feeding increased adipose tissue mass and hepatic fat storage. Consistent with previous data showing considerable variability in the obese and diabetic phenotype (20,21), we observed marked heterogeneity in body weight gain. Additionally, the magnitude of fat storage and NAFLD scoring differed markedly between the mice, giving rise to four well-distinguishable groups. Detailed histological and gene expression analysis indicated that HFH mice exhibit NASH. Accordingly, detailed study of these HFH responders may give novel insight into the development and progression of NAFLD.

Although humans have no epididymal fat pads, we studied epididymal adipose tissue because it represents the most commonly used fat depot in mouse studies, is easily accessible, can be accurately weighed, and is relatively homogenous. Unfortunately, we did not have access to dual-energy X-ray absorptiometry or magnetic resonance imaging to be able to measure fat percentage, lean body mass, or fat distribution. Remarkably, HFH mice, despite showing the highest weight gain, had significantly less epididymal fat after 21 weeks compared with HFL mice, which likely reflects differences in overall adiposity. An important question is why there is an apparent limit to the expansion of adipose tissue in HFH mice and, especially, what is the link with NASH. Obesity-related adipocyte hypertrophy is known to be associated with adipose inflammation characterized by infiltration of macrophages and other leukocytes, appearance of so-called crown-like structures, and increased expression of several inflamma-

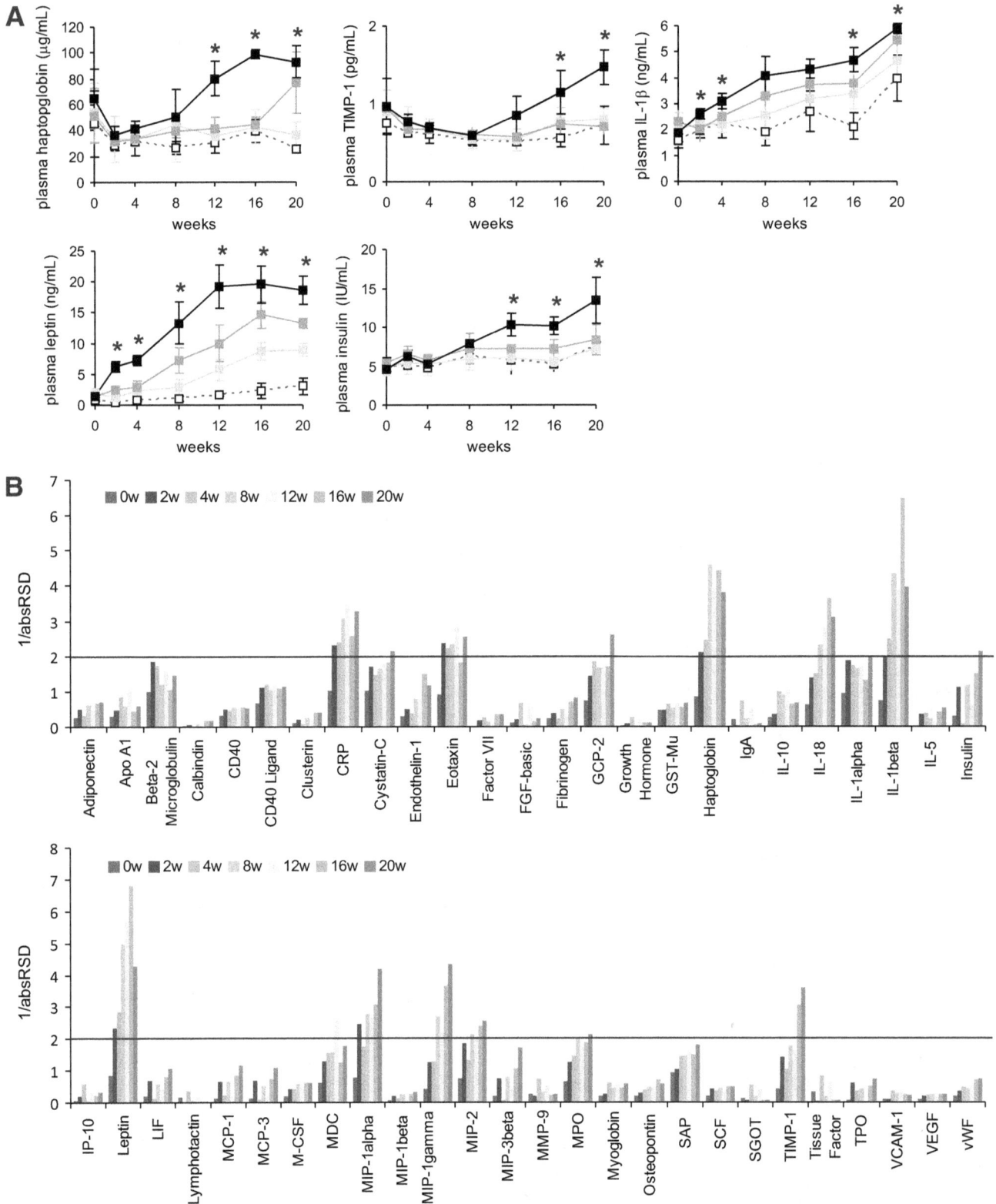

FIG. 6. Plasma proteins as early predictive biomarker for NASH in C57Bl/6 mice. *A*: Plasma concentration of haptoglobin, TIMP-1, IL-1β, leptin, and insulin were determined by multiplex assay at specific time points during the 21 weeks of dietary intervention after a 6-h fast. White squares, LFL; light-gray squares, LFH; dark-gray squares, HFL; black squares, HFH. Error bars reflect SD. *Significantly different from HFL mice according to Student's *t* test (*P* < 0.05). Number of mice per group: *n* = 4 for LFL, HFL, and HFH and *n* = 6 for LFH. *B*: Graphs illustrating the result of multivariate analysis showing the association of protein plasma concentrations at various time points with final liver triglyceride content. The absRSD is the absolute relative standard deviation: the standard deviation of the regression coefficients divided by the absolute mean value of the regression coefficients. Significant proteins display an inverse absRSD value higher than two (bold line indicates the inverse absRSD threshold value of 2). w, weeks.

Diabetes • December 2010 • 59:3181–3191

tory markers (2,3,22,23). How adipose tissue inflammation develops during obesity is not clear, but a role of hypertrophy, hypoxia, and adipocyte cell death has been suggested (23,24). Compared with HFL mice, adipose tissue of HFH mice showed more pronounced inflammation as shown by increased macrophage staining and expression of inflammatory marker genes and increased collagen staining, suggesting fibrosis. Furthermore, decreased adipocyte size and increased cell death were observed in HFH mice. Since HFH mice are classified entirely based on liver histology, these data indicate a strong link between inflammatory and morphological changes in adipose tissue and progression of steatosis to NASH. Consequently, adipose tissue failure or dysfunction may signal progression of hepatic steatosis toward NASH. These data support the previous suggestion that poor expansion of adipose tissue mass due to remodeling contributes to hepatic steatosis induced by high-fat feeding (23) and thereby strengthen an emerging view that obesity starts to cause metabolic problems when adipose tissue cannot fully meet demands for additional storage, leading to fat accumulation in other organs such as muscle, liver, and β-cells and causing lipotoxicity (25–27). The limited expandability of adipose tissue may be related to adipose tissue fibrosis and associated disproportionate accumulation of extracellular matrix components (22).

Multivariate longitudinal analysis of plasma proteins yielded a number of candidates that may serve as prognostic markers for NAFLD and NASH. In addition, these proteins may provide insight into the functional link between adipose tissue dysfunction and NAFLD. Besides leptin, the best predictive markers were the acute phase proteins CRP and haptoglobin and MIP-1α (Ccl3). Plasma CRP was previously proposed as a diagnostic marker for NASH (28). In one study, high-sensitivity CRP was significantly elevated in patients with NASH compared with that in patients with only steatosis (29). Furthermore, high-sensitivity CRP correlated with the severity of fibrosis in NASH. In another study, plasma CRP was not helpful in diagnosis of NASH in severely obese patients, possibly because adipose tissue contributes to plasma CRP in obesity.

Hardly any data exist on the relation between plasma haptoglobin and NASH. Haptoglobin was included in a composite biomarker combining 13 parameters to predict NASH (30). Interestingly, in a recent study plasma haptoglobin showed a negative correlation with fibrosis stage (31). There are no reports on the association between plasma MIP-1α and hepatic steatosis or NASH. However, it was reported that MIP-1α mRNA in human liver is positively associated with liver fat (32).

Another good predictive marker for liver triglycerides was IL-1β. Plasma IL-1β levels were significantly elevated in HFH mice already after 2 weeks of HFD, probably because of elevated production in adipose tissue. Recently, we showed that IL-1β may promote steatosis in mice by inhibiting PPARα activity (33). Whether adipose tissue–derived IL-1β links adipose tissue dysfunction and NASH requires further study.

Recent studies indicate that IL-18 promotes hepatic steatosis in mice (34,35). Interestingly, patients with NAFLD were found to have significantly elevated plasma IL-18 levels (36). According to our multivariate analysis, plasma IL-18 from week eight onward was significantly associated with liver triglycerides. Overall, further research into the potential use of plasma CRP, haptoglobin,

MIP-1α, and possibly IL-1β, eotaxin, and IL-18 as prognostic biomarkers for NAFLD in humans is warranted.

One of the late biomarkers to emerge from our study was TIMP-1. Specifically, plasma TIMP-1 levels started to deviate in the HFH mice after 12 weeks of HFD. Since TIMP-1 expression was increased in HFH mice in both liver and adipose tissue, it is unclear which tissue primarily contributes to increased plasma levels. TIMP-1 is used extensively as a marker of fibrosis related to viral hepatitis (37). However, its use in the context of NAFLD is very limited. According to our data, plasma TIMP-1 levels may have potential as a biomarker for NASH. Consistent with this notion, plasma TIMP-1 was recently shown to be a valuable component of a composite predictive marker of NASH in human (38).

An adipokine that has been extensively linked to NAFLD is adiponectin (37,39). Besides its antisteatotic role (38,40), adiponectin has potent anti-inflammatory effects in liver (39). In humans, plasma adiponectin, either alone or as ratio to plasma leptin (41), has shown promise as a diagnostic marker for NASH, although it should be validated in larger cohorts of patients (9). In the present study, plasma adiponectin was not significantly associated with liver triglycerides.

Overall, the best predictive marker for liver triglycerides, which was also clearly elevated in HFH mice, was leptin. Portal infusion with leptin was shown to increase hepatic triglycerides in rats (42). Furthermore, leptin appears to be one of the key regulators of inflammation and progression to fibrosis in NASH (43–46). Although some studies have found elevated plasma leptin levels in patients with NASH (47,48), other studies have not, thus somewhat questioning the potential of plasma leptin as a noninvasive marker for diagnosis of NASH in humans (49).

Hyperleptinemia in HFH mice is expected to decrease food intake. However, energy intake was higher in HFH compared with that in other subgroups, suggesting existence of leptin resistance, at least centrally in the hypothalamus. In contrast, leptin resistance is expected to be absent from liver, in which chronically elevated leptin levels may promote NASH by stimulating hepatic triglyceride storage, inflammation, and fibrosis (37). Leptin resistance may thus be the basis for hyperleptinemia and hyperphagia in HFH mice, leading to accelerated weight and fat gain and consequent adipose tissue dysfunction.

The significant heterogeneity in the response to HFD in C57Bl/6 mice has been previously reported (20,21). The underlying reason for the large heterogeneity is uncertain but may be related to copy no. variations in the mouse genome (50) and perhaps specifically by differences in the copy no. of the *Ide* gene encoding the insulin-degrading enzyme (51). Alternatively, the variation in phenotype after HFD may be mediated by epigenetic mechanisms (21), giving rise to variable adipose expression of specific genes. However, the importance of epigenetic mechanisms in controlling expression of one of these genes was later discounted (52). Overall, the relative importance of genetic, epigenetic, and environmental factors in the response to high-fat feeding in C57Bl/6 mice is still unclear.

In conclusion, we show that a subset of C57Bl/6 mice fed a HFD composed of palm oil developed NASH. Our data support the existence of a tight relationship between adipose tissue dysfunction and NASH pathogenesis and point to several novel potential predictive biomarkers for NASH.

ACKNOWLEDGMENTS

No potential conflicts of interest relevant to this article were reported.

C.D. designed the research, collected data, analyzed the data, wrote the manuscript, and reviewed and edited the manuscript. U.T. analyzed the data and reviewed and edited the manuscript. S.K. collected and analyzed the data. B.A. collected data and reviewed and edited the manuscript. R.S. collected data and reviewed and edited the manuscript. M.V.B. analyzed the data and reviewed and edited the manuscript. T.R. analyzed the data and reviewed and edited the manuscript. S.K. designed the research, collected data, analyzed the data, wrote the manuscript, and reviewed and edited the manuscript. M.M. designed the research and reviewed and edited the manuscript.

REFERENCES

1. Perlemuter G, Bigorgne A, Cassard-Doulcier AM, Naveau S. Nonalcoholic fatty liver disease: from pathogenesis to patient care. Nat Clin Pract Endocrinol Metab 2007;3:458–469
2. Weisberg SP, McCann D, Desai M, Rosenbaum M, Leibel RL, Ferrante AW Jr.: Obesity is associated with macrophage accumulation in adipose tissue. J Clin Invest 2003;112:1796–1808
3. Xu H, Barnes GT, Yang Q, Tan G, Yang D, Chou CJ, Sole J, Nichols A, Ross JS, Tartaglia LA, Chen H. Chronic inflammation in fat plays a crucial role in the development of obesity-related insulin resistance. J Clin Invest 2003;112:1821–1830
4. Lazar MA. How obesity causes diabetes: not a tall tale. Science 2005;307: 373–375
5. Szendroedi J, Roden M. Ectopic lipids and organ function. Curr Opin Lipidol 2009;20:50–56
6. Yeh MM, Brunt EM. Pathology of nonalcoholic fatty liver disease. Am J Clin Pathol 2007;128:837–847
7. Lalor PF, Faint J, Aarbodem Y, Hubscher SG, Adams DH. The role of cytokines and chemokines in the development of steatohepatitis. Semin Liver Dis 2007;27:173–193
8. Jou J, Choi SS, Diehl AM. Mechanisms of disease progression in nonalcoholic fatty liver disease. Semin Liver Dis 2008;28:370–379
9. Tsochatzis EA, Papatheodoridis GV, Archimandritis AJ. Adipokines in nonalcoholic steatohepatitis: from pathogenesis to implications in diagnosis and therapy. Mediators Inflamm 2009;831670
10. Stienstra R, Mandard S, Patsouris D, Maass C, Kersten S, Muller M. Peroxisome proliferator-activated receptor alpha protects against obesity-induced hepatic inflammations. Endocrinology 2007;148:2753–2763
11. Rakhshandehroo M, Hooiveld G, Muller M, Kersten S. Comparative analysis of gene regulation by the transcription factor PPARalpha between mouse and human. PLoS One 2009;4:e6796
12. Sanderson LM, Degenhardt T, Koppen A, Kalkhoven E, Desvergne B, Muller M, Kersten S. Peroxisome proliferator-activated receptor beta/delta (PPARbeta/delta) but not PPARalpha serves as a plasma free fatty acid sensor in liver. Mol Cell Biol 2009;29:6257–6267
13. Subramanian A, Tamayo P, Mootha VK, Mukherjee S, Ebert BL, Gillette MA, Paulovich A, Pomeroy SL, Golub TR, Lander ES, Mesirov JP. Gene set enrichment analysis: a knowledge-based approach for interpreting genome-wide expression profiles. Proc Natl Acad Sci U S A 2005;102:15545–15550
14. Boulesteix AL, Strimmer K. Partial least squares: a versatile tool for the analysis of high-dimensional genomic data. Brief Bioinform 2007;8:32–44
15. Bro R. Multiway calibration multilinear PLS. J Chemometrics 1996;10: 47–62
16. Smilde AK, Bro R, Geladi P. *Multi-Way Analysis: Applications in the Chemical Sciences*. West Sussex, Wiley, 2004
17. Heidema AG, Thissen U, Boer JM, Bouwman FG, Feskens EJ, Mariman EC. The association of 83 plasma proteins with CHD mortality, BMI, HDL-, and total-cholesterol in men: applying multivariate statistics to identify proteins with prognostic value and biological relevance. J Proteome Res 2009;8:2640–2649
18. Larter CZ, Yeh MM. Animal models of NASH: getting both pathology and metabolic context right. J Gastroenterol Hepatol 2008;23:1635–1648
19. Ito M, Suzuki J, Tsujioka S, Sasaki M, Gomori A, Shirakura T, Hirose H, Ishihara A, Iwaasa H, Kanatani A. Longitudinal analysis of murine steato-

20. Burcelin R, Crivelli V, Dacosta A, Roy-Tirelli A, Thorens B. Heterogeneous metabolic adaptation of C57BL/6J mice to high-fat diet. Am J Physiol Endocrinol Metab 2002;282:E834–E842
21. Koza RA, Nikonova L, Hogan J, Rim JS, Mendoza T, Faulk C, Skaf J, Kozak LP. Changes in gene expression foreshadow diet-induced obesity in genetically identical mice. PLoS Genet 2006;2:e81
22. Khan T, Muise ES, Iyengar P, Wang ZV, Chandalia M, Abate N, Zhang BB, Bonaldo P, Chua S, Scherer PE. Metabolic dysregulation and adipose tissue fibrosis: role of collagen VI. Mol Cell Biol 2009;29:1575–1591
23. Strissel KJ, Stancheva Z, Miyoshi H, Perfield JW 2nd, DeFuria J, Jick Z, Greenberg AS, Obin MS. Adipocyte death, adipose tissue remodeling, and obesity complications. Diabetes 2007;56:2910–2918
24. Trayhurn P, Wang B, Wood IS. Hypoxia in adipose tissue: a basis for the dysregulation of tissue function in obesity? Br J Nutr 2008;100:227–235
25. Tan CY, Vidal-Puig A. Adipose tissue expandability: the metabolic problems of obesity may arise from the inability to become more obese. Biochem Soc Trans 2008;36:935–940
26. Unger RH. The physiology of cellular liporegulation. Annu Rev Physiol 2003;65:333–347
27. Wang MY, Grayburn P, Chen S, Ravazzola M, Orci L, Unger RH. Adipogenic capacity and the susceptibility to type 2 diabetes and metabolic syndrome. Proc Natl Acad Sci U S A 2008;105:6139–6144
28. Uchihara M, Izumi N. [High-sensitivity C-reactive protein (hs-CRP): a promising biomarker for the screening of non-alcoholic steatohepatitis (NASH)]. Nippon Rinsho 2006;64:1133–1138 [in Japanese]
29. Yoneda M, Mawatari H, Fujita K, Iida H, Yonemitsu K, Kato S, Takahashi H, Kirikoshi H, Inamori M, Nozaki Y, Abe Y, Kubota K, Saito S, Iwasaki T, Terauchi Y, Togo S, Maeyama S, Nakajima A. High-sensitivity C-reactive protein is an independent clinical feature of nonalcoholic steatohepatitis (NASH) and also of the severity of fibrosis in NASH. J Gastroenterol 2007;42:573–582
30. Poynard T, Ratziu V, Charlotte F, Messous D, Munteanu M, Imbert-Bismut F, Massard J, Bonyhay L, Tahiri M, Thabut D, Cadranel JF, Le Bail B, de Ledinghen V. Diagnostic value of biochemical markers (NashTest) for the prediction of non alcoholo steato hepatitis in patients with non-alcoholic fatty liver disease. BMC Gastroenterol 2006;6:34
31. Lee HH, Seo YS, Um SH, Won NH, Yoo H, Jung ES, Kwon YD, Park S, Keum B, Kim YS, Yim MJ, Jeen YT, Chun HJ, Kim CD, Ryu HS. Usefulness of non-invasive markers for predicting significant fibrosis in patients with chronic liver disease. J Korean Med Sci 2010;25:67–74
32. Westerbacka J, Kolak M, Kiviluoto T, Arkkila P, Siren J, Hamsten A, Fisher RM, Yki-Jarvinen H. Genes involved in fatty acid partitioning and binding, lipolysis, monocyte/macrophage recruitment, and inflammation are over-expressed in the human fatty liver of insulin-resistant subjects. Diabetes 2007;56:2759–2765
33. Stienstra R, Saudale F, Duval C, Keshtkar S, Groener JE, van Rooijen N, Staels B, Kersten S, Muller M: Kupffer cells promote hepatic steatosis via interleukin-1beta-dependent suppression of peroxisome proliferator-activated receptor alpha activity. Hepatology 51:511–522
34. Chikano S, Sawada K, Shimoyama T, Kashiwamura SI, Sugihara A, Sekikawa K, Terada N, Nakanishi K, Okamura H. IL-18 and IL-12 induce intestinal inflammation and fatty liver in mice in an IFN-gamma dependent manner. Gut 2000;47:779–786
35. Kaneda M, Kashiwamura S, Ueda H, Sawada K, Sugihara A, Terada N, Kimura-Shimmyo A, Fukuda Y, Shimoyama T, Okamura H. Inflammatory liver steatosis caused by IL-12 and IL-18. J Interferon Cytokine Res 2003;23:155–162
36. Li Y, Li-Li Z, Qin L, Ying W. Plasma interleukin-18/interleukin-18 binding protein ratio in Chinese with NAFLD. Hepatogastroenterology 2010;57: 103–106
37. Schaffler A, Scholmerich J, Buchler C. Mechanisms of disease: adipocytokines and visceral adipose tissue–emerging role in nonalcoholic fatty liver disease. Nat Clin Pract Gastroenterol Hepatol 2005;2:273–280
38. Xu A, Wang Y, Keshaw H, Xu LY, Lam KS, Cooper GJ. The fat-derived hormone adiponectin alleviates alcoholic and nonalcoholic fatty liver diseases in mice. J Clin Invest 2003;112:91–100
39. Marra F, Bertolani C. Adipokines in liver diseases. Hepatology 2009;50: 957–969
40. Yamauchi T, Kamon J, Waki H, Terauchi Y, Kubota N, Hara K, Mori Y, Ide T, Murakami K, Tsuboyama-Kasaoka N, Ezaki O, Akanuma Y, Gavrilova O, Vinson C, Reitman ML, Kagechika H, Shudo K, Yoda M, Nakano Y, Tobe K, Nagai R, Kimura S, Tomita M, Froguel P, Kadowaki T. The fat-derived hormone adiponectin reverses insulin resistance associated with both lipoatrophy and obesity. Nat Med 2001;7:941–946
41. Lemoine M, Ratziu V, Kim M, Maachi M, Wendum D, Paye F, Bastard JP,

Poupon R, Housset C, Capeau J, Serfaty L. Serum adipokine levels predictive of liver injury in non-alcoholic fatty liver disease. Liver Int 2009;29:1431–1438

42. Roden M, Anderwald C, Furnsinn C, Waldhausl W, Lohninger A. Effects of short-term leptin exposure on triglyceride deposition in rat liver. Hepatology 2000;32:1045–1049

43. Ikejima K, Honda H, Yoshikawa M, Hirose M, Kitamura T, Takei Y, Sato N. Leptin augments inflammatory and profibrogenic responses in the murine liver induced by hepatotoxic chemicals. Hepatology 2001;34:288–297

44. Ikejima K, Okumura K, Lang T, Honda H, Abe W, Yamashina S, Enomoto N, Takei Y, Sato N. The role of leptin in progression of non-alcoholic fatty liver disease. Hepatol Res 2005;33:151–154

45. Leclercq IA, Farrell GC, Schriemer R, Robertson GR. Leptin is essential for the hepatic fibrogenic response to chronic liver injury. J Hepatol 2002;37: 206–213

46. Saxena NK, Ikeda K, Rockey DC, Friedman SL, Anania FA. Leptin in hepatic fibrosis: evidence for increased collagen production in stellate cells and lean littermates of ob/ob mice. Hepatology 2002;35:762–771

47. Chitturi S, Farrell G, Frost L, Kriketos A, Lin R, Fung C, Liddle C, Samarasinghe D, George J. Serum leptin in NASH correlates with hepatic steatosis but not fibrosis: a manifestation of lipotoxicity? Hepatology 2002;36:403–409

48. Krawczyk K, Szczesniak P, Kumor A, Jasinska A, Omulecka A, Pietruczuk M, Orszulak-Michalak D, Sporny S, Malecka-Panas E. Adipohormones as prognostric markers in patients with nonalcoholic steatohepatitis (NASH). J Physiol Pharmacol 2009;60(Suppl. 3):71–75

49. Tsochatzis E, Papatheodoridis GV, Archimandritis AJ. The evolving role of leptin and adiponectin in chronic liver diseases. Am J Gastroenterol 2006;101:2629–2640

50. Cutler G, Kassner PD. Copy number variation in the mouse genome: implications for the mouse as a model organism for human disease. Cytogenet Genome Res 2008;123:297–306

51. Watkins-Chow DE, Pavan WJ. Genomic copy number and expression variation within the C57BL/6J inbred mouse strain. Genome Res 2008;18: 60–66

52. Koza RA, Rogers P, Kozak LP. Inter-individual variation of dietary fat-induced mesoderm specific transcript in adipose tissue within inbred mice is not caused by altered promoter methylation. Epigenetics 2009;4:512–518

Combined Effect of Nonalcoholic Fatty Liver Disease and Impaired Fasting Glucose on the Development of Type 2 Diabetes

A 4-year retrospective longitudinal study

Ji Cheol Bae, md
Eun Jung Rhee, md, phd
Won Young Lee, md, phd
Se Eun Park, md

Cheol Young Park, md, phd
Ki Won Oh, md, phd
Sung Woo Park, md, phd
Sun Woo Kim, md

OBJECTIVE—To evaluate whether there is a difference in the association between nonalcoholic fatty liver disease (NAFLD) and incident diabetes based on the presence of impaired fasting glucose.

RESEARCH DESIGN AND METHODS—A total of 7,849 individuals (5,409 men and 2,440 women) without diabetes, who underwent comprehensive health check-ups annually for 5 years, were categorized into four groups by the presence of impaired fasting glucose and NAFLD at baseline. The association between NAFLD and incident diabetes was evaluated separately in groups with normal and impaired fasting glucose.

RESULTS—For 4 years, the incidence of diabetes in the NAFLD group was 9.9% compared with 3.7% in the non-NAFLD group, with multivariable-adjusted hazard ratio of 1.33 (95% CI 1.07–1.66). However, this higher risk for diabetes only existed in the impaired fasting glucose group.

CONCLUSIONS—Our study suggests that NAFLD has an independent and additive effect on the development of diabetes under conditions of impaired insulin secretion.

Diabetes Care 34:727–729, 2011

N onalcoholic fatty liver disease (NAFLD) is reported to have an effect on incident diabetes (1–3). NAFLD coexists in a substantial percentage of patients with impaired fasting glucose (IFG) (4). This study was designed to ascertain whether there is a difference in the association between NAFLD and incident diabetes according to the presence of IFG.

RESEARCH DESIGN AND

METHODS—Initial data were obtained from 10,950 individuals who participated in comprehensive health check-ups

annually for 5 years (between January 2005 and December 2009). Among these, 3,101 were excluded for alcohol intake >20 g/day, type 1 or type 2 diabetes, positive serologic markers for hepatitis B or C virus, liver cirrhosis, or missing data. All analyses were performed on 7,849 individuals (5,409 men and 2,440 women) who were aged ≥20 years (mean age, 44.5 years; Supplementary Table 1).

We categorized all participants into four groups according to the presence of IFG and NAFLD in the 2005 records. The hazard ratio (HR) of incipient diabetes associated with NAFLD was estimated

overall and separately in the normal fasting glucose (NFG) and IFG groups using Cox proportional hazards analysis. Also, we evaluated the combined effect of IFG and NAFLD on incident diabetes. Statistical analysis was performed using SPSS 17 software (SPSS, Chicago, IL).

Anthropometric and biochemical variables were measured as described previously (5). Lifestyle information was self-reported.

All subjects had an abdominal ultrasonogram (Logic Q700 MR, GE, Milwaukee, WI), and fatty liver was diagnosed based on known standard criteria, including hepatorenal echo contrast, liver brightness, deep attenuation, and vascular blurring, using a 3.5 MHz probe (6). Several experienced radiologists performed the ultrasound examinations.

IFG was defined as fasting plasma glucose between 100 and 125 mg/dL (7). The development of diabetes was assessed from the annual records of all participants and defined as fasting plasma glucose ≥126 mg/dL or A1C ≥6.5% (7). Also, subjects who had a history of diabetes or currently used insulin or oral antidiabetic drugs based on the self-report questionnaire at each visit were considered to have developed diabetes.

RESULTS—During the mean follow-up of nearly 4 years (47.4 ± 5.0 months), 435 of the 7,849 participants (5.5%) progressed to diabetes. The incidence of diabetes was 9.9% in the NAFLD group and 3.7% in the non-NAFLD group. In a multivariate model adjusted for age, sex, BMI, triglyceride, HDL cholesterol, smoking status, physical activity, alcohol intake, and coexisting IFG, subjects with NAFLD had an HR of 1.33 (95% CI 1.07–1.66) for the development of diabetes compared with the non-NAFLD groups (Supplementary Table 2). However, the significance of this association between NAFLD and incident diabetes was different based on whether IFG was present.

From the Division of Endocrinology and Metabolism, Department of Internal Medicine, Kangbuk Samsung Hospital, Sungkyunkwan University School of Medicine, Seoul, Korea.
Corresponding author: Won Young Lee, drlwy@hanmail.net.
Received 21 October 2010 and accepted 29 December 2010.
DOI: 10.2337/dc10-1991
This article contains Supplementary Data online at http://care.diabetesjournals.org/lookup/suppl/doi:10.2337/dc10-1991/-/DC1.

Table 1—*HRs of incident diabetes for the NAFLD and non-NAFLD groups according to the presence of IFG and combined effects of NAFLD with IFG on the development of diabetes*

Variable	NFG (n = 5,800)			IFG (n = 2,049)		
	Non-NAFLD	NAFLD	P	Non-NAFLD	NAFLD	P
Subjects (N)	4,353	1,447		1,204	845	
Subjects who developed diabetes, n (%)	66 (1.5)	47 (3.2)		142 (11.8)	180 (21.3)	
Person-years of follow-up	17,363	5,773		4,646	3,155	
Incident case of diabetes per 100 person-years (n)	0.4	0.8		3.1	5.7	
Adjusted HR (95% CI)*						
Age and sex	1 (reference)	2.01 (1.35–2.98)	0.001	1 (reference)	1.86 (1.48–2.33)	<0.001
Age, sex, BMI, TG, HDL-C, and systolic BP	1 (reference)	1.37 (0.87–2.18)	0.167	1 (reference)	1.31 (1.02–1.69)	0.035
Multivariate†	1 (reference)	1.39 (0.88–2.23)	0.148	1 (reference)	1.30 (1.02–1.68)	0.037
Adjusted HR (95% CI)*						
Age and sex	1 (reference)	2.03 (1.39–2.97)		7.52 (5.60–10.09)	13.97 (10.43–18.71)	
Age, sex, BMI, TG, HDL-C, and systolic BP	1 (reference)	1.37 (0.92–2.04)		6.68 (4.95–9.00)	8.83 (6.41–12.16)	
Multivariate†	1 (reference)	1.39 (0.93–2.08)		6.79 (5.03–9.16)	8.95 (6.49–12.35)	

BP, blood pressure; HDL-C, HDL cholesterol; TG, triglycerides. *Estimated from Cox proportional hazards analysis. †The multivariate Cox regression model was adjusted for baseline age, sex, BMI, TG, HDL-C, systolic BP, concurrent presence of IFG, smoking status (never smoked, former smoker, or current smoker), physical activity (a minimum of 30 min at least 3 times per week or less), and alcohol consumption (current drinker or not).

Participants with NAFLD had a significantly higher HR for the development of diabetes only if IFG was present, reaching 1.30 (95% CI 1.02–1.68), whereas the HR was 1.39 (95% CI 0.88–2.23) in the NFG groups. After multivariable adjustment, those with IFG alone had an HR of 6.79 (95% CI 5.03–9.16) for the development of diabetes compared with NFG subjects without NAFLD, whereas those with NAFLD alone had an HR of 1.39 (95% CI 0.93–2.08). Among the subjects with IFG and NAFLD, we observed further increased risk of diabetes, with an HR of 8.95 (95% CI 6.49–12.35; Table 1 and Supplementary Fig. 1).

CONCLUSIONS—When we separately analyzed the association between NAFLD and incident diabetes based on the presence of IFG, an independent association was only shown in the subjects with IFG. Early in the natural history of type 2 diabetes, insulin resistance is well established, but glucose tolerance remains normal because of a compensatory increase in insulin secretion (8,9). Although animal studies showed that fat accumulation in the liver inhibited insulin signaling in hepatocytes, which decreased insulin activity to glycogen synthase and increased gluconeogenesis (10,11), the resulting elevation of insulin

concentration can overcome hepatic insulin resistance and cause a nearly normal suppression of hepatic glucose products (9), which could explain our inability to show an independent association between NAFLD and incident diabetes in the individuals with NFG. However, the presence of IFG indicates that β-cells already have impairment of insulin secretion and are unable to maintain a compensatory increase in insulin secretion (12). Our results differed according to the presence of IFG, suggesting that NAFLD has an independent effect on the development of diabetes under conditions of impaired insulin secretion.

The comparison of NAFLD with IFG helps us understand the relative importance of NAFLD in the development of diabetes. Although subjects with NAFLD alone were more obese and insulin resistant than those with IFG alone (Supplementary Table 3), the risk for incident diabetes was much higher in subjects with IFG alone than in those with NAFLD alone. However, the high risk of diabetes among subjects with IFG exaggerated by the presence of NAFLD, even after adjustment for BMI and other risk factors, indicates that IFG and NAFLD have an additive effect on the development of diabetes.

Several limitations to this study should be considered. The lack of a 2-h postload glucose test is a limitation because it might have resulted in inclusion of subjects with undiagnosed diabetes at baseline. The presence of impaired glucose tolerance was not considered, and this might also have an effect on the study results. Ultrasonography was used to diagnose fatty liver. Despite being considerably accurate, ultrasonography cannot identify fatty infiltration of the liver below the threshold of 30% (13). NAFLD is closely associated with abdominal obesity (14). However, our analysis was not adjusted for waist circumference reflecting abdominal obesity. Finally, we did not consider the use of other drugs for dyslipidemia in our analysis, and that might have influenced glucose levels (15).

This study suggests that NAFLD is an independent risk factor for diabetes. This independent association is shown particularly in individuals with IFG, indicating that NAFLD has an independent and additive effect on the development of diabetes under conditions of impaired insulin secretion.

Acknowledgments—This work was partially supported by the Samsung Biomedical Research Institute Grant (SBRI C-A8-223-2).

No potential conflicts of interest relevant to this article were reported.

J.C.B. contributed to study design, statistical analysis, and interpretation of results and wrote the manuscript. E.J.R. contributed to interpretation of results and reviewed and edited the manuscript. W.Y.L. contributed to study design and interpretation of results and reviewed and edited the manuscript. S.E.P. contributed to acquisition of data and discussion. C.Y.P. and K.W.O. reviewed and edited the manuscript. S.W.P. and S.W.K. contributed to discussion.

Parts of this study were presented in abstract form at the 8th International Diabetes Federation-Western Pacific Region Congress, Busan, Korea, 17–20 October 2010.

The authors thank Hyun Il Seo, Kangbuk Samsung Hospital, for help with preparing the manuscript.

References

1. Fraser A, Harris R, Sattar N, Ebrahim S, Davey Smith G, Lawlor DA. Alanine aminotransferase, gamma-glutamyltransferase, and incident diabetes: the British Women's Heart and Health Study and meta-analysis. Diabetes Care 2009;32:741–750
2. Kim CH, Park JY, Lee KU, Kim JH, Kim HK. Fatty liver is an independent risk factor for the development of type 2 diabetes in Korean adults. Diabet Med 2008; 25:476–481
3. Yamada T, Fukatsu M, Suzuki S, Wada T, Yoshida T, Joh T. Fatty liver predicts impaired fasting glucose and type 2 diabetes mellitus in Japanese undergoing a health checkup. J Gastroenterol Hepatol 2010; 25:352–356
4. Jimba S, Nakagami T, Takahashi M, et al. Prevalence of non-alcoholic fatty liver disease and its association with impaired glucose metabolism in Japanese adults. Diabet Med 2005;22:1141–1145
5. Bae JC, Cho YK, Lee WY, et al. Impact of nonalcoholic fatty liver disease on insulin resistance in relation to HbA1c levels in nondiabetic subjects. Am J Gastroenterol 2010;105:2389–2395
6. Saverymuttu SH, Joseph AE, Maxwell JD. Ultrasound scanning in the detection of hepatic fibrosis and steatosis. Br Med J (Clin Res Ed) 1986;292:13–15
7. American Diabetes Association. Standards of medical care in diabetes—2010. Diabetes Care 2010;33(Suppl. 1):S11–S61
8. Kahn SE. The relative contributions of insulin resistance and beta-cell dysfunction to the pathophysiology of type 2 diabetes. Diabetologia 2003;46:3–19
9. DeFronzo RA. Pathogenesis of type 2 diabetes mellitus. Med Clin North Am 2004; 88:787–835, ix
10. Stefan N, Kantartzis K, Häring HU. Causes and metabolic consequences of fatty liver. Endocr Rev 2008;29:939–960
11. Samuel VT, Liu ZX, Qu X, et al. Mechanism of hepatic insulin resistance in nonalcoholic fatty liver disease. J Biol Chem 2004;279:32345–32353
12. Abdul-Ghani MA, DeFronzo RA. Pathophysiology of prediabetes. Curr Diab Rep 2009;9:193–199
13. Bedogni G, Miglioli L, Masutti F, Tiribelli C, Marchesini G, Bellentani S. Prevalence of and risk factors for nonalcoholic fatty liver disease: the Dionysos nutrition and liver study. Hepatology 2005;42:44–52
14. Jakobsen MU, Berentzen T, Sørensen TI, Overvad K. Abdominal obesity and fatty liver. Epidemiol Rev 2007;29:77–87
15. Sattar N, Preiss D, Murray HM, et al. Statins and risk of incident diabetes: a collaborative meta-analysis of randomised statin trials. Lancet 2010;375:735–742

BARIATRIC SURGERY

β-Cell Function in Severely Obese Type 2 Diabetic Patients

Long-term effects of bariatric surgery

STEFANIA CAMASTRA, MD[1,2]
MELANIA MANCO, MD[3]
ANDREA MARI, PHD[4]
ALDO V. GRECO, MD[3]

SILVIA FRASCERRA, PHD[1,2]
GELTRUDE MINGRONE, MD[3]
ELE FERRANNINI, MD[1,2]

Bariatric surgery in severely obese diabetic patients can restore glucose tolerance (1). Malabsorptive bariatric surgery (e.g., bilio-pancreatic diversion [BPD]) in nondiabetic subjects induces an improvement in insulin sensitivity that is greater than predicted by weight loss (2,3); such an effect can be demonstrated early after surgery (4). Impaired β-cell function is the main determinant of glucose intolerance, and modeling of C-peptide responses to graded glucose infusions (5) or oral glucose administration (6) makes it possible to estimate key dynamic parameters of β-cell function such as β-cell glucose sensitivity. The impact of bariatric surgery on β-cell function in diabetic subjects has been investigated using the intravenous glucose tolerance test (7). This test, however, can misjudge β-cell function as compared with more physiological challenges (such as the oral glucose tolerance test or mixed meals) because it explores only one specific aspect of islet function, namely the acute insulin discharge in response to a sudden maximal increment in plasma glucose concentrations (8). Recently, we have applied C-peptide–based modeling to reconstruct insulin secretion and β-cell function during a 24-h multiple-meal test (9). Here, we adopted this approach to analyze the long-term effects

of BPD on glucose metabolism in morbidly obese patients with type 2 diabetes.

RESEARCH DESIGN AND METHODS

We studied 10 morbidly obese (mean ± SE BMI 49.5 ± 2.9 kg/m[2]), non–insulin-treated type 2 diabetic patients (3 men and 7 women) (age 50 ± 2 years) whose weight had been stable (±2 kg) for the preceding 6 months. Oral antidiabetic drugs were discontinued 1 week before the baseline studies. The study protocol was approved by the local ethics committee, and all subjects provided informed written consent to participate.

Following the baseline studies, patients underwent BPD, consisting of a partial gastrectomy with a distal Roux-en-Y reconstruction (2), and were restudied 24 ± 2 months postsurgery.

For the basal study, subjects spent 24 h (starting at 8:00 A.M.) in the metabolic ward. During this period, four meals were administered for a total caloric intake of 30 kcal/kg fat-free mass (20% breakfast, 40% lunch, 10% afternoon snack, and 30% dinner). Diet composition was 17% protein, 35% fat, and 48% carbohydrate. Hourly blood samples were drawn from a central venous catheter for the measurement of glucose, insulin, and C-peptide concentrations. Body

composition was evaluated by measuring total body water with the ^3H_2O technique (10). On another day, a 2-h euglycemic-hyperinsulinemic clamp (240 pmol/min per m[2]) was performed (2). All procedures and measures were repeated in the follow-up study. Eight morbidly obese nondiabetic subjects (BMI 51.1 ± 2.8 kg/m[2]), who were studied with the same protocol before surgery and 24 months after BPD, served as the control group; the complete data on these subjects have been reported (9).

Analytical procedures

Plasma glucose was measured by the glucose oxidase technique on a Beckman Glucose Analyzer (Beckman, Fullerton, CA). Plasma insulin was assayed by a specific radioimmunoassay (Linco Research, St. Charles, MO). C-peptide was assayed by radioimmunoassay (MYRIA; Technogenetics, Milan, Italy).

Modeling

The model used to reconstruct 24-h insulin secretion and its control by glucose has been previously described (11). In brief, it consists of a model for fitting the glucose concentration profile, a model describing the dependence of insulin secretion on glucose concentration, and a model of C-peptide kinetics, in which the model parameters are individually adjusted to the subject's anthropometric data (12). The dependence of insulin release on plasma glucose concentrations is modeled as the sum of two components. The first is the relationship between insulin secretion and glucose concentration, i.e., a dose-response function, whose mean slope (calculated over the individual-observed glycemic range) represents β-cell glucose sensitivity. The dose-response function is modulated by a time-varying factor, the potentiation factor, which encompasses glucose-induced potentiation, incretin potentiation, circadian rhythms, and pulsatility of insulin secretion, and was expressed here as the ratio of the daytime (fed state) to the nighttime (fasting state) value. The second component represents the dependence of insulin secretion on

From the [1]Department of Internal Medicine, University of Pisa School of Medicine, Pisa, Italy; the [2]CNR Institute of Clinical Physiology, University of Pisa School of Medicine, Pisa, Italy; the [3]Department of Medicine, Catholic University, Rome, Italy; and the [4]CNR Institute of Biomedical Engineering, Padua, Italy.

Address correspondence and reprint requests to Ele Ferrannini, MD, Department of Internal Medicine, Via Savi, 8, 56100 Pisa, Italy. E-mail: ferranni@ifc.cnr.it.

Received for publication 4 September 2006 and accepted in revised form 26 December 2006.

Additional information for this article can be found in an online appendix at http://dx.doi.org/10.2337/dc06-1845.

Abbreviations: BPD, bilio-pancreatic diversion.

A table elsewhere in this issue shows conventional and Système International (SI) units and conversion factors for many substances.

DOI: 10.2337/dc06-1845

Table 1—*Anthropometrics, glucose metabolism, and β-cell–function parameters in severely obese patients with type 2 diabetes pre- and postsurgery and in nondiabetic subjects postsurgery*

	Diabetic			Nondiabetic	
	Presurgery	P*	Postsurgery	P†	Postsurgery
Body weight (kg)	136 ± 10	0.01	89 ± 4	NS	87 ± 4
BMI (kg/m^2)	49.5 ± 2.9	0.01	33.1 ± 2.2	NS	33.1 ± 2.8
Fat-free mass (kg)	80 ± 5	0.01	64 ± 3	NS	57 ± 5
Fat mass (kg)	56 ± 5	0.01	26 ± 3	NS	30 ± 5
Fasting glucose (mmol/l)	7.7 ± 0.9	0.03	5.1 ± 0.3	0.01	4.0 ± 0.4
A1C (%)	8.2 ± 0.6	0.01	4.1 ± 0.1	—	—
Mean 24-h glucose (mmol/l)	7.6 ± 0.8	0.03	5.3 ± 0.2	0.01	4.7 ± 0.4
M (μmol · min^{-1} · kg$_{FFM}$$^{-1}$)	26.4 ± 2.7	0.01	55.2 ± 2.1	0.01	68.7 ± 3.3
Fasting insulin (pmol/l)	154 (114)	NS	79 (65)	0.01	20 (20)
Mean 24-h insulin (pmol/l)	233 (182)	NS	136 (125)	0.001	58 (19)
24-h insulin output					
nmol/m^2	228 (83)	0.04	158 (76)	0.01	89 (11)
nmol	608 (214)	0.01	330 (159)	0.01	167 (37)
β-cell glucose sensitivity					
pmol/min per m^2/mmol/l	44 (32)	0.037	76 (89)	NS	65 (47)
pmol · min^{-1} · mmol/l^{-1}	99 (78)	0.1	160 (208)	NS	122 (98)
Rate sensitivity					
nmol/m^2 per mmol/l	0.45 (1.61)	NS	0.01 (0.17)	NS	0.59 (1.20)
nmol/mmol/l	1.3 (3.9)	NS	0.01 (0.4)	NS	1.2 (2.3)
Potentiation factor (day/night)	1.19 (0.40)	NS	0.85 (0.53)	0.02	1.37 (0.57)

Data are means ± SE or median (interquartile range) unless otherwise indicated. NS, not significant. *Presurgery versus postsurgery by Wilcoxon signed-rank test; †diabetic versus nondiabetic by the Mann-Whitney U test.

the rate of change of glucose concentration (rate sensitivity).

Data analysis

Data are given as means ± SE. Insulin parameters, which have a skewed distribution, are presented as median (interquartile range). Wilcoxon's signed-rank test was used to test treatment-induced changes, and the Mann-Whitney U test was used to compare groups. Bivariate regression was carried out by standard techniques, and the results were expressed as partial correlation coefficients.

RESULTS — Two years after BPD, patients had lost 47 ± 9 kg, of which ~2/3 was fat (Table 1). Fasting glycemia, A1C, and day-long glycemia were essentially normalized in all patients (Fig. 1 [available in an online appendix at http://dx.doi.org/10.2337/dc06-1845]), and none needed antidiabetic treatment. On the clamp, insulin sensitivity doubled, while fasting and mean 24-h plasma insulin and C-peptide concentrations were markedly, if not significantly, decreased. There was a 30% decrease in 24-h insulin output. The dose response of glucose-induced insulin release after surgery was shifted to the left and upward of that re-

corded before surgery (Fig. 2 of the online appendix), with a significant increase in the mean slope (Table 1). Potentiation and rate sensitivity were not significantly changed. In comparison with nondiabetic subjects studied 2 years postsurgery with an identical protocol (Table 1), diabetic patients had attained similar body weight and composition, but their fasting and mean plasma glucose and insulin concentrations and 24-h insulin output were still higher (Fig. 1 of the online appendix); insulin sensitivity was slightly, if significantly, lower, but β-cell glucose sensitivity was similar (Fig. 2 of the online appendix).

In the pooled pre- and postsurgery data, mean 24-h glucose was reciprocally related to β-cell glucose sensitivity in a nonlinear fashion ($y = 21 \times x^{-0.31}$, $r = -0.74$, $P < 0.001$). In a multivariate model, treatment-induced changes in 24-h glucose were independently related both to the increase in β-cell glucose sensitivity (partial $r = 0.93$, $P < 0.001$) and to the increase in M (partial $r = 0.71$, $P < 0.001$).

CONCLUSIONS — Two years after malabsorptive surgery, our patients were still obese (BMI 33.1 ± 2.2 kg/m^2), but

their glucose tolerance was back to normal as a result of major changes in both insulin sensitivity and β-cell glucose sensitivity. The notion that bariatric surgery can restore glucose tolerance in the majority (over 75%) of severely obese patients is well established (1). Also established is the fact that bariatric surgery leads to a large improvement in insulin sensitivity, which can be detected early after surgery before any substantial weight loss has occurred (4,13,14). Less information is available on the changes in β-cell function and their time course. Morbid obesity per se is associated with profound insulin resistance and marked insulin hypersecretion, but the dynamics of β-cell function, i.e., β-cell glucose sensitivity, rate sensitivity, and potentiation, are preserved (9). Overt diabetes and impaired glucose tolerance, on the other hand, are characterized by a progressive loss of β-cell glucose sensitivity independent of insulin resistance (6). Polyzogopoulou et al. (7) reported improved first-phase insulin response to intravenous glucose 1 year postsurgery. Here, we show that β-cell glucose sensitivity had fully recovered 2 years postsurgery, despite a fall in absolute insulin secretion, and was quantitatively responsible for restored glucose tolerance during free living regardless of the amount of weight lost. Interestingly, equally obese but nondiabetic subjects studied at the same time distance from surgery showed lower plasma glucose levels and insulin secretion rates and higher insulin sensitivity (Table 1). Because at this time β-cell glucose sensitivity was similar in the two groups, the difference in daylong glycemia between nondiabetic and postdiabetic subjects must have been due to the 20% better insulin sensitivity (and, possibly, better potentiation) of the former versus the latter. Whether this finding is a trace of the inherent (obesity-independent) susceptibility to dysglycemia of postdiabetic subjects (predisposing them to relapsing glucose intolerance) remains to be decided by longer-term follow-up studies.

The mechanisms underlying the dramatic effects of malabsorptive surgery on insulin sensitivity and β-cell function are poorly understood. Because major weight loss achieved by predominantly restrictive bariatric surgery does not lead to the striking changes in insulin sensitivity and β-cell function observed with predominantly malabsorptive surgery (3), some specific consequence of BPD must be involved. Candidate mechanisms span from depletion of intracellular fat depots (2) to attenuation of lipotoxicity to changes in the amount and pattern of gastrointestinal hormonal and neural signals triggered by the new route of food transit (15). This surgical modality certainly represents a very useful tool to gain insight into incretin physiology.

References

1. Buchwald H, Avidor Y, Braunwald E, Jensen MD, Pories W, Fahrbach K, Schoelles K: Bariatric surgery: a systematic review and meta-analysis. *JAMA* 292:1724–1137, 2004
2. Greco AV, Mingrone G, Giancaterini A, Manco M, Morroni M, Cinti S, Granzotto M, Vettor R, Camastra S, Ferrannini E: Insulin resistance in morbid obesity: reversal with intramyocellular fat depletion. *Diabetes* 51:144–151, 2002
3. Muscelli E, Mingrone G, Camastra S, Manco M, Pereira JA, Pareja JC, Ferrannini E: Differential impact of weight loss on insulin resistance: studies in surgically treated obese patients. *Am J Med* 118:51–57, 2005
4. Mari A, Manco M, Guidone C, Nanni G, Castagneto M, Mingrone G, Ferrannini E: Restoration of normal glucose tolerance in severely obese patients after bilio-pancreatic diversion: role of insulin sensitivity and beta cell function. *Diabetologia* 49:2136–2143, 2006
5. Polonsky KS, Given BD, Hirsh L, Shapiro ET, Tillil H, Beebe C, Galloway JA, Frank BH, Karrison T, Van Cauter E: Quantitative study of insulin secretion and clearance in normal and obese subjects. *J Clin Invest* 81:435–441, 1988
6. Ferrannini E, Gastaldelli A, Miyazaki Y, Matsuda M, Mari A, DeFronzo RA: β-Cell function in subjects spanning the range from normal glucose tolerance to overt diabetes: a new analysis. *J Clin Endocrinol Metab* 90:493–500, 2005
7. Polyzogopoulou EV, Kalfarentzos F, Vagenakis AG, Alexandrides TK: Restoration of euglycemia and normal acute insulin response to glucose in obese subjects with type 2 diabetes following bariatric surgery. *Diabetes* 52:1098–1103, 2003
8. Ferrannini E, Mari A: Beta cell function and its relation to insulin action in humans: a critical appraisal. *Diabetologia* 47:943–956, 2004
9. Camastra S, Manco M, Mari A, Baldi S, Gastaldelli A, Greco AV, Mingrone G, Ferrannini E: β-Cell function in morbidly obese subjects during free living: long-term effects of weight loss. *Diabetes* 54:2382–2389, 2005
10. Siri WE: Body composition from fluid spaces and density: analysis of methods. In *Techniques of Measuring Body Composition.* Brozek J, Henschel A, Eds. Washington, DC, Natl. Acad. Sci, Natl. Res. Counc., 1961, p. 107–141
11. Mari A, Tura A, Gastaldelli A, Ferrannini E: Assessing insulin secretion by modeling in multiple-meal tests. *Diabetes* 51 (Suppl. 1):S221–S226, 2002
12. Van Cauter E, Mestrez F, Sturis J, Polonsky KS: Estimation of insulin secretion rates from C-peptide levels: comparison of individual and standard kinetic parameters for C-peptide clearance. *Diabetes* 41:368–377, 1992
13. Wickremesekera K, Miller G, Naotunne TD, Knowles G, Stubbs RS: Loss of insulin resistance after Roux-en-Y gastric bypass surgery: a time course study. *Obes Surg* 15:474–481, 2005
14. Mingrone G, DeGaetano A, Greco AV, Capristo E, Benedetti G, Castagneto M, Gasbarrini G: Reversibility of insulin resistance in obese diabetic patients: role of plasma lipids. *Diabetologia* 40:599–605, 1997
15. Naslund E, Backman L, Holst JJ, Theodorsson E, Hellstrom PM: Importance of small bowel peptides for the improved glucose metabolism 20 years after jejunoileal bypass for obesity. *Obes Surg* 8:253–260, 1998

Incretin Levels and Effect Are Markedly Enhanced 1 Month After Roux-en-Y Gastric Bypass Surgery in Obese Patients With Type 2 Diabetes

BLANDINE LAFERRÈRE, MD[1]
STANLEY HESHKA, PHD[1]
KRYSTLE WANG, BS[1]
YASMIN KHAN, BS[1]

JAMES MCGINTY, MD[2]
JULIO TEIXEIRA, MD[2]
ALLISON B. HART, BS[1]
BLANCA OLIVAN, MD[1]

OBJECTIVE — Limited data on patients undergoing Roux-en-Y gastric bypass surgery (RY-GBP) suggest that an improvement in insulin secretion after surgery occurs rapidly and thus may not be wholly accounted for by weight loss. We hypothesized that in obese patients with type 2 diabetes the impaired levels and effect of incretins changed as a consequence of RY-GBP.

RESEARCH DESIGN AND METHODS — Incretin (gastric inhibitory peptide [GIP] and glucagon-like peptide-1 [GLP-1]) levels and their effect on insulin secretion were measured before and 1 month after RY-GBP in eight obese women with type 2 diabetes and in seven obese nondiabetic control subjects. The incretin effect was measured as the difference in insulin secretion (area under the curve [AUC]) in response to an oral glucose tolerance test (OGTT) and to an isoglycemic intravenous glucose test.

RESULTS — Fasting and stimulated levels of GLP-1 and GIP were not different between control subjects and patients with type 2 diabetes before the surgery. One month after RY-GBP, body weight decreased by 9.2 ± 7.0 kg, oral glucose-stimulated GLP-1 (AUC) and GIP peak levels increased significantly by 24.3 ± 7.9 pmol$\cdot$l$^{-1}\cdot$min^{-1} ($P < 0.0001$) and 131 ± 85 pg/ml ($P = 0.007$), respectively. The blunted incretin effect markedly increased from 7.6 ± 28.7 to 42.5 ± 11.3 ($P = 0.005$) after RY-GBP, at which it time was not different from that for the control subjects ($53.6 \pm 23.5\%$, $P = 0.284$).

CONCLUSIONS — These data suggest that early after RY-GBP, greater GLP-1 and GIP release could be a potential mediator of improved insulin secretion.

Diabetes Care 30:1709–1716, 2007

The prevalence of obesity and type 2 diabetes (1) is increasing in the U.S. More and more patients seek bariatric surgery (surgical weight loss) for treatment of their obesity. Up to 30% of patients presenting for bariatric surgery have type 2 diabetes (2,3). Although weight loss surgery generally results in a loss of 50–70% excess body weight and "cures" diabetes in 77% of patients (4), the rapidity in the onset and the magnitude of the benefits of Roux-en-Y gastric bypass surgery (RY-GBP) on diabetes has thus far baffled clinical scientists.

It has been proposed that the incretins could be some of the key mediators of the antidiabetic effects of certain types of bariatric surgery. The incretins are gut peptides secreted in response to meals, which enhance insulin secretion. The two main incretins are gastric inhibitory peptide (GIP), secreted by the K-cells in the proximal small intestine (5), and glucagon-like peptide-1 (GLP-1), secreted by the L-cells of the distal small intestine (6). Both incretins affect meal-related insulin secretion (7,8). GLP-1 also delays gastric emptying (9), decreases appetite (9–11), inhibits glucagon (12), and may improve insulin sensitivity (13), all effects that are antidiabetogenic. The incretin effect is impaired in patients with type 2 diabetes (14). GLP-1 levels are blunted (15), but the effect of administered GLP-1 on insulin secretion persists (16). Contrary to GLP-1, GIP levels are normal in patients with type 2 diabetes, but the effect of administered GIP on insulin secretion is blunted (17,18). GIP and GLP-1 have additive insulinotropic effects during hyperglycemia. Both GLP-1 and GIP analogs are being developed as antidiabetic agents (19).

Previous data have shown that the significant weight loss observed after various bariatric procedures was accompanied by improvement in diabetes control and increased GLP-1 levels. However, most studies were cross-sectional (20,21), reported fasting (22) rather than postprandial GLP-1 levels, and compared various types of surgery such as jejuno-ileal bypass (JIB) (23,24) or biliopancreatic diversion (BPD) (24), often leading to inconclusive results. Data on fasting GIP levels after bariatric surgery are inconsistent, with reports of either a decrease (22,25,26) or an increase (20,24).

GLP-1 levels increase after a meal in patients after RY-GBP (27) or with oral glucose after BPD (28). Meal-stimulated GIP levels have been reported to increase after JIB (20) or to decrease after GBP or JIB surgery (23,26,29). None of these studies, however, measured GLP-1 and GIP simultaneously, reported the incretin levels and effect on insulin secretion, or were done in diabetic patients.

From the [1]Obesity Research Center, St. Luke's/Roosevelt Hospital Center, Columbia University College of Physicians and Surgeons, New York, New York; and the [2]Bariatric Division, St. Luke's/Roosevelt Hospital Center, Columbia University College of Physicians and Surgeons, New York, New York.

Address correspondence and reprint requests to Blandine Laferrère, MD, Obesity Research Center, St. Luke's/Roosevelt Hospital Center, Columbia University College of Physicians and Surgeons, 1111 Amsterdam Ave., New York, NY 10025. E-mail: bbl14@columbia.edu.

Received for publication 24 July 2006 and accepted in revised form 18 March 2007.

Published ahead of print at http://care.diabetesjournals.org on 6 April 2007. DOI: 10.2337/dc06-1549.

Abbreviations: AUC, area under the curve; BPD, biliopancreatic diversion; DPPIV, dipeptidyl-peptidase IV; GIP, gastric inhibitory peptide; GLP-1, glucagon-like peptide-1; IsoG IVGT, isoglycemic intravenous glucose test; IV, intravenous; JIB, jejunoileal bypass; OGTT, oral glucose tolerance test; RY-GBP, Roux-en-Y gastric bypass surgery.

A table elsewhere in this issue shows conventional and Système International (SI) units and conversion factors for many substances.

Our goal was to investigate the role of incretins as the mechanism for rapid improvement in insulin secretion in obese patients with type 2 diabetes after RY-GBP. Specifically, we wished to measure the changes in GLP-1 and GIP levels in response to oral glucose, as well as the changes in the incretin effect on insulin secretion, in obese patients with type 2 diabetes before and 1 month after RY-GBP.

RESEARCH DESIGN AND METHODS

Obese patients of either sex and all ethnic groups with BMI >35 kg/m^2 who were scheduled for RY-GBP surgery and had type 2 diabetes diagnosed for <5 years, were not taking insulin, had A1C <8%, and were aged <60 years were recruited. They were studied before and within 1 month after the surgery to minimize the amount of weight loss at the time of the second study. A group of obese nondiabetic control subjects was studied for incretin levels and effect. Fat mass was measured by anthropometrics (30).

RY-GBP protocol
All patients underwent a laparoscopic RY-GBP with a 30-ml gastric pouch, 40-cm afferent limb, 150-cm Roux limb, and 12-mm gastrojejunostomy. The post–RY-GBP diet recommendations included a daily intake of 600–800 kcal, 70 g protein, and 64 oz fluid. This was achieved, on an individual basis, with multiple small meals and snacks with various commercial protein supplements. The diet after RY-GBP was monitored by food records but not directly supervised. The diet in the few days preceding the testing in patients before surgery or in control subjects was not controlled.

Measurement of incretin effect
Insulin secretion after oral and isoglycemic intravenous glucose load. Oral glucose tolerance tests (OGTTs) and isoglycemic intravenous glucose tests (IsoG IVGTs) were administered in the morning after a 12-h overnight fast, on two different days, separated by <5 days.
3-h OGTT. All patients underwent first a 3-h OGTT with 50 g glucose (in a total volume of 300 ml). After insertion of an intravenous (IV) catheter, at 8:00 A.M., subjects received 50 g glucose orally. Blood samples, collected in chilled EDTA tubes with added aprotinin (500 kallikrein inhibitory units/ml blood) and dipeptidyl-peptidase IV (DPPIV) inhibi-

tor (Linco, St. Charles, MO) (10 μl/ml blood), were centrifuged at 4°C before storage at −70°C.
IsoG IVGT. The goal of the IsoG IVGT was to expose the pancreas to blood glucose levels matched to the ones obtained during the OGTT in the same subject. Glucose (sterile 20% dextrose solution in water) was infused intravenously over 3 h using a Gemini pump (Gemini). A sample of blood was collected every 5 min using a contralateral antecubital IV catheter and then was transferred in a picofuge tube without any additive and centrifuged immediately for measurement of glucose levels at the bedside. The glucose infusion rate was adjusted to match the glucose concentrations obtained for the same patient during the OGTT at each time point for 3 h. During the OGTT and the IsoG IVGT, the arm used for blood sampling was kept warm with a heating pad.
Incretin effect. The difference in β-cell responses (insulin total area under the curve [INS AUC 0–180 min]) to the oral and the isoglycemic IV glucose stimuli represents the incretin effect (INC), the action of the incretin factor expressed as the percentage of the physiological response to oral glucose, which is taken as the denominator (100%) (14). The formula is

$$INC =$$

$$\frac{INS\ AUC_{oral} - INS\ AUC_{isoglycemic\ IV}}{INS\ AUC_{oral}} \times 100\%$$

Assays. Total GLP-1, an indicator of secretion, was measured by radioimmunoassay (Phoenix Pharmaceutical, Belmont, CA) after plasma ethanol extraction. The intra-assay and interassay coefficients of variation (CVs) were 3–6.5 and 4.7–8.8%, respectively. This assay has 100% specificity for GLP-1(7–36) and GLP-1(9–36), 60% specificity for GLP-1(7–37) and does not cross-react with glucagon (0.2%), GLP-2 (<0.001%), or exendin (<0.01%). Active GLP-1, an indicator of potential action, was measured by ELISA (Linco). The intra-assay and interassay CVs were 3–7 and 7–8%, respectively. The assay is 100% specific for GLP-1(7–36) and GLP-1(7–37) and does not react with GLP-1(9–36), glucagon, or GLP-2. Total GIP was measured by ELISA (Linco). The assay is 100% specific for GIP 1–42 and GIP 3–42 and does not cross-react with GLP-1, GLP-2, oxyntomodulin, or glucagon. The intra-assay and interassay CVs were 3.0−8.8 and

1.8–6.1%, respectively. Plasma insulin and C-peptide concentrations were measured by radioimmunoassay (Linco) with, intra-assay CVs, respectively, of 5–8 and 3–6% and interassay CVs of 7.2 and 5.2–7.7%. The glucose concentration was measured at the bedside by the glucose oxidase method (glucose analyzer; Beckman, Fullerton, CA). All hormonal and metabolites assays were performed at the Hormone and Metabolite Core Laboratory of the New York Obesity Research Center.

Statistical analysis
Outcome variables were serum glucose and plasma insulin, C-peptide, GLP-1, and GIP concentrations. Total AUC 0–180 min for outcome variables were calculated using the trapezoidal method. ANOVA with repeated measures was used to detect hormonal changes over time during the OGTT within each condition and for comparison before and after RY-GBP or between control subjects and patients with type 2 diabetes. Paired t tests were used to compare data from before and after RY-GBP. Statistical significance was set at $P < 0.05$. Statistical analyses were performed with SPSS 13.0 (SPSS, Chicago, IL) (31).

RESULTS
Subject characteristics are shown in Table 1. Eight obese women with type 2 diabetes of 20.1 ± 12.9 months' duration, A1C of 6.9 ± 0.7%, and liver enzymes, thyroid function tests, and blood pressure within normal limits were studied before and 1 month (31 ± 14 days) after RY-GBP. Type 2 diabetes was diagnosed in one patient at the time of screening for surgery. Patients' diabetes medications, sulfonylureas, and/or metformin were discontinued 3 days before they were studied before the surgery. None of the patients were taking insulin, thiazolinediones, or β-blockers before RY-GBP or any diabetes medication after RY-GBP. Seven obese nondiabetic women were studied as control subjects, while consuming their regular diet at stable weight and taking no medications. Control subjects did not differ from patients in terms of age, body weight, or BMI (Table 1).

Side effects
Although a 50-g glucose drink was used rather than 75 g to minimize the risk of dumping syndrome after RY-GBP, three patients experienced stomach cramping and discomfort, nausea, sweating,

Table 1—*Subject characteristics*

	Control subjects	Patients before RY-GBP	P value (vs. control subjects)	Patients after RY-GBP	Δ	P value (Δ)
Age (years)	38.8 ± 7.8	44.8 ± 10.2	0.210			
Weight (kg)	100.4 ± 29.9	113.9 ± 16.4	0.267	104.8 ± 17.1	9.2 ± 7.0	0.008
BMI (kg/m^2)	37.1 ± 11.6	43.6 ± 6.8	0.189	40.1 ± 7.0	3.5 ± 3.6	0.029
Fat mass (%)	41.1 ± 8.3	47.1 ± 1.3	0.06	45.3 ± 3.1	1.8 ± 1.8	0.192
Fasting glucose (mmol/l)	5.4 ± 0.4	8.05 ± 1.82	0.001	6.45 ± 0.84	1.60 ± 1.45	0.017
Fasting insulin (pmol/l)	123 ± 93	171 ± 74	0.303	128 ± 54	43 ± 53	0.057
120-min glucose (mmol/l)	6.04 ± 1.48	11.2 ± 1.72	<0.0001	7.10 ± 1.72	4.10 ± 1.62	<0.0001
Peak insulin (pmol/l)	749 ± 532	507 ± 304	0.301	723 ± 327	216 ± 245	0.042
AUC glucose (mmol $\cdot$ l^{-1} $\cdot$ min^{-1})	1,113 ± 191	2,018 ± 343	<0.0001	1,500 ± 212	517 ± 187	<0.0001
AUC insulin (pmol $\cdot$ l^{-1} $\cdot$ min^{-1})	252 ± 147	356 ± 199	0.294	323 ± 137	32 ± 134	0.514
AUC total GLP-1 (pmol $\cdot$ l^{-1} $\cdot$ min^{-1})	5.26 ± 3.06	7.54 ± 2.79	0.155	31.82 ± 8.10	24.3 ± 7.9	<0.0001
AUC GIP (pmol $\cdot$ l^{-1} $\cdot$ min^{-1})	37.12 ± 20.97	50.96 ± 9.62	0.103	52.66 ± 18.93	1.7 ± 24.3	0.849
Peak GIP (pmol/l)	151 ± 77	213 ± 52	0.088	324 ± 130	111 ± 98	0.015
Incretin effect on insulin (%)	53.6 ± 23.5	7.6 ± 28.7	0.020	42.5 ± 11.3	34.8 ± 24.2	0.005
Incretin effect on C-peptide (%)	49.9 ± 19.4	−17.8 ± 52.8	0.079	26.6 ± 18.1	44.4 ± 43.6	0.024

Data are means ± SD. Control subjects are obese individuals without type 2 diabetes ($n = 7$), and patients are obese individuals with type 2 diabetes ($n = 8$) before and after RY-GBP. Fasting values are the average of two baseline values. Peak (120-min value) and AUC (total area under the curve, 180 min) values were obtained during the OGTT. Δ, difference between pre– and post–RY-GBP.

flushing, and palpitations 5–20 min into the OGTT. No severe adverse effects were observed.

Glucose and insulin levels during the OGTT

Changes in outcome variables after RY-GBP are shown in Table 1. After RY-GBP, body weights and BMIs decreased significantly. Fasting and 120-min glucose levels decreased to the nondiabetic range while peak insulin levels increased significantly.

GLP-1 and GIP levels during the OGTT

Fasting and stimulated GLP-1 and GIP levels were not different between control subjects and patients before RY-GBP (Table 1 and Fig. 1A–C). GLP-1 AUC and peak GIP increased significantly after surgery by factors of 4.2 and 1.6, respectively (Table 1 and Fig. 1A and B). There was no change in GLP-1 or GIP levels during the IsoG IVGT (data not shown). The blunted active GLP-1 levels increased significantly at 15 min during the OGTT after GBP (Fig. 1C). To indirectly assess the activity of the enzyme DPPIV, the ratio of active GLP-1 to total GLP-1 (using OGTT peak values) was calculated. The ratio, which was not statistically different between control subjects and patients before sur-

gery ($P = 0.132$), decreased significantly from 0.70 ± 0.12 to 0.18 ± 0.06 ($P < 0.0001$) after RY-GBP.

Incretin effect

In control subjects, the glucose concentrations were well matched between the IsoG IVGT and the OGTT (mean levels 5.87 ± 0.76 vs. 5.92 ± 0.82 mmol/l, $P = 0.639$). As expected, insulin levels were greater during the OGTT (AUC insulin 252 ± 147 pmol $\cdot$ l^{-1} $\cdot$ min^{-1}) than during the IsoG IVGT (132 ± 101 pmol $\cdot$ l^{-1} $\cdot$ min^{-1}, $P = 0.045$), with a calculated incretin effect on insulin of 53.6 ± 23.5%. In patients before RY-GBP, the glucose levels were well matched between the IsoG IVGT and the OGTT (11.06 ± 1.93 vs. 10.76 ± 1.97 mmol/l, $P = 0.058$) (Fig. 2A). Contrary to results from the control subjects, as expected, the insulin response was not greater after oral glucose (AUC insulin 356 ± 199 pmol $\cdot$ l^{-1} $\cdot$ min^{-1}) than after IV glucose (AUC insulin 305 ± 161 pmol $\cdot$ l^{-1} $\cdot$ min^{-1}, $P = 0.195$) (Fig. 2B), with a resulting blunted incretin effect of 7.6 ± 28.7% (Fig. 1C). After RY-GBP, glucose levels were higher during the IsoG IVGT (mean levels 9.39 ± 1.00 mmol/l) compared with the OGTT (8.42 ± 1.04 mmol/l, $P = 0.046$) (Fig. 2D). However, the insulin response was greater during the oral test (323 ±

137 pmol $\cdot$ l^{-1} $\cdot$ min^{-1}) than during the IV test (184 ± 80 pmol $\cdot$ l^{-1} $\cdot$ min^{-1}, $P = 0.001$) (Fig. 2E), and the incretin effect was markedly increased by a factor of 5 to 42.5 ± 11.3% (mean increase 34.8 ± 24.2%, $P = 0.007$) (Fig. 1C), a level at which it was not significantly different from that for the control subjects (53.6 ± 23.5%, $P = 0.284$) (Fig. 1D). The incretin effect on C-peptide increased significantly after RY-GBP, to a level not statistically different ($P = 0.157$) from that for the control subjects (Table 1). There was a correlation between GIP AUC and the insulin incretin effect in patients before surgery ($r = 0.737$, $P = 0.037$) but not in patients after RY-GBP nor in control subjects. GLP-1 AUC was positively correlated to the C-peptide incretin effect in control subjects and patients after RY-GBP ($r = 0.915$, $P = 0.046$).

CONCLUSIONS — We investigated the changes in incretin levels and effect after RY-GBP in patients with morbid obesity and type 2 diabetes. Our main findings are that the release of incretin after oral glucose is of greater magnitude and the incretin effect on insulin secretion is markedly improved 1 month after RY-GBP.

It has long been hypothesized that the incretins could play a role in the marked

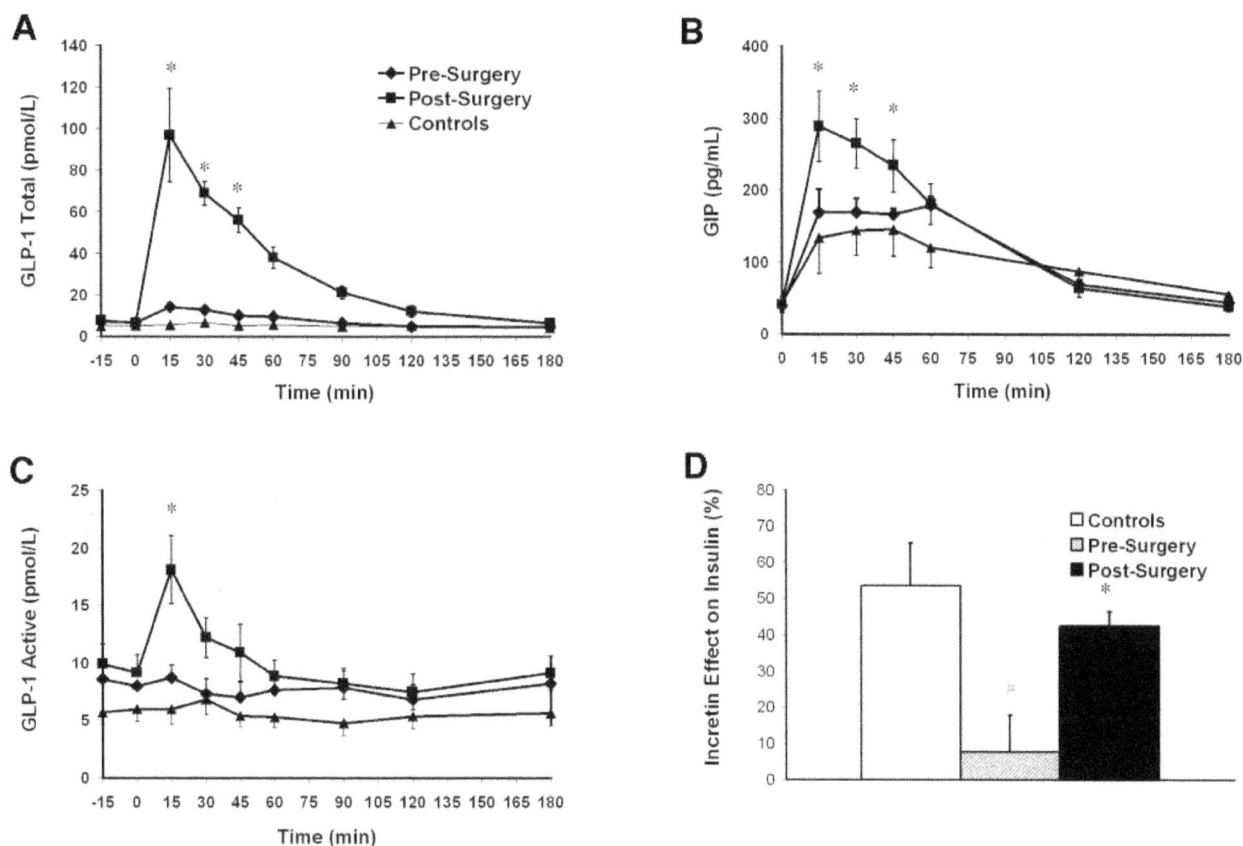

Figure 1—*Total GLP-1 (A), GIP (B), and active GLP-1 (C) levels during OGTTs in patients before (♦) and after (■) RY-GBP (A) and in control subjects (▲) and incretin effect on insulin secretion (D) in control subjects (□), patients before RY-GBP (▨), and patients after RY-GBP (■). The incretin effect was calculated by comparing the insulin response to oral and matched IV glucose loads. Data are means ± SEM. *P < 0.05 compared with patients before RY-GBP. #P < 0.05 compared with control subjects.*

immediate improvements of diabetes control observed after bariatric surgery (32). Limited data (23–25,27,33) suggested that the improvement in insulin secretion after bariatric surgery occurs rapidly. Thus, it may not be wholly accounted for by weight loss but could be a consequence of changes of the enteroinsular axis, particularly in the incretins. However, most of the studies to date have been cross-sectional (20,23,24) or measured only fasting levels of incretins (22,25).

In our study, fasting and glucose-stimulated levels of GLP-1 and GIP were not different between patients before the surgery and control subjects. This is contrary to findings by others showing lower fasting levels and impaired stimulated release of incretins in patients with type 2 diabetes (7,14,17). This discrepancy could be due to different patient populations. Our patients were relatively young (aged 45 years) with recently diagnosed type 2 diabetes (<2 years).

One month after RY-GBP, our data demonstrate a clear and significant increase of GLP-1 (total and active) and GIP release in response to oral glucose in patients with type 2 diabetes. An increase in levels of circulating incretins was previously reported in nondiabetic patients after RY-GBP (27) or BPD (28). Some cross-sectional and longitudinal studies have shown an increase in the stimulated levels of incretins, after a meal or oral glucose, after JIB (24,34) or after RY-GBP (27,35). Our data show that the changes in stimulated incretin levels occur as early as 1 month after RY-GBP, similarly to changes in enteroglucagon obtained after JIB (34). Future studies will address the long-term changes of incretin and help clarify the controversy about β-cell hypertrophy after RY-GBP (36,37).

The mechanisms by which incretin levels increase after surgery are not fully understood. After RY-GBP, as a consequence of the bypass of the upper gut, the lower gut is exposed sooner to the ingested nutrients, thus changing the timing of the physiological release of gut incretins. The time of the peak release of GLP-1 and GIP after oral glucose was at 15 min, although GIP is released by the K-cells of the proximal small intestine and GLP-1 by the more distal L-cells of the small intestine (5,6). More frequent blood sampling could possibly identify different release times for each incretin, according to the anatomical distribution of the secretory cells. Our stimulus was a solution of glucose. Future studies should investigate whether other stimuli, such as amino acids, lipids, or a change in pH, stimulate secretion of the incretins with the same magnitude as a solution of oral glucose. Elegant studies in a rat model of diabetes suggest that the exclusion of the upper gut, rather than weight loss, benefits glucose tolerance (38). Rats after gastrojejunal bypass have better glucose tolerance than sham-operated pair-fed control animals with equivalent body weight (38). Similarly, ileal transposition results in an early improvement in glucose tolerance with an increase of GLP-1 levels in a nonobese type 2 diabetes rat model, com-

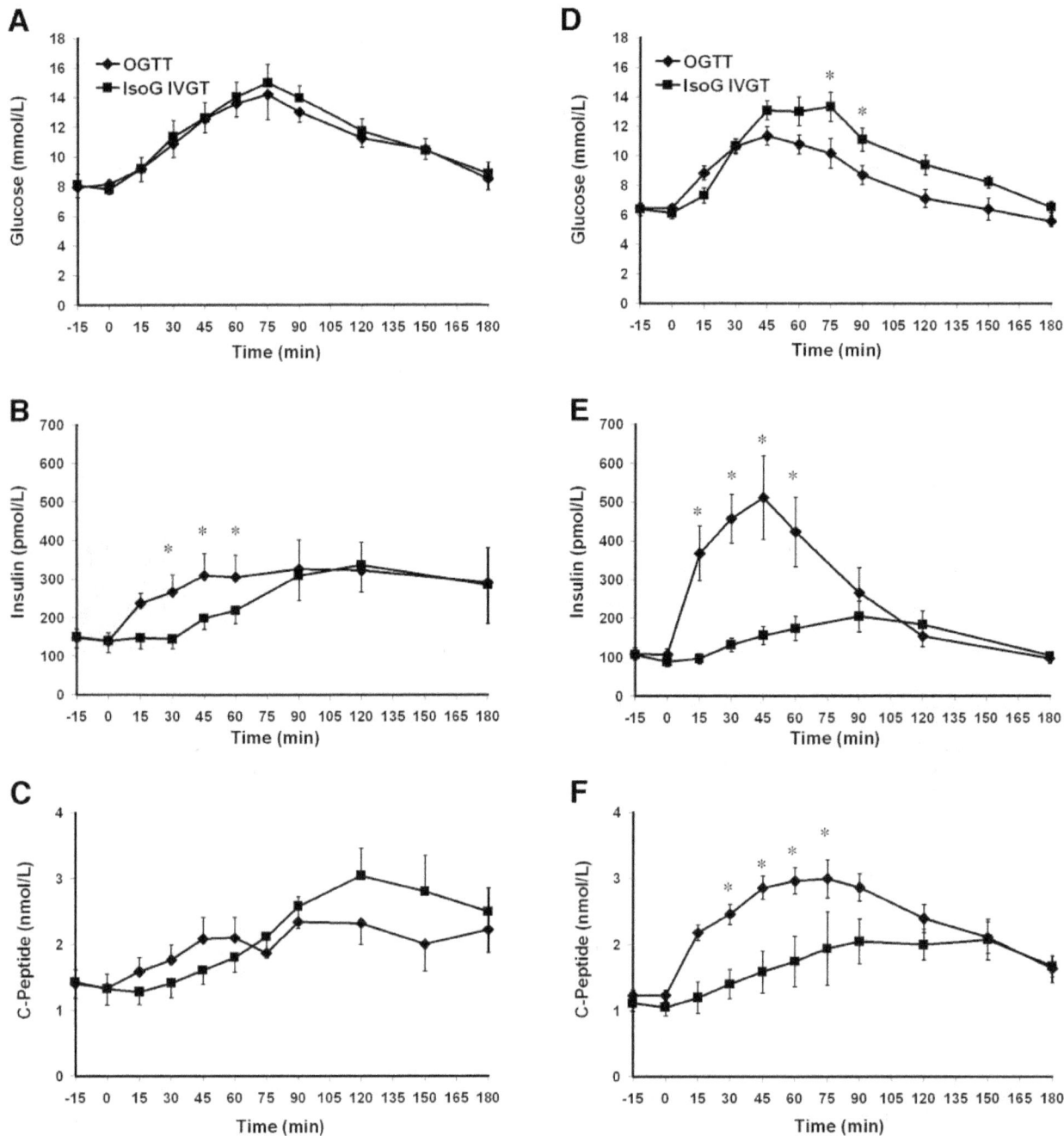

Figure 2—*Glucose (A and D), insulin (B and E), and C-peptide (C and F) concentrations during OGTTs (♦) and IsoG IVGTs (■) before (A–C) and after (D–F) RY-GBP. Data are means ± SEM. *P < 0.05, significant difference between OGTT and IsoG IVGT values within each condition (before or after RY-GBP).*

pared with sham-operated animals (39). The improvement in glucose tolerance was shown to be independent of weight and food intake (40). These rodent studies underline potential mechanisms by which diabetes improves after bariatric surgery and support a role for the gut incretins in glucose tolerance after RY-GBP.

Additionally, the change in circulat-ing incretin levels could result from changes in the level and/or activity of the enzyme DPPIV. Both GLP-1 and GIP are highly susceptible to enzymatic degradation in vivo. The cleavage by DPPIV is an important determinant of incretin action, as it occurs rapidly and generates noninsulinotropic metabolites. DP-PIV inhibitors are used to modulate

incretin levels for the treatment of type 2 diabetes (41). We found that the release of active GLP-1 is also increased after RY-GBP, although the increase is short-lived. The ratio of circulating active GLP-1 levels to total GLP-1 levels decreased after RY-GBP. It is difficult to speculate on the significance of these findings, which could represent a change in levels and/or activity of the enzyme DPPIV. To our knowledge, there are no available data on in vivo DPPIV activity and/or levels in type 2 diabetes or on the effect of diabetes control and/or weight loss on the activity or levels of the enzyme.

As shown by others (14,42), we found that our patients with type 2 diabetes had an impaired incretin effect. After RY-GBP, in addition to increases in the levels of stimulated circulating GLP-1 and GIP levels, the severely impaired incretin effect on insulin and/or C-peptide improved significantly, reaching a magnitude similar to that of the nondiabetic control subjects. To our knowledge, this is the first report of simultaneous increases in stimulated incretin levels and the incretin effect (by comparing the insulin response to the oral and matched IV glucose load) in patients with type 2 diabetes after RY-GBP. Although the incretin effect of the patients normalized to the levels of control subjects after RY-GBP, the magnitude of the increase of stimulated GIP and GLP-1 levels was far greater than that for control subjects, with a fivefold increase for GLP-1. Interestingly, a similar discrepancy between incretin levels and effect occurred in patients before RY-GBP. Stimulated GLP-1 and GIP levels of patients were not different from those of control subjects, yet the incretin effect, normal for the control subjects, was severely impaired for the patients with type 2 diabetes. Other have shown discrepancies between circulating levels of incretins in response to the ingestion of glucose and the incretin effect (43), underlining the importance of looking at both the incretin effect and plasma levels.

The changes in incretin levels and effect, albeit very significant, are probably not the only factor responsible for the improvement in insulin secretion early after RY-GBP. We did find a significant correlation between incretin output during the OGTT and the incretin effect. However, the small sample size does not allow pertinent comments on these findings. Other determinants of impaired insulin secretion in type 2 diabetes, such as glucose toxicity (44,45) and lipotoxicity (46,47), probably improve after weight loss. At 1 month after RY-GBP, the daily calorie intake was minimal (range of 500–700 kcal by 24-h diet recall, data not shown) and the participants had lost about 10 kg. It is known that both caloric restriction and weight loss improve diabetes control (48–51). Diet-induced weight loss also

improves the release of incretins in obese nondiabetic individuals (52,53). However, as all of these events occur simultaneously, it is hard to isolate one factor from the others. Future researchers will have to separate the weight loss effect from the effect of the surgical bypass.

Insulin secretion in diabetes is extremely variable (54,55), depending on, among other factors, the age of the patient (56), the duration of the disease (impossible to measure accurately), the degree of diabetes control (45,46), and the degree of insulin resistance (57). The effects of weight loss will depend upon the prediet β-cell capacity (58). In this study, the mean age of our patients was 45 years, the duration of diagnosed diabetes was <2 years, and the A1C at baseline was <7%. After RY-GBP, the patients discontinued their antidiabetes medications, and fasting and postprandial glucose levels decreased significantly to nondiabetic levels. The changes in insulin and C-peptide (data not shown) levels after the RY-GBP were variable, and changes were not statistically significant. However, the relative amount of insulin secreted in response to glucose (insulin-to-glucose ratio) was greater after the surgery, a marker of improved insulin secretion.

Our study has some weaknesses. Our sample was of small size and ethnically diverse (data not shown) with only women, and, therefore, we could not assess sex or ethnic differences. We did not control for diet before the OGTT testing. Indeed, after the RY-GBP, patients were calorie restricted, and their amount of carbohydrate intake was probably much lower than that before RY-GBP. It has been shown that caloric and carbohydrate restriction could affect the result of the OGTT (59). It is possible that this caloric and carbohydrate restriction could have affected incretin release during the OGTT. Future diet-controlled studies will address this issue. Finally, the matching of the glucose levels was not perfect between OGTTs and IsoG IVGTs in patients after RY-GBP, and the levels of glucose were higher during the IsoG IVGT. However, this does not affect the interpretation of the results. If anything, it strengthens our findings. Although glycemia is greater during the IsoG IVGT, patients still released significantly more insulin during the OGTT than during the IsoG IVGT.

These data clarify the incretin effect on insulin in the early period after RY-GBP. Our main finding is that incretin levels and the incretin effect are markedly

increased 1 month after RY-GBP, in parallel with a significant improvement of diabetes control. The magnitude of the incretin release may be specific to the anatomical changes of the gut resulting from RY-GBP surgery. Further experiments will have to be conducted to separate the effect of the weight loss from the effect of RY-GBP. These results may lead investigators to study other therapeutic maneuvers to alter incretins and develop new treatments for the growing diabetic and prediabetic population. As more obese patients with diabetes undergo RY-GBP, a clear understanding of the mechanism underlying short- and long-term improvements in type 2 diabetes is increasingly important.

Acknowledgments— This work was funded in part by grants from the American Diabetes Association (7-05-CR-18), the National Institutes of Health (R01-DK67561, General Clinical Research Center RR00645, and ORC DK-26687), and Diabetes and Endocrinology Research Center (DK-63068-05).

We thank bariatric surgeons Drs. Christine Ren and Howard Beaton for kindly referring patients for this study, our volunteer participants, and Hao Tran for his help with the figures.

References

1. Mokdad AH, Ford ES, Bowman BA, Nelson DE, Engelgau MM, Vinicor F, Marks JS: Diabetes trends in the U.S.: 1990–1998. *Diabetes Care* 23:1278–1283, 2000
2. Pories WJ, MacDonald KG Jr, Morgan EJ, Sinha MK, Dohm GL, Swanson MS, Barakat HA, Khazanie PG, Leggett-Frazier N, Long SD: Surgical treatment of obesity and its effect on diabetes: 10-y follow-up. *Am J Clin Nutr* 55:582S–585S, 1992
3. Residori L, Garcia-Lorda P, Flancbaum L, Pi-Sunyer FX, Laferrère B: Prevalence of co-morbidities in obese patients before bariatric surgery: effect of race. *Obes Surg* 13:333–340, 2003
4. Buchwald H, Avidor Y, Braunwald E, Jensen MD, Pories W, Fahrbach K, Schoelles K: Bariatric surgery: a systematic review and meta-analysis. *JAMA* 292:1724–1737, 2004
5. Bloom SR, Polak JM: Gut hormones. *Adv Clin Chem* 21:177–244, 1980
6. Kreymann B, Williams G, Ghatei MA, Bloom SR: Glucagon-like peptide-1 7–36: a physiological incretin in man. *Lancet* 2:1300–1304, 1987
7. Perley MJ, Kipnis DM: Plasma insulin responses to oral and intravenous glucose: studies in normal and diabetic subjects. *J Clin Invest* 46:1954–1962, 1967

8. Preitner F, Ibberson M, Franklin I, Binnert C, Pende M, Gjinovci A, Hansotia T, Drucker DJ, Wollheim C, Burcelin R, Thorens B: Gluco-incretins control insulin secretion at multiple levels as revealed in mice lacking GLP-1 and GIP receptors. *J Clin Invest* 113:635–645, 2004

9. Flint A, Raben A, Ersboll AK, Holst JJ, Astrup A: The effect of physiological levels of glucagon-like peptide-1 on appetite, gastric emptying, energy and substrate metabolism in obesity. *Int J Obes Relat Metab Disord* 25:781–792, 2001

10. Gutzwiller JP, Drewe J, Goke B, Schmidt H, Rohrer B, Lareida J, Beglinger C: Glucagon-like peptide-1 promotes satiety and reduces food intake in patients with diabetes mellitus type 2. *Am J Physiol* 276: R1541–R1544, 1999

11. Naslund E, Bogefors J, Skogar S, Gryback P, Jacobsson H, Holst JJ, Hellstrom PM: GLP-1 slows solid gastric emptying and inhibits insulin, glucagon, and PYY release in humans. *Am J Physiol* 277:R910–R916, 1999

12. Drucker DJ: Biological actions and therapeutic potential of the glucagon-like peptides. *Gastroenterology* 122:531–544, 2002

13. D'Alessio DA, Kahn SE, Leusner CR, Ensinck JW: Glucagon-like peptide 1 enhances glucose tolerance both by stimulation of insulin release and by increasing insulin-independent glucose disposal. *J Clin Invest* 93:2263–2266, 1994

14. Nauck M, Stockmann F, Ebert R, Creutzfeldt W: Reduced incretin effect in type 2 (non-insulin-dependent) diabetes. *Diabetologia* 29:46–52, 1986

15. Toft-Nielsen MB, Damholt MB, Madsbad S, Hilsted LM, Hughes TE, Michelsen BK, Holst JJ: Determinants of the impaired secretion of glucagon-like peptide-1 in type 2 diabetic patients. *J Clin Endocrinol Metab* 86:3717–3723, 2001

16. Toft-Nielsen MB, Madsbad S, Holst JJ: Continuous subcutaneous infusion of glucagon-like peptide 1 lowers plasma glucose and reduces appetite in type 2 diabetic patients. *Diabetes Care* 22:1137–1143, 1999

17. Nauck MA, Heimesaat MM, Orskov C, Holst JJ, Ebert R, Creutzfeldt W: Preserved incretin activity of glucagon-like peptide 1 [7–36 amide] but not of synthetic human gastric inhibitory polypeptide in patients with type-2 diabetes mellitus. *J Clin Invest* 91:301–307, 1993

18. Elahi D, McAloon-Dyke M, Fukagawa NK, Meneilly GS, Sclater AL, Minaker KL, Habener JF, Andersen DK: The insulinotropic actions of glucose-dependent insulinotropic polypeptide (GIP) and glucagon-like peptide-1 (7–37) in normal and diabetic subjects. *Regul Pept* 51:63–74, 1994

19. Holst JJ: The Claude Bernard Lecture, 2005: Glucagon-like peptide-1: from extract to agent. *Diabetologia* 49:253–260, 2006

20. Naslund E, Backman L, Holst JJ, Theodorsson E, Hellstrom PM: Importance of small bowel peptides for the improved glucose metabolism 20 years after jejunoileal bypass for obesity. *Obes Surg* 8:253–260, 1998

21. le Roux CW, Aylwin SJ, Batterham RL, Borg CM, Coyle F, Prasad V, Shurey S, Ghatei MA, Patel AG, Bloom SR: Gut hormone profiles following bariatric surgery favor an anorectic state, facilitate weight loss, and improve metabolic parameters. *Ann Surg* 243:108–114, 2006

22. Clements RH, Gonzalez QH, Long CI, Wittert G, Laws HL: Hormonal changes after Roux-en Y gastric bypass for morbid obesity and the control of type-II diabetes mellitus. *Am Surg* 70:1–4, 2004

23. Lauritsen KB, Christensen KC, Stokholm KH: Gastric inhibitory polypeptide (GIP) release and incretin effect after oral glucose in obesity and after jejunoileal bypass. *Scand J Gastroenterol* 15:489–495, 1980

24. Sarson DL, Scopinaro N, Bloom SR: Gut hormone changes after jejunoileal (JIB) or biliopancreatic (BPB) bypass surgery for morbid obesity. *Int J Obes* 5:471–480, 1981

25. Rubino F, Marescaux J: Effect of duodenal-jejunal exclusion in a non-obese animal model of type 2 diabetes: a new perspective for an old disease. *Ann Surg* 239:1–11, 2004

26. Sirinek KR, O'Dorisio TM, Hill D, McFee AS: Hyperinsulinism, glucose-dependent insulinotropic polypeptide, and the enteroinsular axis in morbidly obese patients before and after gastric bypass. *Surgery* 100:781–787, 1986

27. Morinigo R, Moize V, Musri M, Lacy AM, Navarro S, Luis MJ, Delgado S, Casamitjana R, Vidal J: GLP-1, PYY, hunger and satiety following gastric bypass surgery in morbidly obese subjects. *J Clin Endocrinol Metab* 91:1735–1740, 2006

28. Valverde I, Puente J, Martin-Duce A, Molina L, Lozano O, Sancho V, Malaisse WJ, Villanueva-Penacarrillo ML: Changes in glucagon-like peptide-1 (GLP-1) secretion after biliopancreatic diversion or vertical banded gastroplasty in obese subjects. *Obes Surg* 15:387–397, 2005

29. Jorde R, Burhol PG, Johnson JA: The effect of jejunoileal bypass on postprandial release of plasma gastric inhibitory polypeptide (GIP). *Scand J Gastroenterol* 16:313–319, 1981

30. Durnin JV, Womersley J: Body fat assessed from total body density and its estimation from skinfold thickness: measurements on 481 men and women aged from 16 to 72 years. *Br J Nutr* 32:77–97, 1974

31. *SPSS/PC Statistical Program User's Guide. Release 6.1 Edition.* Chicago, SPSS, 1993

32. Fetner R, Pi-Sunyer FX, Russell CD, La-

ferrère B: Incretins, diabetes and bariatric surgery: a review. *Tenn Med* 6:589–597, 2005

33. Service FJ, Rizza RA, Westland RE, Hall LD, Gerich JE, Go VL: Gastric inhibitory polypeptide in obesity and diabetes mellitus. *J Clin Endocrinol Metab* 58:1133–1140, 1984

34. Barry RE, Barisch J, Bray GA, Sperling MA, Morin RJ, Benfield J: Intestinal adaptation after jejunoileal bypass in man. *Am J Clin Nutr* 30:32–42, 1977

35. Morinigo R, Casamitjana R, Moize V, Gomis R, Vidal J: Determinants and relevance of GLP-1 secretion changes following gastric bypass in morbidly obese patients (Abstract). *Int J Obes* 31: S87, 2003

36. Carpenter T, Trautmann ED, Baron AD: Hyperinsulinemic hypoglycemia with nesidioblastosis after gastric bypass surgery. *N Engl J Med* 353:2192–2194, 2005

37. Meier JJ, Butler AE, Galasso R, Butler PC: Hyperinsulinemic hypoglycemia after gastric bypass surgery is not accompanied by islet cell hyperplasia or increased β-cell turnover. *Diabetes Care* 29:1554–1559, 2006

38. Rubino F, Gagner M, Gentileschi P, Kini S, Fukuyama S, Feng J, Diamond E: The early effect of the Roux-en-Y gastric bypass on hormones involved in body weight regulation and glucose metabolism. *Ann Surg* 240:236–242, 2004

39. Patriti A, Facchiano E, Annetti C, Aisa MC, Galli F, Fanelli C, Donini A: Early improvement of glucose tolerance after ileal transposition in a non-obese type 2 diabetes rat model. *Obes Surg* 15:1258–1264, 2005

40. Strader AD, Vahl TP, Jandacek RJ, Woods SC, D'Alessio DA, Seeley RJ: Weight loss through ileal transposition is accompanied by increased ileal hormone secretion and synthesis in rats. *Am J Physiol* 288: E447–E453, 2005

41. Deacon CF: Therapeutic strategies based on GLP-1. *Diabetes* 53:2181–2189, 2004

42. Ebert R, Creutzfeldt W: Gastrointestinal peptides and insulin secretion. *Diabetes Metab Rev* 3:1–26, 1987

43. Henchoz E, D'Alessio DA, Gillet M, Halkic N, Matzinger O, Goy JJ, Chiolero R, Tappy L, Schneiter P: Impaired insulin response after oral but not intravenous glucose in heart- and liver-transplant recipients. *Transplantation* 76:923–929, 2003

44. Rossetti L, Giaccari A, DeFronzo RA: Glucose toxicity. *Diabetes Care* 13:610–630, 1990

45. Leahy JL, Bonner-Weir S, Weir GC: β-Cell dysfunction induced by chronic hyperglycemia: current ideas on mechanism of impaired glucose-induced insulin secretion. *Diabetes Care* 15:442–455, 1992

46. Bergman RN, Ader M: Free fatty acids and

pathogenesis of type 2 diabetes mellitus. *Trends Endocrinol Metab* 11:351–356, 2000

47. Unger RH: Lipotoxicity in the pathogenesis of obesity-dependent NIDDM: genetic and clinical implications. *Diabetes* 44:863–870, 1995

48. Henry RR, Wiest-Kent TA, Scheaffer L, Kolterman OG, Olefsky JM: Metabolic consequences of very-low-calorie diet therapy in obese non-insulin-dependent diabetic and nondiabetic subjects. *Diabetes* 35:155–164, 1986

49. Henry RR, Scheaffer L, Olefsky JM: Glycemic effects of intensive caloric restriction and isocaloric refeeding in noninsulin-dependent diabetes mellitus. *J Clin Endocrinol Metab* 61:917–925, 1985

50. Wing RR, Marcus MD, Salata R, Epstein LH, Miaskiewicz S, Blair EH: Effects of a very-low-calorie diet on long-term glycemic control in obese type 2 diabetic subjects. *Arch Intern Med* 151:1334–1340, 1991

51. Gumbiner B, Polonsky KS, Beltz WF, Griver K, Wallace P, Brechtel G, Henry RR: Effects of weight loss and reduced hyperglycemia on the kinetics of insulin secretion in obese non-insulin dependent diabetes mellitus. *J Clin Endocrinol Metab* 70:1594–1602, 1990

52. Verdich C, Toubro S, Buemann B, Lysgard MJ, Holst JJ, Astrup A: The role of postprandial releases of insulin and incretin hormones in meal-induced satiety—effect of obesity and weight reduction. *Int J Obes Relat Metab Disord* 25:1206–1214, 2001

53. Rask E, Olsson T, Soderberg S, Johnson O, Seckl J, Holst JJ, Ahren B: Impaired incretin release after a mixed meal is associated with insulin resistance in nondiabetic men. *Diabetes Care* 24:1640–1645, 2001

54. DeFronzo RA: Lilly Lecture 1987: The triumvirate: β-cell, muscle, liver: a collusion responsible for NIDDM. *Diabetes* 37:667–687, 1988

55. Porte D Jr: Banting Lecture 1990. β-Cells in type II diabetes mellitus. *Diabetes* 40: 166–180, 1991

56. Kahn SE, Larson VG, Schwartz RS, Beard JC, Cain KC, Fellingham GW, Stratton JR, Cerqueira MD, Abrass IB: Exercise training delineates the importance of B-cell dysfunction to the glucose intolerance of human aging. *J Clin Endocrinol Metab* 74: 1336–1342, 1992

57. Bogardus C: Insulin resistance in the pathogenesis of NIDDM in Pima Indians. *Diabetes Care* 16:228–231, 1993

58. Pi-Sunyer FX: Weight and non-insulin-dependent diabetes mellitus. *Am J Clin Nutr* 63:426S–429S, 1996

59. Conn JW: *Am J Med Sci* 199:555–564, 1940

Bariatric Surgery in Patients With Morbid Obesity and Type 2 Diabetes

Guntram Schernthaner, md[1]
John M. Morton, md[2]

There is an epidemic of obesity throughout the developed and much of the developing world (1–3). Obesity, typically measured as BMI $\geq$30 kg/m^2, has three subclasses: obesity 1 (30–34.9 kg/m^2); obesity 2 (35–39.9 kg/m^2); and extreme obesity (>40 kg/m^2). Extreme or morbid obesity is rapidly increasing in the U.S. and may have the potential of decreasing life expectancy. From 1986 to 2000, the prevalence of BMI >30 kg/m^2 doubled, whereas that of BMI $\geq$40 kg/m^2 quadrupled, and even extreme obesity of BMI $\geq$50 kg/m^2 increased fivefold (2). Of particular concern is the alarming increasing prevalence of obesity among children (1), suggesting that the epidemic will worsen before it improves. Epidemiologic studies have demonstrated that increasing BMI is a causative factor in many life-threatening comorbidities, including type 2 diabetes, cardiovascular disease, and cancer. BMI has been established as an independent risk factor for premature mortality (4). Obesity is a major independent risk factor for the development of type 2 diabetes and is associated with the rapid increase in the prevalence of type 2 diabetes (3). In the U.S., the majority diagnosed with type 2 diabetes are overweight, with 50% obese (i.e., BMI >30 kg/m^2) and 9% morbidly obese (BMI >40 kg/m^2) (5). This twin epidemic of obesity and diabetes carries severe consequence for premature mortality (6).

Lifestyle intervention programs with diet therapy, behavior modification, exercise programs, and pharmacotherapy are widely used in various combinations. Unfortunately, with extremely rare exceptions (7), clinically significant weight loss is generally very modest and transient, particularly in patients with severe obesity. In a recently published study (8), 80 adults with mild to moderate obesity (BMI 30–35 kg/m^2) were randomized to nonsurgical intervention (very-low-calorie diet, orlistat, and lifestyle change) or to surgical intervention (gastric banding); surgical treatment was significantly more effective than nonsurgical therapy in reducing weight, resolving the metabolic syndrome, and improving quality of life during a 24-month treatment program (8). At 2 years, the surgical group had greater weight loss, with a mean of 21.6% of initial weight loss and 87.2% of excess weight loss, whereas the nonsurgical group had a loss of 5.5% of initial weight and 21.8% of excess weight (P = 0.001). When morbidly obese patients with a BMI >40 kg/m^2 were willing to complete an intensive behavioral program, a remarkable weight loss of ~35% of the initial body weight was observed after 40 weeks,. For completers, average weight loss for women was 30.8 kg (23.9%) and for men was 42.6 kg (26.7%) over 39 weeks. However, long-term maintenance of weight loss is difficult for most individuals, as also noted in this particular study (7).

Bariatric surgery includes several surgical procedures that can be performed in obese patients. Per the 1991 National Institutes of Health Consensus Conference Guidelines, patients are considered as surgical candidates only if their BMI is $\geq$40 kg/m^2 or if their BMI is $\geq$35 kg/m^2 and they suffer from other life-threatening comorbidities, such as type 2 diabetes, hypertension, and cardiovascular disease. Presently, the three most common surgical procedures for obesity are the Roux-en-Y gastric bypass, the vertical banded gastroplasty, and the adjustable gastric band with sleeve gastrectomy and duodenal switch, which is less commonly performed. In the Swedish Obesity Study (SOS), the mean changes in weight and risk factors were more favorable among the subjects treated by gastric bypass than among those treated by banding or vertical banded gastroplasty (9). The maintained weight change over 10 years was 25% in the gastric bypass subgroup. In the year 2002–2003, worldwide, 146,301 bariatric surgery operations were performed by 2,839 bariatric surgeons, and 103,000 of these operations were performed in U.S./Canada by 850 surgeons (10).

The outcomes after surgically induced weight loss published in the last years are impressive (9,11,12). In a meta-analysis of 22,094 patients (mean age 47 years, mean BMI 46.9, 72.6% women), the mean percentage of excess weight loss was 61.2% for all patients (12). Excessive weight loss was higher for patients who underwent gastric bypass (61.6%) or gastroplasty (68.2%) compared with those who received gastric banding (47.5%). Remarkably, diabetes was completely resolved in 76.8% of patients and resolved or improved in 86.0%. Hyperlipidemia improved in $\geq$70% of patients, and hypertension was resolved in 61.7% and resolved and improved in 78.5%. Obstructive sleep apnea was resolved in 85.7% of patients and was resolved or improved in 83.6% of patients.

The long-term outcome data of a controlled surgical intervention study of obesity (Swedish Obesity Study) were recently reported by Lars Sjöström at the International Federation of Surgery for Obesity congress in Sydney as well as at the European Association for the Study of Diabetes (EASD) congress in Copenhagen (13). In the Swedish Obesity Study, a surgical group of 2,010 patients (matched by age, sex, BMI, and comorbidities) was compared with a nonsurgical control group consisting of 2,037 patients, and

From the [1]Department of Medicine I, Rudolfstiftung Hospital, Vienna, Austria; and the [2]Department of Surgery, Stanford University, Stanford, California.

Address correspondence and reprint requests to Professor Dr. Guntram Schernthaner, Department of Medicine I, Rudolfstiftung Hospital Vienna, Juchgasse 25, A-1030 Vienna Austria. E-mail: guntram.schernthaner@wienkav.at.

The authors of this article have no relevant duality of interest to declare.

This article is based on a presentation at the 1st World Congress of Controversies in Diabetes, Obesity and Hypertension (CODHy). The Congress and the publication of this article were made possible by unrestricted educational grants from MSD, Roche, sanofi-aventis, Novo Nordisk, Medtronic, LifeScan, World Wide, Eli Lilly, Keryx, Abbott, Novartis, Pfizer, Generx Biotechnology, Schering, and Johnson & Johnson.

Abbreviations: GLP, glucagon-like peptide.

DOI: 10.2337/dc08-s270

both groups were followed for 15 years. Surgically induced weight loss frequently resolved or markedly improved diabetes, reduced myocardial infarction by 43%, and provided a 31% reduction in overall mortality. In this single trial, weight loss induced by bariatric surgery had no effect on incidence of stroke. Interestingly, the benefit in the reduction of myocardial infarction and overall mortality was almost exclusively seen in diabetic patients. The less impressive effects observed in the nondiabetic patients of the Swedish Obesity Study (13) might be explained by the fact that the cardiovascular risk factor profile is frequently quite favorable in morbidly obese subjects despite the accumulation of >40 kg excess fat (14). The postoperative mortality was low and was kept at ~0.25%.

The significant reduction of total mortality in the well-performed randomized Swedish Obesity Study is in line with earlier observational studies reporting a reduced mortality in patients who underwent bariatric surgery (15,16). A retrospective analysis of 232 type 2 diabetic patients with morbid obesity (mean BMI 50 kg/m^2), who underwent either gastric bypass operation ($n = 154$) or did not undergo surgery ($n = 78$), demonstrated a mortality rate of only 9% in the surgical group during the 9-year follow-up compared with 28% in the nonsurgical control group (15). Patients in the control group had 4.5 times the incidence of death of patients in the surgical group. Notably, the improvement in the mortality rate in the surgical group was primarily due to a decrease in the number of cardiovascular deaths. An observational two-cohort study compared the outcome of 1,035 severely obese patients who underwent bariatric surgery with a control group of 5,746 age- and sex-matched severely obese patients who had not undergone weight reduction surgery (16). The mortality rate in the bariatric surgery cohort was 0.68% compared with 6.17% in control subjects, which translated to an impressive 89% reduction in the relative risk of death. Given that this was a retrospective analysis, the impact of the composition of the control group or practice patterns, particularly the use of cardiovascular preventive drugs, might have contributed to the huge difference between the two cohort studies.

It is now generally accepted that weight loss induced by bariatric surgery is the most effective therapy available for people who are extremely obese. It re-

verses, ameliorates, or eliminates major cardiovascular risk factors, including diabetes, hypertension, and lipid abnormalities. However, large epidemiological follow-up studies have shown that obesity per se increases cardiovascular risk, independent of other associated traditional cardiovascular risk factors (17,18). Adipose tissue is the predominant site of fat stores. Increasing obesity results in an overload of lipids within the body's natural storage sink (i.e., the adipocyte) followed by the necessary deposition of fat within ectopic sites such as muscle, liver, and pancreas. The resulting metabolic derangements are associated with insulin resistance, central obesity, and chronic inflammation as adipose tissue acts as an endocrine organ, producing and secreting a host of biologic mediators. There is now increasing evidence that these less well-characterized atherogenic biomarkers or mediators have an important role in obesity-related cardiovascular risk, such as chronic inflammation, endothelial dysfunction, and hypercoagulation (11,19–25). Recent studies have shown that weight loss induced by surgery results in an impressive reduction of insulin resistance (11,21), reduces relevant markers (C-reactive protein, interleukin-6, interleukin-18, and sCD40L) of chronic vascular inflammation (11,21–23), and decreases well-established cardiac risk factors that have been shown to be important predictors of cardiovascular morbidity and mortality (26–30). In addition, surgery improves endothelial dysfunction (24) and reduces key factors responsible for the increased atherothrombotic risk of the morbidly obese patients, such as tissue factor, factor VII, and plasminogen activator inhibitor (PAI)-1 (19,20).

REVERSIBILITY OF DIABETES AFTER BARIATRIC SURGERY — Of considerable interest for morbidly obese patients with diabetes is the observation that euglycemia and normal insulin levels occur within days after surgery, long before there is any significant weight loss (31). Morbid obesity per se is associated with profound insulin resistance and marked insulin hypersecretion, but the dynamics of β-cell function (i.e., β-cell glucose sensitivity, rate sensitivity, and potentiation) are preserved (11,32). On the other hand, overt diabetes and impaired glucose tolerance are characterized by a progressive loss of β-cell glucose sensitivity, independent of insulin resistance (33). It is well

known that bariatric surgery leads to a large improvement in insulin sensitivity (two- to threefold increase), which can be seen early after surgery before any substantial weight loss has occurred (11,34,35). Interestingly, absolute insulin secretion decreases significantly after bariatric surgery, although detailed information in patients with overt and more advanced diabetes is still very limited.

The mechanisms underlying the dramatic effects of malabsorptive surgery on insulin sensitivity and β-cell function are poorly understood. Several mechanisms have been proposed for the early improvement of glucose tolerance after bariatric surgery (36). Among them, caloric restriction and changes in gut hormone release have received the most attention. Glucagon-like peptide (GLP)-1 has emerged as a potential key mediator, since patients after Roux-en-Y gastric bypass had increased postprandial plasma levels of peptide YY and GLP-1 favoring enhanced satiety (37). However, more recent studies have questioned that GLP-1 is responsible for reversal of diabetes after surgery (38,39). Morinigo et al. (38) have demonstrated that GLP-1 response to a meal is not a critical factor for the early amelioration in glucose homeostasis after gastric bypass. Six weeks after surgery, the GLP-1 increase was only significant in patients with normal glucose or impaired glucose tolerance, but not in the diabetic patients. In a longitudinal study (39), fasting GLP-1 concentrations decreased and peptide YY levels increased independently of each other in morbidly obese patients 2 years after dramatic weight loss, indicating that the relationship between these gut hormones seems to be more complicated than assumed before. A very recent three-year follow-up study (40) in diabetic patients has shown that reversibility of diabetes is dependent on the improvement of skeletal muscle insulin sensitivity, mediated by changes in the expression of genes regulating glucose and fatty acid metabolism in response to nutrient availability.

PERIOPERATIVE RISK AND CARE OF BARIATRIC SURGERY — There is clear and convincing evidence that bariatric surgery is a powerful therapy in treating morbid obesity and its health consequences. The ideal target population for bariatric surgery are morbidly obese patients with diabetes and metabolic syndrome because of the enormous benefit derived by surgi-

cal treatment and the large risk of premature mortality engendered by diabetes and the metabolic syndrome (41). Given the paucity of alternative treatments for weight loss in this challenging population, early and prompt surgical referral of the morbidly obese patient with diabetes and metabolic syndrome is needed. Despite the high prevalence of comorbidity in this population, bariatric surgery can provide tertiary prevention of the complications of obesity.

Patient education and selection are important components in long-term success of bariatric surgery. While surgery provides important physiological reinforcement of a healthier lifestyle, patients must still make critical changes in their dietary, exercise, and sleep habits. Preoperative education ensures that patients are prepared to make these substantial changes in lifestyle (42). Surgery remains a tool, not a cure, for morbidly obese patients in their change in lifestyle. These habits are critical given that morbid obesity is a chronic disease and requires lifelong maintenance. Identification of preoperative characteristics of success after surgery remains elusive, and the best determinant of postoperative success is both patient and programmatic commitment (43).

The risk of complications may temper some enthusiasm for bariatric surgery. There are demonstrated differences between surgical techniques and outcomes (44). Randomized trial evidence reveals that the laparoscopic approach shortens time to return to work and decreases wound and pulmonary complications (45). Among the different surgical procedures, the rate of complications is inversely proportional to the amount of weight loss produced by each surgery (44). Beyond the type of procedure, there are identified risk factors for complications after bariatric surgery, including age, sex, BMI, comorbidities, and insurance status (46–50). It should be noted that the best demonstrated and most protective effect against complications is an experienced surgeon and hospital (46,49). In addition, complications may not affect long-term weight loss, which is the outcome that best predicts long-term mortality risk (51).

Age has been repeatedly demonstrated to be a factor influencing outcome after bariatric surgery. In a study examining bariatric surgery outcomes for Medicare patients, the rate of complications for those <65 and >65 years equalized

when patients were treated by experienced surgeons (46). Male sex has also been identified as a risk factor for complications after bariatric surgery. Male sex may lead to more complications due to increased technical difficulty caused by a higher BMI, more visceral fat, and potentially more advanced comorbidities (47–49). In the U.S. (52), in various European countries (53,54), as well as in New Zealand (55), ~80% of bariatric surgery patients are women. The proportion of men undergoing bariatric surgery does not reflect the sex distribution of morbid obesity. Clearly, male morbidly obese patients seek surgical care less often, which may be due to general decreased access to care by men as well as a greater social acceptance of the morbidly obese male. Increased BMI is also recognized as a risk factor for complications due primarily to technical ability to complete the operation and the potential for worsened comorbidity in these patients (49). Finally, certain comorbidities have been demonstrated to increase complication rates including diabetes, chronic obstructive pulmonary disease, sleep apnea, and hypertension (47,49). Studies have substantiated the risk of Medicare insurance status upon bariatric surgery outcomes (46,48). Most likely, Medicare insurance status is a proxy for age, socioeconomic status, and disability. Although patients with the most risk factors carry the greatest risk for surgery, those high-risk patients may also derive the most benefit from bariatric surgery given the disease burden they carry (56).

All of these risk factors are nonmodifiable before surgery. As mentioned previously, the single consistent protective factor for complications is both surgeon and hospital volume. The volume-outcome effect is well established in surgery and, unlike the other risk factors for complications, modifiable. For bariatric surgery, it has been demonstrated that a high-volume surgeon and high-volume hospital leads to decreased morbidity and mortality (46,50). In the U.S., this volume outcome effect has been recognized by the Centers for Medicare and Medicaid Services who now require that Medicare patients only undergo surgery at Bariatric Surgery Centers of Excellence (57). Numerous criteria compose a Bariatric Surgery Center of Excellence, but the primary criteria are surgeon volume >50 cases and hospital volume >125 cases annually. While a referral to a Bariatric Sur-

gery Center of Excellence may lead to decreased morbidity and mortality, this referral pattern must be balanced with appropriate and sufficient access to care for a vulnerable population without other therapeutic options.

Surgical volume is a surrogate measure for a wide expanse of practice patterns that determine best outcomes. More research is required to determine which practice patterns most effect outcomes including preoperative weight loss, advanced surgical training, and surgical assistant status (58,59). Given this need for further research, clinically derived prospectively maintained databases regarding bariatric surgery are required (56,60).

LONG-TERM RESULTS OF BARIATRIC SURGERY: COMPLICATIONS, FAILURES, AND WEIGHT GAIN — The long-term complications and outcomes was recently analyzed in a 12-year follow-up study (53) of 1,791 consecutive patients receiving laparoscopic adjustable gastric banding (LABG) in Italy. Overall, 106 (5.9%) patients required reoperation (band removal in 3.7% and band repositioning in 2.7%). Port-related complications occurred in 200 patients (11.2%), and 41 patients (2.3%) underwent further surgery due to unsatisfactory results. A case-control study involving 821 surgically treated patients versus 821 treated by medical therapy showed a statistically significant difference in survival in favor of the surgically treated group (53). Based on their findings, the authors concluded that LAGB can achieve effective, safe, and stable long-term weight loss with a low complication rate in experienced hands. In contrast, a 10-year long-term follow-up study of 317 patients receiving LAGB in Switzerland (54) showed high long-term complication and failure rates. Overall, 105 (33.1%) of the patients developed late complications, including band erosion in 9.5%, pouch dilatation/slippage in 6.3%, and catheter- or port-related problems in 7.6%. Major reoperation was required in 21.7% of the patients. The mean excess weight loss at 5 years was 58.5% in patients with the band still in place. The failure rate increased from 13.2% after 18 months to 36.9% at 7 years. According to the experience of the Swiss authors with a 5-year failure rate of 37% and 7-year success rate (excess weight loss >50%) in only 43%, LAGB should no longer be con-

sidered as the procedure of choice for obesity (54). On the other hand, a long-term follow-up study of 342 severely obese patients who underwent gastric bypass in New Zealand (55) showed excellent long-term outcomes. BMI and percent excess weight loss after 1, 5, and 10 years were 28.7 and 89%, 31.2 and 70%, and 31 and 75%, respectively. In addition, 62% of individuals with hypertension before surgery were cured and 25% had improved and 85% of those with type 2 diabetes were cured and 10% had improved. Thus, the excellent outcomes, in terms of weight loss and improvement in comorbidities, seen in both the short and medium term after gastric bypass, were well maintained into the longer term. Recently, Christou et al. (61) reported long-term results of 228 gastric bypass patients who were followed up for a mean of 11.4 years (range 4.7–14.9); 63.2% of them were morbidly obese (BMI <50 kg/m^2) and 36.8% were extremely obese (BMI ≥50 kg/m^2). The extremely obese patients lost more rapidly from the preoperative BMI to the lowest BMI and gained more rapidly than the morbid obese patients thereafter ($P < 0.0001$). In the morbidly obese patients, the mean BMI before surgery was 44.3 kg/m^2; the nadir BMI was 26.4 kg/m^2 and occurred 1.9 years after surgery but increased again to 31.0 after 11.4 years after surgery. In the extreme obese patients, the initial mean BMI of 56.2 kg/m^2 decreased to 31.4 kg/m^2 at 2.2 years after surgery, but increased significantly to 38.3 kg/m^2 after 11.6 years after surgery. Satiety is a prominent feature of weight loss after gastric bypass and persists in those patients with an excellent result. Patients who regain large amounts of weight say they are eating almost as much as before the operation. One patient died of pulmonary embolus on the second postoperative day, resulting in a 0.36% 30-day operative mortality. Seven patients died after surgery at 4.8 years of suicide, 5.7 years of suicide, 6.6 years of liver failure, 8 years of unknown cause, 8.8 years of pulmonary embolus, 8.8 years of cardiac failure, and 13 years of cerebrovascular accident, for a 3.2% long-term post-operative mortality. In conclusion, significant weight gain occurred continuously in patients after reaching the nadir weight after gastric bypass. Remarkably, despite this weight gain, the long-term mortality remained low at 3.1%. Other long-term studies (>10-year follow-up) reported much lower late failure rates (31,62,63). Hess et

al. (62) were able to follow 167 of 182 patients (92%) >10 years after biliopancreatic diversion with duodenal switch. They found that 87 (52%) had lost at least 80% of excess weight and that only 6% lost >50% of excess weight. Scopinaro et al. (63) reported excess weight loss of 74% at 10 years, 75% at 12 years, and 77% at 18 years, with no difference between morbid obese and extreme obese patients. Pories et al. (31) showed a remarkable stability of postoperative weight after gastric bypass for up to 14 years. Their study of 608 patients with a 97% follow-up showed a 58% loss of excess weight after 5 years and a BMI of 33.7 kg/m^2. After 10 years, the excess weight loss was 55% and the BMI was 34.7 kg/m^2.

CONCLUSIONS — Even though there are varying degrees of evidence for different surgeries, there is a clear preponderance of evidence for all weight loss surgeries to be vastly superior to traditional weight loss therapies in promoting weight reduction. Obesity is an independent risk factor for cardiovascular disease and contributes strongly to additional risk factors such as hypertension, diabetes, hyperlipidemia, and biochemical inflammatory markers. Cardiac risk among surgically treated morbidly obese patients is greatly diminished by weight loss, comorbidity resolution, and advantageous alteration of biochemical cardiovascular risk factors.

Obesity is a worldwide epidemic with serious medical and economic consequences. The only effective and enduring therapy for morbid obesity is weight loss surgery. Weight loss surgery has the unique ability to solve many different health concerns through a single intervention. Certain risks exist for weight loss surgery that can be mitigated by surgical experience and patient selection, education, and lifelong surveillance. Strong evidence supports the well-known benefits of weight loss surgery including weight loss, comorbidity resolution, quality of life improvement, and increased lifespan. Weight loss surgery is a lifesaving intervention in the right patients and in the right hands.

ADDENDUM — After submission of this review, two important long-term outcome studies (64,65) performed in patients after gastric bypass surgery were published. Sjöström et al. (64) conducted a prospective, controlled study of bari-

atric surgery called the Swedish Obese Subjects (SOS) study, in which 2,010 overweight patients wishing surgery were matched with 2,037 obese patients not desiring surgery. At 10 years, weight losses ranged from 14 to 25% among subjects who had undergone bariatric surgery as compared with only 2% among control subjects. In the surgery group, there was a significant reduction in the adjusted hazard ratio for death (29%) after an average follow-up of 10.9 years. Adams et al. (65) conducted a retrospective cohort study with 7,925 severely obese control subjects obtained from driver's license records that were matched to 7,925 patients who had undergone gastric bypass surgery. During a mean follow-up of 7.1 years, adjusted long-term mortality from any cause in the surgery group decreased by 40%. Cause-specific mortality in the surgery group decreased from diabetes by 92%, from coronary artery disease by 56%, and from cancer by 60%. The reduction of mortality from diabetes and cancer are particularly noteworthy. However, rates of death not caused by disease, such as accidents and suicide, were 58% higher in the surgery group than in the control group.

References
1. Ogden CL, Carroll MD, Curtin LR, McDowell MA, Tabak CJ, Flegal KM: Prevalence of overweight and obesity in the United States 1999–2004. *JAMA* 295:1549–1555, 2006
2. McTigue K, Larson JC, Valoski A, Burke G, Kotchen J, Lewis CE, Stefanick ML, Van Horn L, Kuller L: Mortality and cardiac and vascular outcomes in extremely obese women. *JAMA* 296:79–86, 2006
3. Yoon K, Lee J-H, Kim J-W, Cho JH, Choi Y-H, Ko S-H, Zimmet P, Son HY: Epidemic obesity and type 2 diabetes in Asia. *Lancet* 368:1681–1686, 2006
4. Calle EE, Thun MJ, Petrelli JM: Body-mass index and mortality in a prospective cohort of US adults. *N Engl J Med* 341:1097–1105, 1999
5. Leibson CL, Williamson DF, Melton LJ 3rd, Palumbo PJ, Smith SA, Ransom JE, Schilling PL, Narayan KM: Temporal trends in BMI among adults with diabetes. *Diabetes Care* 24:1584–1589, 2001
6. Olshansky SJ, Passaro DJ, Hershow RC, Layden J, Carnes BA, Brody, Hayflick L, Butler RN, Allison DB, Ludwig DS: A potential decline in life expectancy in the United States in the 21st century. *N Engl J Med* 352:1138–1145, 2005
7. Anderson JW, Grant L, Gotthelf L, Stifler LT: Weight loss and long-term follow-up of severely obese individuals treated with

an intense behavioral program. *Int J Obes* 31:488–493, 2006

8. O'Brien PE, Dixon JB, Laurie C, Skinner S, Proietto J, McNeil J, Strauss B, Marks S, Schachter L, Chapman L, Anderson M: Treatment of mild to moderate obesity with laparoscopic adjustable gastric banding or an intensive medical program: a randomized trial. *Ann Intern Med* 144:625–633, 2006

9. Sjöstrom L, Lindroos AK, Peltonen M, Torgerson J, Bouchard C, Carlsson B, Dahlgren S, Larsson B, Narbro K, Sjostrom CD, Sullivan M, Wedel H, Swedish Obese Subjects Study Scientific Group: Lifestyle, diabetes, and cardiovascular risk factors 10 years after bariatric surgery. *N Engl J Med* 351:2683–2693, 2004

10. Buchwald H, Williams SE: Bariatric surgery worldwide 2003. *Obes Surg* 14:1157–1164, 2004

11. Kopp HP, Kopp CW, Festa A, Krzyzanowska K, Kriwanek S, Minar E, Roka R, Schernthaner G: Impact of weight loss on inflammatory proteins and their association with the insulin resistance syndrome in morbidly obese patients. *Arterioscler Thromb Vasc Biol* 23:1042–1047, 2003

12. Buchwald H, Avidor Y, Braunwald E, Jensen MD, Pories W, Fahrbach K, Schoelles K: Bariatric surgery: a systematic review and meta-analysis. *JAMA* 292:1724–1737, 2004

13. Sjöström L: Bariatric surgery in diabetic patients: what is the evidence? 42nd EASD Meeting, Copenhagen, Denmark, 2006. *Diabetologia* (Suppl. 1) 2006

14. Barakat HA, Mooney N, O'Brien K, Long S, Khazani PG, Pories W, Caro JF: Coronary heart disease risk factors in morbidly obese women with normal glucose tolerance. *Diabetes Care* 16:144–149, 1993

15. MacDonald KG, Long SD, Swanson MS, Brown BM, Morris P, Dohm GL, Pories WJ: The gastric bypass operation reduces the progression and mortality of NIDDM. *J Gastrointest Surg* 1:213–220, 1997

16. Christou NV, Sampalis JS, Liberman M, Look D, Auger S, McLean AP, MacLean LD: Surgery decreases long-term mortality, morbidity, and health care use in morbidly obese patients. *Ann Surg* 240:416–423, 2004

17. Kim KS, Owen WL, Williams D, Adams-Campbell LL: A comparison between BMI and Conicity index on predicting coronary heart disease: the Framingham Heart Study. *Ann Epidemiol* 10:424–431, 2000

18. Jonsson S, Hedblad B, Engstrom G, Nilsson P, Berglund G, Janzon L: Influence of obesity on cardiovascular risk: twenty three-year follow up of 22,025 men from an urban Swedish population. *Int J Obes* 26:1046–1053, 2002

19. Primrose JN, Davies JA, Prentice CR, Hughes R, Johnston D: Reduction in factor VII, fibrinogen and plasminogen activator inhibitor-1 activity after surgical treatment of morbid obesity. *Thromb Haemost* 68:396–399, 1992

20. Kopp CW, Kopp HP, Steiner S, Kriwanek S, Krzyzanowska K, Bartok A, Roka R, Minar E, Schernthaner G: Weight loss reduces tissue factor in morbidly obese patients. *Obes Res* 11:950–960, 2003

21. Hanusch-Enserer U, Cauza E, Spak M, Endler G, Dunky A, Tura A, Wagner O, Rosen HR, Pacini G, Prager R: Improvement of insulin resistance and early atherosclerosis in patients after gastric banding. *Obes Res* 12:284–291, 2004

22. Schernthaner GH, Kopp HP, Kriwanek S, Krzyzanowska K, Satler M, Koppensteiner R, Schernthaner G: Effect of massive weight loss induced by bariatric surgery on serum levels of interleukin-18 and monocyte-chemoattractant-protein-1 in morbid obesity. *Obes Surg* 16:709–715, 2006

23. Schernthaner GH, Kopp HP, Krzyzanowska K, Kriwanek S, Hoellerl F, Koppensteiner R, Schernthaner G: Soluble CD40L in patients with morbid obesity: significant reduction after bariatric surgery. *Eur J Clin Invest* 36:395–401, 2006

24. Krzyzanowska KA, Mittermayer F, Kopp HP, Wolzt M, Schernthaner G: Weight loss reduces circulating asymmetrical dimethylarginine concentrations in morbidly obese women. *J Clin EndocrMetab* 89:6277–6281, 2004

25. Kopp HP, Spranger J, Möhlig M, Krzyzanowska K, Pfeiffer AF, Schernthaner G: Effect of weight loss on plasma levels of adiponectin in association with markers of chronic subclinical inflammation and the insulin resistance syndrome in obese subjects. *Int J Obes (Lond)* 29:766–771, 2005

26. Blankenberg S, Tiret L, Bickel C Peetz D, Cambien F, Meyer J, Rupprecht HJ: Interleukin-18 is a strong predictor of cardiovascular death in stable and unstable angina. *Circulation* 106:24–30, 2002

27. de Lemos JA, Morrow DA, Sabatine MS, Murphy SA, Gibson CM, Antman EM, McCabe CH, Cannon CP, Braunwald E: Association between plasma levels of monocyte chemoattractant protein-1 and long-term clinical outcomes in patients with acute coronary syndromes. *Circulation* 107:690–695, 2003

28. Heeschen C, Dimmeler S, Hamm CW, van den Brand MJ, Boersma E, Zeiher AM, Simoons M: Soluble CD40 ligand in acute coronary syndromes. *N Engl J Med* 348:1104–1111, 2003

29. Williams B, Hagedorn J, Lawson E, Galanko J, Safadi B, Curet M, Morton JM: Gastric bypass reduces biochemical cardiac risk factors, SOARD. *Surg Obes Relat Dis* 3:8–13, 2007

30. Krzyzanowska K, Mittermayer F, Wolzt M, Schernthaner G: Asymmetric dimethylarginine predicts cardiovascular events in patients with type 2 diabetes. *Diabetes Care* 30:1834–1839, 2007

31. Pories WJ, Swanson MS, MacDonald KG, Long SB, Morris PG, Brown BM, Barakat HA, deRamon RA, Israel G, Dolezal JM, et al.: Who would have thought it? An operation proves to be the most effective therapy for adult-onset diabetes mellitus. *Ann Surg* 222:339–350, 1995

32. Camastra S, Manco M, Mari A, Greco AV, Frascerra S, Mingrone G, Ferrannini E: Beta-cell function in severely obese type 2 diabetic patients: long-term effects of bariatric surgery. *Diabetes Care* 30:1002–1004, 2007

33. Ferrannini E, Gastaldelli A, Miyazaki Y, Matsuda M, Mari A, DeFronzo RA: β-Cell function in subjects spanning the range from normal glucose tolerance to overt diabetes: a new analysis. *J Clin Endocrinol Metab* 90:493–500, 2005

34. Wickremesekera K, Miller G, Naotunne TD, Knowles G, Stubbs RS: Loss of insulin resistance after Roux-en-Y gastric bypass surgery: a time course study. *Obes Surg* 15:474–481, 2005

35. Camastra S, Manco M, Mari A, Baldi S, Gastaldelli A, Greco AV, Mingrone G, Ferrannini E: Beta-cell function in morbidly obese subjects during free living: long-term effects of weight loss. *Diabetes* 54:2382–2389, 2005

36. Cummings DE, Overduin J, Foster-Schubert KE, Carlson MJ: Role of the bypassed proximal intestine in the anti-diabetic effects of bariatric surgery. *Surg Obes Relat Dis* 3:109–115, 2007

37. le Roux CW, Aylwin SJ, Batterham RL, Borg CM, Coyle F, Prasad V, Shurey S, Ghatei MA, Patel AG, Bloom SR: Gut hormone profiles following bariatric surgery favor an anorectic state, facilitate weight loss, and improve metabolic parameters. *Ann Surg* 243:108–114, 2006

38. Morinigo R, Lacy AM, Casamitjana R, Delgado S, Gomis R, Vidal J: GLP-1 and changes in glucose tolerance following gastric bypass surgery in morbidly obese subjects. *Obes Surg* 16:1594–1601, 2006

39. Reinehr T, Roth CL, Schernthaner GH, Kopp HP, Kriwanek S, Schernthaner G: Peptide YY and glucagon-like peptide-1 in morbidly obese patients before and after surgically induced weight loss. *Obes Surg* 17:1571–1577, 2007

40. Rosa G, Mingrone G, Manco M, Euthine V, Gniuli D, Calvani R, Calvani M, Favuzzi AM, Castagneto M, Vidal H: Molecular mechanisms of diabetes reversibility after bariatric surgery. *Int J Obes (Lond)* 31:1429–1436, 2007

41. Malik S, Wong N, Franklin S, Kamath TV, L'Italien Gj, Pio JR, Williams GR: Impact of the metabolic syndrome on mortality from coronary heart disease, cardiovascular disease, and all causes in United States adults. *Circulation* 110:1245–1250, 2004

42. Giusti V, DeLucia A, DiVetta, Calmes JM, Heraief E, Gaillard RC, Burckhardt P,

Suter M: Impact of preoperative teaching on surgical option of patients qualifying for bariatric surgery. *Obes Surg* 14:1241–1246, 2004

43. Van Hout GC, Verschure SK, van Heck GL: Psychosocial predictors of success following bariatric surgery. *Obes Surg* 15:552–560, 2005

44. Maggard M, Shugarman L, Suttorp M, Maglione M, Sugerman HJ, Livingston EH, Nguyen NT, Li Z, Mojica WA, Hilton L, Rhodes S, Morton SC, Shekelle PG: Meta-analysis: surgical treatment for obesity. *Ann Intern Med* 142:547–559, 2005

45. Puzziferri N, Austrheim IT, Wolfe BM, Wilson SE, Hguyen NT: Three-year follow-up of a prospective randomized trial comparing laparoscopic versus open gastric bypass. *Ann Surg* 243:181–188, 2006

46. Flum DR, Salem L, Brockel Elrod J, Dellinger EP, Cheadle A, Chan L: Early mortality among Medicare beneficiaries undergoing bariatric surgical procedures. *JAMA* 294:1903–1908, 2005

47. Fernandez AZ, DeMaria EJ, Tichansky DS, Kellum JM, Wolfe LG, Meador J, Sugerman HJ: Multivariate analysis of risk factors for death following gastric bypass for treatment of morbid obesity. *Ann Surg* 239:698–703, 2004

48. Poulose Bk, Griffin MR, Zhu Y, Smalley W, Richards WO, Wright JK, Melvin W, Holzman MD: National analysis of adverse patient safety events in bariatric surgery. *Am Surg* 71:406–413, 2005

49. Livingston EH, Ko CY: Assessing the relative contribution of individual risk factors on surgical outcome for gastric bypass surgery: a baseline probability analysis. *J Surg Rsch* 105:48–52, 2002

50. Liu JH, Zingmond D, Etzioni DA, O'Connell JB, Maggard MA, Livingston EH, Liu CD, Ko CY: Characterizing the performance and outcomes of obesity surgery in California. *Am Surg* 69:823–828, 2003

51. Morton JM, Downey J, Hagedorn JC, Encarnacion BE, Ketchum E, Curet M, Hernandez-Boussard T: Post-operative complications do not affect weight loss. *JACS* 2008. In press

52. Santry HP, Gillen DL, Lauderdale DS: Trends in bariatric surgical procedures. *JAMA* 294:1909–1917, 2005

53. Favretti F, Segato G, Ashton D, Busetto L, De Luca M, Mazza M, Ceoloni A, Banzato O, Calo E, Enzi G: Laparoscopic adjustable gastric banding in 1,791 consecutive obese patients: 12-year results. *Obes Surg* 17:168–175, 2007

54. Suter M, Calmes JM, Paroz A, Giusti V: A 10-year experience with laparoscopic gastric banding for morbid obesity: high long-term complication and failure rates. *Obes Surg* 16:829–835, 2006

55. White S, Brooks E, Jurikova L, Stubbs RS: Long-term outcomes after gastric bypass. *Obes Surg* 15:155–163, 2005

56. Wolfe BM, Morton JM: Weighing in on bariatric surgery: procedure use, readmission rates, and mortality. *JAMA* 294:1960–1963, 2005

57. http://www.cms.hhs.gov/mcd/view decisionmemo.asp?id=160. Accessed December 2006

58. Hsu GP, Morton JM, Jin L, Safadi BY, Satterwhite TS, Curet MJ: Laparoscopic Roux-en-Y gastric bypass: differences in outcome between attendings and assistants of different training backgrounds.

Obes Surg 15:1104–1110, 2005

59. Schauer P, Ikramuddin S, Hamad G, Gourash W: The learning curve for laparoscopic Roux-en-Y gastric bypass is 100 cases. *Surg Endosc* 17(2):212–5. Epub 2002 Dec 4, 2003

60. Nguyen NT, Morton JM, Wolfe BM, Schirmer B, Ali M, Traverso LW: The SAGES bariatric surgery outcome initiative. *Surg Endosc* 19:1429–1438, 2005

61. Christou NV, Look D, Maclean LD: Weight gain after short- and long-limb gastric bypass in patients followed for longer than 10 years. *Ann Surg* 244:734–740, 2006

62. Hess DS, Hess DW, Oakley RS: The biliopancreatic diversion with the duodenal switch: results beyond 10 years. *Obes Surg* 14:408–416, 2005

63. Scopinaro N, Marinari G, Camerini G, Papadia F: 2004 ABS Consensus Conference: Biliopancreatic diversion for obesity: state of the art. *Surg Obes* 1:317–328, 2005

64. Sjöström L, Narbro K, Sjöström CD, Karason K, Larsson B, Wedel H, Lystig T, Sullivan M, Bouchard C, Carlsson B, Bengtsson C, Dahlgren S, Gummesson A, Jacobson P, Karlsson J, Lindroos AK, Lönroth H, Näslund I, Olbers T, Stenlöf K, Torgerson J, Agren G, Carlsson LM: Effects of bariatric surgery on mortality in Swedish obese subjects. *N Engl J Med.* 357:741–52, 2007

65. Adams TD, Gress RE, Smith SC, Halverson RC, Simper SC, Rosamond WD, Lamonte MJ, Stroup AM, Hunt SC: Long-term mortality after gastric bypass surgery. *N Engl J Med.* 357:753–61, 2007

Treatment Modalities of Obesity

What fits whom?

Vojtěch Hainer, md, phd[1]
Hermann Toplak, md, phd[2]
Asimina Mitrakou, md[3]

The prevalence of obesity is increasing in both developed and developing countries, with rates reaching ~10–35% among adults in the Euro-American region. Obesity is associated with increased risks of cardiovascular diseases, type 2 diabetes, arthritis, and some type of cancers. Obesity significantly affects the quality of life and reduces the average life expectancy. The effective treatment of obesity should address both the medical and the social burden of this disease. Obesity needs to be treated within the health care system as any other complex disease, with empathy and without prejudice. Both health care providers and patients should know that the obesity treatment is a lifelong task. They should also set realistic goals before starting the treatment, whereas keeping in mind that even a modest weight loss of 5–15% significantly reduces obesity-related health risks. Essential treatment of obesity includes low-calorie low-fat diets, increased physical activity, and strategies contributing to the modification of lifestyle. Anti-obesity drugs facilitate weight loss and contribute to further amelioration of obesity-related health risks. A short-term weight loss, up to 6 months, is usually achieved easily. However, the long-term weight management is often associated with a lack of compliance, failures, and a high dropout rate. Regular physical activity, cognitive behavioral modification of lifestyle, and administration of anti-obesity drugs improve weight loss maintenance. Bariatric surgery is an effective strategy to treat severely obese patients. Bariatric surgery leads to a substantial improvement of comorbidities as well as to a reduction in overall mortality by 25–50% during the long-term follow-up. Obesity treatment should be individually tailored and the following factors should be taken into account: sex, the degree of obesity, individual health risks, psychobehavioral and metabolic characteristics, and the outcome of previous weight loss attempts. In the future, an evaluation of hormonal and genetic determinants of weight loss could also contribute to a better choice of individual therapy for a particular obese patient. A multilevel obesity management network of mutually collaborating facilities should be established to provide individually tailored treatment. Centers of excellence in obesity management represented by multidisciplinary teams should provide comprehensive programs for the treatment of obesity derived from evidence-based medicine.

Diabetes Care 31 (Suppl. 2):S269–S277, 2008

The prevalence of obesity is increasing worldwide at an alarming rate in both developed and developing countries (1). European obesity prevalences range from 10 to 20% in men and 15 to 25% in women, whereas the prevalence of obesity among U.S. adults has reached 28% in men and 34% in women.

Excess body weight is the sixth most important risk factor contributing to the health burden of the world. Obesity amplifies the risks of type 2 diabetes, hypertension, cardiovascular disease, dyslipidemia, arthritis, and several cancers and is estimated to reduce average life expectancy (2).

A negative energy balance induced by the treatment of obesity should lead to a reduction of fat stores and an appropriate preservation of lean body mass. Among the most important goals of obesity treatment are a preferential reduction of abdominal fat, an amelioration of obesity-related health risks, an improvement in comorbidities and in quality of life, and a reduction in mortality rate (3,4). A successful treatment of obesity should have an important impact on medical resources utilization and health care costs. Physicians and other health care professionals face a great challenge in assisting obese patients not only to lose weight but also to achieve weight loss maintenance.

Obesity treatment should be individually tailored and the age, sex, degree of obesity, individual health risks, metabolic and psychobehavioral characteristics, and outcome of previous weight loss attempts should be taken into account. In the future, hormonal and hereditary factors affecting weight loss should also be considered.

It is necessary to set realistic goals before starting the treatment of obesity. Both physician and the patient should know that a weight loss of 5–15% reduces obesity-related health risks significantly. Unrealistic expectations concerning the weight loss frequently results in weight management failure.

WHAT KIND OF LOW-ENERGY DIET SHOULD BE RECOMMENDED? —

A low-energy diet recommended for the treatment of obesity should be low fat (<30%), high carbohydrate (~55% of daily energy intake), high protein (up to 25% of daily energy intake), and high fiber (25 g/day). A high-carbohydrate low-fat energy-deficient diet is usually recommended for weight management by medical societies and health authorities (3,4). A moderate decrease in energy intake (−2.5 MJ/day) could result in a slow (~2.5 kg/month) and sustained weight loss. Until now, most studies have revealed that the total energy intake and not the macronutrient composition determines the weight loss in response to low-energy diets over a short period of time.

In spite of the generally accepted role of altered fat consumption in influencing an energy balance, an agreement has not been achieved concerning the effects of low-fat diets per se on the weight loss. A meta-analysis of 16 dietary intervention

From the [1]Institute of Endocrinology, Prague, Czech Republic; the [2]Department of Medicine, Diabetes and Metabolism, Medical University Graz, Graz, Austria; and the [3]Department of Internal Medicine, Henry Dunant Hospital, Athens, Greece.

Address correspondence and reprint requests to Dr. Vojtech Hainer, Institute of Endocrinology, Narodni 8, 116 94 Prague 1, Czech Republic. E-mail: vhainer@endo.cz.

The authors of this article have no relevant duality of interest to declare.

This article is based on a presentation at the 1st World Congress of Controversies in Diabetes, Obesity and Hypertension (CODHy). The Congress and the publication of this article were made possible by unrestricted educational grants from MSD, Roche, sanofi-aventis, Novo Nordisk, Medtronic, LifeScan, World Wide, Eli Lilly, Keryx, Abbott, Novartis, Pfizer, Generx Biotechnology, Schering, and Johnson & Johnson.

Abbreviations: PYY, peptide YY; VLCD, very-low-calorie diet.

DOI: 10.2337/dc08-s265

studies demonstrated that a reduction in dietary fat without intentional restriction of energy intake causes weight loss, which is more substantial in heavier subjects (5). A recent lifestyle intervention study of the Diabetes Prevention Program Research Group demonstrated that besides the increased physical activity, the lower percent calories from fat predicted weight loss over 3.2 years of follow-up (6). On the other hand, a meta-analysis of six randomized controlled trials specifically targeting weight loss failed to find significant differences in the effects of low-fat diets and other weight loss diets in obese and overweight subjects (7). It should be considered that the ratio between saturated, monounsaturated, and polyunsaturated fatty acids in ingested fats influences metabolic and cardiovascular risks of obesity including insulin resistance. In a recent statement, the American Diabetes Association recommends to limit an intake of saturated fats to <7% of total calories and to minimize an intake of trans fat (8). Incorporating fish meals rich in n-3 fatty acids in a weight management diet favorably affects cardiometabolic health risks including lipid profile and hypertension (9). However, a high intake of fish oil has been shown to increase moderately blood glucose level and to decrease insulin sensitivity in subjects with type 2 diabetes (10).

Recently, several studies evaluated the role of low-carbohydrate diets in weight management (11). These diets have been advocated because they induce many favorable effects such as a rapid weight loss, a decrease of serum insulin and triglyceride levels, and a reduction of blood pressure as well as a higher suppression of appetite (partly due to ketogenesis, partly due to a higher protein intake). However, several unfavorable effects of low-carbohydrate diet administration have been demonstrated, such as an increased loss of lean body mass, increased levels of LDL cholesterol and uric acid, and an increased urinary calcium excretion. An extremely low intake of carbohydrate may lead to an unwanted energetic efficiency. This energetic efficiency is due to the suppression of the sympathetic nervous activity and to the development of low T_3 syndrome. Long-term studies are needed to evaluate the overall changes in nutritional status, body composition, metabolic health risks, and adverse events in response to low-carbohydrate diets. Without that evalua-

tion, low-carbohydrate diets cannot be recommended (12).

Increased content of protein in a diet contributes to better weight loss maintenance because proteins are more satienting and thermogenic than carbohydrates and fats. Westerterp-Plantenga et al. (13) demonstrated that high protein intake sustained weight maintenance after very-low-calorie diet (VLCD)-induced weight loss.

Studies made on the role of foods with a low glycemic index and the role of increased calcium intake in reducing fat stores in human obesity have so far brought conflicting results (14–16).

VLCDs contain ≤3.5 MJ/day and provide high-quality protein with a minor intake of fat. Vitamins, minerals, and trace elements are added to cover recommended daily allowances. VLCDs may form a part of a comprehensive program undertaken by either an obesity specialist or other physician trained in nutrition and dietetics. Although the short-term weight loss induced by VLCD is greater than that induced by standard low-calorie diets, there is no consensus whether VLCDs per se produce greater long-term weight losses than low-calorie diets (17–19). According to meta-analyses conducted by Saris (18) and Anderson et al. (19), a greater initial weight loss using VLCDs with an active follow-up weight maintenance program, including behavior therapy, nutritional education, and exercise, improves weight loss maintenance. An administration of VLCD should be limited for specific patients (i.e., those in whom rapid weight loss is indicated by a physician) and for short periods of time. Indications and contraindications for VLCD administration should be strictly followed. VLCDs should not be prescribed for patients with kidney and liver disease. On the other hand, an administration of a VLCD is a reasonable approach in obese patients with type 2 diabetes. However, in diabetic patients treated by antidiabetic agents as well as in patients with hypertension treated by antihypertensive drugs, the drug dosage should be modified during the VLCD treatment to avoid hypoglycemia or an inappropriate blood pressure decrease.

Diets with a strict limitation of energy intake leading to semistarvation should be strictly avoided because of serious health hazards that relate to deficiencies of several nutrients. Exaggerated lipid mobilization accompanied by an in-

creased level of free fatty acids, together with a lack of essential amino acids and potassium and magnesium deficiencies might promote life-threatening cardiac arrhythmias (20). It should be taken into account that obesity is frequently associated with a prolongation of the QT interval, which per se predisposes to cardiac arrhythmias. Rapid weight loss results in an increased biliary excretion of cholesterol, which potentiates the formation of biliary stones. An increased production of ketones and ketonuria, which are the results of semistarvation, prevents urinary urate excretion and leads to excessive hyperuricemia, which could result in a gout attack.

It should be kept in mind that diets providing <5 MJ/day might yield deficiencies of several micronutrients, which could exert untoward effects not only on nutritional status but also on the weight management outcome. Meal replacement diets (substitution of one or two daily meal portions by VLCD) may be a useful strategy and have been shown to contribute to nutritionally well-balanced diet and weight loss maintenance (21).

It is recommended to divide the daily food intake into four to five daily meal portions. Nutritional tables with the traffic light system might help an obese patient to choose an appropriate low-energy meal.

PHYSICAL ACTIVITY — Physical activity should be an integral part of the comprehensive obesity management and should be individually tailored to the degree of obesity, age, and presence of comorbidities in each subject. Physical activity not only contributes to an increased energy expenditure and fat loss, but also protects against the loss of lean body mass, improves cardiorespiratory fitness, reduces obesity-related cardiometabolic health risks, and evokes sensations of well-being. Aerobic physical training leads to improvement in oxygen transfer to muscle, which promotes increased utilization of abundant fat stores instead of the limited glycogen stores. Physical activity of a moderate intensity, 30 min in duration, performed 5 days a week is recommended. This activity conducted for a month represents an energy deficit that might contribute to 0.5 kg of weight loss. Patients should be aware of the realistic goals with regard to the expected exercise-induced weight loss as well as of the beneficial effects of exercise per se on cardiometabolic risks. To optimize weight loss, exercise should be increased to 60 min for 5 days a week. Obesity is usually a result of a lack of daily habitual physical activity. Therefore, activities such as walking, cycling, and stair climbing should be encouraged (22). Engagement of physical activity in weight management is positively related to the level of education and, on the other hand, inversely associated with the occurrence of serious comorbidities, with age and with degree of overweight (22). For patients with severe arthritis and problems with mobility, exercising in heated water is recommended. Vigorous physical activity that leads to joints overloading, such as jumping, should be avoided. Strength exercise modalities do not increase lipid oxidation but should be used, especially in less mobile disabled individuals, for protection of lean body mass and amelioration of health risks. Any kind of regular physical activity represents an important factor that contributes to long-term maintenance of weight loss (23). Surprisingly, adding structured exercise to diet counseling does not alleviate metabolic syndrome in obese men better than diet only (24).

PSYCHOLOGICAL FACTORS AND BEHAVIORAL MODIFICATION OF LIFESTYLE — Psychological factors influence both weight loss and, more importantly, long-term weight loss maintenance. Behavioral modification of lifestyle should be included in the weight management strategies. Behavioral management includes several techniques such as self-monitoring, stress management, stimulus control, reinforcement techniques, problem solving, rewarding changes in behavior, cognitive restructuring, social support, and relapse prevention training (25,26). Behavioral therapy can be provided in clinical and commercial settings or as self-help programs. Group counseling results in comparable long-term weight loss as individual counseling. However, initial individual counseling is sometimes preferred for severely obese subjects and for men. Behavioral treatment of obesity in children should address the whole family or at least the mother of an obese child. Data on the efficacy of behavioral programs carried out in controlled settings show that weight losses average nearly 9% in trials lasting ~20 weeks (25). The major limitation of these programs is the high likelihood that individuals will regain weight once the behavioral treatment

is ended. Wing and Hill (27) defined successful weight loss maintainers as "individuals who have intentionally lost at least 10% of their body weight and kept it off at least 1 year." According to the U.S. National Weight Control Registry, a low level of depression and dietary disinhibition and medical triggers for weight loss are associated with successful weight loss maintenance (27). Behavioral modification of lifestyle, especially self-control over daily energy balance, plays a crucial role in long-term success of weight management. Self-monitoring weight, dietary intake, and daily physical activity on a regular basis is an important determinant of weight loss maintenance. Consistent eating patterns, including regularly eating breakfast, also influence the outcome of weight management. It is obvious that special attention should be paid to patients who are prone to failure in long-term weight management. More frequent dietary counseling as well as the use of anti-obesity drugs (see the next paragraph) contribute to a better outcome of long-term weight management. This counseling might be traditional patient visits or can be provided by phone, e-mail, or Internet chat applications (28). Psychological support is necessary for patients with depression or dietary disinhibition. Psychologist should train patients how to cope with situations triggering dietary disinhibition (e.g., stress, anxiety, and depression).

Although meta-analysis of studies done in the U.S. demonstrated that success in weight loss maintenance has improved over the past decade (19), much more research is required to reveal how to sustain the changes in lifestyle behavior. No study thus far has documented long-term maintenance of weight loss with behavior therapy or a maintained positive effect on obesity-associated comorbid conditions. Strategies to achieve better long-term goals are designed to make necessary behavioral changes. Cooper and Fairburn (29) emphasize that long-term adherence to behavioral lifestyle changes should be addressed by a new cognitive behavioral approach to the treatment of obesity that is based in a cognitive conceptualization of weight control. However, it seems that the differences between standard behavior therapy and cognitive-behavioral therapy of obesity are more at the theoretical level than in their practical implementation (30). Therefore, clinicians who are engaged in the long-term treatment of obese patients should use

both cognitive and behavioral strategies within the context of a standard behavioral lifestyle modification program (30).

Two studies that have focused on prevention of type 2 diabetes—the Diabetes Prevention Program (31,32) and the Finnish Diabetes Prevention Study (33,34)—are excellent examples of the implementation and efficacy of behavioral modification of lifestyle. The Diabetes Prevention Program enrolled 3,234 overweight and obese patients with elevated fasting and postload plasma glucose who were randomized to receive placebo, metformin, or intensive lifestyle modification (31). The lifestyle modification program used in the Diabetes Prevention Program (32) resulted in a weight loss of 6.7 kg at 1-year follow-up, compared with weight losses of 2.7 and 0.4 kg in the metformin and placebo groups, respectively. At the 4-year follow-up, lifestyle, metformin, and placebo groups maintained weight losses of 3.5, 1.3, and 0.2 kg, respectively. The average follow-up was 2.8 years. Behavioral modification of lifestyle reduced the incidence of type 2 diabetes by 58% and metformin by 31%, as compared with placebo. Even more interesting are the results of the extended follow-up (34) of the Finnish Diabetes Prevention Study (33). In the initial study (33), lifestyle modification resulted in weight loss of 3.5 ± 5.5 kg compared with 0.8 ± 4.4 kg in the control group and a reduction of 58% in the incidence of diabetes, which was directly related to changes in lifestyle. After a median of 4 years of active intervention period, participants without diabetes were further followed up for a median of 3 years. During the total follow-up, beneficial lifestyle changes achieved by the participants in the intervention group were maintained after discontinuation of the intervention, and the incidence of type 2 diabetes was 4.3 per 100 person-years in the intervention group compared with 7.4 per 100 person-years in the control group (34).

DRUG TREATMENT OF OBESITY — Anti-obesity drugs have been developed to assist weight loss in combination with lifestyle management, to improve weight loss maintenance, and to reduce obesity-related health risks. Pharmacotherapy of obesity should be applied as a part of the comprehensive obesity management, which includes lifestyle modification (3,4).

Anti-obesity drugs affect different targets in the central nervous system or peripheral tissues and aim to normalize regulatory or metabolic disturbances that are involved in the pathogenesis of obesity. Currently, only three anti-obesity drugs have been successfully used in long-term weight management, conducted over period of 1–4 years (35–37). It is expected that lifelong treatment with anti-obesity drugs will be required to specifically target the particular abnormality. Pharmacotherapy of obesity has been indicated for the treatment of obese adults (≤65 years). Several studies have been recently conducted to evaluate efficacy and safety of anti-obesity drugs for children and adolescents (38,39) as well as for the elderly (40). Consequently, the U.S. Food and Drug Administration has approved the drug orlistat for use in children and adolescents.

Our current potential to treat obesity by drugs is limited in comparison to the drug treatment of other complex diseases such as hypertension, diabetes, and dyslipidemia. Sibutramine, as a serotonin and norepinephrine reuptake inhibitor, induces satiety and prevents diet-induced decline in metabolic rate (41). The STORM (Sibutramine Trial on Obesity Reduction and Maintenance) trial data showed that weight loss was achieved with 6 months of treatment with sibutramine and a comprehensive lifestyle management program (35). At 6 months, patients were randomized either to continue with the lifestyle program and sibutramine or to switch to a lifestyle program with placebo in a double-blind design. For those patients switched to placebo, despite the presence of the lifestyle program, weight regain was rapid over the next 18 months. Continued use of sibutramine maintained weight loss almost completely for this period of time (35). In another study, administration of sibutramine facilitated better weight loss maintenance in patients who were treated initially with a VLCD (42). Randomized 1-year trial of lifestyle modification and pharmacotherapy for obesity clearly demonstrated that the combination of sibutramine and lifestyle modification resulted in more weight loss than either medication or lifestyle modification alone (43).

Orlistat, as an inhibitor of lipase, reduces fat absorption in the intestine. The XENDOS (Xenical in the Prevention of Diabetes in Obese Subjects) study compared the weight loss and incidence of diabetes over 4 years in obese subjects who were randomized to lifestyle changes plus either orlistat or placebo (36). Pa-

tients treated with orlistat and lifestyle modification exhibited a greater weight loss and a significant reduction in diabetes incidence compared with those who underwent lifestyle modification and received placebo (36). Toplak et al. (44) recently published the results from the X-PERT study, in which a lifestyle intervention was combined with different dietary interventions and orlistat. Patients showed very good weight loss and exhibited beneficial effects on components of the metabolic syndrome.

Rimonabant, as a selective cannabinoid receptor-1 blocker, reduces food intake and tobacco dependence by blocking cannabinoid receptors in the central nervous system and affects the metabolic profile by targeting the cannabinoid system in adipocytes and hepatocytes (45). Rimonabant administration leads to significant weight reduction and improvement in cardiometabolic risk profile in four randomized double-blind clinical trials conducted in overweight or obese adults (37,45).

Recently, the anti-epileptic drug topiramate was discovered to have beneficial effects on weight control and was investigated as a weight loss drug. It even proved to have a beneficial effect on diabetes control, but because of drug safety issues, a registration for obesity and diabetes seems unlikely (46).

Weight loss induced by currently available anti-obesity drugs is only modest, reaching usually 5–8% of initial body weight. The average weight loss in the drug-treated group is 3–5% higher than in the placebo group. Drug-induced weight loss is associated with improvement in lipid profile and glycemic control. It has been shown that the lipid profile improvement after sibutramine, orlistat, and rimonabant is partly independent of weight loss. Changes in insulin sensitivity observed in patients treated with rimonabant were only attributable to weight loss alone by 49%. Identical effectiveness of both continuous and intermittent drug administration was demonstrated for several anti-obesity drugs (47). Combination treatment with sibutramine and orlistat does not influence weight loss (48). However, in the future, combination therapy with anti-obesity drugs should be expected. Special attention should be paid not only to the efficacy, but also to the potential drug interaction and safety.

Assignment of patients to a particular anti-obesity drug should respect

their licensed indications and contraindications; i.e., sibutramine should not be administered to patients with uncontrolled hypertension, orlistat should not be administered to patients with cholestasis, and centrally acting drugs should be indicated with caution in patients with depression. Drugs should be administered to patients who adequately responded to the initial phase of treatment over a 1.5- to 3-month period. Nonresponders are characterized by a weight loss <1–2 kg after 6 weeks of treatment. However, modest weight loss should be expected in patients with type 2 diabetes and in those who have already lost weight with lifestyle modification. Recently, a weight loss in response to 3 months of treatment by either sibutramine (49) or orlistat (44) in conjunction with diet and exercise has been shown to predict weight loss at 1 year.

Psychological and behavioral predictors of weight loss have also been evaluated in the context of pharmacological treatments of obesity, including fenfluramine, phentermine, mazindol, and caffeine plus ephedrine (50), usually administered as combined therapy (fenfluramine + phentermine, fenfluramine + mazindol). Patients who scored higher on dietary restraint and hunger at baseline were less likely to lose weight over the 6-month period, whereas only high hunger scoring at baseline predicted lower weight loss at 12 months. However, many of the drugs used in the study by Womble et al. (50) have now been withdrawn from the pharmaceutical market.

In our study, obese patients were treated by lifestyle intervention and sibutramine (51). Weight loss at month 12 was predicted by baseline BMI, depression score, restraint score, and total energy intake. These predictive variables accounted for 43.8% of the variance in BMI loss at 12 months. When relationships between the BMI loss and changes in studied psychobehavioral and nutritional parameters were considered after 12 months of treatment, a drop in the disinhibition score of the Eating Inventory appeared the only significant factor that correlated with the BMI decrease.

New anti-obesity drugs possessing novel mechanisms of action are likely to be available in the future. Several potential new agents targeting weight loss in obesity through the central nervous system pathways or peripheral adiposity signals are investigated in clinical trials. Gut hormones and/or their derivatives might contribute to the treatment of obesity and provide the advantage of targeting specific appetite pathways within the brain without producing unacceptable side effects. Future goals for the drug treatment of obesity include evaluation of 1) predictors of drug-induced weight loss and its maintenance (as for example initial weight loss and genetic, metabolic, nutritional, and psychobehavioral factors), 2) primary drug effects on health risks, 3) efficacy and safety of combined drug treatment, and 4) anti-obesity drugs in children, adolescents, and the elderly patients.

BARIATRIC SURGERY — Bariatric surgery is the most effective treatment for morbid obesity in terms of weight loss, health risks, and improvement in quality of life (52,53). It should be considered for patients with BMI $\geq$40.0 kg/m^2 or with BMI between 35.0 and 39.9 kg/m^2 with comorbidities (3,4,52,53). Obesity surgery should be conducted in centers that are able to assess patients before surgery and to offer a comprehensive approach to diagnosis, assessment, treatment, and long-term follow-up (53). Bariatric surgery could be carefully considered in severely obese adolescents who have failed to lose weight in a comprehensive weight management program carried out in a specialized center for at least 6–12 months and who have achieved skeletal and developmental maturity. Centers performing bariatric surgery in adolescents should have extensive experience with such treatment in adults and should be able to provide a multidisciplinary team that possesses pediatric skills related to surgery, dietetics, and psychological management (52,53). In elderly patients (>60 years), the risk-to-benefit ratio should be considered on an individual basis. It is necessary to emphasize that the primary objective of surgery in elderly patients is to improve quality of life, as surgery per se is unlikely to increase lifespan (53).

In bariatric surgery, restrictive procedures as well as procedures limiting absorption of nutrients are currently available. The magnitude of both weight loss and weight loss maintenance is increasing with the following procedures: gastric banding, vertical banded gastroplasty, proximal gastric bypass, biliopancreatic diversion with duodenal switch, and biliopancreatic diversion (53). There are no sufficient evidence-based data to suggest how to assign a particular patient

to a particular bariatric procedure. However, for patients with BMI >50 kg/m^2, gastric bypass or biliopancreatic diversion brings more benefits. Pure restrictive procedures are not recommended for patients with a significant hiatal hernia or severe gastroesophageal reflux disease. Gastric banding cannot contribute to further substantial weight loss in patients in whom a significantly diminished food intake has been verified before the surgery. On the other hand, it should be considered that a laparoscopic adjustable gastric banding is the safest bariatric procedure associated with only minor perioperative surgical risks.

Bariatric surgery has been proved as the most effective way of treating type 2 diabetes in severely obese patients. More than 10 years ago, Pories et al. (54) demonstrated that 83% of patients with diagnosed type 2 diabetes exhibited normal blood glucose and normal glycosylated hemoglobin levels 7.6 years after bariatric surgery. Further, 99% patients with impaired glucose tolerance normalized a glucose tolerance after bariatric surgery (54). The 10-year follow-up in the Swedish Obese Subjects (SOS) study demonstrated that a bariatric surgery is a viable option for the treatment of severe obesity, resulting in long-term weight loss, improvement in lifestyle, and, except for hypercholesterolemia, amelioration of cardiometabolic risk factors (55). After 10 years, the average weight loss from baseline was 25% after gastric bypass, 16% after vertical banded gastroplasty, and 14% after gastric banding. The group that had undergone surgical intervention had lower incidence rates of diabetes, hypertriglyceridemia, and hyperuricemia in comparison to the control group (55). The most important recent finding of the Swedish Obese Subjects study is a reduction of overall mortality by 24.6% in the surgery group versus control subjects (56). However, Adams et al. (57) reported reduction of overall mortality by 50% in comparison with control subjects 8.4 years after gastric bypass surgery. Cause-specific mortality was reduced by 94% for diabetes, 71% for coronary artery disease, 62% for other circulatory diseases, and 55% for cancer (57).

HORMONAL AND HEREDITARY FACTORS AFFECTING WEIGHT LOSS — Whereas substantial attention has been paid to the role of nutritional and psychobehavioral factors in weight man-

agement, the role played by hormonal and hereditary determinants of weight loss and weight loss maintenance has been underestimated.

HORMONAL DETERMINANTS OF WEIGHT LOSS — Several hormones of the central nervous system, adipose tissue, and the gastrointestinal tract involved in the regulation energy balance have been described. The role of baseline hormonal levels and their response to weight management have been studied with regard to both weight loss and weight loss maintenance.

Naslund et al. (58) evaluated the role of leptin, insulin resistance, and thyroid function on weight loss maintenance in obese men who had been followed for a 2-year period of behavioral modification of lifestyle. A high baseline leptin/BMI ratio as a marker of leptin resistance was associated with failure in maintaining achieved weight loss. Multiple regression analysis revealed that 22% of variability in weight loss after the 2-year follow-up was explained by baseline leptin and insulin level together with age. The role of leptin sensitivity in determination of weight loss was confirmed in a subsequent study by Verdich et al. (59). They demonstrated a higher weight loss in response to 24-week weight management in subjects who exhibited lower baseline leptin levels after adjustment for fat mass. On the other hand, inadequately high decreases in serum leptin levels in response to weight management might negatively influence the outcome of weight reduction and predispose to weight regain (60–62) and weight cycling (63).

A recent study by Garcia et al. (64) described association between lower ghrelin levels at baseline and resistance to weight loss. Magnitude of weight loss had also been shown to be influenced by peptide YY (PYY), a hormone secreted in the distal intestine that reduces energy intake and induces weight loss. Low baseline PYY levels and the highest increases in PYY concentrations were associated with the highest weight reduction in children who underwent a 1-year weight management regimen (65). In our study of 67 women (BMI 32.4 ± 4.4 kg/m^2; age 48.7 ± 12.2 years) who had exhibited stable weight on a 7 MJ/day diet during the first week of weight management, the subjects obtained a hypocaloric diet providing 4.5 MJ/day (protein 25.3%, fat 28.7%, carbohydrate 46%) during the subsequent 3-week period (66). The following hormonal parameters were examined both before and after the weight loss, which was on average 3.8 ± 1.6 kg: thyroid-stimulating hormone, fT3, fT4, insulin, C-peptide, prolactin, growth hormone, IGF-I, cortisol, sex hormone–binding globulin, parathormone, ghrelin, leptin, PYY, neuropeptide Y, pancreatic polypeptide, adiponectin, and resistin together with a C-reactive protein as an inflammatory marker. Baseline levels of GH, PYY, neuropeptide Y, and C-reactive protein predicted 49.8% of variability in weight loss. Higher baseline growth hormone levels and lower baseline PYY and neuropeptide Y levels predicted higher weight loss.

HEREDITARY DETERMINANTS OF WEIGHT LOSS

— It is obvious that some obese people can achieve a higher weight loss in response to the same negative energy balance than the others. The role of genetic factors in different capabilities to lose weight was identified in studies conducted in monozygotic twins, i.e., individuals who possess identical genes. The study by Bouchard and Tremblay (67) was focused on responsiveness of slightly overweight identical twins to a negative energy balance as a result of enhanced physical activity. Weight loss was similar in pairs of identical twins but differed significantly between pairs. A subsequent study by Hainer at al. (68) revealed significant similarity in weight loss in response to a 1-month weight management program with a VLCD within the pairs of obese monozygotic twins. Although body weight reduction showed wide interindividual variation, ranging between 5.9 and 12.4 kg, it was similar in pairs of monozygotic twins. Intrapair resemblance in fat loss was 17 times as high as resemblance between pairs.

WEIGHT LOSS IN MONOGENIC FORMS OF OBESITY

— Because the monogenic forms of obesity are rather scarce, only few reports on efficacy of therapy are available. It can be expected that if the therapy of obesity would target the correction of the disorder linked to gene mutation, it should be successful. Until now, there exists only one example of a successful therapy of obesity based on gene mutation. Obesity due to leptin gene mutation was successfully controlled by ad-

ministration of recombinant leptin both in adults (69) and children (70). In view of the known role of genes in the pathogenesis of obesity, some physicians may adopt a nihilist attitude to the treatment of this disorder. Nevertheless, such an approach is unjustified as shown by the last report on body weight, body fat mass, and insulin susceptibility normalization after a 11-month comprehensive weight loss intervention in three children with R236G mutation in the proopiomelanocortin gene (71). The most common monogenic form of human obesity is that caused by mutations in the gene that encodes the melanocortin 4 receptor (MC4R) and is associated with intensive feelings of hunger and hyperphagia in childhood that decreases with aging. No comprehensive clinical studies on weight loss in patients with the MC4R mutation have been published. A pilot study of Hainerova et al. (72) reported a comparable low-energy diet–induced weight loss in carriers of MC4R mutations and in their counterparts with common forms of obesity. This observation is supported by an experimental study of Butler and Cone (73), who described hyperphagia in MC4R-deficient mice fed a high-fat diet. No hyperphagia was observed when low-fat diet was introduced to these mice, thus indicating gene-environment interaction and supporting the role of low-fat diet in weight management, even in strongly genetically determined obesities.

GENETIC COMPONENT OF WEIGHT LOSS IN COMMON FORMS OF OBESITY

— Involvement of genetic factors in the development of obesity is estimated to be 40–70% (74). Almost 600 obesity candidate genes have been described (75). Some of these obesogenic or leptogenic genes might affect weight loss and weight loss maintenance (76). Polymorphisms of several obesity candidate genes have been shown to influence the outcome of weight management (76). Among the genes involved in the outcome of weight management, the ones studied include the genes affecting regulation of energy expenditure (β_3-adrenergic receptor, uncoupling proteins), appetite control (leptin, leptin receptor, serotonin receptor), eating behavior (neuromedin β), adipogenesis (peroxisome proliferator–activated receptor γ2), and development of metabolic syndrome (adiponectin). The ambiguous results observed in several of the studies could be explained by gene-gene interac-

tion that have not been taken into account as well as by the different role of investigated genes in different ethnic, age, and sex cohorts. Moreover, weight loss in response to obesity treatment might also be influenced by changes in obesogenic and/or leptogenic gene expression induced by environmental factors such as the type of ingested nutrients and level of physical activity.

Genotyping could be of relevance in predicting the efficacy of drugs in weight management. Obese individuals with the CC genotype of the G-protein β3 subunit polymorphism (C825T) achieved higher weight loss in response to sibutramine administration compared with individuals with the TT/TC genotypes (77). Polymorphism of phenylethanolamine N-methyltransferase, an enzyme that catalyzes the conversion of norepinephrine to epinephrine, has also been shown to affect sibutramine-induced weight loss. The G-148A polymorphism homozygotes exhibited higher weight loss in response to a 3-month therapy with sibutramine (78).

More comprehensive studies on the interaction between candidate obesity genes, psychobehavioral factors, and environmental factors are needed for a better understanding of the outcome of weight management in our increasingly obesogenic environment.

COMPREHENSIVE MULTILEVEL OBESITY MANAGEMENT NETWORK

— Obesity should be tackled by health care providers as well as by health policy authorities because it is a disease with serious health consequences. The quality of obesity management depends on educating current as well as future health care providers. Effective obesity management requires a comprehensive multilevel obesity management network and the direct involvement of the health and general insurance industries as well as governments. A multilevel obesity management network of mutually collaborating facilities should be established to provide individually tailored treatment (79). A comprehensive obesity management program as a multilevel network includes obesity management centers, obesity specialists and other specialists, primary care physicians, weight loss clubs led by educated counselors and self-assessment, and media. Centers of excellence in obesity management represented by multidisciplinary teams (obesity specialists, dietitians or nutritionists, exercise physiologists or physiatrists, psychologists and/or psychiatrists, bariatric surgeons, specialized trained nurses) should provide comprehensive programs for the treatment of obesity derived from evidence-based medicine. These centers should focus on the care of severely obese patients and those with serious health risks or who failed in their weight control. The centers should also be responsible for eliminating unproven treatment approaches that have been frequently associated with health hazards.

Acknowledgments— This study was partly supported by a grant from the Czech Ministry of Health (IGA NR/7800-4).

References

1. World Health Organization: *Obesity: Preventing and Managing the Global Epidemic: Report of a WHO Consultation.* Geneva, World Health Org., 2000 (Tech. Rep. Ser., no. 894)
2. Haslam DW, James WPT: Obesity. *Lancet* 366:1197–1209, 2005
3. Expert Panel on the Identification, Evaluation, and Treatment of Overweight in Adults: Clinical guidelines on the identification, evaluation, and treatment of overweight and obesity in adults: executive summary. *Am J Clin Nutr* 68: 899–917, 1998
4. Hainer V, Finer N, Tsigos C, Basdevant A, Carruba M, Hancu N, Mathus-Vliegen L, Schutz Y, Zahorska-Markiewicz B: Management of obesity in adults: project for European primary care. *Int J Obes* 28 (Suppl. 1):S226–S231, 2004
5. Astrup A, Grunwald GK, Melanson EL, Saris WH, Hill JO: The role of low-fat diets in body weight control: a meta-analysis of ad libitum dietary intervention studies. *Int J Obes* 24:1545–1552, 2000
6. Hamman RF, Wing RR, Edelstein SL, Lachin JM, Bray GA, Delahanty L, Hoskin M, Kriska AM, Mayer-Davis EJ, Pi-Sunyer X, Regensteiner J, Venditti B, Wylie-Rosett J, for the DPP Group: Effect of weight loss with lifestyle intervention on risk of diabetes. *Diabetes Care* 29:2102–2107, 2006
7. Pirozzo S, Summerbell C, Cameron C, Glasziou P: Should we recommend low-fat diets for obesity? *Obes Rev* 4:83–90, 2003
8. American Diabetes Association: Standards of medical care in diabetes. *Diabetes Care* 29 (Suppl. 1):S4–S42, 2006
9. Mori TA, Bao DQ, Burke V, Puddey IB, Watts GF, Beilin LJ: Dietary fish as a major component of a weight-loss diet: effect on

serum lipids, glucose, and insulin metabolism in overweight hypertensive patients. *Am J Clin Nutr* 70:817–825, 1999
10. Mostad IL, Bjerve KS, Bjorgaas MR, Lydersen S, Grill V: Effects of n-3 fatty acids with type 2 diabetes: reduction of insulin sensitivity and time-dependent alteration from carbohydrate to fat oxidation. *Am J Clin Nutr* 84:540–550, 2006
11. Nordmann AJ, Nordmann A, Briel M, Keller U, Yancy WS Jr, Brehm BJ, Bucher HC: Effects of low-carbohydrate vs low-fat diets on weight loss and cardiovascular risk factors: a metaanalysis of randomized controlled trials. *Arch Intern Med* 166: 285–293, 2006
12. Astrup A, Meinert Larsen T, Harper A: Atkins and other low-carbohydrate diets: hoax or an effective tool for weight loss? *Lancet* 364:897–899, 2004
13. Westerterp-Plantenga MS, Lejeune MP, Nijs I, van Ooijen M, Kovacs EM: High protein intake sustains weight maintenance after body weight loss in humans. *Int J Obes* 28:57–64, 2004
14. Diaz EO, Galgani JE, Aguirre CA: Glycaemic index effects on fuel partitioning in humans. *Obes Rev* 7:219–226, 2006
15. Thompson WG, Holdman NR, Janzow DJ, Slezak JM, Morris KL, Zemel MB: Effect of energy-reduced diets high in dairy products and fiber on weight loss in obese adults. *Obes Res* 13:1344–1348, 2005
16. Zemel MB: Role of calcium and dairy products in energy partitioning and weight management. *Am J Clin Nutr* 79: 907–912, 2004
17. Gilden Tsai A, Wadden T: The evolution of very low calorie diets: an up-date and metaanalysis. *Obesity* 14:1283–1293, 2006
18. Saris WH: Very-low-calorie diets and sustained weight loss. *Obes Res* 9 (Suppl. 4): 295S–301S, 2001
19. Anderson JW, Konz EC, Frederich RC, Wood CL: Long-term weight-loss maintenance: a meta-analysis of US studies. *Am J Clin Nutr* 74:579–584, 2001
20. Fisler JS: Cardiac effects of starvation and semistarvation diets: safety and mechanisms of action. *Am J Clin Nutr* 56 (Suppl. 1):230S–234S, 1992
21. Heymsfield SB, van Mierlo CA, van der Knaap HC, Heo M, Frier HI: Weight management using a meal replacement strategy: meta and pooling analysis from six studies. *Int J Obes* 27:537–549, 2003
22. Wing RR: Physical activity in the treatment of the adulthood overweight and obesity: current evidence and research issues. *Med Sci Sports Exerc* 31:S547–S552, 1999
23. Phalan S, Wyatt HR, Hill JO, Wing RR: Are the eating and exercise habits of successful weight losers changing? *Obesity* 14:710–716, 2006
24. Kukkonen-Harjula KT, Borg PT, Nenonen AM, Fogelholm MG: Effects of a weight

maintenance program with or without exercise on the metabolic syndrome: a randomized trial in obese men. *Prev Med* 41: 784–790, 2005
25. Wadden TA, Foster GD: Behavioral treatment of obesity. *Med Clin North Am* 84: 441–461, 2000
26. Williamson DA, Perrin LA: Behavioral therapy for obesity. *Endocrinol Metab Clin North Am* 25:943–954, 1996
27. Wing RR, Hill JO: Successful weight loss maintenance. *Annu Rev Nutr* 21:323–341, 2001
28. Harvey-Berino J, Pintauro S, Buzzell P, Gold EC: Effect of Internet support on the long-term maintenance of weight loss. *Obes Res* 12:320–329, 2004
29. Cooper Z, Fairburn CG: A new cognitive behavioral approach to the treatment of obesity. *Behav Res Ther* 39:499–511, 2001
30. Fabricatore AN: Behavior therapy and cognitive-behavioral therapy of obesity: Is there a difference? *J Am Diet Assoc* 107: 92–99, 2007
31. Knowler WC, Barrett-Connor E, Fowler SE, Hamman RF, Lachin JM, Walker EA, Nathan DM, Diabetes Prevention Program Research Group: Reduction in the incidence of type 2 diabetes with lifestyle intervention or metformin. *N Engl J Med* 346:393–403, 2002
32. Diabetes Prevention Program (DPP): Description of lifestyle intervention. *Diabetes Care* 25:2165–2171, 2002
33. Tuomilehto J, Lindstrom J, Eriksson JG, Valle TT, Hamalainen H, Ilanne-Parika P, Keinanen-Kiukaanniemi S, Laakso M, Louheranta A, Rastas M, Salminen V, Uusitupa M, Finnish Diabetes Prevention Study Group: Prevention of type 2 diabetes mellitus by changes in lifestyle among subjects with impaired glucose tolerance. *N Engl J Med* 344:1343–1350, 2001
34. Linderstrom J, Ilanne-Perikka P, Peltonen M, Aunola S, Eriksson JG, Hemio K, Hamalainen H, Harkonen P, Keinanen-Kiukaanniemi S, Laasko M, Louheranta A, Mannelin M, Paturi M, Sundvall J, Valle TT, Uusitupa M, Tuomilehto J, Finish Diabetes Prevention Study Group: Sustained reduction in the incidence of type 2 diabetes by lifestyle intervention: follow-up of the Finnish Diabetes Prevention Study. *Lancet* 368:1673–1679, 2006
35. James WP, Astrup A, Finer N, Hilsted J, Kopelman P, Rossner S, Saris WH, van Gaal LF: Effect of sibutramine on weight maintenance after weight loss: a randomised trial: STORM Study Group: Sibutramine Trial of Obesity Reduction and Maintenance. *Lancet* 356:2119–2125, 2000
36. Torgerson JS, Hauptman J, Boldrin MN, Sjostrom L: Xenical in the Prevention of Diabetes in Obese Subjects (XENDOS) study: randomized study of orlistat as an adjunct to lifestyle changes for the pre-

vention of type 2 diabetes in obese patients. *Diabetes Care* 27:155–161, 2004

37. Van Gaal LF, Rissanen AM, Scheen AJ, Ziegler O, Rossner S: Effects of the cannabinoid-1 receptor blocker rimonabant on weight reduction and cardiovascular risk factors in overweight patients: 1-year experience from the RIO-Europe study. *Lancet* 365:1389–1392, 2005

38. Berkowitz RI, Wadden TA, Tershakovec AM, Cronquist JL: Behavior therapy and sibutramine for the treatment of adolescent obesity: a randomized controlled trial. *JAMA* 289:1805–1812, 2003

39. Chanoine JP, Hampl S, Jensen C, Boldrin M, Hauptman J: Effect of orlistat on weight and body composition in obese adolescents: a randomized controlled trial. *JAMA* 293:2873–2883, 2005

40. Mathys M: Pharmacological agents for the treatment of obesity. *Clin Geriatr Med* 21: 735–746, 2005

41. Hansen DL, Toubro S, Stock MJ, Macdonald IA, Astrup A: The effect of sibutramine on energy expenditure and appetite during chronic treatment without dietary restriction. *Int J Obes* 23:1016–1024, 1999

42. Apfelbaum M, Vague P, Ziegler O, Hanotin C, Thomas F, Leutenegger E: Long-term maintenance of weight loss after a very-low-calorie diet: a randomized blinded trial of the efficacy and tolerability of sibutramine. *Am J Med* 106:179–184, 1999

43. Wadden T, Berkowitz R, Womble L, Sarwer D, Phelan S, Cato R, Hesson L, Oser S, Kaplan R, Stunkard A: Randomized trial of lifestyle modification and pharmacotherapy for obesity. *N Engl J Med* 353: 2111–2120, 2005

44. Toplak H, Ziegler O, Keller U, Hamann A, Godin C, Wittert G, Zanella MT, Zuniga-Guajardo S, van Gaal L: X-PERT: weight reduction with orlistat in obese subjects receiving a mildly or moderately reduced-energy diet: early response to treatment predicts weight maintenance. *Diabetes Obes Metab* 7:699–708, 2005

45. Henness S, Robinson DM, Lyseng-Williamson KA: Rimonabant. *Drugs* 66: 2109–2119, 2006

46. Toplak H, Hamann A, Moore R, Masson E, Gorska M, Vercruysse F, Sun X, Fitchet M: Efficacy and safety of topiramate in combination with metformin in the treatment of obese subjects with type 2 diabetes: a randomized, double-blind, placebo-controlled study. *Int J Obes* 31:138–146, 2007

47. Wirth A, Krause J: Long-term weight loss with sibutramine: a randomized controlled trial. *JAMA* 286:1331–1339, 2001

48. Sari R, Balci MK, Cakir M, Altunbas H, Karayalcin U: Comparison of efficacy of sibutramine or orlistat versus their combination in obese women. *Endocr Res* 30: 159–167, 2004

49. Finer N, Ryan DH, Renz CL, Hewkin AC: Prediction of response to sibutramine therapy in obese non-diabetic and diabetic patients. *Diabetes Obes Metab* 8: 206–213, 2006

50. Womble LG, Williamson DA, Greenway FL, Redmann SM: Psychological and behavioral predictors of weight loss during drug treatment for obesity. *Int J Obes Relat Metab Disord* 25:340–345, 2001

51. Hainer V, Kunesova M, Bellisle F, Hill M, Braunerova R, Wagenknecht M, STO-Study Group: Psychobehavioral and nutritional predictors of weight loss in obese women treated with sibutramine. *Int J Obes* 29:208–216, 2005

52. Special Report: Commonwealth of Massachusetts Betsy Lehman Center for Patient Safety and Medical Error Reduction Expert Panel on Weight Loss Surgery. *Obes Res* 13:205–305, 2005

53. Fried M, Hainer V, Basdevant A, Buchwald H, Deitel M, Finer N, Greve JW, Horber F, Mathus-Vliegen E, Scopinaro N, Steffen R, Tsigos C, Weiner R, Widhalm K: Interdisciplinary European guidelines on surgery of severe obesity. *Obes Surg* 17:260–270, 2007

54. Pories WJ, Swanson MS, MacDonald KG, Long SB, Morris PG, Brown BM, Barakat HA, deRamon RA, Israel G, Dolezal JM, Dohm L: Who would have thought it? An operation proves to be the most effective therapy for adult-onset diabetes mellitus. *Ann Surg* 222:339–350, 1995

55. Sjostrom L, Lindroos AK, Peltonen M, Torgerson J, Bouchard C, Carlsson B, Dahlgren S, Larsson B, Narbro K, Sjostrom CD, Sullivan M, Wedel H, Swedish Obese Subjects Study Scientific Group: Lifestyle, diabetes, and cardiovascular risk factors 10 years after bariatric surgery. *N Engl J Med* 351:2683–2693, 2004

56. Sjostrom L: Soft and hard endpoints over 5–18 years in the intervention trial Swedish obese subjects. *Obes Rev* 7 (Suppl. 2): 26, 2006

57. Adams T, Gress R, Smith S, Halverson S, Rosamond W, Simper S, Hunt S: Long-term mortality after gastric bypass surgery. *Obes Rev* 7 (Suppl. 2):94, 2006

58. Naslund E, Andersson I, Degerblad M, Kogner P, Kral JG, Rossner S, Hellstrom PM: Associations of leptin, insulin resistance and thyroid function with long-term weight loss in dieting men. *Intern Med* 248:299–308, 2000

59. Verdich C, Toubro S, Buemann B, Holst JJ, Bulow J, Simonsen L, Sondergaard SB, Christensen NJ, Astrup A: Leptin levels are associated with fat oxidation and dietary-induced weight loss in obesity. *Obes Res* 9:452–461, 2001

60. Geldszus R, Mayr B, Horn R, Geisthovel F, von zur Muhlen A, Brabant G: Serum leptin and weight reduction in female obesity. *Eur J Endocrinol* 135:659–662, 1996

61. Filozof CM, Murua C, Sanchez MP, Brail-

ovsky C, Perman M, Gonzalez CD, Ravussin E: Low plasma leptin concentration and low rates of fat oxidation in weight-stable post-obese subjects. *Obes Res* 8: 205–210, 2000

62. Celi F, Bini V, Papi F, Contessa G, Santilli E, Falorni A: Leptin serum levels are involved in the relapse after weight excess reduction in obese children and adolescents. *Diabetes Nutr Metab* 16:306–311, 2003

63. Benini ZL, Camilloni MA, Scordato C, Lezzi G, Savia G, Oriani G, Bertoli S, Balzola F, Liuzzi A, Petroni ML: Contribution of weight cycling to serum leptin in human obesity. *Int J Obes* 25:721–726, 2001

64. Garcia JM, Iyer D, Poston WSC, Marcelli M, Reeves R, Foreyt J, Balasubramanyam A: Rise of plasma ghrelin with weight loss is not sustained during weight maintenance. *Obesity* 14:1716–1723, 2006

65. Roth CL, Enriori PJ, Harz K, Woelfle J, Cowley MA, Reinehr T: Peptide YY is a regulator of energy homeostasis in obese children before and after weight loss. *J Clin Endocrinol Metab* 90:6386–6391, 2005

66. Hainer V, Kabrnová K, Gojová M, Kunesova M, Klepetar J, Drbohlav J, Kopsky V, Nedvidkova J, Parizkova J, Hill M: Psychobehavioral and hormonal predictors of weight loss in response to a 3-week weight management program. *Obes Res* 13 (Suppl.):A142, 2005

67. Bouchard C, Tremblay Y: Genetic influences on the response of body fat distribution to positive and negative energy balances in human identical twins. *J Nutr* 127:943S–947S, 1997

68. Hainer V, Stunkard AJ, Kunesova M, Parizkova J, Stich V, Allison DB: Intrapair resemblance in very low calorie diet-induced weight loss in female obese identical twins. *Int J Obes* 24:1051–1057, 2000

69. Licinio J, Caglayan S, Ozata M, Yildiz BO, de Miranda PB, O'Kirwan F, Whitby R, Liang L, Cohen P, Bhasin S, Krauss RM, Veldhuis JD, Wagner AJ, De Paoli AM, McCann SM, Wong ML: Phenotypic effects of leptin replacement of morbid obesity, diabetes mellitus, hypogonadism and behavior in leptin-deficient adults. *Proc Natl Acad Sci U S A* 101:4531–4536, 2004

70. O'Rahilly S, Farooqi S, Yeo GHS, Challis BG: Minireview: human obesity lessons from monogenic disorders. *Endocrinology* 144:3757–3764, 2003

71. Santoro N, Perrone L, Cirillo G, Raimondo P, Amato A, Coppola F, Santarpia M, D'Aniello A, Miraglia Del Giudice E: Weight loss in obese children carrying the proopiomelanocortin R236G variant. *J Endocrinol Invest* 29:226–230, 2006

72. Hainerova I, Larsen LH, Holst B, Finková M, Hainer V, Lebl J, Hansen T, Pedersen O: Melanocortin 4 receptor mutations in obese Czech children: studies of preva-

lence, phenotype development, weight reduction response, and functional analysis. *J Clin Endocrinol Metab* 92: 3689–3696, 2007

73. Butler AA, Cone RD: Knockout studies defining different roles for melanocortin receptors in energy homeostasis. *Ann N Y Acad Sci* 994:240–245, 2003

74. Comuzzie AG, Allison DB: The search for human obesity genes. *Science* 280:1374–1377, 1998

75. Rankinen T, Zuberi A, Chagnon YC, Weisnagel SJ, Argyropoulos G, Walts B, Pérusse L, Bouchard C: The human obesity gene map: the 2005 update. *Obesity* 14:529–644, 2006

76. Moreno-Aliaga MJ, Santos JL, Marti A, Martínez JA: Does weight loss prognosis depend on genetic make-up? *Obes Rev* 6:155–168, 2005

77. Hauner H, Meier M, Jockel KH, Frey UH, Siffert W: Prediction of successful weight reduction under sibutramine therapy through genotyping of the G-protein be-ta3 subunit gene (GNB3) C825T polymorphism. *Pharmacogenetics* 13:453–459, 2003

78. Peters WR, Macmurry JP, Walker J Giese RJ Jr, Comings DE: Phenylethanolamine N-methyltransferase G-148A genetic variant and weight loss in obese women. *Obes Res* 11:415–419, 2003

79. Hainer V: How should the obese patient be managed? Possible approaches to a national obesity management network. *Int J Obes* 23 (Suppl. 4):S14–S19, 1999

Impact of Different Bariatric Surgical Procedures on Insulin Action and β-Cell Function in Type 2 Diabetes

ELE FERRANNINI, MD[1]
GELTRUDE MINGRONE, MD[2]

The prevalence of obesity appears to have reached a plateau in the U.S. between 2003 and 2007 (1), but the obesity epidemic is still rampant in many other countries—especially in the developing world (2)—in adults as well as children (http://www.who.int/topics/obesity/en/). A recent analysis of a large prospective cohort of individuals 50–71 years old (3) has generated a precise dose-response gradient for the positive association of BMI and relative risk of death independent of other risk factors (especially smoking and preexisting disease, which cause weight loss). Yet, long-term observational studies have generally found that weight loss, whether spontaneous or intentional, is associated with increased, rather than decreased, overall mortality (rev. in 4).

Lifestyle intervention (diet and exercise), behavioral management, and drug therapy for obesity deliver a degree of weight loss that is usually modest (and therefore unattractive to patients) and short-lived (6 months to 1 year at best) and carry considerable side effects. Moreover, despite the attenuation of risk factors such as diabetes and dyslipidemia, trial evidence for an effect of these weight-control approaches on reducing cardiovascular disease or mortality is still lacking (rev. in 5). On the other hand, and perhaps as a consequence, surgery for the treatment of severe obesity is gaining increasing favor. The annual U.S. frequency of hospital discharges that included bariatric surgery increased sevenfold (from 3.5 to 24.0 per 100,000) between 1996 and 2002 (6). According to a review of 85,048 morbidly obese patients (7), early

(≤30 days) and late (30 days to 2 years) mortality rates for bariatric surgery trend downward (0.28 and 0.35%, respectively). Surgical treatment of massive obesity is being extended to adolescents, seemingly with similar success and risk rates as in adults (8–10). Recently, the 10.9-year follow-up of the Swedish Obese Subjects Study reported a 30% risk reduction for overall mortality in 2,010 obese patients who had undergone bariatric surgery (11). Likewise, in a retrospective cohort of 7,925 surgical patients (12), mortality from any cause was 40% lower than in 7,925 nonsurgical obese patients.

These findings are striking, particularly when considering the high rate of failure of other treatment modalities, such as caloric restriction (13) and antiobesity drugs (14), and may foster a change in the indications for bariatric surgery (15). They also raise a number of questions. The question we address here is the impact of bariatric surgery on type 2 diabetes, its size, and mechanisms.

Bariatric surgery and type 2 diabetes

A systematic review and meta-analysis of the English literature including >22,000 patients (73% women, mean BMI 47 kg/m^2) reported complete resolution of type 2 diabetes (defined as discontinuation of all diabetes-related medications and blood glucose levels within the normal range) in 77% of cases. This percentage increased to 85% when counting patients reporting improvement of glycemic control, and diabetes resolution occurred in concomitance with an average weight loss of 41 kg (~65% of the excess weight) (16). In the analysis by Adams et al. (12),

deaths attributed to diabetes were reduced by a phenomenal 92%. Thus, there can be little doubt that in very obese patients with type 2 diabetes bariatric surgery in general is a highly effective means of curing type 2 diabetes. However, the most frequent kind of type 2 diabetes, i.e., the hyperglycemia surfacing after the fourth decade of life in moderately obese subjects, is a progressive disease (17) that rarely undergoes resolution, whether spontaneously or with treatment. One possibility is that the hyperglycemia of morbid obesity (BMI between 35 and 70 kg/m^2) has a pathogenesis different from that of the hyperglycemia of moderately obese (BMI between 27 and 34 kg/m^2) or lean type 2 diabetes. Another possibility is that bariatric surgery per se interferes with glucose metabolism in ways that none of the other antidiabetes treatments do. Because circulating glucose levels quantitatively result from the insulin sensitivity of glucose uptake (in peripheral tissues) or release (by the liver) and the dynamics (amount and time course) of insulin made available by β-cells, we shall first review the evidence linking surgery-induced weight loss with changes in insulin sensitivity and β-cell function. Next, other potential interactions will be discussed.

Bariatric operations

A number of surgical approaches to induce weight loss have been developed, and several are in current use (cf. ref. 18 for a detailed description). In general, they can be grouped into purely restrictive, mostly restrictive, and mostly malabsorptive procedures. In the first group, the most common procedure is laparoscopic adjustable gastric banding (LAGB), which consists of placing a band around the upper part of the stomach, thereby creating a small pouch that empties into the lower stomach without bypassing the foregut (see Figure A1 in the online appendix available at http://dx.doi.org/10.2337/dc08-1762). In the cited meta-analysis (16), LAGB was associated with the loss of 32–70% of excess weight. Vertical banded gastroplasty is a variant of LAGB, typically leading to the loss of 48–

From the [1]Department of Internal Medicine and C.N.R. (National Research Council) Institute of Clinical Physiology, University of Pisa School of Medicine, Pisa, Italy; and the [2]Department of Medicine, Catholic University, Rome, Italy.
Corresponding author: Ele Ferrannini, ferranni@ifc.cnr.it.
Received 24 September 2008 and accepted 2 December 2008.
DOI: 10.2337/dc08-1762

93% of excess weight. With either of these techniques, the mechanism essentially hinges upon generating effective satiety signals for small amounts of ingested food.

Probably the most common weight-loss surgery is the Roux-en-Y gastric bypass (RYGB), in which the stomach is reduced to a small pouch (<30 ml) that is connected via a tight outlet to the jejunum just past the duodenum while the jejunal stump is anastomosed to the lower jejunum in a Y conformation (Fig. 1). Here, a degree of gastric restriction comparable with that of LAGB (but not adjustable) is coupled with the bypass of the duodenum and upper jejunum, making RYGB a mostly restrictive procedure. Between 33 and 77% of excess weight can be lost following RYGB (16).

With the jejunoileal bypass, the gastric content is emptied directly into the terminal ileum, thereby inducing major malabsorption with no restriction of food intake. Now abandoned, this procedure led to the development of current malabsorptive approaches, the prototype of which is biliopancreatic diversion (BPD). Here, a 60% distal gastric resection with stapled closure of the duodenal stump results in a residual stomach volume of ~300 ml. The small bowel is transected 2.5 m from the ileocecal valve, and its distal end is anastomosed to the remaining stomach. The proximal end of the ileum, comprising the remaining small bowel carrying the biliopancreatic juice and excluded from food transit, is anastomosed to the bowel 50 cm proximal to the ileocecal valve. Consequently, the total length of absorbing bowel is 250 cm, the final 50 cm of which represents the site where ingested food and biliopancreatic juices mix (Fig. 1). This mostly malabsorptive approach is associated with the highest (62–75%) (16) and most durable (19) degree of excess weight loss.

Weight loss and insulin sensitivity: preliminary considerations
Adiposity is one of the physiological determinants of insulin sensitivity (20). Weight loss has been shown to enhance insulin sensitivity under all circumstances (rev. in 21) except wasting, major stress, and HIV infection (22–24). Surgically induced weight loss, in general, appears to take no exception (see below). However, selective surgical removal of fat tissue from subcutaneous depots does not improve insulin resistance. In a well-controlled study of 15 obese women (7 of

whom had diabetes), removal of 9–10 kg of subcutaneous abdominal fat by liposuction did not change insulin-mediated glucose disposal (on a euglycemic-hyperinsulinemic clamp) despite the expected drop in circulating leptin levels (25). Although other studies using liposuction have reported some improvement of insulin sensitivity in the longer term (26), this observation clearly implies that factors other than the sheer mass of subcutaneous adipose tissue have an impact on insulin action. Thus, large adipocytes, such as those that are deposited in subcutaneous depots during weight gain, are less sensitive to insulin than small adipocytes (27); their degree of insulin unresponsiveness in vitro correlates with in vivo insulin insensitivity (28). Ectopic fat, accumulated in abdominal visceral depots, skeletal muscle, and liver, has been specifically linked with the presence of insulin resistance independently of total adiposity. In support of these findings, surgical removal of visceral, but not subcutaneous, fat from aging or diabetic rats restores insulin sensitivity and glucose tolerance (29). In obese humans, the metabolic changes induced by weight loss, i.e., insulin sensitization of both glucose metabolism and lipolysis, have been related to the depletion of ectopic fat stores (30–35). Importantly, whereas fasting for 3 days depresses insulin action in obese subjects (36), caloric restriction enhances it (37), accounting for as much increase in insulin sensitivity as weight loss itself (38). Finally, several peptides expressed and released by adipose tissue are metabolically active. For example, adiponectin upregulates insulin action in liver and skeletal muscle, whereas high circulating levels of some adipocytokines (e.g., tumor necrosis factor-α and retinol binding protein 4) correlate with in vivo insulin resistance (39).

Collectively, these observations suggest the following considerations when interpreting the evidence linking surgically induced weight loss (or, for that matter, any weight change) and insulin sensitivity:

- quality and site are as important as amount of fat gained or lost;
- energy balance matters to insulin action independently of weight changes;
- the endocrine activity of adipose tissue itself may interfere with the relationship between changes in adiposity and insulin sensitivity;
- coordinate changes in body weight and

insulin sensitivity may differ between diabetic and nondiabetic subjects;
- metabolic abnormalities may emerge at different BMI thresholds in individuals of diverse ethnic background (40);
- specifically for bariatric surgery, an understanding of how gastrointestinal transit is altered by the operation may be key to interpreting metabolic effects for any given amount of weight loss.

Bariatric surgery and insulin sensitivity: results
Online appendix Table A1 lists the studies in which data on insulin sensitivity have been reported for obese type 2 diabetic patients undergoing bariatric surgery. With the proviso that our literature search has likely missed diabetic patients included in series that did not provide results separately for diabetic and nondiabetic subjects, the studies in online appendix Table A1 include ~450 type 2 diabetic patients reported over a period of ~25 years. As can be appreciated, type of surgery, duration of follow-up, and methodology vary enough to preclude precise quantitation of the impact of weight loss on insulin sensitivity. Nevertheless, some information can be derived from these data (with no pretense of bona fide meta-analysis). Thus, the weighted mean of preoperative BMI in all 423 patients was 46.4 kg/m^2, which reflects the current indications for bariatric surgery (BMI ≥40 kg/m^2 or ≥35 kg/m^2 in complicated obesity). In the 204 patients in whom homeostasis model assessment (HOMA) (HOMA of insulin resistance, in this case) was used to assess changes in insulin sensitivity ≥4 months after surgery (weighted mean 12 months), insulin sensitivity improved by 51% for a mean BMI drop of 32% (~40 kg). The percent changes in BMI and HOMA across the different studies were loosely related to one another. In the 79 patients in whom HOMA was measured <4 months after surgery (weighted mean 1.5 months), insulin sensitivity improved by 49% for a BMI decrease of 10% (with no correlation between the respective decrements). The few studies in online appendix Table A1 using different methods of estimating insulin sensitivity (insulin sensitivity test, insulin tolerance test, frequently sampled intravenous glucose tolerance test, and clamp [60–65]) do not in general run contrary to this result. Therefore, with all the approximations of this sort of analysis, the notions emerge that 1) bariatric surgery is capable of improving the insu-

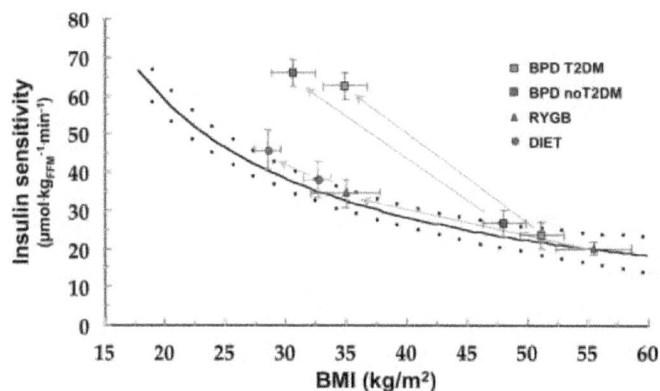

Figure 1—*The results (symbols) are means ± SEM in patients undergoing weight loss by diet (ref. 69), RYGB, or BPD (ref. 68). Green arrows connect pretreatment to posttreatment values. The black line and the black dots are the fitting function and 95% CIs of the data in ref. 68 (same as in online appendix Fig. A2, bottom graph). FFM, fat-free mass; T2DM, type 2 diabetes.*

lin resistance of type 2 diabetes by ~50% while at the same time causing a ~30% decrease in BMI and 2) this improvement of insulin sensitivity may be seen already ~6 weeks following surgery, at which time BMI may be decreased by only 11%. The latter apparent paradox may result from the use of surrogate measures of insulin sensitivity (HOMA). It can also be at least partly explained by the fact that early after surgery, caloric restriction per se (whether achieved by lower intake as per restrictive procedures or reduced absorption as with malabsorptive operations) plays a major role in improving insulin action. Months to years after surgery, weight loss has generally leveled off; a quantitative relationship between the changes in BMI and insulin sensitivity is now usually evident. The weakness of the correlation between the loss of weight and the gain in insulin sensitivity has been repeatedly noted. For example, in a nonrandomized study comparing LAGB and RYGB in a large number of nondiabetic patients (66), HOMA at 30 months postsurgery was similar but RYGB induced a significantly larger weight loss than LAGB (−33 vs. −22%). It should be considered that, in addition to the confounding factors mentioned in the previous section, an important determinant of weight loss is the initial body weight. For example, in a prospective 2-year follow-up of 107 men and women undergoing BPD at one center, there was a strong correlation ($r = 0.68$) between initial weight and achieved weight loss, which was entirely driven by initial fat mass ($r = 0.64$) and not fat-free mass (FFM) (67). This phenomenon is reminiscent of the common clinical observation that with any treatment the re-

sponse is proportional to the initial height of the abnormality (e.g., A1C or arterial blood pressure). As with these other variables, the biology underlying this apparent rule is unclear.

The questions now arise 1) whether insulin sensitivity is fully restored despite the fact that postoperative BMI typically remains in the obese range, 2) whether the heightened insulin sensitivity is alone responsible for the resolution/improvement of hyperglycemia, and 3) whether the different surgical approaches differ from one another in their insulin-sensitizing power.

Some relevant information can be derived from the few studies that have employed the clamp technique to directly measure insulin sensitivity. In two different databases using the same exogenous insulin infusion rate, the dependency of whole-body insulin sensitivity on BMI is best described by curvilinear fits (online appendix Fig. A2). Both in the European Group for the Study of Insulin Resistance (EGIR) cohort (20) and in the study by Muscelli et al. (68), a 30% reduction in BMI (from 46 kg/m^2) predicts a 50% increase in insulin sensitivity. However, both interpolating functions also predict that insulin sensitivity would not be fully restored by a 30% weight decrement (to the level of 42 μmol $\cdot$ kg$_{FFM}^{-1}$ $\cdot$ min^{-1} associated with a BMI of 25 kg/m^2).

We then used these cross-sectional relationships to scale the results of insulin clamp studies in subjects losing weight by different approaches. In nondiabetic subjects on a calorie-restricted diet (69) or undergoing RYGB (68), the data fall well within the 95% CIs of the fit (Fig. 1)—in other words, when weight-stabilized sub-

jects had gained insulin sensitivity in exact proportion to the weight change. Strikingly similar results are obtained when plotting data from two other clamp studies, using caloric restriction (38) or RYGB (70). In contrast, in 107 patients, 35 of whom with type 2 diabetes, undergoing BPD and restudied 2 years later, the increase in insulin sensitivity definitely exceeded the prediction; i.e., insulin resistance was normal or supernormal at BMI values still in the obese range (67). Furthermore, in one study (71) where insulin sensitivity was estimated at variable (but not sequential) time intervals following BPD, completely normal rates of insulin-mediated glucose clearance were found as early as 10 days after surgery; at this time, marked insulin resistance was present in a control group of morbidly obese patients undergoing major nonbariatric abdominal surgery.

With regard to hepatic insulin resistance, we could find no study that measured endogenous glucose production in obese diabetic patients before and after surgery. However, given that hepatic and peripheral insulin resistance correlate with each other, the pattern of results outlined for insulin-mediated glucose uptake can probably be extrapolated to the effects of insulin on endogenous (hepatic) insulin sensitivity. As for fat distribution, in a large cohort of subjects (including type 2 diabetic patients) undergoing LAGB, the ratio of visceral to subcutaneous abdominal fat (measured by ultrasound) was significantly reduced 1 year postoperatively in concomitance with a weight loss of 8 BMI units (43). This finding is consistent with the notion that fat is more rapidly lost from visceral than subcutaneous depots. Whereas this fat redistribution may contribute to the improvement of other metabolic abnormalities, it is doubtful that selective fat removal in very obese subjects who lose substantial portions of excess weight affects insulin action over and above what is engendered by weight loss itself.

Patients with diabetes appear to lose significantly less weight than equally obese nondiabetic subjects following gastric bypass (72). Whether the gain in insulin sensitivity in obese type 2 diabetic patients is any different from that of the nondiabetic obese individuals for the same weight reduction has not been examined systematically. In one series (71), insulin sensitivity was fully restored in subjects with normal glucose tolerance, impaired glucose tolerance, or type 2 diabetes following BPD; because type 2 diabetic patients had lower presurgery levels of insulin sensitivity, their gain was the highest.

The picture emerging from this analysis is as follows: Surgical procedures that greatly restrain food intake (RYGB) or absorption (BPD) may induce some recovery of insulin sensitivity before any large weight loss has occurred. However, when tested under conditions of stable energy balance, insulin resistance is increased by surgically induced weight loss quantitatively. Therefore, long-term–postsurgery morbidly obese patients (nondiabetic and diabetic alike) are likely to retain a degree of insulin resistance if their BMI is still in the overweight/obese range. Malabsorptive procedures take exception in that they may improve insulin sensitivity beyond the effect of weight loss. This fundamental difference between mainly restrictive and malabsorptive procedures needs to be proven by prospective, randomized studies.

Bariatric surgery and β-cell function

Assessing β-cell function is problematic because currently no clinical test has been agreed upon as being the gold standard in the way that the clamp has for the measurement of insulin sensitivity. Furthermore, insulin secretion is intrinsically complex because β-cells must adapt to chronic stimuli (e.g., weight changes) as well as respond to acute challenges (i.e., the succession of fasting and feeding). For the sake of the following discussion, it is important to distinguish between secretory indexes that reflect long-term adaptation from those that result from the dynamic behavior of the β-cell. Basal insulin secretion and total insulin output in response to a standard stimulus are set points of secretory capacity, whereas β-cell glucose sensitivity (or the slope of the insulin secretion/plasma glucose dose-response relationship) is the ability to control glycemia by promptly releasing sufficient hormone. This key function is reflected in empirical indexes such as the acute insulin response (AIR) to intravenous glucose or the insulinogenic index on the oral glucose tolerance test or a mixed meal.

Data on changes in β-cell function with bariatric surgery are few but relatively consistent. Fasting insulin concentrations (44,51) or secretion rates (54) and total insulin output in response to intravenous (47) or oral glucose (71) or mixed meals (54) all have been found to decrease after any bariatric procedure.

This is the expected consequence of the reduced adipose mass and improved insulin sensitivity (73). In contrast, in type 2 diabetic patients, HOMA of β-cell function after LAGB (45), AIR and the insulinogenic index after RYGB (49,52), and AIR after BPD (47) all increased to a variable extent. Model-derived β-cell glucose sensitivity was fully normalized in 10 type 2 diabetic patients 2 years post-BPD in parallel with the normalization of daylong plasma glucose concentrations (54).

Thus, surgical weight loss generally lowers the set point but heightens the dynamic responsivity of the β-cell. Whether β-cell function is fully restored appears to depend principally on the severity of diabetes (relative to duration, degree of metabolic control, and intensity of antidiabetes treatment) (45,55). With purely or mostly restrictive procedures, β-cell function shows progressive improvement over time, paralleling ongoing weight loss. With BPD, almost complete recovery of AIR has been reported in a small group of type 2 diabetic patients as early as 1 month postsurgery (59).

All in all, diabetes in the very obese does not appear to differ in pathophysiology from the more common variety of moderately obese diabetes. Clearly, insulin resistance is more severe because of its quantitative relation to BMI, and drastic increments in insulin action with major weight loss underlie the spectacular remission rates. β-Cell function recovers in large part or in full probably depending on its initial, genetically determined quality.

Mechanisms

Food intake, transit, and absorption are regulated by a complex network including the gastrointestinal system, the liver, and the brain (rev. in 74). Surgical restriction of the stomach may change circulating concentrations of ghrelin, a hormone secreted by endocrine cells in the fundus. When infused into healthy volunteers, ghrelin induces acute insulin resistance (75). However, changes in ghrelin levels after bariatric surgery have been inconsistent and unrelated to the ensuing changes in insulin sensitivity (76). Changes in other gastrointestinal hormones have been analyzed for those bariatric procedures that alter food transit. Glucagon-like peptide-1 (GLP-1) potentiates insulin release in a glucose-dependent manner (74). GLP-1 responses (to glucose or mixed meals) are impaired in association with both type 2 diabetes and obesity

(77), and GLP-1 levels increase early after both RYGB (58,78) and BPD (53) but apparently not after diet (58). Thus, one possibility is that heightened GLP-1 levels contribute to the improvement in β-cell function detectable early after surgery. It is not clear what the precise mechanism is by which GLP-1 release is revved up by anatomical rearrangements that either bypass the duodenum and upper jejunum (RYGB) or exclude the larger part of the entire gastrointestinal tract from food transit (BPD). However, in one study, GLP-1 at 6 weeks postsurgery was increased in normotolerant and impaired glucose-tolerant subjects but not in type 2 diabetic patients despite similar improvements in insulin resistance and β-cell dysfunction (49). Also, infusion of GLP-1 to pharmacological levels fails to stimulate insulin-mediated glucose disposal in healthy volunteers or under experimental conditions where its effects on endogenous insulin release are prevented (as in type 1 diabetic patients) (rev. in 79). Coupled with the current notion that GLP-1 receptors have not been demonstrated in liver, skeletal muscle, or adipose tissue, one can conclude that GLP-1 is an unlikely candidate to explain the remission of insulin resistance in bariatric patients. The involvement of glucose-dependent insulinotropic polypeptide (GIP) is even less clear. GIP resistance has been repeatedly described in type 2 diabetes (e.g., ref. 77), and GIP knockout in mice improves insulin action (80). However, following RYGB, increased (58) or unchanged (81) GIP levels have been reported in type 2 diabetic patients. On the other hand, GLP-1 has been implicated in the dumping syndrome and the reactive hypoglycemia that may follow gastric surgery (82). Its trophic actions on β-cells have been called upon to explain six cases of histologically proven nesidioblastosis after RYGB (83).

Further involvement of the gastrointestinal tract has been inferred from the outcome of novel surgical approaches. In Goto-Kakizaki rats, Rubino et al. (84) found that excluding a short segment of proximal intestine from food passage (via a duodenal-jejunal bypass or a gastrojejunostomy) improved glucose tolerance, whereas restoring duodenal transit reestablished glucose intolerance. This observation has led to a foregut hypothesis, which holds that contact of nutrients with the duodenal mucosa generates signals (hormonal and/or neural) that interfere with glucose metabolism and insulin action; bypassing duodenal passage (as in RYGB and BPD) would remove this inhibition.

In the rat, Strader et al. (85) showed that effects similar to those of duodenal exclusion could be produced by transposing an ileal segment into the upper intestine. In studies in type 2 diabetic patients with a BMI <35 kg/m^2, DePaula et al. (86) reported that ileal interposition with a sleeve gastrectomy (with or without diversion) resulted in weight loss and a drastic fall in A1C, fasting glucose, and HOMA-IR 7 months later. A "hindgut hypothesis" thus proposes that contact with undigested nutrients triggers an ileal brake, i.e., a combination of effects influencing eating behavior and digestion.

Finally, in rats, diversion of the bile flow from the duodenum into the second jejunal loop leads to improved tolerance to oral as well as intravenous glucose compared with sham-operated animals (87). BPD is the only bariatric approach that causes major lipid malabsorption at the same time as it depletes intramyocellular lipids and returns insulin sensitivity to normal or supranormal levels in the longer term (88). Fat starvation in rats reproduces the metabolic picture of BPD with surprising precision (89). Therefore, lipids and lipid signal molecules—and their control by the bile—must be among key messengers released by a subverted gastrointestinal tract.

CONCLUSIONS— Bariatric surgery is a highly effective means of inducing diabetes remission in very obese patients with type 2 diabetes. Rank order of increasing efficacy of the most common surgical procedures progresses from the purely restrictive to the mostly restrictive to the mostly malabsorptive; several new approaches, however, are under very active investigation. Diabetes remission results from the joint improvement of insulin resistance and β-cell dysfunction. Better insulin action on glucose metabolism relieves secretory pressure on the β-cell, resulting in reduced insulin output; dynamic β-cell responses, however, are restored. Rates of complete diabetes remission or glycemic improvement depend essentially on the severity of diabetes (as indexed by duration, A1C levels, presence of complications, and intensity of treatment). Factors such as family history, interaction with previous antidiabetes therapies, or evidence of autoimmunity have not been analyzed specifically.

Caloric restriction and weight loss are the dominant mechanisms of improved glucose metabolism. The former appears to account for the early postsurgical recovery of insulin sensitivity and secretory dynamics; the latter is the final determinant of the outcome once weight and caloric balance have stabilized. When food transit is surgically altered, changes in the pattern of gastrointestinal hormone release may support the early adaptation of β-cell function but are unlikely to make a major contribution to insulin action.

Whether bariatric operations exert an intrinsic antidiabetes action beyond weight loss remains unproven. The best of available evidence indicates that malabsorptive operations presently offer the highest chances of revealing weight-independent mechanisms of diabetes resolution, but smart manipulations of food passage may open entirely new avenues. Experimenting in less obese or nonobese diabetes or minimizing weight loss may provide further evidence. Difficult as they may be, randomized controlled clinical studies using state-of-the-art methodology are required to prove the worth of metabolic surgery.

Acknowledgments— No potential conflicts of interest relevant to this article were reported.

References

1. Ogden CL, Carroll MD, Curtin LR, McDowell MA, Tabak CJ, Flegal KM: Prevalence of overweight and obesity in the United States, 1999–2004. *JAMA* 295: 1549–1555, 2006
2. Hossain P, Kawar B, El NM: Obesity and diabetes in the developing world: a growing challenge. *N Engl J Med* 356:213–215, 2007
3. Adams KF, Schatzkin A, Harris TB, Kipnis V, Mouw T, Ballard-Barbash R, Hollenbeck A, Leitzmann MF: Overweight, obesity, and mortality in a large prospective cohort of persons 50 to 71 years old. *N Engl J Med* 355:763–778, 2006
4. Nilsson PM: Is weight loss beneficial for reduction of morbidity and mortality? *Diabetes Care* 31 (Suppl. 2):S278–S283, 2008
5. Bessesen DH: Update on obesity. *J Clin Endocrinol Metab* 93:2027–2034, 2008
6. Davis MM, Slish K, Chao C, Cabana MD: National trends in bariatric surgery, 1996–2002. *Arch Surg* 141:71–74, 2006
7. Buchwald H, Estok R, Fahrbach K, Banel D, Sledge I: Trends in mortality in bariatric surgery: a systematic review and meta-analysis. *Surgery* 142:621–632, 2007
8. Sugerman HJ, Sugerman EL, DeMaria EJ, Kellum JM, Kennedy C, Mowery Y, Wolfe LG: Bariatric surgery for severely obese adolescents. *J Gastrointest Surg* 7:102–107, 2003
9. Barnett SJ, Stanley C, Hanlon M, Acton R, Saltzman DA, Ikramuddin S, Buchwald H: Long-term follow-up and the role of surgery in adolescents with morbid obesity. *Surg Obes Relat Dis* 1:394–398, 2005
10. Nadler EP, Youn HA, Ren CJ, Fielding GA: An update on 73 US obese pediatric patients treated with laparoscopic adjustable gastric banding: comorbidity resolution and compliance data. *J Pediatr Surg* 43:141–146, 2008
11. Sjöström L, Narbro K, Sjöström CD, Karason K, Larsson B, Wedel H, Lystig T, Sullivan M, Bouchard C, Carlsson B, Bengtsson C, Dahlgren S, Gummesson A, Jacobson P, Karlsson J, Lindroos AK, Lönroth H, Näslund I, Olbers T, Stenlöf K, Torgeson J, Agren G, Carlsson LM, Swedish Obese Subjects Study: Effects of bariatric surgery on mortality in Swedish obese subjects. *N Engl J Med* 357:741–752, 2007
12. Adams TD, Gress RE, Smith SC, Halverson RC, Simper SC, Rosamond WD, Lamonte MJ, Stroup AM, Hunt SC: Long-term mortality after gastric bypass surgery. *N Engl J Med* 357:753–761, 2007
13. Malik VS, Hu FB: Popular weight-loss diets: from evidence to practice. *Nat Clin Pract Cardiovasc Med* 4:34–41, 2007
14. Li Z, Maglione M, Tu W, Mojica W, Arteburn D, Shugarman LR, Hilton L, Suttorp M, Solomon V, Shekelle PG, Morton SC: Meta-analysis: pharmacologic treatment of obesity. *Ann Intern Med* 142:532–546, 2005
15. Ahima RS: Should eligibility for bariatric surgery be expanded? *Gastroenterology* 134:15, 2008
16. Buchwald H, Avidor Y, Braunwald E, Jensen MD, Pories W, Fahrbach K, Schoelles K: Bariatric surgery: a systematic review and meta-analysis. *JAMA* 292:1724–1737, 2004
17. Turner RC, Cull CA, Frighi V, Holman RR: Glycemic control with diet, sulfonylurea, metformin, or insulin in patients with type 2 diabetes mellitus: progressive requirement for multiple therapies (UKPDS 49). UK Prospective Diabetes Study (UKPDS) Group. *JAMA* 281:2005–2012, 1999
18. Crookes PF: Surgical treatment of morbid obesity. *Annu Rev Med* 57:243–264, 2006
19. Scopinaro N, Marinari GM, Camerini GB, Papadia FS, Adami GF: Specific effects of biliopancreatic diversion on the major components of metabolic syndrome: a long-term follow-up study. *Diabetes Care* 28:2406–2411, 2005
20. Ferrannini E, Natali A, Bell P, Cavallo-Perin P, Lalic N, Mingrone G: Insulin resistance and hypersecretion in obesity. European Group for the Study of Insulin Resistance (EGIR). *J Clin Invest* 100:

1166–1173, 1997

21. McAuley K, Mann J: Thematic review series: patient-oriented research. Nutritional determinants of insulin resistance. *J Lipid Res* 47:1668–1676, 2006

22. Pidcoke HF, Wade CE, Wolf SE: Insulin and the burned patient. *Crit Care Med* 35 (Suppl. 9):S524–S530, 2007

23. Brandi LS, Santoro D, Natali A, Altomonte F, Baldi S, Frascerra S, Ferrannini E: Insulin resistance of stress: sites and mechanisms. *Clin Sci* 85:525–535, 1993

24. Grinspoon S: Mechanisms and strategies for insulin resistance in acquired imuune deficiency syndrome. *Clin Infect Dis* 37 (Suppl. 2):S85–S90, 2003

25. Klein S, Fontana L, Young L, Coggan AR, Kilo C, Patterson BW, Mohammed BS: Absence of an effect of liposuction on insulin action and risk factors for coronary heart disease. *N Engl J Med* 350: 2549–2557, 2004

26. Rizzo MR, Paolisso G, Grella R, Barbieri M, Grella E, Ragno E, Grella R, Nicoletti G, D'Andrea F: Is dermolipectomy effective in improving insulin action and lowering inflammatory markers in obese women? *Clin Endocrinol (Oxf)* 63:253–258, 2005

27. Foley JE, Laursen AL, Sonne O, Gliemann J: Insulin binding and hexose transport in rat adipocytes. Relation to cell size. *Diabetologia* 19:234–241, 1980

28. Lundgren M, Svensson M, Lindmark S, Renström F, Ruge T, Eriksson JW: Fat cell enlargement is an independent marker of insulin resistance and 'hyperleptinaemia'. *Diabetologia* 50:625–633, 2007

29. Gabriely I, Ma XH, Yang XM, Atzmon G, Rajala MW, Berg AH, Scherer P, Rossetti L, Barzilai N: Removal of visceral fat prevents insulin resistance and glucose intolerance of aging: an adipokine-mediated process? *Diabetes* 51:2951–2958, 2002

30. Knittle JL, Ginsberg-Fellner F: Effect of weight reduction on in vitro adipose tissue lipolysis and cellularity in obese adolescents and adults. *Diabetes* 21:754–761, 1972

31. Purnell JQ, Kahn SE, Albers JJ, Nevin DN, Brunzell JD, Schwartz RS: Effect of weight loss with reduction of intra-abdominal fat on lipid metabolism in older men. *J Clin Endocrinol Metab* 85:977–982, 2000

32. Goodpaster BH, Theriault R, Watkins SC, Kelley DE: Intramuscular lipid content is increased in obesity and decreased by weight loss. *Metabolism* 49:467–472, 2000

33. Kotronen A, Seppälä-Lindroos A, Bergholm R, Yki-Järvinen H: Tissue specificity of insulin resistance in humans: fat in the liver rather than muscle is associated with features of the metabolic syndrome. *Diabetologia* 51:130–138, 2008

34. Klein S, Luu K, Gasic S, Green A: Effect of weight loss on whole body and cellular lipid metabolism in severely obese humans. *Am J Physiol* 270:E739–E745, 1996

35. Pontiroli AE, Frigé F, Paganelli M, Folli F: In morbid obesity, metabolic abnormalities and adhesion molecules correlate with visceral fat, not with subcutaneous fat: effect of weight loss through surgery. *Obes Surg* 2008 July 16 [Epub ahead of print]

36. DeFronzo RA, Soman V, Sherwin RS, Hendler R, Felig P: Insulin binding to monocytes and insulin action in human obesity, starvation, and refeeding. *J Clin Invest* 62:204–213, 1978

37. Henry RR, Scheaffer L, Olefsky JM: Glycemic effects of intensive caloric restriction and isocaloric refeeding in noninsulin-dependent diabetes mellitus. *J Clin Endocrinol Metab* 61:917–925, 1985

38. Kelley DE, Wing R, Buonocore C, Sturis J, Polonsky K, Fitzsimmons M: Relative effects of calorie restriction and weight loss in noninsulin-dependent diabetes mellitus. *J Clin Endocrinol Metab* 77:1287–1293, 1993

39. Badman MK, Flier JS: The adipocyte as an active participant in energy balance and metabolism. *Gastroenterology* 132:2103–2115, 2007

40. Razak F, Anand S, Vuksan V, Davis B, Jacobs R, Teo KK, Yusuf S: Ethnic differences in the relationships between obesity and glucose-metabolic abnormalities: a cross-sectional, population-based study. *Int J Obes (Lond)* 29:656–667, 2005

41. Hughes TA, Gwynne JT, Switzer BR, Herbst C, White G: Effects of caloric restriction and weight loss on glycemic control, insulin release and resistance, and atherosclerotic risk in obese patients with type II diabetes. *Am J Med* 77:7–17, 1984

42. Gelonese B, Tambascia MA, Pareja JC, Repetto EM, Magna LA: The insulin tolerance test in morbidly obese patients undergoing bariatric surgery. *Obes Res* 9:763–769, 2001

43. Pontiroli AE, Pizzocri P, Librenti MC, Vedani P, Marchi M, Cucchi E, Orena C, Paganelli M, Giacomelli M, Ferla G, Folli F: Laparoscopic adjustable gastric banding for the treatment of morbid (grade 3) obesity and its metabolic complications: a three-year study. *J Clin Endocrinol Metab* 87:3555–3561, 2002

44. Dixon JB, O'Brien PE: Health outcomes of severely obese type 2 diabetic subjects 1 year after laparoscopic adjustable gastric banding. *Diabetes Care* 25:358–363, 2002

45. Dixon JB, Dixon AF, O'Brien PE: Improvements in insulin sensitivity and ß-cell function (HOMA) with weight loss in the severely obese. Homeostatic model assessment. *Diabet Med* 20:127–34, 2003

46. Kopp HP, Kopp CW, Festa A, Krzyzanowska K, Kriwanek S, Minar E, Roka R, Schernthaner G: Impact of weight loss on inflammatory proteins and their associa-tion with the insulin resistance syndrome in morbidly obese patients. *Arterioscler Thromb Vasc Biol* 23:1042–7, 2003

47. Polyzogopoulou EV, Kalfarentzos F, Vagenakis AG, Alexandrides TK: Restoration of euglycemia and normal acute insulin response to glucose in obese subjects with type 2 diabetes following bariatric surgery. *Diabetes* 52:1098–1103, 2003

48. Veronelli A, Laneri M, Ranieri R, Koprivec D, Vardaro D, Paganelli M, Folli F, Pontiroli AE: White blood cells in obesity and diabetes: effects of weight loss and normalization of glucose metabolism. *Diabetes Care* 27:2501–2502, 2004

49. Morinigo R, Lacy AM, Casamitjana R, Delgado S, Gomis R, Vidal J: GLP-1 and changes in glucose tolerance following gastric bypass surgery in morbidly obese subjects. *Obes Surg* 16:1594–1601, 2006

50. Coppini LZ, Bertevello PL, Gama-Rodrigues J, Waitzberg DL: Changes in insulin sensitivity in morbidly obese patients with or without metabolic syndrome after gastric bypass. *Obes Surg* 16: 1520–1525, 2006

51. Ballantyne GH, Farkas D, Laker S, Wasiliewski A: Short-term changes in insulin resistance following weight loss surgery for morbid obesity: laparoscopic adjustable gastric banding versus laparoscopic Roux-en-Y gastric bypass. *Obes Surg* 16: 1189–1197, 2006

52. García-Fuentes E, García-Almeida JM, García-Arnéz J, Rivas-Marín J, Gallego-Perales JL, González-Jiménez B, Cardona I, García-Serrano S, Garriga MJ, Gonzalo M, Ruiz de Adana MS, Soriguer F: Morbidly obese individuals with impaired fasting glucose have a specific pattern of insulin secretion and sensitivity: effect of weight loss after bariatric surgery. *Obes Surg* 16:1179–1188, 2006

53. Guidone C, Manco M, Valera-Mora E, Iaconelli A, Gniuli D, Mari A, Nanni G, Castagneto M, Calvani M, Mingrone G: Mechanisms of recovery from type 2 diabetes after malabsorptive bariatric surgery. *Diabetes* 55:2025–2031, 2006

54. Camastra S, Manco M, Mari A, Greco AV, Frascerra S, Mingrone G, Ferrannini E: ß-cell function in severely obese type 2 diabetic patients. Long-term effects of bariatric surgery. *Diabetes Care* 30:1002–1004, 2007

55. Vidal J, Ibarzabal A, Nicolau J, Vidov M, Delgado S, Martinez G, Balust J, Morinigo R, Lacy A: Short-term effects of sleeve gastrectomy on type 2 diabetes mellitus in severely obese subjects. *Obes Surg* 17: 1069–1074, 2007

56. Gannagé-Yared MH, Yaghi C, Habre B, Khalife S, Noun R, Germanos-Haddad M, Trak-Smayra V: Osteoprotegerin in relation to body weight, lipid parameters insulin sensitivity, adipocytokines, and C-reactive protein in obese and non-obese young individuals: results from

both cross-sectional and interventional study. *Eur J Endocrinol* 158:353–359, 2008

57. Dixon JB, O'Brien PE, Playfair J, Chapman L, Schachter LM, Skinner S, Proietto J, Bailey M, Anderson M: Adjustable gastric banding and conventional therapy for type 2 diabetes: a randomized controlled trial. *JAMA* 299:316–323, 2008

58. Laferrère B, Teixeira J, McGinty J, Tran H, Egger JR, Colarusso A, Kovack B, Bawa B, Koshy N, Lee H, Yapp K, Olivan B: Effect of weight loss by gastric bypass surgery versus hypocaloric diet on glucose and incretin levels in patients with type 2 diabetes. *J Clin Endocrinol Metab* 93:2479–2485, 2008

59. Briatore L, Salani B, Andraghetti G, Danovaro C, Sferrazzo E, Scopinaro N, Adami GF, Maggi D, Cordera R: Restoration of acute insulin response in T2DM subjects 1 month after biliopancreatic diversion. *Obesity* 16:77–81, 2008

60. Shen SW, Reaven GM, Farquhar JW: Comparison of impedance to insulin-mediated glucose uptake in normal subjects and in subjects with latent diabetes. *J Clin Invest* 49:2151–2160, 1970

61. Bonora E, Moghetti P, Zancanaro C, Cigolini M, Querena M, Cacciatori V, Corgnati A, Muggeo M: Estimates of in vivo insulin action in man: comparison of insulin tolerance tests with euglycemic and hyperglycemic glucose clamp studies. *J Clin Endocrinol Metab* 68:374–378, 1989

62. Matthews DR, Hosker JP, Rudenski AS, Naylor BA, Treacher DF, Turner RC: Homeostasis model assessment: insulin resistance and beta-cell function from fasting plasma glucose and insulin concentrations in man. *Diabetologia* 28:412–419, 1985

63. Katz A, Nambi SS, Mather K, Baron AD, Follmann DA, Sullivan G, Quon MJ: Quantitative insulin sensitivity check index: a simple, accurate method for assessing insulin sensitivity in humans. *J Clin Endocrinol Metab* 85:2402–2410, 2000

64. Bergman RN, Ider YZ, Bowden CR, Cobelli C: Quantitative estimation of insulin sensitivity. *Am J Physiol* 236:E667–E677, 1979

65. DeFronzo RA, Tobin JD, Andres R: Glucose clamp technique: a method for quantifying insulin secretion and resistance. *Am J Physiol* 237:E214–E223, 1979

66. Lee W-J, Lee Y-C, Ser K-H, Chen J-C, Chen SC: Improvement of insulin resistance after obesity surgery: a comparison of gastric banding and bypass procedures. *Obes Surg* 18:1119–1125, 2008

67. Valera-Mora ME, Simeoni B, Gagliardi L, Scarfone A, Nanni G, Castagneto M, Manco M, Mingrone G, Ferrannini E: Predictors of weight loss and reversal of comorbidities in malabsorptive bariatric surgery. *Am J Clin Nutr* 81:1292–1297, 2005

68. Muscelli E, Mingrone G, Camastra S, Manco M, Pereira JA, Pareja JC, Ferrannini E: Differential effect of weight loss on insulin resistance in surgically treated obese patients. *Am J Med* 118:51–57, 2005

69. Muscelli E, Emdin M, Natali A, Pratali L, Camastra S, Gastaldelli A, Baldi S, Carpeggiani C, Ferrannini E: Autonomic and hemodynamic responses to insulin in lean and obese humans. *J Clin Endocrinol Metab* 83:2084–2090, 1998

70. Bobbioni-Harsch E, Bongard O, Habicht F, Weimer D, Bounameaux H, Huber O, Chassot G, Morel P, Assimacopoulos-Jeannet F, Golay A: Relationship between sympathetic reactivity and body weight loss in morbidly obese subjects. *Int J Obes Relat Metab Disord* 28:906–911, 2004

71. Mari A, Manco M, Guidone C, Nanni G, Castagneto M, Mingrone G, Ferrannini E: Restoration of normal glucose tolerance in severely obese patients after bilio-pancreatic diversion: role of insulin sensitivity and beta cell function. *Diabetologia* 49:2136–2143, 2006

72. Carbonell AM, Wolfe LG, Meador JG, Sugerman NJ, Kellum JM, Maher JW: Does diabetes affect weight loss after gastric bypass? *Surg Obes Relat Dis* 4:441–444, 2008

73. Ferrannini E, Camastra S, Gastaldelli A, Sironi AM, Natali A, Muscelli E, Mingrone G, Mari A: ß-cell function in obesity: effects of weight loss. *Diabetes* 53 (Suppl. 3):S26–S33, 2004

74. Cummings DE, Overduin J: Gastrointestinal regulation of food intake. *J Clin Invest* 117:13–23, 2007

75. Vestergaard ET, Gormsen LC, Jessen N, Lund S, Hansen TK, Moller N, Jorgensen JO: Ghrelin infusion in humans induces acute insulin resistance and lipolysis independent of growth hormone signaling. *Diabetes* 57:3205–3210, 2008

76. Hanusch-Enserer U, Cauza E, Brabant G, Dunky A, Rosen H, Pacini G, Tüchler H, Prager R, Roden M: Plasma ghrelin in obesity before and after weight loss after laparoscopical adjustable gastric banding. *J Clin Endocrinol Metab* 89:3352–3358, 2004

77. Muscelli E, Mari A, Casolaro A, Camastra S, Seghieri G, Gastaldelli A, Holst JJ, Ferrannini E: Separate impact of obesity and glucose tolerance on the incretin effect in normal subjects and type 2 diabetic patients. *Diabetes* 57:1340–1348, 2008

78. Rubino F, Gagner M, Gentileschi P, Kini S, Fukuyama S, Feng J, Diamond E: The early effect of the Roux-en-Y gastric bypass on hormones involved in body weight regulation and glucose metabolism. *Ann Surg* 240:236–242, 2004

79. Holst JJ: The physiology of glucagon-like peptide 1. *Physiol Rev* 87:1409–1439, 2007

80. Flatt PR: Effective surgical treatment of obesity may be mediated by ablation of the lipogenic gut hormone gastric inhibitory polypeptide (GIP): evidence and clinical opportunity for development of new obesity-diabetes drugs? *Diab Vasc Dis Res* 4:151–153, 2007

81. Whitson BA, Leslie DB, Kellog TA, Maddaus MA, Buchwald H, Billington CJ, Ikramuddin S: Entero-endocrine changes after gastric bypass in diabetic and nondiabetic patients: a preliminary study. *J Surg Res* 141:31–39, 2007

82. Yamamoto H, Mori T, Tsuchihashi H, Akabori M, Naito H, Tani T: A possible role of GLP-1 in the pathophysiology of early dumping syndrome. *Dig Dis Sci* 50:2263–2267, 2005

83. Service GJ, Thompson GB, Service FJ, Andrews JC, Collazo-Clavell ML, Lloyd RV: Hyperinsulinemic hypoglycemia with nesidioblastosis after gastric-bypass surgery. *N Engl J Med* 353:249–254, 2005

84. Rubino F, Forgione A, Cummings DE, Vix M, Gnuli D, Mingrone G, Castagneto M, Marescaux J: The mechanism of diabetes control after gastrointestinal bypass surgery reveals a role of the proximal small intestine in the pathophysiology of type 2 diabetes. *Ann Surg* 244:741–749, 2006

85. Strader AD, Vahl TP, Jandacek RJ, Woods SC, D'Alessio DA, Seeley RJ: Weight loss through ileal transposition is accompanied by increased ileal hormone secretion and synthesis in rats. *Am J Physiol Endocrinol Metab* 288:E447–E453, 2005

86. DePaula AL, Macedo ALV, Rassi N, Machado CA, Schraibman V, Silva LQ, and Halpern, H: Laparoscopic treatment of type 2 diabetes mellitus for patients with a body mass index less than 35. *Surg Endosc* 22:706–716, 2008

87. Manfredini G, Ermini M, Scopsi L, Bonaguidi F, Ferrannini E: Internal biliary diversion improves glucose tolerance in the rat. *Am J Physiol* 249:G519–G527, 1985

88. Greco AV, Mingrone G, Giancaterini A, Manco M, Morroni M, Cinti S, Granzotto M, Vettor R, Camastra S, Ferrannini E: Insulin resistance in morbid obesity: reversal with intramyocellular fat depletion. *Diabetes* 51:144–151, 2002

89. McGarry JD: Banting lecture 2001: dysregulation of fatty acid metabolism in the etiology of type 2 diabetes. *Diabetes* 51:7–18, 2002

First-Phase Insulin Secretion Restoration and Differential Response to Glucose Load Depending on the Route of Administration in Type 2 Diabetic Subjects After Bariatric Surgery

Serenella Salinari, dsc[1]
Alessandro Bertuzzi, dsc[2]
Simone Asnaghi, msc[1]

Caterina Guidone, md[3]
Melania Manco, md[4]
Geltrude Mingrone, md, phd[3]

OBJECTIVE — The purpose of this study was to elucidate the mechanisms of diabetes reversibility after malabsorptive bariatric surgery.

RESEARCH DESIGN AND METHODS — Peripheral insulin sensitivity and β-cell function after either intravenous (IVGTT) or oral glucose tolerance (OGTT) tests and minimal model analysis were assessed in nine obese, type 2 diabetic subjects before and 1 month after biliopancreatic diversion and compared with those in six normal-weight control subjects. Insulin-dependent whole-body glucose disposal was measured by the euglycemic clamp, and glucose-dependent insulinotropic polypeptide (GIP) and glucagon-like peptide-1 (GLP-1) were also measured.

RESULTS — The first phase of insulin secretion after the IVGTT was fully normalized after the operation. The disposition index from OGTT data was increased about 10-fold and became similar to the values found in control subjects, and the disposition index from IVGTT data increased about 3.5-fold, similarly to what happened after the euglycemic clamp. The area under the curve (AUC) for GIP decreased about four times (from $3,000 \pm 816$ to 577 ± 155 pmol$\cdot$l$^{-1}\cdot$min, $P < 0.05$). On the contrary, the AUC for GLP1 almost tripled (from 150.4 ± 24.4 to 424.4 ± 64.3 pmol$\cdot$l$^{-1}\cdot$min, $P < 0.001$). No significant correlation was found between GIP or GLP1 percent changes and modification of the sensitivity indexes independently of the route of glucose administration.

CONCLUSIONS — Restoration of the first-phase insulin secretion and normalization of insulin sensitivity in type 2 diabetic subjects after malabsorptive bariatric surgery seem to be related to the reduction of the effect of some intestinal factor(s) resulting from intestinal bypass.

Diabetes Care 32:375–380, 2009

In 1987, Pories et al. (1) published a stunning observation that 99% of morbidly obese patients with frank type 2 diabetes or impaired glucose tolerance who had undergone Roux-en-Y gastric bypass (RYGB) became and remained euglycemic after surgery. Most interestingly, these authors reported that the patients were converted to euglycemia within 10 days, even if they had required large doses of insulin.

Subsequently, we (2,3) and other authors (4) have found that either restrictive or malabsorptive bariatric surgery is effective in improving/resolving type 2 diabetes. In particular, using the euglycemic hyperinsulinemic clamp we have demonstrated that insulin sensitivity was normalized after malabsorptive bariatric surgery in both obese type 2 diabetic (2) and obese normotolerant subjects.

We theorized that the normalization of insulin sensitivity that occurs very early after biliopancreatic diversion (BPD) before a significant weight loss can occur (2) may be dependent on the hormonal changes related to the nutrient diversion from the duodenum, the entire jejunum, and the proximal portion of the ileum. In fact, the enteroendocrine cells are largely found in these tracts of the small intestine.

Two main hypotheses have been advanced up to now to explain which part of the small intestine is implicated in the reversibility of diabetes. The first, known as the hindgut hypothesis (5), holds that diabetes control results from accelerated delivery of nutrients in the distal small intestine. The second, the so-called foregut hypothesis, states that the exclusion of duodenum and jejunum from nutrient transit might prevent the secretion of a putative signal that promotes insulin resistance (2,6). The balance between the stimulatory action on insulin secretion exerted by incretins and the anti-incretin effect might allow a finer control of glucose disposal.

To test the hypothesis that an imbalance in the release of intestinal hormone(s) can determine insulin resistance and that after BPD secretion of intestinal hormone(s) is reduced, allowing normalization of insulin sensitivity with subsequent β-cell glucose sensitivity improvement, we assessed peripheral insulin sensitivity and β-cell function after either an intravenous or oral glucose tolerance test in nine obese, type 2 diabetic subjects compared with those in six normal-weight age- and sex-matched control subjects. To further support our results, insulin-dependent whole-body glucose disposal was also measured by the euglycemic clamp.

From the [1]Department of Systems Analysis and Informatics, University of Rome "La Sapienza," Rome, Italy; [2]Institute of Systems Analysis and Computer Science, Consiglio Nazionale delle Ricerche, Rome, Italy; [3]Institute of Internal Medicine, Catholic University, School of Medicine, Rome, Italy; and [4]Liver Unit, Bambino Gesù Hospital and Research Institute, Rome, Italy.

Corresponding author: Serenella Salinari, salinari@dis.uniroma1.it.

Received 15 July 2008 and accepted 19 November 2008.

Published ahead of print at http://care.diabetesjournals.org on 25 November 2008. DOI: 10.2337/dc08-1314.

RESEARCH DESIGN AND METHODS

Nine (five women and four men) morbidly obese (BMI 51.7 ± 8.1 kg/m^2, age 41 ± 9 years [mean ± SD]), type 2 diabetic patients and six normotolerant (according to the American Diabetes Association criteria [7]) sex- and age-matched volunteers (three women and three men, BMI 24.6 ± 1.3 kg/m^2, age 39 ± 7 years) were studied. The patients were all characterized as having type 2 diabetes according to the American Diabetes Association criteria. A1C ranged from 7.5 to 9.5%.

At the time of the baseline study, all subjects were consuming a diet with the following average composition: 60% carbohydrate, 30% fat, and 10% protein (~1 g/kg body weight). This dietary regimen was maintained for 1 week before the study. In all patients, an oral glucose tolerance test (OGTT), an intravenous glucose tolerance test (IVGTT), and a euglycemic hyperinsulinemic clamp (EHC) were randomly performed within 1 month before surgery and 1 month after surgery. The healthy volunteers also underwent the same tests. All patients received the same parenteral nutrition regimen (~7,100 kJ/day) during the first 6 days after surgery; then they were free to consume a normal diet.

The study protocol was approved by the institutional ethics committee of the Catholic University of Rome. The nature and purpose of the study were carefully explained to all subjects before they provided their written consent to participate.

Body composition

On a separate day, total body water (TBW) was determined using 0.19 MBq ^{3}H$_2$O in 5 ml of saline administered as an intravenous bolus injection. Blood samples were drawn before and 3 h after the injection. Radioactivity was determined in duplicate on 0.5 ml plasma in a β-scintillation counter (model 1600TR; Canberra-Packard, Meriden, CT). Corrections were made for nonaqueous hydrogen exchange. Water density at body temperature was assumed to be 0.99371 kg/l. TBW (kilograms) was computed as ^{3}H$_2$O dilution space (liters) × 0.95 × 0.99371. Fat-free mass (FFM) was obtained by dividing TBW by 0.732 (8).

OGTT

After an overnight fast, a standard 75-g OGTT was performed in each patient at baseline and within 1 month after surgery as well as in each volunteer, with blood sampling at 0, 30, 60, 90, 120, 150, 180, and 240 min. Samples were placed in chilled tubes, and plasma was separated within 20 min and stored at −70°C.

IVGTT

An IVGTT was performed preoperatively and within 1 month postoperatively. At 8:00–9:00 A.M., after a 12-h overnight fast, an intravenous catheter was placed in one antecubital vein and an intravenous bolus of 0.33 g glucose/kg body weight as 50% water solution was injected in the contralateral antecubital vein. Blood samples were obtained at −15, −5, 2, 4, 6, 8, 10, 12, 14, 16, 18, 20, 25, 30, 40, 50, 60, 70, 80, 100, 120, 140, 160, 180, and 240 min relative to the start of dextrose injection. Samples were placed in chilled tubes, and plasma was separated within 20 min and stored at −70°C.

EHC

Peripheral insulin sensitivity was evaluated by the EHC (9) at baseline and within 4 weeks after surgery. After a cannula was inserted in a dorsal hand vein for sampling arterialized venous blood and another in the antecubital fossa of the contralateral arm for infusions, the subjects rested in the supine position for at least 1 h. They were placed with one hand warmed in a heated-air box set at 60°C to obtain arterialized blood samples. Insulin sensitivity, as the total insulin-mediated glucose uptake, was determined during a primed constant infusion of insulin at the rate of 6 pmol·min^{-1}·kg^{-1}. To maintain the glycemia in a normal range, rapid insulin and potassium phosphate in saline were infused overnight before BPD. The plasma glucose concentration was clamped at 5.1 ± 0.5 mmol/l (mean ± SD) before and at 3.9 ± 0.4 mmol/l after BPD, respectively, throughout the insulin infusion by means of a variable glucose infusion and blood glucose determinations every 5 min. Insulin sensitivity was determined during the last 40 min of the clamp by computing the whole-body glucose uptake (micromoles per minute per kilogram of FFM) or the clearance rate (milliliters per minute per kilogram of FFM) during steady-state euglycemic hyperinsulinemia.

BPD

This malabsorptive surgical procedure (2) consists of an ~60% distal gastric resection with stapled closure of the duodenal stump. The residual volume of the stomach is about 300 ml. The small bowel is transected at 2.5 m from the ileocecal valve, and its distal end is anastomosed to the remaining stomach. The proximal end of the ileum, comprising the remaining small bowel (involved in carrying biliopancreatic juice but excluded from food transit), is anastomosed in an end-to-side fashion to the bowel, 50 cm proximal to the ileocecal valve. Consequently, the total length of absorbing bowel is reduced to 250 cm, the final 50 cm of which, the so-called common channel, represents the site where ingested food and biliopancreatic juices mix.

Analytical procedures

Plasma glucose was measured by the glucose oxidase technique on a Beckman glucose analyzer (Beckman, Fullerton, CA). Plasma insulin was assayed by a microparticle enzyme immunoassay (Abbott, Pasadena, CA) with sensitivity of 1 μU/ml and intra-assay coefficient of variation (CV) of 6.6%. C-peptide was assayed by radioimmunoassay (MYRIA; Technogenetics, Milan, Italy); this assay has a minimal detectable concentration of 17 pmol/l and intra-assay and inter-assay CVs of 3.3–5.7 and 4.6–5.3%, respectively.

Total glucose-dependent insulinotropic polypeptide (GIP) was measured by ELISA (Linco). The assay is 100% specific for GIP 1–42 and GIP 3–42 and does not cross-react with glucagon-like peptide (GLP)-1, GLP-2, oxyntomodulin, or glucagon. The intra-assay and inter-assay CVs were 3.0–8.8 and 1.8–6.1%, respectively. Active GLP-1, an indicator of potential action, was measured by ELISA (Linco). The intra-assay and inter-assay CVs were 3–7 and 7–8%, respectively. The assay is 100% specific for GLP-1(7–36) and GLP-1(7–37) and does not react with GLP-1(9–36), glucagon, or GLP-2.

Mathematical model

The OGTT and IVGTT minimal models (10) were used to compute the insulin sensitivity (S_I). The indexes of β-cell sensitivity to glucose for the IVGTT (the first-phase β-cell sensitivity, Φ_1, and the second-phase sensitivity, Φ_2) and for the OGTT (the dynamic β-cell sensitivity, Φ_d, the static sensitivity, Φ_s, and the total sensitivity, Φ) were computed by the C-peptide minimal model as proposed by Toffolo et al. (11) and Breda et al. (12). The disposition index (DI) was computed as $\Phi \times S_I$. The model parameters were estimated by minimization of a weighted least-squares index using a constrained

Levenberg-Marquardt minimization routine of the MATLAB library. The standard errors of the estimates of individual parameters were evaluated by the Jackknife method (3), and the coefficients of variation were found to be <20%.

Statistics

All of the data are expressed as means ± SEM unless otherwise specified. The Wilcoxon paired-sample test and ANOVA for repeated measurements, followed by the Tukey test, were used for intragroup and intergroup comparisons, respectively. Two-sided $P < 0.05$ was considered significant. Nonparametric Spearman correlations (SPSS for Windows version 10) were used to assess linear relationships between single variables.

RESULTS — A small, but significant, weight loss (from 153.1 ± 34.2 to 143.5 ± 32.8 kg [mean ± SD], $P < 0.01$) was observed 1 month after BPD.

The OGTT glucose incremental area under the curve (ΔAUC) significantly ($P < 0.02$) decreased after BPD from 0.74 ± 0.08 to $0.22 \pm 0.04 \times 10^3$ mmol/l · min, becoming not statistically different from that of control subjects. Insulin ΔAUC decreased from 3.83 ± 0.99 to $1.01 \pm 0.28 \times 10^4$ pmol · l^{-1} · min ($P < 0.02$), reaching a value comparable to that of healthy control subjects (NS). Finally, the C-peptide ΔAUC declined from 2.48 ± 0.35 to $1.10 \pm 0.34 \times 10^2$ nmol/l · min ($P < 0.02$); its value in control subjects was $1.71 \pm 0.36 \times 10^2$ nmol/l · min (NS).

In the IVGTT also, the ΔAUC of glucose significantly decreased from 0.63 ± 0.08 to $0.51 \pm 0.06 \times 10^3$ mmol · l^{-1} min ($P < 0.05$) (control subjects $0.31 \pm 0.02 \times 10^3$ mmol · l^{-1} · min, NS). Similarly, insulin ΔAUC decreased from 3.66 ± 0.65 to $1.90 \pm 0.27 \times 10^4$ pmol · l^{-1} · min ($P < 0.02$) (control subjects $0.50 \pm 0.06 \times 10^4$ pmol · l^{-1} · min). C-peptide ΔAUC did not change significantly (from 1.63 ± 0.28 to $1.54 \pm 0.50 \times 10^2$ nmol · l^{-1} · min, NS); however, the latter was not statistically dissimilar from that in control subjects ($0.85 \pm 0.16 \times 10^2$ nmol · l^{-1} · min, NS), probably as a consequence of a rather large SEM.

The estimates of the indexes computed by the oral and intravenous mathematical models are reported in Table 1. The first phase of insulin secretion was fully normalized after BPD, as shown in Table 1 by the marked increase of the Φ_1

index. Figure 1 shows the recovery of the first phase of the insulin secretion rate in the IVGTT. The dynamic sensitivity index also showed a tendency to increase after BPD.

Before BPD, the insulin sensitivity determined by the OGTT was significantly smaller than that found by the IVGTT or the euglycemic clamp (Table 1), with the M value increasing from 27.7 ± 6.4 to 77.9 ± 20.0 μmol · kg_{FFM}^{-1} · min^{-1} after BPD ($P < 0.0001$). However, 1 month after BPD, insulin sensitivity reached values comparable to those found in control subjects, independently of the glucose administration route. In particular, a threefold increase in the insulin sensitivity estimated by either the IVGTT minimal model or the EHC was observed, whereas the same index computed by the OGTT minimal model was raised six times ($P < 0.05$). The DI, calculated by the OGTT, was increased ~10-fold and became similar to the values found in control subjects, whereas the DI calculated by the IVGTT increased about 3.5 times.

The time courses of GIP and GLP-1 during the OGTT are reported in Fig. 2. GIP peaked earlier after than before BPD, i.e., 30 min compared with 60 min. The ΔAUC_{GIP} (mean ± SEM) decreased about four times, from $3,000 \pm 816$ pmol · l^{-1} · min preoperatively to 577 ± 155 pmol · l^{-1} · min postoperatively ($P < 0.05$). On the contrary, the ΔAUC_{GLP1} was almost tripled, from 150 ± 24 to 424 ± 64 pmol · l^{-1} · min ($P < 0.001$). The ΔAUC of both GLP1 and GIP in control subjects (392 ± 11 and 983 ± 77 pmol · l^{-1} · min, respectively) were not statistically different from the values observed in diabetic patients after BPD.

No significant correlation was found between the percent change in the AUCs of GIP and GLP-1 and the modification of the oral sensitivity index.

CONCLUSIONS — The principal findings of our study are that 1) the first-phase insulin secretion was restored 1 month after BPD (Φ_1), 2) the β-cell glucose sensitivity was fully normalized, 3)

Table 1—Estimates of the indexes computed by the oral and the intravenous mathematical models

	Control subjects	Diabetic subjects before BPD	Diabetic subjects after BPD
Indexes OGTT			
$S_I \times 10^2$ (ml · min^{-1} · kg_{FFM}^{-1} · $pmol^{-1}$ · l)	2.70 ± 0.98	0.64 ± 0.19	3.60 ± 0.97*
$S_{I\,post}/S_{I\,pre}$			6.3 ± 3.1
$\Phi_d \times 10^{-9}$	500 ± 140	203 ± 144	480 ± 365
$\Phi_s \times 10^{-9}$ (min^{-1})	39.2 ± 20.8	23.0 ± 10.0	32.0 ± 16.0
$\Phi \times 10^{-9}$ (min^{-1})	47.7 ± 24.3	25.9 ± 11.2	37.7 ± 12.0#
AUC_{ISR} (nmol · m^{-2})	33.4 ± 12.8	62.3 ± 28.4	37.2 ± 13.3¶
$DI \times 10^{-14}$ (dl · min^{-2} · kg_{FFM}^{-1} · $pmol^{-1}$ · l)	$1,197 \pm 599$	148 ± 51	$1,227 \pm 276$¶
Indexes IVGTT			
$S_I \times 10^2$ (ml · min^{-1} · kg_{FFM}^{-1} · $pmol^{-1}$ · l)	2.10 ± 0.80	1.04 ± 0.28	2.70 ± 0.60§
$S_{I\,post}/S_{I\,pre}$			2.7 ± 1.1
$\Phi_1 \times 10^{-9}$	242 ± 199	27.9 ± 17.1	164 ± 119§
$\Phi_2 \times 10^{-9}$ (min^{-1})	10.2 ± 2.9	10.0 ± 4.8	12.5 ± 8.5
$\Phi \times 10^{-9}$ (min^{-1})	16.6 ± 5.3	10.8 ± 5.2	16.5 ± 9.5#
AUC_{ISR} (nmol · m^{-2})	23.9 ± 3.7	43.9 ± 22.8	41.9 ± 21.7
$DI \times 10^{-14}$ (dl · min^{-2} · kg_{FFM}^{-1} · $pmol^{-1}$ · l)	341 ± 124	118 ± 78	453 ± 318§
Indexes EHC			
$S_I \times 10^2$ (ml · min^{-1} · kg_{FFM}^{-1} · $pmol^{-1}$ · l)		1.4 ± 0.7	4.5 ± 1.5
$S_{I\,post}/S_{I\,pre}$			3.5 ± 1.2

Data are means ± SD. OGTT (after/before): *$P < 0.005$; #$P < 0.05$; ¶$P < 0.02$. Diabetic subjects after BPD/control subjects: NS. IVGTT (after/before): §$P < 0.01$; #$P < 0.05$. Diabetic subjects after BPD/control subjects: NS. EHC: S_I before BPD is significantly different from S_I (OGTT) ($P < 0.001$). S_I (OGTT) and S_I (IVGTT) before BPD are significantly different ($P < 0.05$); S_I (EHC), S_I (OGTT), and S_I (IVGTT) after BPD are not significantly different.

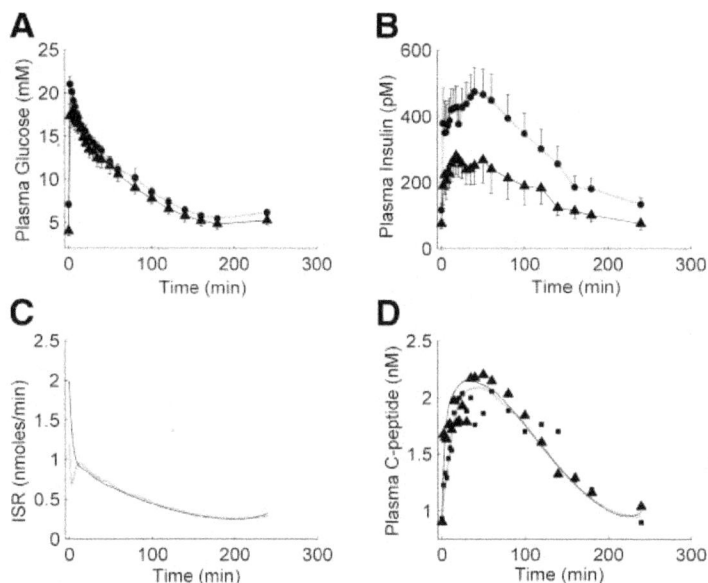

Figure 1— *IVGTT data (mean ± SEM). Glucose (A) and insulin (B) plasma concentrations before (gray shaded line) and after (solid line) BPD. Insulin secretion rate (ISR) (C) and C-peptide data points with the fitting curves superimposed (D). Before BPD: gray shaded lines and ■; after BPD: solid lines and ▲. Because of the overlapping of SEM bars, only mean values of C-peptide data are reported.*

the DI was normalized thanks to the normalization of insulin sensitivity and the consequent reduced requirement of insulin secretion, and 4) the increase in the insulin sensitivity estimated by the OGTT minimal model was larger than that estimated by the IVGTT minimal model.

The association of β-cell dysfunction with insulin resistance represents the main pathophysiological defect responsible for the development of type 2 diabetes. The β-cell function in type 2 diabetes is characterized by a progressive decline, from a net reduction to the disappearance of the first phase of glucose-induced insulin secretion to the impairment of the second-phase insulin secretion. The early insulin response disappears, even in the early stages of the disease, when fasting glucose concentrations

are only slightly higher than normal. This defect is important because first-phase insulin secretion seems to have the greatest impact on postprandial plasma glucose excursions (13), determining postmeal hyperglycemia.

Actually, the causes of this β-cell dysfunction are not completely known. Autopsy studies have shown that <20–50% of the β-cells may have been lost after many years of disease (14). However, there is experimental evidence that a 65% partial pancreatectomy in dogs reduces the maximum secretive pancreatic insulin response, but that the residual pancreatic β-cells become more sensitive to glucose, thus providing partial compensation (15). Therefore, Porte and Kahn (16) noted that "the loss of β-cell function is dispropor-

tionately more important than the degree of β-cell loss." Furthermore, there is more recent evidence from the autopsy of type 2 diabetic patients that the β-cell mass is not significantly diminished in most patients and that β-cells maintain active insulin gene transcription and translation even in amyloid-containing islets. This finding suggests that the main defect resides in an abnormal coupling of insulin secretion to glycemia (17).

It is interesting to note that in the present investigation the first-phase insulin secretion impairment was reversible after BPD, when the body weight was reduced only on the order of ~6%. Briatore et al. (18) have recently reported that the acute insulin response (AIR) after IVGTT was significantly increased after BPD in morbidly obese, type 2 diabetic subjects. However, being based on insulin concentration, AIR does not correspond directly to the first phase of insulin secretion, as it also reflects the hepatic insulin extraction. Because the hepatic extraction differs depending on the pattern and amount of insulin release, AIR does not provide an independent assessment of insulin secretion. Furthermore, insulin clearance appeared to be significantly reduced before BPD, according to recently published findings (19).

Recently, Henquin et al. (20) clearly showed that the first-phase insulin secretion, which was absent in vivo in mice with a double knockout for islet antigen 2 and 2β (21), was fully restored in the islets of the same animals studied in vitro. Thus, these authors (20) suggested the existence of factors, extrinsic to the islets, that can inhibit the in vivo insulin response to an intraperitoneal glucose challenge. In analogy with the hypothesis of Henquin et al. (20), we suggest that a "factor" inhibiting insulin secretion can be produced in the small intestine and that the intestinal bypass, as occurs in BPD, can reduce/suppress its synthesis and/or delivery into the circulatory stream, allowing the restoration of the first-phase insulin secretion.

It has been shown that a 3-h synthetic GLP-1 infusion in type 2 diabetic individuals was able to increase the AIR after an IVGTT from 197 ± 97 to 1,141 ± 409 pmol · l⁻¹ · min, which, however, was still seven times lower than the levels reached in healthy control subjects (22). The corresponding circulating levels of GLP1 were on the order of 40–50 pmol/l. In our series, the

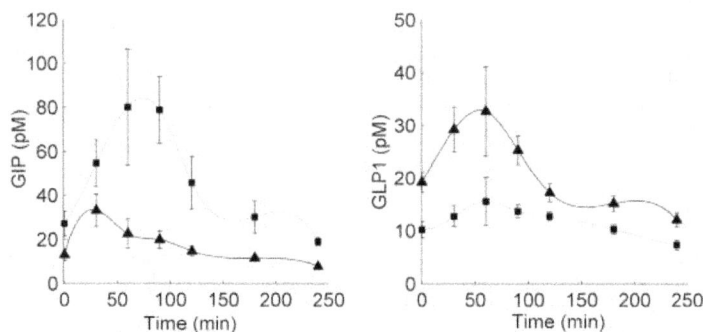

Figure 2— *GIP and GLP-1 concentrations during OGTT in diabetic patients before (■) and after (▲) BPD.*

first-phase insulin secretion was normalized, whereas the circulating GLP1 reached levels of about 35 pmol/l, suggesting that other mechanisms, such as the presence of still unrecognized intestinal factor/s can play a role in normalizing insulin secretion.

This very factor, or even another factor secreted by the small intestine, may also determine the insulin resistance. In fact, insulin sensitivity was fully normalized after BPD when a small but significant weight loss was achieved. In support of this hypothesis, we have found that the insulin-mediated glucose uptake was significantly higher after BPD when the glucose load was administered orally instead of intravenously. Dalla Man et al. (23) have shown that insulin action on glucose disposal estimated by the oral minimal model (S_I^*) was almost identical to that measured by a euglycemic hyperinsulinemic clamp (S_I^{*clamp}), suggesting that the glucose disposal component of the oral glucose minimal model was well described. Therefore, at least in healthy control subjects, the OGTT minimal model of glucose kinetics provides estimates of insulin action equivalent to those with the euglycemic clamp. This observation reinforces our findings that after BPD insulin sensitivity increases much more after an oral than an intravenous glucose challenge. Furthermore, insulin resistance before bariatric surgery was much higher after an oral than after an intravenous glucose load. Therefore, the anatomical changes induced by the operation led to a complete inversion of the insulin sensitivity response, depending on the route of glucose administration.

To our knowledge, very few data are found in the literature for insulin sensitivity after RYGB, and these were measured mostly by empirical methods and thus are not easily comparable to the present results. We reported previously (24) that insulin-mediated glucose uptake, measured by the EHC, did not change significantly after RYGB, whereas it was dramatically increased after BPD in normotolerant, morbidly obese patients, becoming even higher than that reported in healthy subjects. Burstein et al. (25) observed a significant increase in the glucose metabolic clearance rate, from a mean baseline value of 3.0 ± 1.6 to 6.7 ± 3.9 ml · kg^{-1} · min^{-1} after RYGB ($P < 0.02$), which,

however, as noted by the authors, was not completely reversed to normality.

We note that the GLP-1 plasma concentration was increased about threefold after BPD; however, neither the changes in GLP-1 plasma levels nor those in GIP explained the normalization of insulin sensitivity. This fact might suggest the existence of other intestinal factors in the control of insulin action in peripheral tissues, whose secretion is inhibited by surgery-induced nutrient diversion.

In summary, restoration of first-phase insulin secretion as well as normalization of the insulin sensitivity in type 2 diabetic subjects after malabsorptive bariatric surgery seems to be related to a reduction in the effect of some intestinal factor(s) as a consequence of intestinal bypass.

Acknowledgments— No potential conflicts of interest relevant to this article were reported.

References
1. Pories WJ, Caro JF, Flickinger EG, Meelheim HD, Swanson MS: The control of diabetes mellitus (NIDDM) in the morbidly obese with the Greenville gastric bypass. Ann Surg 206:316–323, 1987
2. Guidone C, Manco M, Valera-Mora E, Iaconelli A, Gniuli D, Mari A, Nanni G, Castagneto M, Calvani M, Mingrone G: Mechanisms of recovery from type 2 diabetes after malabsorptive bariatric surgery. Diabetes 55:2025–2031, 2006
3. Salinari S, Bertuzzi A, Iaconelli A, Manco M, Mingrone G: Twenty-four hour insulin secretion and beta cell NEFA oxidation in type 2 diabetic, morbidly obese patients before and after bariatric surgery. Diabetologia 51:1276–1284, 2008
4. Buchwald H, Avidor Y, Braunwald E, Jensen MD, Pories W, Fahrbach K, Schoelles K: Bariatric surgery: a systematic review and meta-analysis. JAMA 292:1724–1737, 2004
5. Strader AD, Vahl TP, Jandacek RJ, Woods SC, D'Alessio DA, Seeley RJ: Weight loss through ileal transposition is accompanied by increased ileal hormone secretion and synthesis in rats. Am J Physiol Endocrinol Metab 288:E447–E453, 2005
6. Rubino F: Is type 2 diabetes an operable intestinal disease? A provocative yet reasonable hypothesis. Diabetes Care 31: S290–S296, 2008
7. Report of the Expert Committee on the Diagnosis and Classification of Diabetes Mellitus. Diabetes Care 26:S5–S20, 2003
8. Sheng HP, Huggins RA: A review of body composition studies with emphasis on to-

tal body water and fat. Am J Clin Nutr 32: 630–647, 1979
9. DeFronzo RA, Tobin JD, Andres R: Glucose clamp technique: a method for quantifying insulin secretion and resistance. Am J Physiol 237:E214–E223, 1979
10. Caumo A, Bergman RN, Cobelli C: Insulin sensitivity from meal tolerance test in normal subjects: a minimal model index. J Clin Endocrinol Metab 85:4396–4402, 2000
11. Toffolo G, Cefalu WT, Cobelli C: β-Cell function during insulin-modified intravenous glucose tolerance test successfully assessed by the C-peptide minimal model. Metabolism 48:1162–1166, 1999
12. Breda E, Cavaghan MK, Toffolo G, Polonsky KS, Cobelli C: Oral glucose tolerance test minimal model indexes of β-cell function and insulin sensitivity. Diabetes 50:150–158, 2001
13. Bruce DG, Chisholm DJ, Storlien LH, Kraegen EW: Physiological importance of deficiency in early prandial insulin secretion in non-insulin-dependent diabetes. Diabetes 37:736–744, 1988
14. Ward WK, Bolgiano DC, McKnight B, Halter JB, Porte D Jr: Diminished B cell secretory capacity in patients with noninsulin-dependent diabetes mellitus. J Clin Invest 74:1318–1328, 1984
15. Ward WK, Wallum BJ, Beard JC, Taborsky GJ Jr, Porte D Jr: Reduction of glycemic potentiation: sensitive indicator of β-cell loss in partially pancreatectomized dogs. Diabetes 37:723–729, 1988
16. Porte D Jr, Kahn SE: β-Cell dysfunction and failure in type 2 diabetes: potential mechanisms. Diabetes 50:S160–S163, 2001
17. Sempoux C, Guiot Y, Dubois D, Moulin P, Rahier J: Human type 2 diabetes: morphological evidence for abnormal β-cell function. Diabetes 50:S172–S177, 2001
18. Briatore L, Salani B, Andraghetti G, Danovaro C, Sferrazzo E, Scopinaro N, Adami GF, Maggi D, Cordera R: Restoration of acute insulin response in T2DM subjects 1 month after biliopancreatic diversion. Obesity 16:77–81, 2008
19. Kotronen A, Juurinen L, Tiikkainen M, Vehavaara S, Yki-Järvinen H: Increased liver fat, impaired insulin clearance, and hepatic and adipose tissue insulin resistance in type 2 diabetes. Gastroenterology 135:122–130, 2008
20. Henquin JC, Nenquin M, Szollosi A, Kubosaki A, Notkins AL: Insulin secretion in islets from mice with a double knockout for the dense core vesicle proteins islet antigen-2 (IA-2) and IA-2β. J Endocrinol 196:573–581, 2008
21. Kubosaki A, Nakamura S, Notkins AL: Dense core vesicle proteins IA-2 and IA-2β: metabolic alterations in double knockout mice. Diabetes 54: S46–S51, 2005
22. Quddusi S, Vahl TP, Hanson K, Prigeon

RL, D'Alessio DA: Differential effects of acute and extended infusions of glucagon-like peptide-1 on first- and second-phase insulin secretion in diabetic and nondiabetic humans. *Diabetes Care* 26:791–798, 2003

23. Dalla Man C, Yarasheski KE, Caumo A, Robertson H, Toffolo G, Polonsky KS, Cobelli C: Insulin sensitivity by oral glucose minimal models: validation against clamp. *Am J Physiol Endocrinol Metab* 289:E954–E959, 2005

24. Muscelli E, Mingrone G, Camastra S, Manco M, Pereira JA, Pareja JC, Ferrannini E: Differential effect of weight loss on insulin resistance in surgically treated obese patients. *Am J Med* 118:51–57, 2005

25. Burstein R, Epstein Y, Charuzi I, Suessholz A, Karnieli E, Shapiro Y: Glucose utilization in morbidly obese subjects before and after weight loss by gastric bypass operation. *Int J Obes Relat Metab Disord* 19: 558–561, 1995

Short-Term Dynamics and Metabolic Impact of Abdominal Fat Depots After Bariatric Surgery

Ram Weiss, md, phd[1]
Liat Appelbaum, md[2]
Chaya Schweiger, msc, rd[3]
Idit Matot, md[4]
Naama Constantini, md[5]

Alon Idan, ms[5]
Noam Shussman, md[6]
Jacob Sosna, md[2]
Andrei Keidar, md[3,6]

OBJECTIVE — Bariatric surgery is gaining acceptance as an efficient treatment modality for obese patients. Mechanistic explanations regarding the effects of bariatric surgery on body composition and fat distribution are still limited.

RESEARCH DESIGN AND METHODS — Intra-abdominal and subcutaneous fat depots were evaluated using computed tomography in 27 obese patients prior to and 6 months following bariatric surgery. Associations with anthropometric and clinical changes were evaluated.

RESULTS — Excess weight loss 6 months following surgery was 47% in male and 42.6% in female subjects. Visceral fat and subcutaneous fat were reduced by 35% and 32%, respectively, in both sexes, thus the visceral-to-subcutaneous fat ratio remained stable. The strongest relation between absolute and relative changes in visceral and subcutaneous fat was demonstrated for the excess weight loss following the operations ($r \sim 0.6-0.7$), and these relations were strengthened further following adjustments for sex, baseline BMI, and fat mass. Changes in waist circumference and fat mass had no relation to changes in abdominal fat depots. All participants met the criteria of the metabolic syndrome at baseline, and 18 lost the diagnosis on follow-up. A lower baseline visceral-to-subcutaneous fat ratio (0.43 ± 0.15 vs. 0.61 ± 0.21, $P = 0.02$) was associated with clinical resolution of metabolic syndrome parameters.

CONCLUSIONS — The ratio between visceral and subcutaneous abdominal fat remains fairly constant 6 months following bariatric procedures regardless of sex, procedure performed, or presence of metabolic complications. A lower baseline visceral-to-abdominal fat ratio is associated with improvement in metabolic parameters.

Diabetes Care 32:1910–1915, 2009

B
ariatric surgery is gaining acceptance as an efficient treatment modality for patients with class 2 and class 3 obesity. Various bariatric procedures have been reported to lead not only to significant weight reduction but also to improvement or disappearance of the typical comorbidities of obese individuals (altered glucose metabolism, hypertension, and dyslipidemia) (1). These results, especially for long-term follow-up (2), seem very promising in comparison with lifestyle modifications and pharmacological interventions, which have limited long-term success against obesity (3,4). Despite these observations, mechanistic

explanations regarding the effects of such procedures on body composition, fat distribution, and hormonal alterations are still limited.

Abdominal fat is composed of subcutaneous fat and intra-abdominal fat (5). These two depots have a major influence on the metabolic phenotype of obese individuals and differ in their hormonal and cytokine secretion profile as well in their anatomical vascular drainage (6). Increased intra-abdominal fat is associated with an adverse metabolic profile and predicts the development of type 2 diabetes (7) and cardiovascular disease (8). The effects of weight loss induced by lifestyle modifications (9) and pharmacotherapy (10) on abdominal fat depots have been described, yet the short-term impact of bariatric procedures on these depots is unknown. Because bariatric procedures are characterized by a significant rapid weight loss that includes a substantial amount of fat during the first months after surgery, our aim was to test the impact of such surgery on abdominal fat depots 6 months after surgery. We further tested the relation of changes in the content of fat in the abdominal depots and improvement of the metabolic phenotype.

RESEARCH DESIGN AND METHODS — Twenty-seven morbidly obese adults undergoing bariatric surgery at the Hadassah Medical Center were recruited for this study. Procedures included laparoscopic gastric banding, sleeve gastrectomy, laparoscopic Roux en Y gastric bypass, and duodenal switch procedures. All patients met the criteria for bariatric operations as recommended by the National Institutes of Health Consensus Conference (11). Pre- and postoperative anthropometric measures included height to the nearest centimeter, weight to the nearest 0.1 kg, and waist (measured at the midpoint between the costal margin and the iliac crest) and hip circumference. Patients were seen at the obesity clinic before surgery and then monthly after surgery in the first month. Blood tests performed before and after surgery at 6 months included a blood count, general chemistry analysis, liver and kidney func-

From the [1]Department of Human Metabolism and Nutrition, Hebrew University School of Medicine, Jerusalem, Israel; the [2]Radiology Department, Hadassah Ein Kerem Medical Center, Jerusalem, Israel; the [3]Bariatric Surgery Service, Hadassah Ein Kerem Medical Center, Jerusalem, Israel; the [4]Department of Anesthesiology and Critical Care Medicine, Sourasky Medical Center, Tel Aviv University, Tel Aviv, Israel; the [5]Department of Orthopedic Surgery, The Hadassah-Hebrew University Medical Center, Jerusalem, Israel; and the [6]General Surgery Department, Hadassah Ein Kerem Medical Center, Jerusalem, Israel.

Corresponding author: Ram Weiss, ram.weiss@ekmd.huji.ac.il.

Received 24 May 2009 and accepted 1 July 2009.

Published ahead of print at http://care.diabetesjournals.org on 8 July 2009. DOI: 10.2337/dc09-0943. Clinical trial reg. no. NCT00431587, clinicaltrials.gov.

R.W. and L.A. contributed equally to this study.

Table 1—*Anthropometric parameters and abdominal fat depots before and after surgery*

	Men (n = 13)			Women (n = 14)		
	Before	After	P	Before	After	P
n		13			14	
Age (years)	49 ± 10			49 ± 11		0.96
Weight (kg)	134 ± 13	103 ± 11	<0.001	104 ± 18	82 ± 14	<0.001
Height (cm)	175 ± 9			157 ± 7		
BMI (kg/m^2)	43.7 ± 4.6	33.5 ± 3.2	<0.001	41.9 ± 5.4	33.1 ± 4.6	<0.001
Excess weight (kg)	66.0 ± 10.5	34.7 ± 8.8	<0.001	52.2 ± 15.1	30.2 ± 12.1	<0.001
Excess weight loss (%)		47 ± 13			42 ± 13	0.36
Fat mass (kg)	48.9 ± 6.1	31.6 ± 5.8	<0.001	51.2 ± 11.7	35.7 ± 9.5	<0.001
Fat mass lost (kg)		17.3			15.5	0.43
Waist circumference (cm)	135 ± 7	115 ± 12	<0.001	123 ± 13	104 ± 11	<0.001
Visceral fat (cm)	163 ± 40	102 ± 30	<0.001	126 ± 36	81 ± 21	<0.001
Subcutaneous fat (cm)	309 ± 52	206 ± 51	<0.001	306 ± 79	218 ± 85	<0.001
Visceral-to-subcutaneous ratio	0.54 ± 0.15	0.50 ± 0.12	0.37	0.44 ± 0.21	0.44 ± 0.27	0.99

Data are means ±SD.

tion tests, and lipid profiles. Abdominal fat depots were evaluated using computed tomography scans before and at 6 months after surgery. Visceral and subcutaneous adipose tissue cross-section areas were calculated using computer software specifically designed for area measurement (12). Body composition was assessed using bioelectrical impedance analysis (Tanita 305 body fat analyzer; Tanita, Tokyo, Japan). Clinical parameters related to the metabolic syndrome were evaluated using the Adult Treatment Panel III criteria (13). Resolution of these parameters was considered as drug discontinuation with normal measurements of fasting glucose, systolic and diastolic blood pressure, and normalization of triglyceride or HDL cholesterol levels. The study was approved by the institutional review board at the Hadassah Hebrew University Medical Center and registered in the National Institutes of Health Protocol Registration System.

Statistical analysis

Data are presented as means ± SD. Group comparisons between men/women and between those who lost the diagnosis of metabolic syndrome were performed using Wilcoxon's rank-sum test. $P < 0.05$ was considered significant. All analyses were performed using SPSS 15.0 for Windows.

RESULTS — Twenty-seven subjects underwent laparoscopic bariatric surgery that included Roux en Y gastric bypass (n = 14), sleeve gastrectomy (n = 7), laparoscopic gastric banding (n = 2), and duodenal switch (n = 4). Baseline and follow-up anthropometric characteristics of the groups according to sex are shown in Table 1. Participants had an excess body weight of 52.2 ± 15.1 kg (women) and 66.0 ± 10.5 kg (men) at baseline. Absolute weight loss and an excess weight loss at 6 months were 31.3 ± 9.6 kg and 47 ± 12% in men and 22.0 ± 8.7 kg and 42 ± 13% in women. In women, fat mass represented 55% of total weight loss, whereas in men it represented 70% of the total weight loss. Visceral fat was ~35% lower on follow-up compared with baseline in both sexes, whereas subcutaneous fat was ~32% lower on follow-up com-

pared with baseline in both sexes. Thus, the visceral-to-subcutaneous fat ratio remained stable after surgically induced weight loss despite the significant weight loss observed.

Clinical characteristics of study participants associated with the metabolic syndrome before and 6 months after surgery are shown in Table 2. All participants met the waist circumference threshold before surgery, and all men kept it on follow-up, whereas two women reduced their waist circumference below the threshold of 88 cm. Diabetes was present in 10 of 13 men and in 11 of 14 women before surgery and only 2 men and 4 women continued to take antihyperglycemic medications on follow-up. Similarly, significant improvements were observed in triglyceride levels and in the presence of hypertension. The prevalence of a low HDL cholesterol level did not change after surgery.

Relations of anthropometric changes and fat depots changes in study participants

The strongest relation between absolute and relative changes in visceral and subcutaneous fat was demonstrated for the excess weight loss after the operations ($r = \sim 0.6 - 0.7$), and this relation was strengthened further for subcutaneous fat after adjustment for sex, baseline BMI, and fat mass (Table 3). Changes in weight and BMI correlated with absolute changes in abdominal fat depots, and the relation with changes in subcutaneous fat were significantly strengthened after adjustment for sex, baseline BMI, and fat mass. Changes in waist circumference and in fat

Table 2—*Presence of metabolic syndrome criteria before and after surgery*

	Before surgery			After surgery		
	Men	Women	P	Men	Women	P
Hypertension	13/0	11/3	0.12	4/9	5/9	0.55
Diabetes	10/3	11/3	0.63	2/11	4/10	0.36
High triglyceride	11/2	10/4	0.36	2/11	3/11	0.53
Low HDL cholesterol	9/4	9/5	0.55	10/3	9/5	0.38
High waist circumference	13/13	14/14	1.0	13/13	12/2	0.25

Data are n.

Table 3—*Correlations between changes in anthropometric indices and changes in abdominal fat depots*

	Δ Weight (%)	Δ BMI (5)	Δ Waist circumference (cm)	Δ Fat mass (kg)	Δ Visceral (cm)	Δ Visceral (%)	Δ Subcutaneous (cm)	Δ Subcutaneous (%)
Excess weight loss (%)	0.75*	0.71*	0.31	0.51†	0.62*	0.63*	0.62*	0.71*
Adjusted	0.96*	0.99*	0.46	0.71†	0.58†	0.57†	0.73†	0.80*
Δ weight (%)		0.91*	0.60†	0.78*	0.50†	0.43†	0.53†	0.37
Adjusted		0.97*	0.48	0.69†	0.51	0.47	0.70*	0.78*
Δ BMI (%)			0.65†	0.77*	0.45†	0.46†	0.51*	0.32
Adjusted			0.48	0.72†	0.55†	0.55†	0.77*	0.82*
Δ waist circumference (cm)				0.38	0.03	0.03	−0.39	−0.11
Adjusted				0.12	−0.01	0.01	−0.38	−0.43
Δ fat mass (kg)					−0.18	−0.07	−0.05	0.13
Adjusted					−0.43	−0.47	−0.42	−0.43
Δ visceral (cm)						0.91*	0.59*	0.66*
Adjusted						0.88*	0.61†	0.47
Δ Visceral (%)							0.59*	0.64*
Adjusted							0.41	0.50
Δ subcutaneous (cm)								0.87*
Adjusted								0.96*

All changes are in their absolute value of change. Adjusted correlations are adjusted for sex, baseline BMI, and baseline fat mass. *$P < 0.001$; †$P < 0.01$.

mass had no relation to changes in abdominal fat depots.

Relation of changes in abdominal fat depots and metabolic parameters

All study subjects met the criteria of the metabolic syndrome before surgery, and 18 of them did not meet these criteria at follow-up. When comparing those who lost the diagnosis on follow-up with those who did not (Table 4), we found no sex or procedure differences between the groups, yet those who did not meet the criteria of the syndrome after surgery were significantly younger (45 ±

9 vs. 57 ± 10 years, $P = 0.01$). The baseline numbers of metabolic syndrome criteria, BMI, fat mass, and excess weight were comparable between the groups. BMI, excess weight loss, and fat mass after the surgery were similar between the groups. As shown in Fig. 1A, excess weight loss on the follow-up was comparable between those who met the criteria of the metabolic syndrome on follow-up and those who did not. The only significant baseline difference between the groups was in the absolute amount of visceral fat (Fig. 1B), which was greater in those who did not lose the diagnosis

(166 ± 49 vs. 132 ± 33 cm, $P = 0.04$). This difference translated to a significantly greater visceral-to-subcutaneous fat ratio (0.61 ± 0.21 vs. 0.43 ± 0.15, $P = 0.02$) (Fig. 1D). Similarly, both groups had similar amounts of subcutaneous (Fig. 1C) abdominal fat at baseline and a comparable reduction after surgery. Thus, all subjects lost a comparable significant amount of fat from both abdominal fat depots yet maintained a constant ratio between these depots.

CONCLUSIONS — This study demonstrates for the first time the early pattern of change in abdominal fat depots 6 months after bariatric procedures in severely obese subjects. The most consistent finding is that the ratio between visceral and subcutaneous abdominal fat remains fairly constant regardless of sex, procedure performed, or the presence of metabolic complications. Excess weight loss was associated with a reduction in fat in both abdominal fat depots more strongly than other anthropometric measures, whereas changes in waist circumference or fat mass had no relation with this reduction. A lower baseline visceral-to-abdominal fat ratio was the determinant of the improvement in metabolic parameters.

Lipid partitioning of specific fat depots in obese subjects is known to be associated with the overall metabolic phenotype (14,15). Specifically, intra-abdominal fat is associated with greater

Table 4—*Anthropometric parameters before surgery and their changes in those who lost the diagnosis of the metabolic syndrome compared with those who did not 6 months after surgery*

	Lost MS	Remained MS	P
n	18	9	
Age (years)	45 ± 9	57 ± 10	0.01
Sex (male/female)	9/9	4/5	0.55
Procedure (RYGB/LAGB/SG/DS)	9/0/5/4	5/2/2/0	0.10
MS score before	3.9 ± 0.2	4.4 ± 0.2	0.11
MS score after	1.8 ± 0.3	3.33 ± 0.5	<0.001
Weight before (kg)	120.7 ± 19.7	115.1 ± 25.7	0.46
Weight after (kg)	92.4 ± 15.1	92.3 ± 19.1	0.86
BMI before (kg/m²)	43.5 ± 5.3	41.2 ± 4.4	0.27
BMI after (kg/m²)	33.3 ± 4.0	33.1 ± 3.9	0.70
Excess weight (kg)	60.5 ± 13.6	55.6 ± 16.9	0.42
Excess weight loss (%)	46.6 ± 14.0	41.4 ± 10.8	0.99
Fat mass before (kg)	52.8 ± 10.2	46.2 ± 9.2	0.17
Fat mass after (kg)	34.9 ± 8.4	33.7 ± 9.3	0.71

Data are means ± SD. DS, duodenal switch; LAGB, laparoscopic gastric banding; MS, metabolic syndrome; RYGB, Roux en-Y gastric bypass; SG, sleeve gastrectomy.

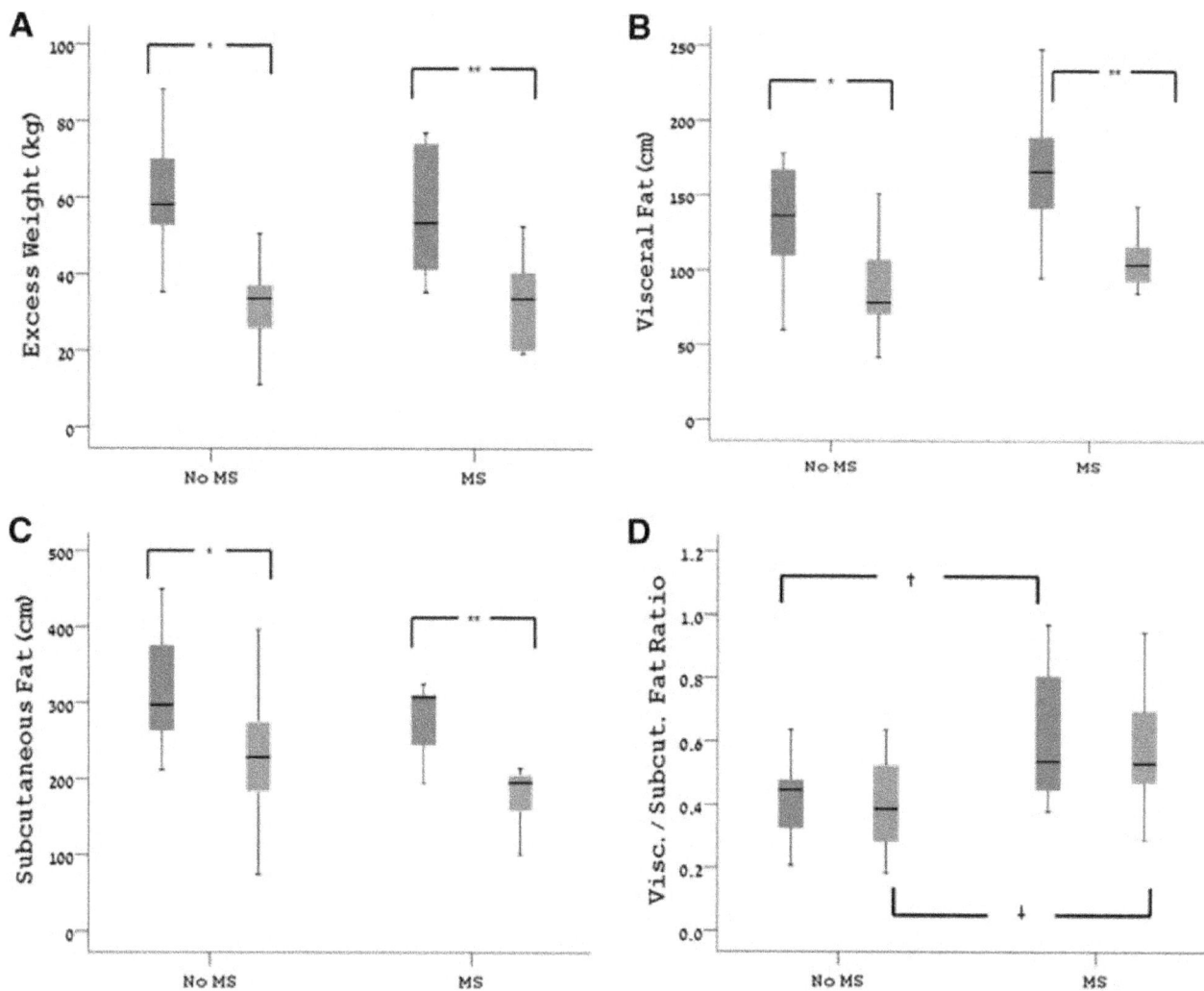

Figure 1—*Comparison of excess weight lost (A), visceral fat change (B), subcutaneous fat change (C), and the visceral-to-subcutaneous fat ratio (D) between those who lost the diagnosis of the metabolic syndrome (No MS) and those who did not (MS). *P < 0.001; **P < 0.01; †P = 0.03.*

insulin resistance and has long been described as a culprit for accelerated atherogenesis and altered glucose metabolism. Standard interventions for obese individuals consist of lifestyle modifications that include dietary changes and physical activity. Diet-induced modest weight loss has been shown to affect visceral fat preferentially, whereas with larger degrees of weight loss the effect was shown to be similar for both visceral and subcutaneous fat (16). For every 1 kg of diet-induced weight loss, the corresponding reduction in visceral fat expressed in absolute terms is $\sim$3–4 cm^2, and a 1-cm reduction in waist circumference corresponds to a 5-cm^2 reduction in visceral fat area (17). In our subjects, mean visceral fat area reduction was 53.1 ± 35 cm^2 (a reduction of $34.5 \pm 17.1\%$). Mean weight loss in 6 months was 26.4 ± 10.2 kg ($\sim$2

cm^2 or 1.32% of visceral fat/kg weight lost), whereas mean waist circumference reduction was 18.5 ± 9.2 cm ($\sim$ 3 cm^2 or 1.85% of visceral fat per cm waist circumference reduction). Importantly, the strongest relation of visceral fat changes was with the excess weight lost, whereas changes in waist circumference had no relation whatsoever with the reduction in visceral fat or subcutaneous fat. Our subjects were more severely obese and had a greater absolute weight loss than those described in the previous references, which may provide some explanation for the seemingly lower visceral fat reduction in relation to weight loss. Whereas previous studies have shown a preferential loss of visceral fat in the early phases after bariatric surgery (8–10 weeks) (18,19), minimal changes in peripheral insulin sensitivity were observed. These results

suggest that the ratio between abdominal and subcutaneous fat, which according to our data is rather stable, is one of the determinants of overall insulin sensitivity and of its clinical consequences.

Whether the absolute amount of visceral fat has a threshold above which metabolic derangements tend to occur or whether the ratio of visceral-to-subcutaneous fat is the main determinant of such derangements (or maybe both) is debatable. In both men and women, a value of 100 cm^2 of visceral fat has been shown to be associated with significant alterations in cardiovascular disease risk profile and a further deterioration in the metabolic profile was observed with values >130 cm^2 of visceral adipose tissue (20). Participants in our study had greater visceral fat before surgery than those described in previous studies, yet a significant number had an area of <100 cm^2 after the bariatric procedure, correlating well with the significant improvement in metabolic parameters (the mean visceral fat area in the group who lost the diagnosis of metabolic syndrome was 86.6 ± 26.5 cm^2).

On the other hand, a ratio of visceral-to-subcutaneous fat of 0.4 has been suggested to be a threshold value that signifies metabolic risk (21). Indeed, the patients who did not lose the diagnosis of the metabolic syndrome had a high visceral-to-subcutaneous fat ratio to begin with, and this ratio did not change despite significant weight loss. In comparison with exercise regimens, which have been reported to reduce the visceral-to-subcutaneous ratio by up to 33% (22), treatment with metformin showed no change in the relation of abdominal fat depots despite a significant weight loss (23) and thiazoladinediones reduced this ratio by way of increasing the amount of subcutaneous fat (24). It seems that rapid weight loss induced by bariatric surgical procedures, which can be considered a period of a very low calorie diet, induces a proportional decrease in both abdominal fat depots, resulting in a maintained ratio between them. Because both the absolute amount of visceral fat and the visceral-to-subcutaneous fat ratio are determinants of the clinical metabolic characteristics of obese individuals, a lower ratio at baseline probably raises the chances of clinical improvement because the ratio remains fairly constant due to proportional fat loss from both depots. However, the "visceral threshold" is probably crossed back to the tolerable range (25).

This study is limited by the modest sample size, short follow-up period, and the variability of procedures performed, which differ in their malabsorption component and may thus have a different impact on lipid partitioning after surgery. Therefore, although we were interested in the impact of surgically induced rapid weight loss on lipid depot distribution in general, specific procedures at different ages may differ in their overall impact. The findings raise the possibility of adding parameters in addition to BMI as indications and predictors of the metabolic response to bariatric procedures. Present indications for bariatric surgery are based (11) only on BMI and obesity-related comorbidity and disregard lipid partitioning patterns. Our findings suggest that baseline assessment of abdominal fat depots may add information regarding the

expected early clinical response, whereas changes in waist circumference correlate poorly with visceral fat reduction. Longer follow-up is still needed to determine whether the observed changes remain stable over longer periods.

Acknowledgments— No potential conflicts of interest relevant to this article were reported.

References

1. Buchwald H, Avidor Y, Braunwald E, Jensen MD, Pories W, Fahrbach K, Schoelles K. Bariatric surgery: a systematic review and meta-analysis. JAMA. 2004;292:1724–1737
2. Sjöström L, Narbro K, Sjöström CD, Karason K, Larsson B, Wedel H, Lystig T, Sullivan M, Bouchard C, Carlsson B, Bengtsson C, Dahlgren S, Gummesson A, Jacobson P, Karlsson J, Lindroos AK, Lönroth H, Näslund I, Olbers T, Stenlöf K, Torgerson J, Agren G, Carlsson LM, Swedish Obese Subjects Study. Effects of bariatric surgery on mortality in Swedish obese subjects. N Engl J Med 2007;357:741–752
3. Norris SL, Zhang X, Avenell A, Gregg E, Brown TJ, Schmid CH, Lau J. Long-term non-pharmacologic weight loss interventions for adults with type 2 diabetes. Cochrane Database Syst Rev 2005;2:CD004095
4. Li Z, Maglione M, Tu W, Mojica W, Arterburn D, Shugarman LR, Hilton L, Suttorp M, Solomon V, Shekelle PG, Morton SC. Meta-analysis: pharmacologic treatment of obesity. Ann Intern Med 2005;142:532–546
5. Wajchenberg BL. Subcutaneous and visceral adipose tissue: their relation to the metabolic syndrome. Endocr Rev 2000;21:697–738
6. Mårin P, Andersson B, Ottosson M, Olbe L, Chowdhury B, Kvist H, Holm G, Sjöström L, Björntorp P. The morphology and metabolism of intraabdominal adipose tissue in men. Metabolism 1992;41:1242–1248
7. Bray GA, Jablonski KA, Fujimoto WY, Barrett-Connor E, Haffner S, Hanson RL, Hill JO, Hubbard V, Kriska A, Stamm E, Pi-Sunyer FX, Diabetes Prevention Program Research Group. Relation of central adiposity and body mass index to the development of diabetes in the Diabetes Prevention Program. Am J Clin Nutr 2008;87:1212–1218
8. Fox CS, Massaro JM, Hoffmann U, Pou KM, Maurovich-Horvat P, Liu CY, Vasan RS, Murabito JM, Meigs JB, Cupples LA, D'Agostino RB Sr, O'Donnell CJ. Abdominal visceral and subcutaneous adipose tissue compartments: association with metabolic risk factors in the Framingham Heart Study. Circulation 2007;116:39–48
9. Ross R, Dagnone D, Jones PJ, Smith H, Paddags A, Hudson R, Janssen I. Reduc-

tion in obesity and related comorbid conditions after diet-induced weight loss or exercise-induced weight loss in men: a randomized, controlled trial. Ann Intern Med 2000;133:92–103
10. Després JP, Ross R, Boka G, Alméras N, Lemieux I, ADAGIO-Lipids Investigators. Effect of rimonabant on the high-triglyceride/low-HDL-cholesterol dyslipidemia, intraabdominal adiposity, and liver fat: the ADAGIO-Lipids trial. Arterioscler Thromb Vasc Biol 2009;29:416–423
11. NIH Consensus Development Panel. Gastrointestinal surgery for severe obesity. Ann Intern Med 1991;115:956–961
12. Chowdhury B, Sjöström L, Alpsten M, Kostanty J, Kvist H, Löfgren R. A multicompartment body composition technique based on computerized tomography. Int J Obes Relat Metab Disord 1994;18:219–234
13. National Institutes of Health. *Third Report of the National Cholesterol Education Program Expert Panel on Detection, Evaluation, and Treatment of High Blood Cholesterol in Adults (Adult Treatment Panel III).* Bethesda, MD, National Institutes of Health; 2001 (NIH publ. no. 01-3670)
14. Després JP, Lemieux I. Abdominal obesity and metabolic syndrome. Nature 2006;444:881–887
15. Weiss R. Fat distribution and storage: how much, where, and how? Eur J Endocrinol 2007;157(Suppl. 1):S39–S45
16. Chaston TB, Dixon JB. Factors associated with percent change in visceral versus subcutaneous abdominal fat during weight loss: findings from a systematic review. Int J Obes (Lond) 2008;32:619–628
17. Ross R. Effects of diet- and exercise-induced weight loss on visceral adipose tissue in men and women. Sports Med 1997;24:55–64
18. Phillips ML, Lewis MC, Chew V, Kow L, Slavotinek JP, Daniels L, Valentine R, Toouli J, Thompson CH. The early effects of weight loss surgery on regional adiposity. Obes Surg 2005;15:1449–1455
19. Busetto L, Tregnaghi A, Bussolotto M, Sergi G, BeninCà P, Ceccon A, Giantin V, Fiore D, Enzi G. Visceral fat loss evaluated by total body magnetic resonance imaging in obese women operated with laparoscopic adjustable silicone gastric banding. Int J Obes Relat Metab Disord 2000;24:60–69
20. Lamarche B. Effects of diet and physical activity on adiposity and body fat distribution: implications for the prevention of cardiovascular disease. Nutr Res Rev 1993;6:137–159
21. Fujioka S, Matsuzawa Y, Tokunaga K, Tarui S. Contribution of intra-abdominal fat accumulation to the impairment of glucose and lipid metabolism in human obesity. Metabolism 1987;36:54–59
22. Boudou P, de Kerviler E, Erlich D, Vexiau

P, Gautier JF. Exercise training-induced triglyceride lowering negatively correlates with DHEA levels in men with type 2 diabetes. Int J Obes Relat Metab Disord 2001;25:1108–1112

23. Lord J, Thomas R, Fox B, Acharya U, Wilkin T. The effect of metformin on fat distribution and the metabolic syndrome in women with polycystic ovary syndrome—a randomised, double-blind, placebo-controlled trial. BJOG 2006;113: 817–824

24. Yang X, Smith U. Adipose tissue distribution and risk of metabolic disease: does thiazolidinedione-induced adipose tissue redistribution provide a clue to the answer? Diabetologia 2007;50:1127–1139

25. Kral JG. Surgical treatment of regional adiposity: lipectomy versus surgically induced weight loss. Acta Med Scand Suppl 1988;723:225–231

Bariatric Surgery Reduces Oxidative Stress by Blunting 24-h Acute Glucose Fluctuations in Type 2 Diabetic Obese Patients

Raffaele Marfella, md, phd[1]
Michelangela Barbieri, md, phd[1]
Roberto Ruggiero, md[2]
Maria Rosaria Rizzo, md, phd[1]

Rodolfo Grella, md, phd[1]
Anna Licia Mozzillo, md[2]
Ludovico Docimo, md[2]
Giuseppe Paolisso, md, phd[1]

OBJECTIVE — We evaluated the efficacy of malabsorptive bariatric surgery on daily blood glucose fluctuations and oxidative stress in type 2 diabetic obese patients.

RESEARCH DESIGN AND METHODS — The 48-h continuous subcutaneous glucose monitoring was assessed in type 2 diabetic patients before and 1 month after biliopancreatic diversion (BPD) ($n = 36$), or after diet-induced equivalent weight loss ($n = 20$). The mean amplitude of glycemic excursions and oxidative stress (nitrotyrosine) were evaluated during continuous subcutaneous glucose monitoring. During a standardized meal, glucagon-like peptide (GLP)-1, glucagon, and insulin were measured.

RESULTS — Fasting and postprandial glucose decreased equally in surgical and diet groups. A marked increase in GLP-1 occurred during the interprandial period in surgical patients toward the diet group ($P < 0.01$). Glucagon was more suppressed during the interprandial period in surgical patients compared with the diet group ($P < 0.01$). Mean amplitude of glycemic excursions and nitrotyrosine levels decreased more after BPD than after diet ($P < 0.01$).

CONCLUSIONS — Oxidative stress reduction after biliopancreatic diversion seems to be related to the regulation of glucose fluctuations resulting from intestinal bypass.

Diabetes Care 33:287–289, 2010

C ogent evidence suggests that acute fluctuations of glucose around a mean value over a daily period of intermittent hyperglycemia and obesity, activating oxidative stress, might play an important role in cardiovascular disease in type 2 diabetic patients (1–3). As a consequence, it is strongly suggested that a global antidiabetic strategy should be aimed at reducing the different components of dysglycemia (A1C, fasting and postprandial glucose, and glucose variability). Although improvements in glycemic control have been observed in subjects with type 2 diabetes after malabsorptive bariatric surgery

(4), there are no studies that have examined the surgery effects on the glucose fluctuations over a daily period and on oxidative stress production. Because the regulation strategy of daily glucose fluctuations attempts to normalize incretin secretions over a daily period (5), this study was conducted to evaluate the efficacy of biliopancreatic diversion (BPD), as malabsorptive bariatric surgery, on glucagon-like peptide (GLP)-1 and glucagon as well as on oxidative stress activation (nitrotyrosine) and daily blood glucose fluctuations during continuous subcutaneous glucose monitoring in type 2 diabetic obese patients.

RESEARCH DESIGN AND METHODS —
A total of 56 obese type 2 diabetic patients (BMI >40 kg/m^2), eligible candidates for BPD, not on insulin, exenatide, or dipeptidyl peptidase 4 inhibitors, were studied. All participants signed an informed consent, approved by our institution. One group was studied before and 1 month after GBP (surgical group, $n = 36$). A second group, fulfilling the same recruitment criteria, was studied before and after a 10-kg diet-induced weight loss (diet group, $n = 20$). All participants have voluntarily chosen to undergo to surgery or dietary intervention. In the diet group, the mean recommended daily caloric intake was 1,100 kcal (from 1,050 to 1,250 kcal). The recommended dietary regimen was 55% carbohydrates, 30% lipid, and 15% protein, and this regimen was followed on an outpatient basis until 10-kg weight loss. The surgical group had undergone BPD that was performed as previously described (6). All patients received the same parenteral nutrition regimen (1,400 kcal/day) during the first 6 days after surgery; then the same daily caloric intake of the diet group was recommended. Continuous subcutaneous glucose monitoring measurements (Glucoday, Menarini, Italy) were monitored, over a period of 3 consecutive days, at baseline and within 1 month after surgery in the surgical group and after a 10-kg diet-induced weight loss in the diet group. The mean amplitude of glycemic excursions (MAGE), which has been described by Service et al. (7), was used for assessing glucose fluctuations during the fasting plasma glucose (FPG), postprandial plasma glucose (PPG), diurnal and nocturnal interprandial periods on study days 1 and 2. Standardized meal tests with 24-h sampling comprising three mixed meals were performed on days 1, 2, and 3 (breakfast: 310 kcal; lunch: 440 kcal; dinner: 350 kcal). During the standardized meal, glucose, GLP-1 (enzyme-linked immunosorbent assay [ELISA], D.B.A., Santa Cruz Biotechnology, Milan, Italy), glucagon

From the [1]Department of Geriatrics and Metabolic Diseases, Second University of Naples, Naples, Italy; and the [2]Department of Surgery, Second University of Naples, Naples, Italy.

Corresponding author: Raffaele Marfella, raffaele.marfella@unina2.it.

Received 22 July 2009 and accepted 24 October 2009. Published ahead of print at http://care.diabetesjournals.org on 4 November 2009. DOI: 10.2337/dc09-1343.

Table 1—*Clinical characteristics and metabolic profile before and after 1 month after biliopancreatic diversion or 10-kg weight loss*

	Biliopancreatic diversion group			Diet group		
	Baseline	After 1 month	P	Baseline	After 10-kg weight loss	P
Age (years)	45 ± 8	—	—	46 ± 6	—	—
Male/female sex (n)	16/20	16/20	—	9/11	9/11	—
BMI (kg/m^2)	43.7 ± 2.9	39.1 ± 3.2	0.01	43.6 ± 3.1	38.9 ± 3.3	0.01
Systolic blood pressure (mmHg)	120 ± 12	119 ± 13	NS	121 ± 13	120 ± 10	NS
Diastolic blood pressure (mmHg)	79 ± 5	78 ± 3	NS	80 ± 4	79 ± 3	NS
Diabetes duration (years)	3.2 ± 4	—	—	3.1 ± 6	—	—
Risk factors						
Hypertension	9 (25)	—	—	5 (25)	—	—
Hypercholesterolemia	4 (11)	—	—	2 (10)	—	—
Smokers	4 (11)	—	—	2 (10)	—	—
Laboratory						
Fasting glycemia (mg/dl)	129 ± 19	109 ± 12	0.01	128 ± 13	106 ± 14	0.01
2-h postprandial glycemia (mg/dl)	186 ± 23	164 ± 16	0.01	185 ± 21	165 ± 15	0.01
A1C (%)	7.1 ± 0.4	6.8 ± 0.3	0.01	7.0 ± 0.5	6.6 ± 0.4	0.01
MAGE (mg/dl glucose)	61 ± 13	35 ± 12*	0.01	60 ± 21	55 ± 14	NS
Nitrotyrosine (μmol/l)	0.81 ± 0.04	0.44 ± 0.03*	0.01	0.79 ± 0.03	0.76 ± 0.06	NS
Fasting insulin (pmol/l)	170 ± 55	131 ± 48	0.01	178 ± 68	127 ± 50	0.01
Postmeal insulin AUC (pmol/l)	498 ± 179	669 ± 135	0.01	505 ± 157	655 ± 122	0.01
Interprandial insulin AUC (pmol · l^{-1} · min^{-1})	325 ± 124	290 ± 108	0.01	339 ± 111	301 ± 122	0.01
Fasting glucagon (ng/l)	71.9 ± 12	65.3 ± 11.6	NS	69.9 ± 13	66.2 ± 11	NS
Postmeal glucagon AUC (ng/l)	68.3 ± 14	50 ± 9	0.01	66.7 ± 10	53 ± 12	0.01
Interprandial glucagon AUC (ng · l^{-1} · min^{-1})	70.7 ± 13	53.6 ± 12*	0.01	69.3 ± 12	68.6 ± 13	NS
Fasting GLP-1 (pmol/l)	6.5 ± 1.2	7.1 ± 1.1	NS	6.6 ± 1.8	6.9 ± 1.5	NS
Postmeal GLP-1 AUC (pmol/l)	9.9 ± 2.1	18.7 ± 3.2	0.01	10.2 ± 2.9	19.3 ± 2.6	0.01
Interprandial GLP-1 AUC (pmol · l^{-1} · min^{-1})	6.2 ± 1.1	11.7 ± 2.5*	0.01	6.5 ± 1.3	7.2 ± 1.4	NS
Active therapy						
ACE inhibitors	5 (14)	5 (14)	—	3 (15)	3 (15)	—
Angiotensin II antagonists	4 (11)	4 (11)	—	2 (10)	2 (10)	—
Diuretics	4 (11)	4 (11)	—	2 (10)	2 (10)	—
Aspirin	10 (28)	10 (28)	—	6 (30)	6 (30)	—
Statins	8 (22)	8 (22)	—	5 (25)	5 (25)	—
Metformin	32 (89)	32 (89)	—	18 (90)	18 (90)	—
Thiazolinediones	10 (28)	10 (28)	—	6 (30)	6 (30)	—

Data are means ± SD or n (%) unless otherwise indicated. Postmeal (0–120 min) and interprandial (120–300 min after meal) areas under the curve (AUCs) for outcome variables were calculated using the trapezoidal method. *$P < 0.05$ compared with the diet group. Nitrotyrosine was assayed as described previously (8): the standard curve was constructed with serial dilution of a nitrated protein solution; the limit of detection of the assay was 10 nmol/l, with intra- and interassay coefficients of variation of 4.5 and 8%, respectively.

(ELISA, D.B.A., Santa Cruz Biotechnology), and insulin (Ares, Serono, Italy) were evaluated at the following times: 0, 60, 120, 180, 240, and 300 min, with the meal beginning immediately after time 0 and consumed within 15 min. Nitrotyrosine (anti-nitrotyrosine rabbit polyclonal antibody; D.B.A., Santa Cruz Biotechnology) (8) was assessed at baseline and after 1 month in the surgical group and after a 10-kg diet-induced weight loss in the diet group. A P value <0.05 defined as statistical significance. Simple Pearson

correlation was used to assess linear relationships between single variables.

RESULTS — At baseline, patients were matched for anthropometric, physical activity, metabolic, and hormonal variables (Table 1). Duration of weight loss was shorter for the surgical group (30.2 ± 11.9 days) than the diet group (60.2 ± 10.1 days; $P < 0.001$). BMI, A1C, FPG, and PPG decreased significantly and equally in surgical and diet groups (Table 1). Despite similar data in A1C, FPG, and

PPG during weight loss in the surgical and diet groups, pattern of daily glucose fluctuations (MAGE) improved after BPD ($P < 0.01$), but not in the diet group, despite a similar weight loss (Table 1). Focusing on hormone profiles during a standard meal and interprandial periods, one can highlight that increase in GLP-1 after food intake was substantially identical in the two groups, whereas a significant ($P < 0.05$) and sustained increase during the interprandial period (from 120 to 300 min after a meal) of active GLP-1 in

BPD toward diet patients occurred (Table 1). In addition, plasma glucagon levels were more suppressed during the interprandial period in surgical patients compared with diet patients (Table 1), but such differences did not reach statistical significance during the postprandial period. Finally, both fasting and postmeal plasma insulin level changes were similar in the two groups (Table 1). Nitrotyrosine levels were significantly lower after BPD compared with diet ($P < 0.01$) (Table 1). Interestingly enough, nitrotyrosine reductions were directly related to MAGE changes in the surgery group ($r = 0.55, P < 0.01$). Moreover, MAGE changes were directly related to interprandial GLP-1 increases ($r = 0.45, P < 0.01$). Finally, the GLP-1 changes were inversely correlated with the glucagon changes ($r = -0.42, P < 0.01$) and directly correlated with insulin changes ($r = 0.52, P < 0.01$).

CONCLUSIONS— BPD, when performed in obese diabetic patients, is effective in improving glycemic control (6). In this study, the efficacy of BPD on A1C, FPG, and PPG reductions was comparable to the diet intervention. Nevertheless, our study shows evidence that the effects of BPD on daily glucose fluctuations, as estimated from MAGE indexes that reflect both upward and downward glucose changes, were more pronounced in the BPD group than in the diet group, which could be due to different effects on incretin secretion. Although the well-matched surgical and diet groups lost the same amount of weight, their changes in incretin levels were strikingly different. According to the previous data (9,10), both GLP-1 and glucagon responses to standardized meals markedly increased 1 month after BPD and 10-kg diet-induced weight loss, without significant differences among the groups. However, BPD patients showed a significantly better daily GLP-1 and glucagon profiles in interprandial periods, which could be responsible for a MAGE within a shorter range. From a more practical point of view, since BPD, by blunting the daily fluctuations of glucose, is associated with a reduction of oxidative stress, the malabsorptive surgery may have an important role not only in the normalization of glycemic variability but also in reducing the impact of diabetes in vascular health.

Acknowledgments— No potential conflicts of interest relevant to this article were reported.

References
1. Monnier L, Mas E, Ginet C, Michel F, Villon L, Cristol JP, Colette C. Activation of oxidative stress by acute glucose fluctuations compared with sustained chronic hyperglycemia in patients with type 2 diabetes. JAMA 2006;295:1681–1687
2. Piconi L, Quagliaro L, Assaloni R, Da Ros R, Maier A, Zuodar G, Ceriello A. Constant and intermittent high glucose enhances endothelial cell apoptosis through mitochondrial superoxide overproduction. Diabete Metab Res Rev 2006;22:198–203
3. Dandona P, Mohanty P, Ghanim H, Aljada A, Browne R, Hamouda W, Prabhala A, Afzal A, Garg R. The suppressive effect of dietary restriction and weight loss in the obese on the generation of reactive oxygen species by leukocytes, lipid peroxidation, and protein carbonylation. J Clin Endocrinol Metab 2001;86:355–362
4. Garrido-Sánchez L, García-Almeida JM, García-Serrano S, Cardona I, García-Arnes J, Soriguer F, Tinahones FJ, García-Fuentes E. Improved carbohydrate metabolism after bariatric surgery raises antioxidized LDL antibody levels in morbidly obese patients. Diabetes Care 2008;31:2258–2264
5. Monnier L, Colette C. Glycemic variability: should we and can we prevent it? Diabetes Care 2008;31 (Suppl. 2):S150–S154
6. Salinari S, Bertuzzi A, Asnaghi S, Guidone C, Manco M, Mingrone G. First-phase insulin secretion restoration and differential response to glucose load depending on the route of administration in type 2 diabetic subjects after bariatric surgery. Diabetes Care 2009;32:375–380
7. Service FJ, Molnar GD, Rosevear JW, Ackerman E, Taylor WF, Cremer GM, Moxness KE. Mean amplitude of glycemic excursions, a measure of diabetic instability. Diabetes 1970;19:644–655
8. Ceriello A, Mercuri F, Quagliaro L, Assaloni R, Motz E, Tonutti L, Taboga C. Detection of nitrotyrosine in the diabetic plasma: evidence of oxidative stress. Diabetologia 2001;44:834–838
9. Laferrère B, Teixeira J, McGinty J, Tran H, Egger JR, Colarusso A, Kovack B, Bawa B, Koshy N, Lee H, Yapp K, Olivan B. Effect of weight loss by gastric bypass surgery versus hypocaloric diet on glucose and incretin levels in patients with type 2 diabetes. J Clin Endocrinol Metab 2008; 93:2479–2485
10. Verdich C, Toubro S, Buemann B, Lysgard Madsen J, Juul Holst J, Astrup A. The role of postprandial releases of insulin and incretin hormones in meal-induced satiety: effect of obesity and weight reduction. Int J Obes Relat Metab Disord 2001; 25:1206–1214

The Importance of Caloric Restriction in the Early Improvements in Insulin Sensitivity After Roux-en-Y Gastric Bypass Surgery

James M. Isbell, md, msci[1]
Robyn A. Tamboli, phd[1]
Erik N. Hansen, md, mph[1]
Jabbar Saliba, md[1]
Julia P. Dunn, md[2]
Sharon E. Phillips, msph[3]
Pamela A. Marks-Shulman, ms, rd[1]
Naji N. Abumrad, md[1]

OBJECTIVE — Many of the metabolic benefits of Roux-en-Y gastric bypass (RYGB) occur before weight loss. In this study we investigated the influence of caloric restriction on the improvements in the metabolic responses that occur within the 1st week after RYGB.

RESEARCH METHODS AND DESIGN — A mixed meal was administered to nine subjects before and after RYGB (average 4 ± 0.5 days) and to nine matched, obese subjects before and after 4 days of the post-RYGB diet.

RESULTS — Weight loss in both groups was minimal; the RYGB subjects lost 1.4 ± 5.3 kg ($P = 0.46$) vs. 2.2 ± 1.0 kg ($P = 0.004$) in the calorically restricted group. Insulin resistance (homeostasis model assessment of insulin resistance) improved with both RYGB (5.0 ± 3.1 to 3.3 ± 2.1; $P = 0.03$) and caloric restriction (4.8 ± 4.1 to 3.6 ± 4.1; $P = 0.004$). The insulin response to a mixed meal was blunted in both the RYGB and caloric restriction groups (113 ± 67 to 65 ± 33 and 85 ± 59 to 65 ± 56 nmol $\cdot$ l^{-1} $\cdot$ min^{-1}, respectively; $P < 0.05$) without a change in the glucose response. Glucagon-like peptide 1 levels increased (9.2 ± 8.6 to 12.2 ± 5.5 pg $\cdot$ l^{-1} $\cdot$ min^{-1}; $P = 0.04$) and peaked higher (45.2 ± 37.3 to 84.8 ± 33.0 pg/ml; $P = 0.01$) in response to a mixed meal after RYGB, but incretin responses were not altered after caloric restriction.

CONCLUSIONS — These data suggest that an improvement in insulin resistance in the 1st week after RYGB is primarily due to caloric restriction, and the enhanced incretin response after RYGB does not improve postprandial glucose homeostasis during this time.

Diabetes Care 33:1438–1442, 2010

Bariatric surgical procedures achieve a large and sustained improvement in insulin sensitivity and a high resolution rate in type 2 diabetes. The metabolic benefits of Roux-en-Y gastric bypass surgery (RYGB) are observed very early and precede substantial weight loss (1). It has been proposed that the long-term improvements are related to a reduction in fat mass (2); however, the mechanisms for the early improvements remain uncertain. The surgical bypass of the foregut and/or rapid nutrient exposure of the distal gut alters enterokine release, which has been proposed to result in metabolic improvements (3) and in particular glucose homeostasis. However, caloric restriction in the absence of weight loss has metabolic benefits (4) and could also contribute to the early improvements in glucose homeostasis.

The incretins, namely glucagon-like peptide 1 (GLP-1) and gastric inhibitory peptide (GIP), are gut hormones that contribute to postprandial insulin secretion (5). RYGB augments GLP-1 secretion, whereas its impact on GIP is less consistent (3). In contrast, bariatric procedures that induce weight loss by caloric restriction in the absence of intestinal bypass, such as adjustable gastric banding, do not alter postprandial incretin levels (3). Ghrelin is another enterokine that has a primary role in appetite stimulation but also has glucose and insulin modulatory effects (6). The presence of an acyl group is considered necessary for biological activity of ghrelin, although the desacyl form probably has biological functions as well (7). Ghrelin levels are abnormally low in obese individuals and remain suppressed after RYGB, whereas weight loss by diet enhances ghrelin levels (8). Leptin and adiponectin, adipocyte-derived hormones, are thought to be mediators of weight-related improvements in insulin resistance. The concentrations of these hormones are aberrant in obesity and normalize after RYGB. A recent study indicated that >5% weight loss by consumption of a hypocaloric diet (~40% energy restriction) is required to favorably change circulating adipokines and metabolic parameters (9).

A limited number of reports have directly compared the contribution of duodenal bypass versus caloric restriction on enterokine responses and hormone levels after RYGB (10–12). These studies all incorporated moderate weight loss (~10 kg) and were conducted 2–4 weeks postoperatively. In the present study, we compared the immediate, weight loss–independent effects of RYGB and caloric restriction on fasting hormone levels and meal-stimulated enterokine release. RYGB were evaluated within the 1st week after surgery, and a matched group of subjects were evaluated after 4 days of the equivalent post–bariatric surgery diet.

RESEARCH DESIGN AND METHODS

— RYBG subjects were recruited from the Center for Surgical Weight Loss at Vanderbilt University Medical Center after approval for surgery. Diet control were matched to the surgery group (Table 1) for age ($P = 0.37$), weight ($P = 0.09$), diabetes status and duration ($P = 0.80$), and A1C ($P = 0.56$). All subjects provided written, informed

From the [1]Department of Surgery, Vanderbilt University School of Medicine, Nashville, Tennessee; the [2]Department of Medicine, Vanderbilt University School of Medicine, Nashville, Tennessee; and the [3]Department of Biostatistics, Vanderbilt University School of Medicine, Nashville, Tennessee.
Corresponding author: Naji N. Abumrad, naji.abumrad@vanderbilt.edu.
Received 16 November 2009 and accepted 25 March 2010. Published ahead of print at http://care.diabetesjournals.org on 5 April 2010. DOI: 10.2337/dc09-2107. Clinical Trial reg. no. NCT00765596, clinicaltrials.gov.
J.M.I. and R.A.T. contributed equally to this study.

Table 1—*Baseline subject characteristics*

	RYGB	Diet
n	9	9
Age (years)	41.1 ± 11.5	46.6 ± 6.7
Sex (male/female)	3/6	2/7
Weight (kg)	153.2 ± 32.2	127.0 ± 36.5
Type 2 diabetes (yes/no)	5/4	4/5
Diabetes duration (years)	3.7 ± 4.7	2.6 ± 1.5
A1C (%)	6.5 ± 1.3	6.2 ± 1.0

Data are means ± SD or count. All comparisons between groups were nonsignificant (*P* > 0.05).

consent to participate in the study. The study protocol was approved by the Vanderbilt University Institutional Review Board.

Subjects were studied at baseline and then after RYGB (surgery group) or after caloric restriction (diet group). After the baseline study, subjects in the surgery group underwent either open or laparoscopic RYGB (13). The average time for the postoperative study was 4 ± 0.5 days (range 2–7 days). The diet group was studied after 4 days of caloric restriction that replicated the post-RYGB diet. The diet consisted of 2.5 liters of fluid/day for 3 days; the 1st day included water only, followed by water and sugar-free clear liquids (e.g., gelatin, juices, and/or broths equivalent to 200–300 kcal/day) on days 2 and 3. For each study visit, subjects were admitted after a 12-h overnight fast for measurement of fasting and meal-induced metabolic and hormonal responses. Blood samples were collected from a heated forearm vein at 0700 h (time 0), immediately after completion of a meal (time 20), and every subsequent hour for 4 h. Subjects were asked to take 15–20 min to complete the meal to account for the reduced stomach capacity after RYGB. The meal was a standardized 250-kcal liquid mixed-meal containing 40 g carbohydrates, 6 g fat, and 9 g protein (8 oz of Ensure).

Sample collection and analysis
Blood was collected in chilled EDTA tubes and immediately centrifuged, and plasma was stored at −80°C until analysis. Glucose was measured via the glucose oxidase method (Beckman glucose analyzer). The plasma designated for GLP-1 measurement was supplemented with aprotinin (1,000 kIU/ml) and dipeptidyl peptidase 4 inhibitor (20 μl/ml plasma). Plasma designated for acylated ghrelin measurement was treated with 1 N hydrochloric acid (50 μl/ml plasma) and

phenylmethylsulfonyl fluoride (0.1 mg/ml plasma). Plasma insulin, leptin, adiponectin, and active GLP-1 were measured using multiplex immunoassays (Luminex xMAP). Total (acylated and desacyl) and acylated ghrelin were determined by radioimmunoassay. Plasma concentrations of total GIP were measured by enzyme-linked radioimmunoassay. A1C was assayed using high-pressure liquid chromatography.

Calculations
The homeostasis model assessment of insulin resistance index (HOMA-IR) is derived from the inverse of insulin sensitivity based on Levy's nonlinear computer model (14). Total area under the curve (AUC) was calculated according to the trapezoidal rule in GraphPad Prism (version 5.02).

Statistical analyses
The Wilcoxon signed rank test was performed to compare data from the same subjects. The nonparametric Mann-Whitney test was used for comparisons between RYGB and diet groups. All analyses were performed in R 2.6.2 (www.

r-project.org). Data are means ± SD, except for graphs which are presented as means ± SEM.

RESULTS

Weight loss
RYGB subjects lost 1.4 ± 5.3 kg or 1.0 ± 3.4% of initial body weight (*P* = 0.46) in the 1st week postoperatively. Caloric-restricted control subjects lost 2.2 ± 1.0 kg or 2.2 ± 1.0% of initial body weight (*P* = 0.004). Comparison of the weight changes with RYGB and diet was not significant (*P* = 0.09) (Table 2).

Fasting measures of insulin resistance
Within 1 week after RYGB, fasting glucose levels were similar to preoperative levels (−6%; *P* = 0.14); however, a decrease in insulin levels was observed (−25%; *P* = 0.04). HOMA-IR also decreased by 25% (*P* = 0.03). Diet control subjects exhibited a disparate decrease in glucose levels (−20%; *P* = 0.004) but a similar decrease in fasting insulin levels (−27%; *P* = 0.07) and improvement in the HOMA-IR index (−30%; *P* = 0.004). Changes in HOMA-IR with RYGB and diet were not different (*P* = 0.45) (Table 2).

Fasting levels of enterokines and adipokines
Fasting plasma levels of GLP-1 and GIP were not altered either by RYGB (*P* = 0.65 and 0.16, respectively) or after caloric restriction (*P* = 0.73 and 0.13, respectively). On the other hand, there were decreases in the fasting levels of acylated (−21%; *P* = 0.03) and total ghrelin (−20%; *P* = 0.05) after RYGB, with no changes in the caloric-restricted group

Table 2—*Early effects of RYGB and short-term diet restriction on body weight and fasting metabolic parameters*

	Before RYGB	After RYGB	Before diet	After diet
Weight (kg)	153.2 ± 32.2	151.8 ± 33.1	127.0 ± 36.5	124.2 ± 36.5*
BMI (kg/m^2)	51.9 ± 6.0	51.4 ± 6.6	44.2 ± 9.9	43.2 ± 10.0*
Glucose (mmol/l)	6.4 ± 1.5	6.0 ± 1.8	6.8 ± 1.8	5.4 ± 1.1*
Insulin (pmol/l)	236 ± 159	155 ± 102*	220 ± 196	178 ± 217
HOMA-IR	5.0 ± 3.1	3.3 ± 2.1*	4.8 ± 4.1	3.6 ± 4.1*
GLP-1 (pg/ml)	34.9 ± 32.4	36.5 ± 32.6	39.4 ± 14.9	39.3 ± 32.8
GIP (pg/ml)	58.0 ± 31.6	42.4 ± 21.1	53.3 ± 29.0	33.7 ± 25.5
Leptin (ng/ml)	72.4 ± 15.3	49.5 ± 15.1*	61.1 ± 30.6	38.0 ± 21.9
Adiponectin (μg/ml)	7.3 ± 3.0	6.4 ± 2.0	4.5 ± 2.6	4.7 ± 2.6
Acylated ghrelin (pg/ml)	68.2 ± 33.6	48.5 ± 26.9*	34.7 ± 23.5	26.1 ± 20.2
Total ghrelin (pg/ml)	585 ± 272	414 ± 107	623 ± 205	559 ± 268

Data are means ± SD. *P* < 0.05 compared with baseline within each group (RYGB or Diet).

($P > 0.2$). The fasting levels of leptin declined 1 week after RYGB (-31%; $P = 0.004$) and after caloric restriction (-26%; $P = 0.05$), whereas adiponectin levels were not altered in either group ($P > 0.1$) (Table 2).

Metabolic response to a mixed meal

RYGB did not result in differences in the glucose AUC ($P = 0.13$) or peak glucose levels ($P = 0.21$) achieved after a mixed meal. The insulin response was reduced after RYGB, evidenced by decreases in AUC ($P = 0.004$) and peak levels of insulin ($P = 0.02$). Conversely, there were increases in the AUC ($P = 0.04$) and peak ($P = 0.01$) GLP-1 levels postoperatively. Whereas the AUC and peak levels of GIP were not altered in response to a mixed meal after RYGB, the peak in GIP occurred earlier. Despite a decrease in the AUC and nadir for total ghrelin in the early postoperative period ($P = 0.004$ for both), ghrelin remained at fasting levels throughout the study (Fig. 1, Table 3).

The subjects who underwent caloric restriction similar to that for the subjects undergoing RYGB displayed similar changes in meal-stimulated glucose and insulin release after the diet; the AUC ($P = 0.13$) and peak ($P = 0.34$) glucose concentrations did not change and the AUC ($P = 0.02$) and peak ($P = 0.04$) insulin concentrations decreased. Although the AUC for insulin was decreased in both the RYGB and diet groups, the change in the RYGB group was greater ($P = 0.04$). Caloric restriction alone did not induce any changes in enterokine responses to a mixed meal (all $P > 0.05$), with the exception of a decreased nadir in ghrelin release after diet ($P = 0.05$). Interestingly, caloric restriction altered the pattern of ghrelin release. At baseline, ghrelin levels did not vary after the mixed meal similar to that in the RYGB subjects; however, after the diet, ghrelin release was suppressed after the mixed meal followed by a steady increase in ghrelin release above fasting levels.

CONCLUSIONS — It is well established that RYGB is effective in improving insulin resistance and ameliorating type 2 diabetes. The beneficial metabolic effects of RYGB were initially attributed to the substantial weight reduction achieved with surgery; however, subsequent investigations revealed an improvement in insulin sensitivity at 6 days after RYGB without appreciable weight loss (15). We have confirmed these findings by demon-

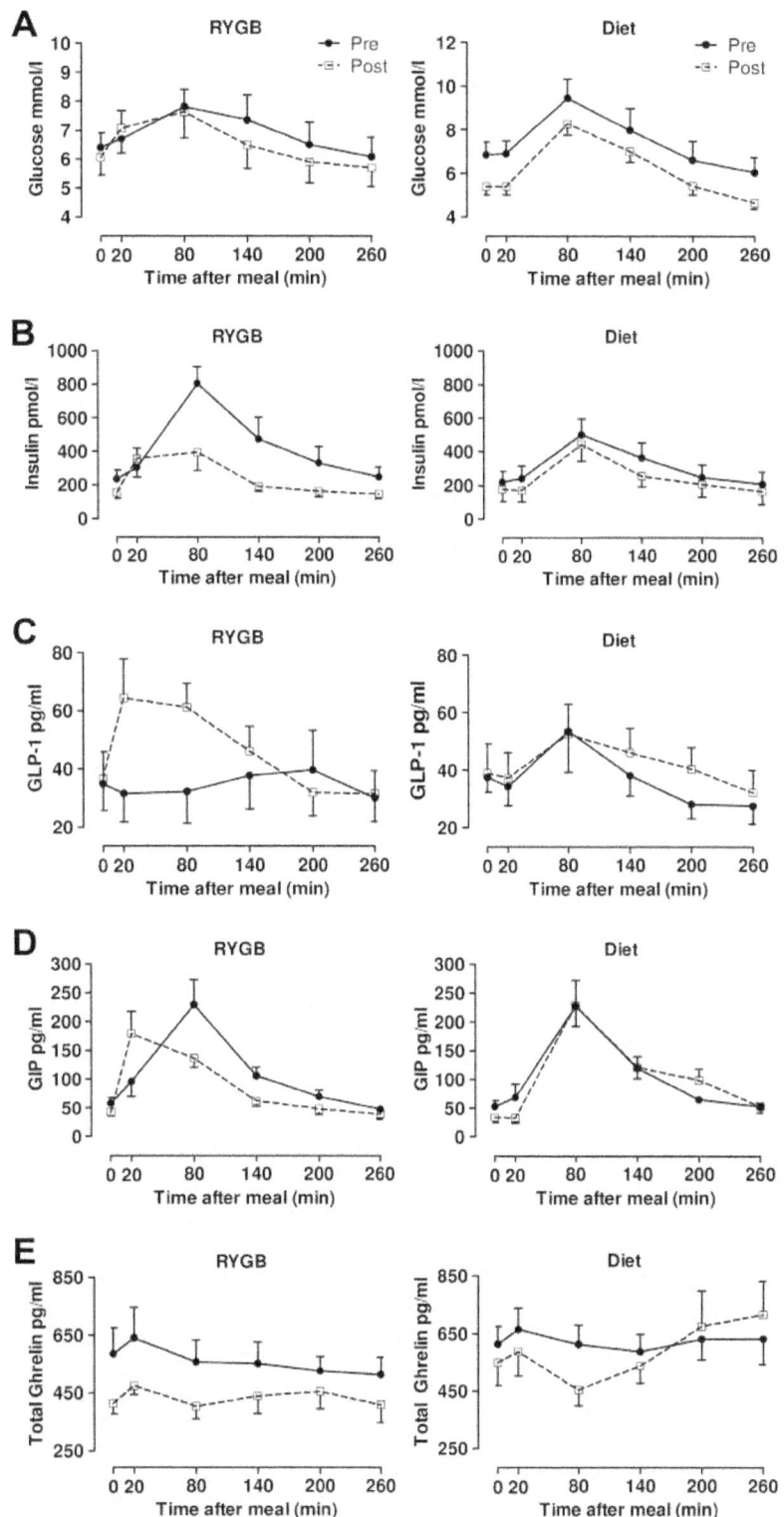

Figure 1—*Metabolic responses during a mixed-meal before and after RYGB and diet. Blood was drawn before (time 0), immediately after the ingestion of a mixed-meal (time 20), and every subsequent hour for 4 h. Plasma levels of glucose (A), insulin (B), GLP-1 (C), GIP (D), and total ghrelin (E) were measured at each time point at baseline (●) and 4 days after RYGB (□) or 3 days after a post–bariatric surgery diet (□). Data are means ± SEM.*

Table 3—*Metabolic responses to a mixed-meal before and after RYGB and diet*

	Before RYGB	After RYGB	Before diet	After diet
Glucose AUC (mmol · l^{-1} · min^{-1})	1,829 ± 510	1,714 ± 568	1,966 ± 641	1,637 ± 297
Peak glucose (mmol/l)	8.4 ± 2.1	7.9 ± 2.5	9.4 ± 2.6	8.2 ± 1.5
Insulin AUC (mmol · l^{-1} · min^{-1})	113 ± 67	65 ± 33*	85 ± 59	65 ± 56*
Peak insulin (pmol/l)	742 ± 347	485 ± 307*	532 ± 287	406 ± 307*
GLP-1 AUC (pg · l^{-1} · min^{-1})	9.2 ± 8.4	12.2 ± 5.5*	10.2 ± 5.9	11.6 ± 6.4
Peak GLP-1 (pg/ml)	45.2 ± 37.3	84.8 ± 33.0*	58.8 ± 43.2	57.2 ± 28.4
GIP AUC (pg · l^{-1} · min^{-1})	28.7 ± 12.3	23.5 ± 8.6	29.5 ± 13.5	30.1 ± 13.8
Peak GIP (pg/ml)	227 ± 115	193 ± 111	235 ± 128	228 ± 105
Ghrelin AUC (pg · l^{-1} · min^{-1})	145 ± 53	112 ± 36*	162 ± 58	142 ± 52
Nadir ghrelin (pg/ml)	456 ± 165	341 ± 84*	543 ± 217	393 ± 201

Data are means ± SD. *$P < 0.05$ compared with baseline within each group (RYGB and diet).

strating a 25% improvement in insulin sensitivity (HOMA-IR) within 1 week after RYGB before any apparent weight loss. Interestingly, obese subjects, albeit with a nonsignificantly lower body weight, who consumed a post–bariatric surgery liquid diet for 4 days replicated the improved insulin sensitivity observed in the RYGB subjects. The parallel improvements occurred with minimal noticeable differences in weight loss between the two groups. HOMA-IR is a fasting measure of whole-body insulin resistance that has been shown to correlate with other dynamic measures of insulin sensitivity in obese subjects, such as the hyperinsuline-mic-euglycemic clamp (16). Such studies suggest that a short duration, very-low-calorie diet can reduce hepatic glucose production (17) and improve skeletal muscle insulin sensitivity (4). Our data demonstrate that the improvement in insulin sensitivity, as measured by HOMA-IR, precedes appreciable weight loss and is largely achieved with caloric restriction. However, we must consider the possibility that the immediate improvements in insulin sensitivity after RYGB could have been blunted consequent to the associated stress/inflammatory responses of surgery, thus masking a greater improvement in insulin sensitivity with RYGB than with caloric restriction.

Fasting levels of GLP-1 have been reported to remain stable 2–10 weeks after RYGB (1,11,18,19), consistent with our current observations within the 1st postoperative week. Our data show increases in peak GLP-1 levels and total GLP-1 release after ingestion of a mixed meal 1 week after RYGB, in agreement with previous short-term follow-up investigations (11,19–21). This increase in GLP-1 could not be attributed to the restrictive nature of the surgical procedure, because the ca-

loric-restricted diet group did not show enhanced an GLP-1 release in response to the mixed meal. The findings with GIP are novel; GIP is released sooner but not to a greater extent with a meal within the 1st week after RYGB. Laferrère et al. (11) and Campos et al. (10) compared incretin levels in two groups of subjects after a 10-kg weight loss via RYGB or diet and reported an increase in GLP-1 only after RYGB; their findings for GIP were disparate, with one reporting an increase (11) and the other reporting no change (10). Our results, however, show altered incretin release after RYGB before substantial weight loss. The proposed mechanism of enhanced incretin release after RYGB is most likely related to the increased and more rapid nutrient stimulus to the intestinal neuroendocrine cells.

The effects of the changes in incretin levels on the improved metabolic responses after RYGB remain controversial. In our study, the observed increase in GLP-1 and shift to an earlier GIP peak within 1 week after RYGB was accompanied by improved insulin sensitivity, whereas the improvement in insulin sensitivity after caloric restriction occurred without alterations in either GLP-1 or GIP. Thus, the improvements in insulin sensitivity in our study are unlikely to be due to altered incretin-induced insulin release but rather to the caloric restriction. In fact, in both surgical and caloric-restricted diet groups we observed similar decreases in insulin release (Fig. 1) accompanied by improved insulin sensitivity. These findings contrast with previous reports of either no early changes in insulin release (10) or an increase in insulin release (11) after RYGB. The discrepancy with our findings may be related to the associated losses (10 kg) in body weight in these studies (10,11). In addition,

GLP-1 could exert extrapancreatic effects on improving insulin sensitivity (22), which in our RYGB group could have been blunted as a result of the associated inflammatory responses immediately after surgery. Lastly, perhaps the improved GLP-1 response in the 1st week after RYGB is not robust enough to elicit increased insulin secretion and glucose-lowering effects and may take longer to exert such effects.

Levels of the orexiogenic hormone ghrelin are diminished in obesity (23), perhaps indicating a positive energy balance. The short-term effect of RYGB on fasting total ghrelin is controversial. We observed 20% decreases in fasting levels of acylated and total ghrelin within 1 week after RYGB; these are consistent with previously reported decreases in fasting total ghrelin at 6 weeks (24) but different from another report showing no change 1 month after RYGB (12). Whether the decreased levels of acylated and total ghrelin levels play a role in the improvement in insulin sensitivity after RYGB remains to be determined. Vestergaard et al. (6) demonstrated that exogenous infusion of a pharmacological dose of acyl-ghrelin acutely induced insulin resistance independent of growth hormone and cortisol.

Alterations in adipokines, such as leptin and adiponectin, after RYGB have been attributed to fat mass loss and are responsible for the long-term improvements in insulin resistance (2). The similarities in the decrease in plasma leptin in the RYGB and diet groups suggest that this immediate change in leptin after surgery can be accounted for by caloric restriction. A similar finding was reported 1 month after RYGB and diet, coinciding with a 10-kg weight loss (12). The stable adiponectin concentrations during caloric restriction via RYGB and diet could indicate dissociation in the regulation of these two adipokines between nutrient exposure and fat mass.

In summary, our present data suggest that caloric restriction without substantial weight loss is of primary importance in the rapid improvement of insulin sensitivity within the 1st week after RYGB. Early alterations in the incretin response can be attributed to the surgery; however, the enhanced incretin response does not seem to have any additional benefit beyond caloric restriction on glucose homeostasis and insulin sensitivity. It is important to note that our cohorts of obese subjects were balanced for type 2 diabetes, and the measured parameters were similar at baseline (except for HOMA-IR, which was higher in the subjects with type 2 diabetes) and changed similarly after intervention. Further investigations in the immediate postoperative period with more dynamic measures of insulin resistance are also warranted to determine the mechanisms/site of improved insulin sensitivity, along with a direct assessment of the incretin effect on insulin production.

Acknowledgments— This work was supported by the following National Institutes of Health grants: National Institute of Diabetes and Digestive and Kidney Diseases grant R01-DK-070860 (to N.N.A.), Vanderbilt Clinical and Translational Science Award grant 1-UL1-RR-024975 from the National Center for Research Resources, grant DK-20593 to the Vanderbilt Diabetes Research and Training Center, grant DK-058404 to the Vanderbilt Digestive Disease Research Center, and grant T32-DK-007061-31A1 (to J.M.I.).

No potential conflicts of interest relevant to this article were reported.

We thank Marcy Buckley for nursing support and Kareem Jabbour and Nadine Saliba for laboratory assistance.

References

1. Rubino F, Gagner M, Gentileschi P, Kini S, Fukuyama S, Feng J, Diamond E. The early effect of the Roux-en-Y gastric bypass on hormones involved in body weight regulation and glucose metabolism. Ann Surg 2004;240:236–242
2. Gumbs AA, Modlin IM, Ballantyne GH. Changes in insulin resistance following bariatric surgery: role of caloric restriction and weight loss. Obes Surg 2005;15:462–473
3. Bose M, Oliván B, Teixeira J, Pi-Sunyer FX, Laferrère B. Do incretins play a role in the remission of type 2 diabetes after gastric bypass surgery: what are the evidence? Obes Surg 2009;19:217–229
4. Lara-Castro C, Newcomer BR, Rowell J, Wallace P, Shaughnessy SM, Munoz AJ, Shiflett AM, Rigsby DY, Lawrence JC, Bohning DE, Buchthal S, Garvey WT. Effects of short-term very low-calorie diet on intramyocellular lipid and insulin sensitivity in nondiabetic and type 2 diabetic subjects. Metabolism 2008;57:1–8
5. Preitner F, Ibberson M, Franklin I, Binnert C, Pende M, Gjinovci A, Hansotia T, Drucker DJ, Wollheim C, Burcelin R, Thorens B. Gluco-incretins control insulin secretion at multiple levels as revealed in mice lacking GLP-1 and GIP receptors. J Clin Invest 2004;113:635–645
6. Vestergaard ET, Gormsen LC, Jessen N, Lund S, Hansen TK, Moller N, Jorgensen JO. Ghrelin infusion in humans induces acute insulin resistance and lipolysis independent of growth hormone signaling. Diabetes 2008;57:3205–3210
7. Soares JB, Leite-Moreira AF. Ghrelin, desacyl ghrelin and obestatin: three pieces of the same puzzle. Peptides 2008;29:1255–1270
8. Cummings DE, Weigle DS, Frayo RS, Breen PA, Ma MK, Dellinger EP, Purnell JQ. Plasma ghrelin levels after diet-induced weight loss or gastric bypass surgery. N Engl J Med 2002;346:1623–1630
9. Varady KA, Tussing L, Bhutani S, Braunschweig CL. Degree of weight loss required to improve adipokine concentrations and decrease fat cell size in severely obese women. Metabolism 2009;58:1096–1101
10. Campos GM, Rabl C, Peeva S, Ciovica R, Rao M, Schwarz JM, Havel P, Schambelan M, Mulligan K. Improvement in peripheral glucose uptake after gastric bypass surgery is observed only after substantial weight loss has occurred and correlates with the magnitude of weight lost. J Gastrointest Surg 2010;14:15–23
11. Laferrère B, Teixeira J, McGinty J, Tran H, Egger JR, Colarusso A, Kovack B, Bawa B, Koshy N, Lee H, Yapp K, Olivan B. Effect of weight loss by gastric bypass surgery versus hypocaloric diet on glucose and incretin levels in patients with type 2 diabetes. J Clin Endocrinol Metab 2008;93:2479–2485
12. Oliván B, Teixeira J, Bose M, Bawa B, Chang T, Summe H, Lee H, Laferrère B. Effect of weight loss by diet or gastric bypass surgery on peptide YY3–36 levels. Ann Surg 2009;249:948–953
13. Saliba J, Wattacheril J, Abumrad NN. Endocrine and metabolic response to gastric bypass. Curr Opin Clin Nutr Metab Care 2009;12:515–521
14. Levy JC, Matthews DR, Hermans MP. Correct homeostasis model assessment (HOMA) evaluation uses the computer program. Diabetes Care 1998;21:2191–2192
15. Wickremesekera K, Miller G, Naotunne TD, Knowles G, Stubbs RS. Loss of insulin resistance after Roux-en-Y gastric bypass surgery: a time course study. Obes Surg 2005;15:474–481
16. Wallace TM, Levy JC, Matthews DR. Use and abuse of HOMA modeling. Diabetes Care 2004;27:1487–1495
17. Jazet IM, Pijl H, Frölich M, Romijn JA, Meinders AE. Two days of a very low calorie diet reduces endogenous glucose production in obese type 2 diabetic patients despite the withdrawal of blood glucose-lowering therapies including insulin. Metabolism 2005;54:705–712
18. Clements RH, Gonzalez QH, Long CI, Wittert G, Laws HL. Hormonal changes after Roux-en Y gastric bypass for morbid obesity and the control of type-II diabetes mellitus. Am Surg 2004;70:1–4; discussion 4–5
19. Laferrère B, Heshka S, Wang K, Khan Y, McGinty J, Teixeira J, Hart AB, Olivan B. Incretin levels and effect are markedly enhanced 1 month after Roux-en-Y gastric bypass surgery in obese patients with type 2 diabetes. Diabetes Care 2007;30:1709–1716
20. le Roux CW, Welbourn R, Werling M, Osborne A, Kokkinos A, Laurenius A, Lönroth H, Fändriks L, Ghatei MA, Bloom SR, Olbers T. Gut hormones as mediators of appetite and weight loss after Roux-en-Y gastric bypass. Ann Surg 2007;246:780–785
21. Morínigo R, Lacy AM, Casamitjana R, Delgado S, Gomis R, Vidal J. GLP-1 and changes in glucose tolerance following gastric bypass surgery in morbidly obese subjects. Obes Surg 2006;16:1594–1601
22. Vella A, Rizza RA. Extrapancreatic effects of GIP and GLP-1. Horm Metab Res 2004;36:830–836
23. Tschöp M, Weyer C, Tataranni PA, Devanarayan V, Ravussin E, Heiman ML. Circulating ghrelin levels are decreased in human obesity. Diabetes 2001;50:707–709
24. Morínigo R, Casamitjana R, Moizé V, Lacy AM, Delgado S, Gomis R, Vidal J. Short-term effects of gastric bypass surgery on circulating ghrelin levels. Obes Res 2004;12:1108–1116

Cost-Effectiveness of Bariatric Surgery for Severely Obese Adults With Diabetes

Thomas J. Hoerger, phd[1]
Ping Zhang, phd[2]
Joel E. Segel, ba[3]

Henry S. Kahn, md[2]
Lawrence E. Barker, phd[2]
Steven Couper, bs, ba[1]

OBJECTIVE — To analyze the cost-effectiveness of bariatric surgery in severely obese (BMI ≥35 kg/m²) adults who have diabetes, using a validated diabetes cost-effectiveness model.

RESEARCH DESIGN AND METHODS — We expanded the Centers for Disease Control and Prevention–RTI Diabetes Cost-Effectiveness Model to incorporate bariatric surgery. In this simulation model, bariatric surgery may lead to diabetes remission and reductions in other risk factors, which then lead to fewer diabetes complications and increased quality of life (QoL). Surgery is also associated with perioperative mortality and subsequent complications, and patients in remission may relapse to diabetes. We separately estimate the costs, quality-adjusted life-years (QALYs), and cost-effectiveness of gastric bypass surgery relative to usual diabetes care and of gastric banding surgery relative to usual diabetes care. We examine the cost-effectiveness of each type of surgery for severely obese individuals who are newly diagnosed with diabetes and for severely obese individuals with established diabetes.

RESULTS — In all analyses, bariatric surgery increased QALYs and increased costs. Bypass surgery had cost-effectiveness ratios of $7,000/QALY and $12,000/QALY for severely obese patients with newly diagnosed and established diabetes, respectively. Banding surgery had cost-effectiveness ratios of $11,000/QALY and $13,000/QALY for the respective groups. In sensitivity analyses, the cost-effectiveness ratios were most affected by assumptions about the direct gain in QoL from BMI loss following surgery.

CONCLUSIONS — Our analysis indicates that gastric bypass and gastric banding are cost-effective methods of reducing mortality and diabetes complications in severely obese adults with diabetes.

Diabetes Care 33:1933–1939, 2010

In recent years, bariatric surgery has emerged as a popular treatment to reduce body weight and improve obesity-related complications, particularly in the diabetic population. Several studies have shown that surgery can lead to significant weight loss, with excess body weight reduced by >50% (1,2). Although weight loss declines over time, the Swedish Obese Subjects (SOS) Study found significant weight loss even 10 years after surgery (3,4). In addition to sustained weight loss, bariatric surgery may provide additional benefits to people with diabetes. Among severely obese patients with diabetes, bariatric surgery often leads to diabetes remission, with remission rates that are as high as 80% in the short run (1) and that remain significant in the long run (3,4).

Although the evidence suggests that bariatric surgery is a successful long-term treatment of obesity for people with diabetes, it is an expensive procedure. The average cost of surgery exceeds $13,000 (5), with additional costs possible in the months following surgery (6). This raises the question of whether bariatric surgery is cost-effective for severely obese people with diabetes.

Several studies have estimated the cost-effectiveness of bariatric surgery and found that surgery is either cost-effective (7–10) or that it leads to cost savings over time (6,11–13). The existing studies tend to be relatively simple, and only two (10,13) focus on people with diabetes. The studies generally do not model the microvascular complications associated with diabetes, the effect of surgery on blood pressure and cholesterol levels, or the resulting outcomes.

This study used the Centers for Disease Control and Prevention (CDC)-RTI Diabetes Cost-Effectiveness Model to analyze the cost-effectiveness of bariatric surgery in severely obese adults with diabetes. We separately estimated the cost-effectiveness of gastric bypass surgery relative to usual diabetes care and the cost-effectiveness of gastric banding surgery relative to usual diabetes care. Gastric bypass and gastric banding are the two forms of bariatric surgery most commonly studied (1). We examined the cost-effectiveness of each type of surgery for severely obese people who are newly diagnosed with diabetes (no more than 5 years after diagnosis) and for people with established diabetes (at least 10 years after diagnosis).

RESEARCH DESIGN AND METHODS — The CDC-RTI Diabetes Cost-Effectiveness Model is a Markov simulation model of disease progression and cost-effectiveness for type 2 diabetes that follows patients from diagnosis to either death or age 95 years. The model simulates development of diabetes-related complications on three microvascular disease paths (nephropathy, neuropathy, and retinopathy) and two macrovascular disease paths (coronary heart disease [CHD] and stroke). Model outcomes include disease complications, deaths, costs, and quality-adjusted life-years (QALYs). In the model, progression between disease states is governed by transition probabilities that depend on risk

From ¹RTI-UNC Center of Excellence in Health Promotion Economics, RTI International, Research Triangle Park, North Carolina; the ²Division of Diabetes Translation, Centers for Disease Control and Prevention, Atlanta, Georgia; and ³School of Public Health, University of Michigan, Ann Arbor, Michigan.
Corresponding author: Thomas J. Hoerger, tjh@rti.org.
Received 29 March 2010 and accepted 10 June 2010.
The findings and conclusion in this article are those of the authors and do not necessarily reflect the views of the Centers for Disease Control and Prevention.
DOI: 10.2337/dc10-0554

See accompanying editorial, p. 2126.

factors and duration of diabetes. Interventions affect the transition probabilities and resulting complications. The model has been used to estimate the cost-effectiveness of interventions for patients with diagnosed diabetes or prediabetes (14,15). Details about the model and its validation are presented elsewhere (14–16).

Bariatric surgery is incorporated in the following ways. First, the model allows for diabetes remission and improvement, important results of bariatric surgery. We defined remission as normal glycemic levels following surgery without antidiabetes medications. This was incorporated in the model as no progression along the microvascular paths, no diabetes treatment costs, elimination of the diabetes indicator variable in the CHD and stroke equations, and elimination of the diabetes other-cause mortality multiplier. We created an "improved diabetes" state for people who reduced the use of antidiabetes medications but did not achieve full diabetes remission. The rates of diabetes remission and improvement following bariatric surgery procedures are shown in Table 1 with values based on a meta-analysis (1). The reduction in costs for improvement is based on two smaller studies (17,18). The online appendix (available at http://care.diabetesjournals.org/cgi/content/full/dc10-0554/DC1) provides additional details on sources and parameter derivation for the variables described in this section.

Second, the model includes an annual probability of relapse from remission to diabetes. Because few studies examine the long-term effects of bariatric surgery, we focused on the SOS study, which followed patients for 10 years after bariatric surgery (3). We used the diabetes remission rates reported at 2 and 10 years to calculate the probability of relapse in Table 1.

Third, the model accounts for perioperative mortality and the long-term effects of surgery on mortality. For perioperative mortality, we used separate rates for bypass and banding surgery (19). The model calculates future changes in mortality based on surgery's effects on blood pressure, cholesterol, and the remission or improvement of diabetes. We used multiple literature sources to estimate the effect of surgery on blood pressure and cholesterol values. Remission or improvement in diabetes stops or slows progression of diabetes complications, which reduces mortality. For people in diabetes remission, we also lowered other-cause

mortality to the baseline rate among people with no diabetes. These effects are listed in Table 1.

Fourth, the model includes the costs of bariatric surgery. First-year bypass and banding surgery costs are based on an analysis of Medstat claims by Eric A. Finkelstein et al. (2008, unpublished data). The analysis calculated the costs attributable to surgery, including the surgery costs and any complication costs in the first year. For costs in subsequent years, we included costs of follow-up care visits; nutritional supplements; long-term complications, such as revisional surgery, cholelithiasis, abdominoplasty, and nonoperative leaks; and band removal (for gastric banding). Table 1 lists the complication costs by year after surgery.

Finally, in addition to changes in quality of life (QoL) following surgery that result from reductions in diabetes complications, the model includes changes in QoL directly associated with bariatric surgery. We included a change in QoL associated with bariatric surgery that was the product of the change in utility for a 1–BMI unit change in weight and the change in BMI associated with surgery.

To analyze the cost-effectiveness of bariatric surgery, we focused on the population with BMI $\geq$35 kg/m^2 and diabetes. We defined the characteristics of this population by estimating the distribution of age, sex, race, hypertension status, cholesterol status, and smoking status as well as systolic blood pressure, total cholesterol, and HDL levels within the National Health and Nutrition Examination Survey for the subset of the obese population (BMI $\geq$30 kg/m^2) with self-reported diabetes. Values for the population with BMI $\geq$35 kg/m^2 were similar, so we used data from the full obese population with its larger sample size.

Within the severely obese diabetic population, we separately analyzed the newly diagnosed diabetic population and the established diabetic population. We distinguished between these two groups because studies have shown that surgery leads to significantly less weight loss and lower rates of diabetes remission in people with longer diabetes duration (17,18). The primary differences between the populations are that the newly diagnosed diabetic population is younger (aged 35–74 years) than the established diabetic population (aged 45–74 years) to represent the 10-year difference in duration, and the diabetes remission rate is lower for the

established diabetic population (18). We adjusted diabetes duration to 10 years in the model to reflect changes in glycemic control and complications in the established diabetic population.

Using these two severely obese diabetic populations, we estimated the cost-effectiveness of gastric bypass and gastric banding surgery. The two surgeries differ in several factors, including diabetes remission rate, diabetes improvement rate, perioperative mortality rate, first-year and following-year costs, and effect on blood pressure, cholesterol, and QoL. Table 1 includes the specific parameter values for each surgery type. For our baseline analyses for each type of surgery, we compared the surgery to usual diabetes care that included tight glycemic control similar to that provided in the UK Prospective Diabetes Study (20). We assumed that patients who were not in diabetes remission would also receive tight glycemic control. In total, our baseline analyses included four model runs, with separate runs for each type of surgery and for each diabetic population (newly diagnosed and established).

We converted all costs to 2005 U.S. dollars using the medical-care component of the Consumer Price Index (21). We discounted costs and QALYs by a 3% annual rate, and we estimated incremental cost-effectiveness ratios that were rounded to the nearest $1,000/QALY. We also report undiscounted remaining life-years.

We ran one-way sensitivity analyses to determine how key factors affected the cost-effectiveness ratios. When possible, we used end points of the published 95% (90% for surgery costs) CI of the model parameter to determine upper and lower values to input into the model. For most parameters where CIs were unavailable, we halved and doubled the baseline values. We varied the change in QoL per unit BMI change from 0 (i.e., surgery-related weight loss has no direct effect on QoL) to 0.017. We also analyzed the effect of surgery on the diabetic population with a BMI between 30 and 34 kg/m^2. We assumed a similar percentage change in excess weight loss (22) as in our main analysis, which leads to a smaller change in BMI and QoL improvement.

To examine how conjoint parameter uncertainty affected the model results, we conducted probabilistic sensitivity analysis (PSA) on key parameters involved in estimating the cost-effectiveness ratios. Applying distributions for surgery costs,

Table 1—Key surgery-related model parameter values

Variable	Bypass	Banding	Parameter value	Range for sensitivity analysis
Parameter values for people with newly diagnosed diabetes				
Diabetes remission rate	√		80.3%	74.4–86.1%
		√	56.7%	46.7–66.8%
Glycemic level after remission	√	√	6.0%	
Diabetes improvement rate	√		0.0%	
		√	24.0%	19.8–28.3%
Glycemic level after improvement	√	√	5.9%	
Reduction in oral medications usage due to diabetes improvement	√	√	51.8%	
Annual probability of relapse	√	√	8.3%	
Perioperative mortality rate	√		0.253%	0.143–0.365%
		√	0.068%	0.009–0.136%
Effect of surgery on systolic blood pressure	√		11.25% reduction first 2 years Effect then reduced by 1.4% each year until no reduction in year 10	
		√	3.2% reduction first 2 years then reduction to 0	
Effect of surgery on total cholesterol	√		16.1% reduction first 2 years Effect then reduced by 1.2% each year until no reduction in year 10	
		√	5.0% reduction first 2 years then reduction to 0	
Effect of surgery on HDL	√		No effect first 2 years Effect then increased by 1.7% each year until year 10	
		√	10.0% increase first 2 years Effect then decreased by 0.05% each year until year 10	
Effect of surgery on QoL (equals utility improvement per 1 unit BMI decline times BMI loss following surgery)	√		0.0899	0–0.275
		√	0.0668	0–0.204
Mean utility improvement per 1 unit BMI decline	√	√	0.0056	0–0.017
Mean BMI loss following surgery	√		16.17	14.07–18.27
		√	12.01	10.78–13.24
Surgery and first year costs	√		$23,871	$6,612–55,261
		√	$15,169	$2,857–30,186
Year 2 costs	√		$3,207	$1,603–6,414
Year 3 costs	√		$1,990	$995–3,981
Year 4 costs	√		$1,469	$734–2,938
Year 5 costs	√		$1,469	$734–2,938
Year ≥6 costs	√		$330	$165–661
Year 2 costs		√	$3,300	$1,650–6,600
Year 3 costs		√	$1,940	$970–3,880
Year 4 costs		√	$1,940	$970–3,880
Year 5 costs		√	$1,940	$970–3,880
Year ≥6 costs		√	$802	$401–1,604
Parameter values that differ for people with established diabetes				
Diabetes remission rate	√	√	40%	37.2–43.1%
Diabetes improvement rate	√	√	40%	37.2–43.1%
Glycemic level after improvement	√	√	7.0%	
Reduction in oral medication usage due to diabetes improvement	√	√	24.9%	12.45%
Reduction in insulin usage due to diabetes improvement	√	√	62.5%	31.25%

See online appendix for details on sources and parameter derivation.

Table 2—*Life-years gained and cost-effectiveness ratios (relative to no surgery) for baseline analyses*

	Total costs*	Remaining life-years	QALYs*	Cost-effectiveness ratio ($/QALY)†
Patients with newly diagnosed diabetes				
No surgery (standard care)	$71,130	21.62	9.55	
Bypass surgery	$86,665	23.34	11.76	
Incremental (vs. no surgery)	$15,536	1.72	2.21	$7,000
Banding surgery	$89,029	22.76	11.12	
Incremental (vs. no surgery)	$17,900	1.14	1.57	$11,000
Patients with established diabetes				
No surgery	$79,618	16.86	7.68	
Bypass surgery	$99,944	17.95	9.38	
Incremental (vs. no surgery)	$20,326	1.09	1.70	$12,000
Banding surgery	$96,921	17.80	9.02	
Incremental (vs. no surgery)	$17,304	0.94	1.34	$13,000

*Costs and QALYs are discounted at a 3% annual rate. †Cost-effectiveness ratios are rounded to the nearest $1,000/QALY.

remission rates, BMI loss, and other input parameters (see online appendix), we drew 1,000 parameter combinations and ran the model separately for each combination for newly diagnosed patients undergoing bypass surgery. We repeated the process for newly diagnosed patients undergoing banding surgery. Due to run time constraints, we only looked at patients in the 45- to 54-year age-group, which had a cost-effectiveness ratio that was close to the cost-effectiveness ratio for the entire population.

RESULTS — Based on the model assumptions, bariatric surgery leads to diabetes remission, and the share of patients in remission declines over time as patients relapse or die. Surgery also reduced the incidence of many diabetes-related complications for people with newly diagnosed diabetes (see online appendix).

In each of our main analyses, bariatric surgery had cost-effectiveness ratios between $7,000 and $13,000/QALY. Table 2 shows total costs, life-years, QALYs, and cost-effectiveness ratios (cost/QALY gained) by surgery type and patient group. Within the newly diagnosed diabetic population, gastric bypass led to 1.72 life-years gained, 2.21 QALYs gained, and a cost-effectiveness ratio of $7,000/QALY; gastric banding led to 1.14 life-years gained, 1.57 QALYs gained, and a cost-effectiveness ratio of $11,000/QALY. Relative to the newly diagnosed diabetic population, bariatric surgery led to fewer life-years gained and higher incremental cost-effectiveness ratios within the established diabetic population. Gas-

tric bypass led to 1.09 life-years gained, 1.70 QALYs gained, and a cost-effectiveness ratio of $12,000/QALY, whereas gastric banding led to 0.94 life-years gained, 1.34 QALYs gained, and a cost-effectiveness ratio of $13,000/QALY in the established diabetic population.

One-way sensitivity analyses
Fig. 1 shows the effect on the cost-effectiveness ratio of varying each parameter in one-way sensitivity analyses. The figure includes separate panels for each baseline analysis group (i.e., bypass and banding surgery for the newly diagnosed and established diabetic populations). For each analysis population, varying the effects of surgery on remission rates, perioperative mortality, and relapse rate had relatively small effects on the cost-effectiveness ratios. Varying the change in BMI from surgery also had little effect, but varying the direct QoL improvement per unit of BMI loss from 0.017 (which reduces the cost-effectiveness ratio) to 0 (which increases the cost-effectiveness ratio) had the biggest impact on the cost-effectiveness ratios. Doubling the cost of tight glycemic control (i.e., increasing the cost of treating active diabetes) produces the lowest or second lowest cost-effectiveness ratio in each analysis population. Varying surgery costs had a bigger impact on the bypass cost-effectiveness ratios than on the banding ratios, while varying follow-up costs had a bigger impact on the banding cost-effectiveness ratios than on the bypass ratios. Halving the reduction in medication usage associated with diabetes improvement increased the

cost-effectiveness ratios by <$1,000/QALY for each analysis population (not shown).

In addition, we ran analyses for different subpopulation groups. Running the analysis for a diabetic population with a BMI of 30–34 kg/m^2 approximately doubled the cost-effectiveness ratios, due primarily to the lower BMI loss and consequently smaller change in QoL. We also ran analyses with each 10-year age-group (not shown). Within the newly diagnosed diabetic population, cost-effectiveness ratios ranged from $5,000/QALY at ages 35–44 years to $12,000/QALY at ages 65–74 years for bypass surgery and from $9,000 to $17,000/QALY for the same ages for banding surgery. Within the established diabetic population, cost-effectiveness ratios ranged from $9,000/QALY at ages 45–54 years to $18,000/QALY at ages 65–74 years for bypass surgery and from $11,000 to $19,000/QALY for the same ages for banding surgery. The age-group analyses assumed (due to lack of age-specific data) that remission, perioperative mortality, and other direct surgical outcome rates and costs did not vary by age. Therefore, the age-group results were driven by higher mortality rates in older populations.

PSA
For bypass surgery, the median cost-effectiveness ratio for the 1,000 simulations on newly diagnosed patients aged 45–54 years was $6,000/QALY, and 95% of the values fell between −$2,000 and $23,000/QALY. All simulations with a negative cost-effectiveness ratio had lower costs and higher QALYs. For banding, the median cost-effectiveness ratio for the 1,000 simulations was $10,000/QALY, and 95% of the estimates fell between just under $0 and $30,000/QALY. Again, all simulations with a negative cost-effectiveness ratio had lower costs and higher QALYs. For detailed PSA results, including cost-effectiveness acceptability curves, see the online appendix.

CONCLUSIONS — Overall, we find that gastric bypass and gastric banding appear to be relatively cost-effective treatments in the severely obese diabetic population, with cost-effectiveness ratios ranging from $7,000 to $13,000/QALY. These cost-effectiveness ratios are lower than the cost-effectiveness ratios for commonly applied diabetes interventions and well below the $50,000/QALY benchmark sometimes applied (23) as a mea-

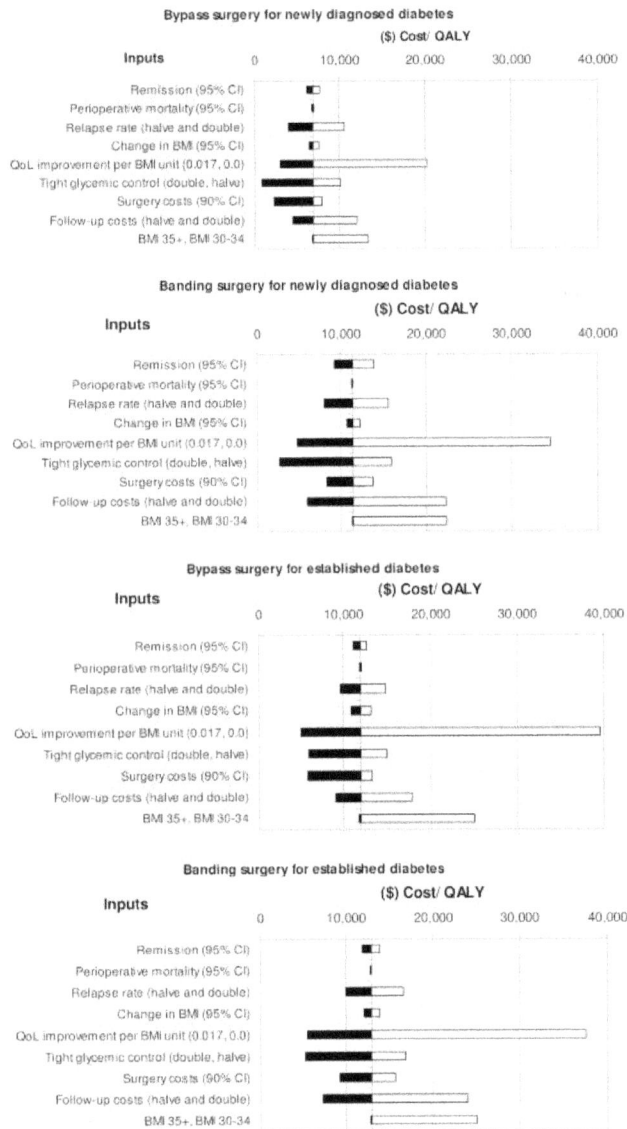

Figure 1—Sensitivity analyses: cost-effectiveness ratios for lower and upper bound of input values. The range of cost-effectiveness ratios after varying input parameters. For example, using the 95% CI values of remission for bariatric surgery in newly diagnosed patients, we find cost-effectiveness ratios ranging from $6,000 to $8,000/QALY. A QoL improvement of 0.017 leads to a lower cost-effectiveness ratio, and an improvement of 0 leads to a higher cost-effectiveness ratio. Doubling tight glycemic control costs leads to a lower cost-effectiveness ratio, and halving them leads to a higher cost-effectiveness ratio.

to surgery and that savings in the years following surgery would persist. The second study (12) estimated cost differences related to BMI in cross-sectional data and then calculated the effect of surgery on costs based on the decrease in BMI following surgery. It also assumed that cost reductions after surgery would persist. We explicitly model relapse to diabetes, which leads to decreasing cost savings over time. Third, our approach only includes diabetes-related costs that are saved as a result of diabetes remission and the reduction of micro- and macrovascular complications; this could result in lower savings than those found by the two U.S. studies, which considered all obesity-related costs.

In our analysis, bypass surgery leads to greater gains in QALYs and has lower costs than banding surgery for patients with newly diagnosed diabetes. The principal parameters that led to this result are the higher diabetes remission rate in bypass surgery and the larger BMI loss and therefore larger QoL improvement associated with bypass surgery. The two parameters favoring banding surgery—bypass surgery has higher first-year costs and higher perioperative mortality—do not offset the parameters favoring bypass surgery. The difference in cost-effectiveness ratios between the two surgeries is less pronounced in the established diabetic population than in the newly diagnosed diabetic population. In the established diabetic population, bypass and banding were assumed to have the same rates of remission and improvement.

Although the model parameters appear to favor bypass surgery, there have not been direct trials of the two types of surgeries. The more favorable bypass surgery parameters may be due to the different characteristics of people who opt for bypass surgery. This population tends to have a higher initial BMI and a greater prevalence of comorbidities (1). A randomized trial comparing bypass and banding would provide more compelling evidence on the relative cost-effectiveness of the two procedures than our simulation provides.

Current National Institutes of Health (24) guidelines state that patients with a BMI ≥ 40 kg/m^2 or a BMI between 35 and 40 kg/m^2 plus a comorbidity such as diabetes may be candidates for bariatric surgery. Most key model parameters are based on surgery for extremely obese individuals (in a key meta-analysis [1], the mean BMI is 47.9). One study (25), how-

sure of society's willingness to pay for health interventions. The cost-effectiveness ratios are lower for the newly diagnosed diabetic population than for the established diabetic population because the diabetes remission rate is higher for those newly diagnosed.

Although our cost-effectiveness ratios are in a similar range as several studies that found that bariatric surgery increases costs and QALYs (7–10), we do not find cost savings from either gastric bypass or gastric banding surgery as several other

studies have reported (6,11–13). There are at least three reasons why we did not find cost savings. First, the two cost-effectiveness models that find cost savings (11,13) are set outside of the U.S. Because our model reflects U.S. treatment costs, our results may not be comparable. Second, neither U.S.-based study that found cost savings (6,12) used a cost-effectiveness model. One study (6) compared total costs for a surgery population and a nonsurgery population; it assumed that any cost differences were attributable

ever, shows good results for diabetes remission in people with relatively low BMI. In our sensitivity analysis for people with a BMI between 30 and 34 kg/m^2, we estimated higher cost-effectiveness ratios than those for more obese patients, but the ratios are still reasonably attractive.

Our analysis has several limitations. First, our model is limited by the health parameters included in the model. We only measure the benefits of bariatric surgery arising from its effect on diabetes remission, blood pressure, and cholesterol levels—which in turn affect diabetes micro- and macrovascular complications—and the effect of BMI loss on QoL. These benefits include reduced rates of coronary heart disease and stroke, important drivers of morbidity and mortality in people with diabetes. Second, limited data are available on the long-term effects of bariatric surgery. Sensitivity analyses on the diabetes remission rate and diabetes relapse rate—two important long-term effects—suggest that varying these parameters may not change the general conclusion that bariatric surgery is cost-effective. More broadly, the long-term impacts of surgery on diabetes complications, costs, and QALYs are generated by our simulation model. There are little or no direct data on surgery's long-term impact on these variables. In the absence of long-term study data, a simulation model may provide policy makers with useful information about the possible effects of interventions. Third, we assumed a QoL improvement directly associated with BMI loss based on cross-sectional data due to limited data on QALYs per BMI unit loss following surgery. Fourth, few studies examine diabetes remission in the population with longer-term diabetes. Based on a single study (18), we assumed rates of 40% remission and 40% improvement for bypass and banding in the established diabetic population.

Fifth, data on surgical outcomes for patients with established diabetes are limited. We incorporated lower rates of remission in established patients in our analysis, but we assumed (due to lack of data) that surgical costs and perioperative mortality rates were the same for established patients as for newly diagnosed patients. If the outcomes are less favorable for established patients, their cost-effectiveness ratios would increase. Data on surgical outcomes for older patients are also limited, with similar implications for the cost-effectiveness ratios.

Finally, our model assumes that diabetes progression rates are homogeneous, in the sense that a severely obese person with active diabetes and an A1C of 8.0% has the same progression rates for diabetes complications as a nonobese person with active diabetes and an A1C of 8.0%. This assumption is reasonable given current evidence, but it ignores alternative possibilities.

Subject to these limitations, our analysis indicates that gastric bypass and gastric banding surgery appear to provide a cost-effective method of reducing mortality and diabetes complications in severely obese adults with diabetes. We do not find that bariatric surgery is cost-saving. Therefore, health care costs will increase if more individuals receive bariatric surgery, but the increased costs appear to offer good value. As trials directly comparing bypass and banding surgery emerge and more studies examine the long-term effects of bariatric surgery, estimates of the cost-effectiveness of surgery can become more fine tuned, helping to guide future policy decisions.

Acknowledgments— T.J.H., J.E.S., and S.C. received support from the Centers for Disease Control and Prevention (CDC) under contract no. 200-2008-F-26817.

No potential conflicts of interest relevant to this article were reported.

T.J.H., P.Z., J.E.S., and S.C. researched data. T.J.H., P.Z., J.E.S., H.S.K., L.E.B., and S.C. contributed to discussion. T.J.H. and J.E.S. wrote the manuscript. P.Z., H.S.K., L.E.B., and S.C. reviewed/edited the manuscript.

We received assistance from an Expert Panel that included Drs. Edward H. Livingston, E. Patchen Dellinger, Myrlene Staten, and Eric A. Finkelstein. We thank Susan Murchie from RTI International for editorial assistance.

References
1. Buchwald H, Estok R, Fahrbach K, Banel D, Jensen MD, Pories WJ, Bantle JP, Sledge I. Weight and type 2 diabetes after bariatric surgery: systematic review and meta-analysis. Am J Med 2009;122:248–256
2. Maggard MA, Shugarman LR, Suttorp M, Maglione M, Sugarman HJ, Livingston EH, Nguyen NT, Li Z, Mojica WA, Hilton L, Rhodes S, Morton SC, Shekelle PG. Meta-analysis: surgical treatment of obesity. Ann Intern Med 2005;142:547–559
3. Sjostrom L, Lindroos AK, Peltonen M, Torgerson J, Bouchard C, Carlsson B, Dahlgren S, Larsson B, Narbro K, Sjostrom CD, Sullivan M, Wedel H. Lifestyle, diabetes, and cardiovascular risk factors 10 years after bariatric surgery. N Engl J Med 2004;351:2683–2693
4. Sjostrom L, Narbro K, Sjostrom D, Karason K, Larsson B, Wedel H, Lystig T, Sullivan M, Bouchard C, Carlsson B, Bengtsson C, Dahlgren S, Gummesson A, Jacobson P, Karlsson J, Lindross AK, Lonroth H, Naslund I, Olbers T, Stenlof K, Torgerson J, Agren G, Carlsson LMS. Effects of bariatric surgery on mortality in Swedish obese subjects. N Engl J Med 2007;357:741–752
5. Encinosa WE, Bernard DM, Steiner CA, Chen CC. Use and costs of bariatric surgery and prescription weight-loss medications. Health Affairs 2005;24:1039–1046
6. Cremieux PY, Buchwald H, Shikora SA, Ghosh A, Yang HE, Buessing M. A study on the economic impact of bariatric surgery. Am J Manag Care 2008;14:589–596
7. Clegg A, Colquitt J, Sidhu M, Royle P, Walker A. Clinical and cost effectiveness of surgery for morbid obesity: a systematic review and economic evaluation. Int J Obes Relat Metab Disord 2003;27:1167–1177
8. Craig BM, Tseng DS. Cost-effectiveness of gastric bypass for severe obesity. Am J Med 2002;113:491–498
9. Salem L, Devlin A, Sullivan SD, Flum DR. Cost-effectiveness analysis of laparoscopic gastric bypass, adjustable gastric banding, and nonoperative weight loss interventions. Surg Obes Relat Dis 2008;4:26–32
10. Ikramuddin S, Klingman D, Swan T, Minshall ME. Cost-effectiveness of Roux-en-Y gastric bypass in type 2 diabetes patients. Am J Manag Care 2009;15:607–615
11. Ackroyd R, Mouiel J, Chevallier JM, Daoud F. Cost-effectiveness and budget impact of obesity surgery in patients with type-2 diabetes in three European countries. Obes Surg 2006;16:1488–1503
12. Finkelstein EA, Brown DS. A cost-benefit simulation model of coverage for bariatric surgery among full-time employees. Am J Manag Care 2005;11:641–646
13. Keating CL, Dixon JB, Moodie ML, Peeters A, Bulfone L, Maglianno DJ, O'Brien PE. Cost-effectiveness of surgically induced weight loss for the management of type 2 diabetes: modeled lifetime analysis. Diabetes Care 2009;32:567–574
14. CDC Diabetes Cost-Effectiveness Group (Corresponding Author: T.J. Hoerger). Cost-effectiveness of intensive glycemic control, intensified hypertension control, and serum cholesterol level reduction for type 2 diabetes. JAMA 2002;287:2542–2551
15. Herman WH, Hoerger TJ, Brandle M, Hicks K, Sorensen S, Zhang P, Hamman RF, Ackermann RT, Engelgau MM, Ratner RE. Diabetes Prevention Program Research Group. The cost-effectiveness of

lifestyle modification or metformin in preventing type 2 diabetes in adults with impaired glucose tolerance. Ann Intern Med 2005;142:323–332

16. Hoerger TJ, Segel JE, Zhang P, Sorensen SW. *Validation of the CDC-RTI Diabetes Cost-Effectiveness Model*. RTI Press Methods Report, Research Triangle Part, NC, RTI International, 2009

17. Brancatisano A, Wahlroos S, Matthews S, Brancatisano R. Gastric banding for the treatment of type 2 diabetes mellitus in morbidly obese. Surg Obes Relat Dis 2008;4:423–429

18. Schauer PR, Burguera B, Ikramuddin S, Cottam D, Gourash W, Hamad G, Eid GM, Mattar S, Ramanathan R, Barinas-Mitchel E, Rao RH, Kuller L, Kelley D. Effect of laparoscopic Roux-en-Y gastric bypass on type 2 diabetes mellitus. Ann Surg 2003;238:467–485

19. Buchwald H, Estok R, Fahrbach K, Banel D, Sledge I. Trends in mortality in bariatric surgery: a systematic review and meta-analysis. Surgery 2007;142:621–635

20. UK Prospective Diabetes Study (UKPDS) Group. Intensive blood-glucose control with sulphonylureas or insulin compared with conventional treatment and risk of complications in patients with type 2 diabetes. Lancet 1998;352:837–853

21. U.S. Department of Labor, Bureau of Labor Statistics. Consumer Price Index, [article online]. Available from http://data.bls.gov/cgi-bin/surveymost?cu. Accessed 15 April 2009

22. Angrisani L, Di Lorenzo N, Favretti F, Furbetta F, Iuppa A, Doldi SB, Paganelli M, Basso N, Lucchese M, Zappa M, Lesti G, Capizzi FD, Giardiello C, Paganini A, Di Cosmo L, Veneziani A, Lacitignola S, Silecchia G, Alkilani M, Forestieri P, Puglisi F, Gardinazzi A, Toppino M, Campanile F, Marzano B, Bernante P, Perrotta G, Borrelli V, Lorenzo M, the Italian Collaborative Study Group for LAP-BAND. Predictive value of initial body mass index for weight loss after 5 years of follow-up Surg Endosc 2004;18:1524–1527

23. Grosse SD. Assessing cost-effectiveness in healthcare: history of the $50,000 per QALY threshold. Expert Rev Pharmacoeconomics Outcomes Res 2008;8:165–178

24. National Institutes of Health (NIH). *Clinical Guidelines on the Identification, Evaluation, and Treatment of Overweight and Obesity in Adults: The Evidence Report*. Bethesda, MD, NIH, 1998 [NIH publication no. 98-4083]

25. Dixon JB, O'Brien PE, Playfair J, Chapman L, Schachter LM, Skinner S, Proietto J, Bailey M, Anderson M. Adjustable gastric banding and conventional therapy for type 2 diabetes: a randomized controlled trial. JAMA 2008;299(3):316–323

Differential Adaptation of Human Gut Microbiota to Bariatric Surgery–Induced Weight Loss

Links With Metabolic and Low-Grade Inflammation Markers

Jean-Pierre Furet,[1] Ling-Chun Kong,[2,3] Julien Tap,[1] Christine Poitou,[2,3] Arnaud Basdevant,[2,3] Jean-Luc Bouillot,[4] Denis Mariat,[1] Gérard Corthier,[1] Joël Doré,[1] Corneliu Henegar,[2] Salwa Rizkalla,[2,3] and Karine Clément[2,3]

OBJECTIVE—Obesity alters gut microbiota ecology and associates with low-grade inflammation in humans. Roux-en-Y gastric bypass (RYGB) surgery is one of the most efficient procedures for the treatment of morbid obesity resulting in drastic weight loss and improvement of metabolic and inflammatory status. We analyzed the impact of RYGB on the modifications of gut microbiota and examined links with adaptations associated with this procedure.

RESEARCH DESIGN AND METHODS—Gut microbiota was profiled from fecal samples by real-time quantitative PCR in 13 lean control subjects and in 30 obese individuals (with seven type 2 diabetics) explored before (M0), 3 months (M3), and 6 months (M6) after RYGB.

RESULTS—Four major findings are highlighted: *1*) *Bacteroides/ Prevotella* group was lower in obese subjects than in control subjects at M0 and increased at M3. It was negatively correlated with corpulence, but the correlation depended highly on caloric intake; *2*) *Escherichia coli* species increased at M3 and inversely correlated with fat mass and leptin levels independently of changes in food intake; *3*) lactic acid bacteria including *Lactobacillus/Leuconostoc/Pediococcus* group and *Bifidobacterium* genus decreased at M3; and *4*) *Faecalibacterium prausnitzii* species was lower in subjects with diabetes and associated negatively with inflammatory markers at M0 and throughout the follow-up after surgery independently of changes in food intake.

CONCLUSIONS—These results suggest that components of the dominant gut microbiota rapidly adapt in a starvation-like situation induced by RYGB while the *F. prausnitzii* species is directly linked to the reduction in low-grade inflammation state in obesity and diabetes independently of calorie intake. *Diabetes* **59: 3049–3057, 2010**

From the [1]French National Institute for Agricultural Research, U910, Unité d'Ecologie et de Physiologie du Système Digestif, Jouy-en-Josas, France; the [2]Assistance Publique-Hôpitaux de Paris, Hôpital Pitié-Salpêtrière, Département de Nutrition et d'Endocrinologie, Paris, France, and the Centre de Recherche Nutrition Humaine, Ile de France, Paris, France; [3]INSERM, U872, équipe 7 Nutriomique, Paris, France, and the Université Pierre et Marie Curie-Paris, Centre de Recherche des Cordeliers, UMR S 872, Paris, France; and the [4]Assistance Publique-Hôpitaux de Paris, Département de Chirurgie, Hôpital Hôtel-Dieu, Paris, France.

Corresponding author: Karine Clément, karine.clement@psl.aphp.fr.

Received 22 February 2010 and accepted 21 August 2010. Published ahead of print at http://diabetes.diabetesjournals.org on 28 September 2010. DOI: 10.2337/db10-0253. Clinical trial reg. no. NCT0047658, www.clinicaltrials.gov.

J.-P.F. and L.-C.K. contributed equally to this work.

besity is characterized by increased fat mass accumulation and the development of comorbidities including other metabolic and cardiovascular diseases. Even though some but not all environmental factors have been elucidated, the increasing epidemic of obesity appears virtually impossible to control, and the mechanisms associated with fat mass expansion need to be identified. Obesity is considered a low-grade inflammatory disease with adipose tissue contributing to this state via the secretion of molecules capable of altering metabolic homeostasis (1,2). A novel factor identified to play a role in human obesity and associated metabolic risks is the commensal microbiota of the intestine (3).

A role for the intestinal microbiota in harvesting energy from food (4) and regulating body fat storage (5) was proposed in rodents. Germ-free mice colonized by microbiota increase their body fat and develop insulin resistance in spite of a 30% decrease in food intake. These changes were associated with a dysbiosis in obese mice: an increased representation of the Firmicutes phylum and a reduced representation of the Bacteroidetes phylum (6). Other studies suggested a contribution of the gut microbiota-produced lipopolysaccharides to inflammation and development of metabolic syndrome (7–9). In humans, increased endotoxemia (circulating lipopolysaccharides) was found to be associated with increased fat consumption (10). In obese patients losing weight throughout low calorie diets, diminished Bacteroidetes and increased Firmicutes were found trended to that of lean control subjects at the end of the dietary intervention (11). However, modification of the Firmicutes-to-Bacteroidetes ratio observed in obese individuals was not confirmed in other studies (12). No study has clearly explored the association between these bacterial changes and improvement of metabolic or inflammatory phenotypes associated with weight modification over time.

Roux-en-Y gastric bypass (RYGB) surgery is an increasingly effective model to study in this context. RYGB leads to major improvements in metabolic and inflammatory markers (13). This procedure allows for an understanding of the molecular adaptations underlying the observed health benefits and the potential role of calorie restriction in changes in gut microbiota pattern.

Our present work analyzed the microbiota profiles in the feces of morbidly obese subjects before and after RYGB.

We examined the association between gut microbiota changes and a range of body composition, metabolic, and inflammatory markers. These results provide new insight regarding gut microbiota changes in obese subjects after RYGB and highlight some bacterial groups as possible factors associated with changes in nutritional status and others with metabolic and inflammatory parameters.

RESEARCH DESIGN AND METHODS

Thirty obese subjects (27 women and 3 men) enrolled in a bariatric surgery program were recruited at the Center of Reference for Medical and Surgical Care of Obesity (Pitié-Salpêtrière Hospital, Paris, France). The patients had the criteria for obesity surgery: BMI ≥ 40 kg/m^2 with at least two comorbidities (hypertension, type 2 diabetes, dyslipidemia, or obstructive sleep apnea syndrome). The subjects' weight was stable (± 2 kg) for at least 3 months prior to surgery. Subjects were exempted from acute or chronic inflammatory diseases, infectious diseases, viral infection, cancer, and/or known alcohol consumption. No antibiotics were taken before surgery or during the postsurgery follow-ups. Clinical and biological parameters were assessed prior to RYGB surgery (i.e., basal or M0) and at 3- and 6-months postsurgery (M3 and M6, respectively). The oral glucose tolerance test was performed in the 23 nondiabetic subjects (OB/nD subgroup). All had a glycemia <11 mmol/l 2 h after 75-g oral glucose. Seven subjects had type 2 diabetes (OB/D subgroup) with a fasting glycemia over 7 mmol/l and/or the use of an antidiabetic drug. Two individuals necessitated insulin therapy while the other five subjects were treated with metformin and hypolipidemic drugs (either fibrate or statins). Thirteen normal weight, healthy women volunteers living in the same area as the obese subjects were recruited as a lean control subject group. The Ethics Committee of the Hôtel-Dieu Hospital approved the clinical protocol. All subjects gave written informed consent.

Dietary assessment. At each visit, caloric intake and macronutrient portions were evaluated by a registered dietitian during a 1-h questioning period. Multivitamins and iron supplements were provided to avoid deficiencies, a well-known secondary effect of bariatric surgery (14). Serum iron, ferritin, the coefficient of saturation of iron in transferrin, vitamins (A, D, E, B1, B12, and B9), micronutrients, and calcium were measured using routine bio-clinical tests. Serum analyses showed that these parameters were in the normal range at all time points (data not shown).

Body composition, metabolic, and inflammatory parameters. Body composition was determined before and after the surgery by dual-energy X-ray absorptiometry (GE Lunar Prodigy Corporation, Madison, WI), and resting energy expenditure was measured by indirect calorimetry (Deltatrac, Datex, France). Periumbilical surgical biopsies of subcutaneous adipose tissues were obtained and adipocyte diameter was measured as described (15). Blood samples were obtained at each time point after 12-h fasting to measure plasma lipids (total cholesterol, HDL cholesterol, and triglycerides), insulin, glucose, leptin, adiponectin, and inflammatory markers (high-sensitivity C-reactive protein [hs-CRP], interleukin [IL]-6, orosomucoid).

Fecal samples. Fecal samples were obtained in the morning before breakfast. Whole stools were self-collected in sterile boxes and stored at $-20°C$ within 4 h. Samples were treated in the laboratory as 200-mg aliquots and stored at $-80°C$ until further analysis. The 30 obese subjects and 13 healthy control subjects delivered samples at M0. During follow-ups, fecal samples were obtained for 26 subjects (including 6 diabetic subjects) at M3 and for 15 subjects (including 5 diabetic subjects) at M6. A complete course of stool samples (M0, M3, and M6) was finally obtained for 10 individuals.

DNA extraction from fecal samples. DNA was extracted from (200-mg aliquots) feces as previously described (16). After the final precipitation, DNA was resuspended in 150 ml of TE buffer and stored at $-20°C$ prior to further analysis.

Oligonucleotide primers and probes. The primers and probes used in this study are presented in supplementary Table 6, available in an online appendix at http://diabetes.diabetesjournals.org/cgi/content/full/db10-0253/DC1. TaqMan qPCR was adapted to quantify the total bacteria population in addition to the dominant (>1% of fecal bacteria) bacterial species *Clostridium leptum* (*C. leptum*), *Clostridium coccoides* (*C. coccoides*), *Bacteroides/Prevotella*, and *Bifidobacterium*. Real-time qPCR using SYBR Green was performed for the *Lactobacillus/Leuconostoc/Pediococcus* and for the subdominant bacterial species *Escherichia coli* (*E. coli*), as well as for the *Faecalibacterium prausnitzii* (*F. prausnitzii*). The TaqMan probes were synthesized by Applied Biosystems Applera-France (Courtaboeuf, France). Primers were purchased from MWG (MWG-Biotech AG, Ebersberg, Germany).

Real-time qPCR. Real-time qPCR was performed using an ABI 7000 Sequence Detection System with software version 1.2.3 (Applied Biosystems, Foster City, CA). Amplification and detection were carried out in 96-well plates with

TaqMan Universal PCR 2× MasterMix (Applied Biosystems) or with SYBR Green PCR 2× Master Mix (Applied Biosystems). Each reaction was run in duplicate in a final volume of 25 ml with 0.2 mmol/l final concentration of each primer, 0.25 mmol/l final concentration of each probe, and 10 µl of appropriately diluted DNA samples. Amplifications were carried out using the following ramping profile: one cycle at 95°C for 10 min, followed by 40 cycles of 95°C for 30 s, 60°C for 1 min. For SYBR Green amplifications, a melting step was added to improve amplification specificity. The total numbers of bacteria were inferred from averaged standard curves as described (17).

Normalization of qPCR data. All bacteria results were presented as the mean of the $\log_{10}$ value $\pm$ SEM. To recount for water content in fecal samples, data for each fecal sample was normalized as previously described (16). The level for each bacterial species or group was subtracted from all bacteria content. The data are presented as log number of bacteria per gram of stool.

Day-to-day variations. To evaluate the stability of results of microbiota, we added a supplementary experiment to estimate day-to-day variations of fecal samples. Five healthy lean women (BMI: 23 ± 1; age 28 years ± 0.3) were included in this study. Fecal samples were collected during two consecutive days in the same conditions and with the same method of collection and treatment as cited above (supplementary Table 5).

Biochemical assays. Plasma glucose was measured by the glucose oxidase method (Beckman Fullerton, Palo Alto, CA). Plasma insulin was determined by using the reactive kit from Abbott (Rungis, France). Plasma triglycerides and free fatty acids were measured with Biomérieux kits (Marcy l'Etoile, France), and total cholesterol, HDL cholesterol, and LDL cholesterol with Labintest kits (Aix-en-Provence, France). Leptin, adiponectin, hs-CRP, IL-6, and TNF-α were determined by using ELISA kits from R&D Systems (Minneapolis, MN).

Statistical analysis. All values are expressed as mean ± SEM. Homeostasis model assessment of insulin resistance (HOMA-IR), insulin sensitivity (HOMA-S%), and β-cell function (HOMA-B%) provided in supplementary Table 2 were estimated. The composition of microbiota is expressed as mean of the $\log_{10}$ of the normalized PCR values. Wilcoxon rank sum tests were used to assess statistical significance of differences between lean control subjects and OB/nD and OB/D subjects at baseline. Paired Wilcoxon tests were performed to analyze changes in these parameters between various time points after surgery.

Principal component analysis (PCA) combined with co-inertia analysis was used to explore complex and potentially redundant relationships involving a relatively large number of clinical, biological, and microbiological variables at baseline and following RYGB. Co-inertia analysis is a coupling method for comparing different types of parameters presenting different variances. The significances of the associated variations of biological and clinical parameters and of bacterial counts during the follow-up after surgery were evaluated by Monte Carlo tests. Significant associations were visualized by a circle of correlations while their intensity was expressed by computing Spearman correlation coefficients (Rs).

The significances of the strongest dynamic associations of clinical-biological parameters and of bacterial counts after surgery among those identified by PCA and co-inertia analysis were further evaluated by building linear mixed-effects (LME) models to test for inter-variable redundancies and to adjust for potential confounding factors. All LME models were fit by maximizing the restricted log-likelihood (REML) of their estimated coefficients. All statistical analyses were performed using the R software (http://www.r-project.org). PCA and co-inertia analyses were performed with ADE-4 package (18). LME modeling was performed by relying on statistical functions available in the nlme package (19). All statistical computations were considered significant when resulting P values were <0.05 threshold.

RESULTS

Clinical and biological characteristics before RYGB. The clinical characteristics of lean and OB/D or OB/nD subjects are presented in supplemental Table 1. While mean age between control subjects and OB/nD subjects were not statistically different, OB/D subjects were older. **RYGB improves markedly clinical, metabolic, and inflammatory phenotypes.** Along with the drastic reduction in food consumption, RYGB resulted in significant changes in body weight and fat mass from M0 to M3 and M6 (Table 1). For the majority of parameters, improvements occurred rapidly in the first 3 months. At M6, the subjects had lost 22% of their initial weight ($P < 0.01$). Fat mass decreased and the percentage of fat-free mass increased. These changes were associated with a decrease

TABLE 1
Clinical and biological characteristics of obese subjects before, and 3 and 6 months after gastric surgery

	Before bypass	After bypass 3 months	6 months
Food intake			
Food intake (kcal)	$1{,}933 \pm 101^A$	$1{,}080 \pm 87^B$	$1{,}355 \pm 54^C$
Adiposity markers			
Body weight (kg)	126 ± 4.2^A	107 ± 3.9^B	98 ± 3.8^C
BMI (kg/m^2)	47.6 ± 1.5^A	40.6 ± 1.3^B	37.1 ± 1.3^C
Adipocyte diameter (μm)	116.7 ± 1.5^A	110.7 ± 1.0^B	103.3 ± 3.2^C
REE (kcal)	$1{,}814.4 \pm 54.8^A$	$1{,}842.5 \pm 53.6^A$	$1{,}551.1 \pm 42.9^B$
Fat mass %	47.9 ± 1.0^A	44.5 ± 1.0^B	41.3 ± 1.2^C
Fat-free mass %	50.0 ± 1.0^A	53.0 ± 0.9^B	55.9 ± 1.1^C
Leptin (ng/ml)	50.8 ± 3.7^A	25.6 ± 2.5^B	24.9 ± 2.8^B
Plasma glucose homeostasis and insulin sensitivity			
Glycemia (mmol/l)	6.4 ± 0.5^A	5.1 ± 0.2^B	4.8 ± 0.1^B
A1C (%)	6.4 ± 0.3^A	5.7 ± 0.1^B	5.8 ± 0.1^B
Insulinemia (μU/ml)	17.1 ± 1.6^A	10.7 ± 0.9^B	6.9 ± 0.7^C
HOMA-IR	0.88 ± 0.09^A	0.63 ± 0.03^B	0.78 ± 0.09^A
Adiponectin (μg/ml)	6.4 ± 0.5^A	7.8 ± 0.7^A	8.3 ± 0.7^B
Plasma lipid homeostasis			
Total cholesterol (mmol/l)	4.54 ± 0.16^A	4.23 ± 0.16^A	4.34 ± 0.15^A
Triglycerides (mmol/l)	1.57 ± 0.19^A	1.54 ± 0.17^A	1.48 ± 0.17^A
HDL cholesterol (mmol/l)	1.22 ± 0.05^A	1.17 ± 0.06^A	1.30 ± 0.06^B
Inflammatory markers			
Plasma hs-CRP (mg/dl)	3.1 ± 0.8^A	2.5 ± 0.9^B	2.7 ± 0.8^B
Plasma IL-6 (pg/ml)	4.4 ± 0.4^A	4.2 ± 0.4^A	3.4 ± 0.4^A
Plasma orosomucoid (g/l)	$1.02 \pm 0.04^{A,B}$	0.94 ± 0.04^A	0.86 ± 0.03^B

Values are expressed as mean $\pm$ SE ($n = 30$). Fat mass %, fat-free mass %: values expressed as a percentage of body weight. Paired Wilcoxon stands for analyzing parameters changes between various time points. Data not sharing the same letter within a horizontal line are significantly different ($P < 0.05$). REE: resting energy expenditure.

in adipocyte cell diameter ($P < 0.05$) and leptin serum concentrations ($P < 0.01$). These improvements were observed in both groups (OB/nD and OB/D) when considered separately (supplementary Table 2). However, the improvements found in inflammatory parameters (hs-CRP, orosomucoid) in the whole group of obese subjects (Table 1) disappeared when considered separately (supplementary Table 2). A slight decrease in orosomucoid remained in the OB/nD group.

Plasma glucose, insulin levels, glycosylated hemoglobin (A1C) and HOMA-IR decreased significantly post-RYGB, however adiponectin concentration did not change significantly at M3 (Table 1). An improvement in insulin sensitivity (HOMA-S%) of the OB/nD group and an amelioration of blood glucose homeostasis were found in the seven diabetic subjects (supplementary Table 2). Antidiabetic drugs were stopped in diabetic subjects as well as hypolipidemic treatment in all obese individuals.

Basal bacterial groups counts: decreased amount of Bacteroides/Prevotella in obesity and of F. prausnitzii in diabetes. Average counts for each bacterial group of control, OB/nD, and OB/D subjects are presented in Table 2 and Fig. 1. The Bacteroides/Prevotella group was lower in obese subjects (OB/nD: $P = 0.039$ and OB/D: $P = 0.038$) compared with lean subjects. However, while the population of C. leptum tended to be lower in obese subjects, the differences did not reach statistical significance probably due to the high interindividual variability in this bacterial population subgroup. F. prausnitzii species qPCR system could reliably distinguish between the control and OB/D microbiota. Their counts in the OB/D microbiota were significantly lower when compared with

those of the control group ($P < 0.01$) and OB/nD subjects ($P < 0.05$). These results suggest that while obesity leads to modification in the Bacteroides/Prevotella group, diabetes seems to influence the abundance of F. prausnitzii (supplementary Fig. 1).

Bacterial changes after RYGB: increased amount of Bacteroides/Prevotella and E. coli, decreased Bifidobacterium and Lactobacillus/Leuconostoc/Pediococcus groups. Changes of bacteria amounts were observed in the obese group (OB/nD and OB/D together) after surgery but with a different pattern depending on the bacterial group (Fig. 1). Supplementary Table 3 illustrates the progression of all bacterial populations within the microbiota before (M0) and after RYGB (M3 and M6) in each obese group and separated by the diabetic status. In the OB/D subjects, a similar pattern of changes as the one characterizing the OB/nD subjects was observed, but changes for certain bacterial groups did not reach statistical significance. The Bacteroides/Prevotella population, whose level was lower in obese subjects before RYGB, increased at M3 and remained stable until M6 (Fig. 1) at a level close to that of the control subjects. Importantly, the obese subjects remained obese at M6 (BMI 37.1 $\pm$ 1.3 vs. 21.1 $\pm$ 0.4, obese and lean subjects, respectively). At M3, E. coli showed a rapid and significant increase reaching a level higher than that of the control subjects. An opposite pattern was observed for both the Bifidobacterium and Lactobacillus/Leuconostoc/Pediococcus groups. Levels of both populations decreased at M3 and M6 and reached, in the case of Bifidobacterium, a level lower than that measured in the control subjects.

Interestingly, the level of F. prausnitzii, which was

TABLE 2
Composition of microbiota compared in lean control subjects, obese diabetic (OB/D) subjects, and nondiabetic (OB/nD) subjects before gastric surgery

			Firmicutes				Bacteroidetes		
	n	All bacteria*	Clostridium Coccoides group†	Lactobacillus/ Leuconostoc/ Pediococcus group†	Clostridium leptum group†	Faecalibacterium prausnitzii species†‡	Bifidobacterium genus†	Bacteroides/ Prevotella group†	E. coli species†
Control subject	13	11.74 ± 0.1	-1.58 ± 0.1^A	-3.46 ± 0.2^A	-0.31 ± 0.1^A	-1.06 ± 0.2^A	-2.47 ± 0.4^A	-1.11 ± 0.1^A	-3.43 ± 0.3^A
OB/nD	23	11.29 ± 0.1	-1.58 ± 0.2^A	-2.75 ± 0.3^A	-0.86 ± 0.3^A	-1.45 ± 0.2^A	-2.37 ± 0.2^A	-1.61 ± 0.1^B	-3.42 ± 0.3^A
OB/D	7	11.17 ± 0.1	-1.46 ± 0.4^A	-2.62 ± 0.5^A	-1.63 ± 0.8^A	-2.79 ± 0.5^B	-2.22 ± 0.4^A	-1.61 ± 0.2^B	-2.49 ± 0.3^A

Data not sharing the same letter within a column are significantly different ($P < 0.05$). n: represents the numbers of studied samples. *All bacteria results obtained by qPCR were expressed as mean of the $\log_{10}$ value $\pm$ SE. †Results were expressed as mean of the $\log_{10}$ value $\pm$ SE of normalized data, calculated as the log number of targeted bacteria minus the log number of all bacteria. ‡Faecalibacterium prausnitzii is the major component of the Clostridium leptum group.

lower in OB/D subjects before RYGB, increased at M3 and remained stable at M6 (supplementary Table 3). The populations of Clostridium (C. leptum and C. coccoides) were stable post-RYGB.

Association between microbiota composition and clinical phenotypes before RYGB. In OB/nD and OB/D subjects, we observed significant relationships between the amount of F. prausnitzii, E. coli, and Bacteroides/ Prevotella and metabolic and inflammatory parameters (supplementary Table 4A). The strongest associations were found for the amount of F. prausnitzii, which was negatively correlated with serum concentrations of inflammatory circulating markers (hs-CRP Rs -0.54, $P < 0.01$ and IL-6 Rs -0.65, $P < 0.001$). This negative correlation was consistently significant when analyzed alone in the OB/nD subjects. No significant association was correlated with age for any analysis.

Time-dependant associations between metabolic phenotypes and bacterial populations. Statistical LME models were used to distinguish within-subject from between-subject sources of variation and to describe how trajectories in clinical and bacterial population mean responses showed related changes over time. Analyses firstly included the entire population of obese subjects regardless of their diabetic status, and secondly in the OB/nD group or the OB/D group alone. The corpulence parameters, including body weight, BMI, body fat mass, and serum leptin concentrations, were correlated negatively with the counts of Bacteroides/Prevotella and E. coli, while positively with the amounts of Bifidobacterium population, independent of the diabetic states.

In the OB/nD group, Bacteroides/Prevotella counts correlated negatively with calorie intake ($P < 0.01$), which drastically changed after the bypass (supplementary Table 4B). Analysis, performed in the OB/nD group and associating calorie intake and each of the adiposity-related parameters as fixed-effects in a combined LME model, confirmed the negative relationship between Bacteroides/ Prevotella counts and the decrease in food consumption post-RYGB ($P < 0.05$). This result was independent of corpulence. The combined model could not demonstrate significant independent relationships with any of the adiposity-related parameters, thus indicating that variations in Bacteroides/Prevotella population after surgery are related mostly to calorie intake in this cohort.

Unlike the Bacteroides/Prevotella population, the relationship between calorie intake and E. coli counts lost statistical significance in the combined model. This suggests that E. coli could be considered as a marker of corpulence variation after surgery, independent of energy intake. The relationships between the microbiota and these clinical parameters, explored through PCA, is illustrated in Fig. 2A, which displays the strong negative correlation between E. coli counts and leptin serum concentration (Rs -0.53, $P < 0.001$). This correlation is reinforced in Fig. 2B, which concomitantly illustrates the kinetic evolution between E. coli population and leptin as a mirror image.

Time-dependant associations between inflammatory parameters and changes in bacterial populations: importance of F. prausnitzii. F. prausnitzii showed a consistent correlation with low-grade inflammation. After the surgery, the circulating inflammatory parameters (hs-CRP, IL-6, and orosomucoid) were reduced and an association was found with an increase in F. prausnitzii. F. prausnitzii variation was strongly and negatively corre-

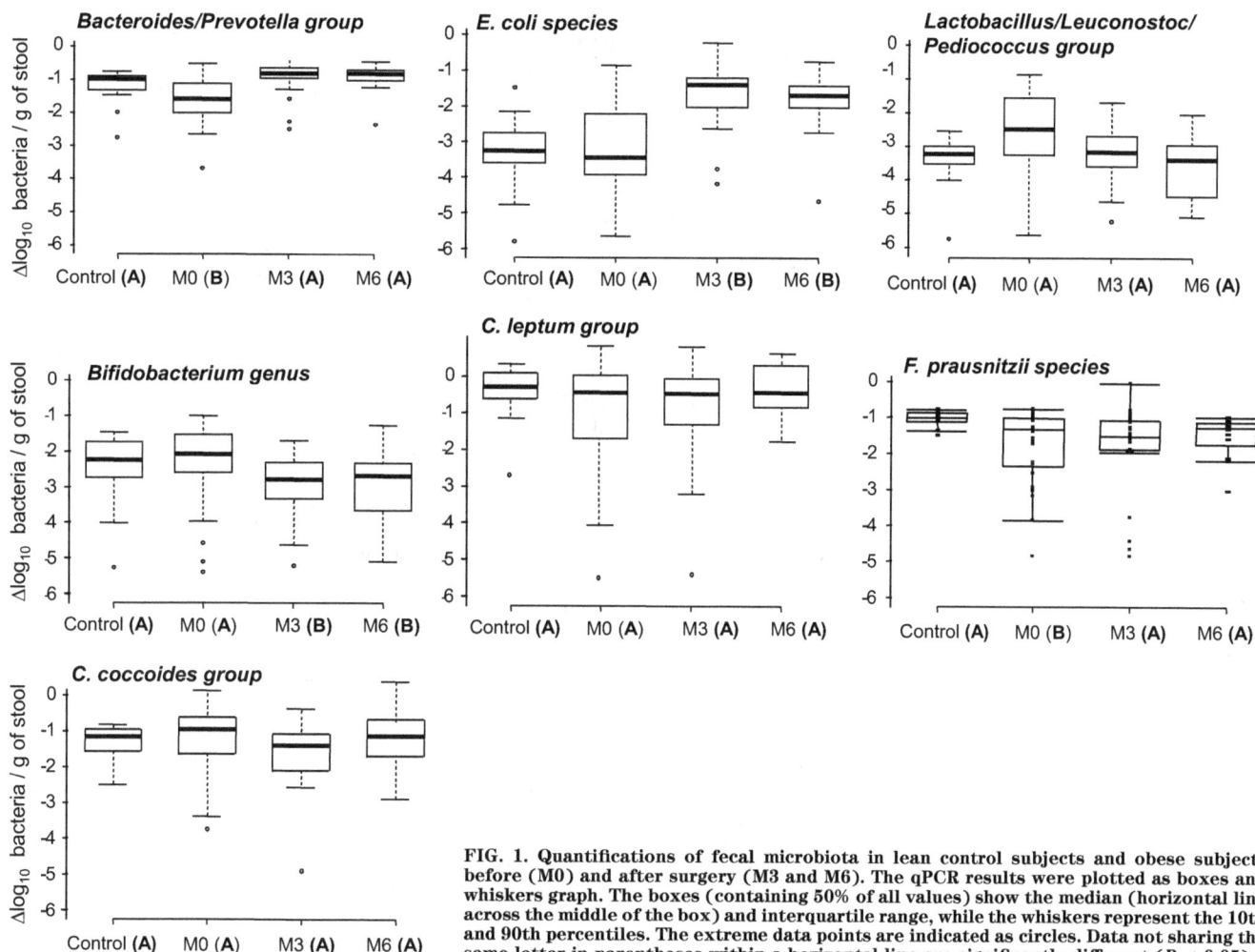

FIG. 1. Quantifications of fecal microbiota in lean control subjects and obese subjects before (M0) and after surgery (M3 and M6). The qPCR results were plotted as boxes and whiskers graph. The boxes (containing 50% of all values) show the median (horizontal line across the middle of the box) and interquartile range, while the whiskers represent the 10th and 90th percentiles. The extreme data points are indicated as circles. Data not sharing the same letter in parentheses within a horizontal line are significantly different ($P < 0.05$).

lated with changes in hs-CRP, IL-6, and orosomucoid serum levels when nondiabetic and diabetic obese subjects were grouped together. The correlations with hs-CRP and IL-6 were maintained in the OB/nD group (supplementary Table 4B). These relationships were independent of calorie intake.

DISCUSSION

Analysis of the dynamic changes post-RYGB provided important information regarding potential associations between gut microbiota composition, food intake, metabolic adaptations, and inflammation. In spite of the relatively sample size of the diabetic group and some incompletion in the collection of fecal samples, this study compared not only the different profile of gut microbiota between lean and obese diabetic or nondiabetic subjects, but revealed for the first time that changes of gut microbiota in the same individual before and after RYGB associate with a series of phenotypes. While some gut bacteria groups correlated with energy intake, body corpulence, and metabolic changes, others, such as *F. prausnitzii*, associated with changes in the inflammatory state and diabetes.

Our observation was made in severely obese subjects and might not be extended to moderately obese subjects. However, the lower proportion of *Bacteroides/Prevotella* in obese subjects before RYGB and their increase after

weight loss are in agreement with landmark studies in less obese populations (11,20). Correlation studies in LME kinetic models provide important information showing that these populations of bacteria were strongly associated with body composition and metabolic parameters. After RYGB, the higher the increase in the proportions of *Bacteroides/Prevotella*, the better the reduction in body fat mass and plasma leptin. These associations were dependent on energy intake. The estimated Firmicutes-to-Bacteroidetes ratio diminished substantially during weight loss, an observation also made in our study mostly due to the increase in *Bacteroides/Prevotella*. A degree of controversy was raised with regard to this result. No changes in the proportion of Bacteroidetes or Firmicutes-to-Bacteroidetes ratio were found, while the total numbers of bacteria decreased in other studies (12,21). These discrepancies could be attributed to substantial differences in clinical protocols with varying levels and duration of calorie restriction and fat mass loss. RYGB could be considered as a unique model that can be clinically followed over time in the same individual. RYGB was found to be associated with a decrease in Firmicutes together with an increase in γ-Proteobacteria in three adults (22). In this first study, the individual fecal samples before and after weight loss were not paired, and no information was

A

B

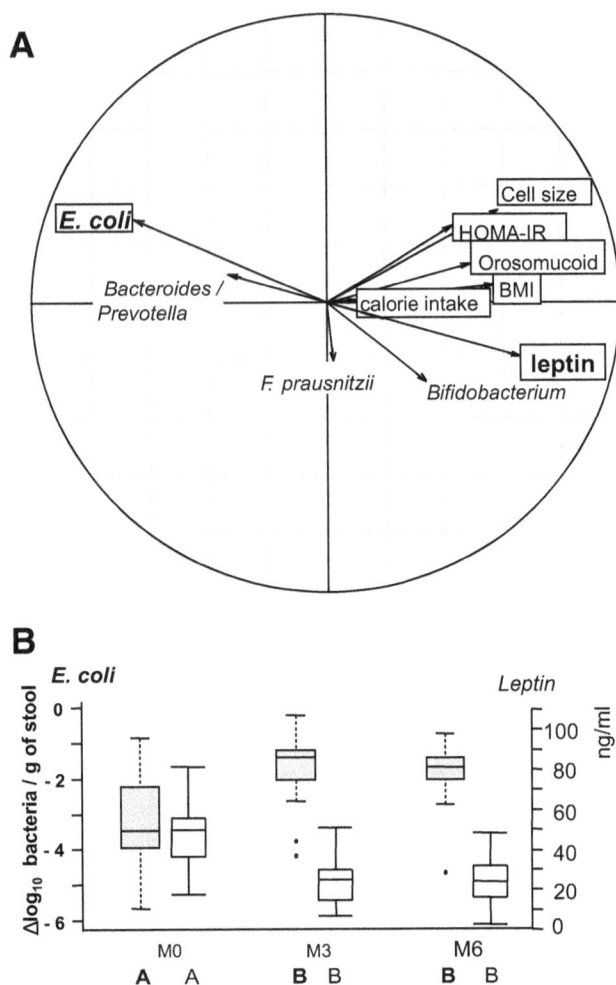

FIG. 2. Relationship between changes in fecal microbiota composition and clinical parameters in obese patients following RYGB surgery. Real-time qPCR quantifications were used to determine the fecal microbiota composition for the bacterial groups indicated in supplementary Table 6. Clinical parameters included adipocyte cell size, BMI, calorie intake, HOMA-IR, leptin, and orosomucoid. A: Principal component analysis (between class analyses). Bold arrows indicate the marked inverse relationship between changes in E. coli population and leptin serum concentrations. B: Dynamics of E. coli population evolution and leptin concentration during the study. E. coli population levels are expressed as mean ± SEM of the $\Delta\log_{10}$ value of normalized data calculated as the log number of targeted bacteria minus the log number of all bacteria. Leptin results were expressed as mean ± SEM of serum concentrations.

provided about the amount weight lost and associated phenotypic changes.

Here our patients were followed for 6 months with a marked reduction in food intake at M3 and M6 post-RYGB. It is important to note that there is a well-known uncertainty and possible underestimation of food intake in obese subjects (23). Nevertheless, after a short fasting period (1–3 days), the subjects started to increase their food intake that was composed of liquid or semi-liquid foods for 1 week. During the 3 months after RYGB, starch-based foods are often the principal food items with solid foods being progressively reintroduced. With reduced calorie intake and changes in body composition, leptin dropped and its variations were negatively associated with the amount of Bacteroides/Prevotella and E. coli, while positively associated with Bifidobacterium and

Lactobacillus/Leuconostoc/Pediococcus. Among its diverse physiological functions, the major adipocyte-secreted hormone, leptin, has a critical role in the initiation of adaptation responses to starvation (24). In the present study, leptin levels fell rapidly with the onset of energy deprivation at M3 (−50% of basal values) and relatively stabilized at M6 while BMI, fat mass, and adipocyte sizes continued to shrink, which is in line with the results found in other studies (25). This phenomenon is recognized as signaling the shift between sufficient and insufficient body energy. The ability of sustained fasting to induce dissociation between circulating leptin levels and adipose tissue mass could also reflect a permissive effect of insulin on leptin secretion. This may have conferred a survival advantage during evolution as leptin stimulates energy expenditure and inhibits appetite (26). In agreement with Bajzer and Seeley (27), changes in gut microbiota post-RYGB could be linked to maximizing energy harvest as a host adaptation to the starvation-like condition. The fact that for most gut bacteria, changes were observed at M3 and remained stable at M6 (supplementary Table 3) while corpulence and metabolic factors continued to improve favors this particular interpretation. This is also strengthened by the results of another study (L.-C. Kong, S. Rizkalla, K. Clément, et al.) from our laboratory that demonstrates early changes in fecal bacteria population, which started 1 week after caloric restriction. Interestingly, compared with germ-free animals, hepatic ketogenesis is enhanced during 24-h fasting in mice (CONV-D) after a microbiota transplant from the distal gut of conventionally raised lean counterparts fed with carbohydrates (28). The CONV-D mice showed an increase of short-chain fatty acids, and the proportion of Bacteroidetes switched from 20.6% at the fed state to 42.3% at the fasted state, while the proportion of Firmicutes reduced from 77.1 to 52.6%. We also found that the relationship between some gut microbiota changes and corpulence and metabolic parameters might not be statistically dependent on dietary changes as in the case of E. coli and Bifidobacterium. This is an indirect indication that microbiota components could participate in metabolic changes associated with this surgical procedure.

RYGB procedure per se may contribute to changes in gut microbiota composition. RYGB creates a small gastric pouch and the distal stomach and proximal small intestine are bypassed by attaching the distal end of the midjejunum to the proximal gastric pouch. The bile and pancreatic limb is attached along the Roux limb. Gastric acidity is bypassed leading to a reduction of chloride acid flux in the gut. Patients were also under the proton pump inhibitor therapy during the first 3 months, which can also influence the gastric pH. The resulting increased pH, together with the downstream delivery of bile acids, could contribute to modify fecal bacteria population. In in vitro culture studies, the growth of Bacteroidetes was found to be inhibited when reducing pH, while the growth of E. coli was facilitated by increased pH (29). We did not measure the pH in our subjects' fecal samples, but the decreased acidity in the gut after RYGB could favor an increase in Bacteroides/Prevotella and E. coli counts. The changes in E. coli strongly correlated negatively with leptin variation (Fig. 2A). However, leptin can also be secreted by cells in the lower half of the stomach glands (30). The signaling molecules mechanistically involved in driving these links need to be elucidated. Another consequence of pH change post-RYGB could be the decrease in Lactobacillus/Leuconostoc/*Pediococcus* and *Bifidobacterium* (31). This is not consistent with the studies in mice that suggest a beneficial effect of *Bifidobacterium* species in the improvement of obesity-related metabolic and inflammatory condition (8). The *Bifidobacterium* genus, however, is complex. In adolescents losing moderate amounts of weight, the counts of *B. bifidum* and of *B. breve* diminished while *B. catenulatum* increased (32). Information on the intake of prebiotic or probiotic are not available in this study; hence, we cannot exclude a possible influence of functional ingredients included in foods (e.g., yogurts) on these bacteria.

Shorter- and longer-term studies are needed to explore the dynamics of subjects undergoing bypass surgery with attention given to food intake behavior, measures of metabolic mediators (such as short-chain fatty acids and free fatty acids), measures of fecal pH to explore the dependency between changes in food intake, the influence of the surgery per se, and gut bacterial groups. A comparison with patients only subjected to a restrictive surgical procedure (i.e., gastroplasty) would be useful in this respect.

The other important information provided here was that *F. prausnitzii* was associated with inflammatory markers. *F. prausnitzii* has been identified as a conserved and dominant species of the human fecal microbiota of healthy individuals (33). *F. prausnitzii* might play a role in preventing local bowel inflammation and infection in acute inflammatory disease. A reduction of *F. prausnitzii* has been described in inflammatory bowel disease and in infectious colitis (34). Our study suggests that *F. prausnitzii* could also play a role in low-grade inflammation pathologies like obesity and diabetes (35–37). The relationship between *F. prausnitzii* and inflammatory markers was observed both in OB/nD and OB/D patients and remained after adjustment for BMI. The proportions of *F. prausnitzii* were lower in type 2 diabetic subjects displaying a worsening of their low-grade inflammation (38) and higher insulin resistance. A negative association was also seen between *F. prausnitzii* and HOMA-IR, which could be explained by the amelioration of glucose metabolism in the diabetic group. However in the present study, this was not true for adiponectin, another marker of insulin sensitivity. The discrepancy between HOMA-IR and adiponectin during weight loss has been well documented (39).

F. prausnitzii population variation was associated with modulation of urinary metabolites of diverse structure indicating that this species is a highly active member of the microbiome, influencing host pathways (40). *F. prausnitzii* exhibits anti-inflammatory effects, partly due to secreted metabolites able to block nuclear factor-κB activation and the secretion of proinflammatory mediators (41). Oral administration of *F. prausnitzii* or of supernatant from *F. prausnitzii* cultures increased the production of IL-10 by blood mononuclear cells and reduced the production of the proinflammatory mediator-like IL-12 in the colon. The modulation of nuclear factor-κB by pharmacological agents such as statins or salicylates has been proposed as a tool to improve insulin sensitivity in type 2 diabetic patients (42,43). Our study raises the question regarding the role of *F. prausnitzii* as a mediator of low-grade inflammation in obesity and diabetes and open avenues for future investigation exploring its contribution to insulin resistance.

Because of an increasing interest in treating type 2 diabetes with gastric bypass surgery, the improvement of insulin sensitivity and the reduction of diabetes in subjects postsurgery has become a primary axis of interest (44). Unraveling the immediate and long-term adaptations associated with gastric bypass surgery has proved challenging predominantly because the consequences of this procedure include caloric restriction, diminished nutrient absorption, reduced adipose mass, modified gut hormone signaling, and changes in whole-body glucose metabolism, which can each cause numerous physiological and metabolic adaptations (45,46). Hypotheses have been postulated to explain the improved insulin sensitivity witnessed postsurgery and include the altered secretion of gut hormones (47,48), modifications in intestinal gluconeogenesis (49), and changes in intramyocellular lipid content (50). While the definitive explanation for improved insulin sensitivity post-RYGB remains unclear, it is most probably a combination of the aforementioned hypotheses. Components of gut microbiota and possibly the relationship between gut hormones and *F. prausnitzii* should also be considered in this context. Taken together, the applicability of *F. prausnitzii* as a valuable therapeutic tool for the improvement of inflammation, blood glucose tolerance, and insulin sensitivity, calls for more investigations.

ACKNOWLEDGMENTS

This work was funded in part by the French National Agency for Research under project MicroObes (ANR-07-GMGE-002.1-01). L.-C.K. received support from Danone (France), and C.H. received support from sanofi-aventis/French Association for the Research on Obesity. No other potential conflicts of interest relevant to this article were reported.

J.-P.F. researched data, contributed to the discussion, wrote the manuscript, and reviewed/edited the manuscript. L.-C.K. researched data, contributed to the discussion, wrote the manuscript, and reviewed/edited the manuscript. J.T. researched data, contributed to the discussion, and reviewed/edited the manuscript. C.P. researched data and reviewed/edited the manuscript. A.B. researched data and reviewed/edited the manuscript. J.-L.B. researched data and reviewed/edited the manuscript. D.M. researched data. G.C. researched data, contributed to the discussion, and reviewed/edited the manuscript. J.D. contributed to the discussion and reviewed/edited the manuscript. C.H. contributed to the discussion and reviewed/edited the manuscript. S.R. researched data, contributed to the discussion, wrote the manuscript, and reviewed/edited the manuscript. K.C. researched data, contributed to the discussion, wrote the manuscript, and reviewed/edited the manuscript.

Parts of this study were presented at the 70th Scientific Sessions of the American Diabetes Association, Orlando, Florida, 25–29 June 2010.

We appreciate the support from the Assistance Publique-Hôpitaux de Paris and the Department of Clinical Research, which promoted and supported the clinical investigation (CRIC NCT 0047658). We thank Christine Baudouin, Dr. Florence Marchelli, and Patricia Ancel (Center of Research on Human Nutrition, Pitié-Salpêtrière Hospital, Paris, France) who were involved in patient recruitment, data collection, and sampling at the Center of Research on Human Nutrition, Pitié-Salpêtrière Hospital. We thank Dr. Sean P. Kennedy (Unit of Digestive System

Ecology and Physiology, French National Institute for Agricultural Research, Jouy-en-Josas, France) for the critical reading of the manuscript.

REFERENCES

1. Clement K, Langin D. Regulation of inflammation-related genes in human adipose tissue. J Intern Med 2007;262:422–430
2. Pradhan A. Obesity, metabolic syndrome, and type 2 diabetes: inflammatory basis of glucose metabolic disorders. Nutr Rev 2007;65:S152–156
3. DiBaise JK, Zhang H, Crowell MD, Krajmalnik-Brown R, Decker GA, Rittmann BE. Gut microbiota and its possible relationship with obesity. Mayo Clin Proc 2008;83:460–469
4. Turnbaugh PJ, Ley RE, Mahowald MA, Magrini V, Mardis ER, Gordon JI. An obesity-associated gut microbiome with increased capacity for energy harvest. Nature 2006;444:1027–1131
5. Bäckhed F, Ding H, Wang T, Hooper LV, Koh GY, Nagy A, Semenkovich CF, Gordon JI. The gut microbiota as an environmental factor that regulates fat storage. Proc Natl Acad Sci U S A 2004;101:15718–15723
6. Ley RE, Bäckhed F, Turnbaugh P, Lozupone CA, Knight RD, Gordon JI. Obesity alters gut microbial ecology. Proc Natl Acad Sci U S A 2005;102: 11070–11075
7. Cani PD, Delzenne NM. Gut microflora as a target for energy and metabolic homeostasis. Curr Opin Clin Nutr Metab Care 2007;10:729–734
8. Cani PD, Neyrinck AM, Fava F, Knauf C, Burcelin RG, Tuohy KM, Gibson GR, Delzenne NM. Selective increases of bifidobacteria in gut microflora improve high-fat-diet-induced diabetes in mice through a mechanism associated with endotoxaemia. Diabetologia 2007;50:2374–2383
9. Cani PD, Bibiloni R, Knauf C, Waget A, Neyrinck AM, Delzenne NM, Burcelin R. Changes in gut microbiota control metabolic endotoxemia-induced inflammation in high-fat diet-induced obesity and diabetes in mice. Diabetes 2008;57:1470–1481
10. Amar J, Burcelin R, Ruidavets JB, Cani PD, Fauvel J, Alessi MC, Chamontin B, Ferriéres J. Energy intake is associated with endotoxemia in apparently healthy men. Am J Clin Nutr 2008;87:1219–1223
11. Ley RE, Turnbaugh PJ, Klein S, Gordon JI. Microbial ecology: human gut microbes associated with obesity. Nature 2006;444:1022–1023
12. Duncan SH, Lobley GE, Holtrop G, Ince J, Johnstone AM, Louis P, Flint HJ. Human colonic microbiota associated with diet, obesity and weight loss. Int J Obes (Lond) 2008;32:1720–1724
13. Poitou C, Lacorte JM, Coupaye M, Bertrais S, Bedel JF, Lafon N, Bouillot JL, Galan P, Borson-Chazot F, Basdevant A, Coussieu C, Clément K. Relationship between single nucleotide polymorphisms in leptin, IL6 and adiponectin genes and their circulating product in morbidly obese subjects before and after gastric banding surgery. Obes Surg 2005;15:11–23
14. Kushner RF, Noble CA. Long-term outcome of bariatric surgery: an interim analysis. Mayo Clin Proc 2006;81:S46–S51
15. Clément K, Vega N, Laville M, Pelloux V, Guy-Grand B, Basdevant A, Vidal H. Adipose tissue gene expression in patients with a loss of function mutation in the leptin receptor. Int J Obes Relat Metab Disord 2002;26:1533–1538
16. Furet JP, Firmesse O, Gourmelon M, Bridonneau C, Tap J, Mondot S, Doré J, Corthier G. Comparative assessment of human and farm animal faecal microbiota using real-time quantitative PCR. FEMS Microbiol Ecol 2009;68: 351–362
17. Lyons SR, Griffen AL, Leys EJ. Quantitative real-time PCR for Porphyromonas gingivalis and total bacteria. J Clin Microbiol 2000;38:2362–2365
18. Chessel D, Dufour AB, Dray S. *Analysis of Ecological Data: Exploratory and Euclidean Methods in Environmental Sciences. Version 1.4–14.* 2 October 2010;1:4–11
19. Pinheiro J, Bates B, DebRoy S, Sarkar D. *Linear and Nonlinear Mixed Effects Models, R Package. Version 3.1–97.* 9 December 2009;3:1–1.93
20. Turnbaugh PJ, Hamady M, Yatsunenko T, Cantarel BL, Duncan A, Ley RE, Sogin ML, Jones WJ, Roe BA, Affourtit JP, Egholm M, Henrissat B, Heath AC, Knight R, Gordon JI. A core gut microbiome in obese and lean twins. Nature 2009;457:480–484
21. Nadal I, Santacruz A, Marcos A, Warnberg J, Garagorri M, Moreno LA, Martin-Matillas M, Campoy C, Marti A, Moleres A, Delgado M, Veiga OL, Garcia-Fuentes M, Redondo CG, Sanz Y. Shifts in clostridia, bacteroides and immunoglobulin-coating fecal bacteria associated with weight loss in obese adolescents. Int J Obes (Lond) 2009;33:758–767
22. Zhang H, DiBaise JK, Zuccolo A, Kudrna D, Braidotti M, Yu Y, Parameswaran P, Crowell MD, Wing R, Rittmann BE, Krajmalnik-Brown R. Human gut microbiota in obesity and after gastric bypass. Proc Natl Acad Sci U S A 2009;106:2365–2370
23. Heitmann BL, Lissner L. Dietary underreporting by obese individuals: is it specific or non-specific? BMJ 1995;311:986–989
24. Ahima RS, Prabakaran D, Mantzoros C, Qu D, Lowell B, Maratos-Flier E, Flier JS. Role of leptin in the neuroendocrine response to fasting. Nature 1996;382:250–252
25. Korner J, Inabnet W, Febres G, Conwell IM, McMahon DJ, Salas R, Taveras C, Schrope B, Bessler M. Prospective study of gut hormone and metabolic changes after adjustable gastric banding and Roux-en-Y gastric bypass. Int J Obes(Lond) 2009;33:786–95
26. Weigle DS, Duell PB, Connor WE, Steiner RA, Soules MR, Kuijper JL. Effect of fasting, refeeding, and dietary fat restriction on plasma leptin levels. J Clin Endocrinol Metab 1997;82:561–565
27. Bajzer M, Seeley RJ. Physiology: obesity and gut flora. Nature 2006;444: 1009–1010
28. Crawford PA, Crowley JR, Sambandam N, Muegge BD, Costello EK, Hamady M, Knight R, Gordon JI. Regulation of myocardial ketone body metabolism by the gut microbiota during nutrient deprivation. Proc Natl Acad Sci U S A 2009;106:11276–11281
29. Duncan SH, Louis P, Thomson JM, Flint HJ. The role of pH in determining the species composition of the human colonic microbiota. Environ Microbiol 2009;11:2112–2122
30. Cinti S, Matteis RD, Pico C, Ceresi E, Obrador A, Maffeis C, Oliver J, Palou A. Secretory granules of endocrine and chief cells of human stomach mucosa contain leptin. Int J Obes 2000;24:789–793
31. Mason EE, Munns JR, Kealey GP, Wangler R, Clarke WR, Cheng HF, Printen KJ. Effect of gastric bypass on gastric secretion: 1977. Surg Obes Relat Dis 2005;1:155–160
32. Santacruz A, Marcos A, Warnberg J, Marti A, Martin-Matillas M, Campoy C, Moreno LA, Veiga O, Redondo-Figuero C, Garagorri JM, Azcona C, Delgado M, Garcia-Fuentes M, Collado MC, Sanz Y. Interplay between weight loss and gut microbiota composition in overweight adolescents. Obesity (Silver Spring) 2009;17:1906–1915
33. Tap J, Mondot S, Levenez F, Pelletier E, Caron C, Furet JP, Ugarte E, Muñoz-Tamayo R, Paslier DL, Nalin R, Dore J, Leclerc M. Towards the human intestinal microbiota phylogenetic core. Environ Microbiol 2009; 11:2574–2584
34. Sokol H, Seksik P, Furet JP, Firmesse O, Nion-Larmurier I, Beaugerie L, Cosnes J, Corthier G, Marteau P, Doré J. Low counts of Faecalibacterium prausnitzii in colitis microbiota. Inflamm Bowel Dis 2009;15:1183–1189
35. Hotamisligil GS, Shargill NS, Spiegelman BM. Adipose expression of tumor necrosis factor-alpha: direct role in obesity-linked insulin resistance. Science 1993;259:87–91
36. Sartipy P, Loskutoff DJ. Monocyte chemoattractant protein 1 in obesity and insulin resistance. Proc Natl Acad Sci U S A 2003;100:7265–7270
37. Maachi M, Piéroni L, Bruckert E, Jardel C, Fellahi S, Hainque B, Capeau J, Bastard JP. Systemic low-grade inflammation is related to both circulating and adipose tissue TNFalpha, leptin and IL-6 levels in obese women. Int J Obes Relat Metab Disord 2004;28:993–997
38. Akbay E, Yetkin I, Ersoy R, Kulaksizoğlu S, Törüner F, Arslan M. The relationship between levels of alpha1-acid glycoprotein and metabolic parameters of diabetes mellitus. Diabetes Nutr Metab 2004;17:331–335
39. Keogh JB, Brinkworth GD, Noakes M, Belobrajdic DP, Buckley JD, Clifton PM. Effects of weight loss from a very-low-carbohydrate diet on endothelial function and markers of cardiovascular disease risk in subjects with abdominal obesity. Am J Clin Nutr 2008;87:567–76
40. Li M, Wang B, Zhang M, Rantalainen M, Wang S, Zhou H, Zhang Y, Shen J, Pang X, Zhang M, Wei H, Chen Y, Lu H, Zuo J, Su M, Qiu Y, Jia W, Xiao C, Smith LM, Yang S, Holmes E, Tang H, Zhao G, Nicholson JK, Li L, Zhao L. Symbiotic gut microbes modulate human metabolic phenotypes. Proc Natl Acad Sci U S A 2008;105:2117–2122
41. Sokol H, Pigneur B, Watterlot L, Lakhdari O, Bermúdez-Humarán LG, Gratadoux JJ, Blugeon S, Bridonneau C, Furet JP, Corthier G, Grangette C, Vasquez N, Pochart P, Trugnan G, Thomas G, Blottière HM, Doré J, Marteau P, Seksik P, Langella P. Faecalibacterium prausnitzii is an anti-inflammatory commensal bacterium identified by gut microbiota analysis of Crohn disease patients. Proc Natl Acad Sci U S A 2008;105:16731–16736
42. Weitz-Schmidt G. Statins as anti-inflammatory agents. Trends Pharmacol Sci 2002;23:482–486
43. Fleischman A, Shoelson SE, Bernier R, Goldfine AB. Salsalate improves glycemia and inflammatory parameters in obese young adults. Diabetes Care 2008;31:289–294
44. Couzin J. Medicine: bypassing medicine to treat diabetes. Science 2008; 320:438–440
45. Buchwald H, Avidor Y, Braunwald E, Jensen MD, Pories W, Fahrbach K, Schoelles K. Bariatric surgery: a systematic review and meta-analysis. JAMA 2004;292:1724–1737
46. Buchwald H, Estok R, Fahrbach K, Banel D, Jensen MD, Pories WJ, Bantle JP, Sledge I. Weight and type 2 diabetes after bariatric surgery: systematic review and meta-analysis. Am J Med 2009;122:248–256.e5

47. Korner J, Bessler M, Cirilo LJ, Conwell IM, Daud A, Restuccia NL, Wardlaw SL. Effects of Roux-en-Y gastric bypass surgery on fasting and postprandial concentrations of plasma ghrelin, peptide YY, and insulin. J Clin Endocrinol Metab 2005;90:359–365

48. Morínigo R, Moizé V, Musri M, Lacy AM, Navarro S, Marín JL, Delgado S, Casamitjana R, Vidal J. Glucagon-like peptide-1, peptide YY, hunger, and satiety after gastric bypass surgery in morbidly obese subjects. J Clin Endocrinol Metab 2006;91:1735–1740

49. Isbell JM, Tamboli RA, Hansen EN, Saliba J, Dunn JP, Phillips SE, Marks-Shulman PA, Abumrad NN. The importance of caloric restriction in the early improvements in insulin sensitivity after Roux-en-Y gastric bypass surgery. Diabetes Care 2010;33:1438–1442

50. Houmard JA, Tanner CJ, Yu C, Cunningham PG, Pories WJ, MacDonald KG, Shulman GI. Effect of weight loss on insulin sensitivity and intramuscular long-chain fatty acyl-CoAs in morbidly obese subjects. Diabetes 2002;51:2959–2963

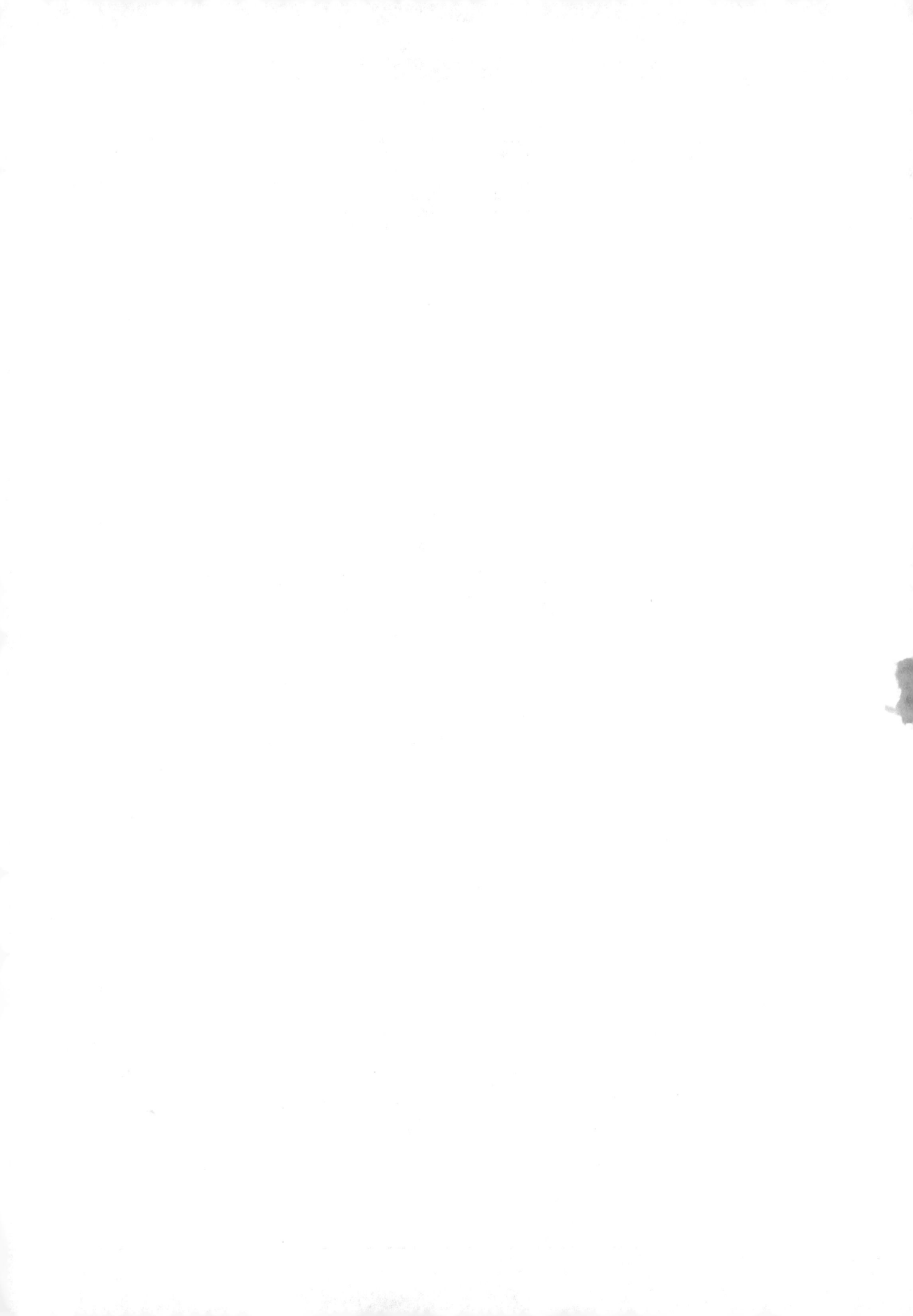

GUT INFLAMMATION AND CELIAC DISEASE

β-Cell Autoimmunity in Pediatric Celiac Disease: The Case for Routine Screening?

Giuseppe d'Annunzio, md[1]
Alessandro Giannattasio, md[1]
Elena Poggi, md[1]
Emanuela Castellano, md[2]

Angela Calvi, md[2]
Angela Pistorio, md[3]
Arrigo Barabino, md[2]
Renata Lorini, md[1]

OBJECTIVE — To evaluate the prevalence of β-cell autoimmunity and the usefulness of a type 1 diabetes screening in patients with celiac disease.

RESEARCH DESIGN AND METHODS — We measured GAD antibodies (GADAs), insulinoma-associated protein 2 antigens (IA-2As), and insulin autoantibodies (IAAs) in 188 young Italian patients with celiac disease (66 male [35.1%]). Mean age at celiac disease diagnosis was 5.4 years (0.5–17.1), and mean celiac disease duration was 4.2 years (0–28.8). Celiac disease was diagnosed by jejunal biopsy after positivity for endomysial and tissue transglutaminase antibody was confirmed.

RESULTS — GADAs were positive in seven patients (3.7%), and IA-2As were positive in two patients. IAAs were negative in all cases. Metabolic evaluation was normal, and no patients developed diabetes during follow-up. There was no significant association among β-cell autoimmunity and sex, age, pubertal stage, family history, or coexistence of other autoimmune disorders; compliance to a gluten-free diet was confirmed.

CONCLUSIONS — Our results showed a low prevalence of β-cell autoimmunity and do not support a precocious screening for β-cell autoimmunity in young celiac disease patients.

Diabetes Care 32:254–256, 2009

Celiac disease, whose prevalence in the general Western population is about 1%, is associated with other autoimmune disorders (1). Type 1 diabetes and celiac disease share a prodromic period, with autoantibodies to islet or gut antigens. Antibodies to GAD (GADAs), to insulinoma-associated protein 2 antigen (IA-2A), and anti-insulin (insulin autoantibody [IAA]) are used for type 1 diabetes screening; antiendomysial antibodies (EMAs) and endomysial tissue transglutaminase antibodies (tTGAs) are recommended for celiac disease screening (2,3). Few reports investigated β-cell autoimmunity in celiac disease patients (4,5). We evaluated the frequency of β-cell autoimmunity and the usefulness of type 1 diabetes screening in young celiac disease patients.

RESEARCH DESIGN AND METHODS

— We measured β-cell autoantibodies in 188 Italian patients with celiac disease diagnosed by jejunal biopsy according to Marsh staging criteria after confirmation of EMA and tTGA positivity and presentation of various degrees of symptoms. Gluten-free diet (GFD) compliance was evaluated by means of EMA and tTGA.

IgA tTGA was detected using enzyme-linked immunosorbent assay, and IgA EMA by indirect immunofluorescence. All samples were analyzed for GADA, IA-2A, and IAA with radiobinding assays (6). Personal and family histories for other autoimmune disorders were recorded.

Comparison of qualitative data among various groups was made by a χ^2 test or Fisher's exact test. All tests were two sided; a

P value <0.05 was significant. Statistica (release 6; StatSoft, Tulsa, OK) was used for all of the analyses. Comparison of celiac disease duration between the two groups of patients (positive vs. negative to β-cell autoantibodies) was performed by means of the parametric Mann-Whitney U test because the normality assumption of the evaluable variable was not fulfilled.

RESULTS — Characteristics of the study population are reported in Table 1. Celiac disease was diagnosed in 78.7% of children with classical symptoms, in 7.5% with atypical symptoms, and in 13.8% after the screening procedure.

We found concomitant autoimmune thyroid disease (ATD) in 5.6% of the patients. No patients had juvenile idiopathic arthritis, atrophic gastritis, Addison's disease, or vitiligo. A positive history of one or more autoimmune disorders was found in 35.6% of the families (celiac disease in 26.6, ATD in 9.6, and both type 1 diabetes and juvenile idiopathic arthritis in 2.3%).

We found positivity for diabetes-related autoantibodies in nine patients (4.8% [95% CI 2.2–8.9]): seven patients showed positivity for GADA (3.7% [1.5–7.5]) and two patients for IA-2A (1.1% [0.1–3.8]), whereas no patients presented with IAA or were positive for two autoantibodies. All nine positive patients had normal fasting plasma glucose, A1C levels, and + 120′ plasma glucose after the oral glucose tolerance test. The intravenous glucose tolerance test showed first-phase insulin response less than the first percentile only in three of nine cases. No patients developed clinical type 1 diabetes after a 3-year follow-up.

We found no significant association among β-cell autoimmunity and sex, age at diagnosis (<10 vs. ≥10 years), family history of autoimmune disorders, concomitant ATD, GFD compliance, and Tanner pubertal stage. No relationships were observed between celiac disease duration and positivity to β-cell autoantibodies (P = 0.79).

HLA class II typing (DQ2 and DQ8 alleles) was performed in 80 of 188 celiac disease patients (42.5%). Among the nine patients with β-cell autoantibodies, HLA typing was performed in eight cases. We

From the [1]Department of Pediatrics, University of Genoa, IRCCS G. Gaslini Institute, Genoa, Italy; the [2]Department Service of Gastroenterology, IRCCS G. Gaslini Institute, Genoa, Italy; and the [3]Epidemiology and Biostatistics Unit, IRCCS G. Gaslini Institute, Genoa, Italy.
Corresponding author: Giuseppe d'Annunzio, giuseppedannunzio@ospedale-gaslini.ge.it.
Received 13 August 2008 and accepted 4 November 2008.
Published ahead of print at http://care.diabetesjournals.org on 18 November 2008. DOI: 10.2337/dc08-1487.

Table 1—Clinical characteristics of celiac disease patients (n = 188)

Sex		
Male	66 (35.1)	
Female	122 (64.9)	
Tanner pubertal stage		
I	103 (54.8)	
II	26 (13.8)	
III	18 (9.6)	
IV	10 (5.3)	
V	31 (16.5)	
Age at celiac disease diagnosis (years)	5.4 ± 4.2	4.0 (0.5–17.1)
Age at study visit (years)	10.4 ± 6.8	9.0 (1.5–48.2)
Celiac disease duration (years)	4.2 ± 5.9	2.1 (0.0–28.8)

Data are n (%), means ± SD, or median (minimum–maximum) unless otherwise indicated.

found HLA-DQ2 in six cases, HLA-DQ8 in one case, and HLA-DQ2/DQ8 in one case. Among the remaining 72 patients without β-cell autoantibodies, we found HLA-DQ2 in 69 cases, HLA-DQ8 in two cases, and HLA-DQ2/DQ8 in one case.

CONCLUSIONS — A low prevalence of diabetes-related antibodies was observed, as well as no association with other autoimmune disorders. In adults, celiac disease is associated with several autoimmune disorders (mostly type 1 diabetes and thyroid diseases). Otherwise, in pediatric celiac disease patients, the rate and significance of diabetes-related antibodies yielded conflicting results (7).

Di Mario et al. (8) evaluated IAAs and islet cell antibodies (ICAs) in children with newly diagnosed celiac disease on a gluten-containing diet, in those with long-standing celiac disease following GFD, and in control groups and raised the question as to whether they are predictive of subclinical diabetes or whether they are indicators of a general autoimmune diathesis. Karagiozoglou-Lampoudi et al. (9) reported no positivity for ICA in pediatric celiac disease patients. Galli-Tsinopoulou et al. (10) showed GADA and IA-2A in 23% of celiac disease patients and recommended screening for β-cell autoimmunity.

In a retrospective study of 90 young Italian patients with celiac disease, the prevalence of diabetes-related autoantibodies was 11.1% and related to gluten exposure (7). Similarly, in an Italian large case series of adult celiac disease patients, a high prevalence (9%) of one diabetes-related autoantibody (ICA, IA-2A, or GADA) was observed independently of GFD compliance (11). Despite this high rate of diabetes-related autoimmunity, no incident cases of diabetes were reported, supporting the role of common genetic

susceptibility to both diseases and factors involved in gut permeability (7).

Conflicting data about prevalence of diabetes-related autoantibodies in celiac disease patients could be due to the improvement of laboratory methods, which excluded false-positive data.

In young celiac disease patients, the length of gluten exposure could influence the development of other autoimmune disorders (7). Bonamico et al. (12) reported at least one endocrine-related serum autoantibody (either ICA or anti-thyroid microsomal antibody) in 50% of adolescents with undiagnosed celiac disease but in only 12% of celiac disease patients on GFD, suggesting that these autoantibodies could be partly gluten dependent.

Abnormal regulation of intestinal permeability and increased autoantibody production in the setting of chronic gut inflammation are trigger factors for the development of autoimmune response (12). Recent evidence suggests that gluten-induced upregulation of zonulin, an intestinal peptide involved in the regulation of gut tight junctions, could be responsible for the aberrant increase in gut permeability otherwise found in type 1 diabetes (13). The gut immune system includes the majority of the total lymphoid tissue in humans; therefore, a detrimental response to dietary components would have repercussions throughout the organism, carried either by immune cells or immune mediators released from the gut (14).

Laadhar et al. (4) did not find differences in prevalence of β-cell autoantibodies between children with newly diagnosed celiac disease and control groups and concluded that screening for diabetes-related autoantibodies is not justified. This opinion has been shared by Fanciulli et al. (5), who did not recommend regular screening for

β-cell autoimmunity in all celiac disease patients because of low prevalence of diabetes-related autoimmunity in young celiac disease patients.

Acknowledgements— No potential conflicts of interest relevant to this article were reported.

We thank Andrea Mascagni, from the Department of Pediatrics, IRCCS G. Gaslini Institute, Genoa, Italy, for GADA, IA2-A, and IAA measurements.

References
1. Collin P, Kaukinen K, Välimäki M, Salmi J: Endocrinological disorders and celiac disease. *Endocr Rev* 23:464–483, 2002
2. Bingley PJ, Bonifacio E, Williams AJ, Genovese S, Bottazzo GF, Gale EA: Prediction of IDDM in the general population: strategies based on combinations of autoantibody markers. *Diabetes* 46:1701–1710, 1997
3. Lorini R, Avanzini MA, Lenta E, Cotellessa M, De Giacomo C, d'Annunzio G: Antibodies to tissue transglutaminase C in newly diagnosed and long-standing type I diabetes mellitus. *Diabetologia* 43:815–816, 2000
4. Laadhar L, Ben Hariz M, Zitouni M, Sellami-Kallel M, Toumi A, Mehrezi A, Makni S: Prevalence of diabetes-related autoantibodies in celiac disease. *Ann Endocrinol (Paris)* 67:588–590, 2006
5. Fanciulli G, Meloni G, Locatelli M, Bottazzo GF, Delitala G: Diabetes-related autoantibodies in schoolchildren with celiac disease. *Ann Endocrinol (Paris)* 68:212–213, 2007
6. Lorini R, Alibrandi A, Vitali L, Klersy C, Martinetti M, Betterle C, d'Annunzio G, Bonifacio E, Pediatric Italian Study Group of Prediabetes: Risk of type 1 diabetes development in children with incidental hyperglycemia: a multicenter Italian study. *Diabetes Care* 24:1210–1216, 2001
7. Ventura A, Neri E, Ughi C, Leopaldi A, Città A, Not T: Gluten-dependent diabetes-related and thyroid-related autoantibodies in patients with celiac disease. *J Pediatr* 137:263–265, 2000
8. Di Mario U, Anastasi E, Mariani P, Ballati G, Perfetti R, Triglione P, Morellini M, Bonamico M: Diabetes-related autoantibodies do appear in children with coeliac disease. *Acta Paediatr* 81:593–597, 1992
9. Karagiozoglou-Lampoudi T, Nousia-Arvanitaki S, Augoustidou-Savopoulou P, Salem N, Polymenidis Z, Kanakoudi-Tsakalidou F: Insulin secretion decline unrelated to jejunal morphology or exocrine pancreatic function in children with celiac disease. *J Pediatr Endocrinol Metab* 9:585–591, 1996
10. Galli-Tsinopoulou A, Nousia-Arvanitakis S, Dracoulacos D, Xefteri M, Karamouzis M: Autoantibodies predicting diabetes mellitus type 1 in celiac disease. *Horm Res* 52:119–124, 1999

11. Bruno G, Pinach S, Martini S, Cassader M, Pagano G, Guidetti CS: Prevalence of type 1 diabetes-related autoantibodies in adults with celiac disease. *Diabetes Care* 26:1644–1645, 2003

12. Bonamico M, Anastasi E, Calvani L: Endocrine autoimmunity and function in adolescent coeliac patients: importance of the diet. *J Pediatr Gastroenterol Nutr* 24:463, 1997

13. Fasano A, Not T, Wang W, Uzzau S, Berti I, Tommasini A, Goldblum SE: Zonulin, a newly discovered modulator of intestinal permeability, and its expression in coeliac disease. *Lancet* 355:1518–1519, 2000

14. Tiittanen M, Westerholm-Ormio M, Verkasalo M, Savilahti E, Vaarala O: Infiltration of forkhead box P3-expressing cells in small intestinal mucosa in coeliac disease but not in type 1 diabetes. *Clin Exp Immunol* 152:498–507, 2008

Majority of Children With Type 1 Diabetes Produce and Deposit Anti-Tissue Transglutaminase Antibodies in the Small Intestine

Mariantonia Maglio,[1] Fiorella Florian,[2] Monica Vecchiet,[2] Renata Auricchio,[1] Francesco Paparo,[1] Raffaella Spadaro,[1] Delia Zanzi,[1] Luciano Rapacciuolo,[1] Adriana Franzese,[1] Daniele Sblattero,[3] Roberto Marzari,[2] and Riccardo Troncone[1]

OBJECTIVE—Anti-tissue transglutaminase (TG2) antibodies are the serological marker of celiac disease. Given the close association between celiac disease and type 1 diabetes, we investigated the production and deposition of anti-TG2 antibodies in the jejunal mucosa of type 1 diabetic children.

RESEARCH DESIGN AND METHODS—Intestinal biopsies were performed in 33 type 1 diabetic patients with a normal mucosal architecture: 14 had high levels (potential celiac disease patients) and 19 had normal levels of serum anti-TG2 antibodies. All biopsy specimens were investigated for intestinal deposits of IgA anti-TG2 antibodies by double immunofluorescence. In addition, an antibody analysis using the phage display technique was performed on the intestinal biopsy specimens from seven type 1 diabetic patients, of whom four had elevated and three had normal levels of serum anti-TG2 antibodies.

RESULTS—Immunofluorescence studies showed that 11 of 14 type 1 diabetic children with elevated levels and 11 of 19 with normal serum levels of anti-TG2 antibodies presented with mucosal deposits of such autoantibodies. The phage display analysis technique confirmed the intestinal production of the anti-TG2 antibodies; however, whereas the serum-positive type 1 diabetic patients showed a preferential use of the VH5 antibody gene family, in the serum-negative patients the anti-TG2 antibodies belonged to the VH1 and VH3 families, with a preferential use of the latter.

CONCLUSIONS—Our findings demonstrate that there is intestinal production and deposition of anti-TG2 antibodies in the jejunal mucosa of the majority of type 1 diabetic patients. However, only those with elevated serum levels of anti-TG2 antibodies showed the VH usage that is typical of the anti-TG2 antibodies that are produced in patients with celiac disease. *Diabetes* **58:1578–1584, 2009**

Insulin-dependent diabetes (type 1 diabetes) is characterized by an autoimmune destruction of the pancreatic islet β-cells that results in a loss of insulin secretion. T-cells that are reactive against specific β-cell antigens infiltrate the endocrine pancreas and destroy the β-cells (1). Both genetic susceptibility and environmental factors contribute to the pathogenesis of type 1 diabetes.

Mounting evidence suggests that the gut immune system is involved in the development of autoimmune diabetes. An inflammatory state has been demonstrated to be present in the structurally normal intestine of patients with type 1 diabetes (2,3), and the abnormal intestinal permeability that has been found in these patients could represent a contributing factor (4). Higher intestinal levels of proinflammatory cytokines, such as interleukin-1α and also interleukin-4, have been reported (3). Recently, we used immunohistochemistry to demonstrate signs of activated cell-mediated mucosal immunity in the lamina propria of the small intestine of type 1 diabetic patients (5); furthermore, the epithelial compartment shows signs of increased infiltration by CD3$^+$ and γδ$^+$ cells (5).

Type 1 diabetes has been found to be associated with other autoimmune diseases, including celiac disease (6–8). Celiac disease is an immune-mediated disease that is triggered by the ingestion of gliadin and other toxic prolamines. It is characterized by a dysregulated immune response at the gut level (9) that results in enteropathy. Several autoantibodies, of which anti-tissue transglutaminase (TG2) autoantibodies are the most frequently observed, are present in the serum of patients with untreated celiac disease. Several studies that have used phage display libraries suggest that these autoantibodies are primarily produced in the small bowel mucosa and that there is a preferential use of heavy-chain variable regions belonging to the VH5 gene family in patients with celiac disease (10). At the mucosal level, anti-TG2 antibodies are found to be deposited on extracellular TG2 (11).

It is possible that type 1 diabetes and celiac disease are more than simply associated; gluten may also have a causative role in type 1 diabetes. This hypothesis has been suggested by the observation of an altered intestinal immune response to gluten in type 1 diabetes. In type 1 diabetic patients, we reported that there is local mucosal recruitment of lymphocytes after rectal instillation of gliadin (12); we also observed an enhanced immune response to gliadin after in vitro gluten challenge in biopsy specimens from type 1 diabetic patients negative for

From the [1]Department of Pediatrics and European Laboratory for the Investigation of Food-Induced Diseases, University "Federico II," Naples, Italy; the [2]Department of Health Sciences, University of Trieste, Trieste, Italy; and the [3]Department of Medical Sciences and Research Centre on Autoimmune Diseases, University of Eastern Piedmont, Novara, Italy.

Corresponding author: Riccardo Troncone, troncone@unina.it.

Received 18 July 2008 and accepted 8 April 2009.

Published ahead of print at http://diabetes.diabetesjournals.org on 28 April 2009. DOI: 10.2337/db08-0962.

serum anti-human TG2 antibodies (5). These subjects with signs of a deranged immune response to gliadin may be considered potential celiac disease patients (13); in fact, some of the type 1 diabetic patients who are negative for celiac disease–associated autoantibodies may later become seropositive and may eventually develop frank enteropathy (14).

It has recently been shown that specific celiac disease autoantibodies against TG2 are deposited in the normal jejunal mucosa before they can be detected in the circulation and that their deposition precedes the gluten-induced jejunal lesion (15). This finding raises the possibility that the anti-TG2 antibodies might be located only at the small mucosal level in some type 1 diabetic patients.

In this study, we investigated the production and deposition of anti-TG2 autoantibodies in the small intestinal mucosa of type 1 diabetic children, irrespective of the presence of this autoantibody in their serum, with the aim of elucidating both the full spectrum of intestinal immunological derangement in type 1 diabetes and the possible relation with dietary gluten.

RESEARCH DESIGN AND METHODS

We studied 33 patients with type 1 diabetes who were consuming a gluten-containing diet at the time of biopsy (median age 11 years, range 3–22 years). All diabetic patients presented with normal jejunal architecture (stage T0/T1 according to the Marsh classification modified by Oberhuber et al. [16]) and were divided into two groups. Group A consisted of 14 patients with raised serum levels of anti-TG2 antibodies (TG2$^+$), and group B consisted of 19 patients with normal serum levels of specific celiac disease autoantibodies (TG2$^-$).

Twelve patients with untreated celiac disease, who had the diagnosis of celiac disease on the basis of biopsy findings, high serum levels of anti-TG2 antibodies, and a positive response to a gluten-free diet, were included. Twenty-eight subjects without celiac disease (final diagnoses: iron deficiency anemia, failure to thrive, gastroesophageal reflux, and recurrent abdominal pain) were enrolled as the control group. Finally, 18 patients with inflammatory bowel diseases (IBDs) and 9 with food allergies were enrolled to form an additional control group that represented subjects with other conditions characterized by gut inflammation.

The patients or the parents, where appropriate, gave their consent for the biopsy sampling for the study. The University Ethics Committee approved the use of the biopsy specimens in the study.

HLA typing. DNA extracted from blood samples was used to genotype for HLA-II DQ2 and DQ8 haplotypes in the type 1 diabetic patients. In control subjects, DNA was extracted from the biopsy specimens using PrepMan Ultra Sample Preparation Reagent (Applied Biosystems). The Eu-DQ kit (Eurospital) was used for typing.

Jejunal biopsy and immunohistochemical analysis. Jejunal biopsy specimens were obtained with a gastroscope from all of the patients. One fragment was treated for histological analysis as described previously (17); a second fragment was immediately embedded in an optimal cutting temperature compound (BioOptica) and used in the detection of mucosal anti-TG2 antibody deposits. From seven of the diabetic patients, we obtained a third fragment used for total RNA purification. Immunohistochemistry, staining, and morphometric analyses were performed as described previously (17).

Serum IgA anti-TG2 antibodies. Serum levels of IgA anti-TG2 antibodies were determined by an enzyme-linked immunosorbent assay (ELISA) using a kit based on recombinant human TG2 (Eu-tTg IgA kit; Eurospital) as described previously (17). Values were considered positive if they were ≥7 arbitrary units/ml.

Intestinal anti-TG2 antibody IgA deposits by double immunofluorescence and confocal analysis. All the of patients were investigated for mucosal deposition of anti-TG2 antibody IgA. The technique described by Korponay-Szabo et al. (11) was implemented with minor modifications. Acetone-fixed, 5-μm frozen sections from each patient were examined by double immunofluorescence. After a 15-min preincubation with normal rabbit serum (1:100; Dako), the sections were covered with a monoclonal mouse antibody against guinea pig TG2 (CUB 7402, 1:200; NeoMarkers) for 1 h at room temperature in a humidified chamber. The sections were washed with PBS and then incubated with a mixture of a fluorescein isothiocyanate–labeled rabbit antibody against human IgA (1:100; Dako) to detect (in green)

IgA and an R-phycoerythrin–labeled rabbit anti-mouse antibody (1:40; Dako) to detect (in red) TG2 for 30 min in the dark. Finally, the sections were washed in PBS and mounted with glycerol/PBS (1:10). The preparations were analyzed with an Axioscope2 (Zeiss) microscope linked to an analysis image system (Siemens). The colocalization of IgA mucosal deposits and TG2 resulted in a yellow image at the fluorescence microscope. The colocalization was confirmed by confocal microscopy (LSM510; Zeiss).

Phage display antibody libraries. Jejunal specimens from seven of the type 1 diabetic patients (three with normal levels of serum anti-TG2 autoantibodies) were used for the purification of tissue total RNA using TRIzol (Gibco Life Technologies). cDNA was synthesized using random hexamers and SuperScript III reverse transcriptase (Gibco Life Technologies). Two types of intestinal B-lymphocyte phage display antibody libraries were constructed: an IgA-VH5 gene family library and an IgA-whole gene family library. Ig VH5 regions were amplified using a specific V-region primer designed against the first 36 nucleotide bases of the VH5 family (18). Conversely, in the IgA whole gene family library, VH and VL regions were amplified using a 3′- and 5′-primer set as described previously (19). In the first library, the PCR fragments were gel purified and digested with *Xho*I and *Nhe*I (New England Biolabs) for cloning into pDAN5 that had been modified with a VL region. In the latter library, the PCR fragments were assembled in a single-chain fragment variable (scFv) and digested with *Bssh*II and *Nhe*I before cloning into the same vector. The phage propagation was carried out in the strain *Escherichia coli* DH5αF′. Rescue of phagemid particles was carried out as described previously (20). Panning was performed by adding phages diluted in 2% nonfat milk/PBS to immunotubes (Nunc) coated with purified recombinant human TG2 and α-gliadin (10 μg/ml); the next steps were performed as reported previously (18). After two rounds of panning, up to 93 individual clones were screened for reactivity to the antigens. Phages from individual colonies were grown in 96-well plates (20). ELISAs were performed in microtiter plates coated with antigens at 10 μg/ml (18). Purified α-gliadin was prepared as described previously (21). Recombinant human TG2 was obtained by amplifying as described previously (22). The V genes from the different anti-TG2 scFv clones were sequenced (BigDye Terminator v3.1 Cycle Sequencing kit; Applied Biosystems), and the VH gene families used were assessed by screening against the V BASE (http://vbase.mrc-cpe.cam.ac.uk) database (23). Immunofluorescence analysis with the different gene family anti-TG2 scFvs was performed on histological sections of monkey esophagus (MeDiCa, Encinitas, CA).

Statistical analysis. A χ^2 test was used to compare percentage values. $P < 0.05$ was considered significant.

RESULTS

Immunohistochemical analysis of type 1 diabetic jejunal biopsy specimens. All of the type 1 diabetic patients were observed to be HLA-DQ2 and/or -DQ8 positive. Signs of activated cell-mediated mucosal immunity were present in approximately one-third of the type 1 diabetic subjects. In group A (TG2$^+$), 4 of 14 patients (29%) showed an increased density of CD25$^+$ mononuclear cells (>4 CD25$^+$ cells/mm^2) in the lamina propria. Crypt epithelium HLA-DR and intercellular adhesion molecule (ICAM)-1 expressions were enhanced in 10 of 14 (71%) and 4 of 14 (29%) patients, respectively. In the epithelial compartment, 6 of 14 patients (43%) presented with a density of CD3$^+$ intraepithelial lymphocytes (IELs) that was higher than the cutoff (>34 cells/mm epithelium), and 9 of 14 patients (64%) presented with a density of γδ$^+$ IELs that was higher than the cutoff (>3.4 cells/mm epithelium). In addition, 5 of 14 patients (36%) presented with three or more of these above-mentioned altered values.

In group B (TG2$^-$), 7 of 19 patients (37%) showed an increased density of CD25$^+$ mononuclear cells and 11 of 19 (58%) and 6 of 19 (31%) presented with increased HLA-DR and ICAM-1 expression, respectively. With respect to the epithelial compartment, 4 of 19 (21%) and 5 of 19 patients (26%) presented with an increased density of CD3$^+$ and γδ$^+$ IELs, respectively (Table 1). Again, 5 of 19 patients (26%) presented with three or more of the above-mentioned altered values. Only the percentage of subjects

TABLE 1

Immunohistochemical findings in the small intestine of type 1 diabetic patients enrolled in this study

	Group A	Group B	P
$CD3^+$ >34/mm	6/14 (43)	4/19 (21)	NS
$\gamma\delta^+$ >3.4/mm	9/14 (64)	5/19 (26)	<0.05
$CD25^+$ >4/mm^2	4/14 (29)	7/19 (37)	NS
HLA-DR (++/+++)	10/14 (71)	11/19 (58)	NS
ICAM-1 (++/+++)	4/14 (29)	6/19 (31)	NS

Group A consisted of type 1 diabetic patients with elevated serum levels of anti-TG2 antibodies (TG2$^+$). Group B consisted of type 1 diabetic patients with normal serum levels of anti-TG2 antibodies (TG2$^-$). $CD3^+$ and $\gamma\delta^+$ IELs are expressed per millimeter of epithelium; $CD25^+$ cells are expressed per square millimeter of lamina propria. The expression of crypt epithelial HLA-DR and the expression of lamina propria ICAM-1 were evaluated in terms of their staining intensity and graded on an arbitrary scale of staining level, where − = no staining, + = weak staining, ++ = strong staining, and +++ = very strong staining. The data were analyzed by a χ^2 test. $P < 0.05$ was considered significant.

with an increased number of $\gamma\delta^+$ IELs was significantly higher in group A than in group B ($P < 0.05$).

Immunofluorescence studies. Jejunal mucosa from most of the control subjects without celiac disease showed IgA antibodies, only inside the plasma cells and the epithelial cells, which were labeled in green (Fig. 1A), and only 4 of 28 subjects had patchy IgA mucosal deposits. With regard to HLA status, 9 of the 28 (32%) control subjects were HLA-DQ2 and/or -DQ8 positive, but only one of the four individuals who were positive for mucosal deposits was HLA-DQ2 positive. In the group of patients with other inflammatory conditions of the gut, only three of the subjects with IBD (16.6%) showed patchy deposits.

All 12 patients with untreated celiac disease showed evident IgA deposits below the villous and crypt basement membranes and around the mucosal vessels, corresponding to the intestinal localization of TG2 (in red), apart from the IgA inside the plasma cells. IgA-specific anti-TG2 antibody deposits appeared in yellow-orange because of colocalization with TG2 (Fig. 1E).

Not unexpectedly, in group A (TG2$^+$), 11 of the patients (78%) were observed to have IgA anti-TG2 antibody mucosal deposits that had a patchy distribution. Surprisingly, we found that a high percentage of patients in group B (TG2$^-$) exhibited an IgA deposit–positive pattern; in fact, 11 of the 19 (58%) group B subjects showed IgA anti-TG2 antibody mucosal deposits (Fig. 1C). Four of these 11 patients (36%) presented with a density of $\gamma\delta^+$ IELs that was higher than the cutoff.

Most of the specimens with a patchy IgA deposit pattern, all biopsy specimens from patients with untreated celiac disease, and several normal biopsy specimens were analyzed by confocal microscopy to further assess the colocalization of IgA deposits with TG2 (Fig. 1,B, D, and F). In all of the specimens, confocal analysis confirmed the observations described previously. All data are summarized in Table 2.

Phage display antibody libraries. To further confirm the presence of anti-TG2 antibodies in the IgA deposits that colocalized with TG2 in the jejunal specimens of type 1 diabetic patients, we performed an analysis based on antibody phage display. In a previous article, we demonstrated the prevalent use of the VH5 segment to make antibodies against TG2 by the intestinal lymphocytes of patients with celiac disease (10). Also, the reactivity to

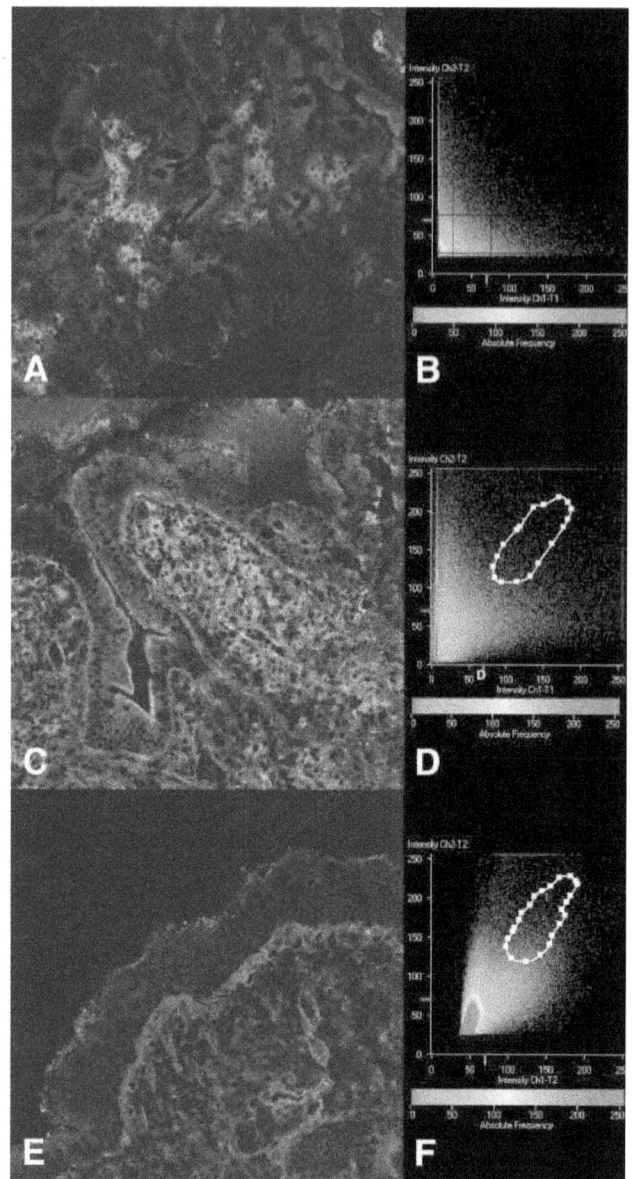

FIG. 1. A and B: Jejunal section from a subject without celiac disease. It is a negative sample. In A, IgA deposits (in green) are detected only inside plasma cells, whereas tissue transglutaminase (in red) is evident around the crypts and in the subepithelial area. B: Confocal analysis with a scatter plot of the image. In this plot, no area of colocalization is evident around the diagonal of the Cartesian graphic. C and D: Jejunal section from a type 1 diabetic patient with a high serum level of anti-TG2 autoantibodies. In C, IgA deposits (in yellow-orange) are present in a patchy distribution in the subepithelial area and around mucosal vessels. These IgA/anti-TG2 antibody colocalization areas have been analyzed by confocal microscopy. The related scatter plot is shown in D, and the image of this area of colocalization is represented by orange dots. E and F: Jejunal section from a patient with untreated celiac disease with positive serum anti-TG2 antibodies and EMAs, in which thick IgA anti-TG2 antibody deposits are evident just under the superficial epithelium and around the vessels (E). This subepithelial area has been studied by confocal microscopy, and the related scatter plot (F) shows an extensive area of IgA deposits/TG2 colocalization. (A high-quality digital representation of this figure is available in the online issue.)

TG2 was demonstrated to be restricted to the VH chain alone because shuffling of the VL chain with unrelated genes did not affect the antibody reactivity. This feature was shared by the antibodies to TG2 from all of the patients with celiac disease examined (18). For this rea-

TABLE 2
Prevalence of IgA anti-TG2 mucosal deposits in the study population

Patients	Presence of anti-TG2 mucosal deposits	% Positivity
Type 1 diabetic patients		
$TG2^+$	11/14	78
TG^-	11/19	58
Patients with untreated celiac disease	12/12	100
Control subjects	4/28	14
Patients with IBD	3/18	16.6
Patients with food allergies	0/9	0

$TG2^+$ type 1 diabetic patients had increased serum levels of anti-TG2 antibodies; $TG2^-$ type 1 diabetic patients had normal serum levels of anti-TG2 antibodies.

son, we are inclined to think that the antibodies to TG2 belonging to the VH5 family are a distinctive marker of celiac disease. Thus, in the present study, a first analysis was performed on intestinal biopsy cDNAs by cloning the VH5 family alone.

Seven IgA-VH5 gene family phage display libraries from type 1 diabetic patients (three with normal levels of anti-TG2 serum autoantibodies and four with elevated levels, here reported as $TG2^-$ and $TG2^+$ type 1 diabetic patients, respectively) were constructed using a phagemid vector with resident VL genes compatible with TG2 recognition (18). In all cases, the library diversity resulted in at least 10^6 clones expressing human antibody fragments. After two rounds of selection at a high level of stringency, 45 individual clones were analyzed for their reactivity to recombinant human TG2 by a phage ELISA. In the libraries obtained from the intestinal biopsy lymphocytes of $TG2^+$ patients, the number of positive clones ranged from 28 to 84% (Table 3). Conversely, using the three libraries constructed from the lymphocytes of $TG2^-$ patients, the number of clones recognizing TG2 was rather low, comprising between 0 and 6% of the tested clones. Because the same antibody might be represented many times within the selected clones, the diversity of the positive clones was assessed by fingerprinting the PCR-amplified VH5 region. The diversity was confirmed for the large majority of the clones, attesting to the polyclonal IgA response to TG2.

Considering the high percentage of $TG2^-$ patients who were observed to have intestinal deposits of anti-TG2 antibodies, we decided to determine whether an anti-TG2 antibody response could be ascribed to non-VH5 antibodies, which were not present in the first version of the antibody libraries. The whole antibody repertoire of the

seven type 1 diabetic patients and three control subjects without celiac disease was cloned, assembling all of the VH and VL gene family sequences. The results of the library selections for TG2, reported in Table 4, show a significant number of clones that are positive for recombinant human TG2 isolated from the four libraries of type 1 diabetic patients with anti-TG2 serum antibodies (values ranging from 46 to 88%). Unexpectedly, a comparable result was obtained with the three libraries from the type 1 diabetic patients who did not have peripheral antibodies to TG2, with a number of bacterial clones ranging from 71 to 86%. The antibody diversity, measured by fingerprinting, was high in all of the clusters, attesting to the humoral response to TG2 involving different antibodies. Very few positive clones were found in the control subjects without celiac disease, with 0, 10, and 3 anti-TG2 antibody-positive clones of 90 tested.

Furthermore, the whole IgA antibody libraries were selected on native gliadin. Both $TG2^+$ and $TG2^-$ type 1 diabetic patients showed an elevated number of anti-gliadin antibodies, with a positivity ranging from 53 to 97% of the tested clones. In addition, the antibody diversity was high in all cases. All data are summarized in Table 4.

Finally, assignment to the seven VH gene family members of the positive antibodies to TG2 that were selected from the whole libraries was determined by DNA sequencing. As reported in Fig. 2, >50% of the phage antibodies from the type 1 diabetic patients belonged to the VH3 family, with minor usage of the other gene families. For comparison, the antibodies to TG2 selected from the phage display libraries from the intestinal B lymphocyte of three patients with celiac disease that were constructed previously were sequenced for gene family assignment. As reported in Fig. 2, the results showed a more distributed usage of the VH gene families with a stronger trend for VH1 and VH5.

To further confirm the specificity of the anti-TG2 antibodies from the intestinal biopsy specimens of the type 1 diabetic patients, four soluble antibody fragments belonging to VH3, VH1, and VH4 families were assayed for anti-endomysium structure reactivity in monkey esophagus specimens. As shown in Fig. 3, the VH5 antibody (bottom right) showed a pattern that is typical of anti-endomysium antibodies (EMAs), and of all the other antibodies, attesting to their specificity to TG2.

DISCUSSION

In this study, given the reported derangement of the intestinal immunity in type 1 diabetic patients (2,3,5) and the association of type 1 diabetes and celiac disease (6–8), we investigated the production and presence of anti-TG2 antibodies, which are a hallmark of celiac disease, in the

TABLE 3
VH5 gene family–restricted IgA phage display libraries

	VH5 gene family IgA phage display libraries						
	Type 1 diabetic $TG2^+$			Type 1 diabetic $TG2^-$			
Library code	N1	N2	N3	N4	N5	N6	N7
Library size	3.1×10^6	3.2×10^6	1.6×10^6	4.1×10^6	6.3×10^6	4.6×10^6	2.6×10^6
Anti-TG2 antibodies	84	28	73	42	2	0	6

Data are the percentage of positive clones. VH5 gene family–restricted IgA phage display libraries from type 1 diabetes patient lymphocytes were selected for human TG2. The library size represents the number of bacterial clones expressing an antibody fragment. After two rounds of panning, 45 clones for each library were individually tested by ELISA for TG2. Only serologically $TG2^+$ type 1 diabetic patients have a significant number of recombinant α-human TG2 antibodies using the VH5 gene family.

TABLE 4
Whole VH gene family IgA phage display libraries

	Whole VH gene family IgA phage display libraries									
	Type 1 diabetic TG2$^+$				Type 1 diabetic TG2$^-$			Control subjects without celiac disease		
Library code	N1	N2	N3	N4	N5	N6	N7	H1	H2	H3
Library size	8.6×10^7	8.8×10^8	3.8×10^8	7.5×10^7	6.9×10^7	1.8×10^7	2.8×10^7	5.7×10^7	5.7×10^7	6×10^7
Anti-TG2 antibodies	86	88	73	46	71	68	86	10	3	0
Anti–α-gliadin antibodies	80	97	77	53	57	93	82	3	11	0

Data are the percentage of positive clones. IgA phage display libraries from the lymphocytes isolated from type 1 diabetes patients and control subjects without celiac disease were constructed using all of the VH gene families. The libraries were selected for human TG2 and α-gliadin. After two rounds of selection, 45 clones for each type 1 diabetes library and 90 clones for each control library were individually tested by ELISA for the corresponding antigen. All of the libraries from type 1 diabetic patients who were either serologically positive or negative for TG2 show a high percentage of positive clones.

intestine of type 1 diabetic patients (24). Only patients with normal jejunal architecture were included in this study, which excluded patients with villous atrophy and a diagnosis of overt celiac disease. The results obtained show the presence of anti-TG2 antibodies in the jejunal mucosa of most patients with type 1 diabetes. However, a more precise analysis of the features of these antibodies, particularly the use of the VH genes, has shown that only in type 1 diabetic patients with serum titers of anti-TG2 antibodies that are higher than the cutoff do the anti-TG2 antibodies have the same features that they have in patients with celiac disease.

The immunofluorescence technique we used to detect intestinal deposits of anti-TG2 antibodies (11) is based on the colocalization of antibodies to IgA and to TG2; in this study, we validated this immunofluorescence technique with the use of confocal microscopy to confirm the colocalization. We have previously shown the presence of these deposits (25) in patients with villous atrophy as well as in subjects who had normal mucosa but other signs suggestive of potential celiac disease, such as the presence of EMAs in the serum (17) or an increased density of IELs expressing the γδ receptor (17). In the latter patients, these deposits have been shown by others to predict the future evolution to frank disease (15). In the potential celiac disease patients, we observed that these deposits were often observed in a patchy distribution and were less thick (25). The patchy pattern has also been observed in

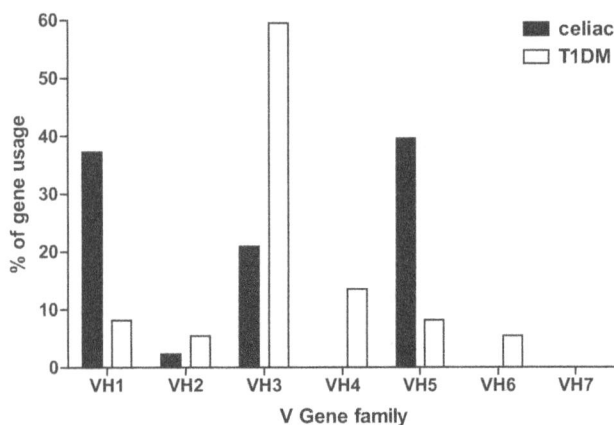

FIG. 2. Percentage of VH gene family usage in the recombinant anti-TG2 antibodies selected from seven intestinal B lymphocytes of type 1 diabetic patients (T1DM) and three intestinal B lymphocytes of patients with celiac disease.

the patients with type 1 diabetes in this study. In fact, in the type 1 diabetic patients with normal mucosa and a high serum titer of anti-TG2 antibodies, these titers were still lower than those in subjects with villous atrophy; these lower titers and probably the lower antibody affinity might explain the patchy distribution and the thinner line of intestinal deposits.

The presence of these antibodies at the intestinal level strongly suggests that they are locally produced. As a matter of fact, the intestinal production of these antibodies has been demonstrated in patients with celiac disease by means of organ culture (26) and by the detection and measurement of these antibodies in intestinal juices (27) and feces (26). The results obtained with the phage display antibody libraries definitely support the above data on the presence of deposits and local production of anti-TG2 antibodies in the intestine of type 1 diabetic patients. The first attempt, in which we aimed to construct and select antibody libraries that used only the VH5 gene family, yielded many clones isolated from type 1 diabetic patients with a detectable serum titer of antibodies to TG2, whereas very few VH5 antibodies were selected from type 1 diabetic patients without elevated serum antibodies to TG2. This result is not in contrast with our previous studies on celiac disease anti-TG2 antibody profiling, in which we found that all the patients shared an atypical VH5 gene family usage in making antibodies to TG2 (10). However, in these patients, other antibodies belonging to the VH1 and VH3 families that recognize a different epitopic region are also produced. In this respect, the TG2 serologically negative type 1 diabetic patients do not correspond to patients with celiac disease because very few VH5 antibodies were selected. On the other hand, the remarkable intestinal antibody response to TG2 revealed by the whole antibody libraries from the TG2$^-$ type 1 diabetic patients, although with a preferential use of the VH3 family, again suggests a relationship with celiac disease. Moreover, these antibodies, along with the VH1 and VH4 antibodies, were shown to recognize the endomysial TG2 according to the EMA pattern that is typical for the VH5 antibodies. The interpretation that this antibody production might be gluten dependent is strengthened by the number of antibodies to gliadin that were isolated from all of the type 1 diabetic patient libraries but not from the control subjects without celiac disease. We cannot predict whether type 1 diabetic patients with a normal serum level of anti-TG2 antibodies who show a strong anti-TG2 antibody intestinal response either are in a very early stage of

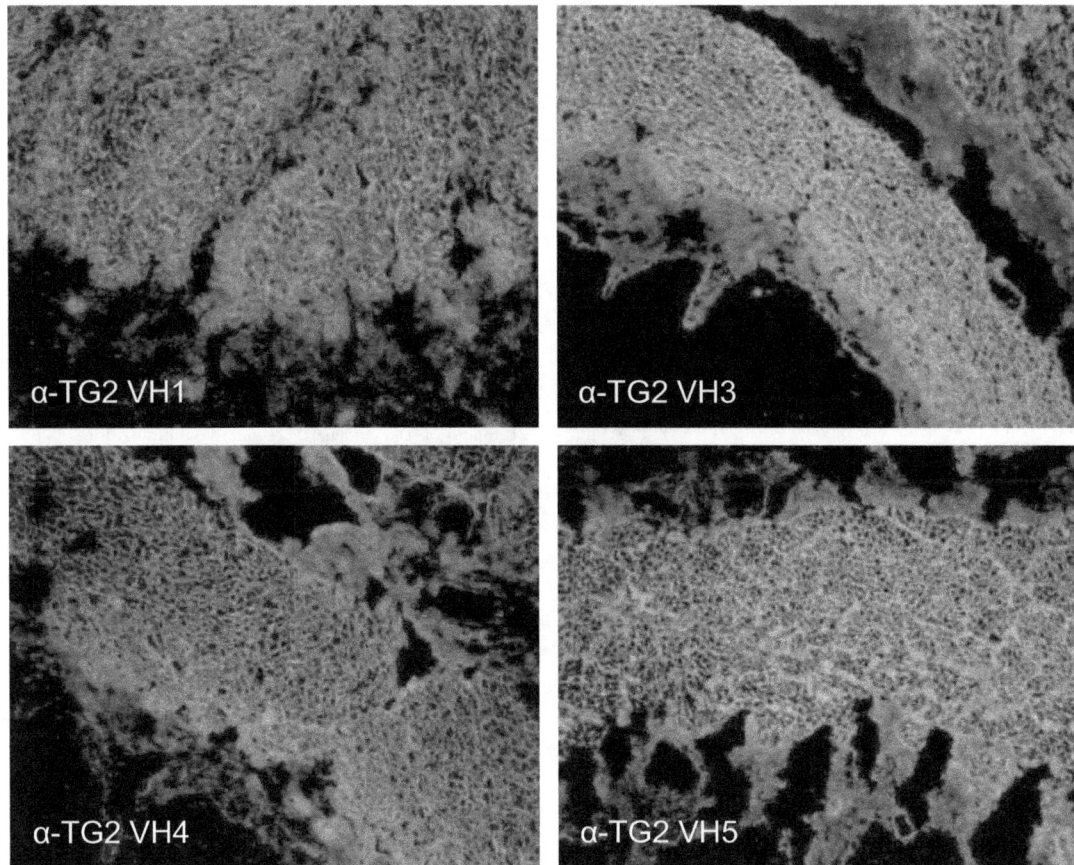

FIG. 3. Monkey esophagus sections stained with anti-TG2 scFv containing a VH1, VH3, and VH4 gene segment. An anti-TG2 VH5 scFv is shown as a control. All of the scFvs recognize native TG2–anti-endomysium structures in the oesophagus muscularis mucosa according to the reticular motif, which is similar to the results observed for serum anti-endomysium antibodies. (A high-quality digital representation of this figure is available in the online issue.)

celiac disease or will never progress toward the disease. In addition, we do not know whether a possible shift in the VH3-based antibody response to a VH5 response may be a significant step in the progression of the illness. Antigen spreading by both antibody and T-cell epitopes is a well-known feature of autoimmune diabetes, and we wonder whether this is a characteristic of the anti-TG2 antibody response as well. If the results that have been reported here are confirmed, the cloning of intestinal antibodies could be considered a useful tool for investigating the immunological background of both type 1 diabetes and celiac disease. In a preliminary study (28), we found that consumption of a gluten-free diet was beneficial for type 1 diabetic patients and was paralleled by a change in the profile of the intestinal antibody response. In this respect, the present study provides a more comprehensive interpretation of the possible immunotoxic effect of gluten.

Intestinal anti-TG2 antibodies have also been noted in the intestines of NOD mice (29). In NOD mice, the presence of the antibodies in the gut is accompanied by high antibody levels in the serum, but their presence is not dependent on the presence of gluten in the diet. The same could apply to type 1 diabetic patients who do not show the same special use of the VH genes. We have not investigated other autoimmune conditions, but we can exclude the notion that the finding of the intestinal anti-TG2 autoantibodies is simply related to HLA status or is merely a consequence of intestinal inflammation.

It is difficult to predict which functional effect could be exerted by the anti-TG2 antibodies present in the gut of type 1 diabetic patients. Studies conducted on antibodies derived from patients with celiac disease suggest that they at least partly inhibit enzymatic activity (30); furthermore, it was recently found that they favor proliferation in the epithelial compartment (31).

In conclusion, we have shown that the majority of patients with type 1 diabetes have anti-TG2 antibodies in their intestinal mucosa. The special use of the VH5 genes in type 1 diabetic patients with serum positivity for anti-endomysium suggests a gluten-dependent phenomenon analogous to what has been found in celiac disease. These patients belong to the spectrum of gluten sensitivity that ranges from an abnormal immune response to frank villous atrophy. More difficult is the interpretation of the finding of the intestinal anti-TG2 antibodies, not necessarily using the VH5 genes, in those with an absence of a high titer of these antibodies in the serum; in these patients, the relationship with gluten is uncertain. It could be an expression of autoimmunity, analogous to what has been observed in NOD mice, and be included in the more general derangement of the intestinal mucosal immunity observed in type 1 diabetes. In addition, the raised density of $\gamma\delta^+$ IELs that has been observed in type 1 diabetes, irrespective of the presence of high serum titers of anti-TG2 antibodies, could be a feature of autoimmunity that has also been observed in other autoimmune conditions

(32,33). Current studies with the aim of defining the molecular basis of the antibody response to TG2 will help to interpret the observations reported here and, in particular, to understand to what extent the presence of these antibodies and, in general, the derangement of the mucosal immunity is related to dietary gluten in type 1 diabetes.

ACKNOWLEDGMENTS

This work was supported by Fondazione Cariplo, Compagnia Sanpaolo, and the Italian Ministry of University and Research (project "Intestino e autoimmunità").

No potential conflicts of interest relevant to this article were reported.

REFERENCES

1. Mallone R, van Ender P. T cells in the pathogenesis of type 1 diabetes. Curr Diab Rep 2008;8:101–106
2. Savilahti E, Ormala T, Sukkonen T, Sandini-Pohjavouri U, Kantele JM, Arato A, Ilonen J, Åkerblom HK. Jejuna of patients with insulin-dependent diabetes mellitus (IDDM) shows signs of immune activation. Clin Exp Immunol 1999;116:70–77
3. Westerholm-Ormio M, Vaarala O, Pihkala P, Ilonen J, Savilahti E. Immunologic activity in the small intestinal mucosa of pediatric patients with type 1 diabetes. Diabetes 2003;52:2287–2295
4. Carratù R, Secondulfo M, De Magistris L, Iafusco D, Urio A, Cardone MG, Pontoni G, Cartenì M, Prisco F. Altered intestinal permeability to mannitol in diabetes mellitus type 1. J Pediatr Gastroenterol Nutr 1999;28:264–269
5. Auricchio R, Paparo F, Maglio M, Franzese A, Lombardi F, Valerio G, Nardone G, Percopo S, Greco L, Troncone R. In vitro-deranged intestinal immune response to gliadin in type 1 diabetes. Diabetes 2004;53:1680–1683
6. Maki M, Hallstrom O, Huupponen T, Vesikari T, Visakorpi JK. Increased prevalence of coeliac disease in diabetes. Arch Dis Child 1984;59:739–742
7. Savilahti E, Simell O, Koskimies S, Rilva A, Akerblom HK. Coeliac disease in insulin dependent diabetes mellitus. J Pediatr 1986;108:690–693
8. Sategna-Guidetti C, Grossa S, Pulitano R, Benaduce E, Dani F Carta Q. Celiac disease and insulin dependent diabetes mellitus: screening in adult population. Dig Dis Sci 1994;39:1633–1637
9. Sollid LM. Coeliac disease: dissecting a complex inflammatory disorder. Nat Rev Immunol 2002;2:647–655
10. Marzari R, Sblattero D, Florian F, Tongiorgi E, Not T, Tommasini A, Ventura A, Bradbury A. Molecular dissection of the tissue transglutaminase autoantibody response in celiac disease. J Immunol 2001;166:4170–4176
11. Korponay-Szabo IR, Halttunen T, Szalai Z, Laurila K, Kiraly R, Kovacs JB, Fesus L, Maki M. In vivo targeting of intestinal and extraintestinal transglutaminase 2 by coeliac autoantibodies. Gut 2004;53:641–648
12. Troncone R, Franzese A, Mazzarella G, Paparo F, Auricchio R, Coto I, Mayer M, Greco L. Gluten sensitivity in a subset of children with insulin dependent diabetes mellitus. Am J Gastroenterol 2003;98:590–595
13. Troncone R, Paparo F, Mazzarella G, Maglio M, Iovine G, Mayer M, Greco L, Auricchio S. The spectrum of gluten sensitivity. In Coeliac disease. Auricchio S, Greco L, Maiuri L, Troncone R, Eds. Naples, Jean Gilder Editions, 2000, p. 151–155
14. Maki M, Huopponen T, Holm K, Hallstrom O. Seroconversion of reticulin autoantibodies predicts coeliac disease in insulin dependent diabetes mellitus. Gut 1995;36:239–242
15. Salmi TT, Collin P, Jarvinen O, Haimila K, Partanen J, Laurila K, Korponay-Szabo IR, Huhtala H, Reunala T, Maki M, Kaukinen K. Immunoglobulin A autoantibodies against transglutaminase 2 in the small intestinal mucosa

16. Oberhuber G, Granditsch G, Vogelsang H. The histopathology of celiac disease: time for a standardized report scheme for pathologists. Eur J Gastroenterol Hepatol 1999;11:1185–1194
17. Paparo F, Petrone E, Tosco A, Maglio M, Borrelli M, Salvati VM, Miele E, Greco L, Auricchio S, Troncone R. Clinical, HLA, and small bowel immunohistochemical features of children with positive serum anti-endomysium antibodies and architecturally normal small intestinal mucosa. Am J Gastroenterol 2005;100:2294–2298
18. Sblattero D, Florian F, Azioni E, Ziberna F, Tommasini A, Not T, Ventura A, Bradbury A, Marzari R. One-step cloning of anti tissue transglutaminase scFv from subjects with celiac disease. J Autoimmun 2004;22:65–72
19. Sblattero D, Bradbury A. A definitive set of oligonucleotide primers for amplifying human V regions. Immunotechnology 1998;3:271–278
20. Marks JD, Hoogenboom HR, Bonnert TP, McCafferty J, Griffiths AD, Winter G. By-passing immunization: human antibodies from V-gene libraries displayed on phage. J Mol Biol 1991;222:581–597
21. Silano M, De Vincenzi M. Bioactive antinutritional peptides derived from cereal prolamins: a review. Nahrung 1999;43:175–184
22. Sblattero D, Berti I, Trevisiol C, Marzari R, Tommasini A, Bradbury A, Fasano A, Ventura A, Not T. Human recombinant tissue transglutaminase ELISA: an innovative diagnostic assay for celiac disease. Am J Gastroenterol 2000;95:1253–1257
23. Tomlinson IM, Williams SC, Corbett SJ, Cox JPL, Winter G: V BASE Sequence Directory. Cambridge, U.K., Medical Research Council Centre for Protein Engineering, 1996
24. Dieterich W, Ehnis T, Bauer M, Donner P, Volta U, Riecken EO, Schuppan D. Identification of tissue transglutaminase as the autoantigen of celiac disease. Nat Med 1997;3:797–801
25. Tosco A, Maglio M, Paparo F, Rapacciuolo L, Sannino A, Miele E, Barone MV, Auricchio R, Troncone R. Immunoglobulin A anti-tissue transglutaminase antibody deposits in the small intestinal mucosa of children with no villous atrophy. J Pediatr Gastroenterol Nutr 2008;47:293–298
26. Picarelli A, Sabbatella L, Di Tola M, Di Cello T, Vetrano S, Anania MC. Antiendomysial antibody detection in fecal supernatants: in vivo proof that small bowel mucosa is the site of antiendomysial antibody production. Am J Gastroenterol 2002;97:95–98
27. Mawhinney H, Love AH. Anti-reticulin antibody in jejunal juice in coeliac disease. Clin Exp Immunol 1975;21:394–398
28. Sblattero D, Ventura A, Tommasini A, Cattin L, Martelossi S, Florian F, Marzari R, Bradbury A, Not T. Cryptic gluten intolerance in type 1 diabetes: identifying suitable candidates for a gluten free diet. Gut 2006;55:133
29. Sblattero D, Maurano F, Mazzarella G, Rossi M, Auricchio S, Florian F, Ziberna F, Tommasini A, Not T, Ventura A, Bradbury A, Marzari R, Troncone R. Characterization of the anti-tissue transglutaminase antibody response in nonobese diabetic mice. J Immunol 2005;174:5830–5836
30. Esposito C, Paparo F, Caputo I, Rossi M, Maglio M, Sblattero D, Not T, Porta R, Auricchio S, Marzari R, Troncone R. Anti-tissue transglutaminase antibodies from coeliac patients inhibit transglutaminase activity both in vitro and in situ. Gut 2002;5:177–181
31. Barone MV, Caputo I, Ribecco MT, Maglio M, Marzari R, Sblattero D, Troncone R, Auricchio S, Esposito C. Humoral immune response to tissue transglutaminase is related to epithelial cell proliferation in celiac disease. Gastroenterology 2007;132:1245–1253
32. Valentino R, Savastano S, Maglio M, Paparo F, Ferrara F, Dorato M, Lombardi G, Troncone R. Markers of potential coeliac disease in patients with Hashimoto's thyroiditis. Eur J Endocrinol 2002;146:479–483
33. Iltanen S, Holm K, Partanen J, Laippala P, Mäki M. Increased density of jejunal $\gamma\delta^+$ T cells in patients having normal mucosa—marker of operative autoimmune mechanisms? Autoimmunity 1999;29:179–187

Diabetes-Specific HLA-DR–Restricted Proinflammatory T-Cell Response to Wheat Polypeptides in Tissue Transglutaminase Antibody–Negative Patients With Type 1 Diabetes

Majid Mojibian,[1,2] Habiba Chakir,[1,2] David E. Lefebvre,[1,2] Jennifer A. Crookshank,[1] Brigitte Sonier,[1,2] Erin Keely,[3] and Fraser W. Scott[1,2,3]

OBJECTIVE—There is evidence of gut barrier and immune system dysfunction in some patients with type 1 diabetes, possibly linked with exposure to dietary wheat polypeptides (WP). However, questions arise regarding the frequency of abnormal immune responses to wheat and their nature, and it remains unclear whether such responses are diabetes specific.

RESEARCH DESIGN AND METHODS—In type 1 diabetic patients and healthy control subjects, the immune response of peripheral $CD3^+$ T-cells to WPs, ovalbumin, gliadin, α-gliadin 33-mer peptide, tetanus toxoid, and phytohemagglutinin was measured using a carboxyfluorescein diacetate succinimidyl ester (CFSE) proliferation assay. T–helper cell type 1 (Th1), Th2, and Th17 cytokines were analyzed in WP-stimulated peripheral blood mononuclear cell (PBMNC) supernatants, and HLA was analyzed by PCR.

RESULTS—Of 42 patients, 20 displayed increased $CD3^+$ T-cell proliferation to WPs and were classified as responders; proliferative responses to other dietary antigens were less pronounced. WP-stimulated PBMNCs from patients showed a mixed proinflammatory cytokine response with large amounts of IFN-γ, IL-17A, and increased TNF. HLA-DQ2, the major celiac disease risk gene, was not significantly different. Nearly all responders carried the diabetes risk gene HLA-DR4. Anti-DR antibodies blocked the WP response and inhibited secretion of Th1 and Th17 cytokines. High amounts of WP-stimulated IL-6 were not blocked.

CONCLUSIONS—T-cell reactivity to WPs was frequently present in type 1 diabetic patients and associated with HLA-DR4 but not HLA-DQ2. The presence of an HLA-DR–restricted Th1 and Th17 response to WPs in a subset of patients indicates a diabetes-related inflammatory state in the gut immune tissues associated with defective oral tolerance and possibly gut barrier dysfunction. *Diabetes* **58:1789–1796, 2009**

From the [1]Chronic Disease Program, Ottawa Hospital Research Institute, Ottawa, Canada; the [2]Department of Biochemistry, Microbiology and Immunology, University of Ottawa, Ottawa, Canada; and the [3]Department of Medicine, University of Ottawa, Ottawa, Canada.
Corresponding author: Fraser W. Scott, fscott@ohri.ca.
Received 12 November 2008 and accepted 20 April 2009.
Published ahead of print at http://diabetes.diabetesjournals.org on 28 April 2009. DOI: 10.2337/db08-1579.

See accompanying commentary, p. 1723.

The gastrointestinal tract contains the largest collection of immune cells in the body. In healthy individuals, the gut immune system does not normally mount an immune response against molecules from foods and commensal bacteria, preferring a default state of immune unresponsiveness called oral tolerance (1).

When oral tolerance is broken, an immune imbalance results that can lead to increased gut permeability, inflammation, and tissue damage. The best understood example of this is celiac disease, which is the classic food-induced autoimmune disorder and the only autoimmune disease for which the autoantigen (tissue transglutaminase) and the inciting environmental factors (gluten proteins) are known (2). In celiac disease, specific wheat gliadin peptides undergo deamidation by gut mucosal tissue transglutaminase and are presented to T-cells on HLA-DQ2 or HLA-DQ8 molecules, resulting in the stimulation of a T–helper cell type 1 (Th1)-biased proinflammatory attack that causes villous atrophy (2). It has also been proposed that the gut and dietary antigens play an important role in human type 1 diabetes, based on animal studies, epidemiological reports, and a small number of studies on human tissue (3–5).

The gut barrier and immune system in diabetes-prone rodents display abnormalities similar to those of celiac disease. For example, there are signs of enteropathy in BBdp rats (6) and NOD mice (7) and inflammatory cytokines in the gut are increased (8,9), as is permeability before islet inflammation (10–12). Closing gut-tight junctions prevents diabetes in the rat (12), there is increased antibody and T-cell response to dietary antigens (13,14), and wheat-based diets are major promoters of diabetes in rats and mice (4). Diabetes appearance can be partly inhibited by early neonatal feeding of small amounts of wheat proteins to BBdp rats by dampening the proinflammatory state of the gut (8). There are also indications that a gluten-free diet can enhance islet mass in BB rats (15). High-risk children on a gluten-free diet for 6 months showed enhanced first-phase insulin response during an intravenous glucose tolerance test, which could be an indication of increased β-cell mass and/or function (16,17). Thus, wheat is one external factor that could influence the development of diabetes.

Normal regulation of the gut immune system depends on maintaining the integrity of the gut barrier (18). There are now several reports of gut inflammation and signs of gut damage or leakage in humans with type 1 diabetes (19–24). T-cells from human diabetic pancreas display gut mucosal homing properties (25), and T-cells reactive against the diabetes autoantigen GAD express the gut-associated homing receptor $\alpha4\beta7$-integrin (26). In two prospective analyses of high-risk children, early exposure to cereals including wheat increased the risk of islet autoimmunity (27,28). Another study showed increased T-cell proliferation in response to high concentrations of wheat gluten in 24% of patients (29). Auricchio et al. (30) reported inflammation and increased immune response to gliadin in jejunal biopsies from patients. Approximately 2–6% of patients with type 1 diabetes have celiac disease, a rate that is several times higher than in the general population, and a recent report indicated that celiac disease patients on a gluten-free diet were protected from later development of type 1 diabetes (31). These findings point to both a loss of barrier integrity and dysregulation in the gut immune system.

Thus, questions arise regarding the frequency of abnormal immune responses to wheat and their nature, and it remains unclear whether such responses are diabetes related, reflect a separate gut dysfunction, or are simply due to shared celiac risk genes, such as HLA-DQ2, HLA-DQ8, and HLA-DR3. The number of studies examining the response of immune cells to wheat proteins in type 1 diabetic patients is limited (20,29,30), and it remains unclear whether there is a genetically determined abnormal immune response to wheat in humans at risk for type 1 diabetes. We favor the view that there is a diabetes-specific abnormal immune response to wheat in some patients that is not explained by shared celiac disease risk genes.

We hypothesize that in some type 1 diabetic patients, excessive amounts of wheat proteins/polypeptides enter the body through a leaky gut barrier and promote an abnormal immune response that breaks oral tolerance and stimulates immune cells that are involved in type 1 diabetes pathogenesis (4). As a first step, it is important to clarify what proportion of patients with type 1 diabetes display abnormal immune reactivity to dietary wheat polypeptides (WPs) and to characterize this abnormal response. The objectives of the present study were to determine whether patients with type 1 diabetes display increased T-cell proliferation in response to a mixture of WPs, to analyze the pattern of cytokines produced, and to determine whether this reactivity is associated with specific HLA alleles.

RESEARCH DESIGN AND METHODS

Type 1 diabetic patients were recruited through physicians at The Ottawa Hospital and the Children's Hospital of Eastern Ontario, Ottawa, Canada. All patients have clinically proven type 1 diabetes. The majority of the 42 subjects were young adults of both sexes, with one child included. A total of 22 unrelated control subjects of a similar age range and ethnic group (Caucasian) without acute infection or autoimmune disease were recruited (Table 1). All individuals included in the study were negative for tissue transglutaminase antibody, as measured by the Ottawa Hospital Clinical Laboratory. Blood was obtained by venepuncture from patients and healthy control subjects with informed consent. The local ethics committees approved the study.

Isolation of mononuclear cells, tissue culture, and antigen response. Peripheral blood mononuclear cells (PBMNCs) were isolated by density gradient centrifugation over Ficoll (Histopaque 1.077; Sigma Aldrich, Oakville, ON, Canada). Cells were washed twice with Hank's buffer (Invitrogen, Burlington, ON, Canada) containing 20 mmol/l HEPES (Invitrogen). PBMNCs (20×10^6/ml) were labeled with 2 mmol/l carboxyfluorescein diacetate succinimidyl ester (CFSE) (Invitrogen) for 20 min and incubated at 37°C in 5% CO_2. Cells were washed twice with Hank's buffer containing 5% pooled human

TABLE 1
Description of control subjects and patients with type 1 diabetes

Group	n	Sex ratio (female/male)	Age	Duration of diabetes (years)
Type 1 diabetic patients	42	28/14	26.7 (8–41)	11.2 ± 7
Healthy control subjects	22	11/11	24.5 (18–32)	NA

Data are means (range) or means ± SD unless otherwise indicated. NA, not applicable.

AB$^+$ serum (Bioreclamation, Hicksville, NY) and finally diluted in RPMI-1640 (Sigma Aldrich) containing 5% human AB$^+$ serum, 2 mmol/l L-glutamine (Invitrogen), 25 mmol/l HEPES (Invitrogen), 50 μmol/l β-mercaptoethanol (Sigma Aldrich), and 1% antibiotic/antimycotic (Invitrogen). Cells were cultured with various concentrations of wheat protein/peptides (chymotrypsin-treated, heat-inactivated WP; ICN Biochemicals, Cleveland, OH [32]) (3.1–12.4 μg/ml), 10 μg/ml gliadin (Sigma Aldrich), 10 μg/ml α-gliadin 33-mer peptide (a generous gift from Dr. Chaitan Khosla, Stanford University, Stanford, CA, and Dr. Hubert Kolb, German Diabetes Center, Düsseldorf, Germany), 10 μg/ml insulin (Sigma Aldrich), 1 μmol ovalbumin (Sigma Aldrich), 2.7 LF/ml tetanus toxoid (Connaught Laboratory, Toronto, ON, Canada), or 5 μg/ml phytohemagglutinin (Sigma Aldrich). 1.2×10^6 cells in 1 ml/well were cultured in 24-well plates (Falcon; VWR, Mississauga, ON, Canada). After 3 days of culture, 10 IU/ml recombinant human interleukin (IL)-2 (PeproTech, Rocky Hill, NJ) was added to each well. On day 8, supernatants were harvested and cell proliferation was assessed using a CFSE-based, flow cytometric assay with results expressed as the cell division index (CDI) (defined as the number of CD3$^+$ CFSE^{dim} cells cultured with antigen/number of CD3$^+$ CFSE^{dim} cells without antigen; the number of CFSE^{dim} events was the number corresponding to 5,000 CFSE^{bright} cells) (33).

Wheat protein preparations were analyzed for lipopolysaccharide (LPS). The concentration was low and comparable with other recombinant proteins. The addition of the LPS inhibitor polymyxin B (Sigma) had no effect on WP-induced T-cell proliferation but blocked LPS-induced T-cell proliferation (supplementary Fig. S1, available in an online appendix at http://diabetes.diabetesjournals.org/cgi/content/full/db08-1579/DC1).

Blocking of HLA-DR with anti-DR antibody. Inhibition of the proliferation of PBMNCs to wheat protein was studied by adding monoclonal anti-DR antibodies (clone G46-6 and mouse IgG$_{2a}$,κ; BD Biosciences, Mississauga, ON, Canada) to the culture 30 min before adding wheat protein to the cell culture wells. The mouse IgG$_{2a}$,κ isotype antibody (BD Biosciences) was used as a control. Both antibodies were used at a concentration of 5 μg/ml.

Cytokine evaluation in culture supernatants. Cytokines including IL-4, IL-6, IL-10, tumor necrosis factor (TNF), and γ-interferon (IFN-γ) were quantified simultaneously using a human Th1/Th2 cytokine cytometric bead array (CBA) kit. The CBA kit and CBA software were purchased from BD Biosciences. All assays were performed according to the manufacturer's protocol, and samples were read in a Coulter FC500 flow cytometer after appropriate calibration. Quantification of cytokine levels was performed by comparison with standards provided in the kit using CBA software. IL-17A was analyzed in supernatants of PBMNC from a subset of patients and healthy control subjects in the presence or absence of anti-DR antibodies using an enzyme-linked immunosorbent assay (ELISA) kit purchased from eBioscience (San Francisco, CA).

HLA typing. HLA-DR and -DQ haplotypes of subjects were characterized by PCR-based HLA class II tissue typing using low resolution Olerup SSP typing kits for HLA-DR and -DQ (Genovision, West Chester, PA) or by the Ottawa Hospital Clinical Laboratory.

Statistical analysis. Differences in CDI among patients and control subjects were analyzed by the nonparametric Mann-Whitney U test using GraphPad Prism (version 4.03 for Windows; GraphPad Software, San Diego, CA). Significance of differences in frequencies was evaluated using Fisher's exact two-tailed test. Spearman's correlation was used to analyze the correlation between WP T-cell response and the other dietary or autoantigens using STATISTICA (version 6; Statsoft, Tulsa, OK).

RESULTS

CD3$^+$ T-cell response to WPs in control and type 1 diabetic subjects. The CFSE assay permitted evaluation of T-cell proliferation to low, nontoxic concentrations of

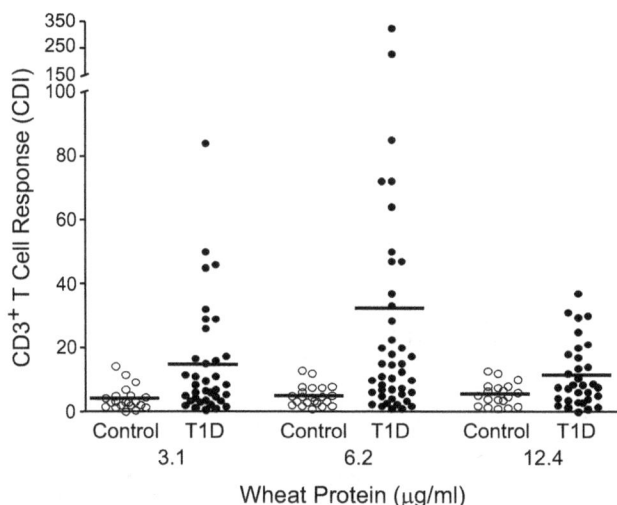

FIG. 1. Antigen-specific CD3[+] T-cell proliferation. 1.2×10^6 CFSE-labeled PBMNCs from patients with type 1 diabetes (T1D) or healthy control subjects were cultured for 8 days in the absence or presence of different concentrations of WPs. On day 8, cells were stained with Cy-chrome conjugated anti-CD3 monoclonal antibody. CDI was calculated based on a fixed number of 5,000 CD3[+] CFSE[bright] cells using the following formula: CDI = number of CD3[+], CFSE[dim] cells with antigen/number of CD3[+], CFSE[dim] cells without antigen (medium). The horizontal line indicates the mean.

WP (Fig. 1). CD3[+] T-cell proliferation in the presence of 3.1 and 6.2 μg/ml WP was significantly higher in the type 1 diabetic patient group compared with control subjects (Fig. 1). At 12.4 μg/ml, CDI was still higher in the type 1 diabetic patient group but the response was less than at 6.2 μg/ml, suggesting inhibition. Therefore, 6.2 μg/ml was chosen as the optimum concentration. To identify patients with a positive proliferation response to WP, the mean + 3 SD of the control group CDI (CDI ≥14.6) was chosen as the cutoff. Of the 42 patients with type 1 diabetes, 20 (47%) had a positive proliferation response to WP. In an expanded analysis of two responders, the proliferative response to WP was mainly from CD4[+] T-cells with only a weak CD8[+] T-cell response (data not shown). The distribution of CDI to WP was significantly different between patients ($n = 42$) and control subjects ($n = 22$); for patients, the median was 11.8 (range 1.0–323) and for

control subjects 4.5 (0.8–12.8) ($P = 0.0004$; Mann-Whitney U test) (Fig. 1).

The mean ± SD CDI was 32 ± 60 for patients and 4.9 ± 3.2 for control subjects. WP response was not correlated with duration of disease, but there was a moderate inverse correlation with age ($r = -0.35$, $P = 0.025$; data not shown). When a subgroup of six control subjects was matched with 19 patients for HLA-DR4, age, and sex, the increased T-cell proliferation in response to WP in the type 1 diabetic patient group remained significant ($P = 0.038$) (supplementary Fig. S2).

T-cell responses to other dietary antigens moderately increased in type 1 diabetic patients. Some patients displayed increased T-cell responses to other dietary antigens including ovalbumin, an irrelevant dietary antigen, and to the celiac-related antigens (wheat gliadin and α-gliadin 33-mer peptide) as well as the type 1 diabetes autoantigen insulin ($P = 0.02$, $P = 0.03$, $P = 0.001$, and $P = 0.03$, respectively) (Fig. 2). We did not find significant differences between type 1 diabetic patients and control subjects in response to the recall antigen, tetanus toxoid, or the T-cell mitogen phytohemagglutinin ($P = 0.2$) (Fig. 2). There was a positive correlation between WP T-cell responses and T-cell responses to ovalbumin, gliadin, and α-gliadin 33-mer peptide in type 1 diabetic patients ($P = 0.01$, $P = 0.002$, and $P = 0.0001$; data not shown). In contrast, we detected a weak, nonsignificant correlation between WP T-cell response and insulin T-cell response in type 1 diabetic patients ($P = 0.06$; data not shown).

High concentration of IFN-γ, IL-6, and IL-17A in supernatants of WP-stimulated PBMNC. Cytokines secreted by WP-stimulated PBMNC were analyzed in the culture supernatant using flow CBAs or ELISA (IL-17A) (Fig. 3). The concentration of the proinflammatory cytokines IFN-γ, TNF, and IL-6 was higher in WP-stimulated PBMNC from type 1 diabetic patients ($P = 0.03$, $P = 0.008$, and $P = 0.001$, respectively), whereas the counter inflammatory cytokines IL-4 and IL-10 were not different. Removing one control subject from the IL-4 group analysis (circled symbol, Fig. 3) revealed significantly higher IL-4 concentration in the type 1 diabetic patient supernatants. However, the concentration of IL-4 was much lower than that of IFN-γ. The concentration of IL-17A in WP-stimulated PBMNC culture supernatants from pa-

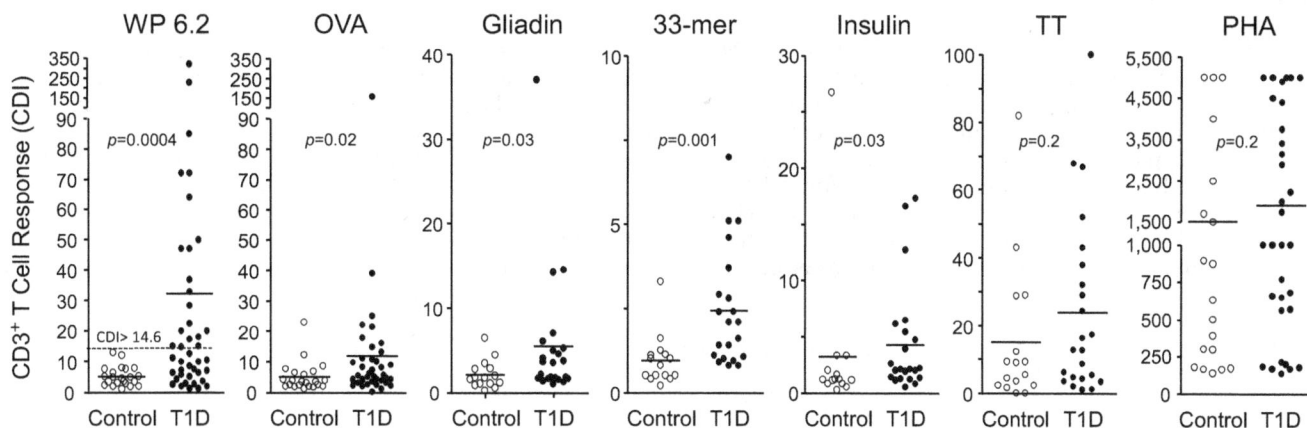

FIG. 2. T-cell proliferation in response to WPs and other antigens or mitogen. 1.2×10^6 CFSE-labeled PBMNCs from patients with type 1 diabetes (T1D) or healthy control subjects were cultured for 8 days in the absence or presence of WP, ovalbumin (OVA), gliadin, 33-mer, insulin, tetanus toxoid (TT), or phytohemagglutinin (PHA) (see RESEARCH DESIGN AND METHODS for details). On day 8, cells were stained with Cy-chrome–conjugated anti-CD3 monoclonal antibody. CDI was calculated. A CDI value greater than the control mean + 3 SD (CDI >14.6) was used to define a positive response to WP. *P* values indicate statistical difference compared with control subjects. The horizontal lines indicate the means.

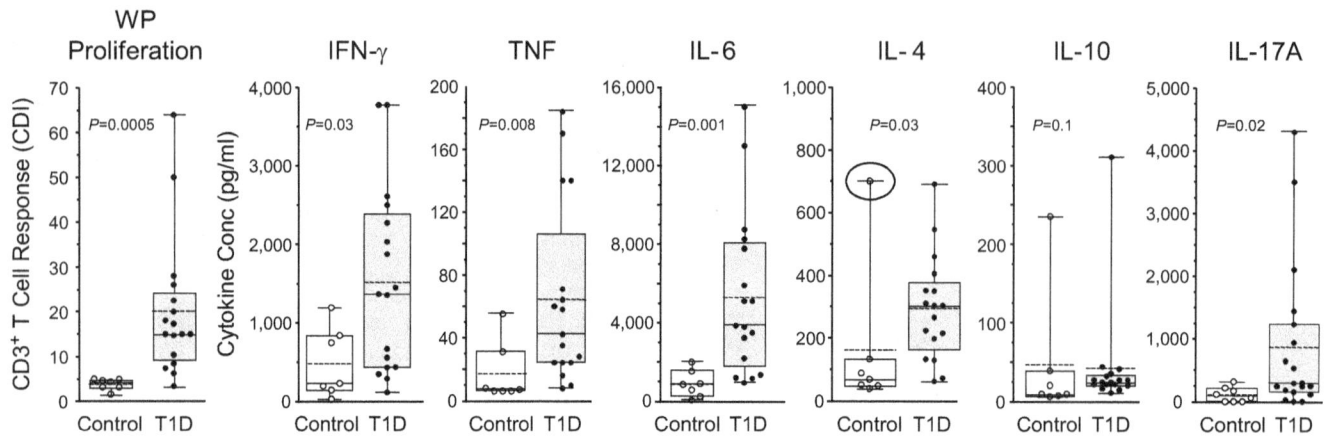

FIG. 3. WP-stimulated cytokine secretion by PBMNC at day 8 of culture. Box and Whisker plots with individual values for control and diabetic subjects. IFN-γ, TNF, IL-6, IL-4, and IL-10 were measured by flow CBA. IL-17A was measured by ELISA. Each plot includes the mean (dashed line), median (solid line), distribution, and range. (For IL-4, the difference between control and type 1 diabetic [T1D] subjects is significant when the circled outlier value in the control group is removed [P = 0.03].)

tients was increased compared with control subjects (P = 0.02) (Fig. 3).

Association of HLA-DR4 risk alleles for type 1 diabetes with immunity to WPs. We analyzed HLA-DR and -DQ haplotypes in patients with type 1 diabetes and control subjects. The frequency of HLA haplotypes in the control group was similar to previously published reference populations (34) (data not shown). HLA-DRB1*03 and -DRB1*04, which are associated with type 1 diabetes, were more frequent in type 1 diabetic patients compared with control subjects. Heterozygous DR3/DR4 individuals represented 29% of our type 1 diabetic patients, but none of our control subjects was heterozygous for HLA-DR3/DR4 (data not shown). In addition, we compared the frequency of risk alleles in type 1 diabetic patients who were either responders or nonresponders to WP (Table 2). Type 1 diabetic responders to WP carried HLA-DRB1*04 in 95% of cases, which was significantly higher than in the nonresponders (59%; P = 0.01) (Table 2). Distribution of T-cell proliferation (CDI) to WP in type 1 diabetic patients with HLA-DRB1*03 or HLA-DRB1*04 or in those heterozygous for HLA-DRB1*03/*04 is shown in Fig. 4. One of seven type 1 diabetic patients with HLA-DRB1*03$^+$/*04$^-$ showed positive responses to WP. In contrast, 10 of 20 type 1 diabetic patients who carried one risk allele HLA-DRB1*04 or 9 of 12 patients who carried both risk genes HLA-DRB1*03/*04 showed positive reactivity to WP.

The frequency of HLA-DQ2, the major celiac disease–associated allele, was not significantly different between type 1 diabetic patients and control subjects (P = 0.6; data not shown). Importantly, the difference for HLA-DQ2 between responders and nonresponders was not significant (P = 0.75) (Table 2). We also evaluated the HLA-DR and -DQ haplotypes by high-resolution analysis in type 1

diabetic patients. A positive response to WP in patients was more frequently associated with the HLA-DR4 (DRB1*0401/4) DQB1*0301/2 haplotype, and HLA-DR3/DQB1*0201 appeared to magnify the response (Fig. 4). Patients who were HLA-DQ3$^+$ were also more likely to be responders (Table 2).

T-cell responses to WP inhibited by monoclonal anti-DR antibodies. To confirm the role of HLA-DR in the T-cell response to WP, we evaluated the blocking effect of anti–HLA-DR monoclonal antibodies on PBMNC of 14 type 1 diabetic patients. Monoclonal anti-DR antibodies blocked T-cell responses to WPs in type 1 diabetic patients, whereas isotype control antibody did not prevent the T-cell response (Fig. 5A). Anti–HLA-DR4 antibody had only a small inhibitory effect on T-cell response to tetanus toxoid (supplementary Fig. S3). CBA cytokine analysis of the culture supernatants from WP-stimulated PBMNC of type 1 diabetic patients showed that monoclonal anti-DR antibody significantly inhibited secretion of Th1 cytokines but not Th2 cytokines (Fig. 5B). WP-induced production of IL-17A was also blocked by the addition of anti-DR (P = 0.008) (Fig. 5B).

DISCUSSION

The foods we eat contain numerous nonself molecules that do not normally stimulate a proinflammatory immune response in healthy individuals (35). In some diabetes-prone rodents (6,7,10) and humans (19,21–23), there is evidence that the gut mucosa is mildly inflamed and the epithelial barrier is leaky, providing a potential entry point for nonself antigens in the context of a proinflammatory cytokine imbalance that could promote autoimmunity (4,18). The present results support this view. Although the

TABLE 2
HLA-DR and -DQ in type 1 diabetic responders and nonresponders

	n	DR3	DR4	DR3/DR4	DQ2	DQ3
Nonresponders	22	41	59	14	41	64
Responders	20	50	95 (P = 0.01)	45 (P = 0.04)	50 (P = 0.75)	95 (P = 0.02)

Data are % unless otherwise indicated. T-cell proliferation (CDI) to WP was evaluated in type 1 diabetic patients. Patients with a CDI value greater than mean + 3 SD of the control group (CDI >14.6) were classified as responders. Those below were classified as nonresponders. The percentage of individuals with the indicated HLA haplotypes in these groups was calculated.

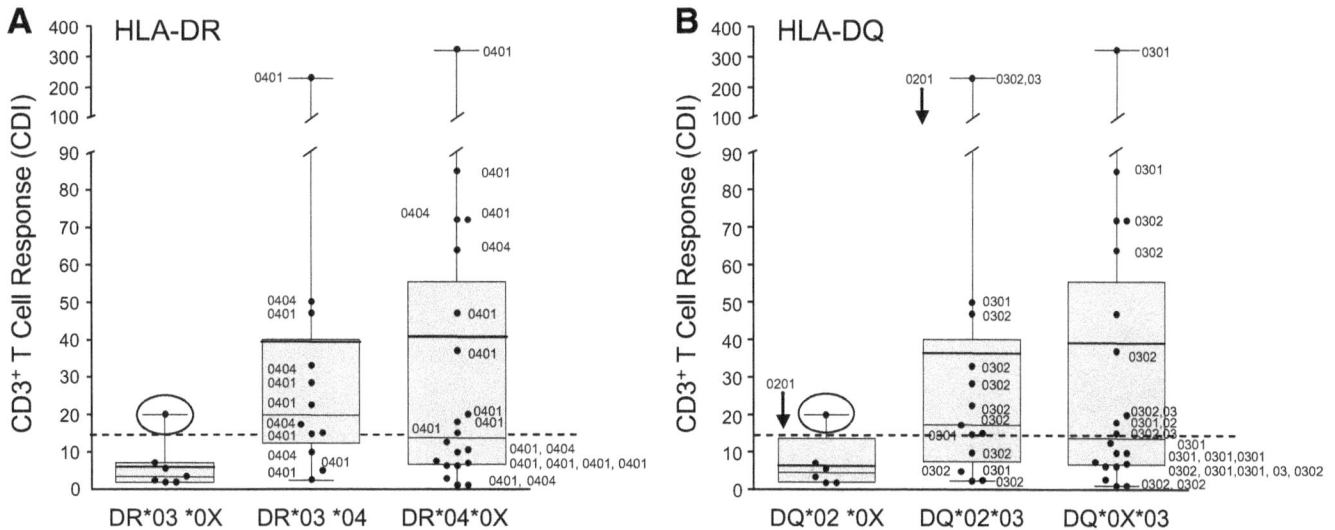

FIG. 4. Graphic representation of the relationship between wheat-induced T-cell response and high-resolution HLA diabetes risk alleles. Box and Whisker plots with individual values for diabetic subjects. Each plot includes the mean (bold line), median (solid thin line), distribution, and range. *A*: Distribution of T-cell proliferation (CDI) to WP in type 1 diabetic patients with HLA-DRB1*03 and HLA-DRB1*04 or in those heterozygous for HLA-DRB1*03/*04. A CDI value greater than mean + 3 SD of the control group (CDI >14.6, dashed line) was used to define a positive proliferation response. One of the type 1 diabetic patients with HLA-DRB1*03⁺/*04⁻ showed positive responses to WP (○). Type 1 diabetic patients who carried one risk allele HLA-DRB1*04 (10 of 20) or patients who carried both risk genes HLA-DRB1*03/*04 (9 of 12) showed positive reactivity to WP. High-resolution results of HLA-DR are labeled beside each individual. *B*: Distribution of T-cell proliferation (CDI) to WP in type 1 diabetic patients with HLA-DQB1*02 and HLA-DQB1*03 or in those heterozygous for HLA-DQB1*02/*03. High-resolution analyses for HLA-DQB1*02 and *03 are labeled beside each symbol. ↓ (beside 0201) means all individuals in the column carry HLA-DQB1*0201. (Three of the 42 type 1 diabetic individuals are neither DR3 nor DR4, and therefore they are not included in this figure. One of the seven individuals with DR3/non-DR4 in the *left panel* is heterozygous for DQ*02/*03 and was therefore placed in the middle column in the *right panel* [DQ*02*03]. Differences in high-resolution haplotypes between responders and nonresponders were not evaluated statistically because of the small sample size.)

origin of the antigens and immune cells that initiate or drive the β-cell–specific autoimmune response is not known, diet is an important factor influencing diabetes outcome, possibly by supplying a constant source of stimulatory antigens to the gut immune system (4).

There was moderately increased T-cell proliferative response to other dietary antigens such as ovalbumin, gliadin, and the celiac toxic gliadin 33-mer peptide (Fig. 2), but this was less pronounced than the response to WP. These data suggest a general impairment of oral tolerance in some type 1 diabetic patients (36), with the strongest and most frequent abnormal proliferative response induced by the mixture of WPs.

We are aware of only one other study of WP response in patient PBMNCs (29). Klemetti et al. (29) showed an increased cell-mediated immune response to high concentrations of wheat gluten (400 μg/ml) in 24% of newly diagnosed type 1 diabetic patients. The proliferative responses in this study were low compared with those in the present study, possibly as a result of the high polypeptide concentration, different gluten fractions, culture conditions, proliferation assay, and/or different genetic background of the subjects as well as different duration of diabetes. In keeping with reports that high concentrations of gliadin are cytotoxic (37), we found that 25 μg/ml of wheat protein extract inhibited response of PBMNC, whereas 6.2 μg/ml was optimum for our assay (29). The CFSE assay used here not only permits identification of individual cell populations by flow cytometry but is also more sensitive than the thymidine assay (33). Therefore, the present analysis permitted us to detect wheat-specific CD3⁺ T-cell proliferation using a low, noninhibitory dose of WP.

Additional evidence linking the development of diabetes in humans to wheat comes from epidemiological studies

(27,28) and reports of immune responses of patient tissues to WP (29,30). Anti-gliadin antibodies have been reported in newly diagnosed children with type 1 diabetes (38), and prospective studies of infants at high risk indicate that early exposure to cereals, particularly wheat, was linked to appearance of islet autoantibodies (27,28). Furthermore, a significant subset of type 1 diabetic patients displays celiac disease autoantibodies (39). CD3⁺ lamina propria and intestinal epithelial lymphocytes were increased in 20% of type 1 diabetic patients receiving rectally instilled gliadin (40). Immunohistochemical evaluation and culture of jejunal biopsies from tissue transglutaminase antibody–negative type 1 diabetic children with WP increased frequency of activated CD25⁺ cells in the lamina propria as well as expression of HLA-DR in the crypts in association with enhanced infiltration of the epithelium by CD3⁺ cells (30). Therefore, the present results are consistent with those of Auricchio et al. (30) showing that a subset of type 1 diabetic patients displayed signs of inflamed gut mucosa and increased immune reactivity to WPs.

Type 1 diabetes has been traditionally thought of as a T-cell–mediated disease associated with high levels of the Th1 cytokine IFN-γ. It now seems likely that type 1 diabetes is the result of dysregulation within a broader network of immune cell types (41). For example, the role of the recently discovered Th17 cells and the extent to which there is a dysregulation of communication between Th1, Th2, and Th17 cells in human diabetes remain unclear. We observed WP-induced T-cell proliferation in nearly half of our type 1 diabetic patients but not in healthy control subjects. This response was mixed in nature, accompanied by increased production of proinflammatory cytokines IFN-γ, TNF, IL-6, and IL-17A as well

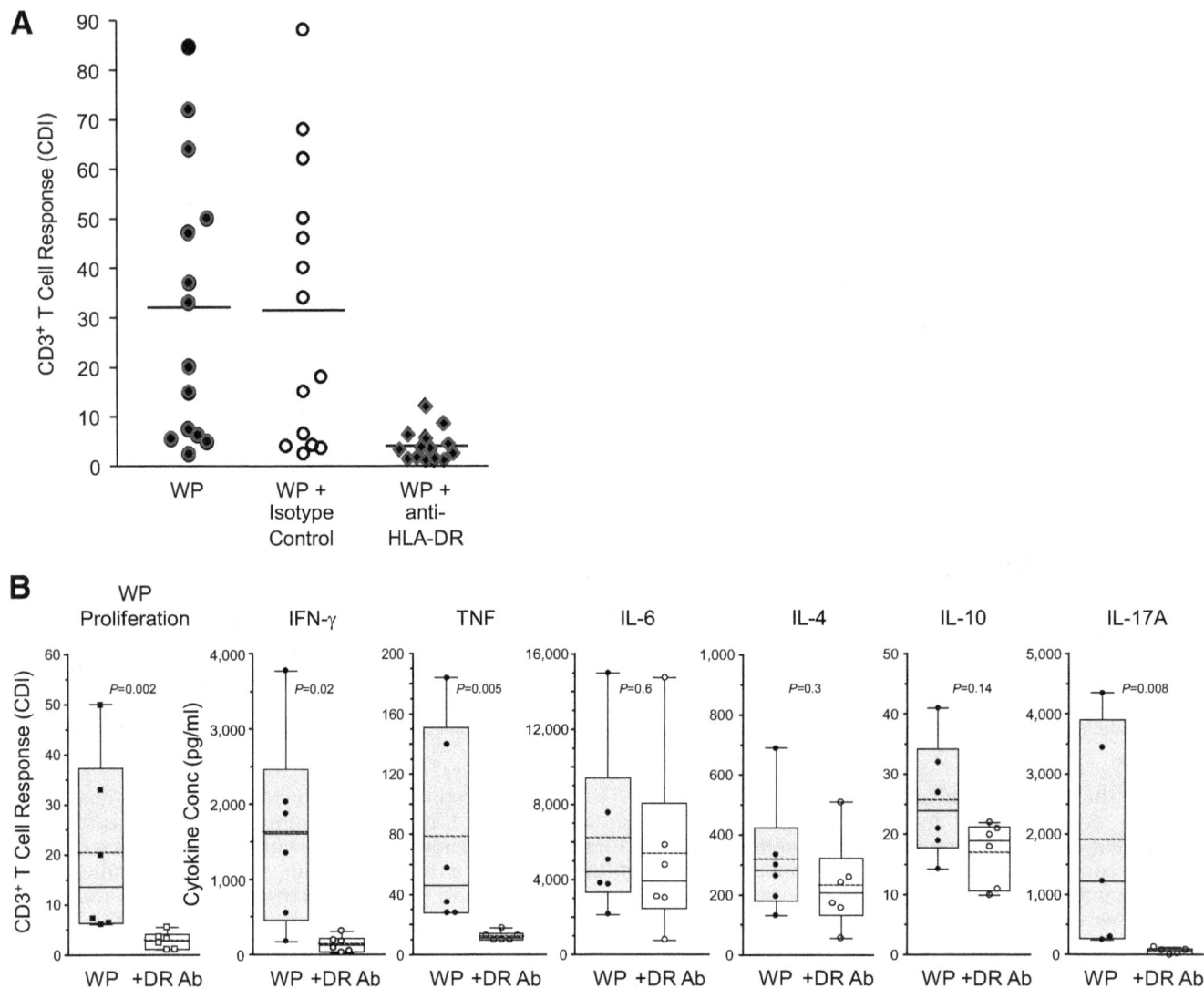

FIG. 5. Role of HLA-DR in the type 1 diabetes T-cell and cytokine response to WPs. *A*: The T-cell response to wheat protein (6.2 μg/ml) was calculated as CDI in 14 patients and compared with cells cultured in the presence of anti–HLA-DR monoclonal antibody (5 μg/ml) or with isotype control antibody. *B*: Cytokine profiles of supernatants from WP-stimulated PBMNC of patients were evaluated in the absence and presence of monoclonal HLA-DR antibodies using Th1/Th2 CBAs for IFN-γ, IL-4, TNF, IL-10, and IL-6 or an ELISA kit for IL-17A.

as the counterinflammatory Th2 cytokine IL-4. The high concentrations of IFN-γ and IL-17A suggest that Th1 and Th17 cytokine–producing, WP-responsive CD3⁺ cells were activated in association with a proinflammatory condition in the gut (6,30). IL-6 was present in WP culture supernatants at very high levels, four to six times those of IFN-γ. TNF was also increased but to a much lesser extent. IL-6 and TNF are proinflammatory cytokines that promote the secretion of IL-17 by Th17 cells and block the production of Foxp3⁺ regulatory T-cells (42). We did not observe a significant increase in IL-10 in response to WP, making it unlikely that IL-17 originated from Th17 regulatory cells that produce both IL-10 and IL-17. It seems unlikely that such high amounts of IL-17 could originate from CD8⁺ T-cells because expansion of WP-responsive T-cells was predominantly from CD4⁺ cells and IL-17A production was blocked by anti-DR antibody.

High levels of IFN-γ were produced in response to WP, whereas the concentration of the Th2 cytokine IL-4, although significantly increased, was only one-third that of

IFN-γ, suggesting a predominance of Th1 over Th2 cells. Although both of these cytokines can inhibit development of Th17 cells from naive precursors (42), it has been suggested that committed Th17 cells are not affected (41). Therefore, we favor the interpretation that WP stimulates the production of IL-17A from previously committed Th17 cells. While IL-17A can be produced under certain circumstances by CD8⁺ T-cells and members of the innate immune system (γδT-cells and natural killer T-cells), Th17 cells are the major producers of IL-17A. Thus, the overall cytokine pattern observed in WP-stimulated PBMNC from type 1 diabetic patients suggests a predominant Th1 and Th17 proinflammatory state consistent with the speculation that autoimmunity can occur when there is inappropriate cross-regulation between Th1 and Th17 cytokine networks (42).

The role of IL-6 in type 1 diabetes remains controversial (43). In the present study, patient PBMNC cultured with WP secreted large amounts of IL-6, the origin of which is presently unclear. Nonetheless, some points are worth noting: WP response was mainly from $CD4^+$ and not $CD8^+$ cells, most responders were HLA-DR4$^+$, and treatment with anti-DR did not block production of IL-6. These results suggest that IL-6 originated from non–T-cells. Others report that IL-6 gene expression was upregulated threefold in monocytes from adult-onset type 1 diabetic subjects (44). Furthermore, overexpression of IL-6 in pancreas was correlated with islet inflammation, which could contribute to the development of autoimmune disease (43). The high concentration of WP-induced IL-6 further supports our previous proposal of a potential mechanism by which wheat can promote the development of diabetes involving induction of proinflammatory cytokines such as IL-6, IFN-γ, and TNF-α by wheat antigens (4,9,13,45).

The HLA genes are the major genetic determinant of type 1 diabetes. More than 90% of Caucasian type 1 diabetic patients carry either HLA-DR3 or HLA-DR4 haplotype, and a synergistic effect on type 1 diabetes risk is observed in HLA-DR3/4 heterozygous individuals (46). Patients with type 1 diabetes and celiac disease share some HLA-associated risk genes such as HLA-DQ2 (HLA-DQB1*02) and HLA-DQ8 (HLA-DQB1*0302). The frequency of HLA risk genes is different between the two diseases: 90–95% of celiac disease patients are HLA-DQ2 and 5–10% are HLA-DQ8 (47), whereas up to 50% of diabetic patients are HLA-DQ8/DQ2 heterozygous (48). In our type 1 diabetic population, increased immune response to WPs was not explained by shared genetic risk for celiac disease. The frequency of HLA-DQB1*02 was not significantly different between type 1 diabetic patients and control subjects ($P = 0.6$), and we did not detect any significant differences for HLA-DQB1*02 between WP responders and nonresponders ($P = 0.75$) (Table 2). We also evaluated the HLA-DR and -DQ haplotype by high-resolution analysis in type 1 diabetic patients. A positive response to WP in patients was more frequently associated with the HLA-DR4 (DRB1*0401/4) DQB1*0301/2 haplotype, and HLA-DR3/DQB1*0201 appeared to magnify the response (Table 2, Fig. 4).

A genetic basis for WP response in type 1 diabetic patients is suggested by the finding that T-cell proliferation and inflammatory cytokine production were blocked by anti-DR antibodies and responders were nearly all HLA-DR4$^+$. Others have observed enhanced expression of HLA-DR in the intestinal mucosa of children with type 1 diabetes (20,30), and gluten-induced T-cell proliferation was blocked by anti-DR antibodies in two patients in a previous study (29). Importantly, WP-induced T-cell proliferation was not explained by an overrepresentation of the major celiac disease risk gene HLA-DQ2. HLA-DQ2 prevalence was not different between patients and control subjects or between WP responder and nonresponder patient groups, and the T-cell response was not attributable to the presence of subclinical celiac disease given that all our patients with type 1 diabetes were negative for antibodies against the pathognomic celiac disease autoantigen, tissue transglutaminase. These findings are consistent with other reports showing that the gut inflammation observed in type 1 diabetic patients is different from that seen in patients with celiac disease (20,49) and not necessarily related to HLA-DQ2 or HLA-DQ8 (30). Therefore, the tolerogenic function of the gut immune system with respect to WPs was compromised in a large subset of patients with type 1 diabetes in an HLA-DR–restricted, diabetes-specific manner.

In summary, almost half of our type 1 diabetic patients displayed increased proliferation when PBMNCs were cultured in vitro with nontoxic concentrations of WP. The cytokine pattern was mixed having characteristics of a predominant Th1 and Th17 response with a lesser contribution of the Th2 cytokine IL-4. The WP proliferative response occurred mainly in HLA-DR4 individuals and was blocked with anti-DR antibodies but was not due to the major celiac disease gene HLA-DQ2. This demonstrated the presence of a mixed proinflammatory Th1/Th17 response to dietary WPs that appeared to be diabetes specific.

ACKNOWLEDGMENTS

This work was supported by the Juvenile Diabetes Research Foundation and Canadian Institutes of Health Research.

No potential conflicts of interest relevant to this article were reported.

Parts of this study were presented in abstract form at the 65th Scientific Sessions of the American Diabetes Association, San Diego, California, 10–14 June 2005, and at the First Nordic Meeting on Genetics and Pathogenesis of Immunological Diseases, Helsinki, Finland, 4–5 September 2006.

We are indebted to the volunteers and the following physicians: Drs. Rene Wong and Janine Malcolm (The Ottawa Hospital) and Dr. Sarah Lawrence (the Children's Hospital of Eastern Ontario). We thank Nancy Hampton (The Ottawa Hospital) for HLA typing and helpful discussions. Dr. Chaitan Khosla (Stanford University) and Dr. Hubert Kolb (German Diabetes Center, Düsseldorf, Germany) provided the α-gliadin 33-mer peptide. We thank Drs. Hubert Kolb and Nanette Schloot (German Diabetes Center, Düsseldorf, Germany) and Dr. William Cameron (the Ottawa Hospital Research Institute) for reviewing the manuscript.

REFERENCES

1. Solly NR, Honeyman MC, Harrison LC. The mucosal interface between 'self' and 'non-self' determines the impact of environment on autoimmune diabetes. Curr Dir Autoimmun 2001;4:68–90
2. Sollid LM. Coeliac disease: dissecting a complex inflammatory disorder. Nat Rev Immunol 2002;2:647–655
3. Courtois P, Nsimba G, Jijakli H, Sener A, Scott FW, Malaisse WJ. Gut permeability and intestinal mucins, invertase and peroxidase in control and diabetes-prone BB rats fed either a protective or diabetogenic diet. Dig Dis Sci 2005;50:266–275
4. Lefebvre DE, Powell KL, Strom A, Scott FW. Dietary proteins as environmental modifiers of type 1 diabetes mellitus. Annu Rev Nutr 2006;26:175–202
5. Vaarala O, Atkinson MA, Neu J. The "perfect storm" for type 1 diabetes: the complex interplay between intestinal microbiota, gut permeability, and mucosal immunity. Diabetes 2008;57:2555–2562
6. Graham S, Courtois P, Malaisse WJ, Rozing J, Scott FW, Mowat AM. Enteropathy precedes type 1 diabetes in the BB rat. Gut 2004;53:1437–1444
7. Maurano F, Mazzarella G, Luongo D, Stefanile R, D'Arienzo R, Rossi M, Auricchio S, Troncone R. Small intestinal enteropathy in non-obese diabetic mice fed a diet containing wheat. Diabetologia 2005;48:931–937
8. Scott FW, Rowsell P, Wang GS, Burghardt K, Kolb H, Flohe S. Oral exposure to diabetes-promoting food or immunomodulators in neonates alters gut cytokines and diabetes. Diabetes 2002;51:73–78
9. Flohe SB, Wasmuth HE, Kerad JB, Beales PE, Pozzilli P, Elliott RB, Hill JP, Scott FW, Kolb H. A wheat-based, diabetes-promoting diet induces a Th1-type cytokine bias in the gut of NOD mice. Cytokine 2003;21:149–154
10. Meddings JB, Jarand J, Urbanski SJ, Hardin J, Gall DG. Increased gastrointestinal permeability is an early lesion in the spontaneously diabetic BB rat. Am J Physiol 1999;276:G951–G957
11. Neu J, Reverte CM, Mackey AD, Liboni K, Tuhacek-Tenace LM, Hatch M,

Li N, Caicedo RA, Schatz DA, Atkinson M. Changes in intestinal morphology and permeability in the biobreeding rat before the onset of type 1 diabetes. J Pediatr Gastroenterol Nutr 2005;40:589–595

12. Watts T, Berti I, Sapone A, Gerarduzzi T, Not T, Zielke R, Fasano A. Role of the intestinal tight junction modulator zonulin in the pathogenesis of type I diabetes in BB diabetic-prone rats. Proc Natl Acad Sci U S A 2005;102:2916–2921

13. Chakir H, Lefebvre DE, Wang H, Caraher E, Scott FW. Wheat protein-induced proinflammatory T helper 1 bias in mesenteric lymph nodes of young diabetes-prone rats. Diabetologia 2005;48:1576–1584

14. MacFarlane AJ, Burghardt KM, Kelly J, Simell T, Simell O, Altosaar I, Scott FW. A type 1 diabetes-related protein from wheat (Triticum aestivum). cDNA clone of a wheat storage globulin, Glb1, linked to islet damage. J Biol Chem 2003;278:54–63

15. Wang GS, Kauri L, Wang G-S, Patrick C, Scott FW. Enhanced islet neogenesis and beta cell proliferation in pre-insulitic diabetes-prone rats fed a hydrolyzed casein diet. FASEB J 2007;21:A771

16. Pastore MR, Bazzigaluppi E, Belloni C, Arcovio C, Bonifacio E, Bosi E. Six months of gluten-free diet do not influence autoantibody titers, but improve insulin secretion in subjects at high risk for type 1 diabetes. J Clin Endocrinol Metab 2003;88:162–165

17. Kahn SE, Carr DB, Faulenbach MV, Utzschneider KM. An examination of beta-cell function measures and their potential use for estimating beta-cell mass. Diabetes Obes Metab 2008;10(Suppl.4):63–76

18. Fasano A, Shea-Donohue T. Mechanisms of disease: the role of intestinal barrier function in the pathogenesis of gastrointestinal autoimmune diseases. Nat Clin Pract Gastroenterol Hepatol 2005;2:416–422

19. Mooradian AD, Morley JE, Levine AS, Prigge WF, Gebhard RL. Abnormal intestinal permeability to sugars in diabetes mellitus. Diabetologia 1986; 29:221–224

20. Westerholm-Ormio M, Vaarala O, Pihkala P, Ilonen J, Savilahti E. Immunologic activity in the small intestinal mucosa of pediatric patients with type 1 diabetes. Diabetes 2003;52:2287–2295

21. Carratu R, Secondulfo M, de Magistris L, Iafusco D, Urio A, Carbone MG, Pontoni G, Carteni M, Prisco F. Altered intestinal permeability to mannitol in diabetes mellitus type I. J Pediatr Gastroenterol Nutr 1999;28:264–269

22. Damci T, Nuhoglu I, Devranoglu G, Osar Z, Demir M, Ilkova H. Increased intestinal permeability as a cause of fluctuating postprandial blood glucose levels in Type 1 diabetic patients. Eur J Clin Invest 2003;33:397–401

23. Secondulfo M, Iafusco D, Carratu R, deMagistris L, Sapone A, Generoso M, Mezzogiomo A, Sasso FC, Carteni M, De Rosa R, Prisco F, Esposito V. Ultrastructural mucosal alterations and increased intestinal permeability in non-celiac, type I diabetic patients. Dig Liver Dis 2004;36:35–45

24. Sapone A, de Magistris L, Pietzak M, Clemente MG, Tripathi A, Cucca F, Lampis R, Kryszak D, Carteni M, Generoso M, Iafusco D, Prisco F, Laghi F, Riegler G, Carratu R, Counts D, Fasano A. Zonulin upregulation is associated with increased gut permeability in subjects with type 1 diabetes and their relatives. Diabetes 2006;55:1443–1449

25. Hanninen A, Jalkanen S, Salmi M, Toikkanen S, Nikolakaros G, Simell O. Macrophages, T cell receptor usage, and endothelial cell activation in the pancreas at the onset of insulin-dependent diabetes mellitus. J Clin Invest 1992;90:1901–1910

26. Paronen J, Klemetti P, Kantele JM, Savilahti E, Perheentupa J, Akerblom HK, Vaarala O. Glutamate decarboxylase-reactive peripheral blood lymphocytes from patients with IDDM express gut-specific homing receptor α4β7- integrin. Diabetes 1997;46:583–588

27. Norris JM, Barriga K, Klingensmith G, Hoffman M, Eisenbarth GS, Erlich HA, Rewers M. Timing of initial cereal exposure in infancy and risk of islet autoimmunity. JAMA 2003;290:1713–1720

28. Ziegler AG, Schmid S, Huber D, Hummel M, Bonifacio E. Early infant feeding and risk of developing type 1 diabetes-associated autoantibodies. JAMA 2003;290:1721–1728

29. Klemetti P, Savilahti E, Ilonen J, Akerblom HK, Vaarala O. T-cell reactivity to wheat gluten in patients with insulin-dependent diabetes mellitus. Scand J Immunol 1998;47:48–53

30. Auricchio R, Paparo F, Maglio M, Franzese A, Lombardi F, Valerio G, Nardone G, Percopo S, Greco L, Troncone R. In vitro-deranged intestinal immune response to gliadin in type 1 diabetes. Diabetes 2004;53:1680–1683

31. Cosnes J, Cellier C, Viola S, Colombel JF, Michaud L, Sarles J, Hugot JP, Ginies JL, Dabadie A, Mouterde O, Allez M, Nion-Larmurier I. Incidence of autoimmune diseases in celiac disease: protective effect of the gluten-free diet. Clin Gastroenterol Hepatol 2008;6:753–758

32. Arentz-Hansen EH, McAdam SN, Molberg O, Kristianson C, Sollid LM. Production of a panel of recombinant gliadins for the characterisation of T cell reactivity in coeliac disease. Gut 2000;46:46–51

33. Mannering SI, Morris JS, Jensen KP, Purcell AW, Honeyman MC, van Endert PM, Harrison LC. A sensitive method for detecting proliferation of rare autoantigen-specific human T cells. J Immunol Methods 2003;283:173–183

34. Svejgaard A, Platz P, Ryder LP. HLA and disease 1982—a survey. Immunol Rev 1983;70:193–218

35. Mowat AM. The regulation of immune responses to dietary antigens. Immunol Today 1987;8:93–98

36. Atkinson MA, Bowman MA, Kao KJ, Campbell L, Dush PJ, Shah SC, Simell O, Maclaren NK. Lack of immune responsiveness to bovine serum albumin in insulin- dependent diabetes. N Engl J Med 1993;329:1853–1858

37. Elli L, Dolfini E, Bardella MT. Gliadin cytotoxicity and in vitro cell cultures. Toxicol Lett 2003;146:1–8

38. Catassi C, Guerrieri A, Bartolotta E, Coppa GV, Giorgi PL. Antigliadin antibodies at onset of diabetes in children. Lancet 1987;2:158

39. Lampasona V, Bonfanti R, Bazzigaluppi E, Venerando A, Chiumello G, Bosi E, Bonifacio E. Antibodies to tissue transglutaminase C in type I diabetes. Diabetologia 1999;42:1195–1198

40. Troncone R, Franzese A, Mazzarella G, Paparo F, Auricchio R, Coto I, Mayer M, Greco L. Gluten sensitivity in a subset of children with insulin dependent diabetes mellitus. Am J Gastroenterol 2003;98:590–595

41. Nikoopour E, Schwartz JA, Singh B. Therapeutic benefits of regulating inflammation in autoimmunity. Inflamm Allergy Drug Targets 2008;7:203–210

42. Bettelli E, Oukka M, Kuchroo VK. T(H)-17 cells in the circle of immunity and autoimmunity. Nat Immunol 2007;8:345–350

43. Kristiansen OP, Mandrup-Poulsen T. Interleukin-6 and diabetes: the good, the bad, or the indifferent? Diabetes 2005;54(Suppl.2):S114–S124

44. Padmos RC, Schloot NC, Beyan H, Ruwhof C, Staal FJ, de Ridder D, Aanstoot HJ, Lam-Tse WK, de Wit H, de Herder C, Drexhage RC, Menart B, Leslie RD, Drexhage HA. Distinct monocyte gene-expression profiles in autoimmune diabetes. Diabetes 2008;57:2768–2773

45. Nikulina M, Habich C, Flohe SB, Scott FW, Kolb H. Wheat gluten causes dendritic cell maturation and chemokine secretion. J Immunol 2004;173:1925–1933

46. Onengut-Gumuscu S, Concannon P. Mapping genes for autoimmunity in humans: type 1 diabetes as a model. Immunol Rev 2002;190:182–194

47. Margaritte-Jeannin P, Babron MC, Bourgey M, Louka AS, Clot F, Percopo S, Coto I, Hugot JP, Ascher H, Sollid LM, Greco L, Clerget-Darpoux F. HLA-DQ relative risks for coeliac disease in European populations: a study of the European Genetics Cluster on Coeliac Disease. Tissue Antigens 2004;63:562–567

48. Melanitou E, Fain P, Eisenbarth GS. Genetics of type 1A (immune mediated) diabetes. J Autoimmun 2003;21:93–98

49. Tiittanen M, Westerholm-Ormio M, Verkasalo M, Savilahti E, Vaarala O. Infiltration of forkhead box P3-expressing cells in small intestinal mucosa in coeliac disease but not in type 1 diabetes. Clin Exp Immunol 2008;152:498–507

Age at Development of Type 1 Diabetes- and Celiac Disease-Associated Antibodies and Clinical Disease in Genetically Susceptible Children Observed From Birth

Satu Simell, md[1,2]
Sanna Hoppu, md, phd[1,3]
Tuu Simell, mph, phd[1,2]
Marja-Riitta Ståhlberg, md, phd[2]
Markku Viander, md, phd[4]
Taina Routi, md, phd[2]

Ville Simell, msc[1,2]
Riitta Veijola, md, phd[1,5]
Jorma Ilonen, md, phd[1,6,7]
Heikki Hyöty, md, phd[1,8]
Mikael Knip, md, phd[1,3,9]
Olli Simell, md, phd[1,2]

OBJECTIVE — To compare the ages and sequence in which antibodies associated with type 1 diabetes and celiac disease appear and overt diseases develop in children with an HLA-conferred susceptibility to both diseases.

RESEARCH DESIGN AND METHODS — We observed 2,052 children carrying genetic risks for both type 1 diabetes and celiac disease from birth until the median age of 5.7 years and analyzed diabetes- and celiac disease–associated antibodies in serum samples collected at 3- to 12-month intervals. Diabetes was confirmed by World Health Organization criteria and celiac disease by duodenal biopsies.

RESULTS — Altogether 342 children seroconverted to positivity for at least one diabetes-associated autoantibody and 88 to positivity for at least one celiac disease–associated antibody at the median ages of 3.0 and 1.5 years, respectively ($P < 0.001$). If only children with biochemically defined diabetes-associated autoantibodies against insulin, GAD, or IA-2A protein ($n = 146$) and children with tissue transglutaminase autoantibodies were compared ($n = 86$), the median seroconversion ages were 2.5 and 3.0 years ($P = 0.011$). Fifty-one children progressed to overt diabetes at 4.5 years and 44 children to celiac disease at 4.3 years ($P = 0.257$). Of the 19 children who developed both diabetes- and celiac disease–associated antibodies, 3 progressed to both diabetes and celiac disease.

CONCLUSIONS — Children with HLA-conferred susceptibility to type 1 diabetes and celiac disease develop celiac disease–associated antibodies mostly at a younger age or the same age at which they develop diabetes-associated autoantibodies. Clinical diabetes and celiac disease are commonly diagnosed at the same median age.

Diabetes Care 33:774–779, 2010

T he incidences of type 1 diabetes and celiac disease are increasing rapidly (1). These autoimmune diseases often occur together, as ~4.5% of subjects with recent-onset type 1 diabetes also have celiac disease, and the coexistence is even more common in subjects with long-standing type 1 diabetes (2,3). Shared susceptibility alleles in the HLA region probably contribute to this coexistence (4). Although appearance of diabetes- and celiac disease–specific antibodies strongly indicates commencement of autoimmunity (5), antibodies also predict progression to the respective clinical diseases. However, in the case of diabetes, in particular, the time from autoimmunity to overt disease may vary from months to years. Interestingly, clinical type 1 diabetes is usually diagnosed first and celiac disease within the following few years (6,7). The order is rarely reversed (8).

Although coexistence of type 1 diabetes and celiac disease has been studied mainly in clinical patients, Williams et al. (9) showed in a cross-sectional study that 5.4% of nondiabetic first-degree relatives of type 1 diabetic patients who were positive for diabetes-associated autoantibodies were positive also for tissue transglutaminase autoantibody (TGA). However, the findings of the Diabetes Autoimmunity Study in the Young (DAISY) indicated that the two types of antibodies rarely appeared simultaneously (10), whereas the German BabyDiab study suggested that celiac disease–associated antibodies invariably develop later than diabetes-associated autoantibodies (11,12).

Here we report the age and order in which the diabetes- and celiac disease–associated antibodies and the two clinical diseases developed in children who carried genetic type 1 diabetes and celiac disease susceptibility and participated in the type 1 Diabetes Prediction and Prevention (DIPP) study.

RESEARCH DESIGN AND METHODS — All study children were participants in the ongoing population-based DIPP study, which is a survey of the natural course of preclinical type 1 diabetes in genetically susceptible individuals born in the cities of Turku, Oulu, and Tampere in Finland (13). After parental consent, the newborns carrying HLA-DQB1 genotypes conferring susceptibility to type 1 diabetes (*02/*0302; *0302/x

From the [1]Juvenile Diabetes Research Foundation Center for Prevention of Type 1 Diabetes in Finland, Turku, Oulu, and Tampere, Finland; the [2]Department of Pediatrics, University of Turku, Turku, Finland; the [3]Pediatric Research Center, Medical School, University of Tampere, and the Department of Pediatrics, Tampere University Hospital, Tampere, Finland; the [4]Department of Medical Microbiology, University of Turku, Turku, Finland; the [5]Department of Pediatrics, University of Oulu, Oulu, Finland; the [6]Department of Clinical Microbiology, University of Kuopio, Kuopio, Finland; the [7]Immunogenetics Laboratory, University of Turku, Turku, Finland; the [8]Department of Virology, University of Tampere Medical School and Tampere University Hospital, Tampere, Finland; and the [9]Hospital for Children and Adolescents and Folkhälsan Research Institute, University of Helsinki, Helsinki, Finland.
Corresponding author: Satu Simell, satu.simell@tyks.fi.
Received 3 July 2009 and accepted 22 December 2009. Published ahead of print at http://care. diabetesjournals.org on 7 January 2010. DOI: 10.2337/dc09-1217.

[x ≠ *02, *0301, *0602, or *0603] and male infants in Turku with HLA-DQB1*02/x) (13) were observed from birth for the appearance of diabetes-associated antibodies. The at-risk children in Turku were examined at 3-month intervals until 2 years of age and then at 6-month intervals. In Oulu and Tampere, the children were examined at 3, 6, 12, 18, and 24 months and then at 12-month intervals. At every examination, a blood sample was drawn, processed, and stored as described (13).

For this study, we chose an 11-year cohort of DIPP study children carrying HLA alleles DQB1*02/DQB1*0302 or DQA1*05-DQB1*02 and born between November 1994 and December 2005. The HLA alleles were determined from cord blood spots dried on filter paper using a semiautomated technique (14). To document when diabetes autoimmunity began, islet cell autoantibody (ICA) was first measured from every blood sample drawn. If the sample was ICA-positive, autoantibodies against biochemically characterized autoantigens (insulin [IAA], GAD [GADA], and protein tyrosine phosphatase-related IA-2 protein [IA-2A]) were also analyzed in all samples drawn from that child since birth. To evaluate which proportion of children remaining ICA-negative but developing other diabetes-associated autoantibodies were missed when ICA alone was measured, we analyzed the four diabetes-associated autoantibodies in all samples drawn from a time-restricted cohort of 1,006 DIPP study children (15), in all samples drawn from children born to autoantibody-positive mothers, and in all samples drawn from children born on or after 1 January 2003. All children who developed diabetes-associated autoantibodies were permanently observed at 3-month intervals (13).

We used IgA-class TGA as the primary marker of celiac disease autoimmunity. We first measured TGA in the samples drawn during the year 2000 from all children with HLA-conferred diabetes and celiac disease susceptibility. The age of the oldest child in the year 2000 screening was 5.2 years. Later, TGA was first analyzed at the age of 1 year in the children with genetic celiac disease susceptibility. Taking into account all samples analyzed, the first assessment of TGA was made from samples collected at a median age (range) of 1.8 years (0.1–9.1). The children were retested annually until the end of March 2007, when the oldest

children were 12.3 years. When a child became TGA positive, antibodies against endomysium (EMA), reticulin (ARA), and gliadin (AGA-IgA and AGA-IgG) were also analyzed in all of the child's previous and forthcoming samples (5). TGA was also measured in the last available samples from the six children who withdrew from the follow-up before the year 2000. The age at seroconversion to antibody positivity was defined as the age when the first positive blood sample was drawn, irrespective of the slight variation in the intervals between the last autoantibody-negative and the first autoantibody-positive sample.

The diagnosis of type 1 diabetes was based on the World Health Organization criteria (16). Duodenal biopsies were recommended for all TGA-positive children. If biopsies showed villous atrophy, celiac disease was diagnosed and a gluten-free diet was recommended.

The ethics committees of the participating university hospitals approved the study. Written informed consent was obtained from the parents for autoantibody analysis and intestinal biopsies. The child's consent was also requested for children aged >7 years.

Type 1 diabetes–associated antibodies and celiac disease–associated antibodies

ICA was quantified using a standard indirect immunofluorescence method, and biochemical autoantibodies (IAA, GADA, and IA-2A) were quantified using radiobinding assays (17). TGA was measured with a recombinant human TGA kit (Celikey; Pharmacia Diagnostics, Freiburg, Germany) (18). EMA and ARA were determined by indirect immunofluorescence (19,20). Serum AGA-IgG and AGA-IgA were analyzed by an enzyme-linked immunosorbent assay (ELISA) (21).

Serum IgA was analyzed when a child's antibodies were measured for the first time. If the concentration was <0.05 g/l, IgG class TGA and AGA were analyzed by ELISA (21).

Positivity for diabetes-associated antibodies and celiac disease–associated antibodies

We measured ICA in all samples, and if the result was positive, we also analyzed IAA, GADA, and IA-2A in all previous and forthcoming samples for that child. We defined the age at seroconversion to positivity for diabetes-associated autoantibodies as the age when any of the

autoantibodies was positive for the first time and positivity for a biochemically defined diabetes-associated autoantibody as the age when the first of at least two consecutive samples positive for IAA, GADA, or IA-2A was drawn.

Because TGA was used for the primary screening of celiac disease autoimmunity, all children with celiac disease–associated autoantibodies were positive in at least one sample for TGA. The age at seroconversion to positivity for celiac disease–associated antibodies (TGA, AGA-IgA, AGA-IgG, EMA, or ARA) was defined as the age when the first one of these antibodies was positive, alone or in any combination. For IgA-deficient children, AGA-IgG and TGA-IgG were measured to determine the age at seroconversion.

Statistical analysis

We used Wilcoxon's test to compare differences between the median seroconversion ages and Cox's regression analysis to compare the development of diabetes-associated and celiac disease–associated antibodies. Tests were considered significant if two-sided $P < 0.05$. The statistical analyses were performed using SAS (version 9.2; SAS Institute, Cary, NC).

RESULTS

Children positive for diabetes-associated or celiac disease–associated antibodies

We first analyzed HLA-conferred type 1 diabetes susceptibility in 100,846 consecutive newborns (Fig. 1) and formed the cohort of this study by selecting from the diabetes-susceptible infants those 2,052 who also were at high genetic risk for celiac disease. The median age of the cohort children at the end of this study was 5.7 years (range 1.0–12.3 years). Boys made up 65% ($n = 1,332$) of the cohort because of the inclusion criteria of the DIPP study (13).

At least one sample in 342 children was positive for ICA (Fig. 1), whereas 146 children tested positive for at least one biochemical diabetes-associated autoantibody in at least two consecutive samples. These children included 19 who were continuously ICA-negative. Altogether 215 children were positive only for ICA, and 17 were positive in only one sample. At least one sample in 86 children was positive for TGA, and 2 children with IgA deficiency were positive for AGA-IgG. Consequently, 88 children were regarded

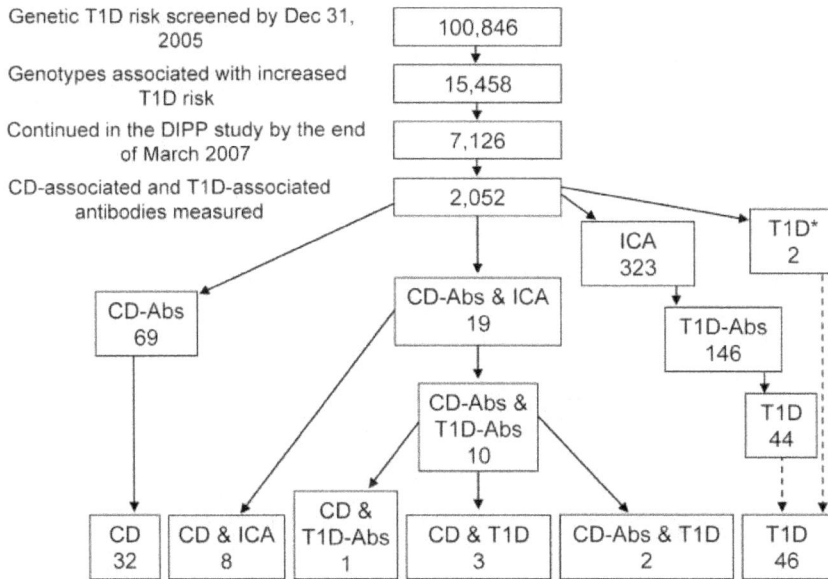

Figure 1—*Flow chart of the children in the DIPP study. CD-Abs, at least one sample positive for TGA (IgA or IgG) and/or AGA-IgA, AGA-IgG, EMA, or ARA; ICA, at least one sample positive for ICA, or ICA and IAA, GADA, and/or IA-2A; T1D-Abs, two consecutive samples positive for IAA, GADA, and/or IA-2A. *Two children were negative for type 1 diabetes (T1D)-associated autoantibodies in the last follow-up sample drawn, but were positive in a sample drawn at the time of type 1 diabetes diagnosis.*

as positive for celiac disease–associated antibodies.

Seroconversion to positivity for the first-appearing celiac disease–associated antibody occurred at the median age of 1.5 years (range 0.5–7.5), i.e., at a markedly younger age than the seroconversion to positivity for the first diabetes-associated autoantibody (3.0 years, range 0.4–11.1; $P < 0.001$) (Fig. 2). If only persisting biochemical diabetes-associated autoantibodies were accepted for analysis, the children seroconverted at a median age of 2.5 years (0.5–10.1), also clearly later than the children seroconverted to celiac disease–associated antibody positivity ($P = 0.007$). Restricting celiac disease–associated antibodies to TGA, the children seroconverted at a median age of 3.0 years (1.0–9.0), i.e., at the same age as the children seroconverted to positivity for diabetes-associated autoantibodies but later than they seroconverted to positivity for the first biochemically defined diabetes-associated autoantibody ($P = 0.011$) (Table 1). If we omit AGA-IgG and AGA-IgA from the analysis, the median age at seroconversion to positivity for TGA, EMA, or ARA was 2.5 years.

Of the 86 TGA-positive children, 66 children seroconverted first to AGA-IgG positivity. In 40 of them, the first sample positive for a celiac disease–associated autoantibody was for AGA-IgG alone. The

time from seroconversion to AGA-IgG positivity to positivity for another celiac disease–associated antibody (TGA, EMA, ARA, or AGA-IgA) was 0.8 years (range 0.2–6.1).

Interestingly, among the 86 children who seroconverted to TGA positivity, 39 (45%) reverted spontaneously to negativity, or the values fluctuated at least twice from negativity to positivity without dietary intervention. Although 23 children were TGA-positive in only one sample, all except one showed positivity in the same sample for AGA-IgG, AGA-IgA, EMA, and/or ARA. Antibody transience and fluctuation were common also among AGA-IgA (24 of 50 [48%]), AGA-IgG (22 of 78 [28%]), EMA (29 of 85 [34%]), and ARA (26 of 74 [35%]).

During the follow-up, 51 of the 342 children positive for diabetes-associated autoantibodies progressed to overt diabetes, and 43 of the 88 children positive for celiac disease–associated antibodies progressed to biopsy-proven celiac disease. One additional child developed skin biopsy–confirmed dermatitis herpetiformis at age 4.3 years. Although celiac disease–associated antibodies developed, on average, at a slightly younger age than the diabetes-associated autoantibodies, overt diabetes and celiac disease were diagnosed at the ages of 4.5 years (range 1.4–11.6) and 4.3 years (1.6–9.8),

respectively ($P = 0.257$). Twenty-five children lost TGA spontaneously before endoscopy, the parents of three children refused the procedure, and four children were on the endoscopy waiting list at the end of the follow-up.

Children with both diabetes-associated antibodies and celiac disease–associated antibodies

Nineteen (5.6%) children developed both diabetes-associated and celiac disease–associated antibodies. Eight children seroconverted first to positivity for diabetes-associated autoantibodies, eight first to positivity for celiac disease–associated antibodies, and three to positivity for both types of antibodies. The median ages of the 19 children who seroconverted to positivity for the first diabetes-associated autoantibody and the first celiac disease–associated antibody were 1.6 years (range 0.5–6.5) and 1.5 years (0.8–7.2), respectively. Accordingly, the children who seroconverted to positivity for both diabetes- and celiac disease–associated antibodies seroconverted at a younger age than those who were positive only for diabetes-associated antibodies (1.6 vs. 3.0 years; $P = 0.026$).

Of the 19 children with both diabetes-associated and celiac disease–associated antibodies, 10 were positive for the biochemical autoantibodies. Four of them developed first IAA, GADA, or IA-2A; four developed celiac disease–associated antibodies; and two developed both types of antibodies at the same age. The children seroconverted to positivity for biochemical autoantibodies and celiac disease–associated antibodies at the median ages of 1.4 years (range 0.5–8.9) and 1.4 years (0.8–2.6), respectively. The 3 children who progressed to clinical type 1 diabetes and celiac disease during the follow-up developed autoantibodies and overt diseases in random order (supplemental Fig. 3, available in an online appendix at http://care.diabetesjournals.org/cgi/content/full/dc09-1217/DC1).

CONCLUSIONS — Our findings suggest that celiac disease–associated antibodies often develop earlier than or at the same age as diabetes-associated autoantibodies in children with an HLA-conferred risk for both diseases, assuming that the children are followed up from birth at frequent intervals. The children who developed both diabetes- and celiac disease–associated antibodies generated

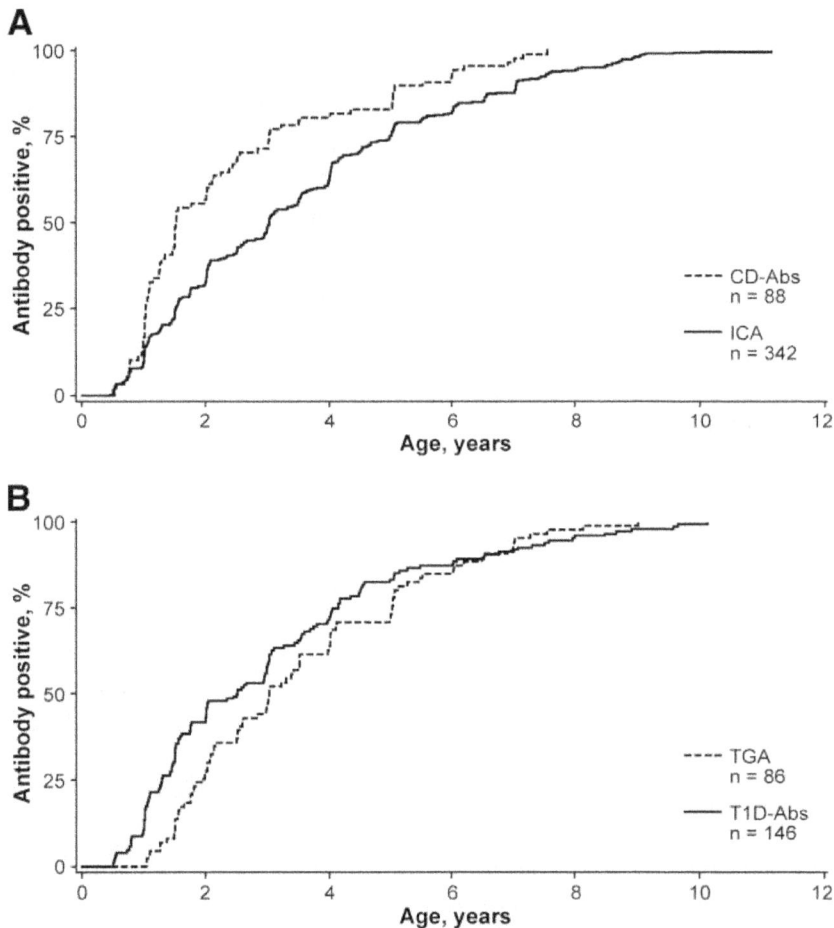

Figure 2—*Cumulative seroconversion to positivity for type 1 diabetes (T1D)- and celiac disease (CD)-associated antibodies in the DIPP study children with HLA-conferred genetic type 1 diabetes and celiac disease susceptibility. A: Cumulative seroconversion to positivity for diabetes-associated and celiac disease–associated antibodies (P < 0.001). B: Cumulative seroconversion to positivity for one or more of the persisting biochemical diabetes-associated autoantibodies and to positivity for TGA (P = 0.011). TGA, at least one sample positive for TGA. For other abbreviations, see Fig. 1.*

ples in the DIPP study were still collected at 3- to 6-month intervals.

When we measured all diabetes- and celiac disease–associated antibodies to determine the median ages of commencement of the two autoimmune diseases in the DIPP study cohort, biochemical diabetes-associated autoantibodies developed slightly later than celiac disease–associated antibodies (2.5 vs. 1.5 years). In the BabyDiab study, celiac disease autoimmunity was defined as being positive for TGA in at least one sample, but the positivity had to be confirmed using both an ELISA and a radiobinding assay. In the DIPP study, we also defined celiac disease autoimmunity as being positive for TGA with an ELISA in at least one sample; this was obviously appropriate, because all children except one were simultaneously positive also for AGA-IgA, AGA-IgG, EMA, and/or ARA. In the BabyDiab study, the prevalence of celiac disease–associated antibody positivity among the children positive also for diabetes-associated autoantibodies was 3 of 107 (2.8%). All 3 of these children first developed diabetes-associated autoantibodies. In our DIPP study cohort, 10 of 146 (6.8%) of the children were positive for both types of antibodies, closely resembling British data (5.4%), but markedly exceeding the values obtained in the BabyDiab study (9,12). Differences in the study populations may have influenced these results, because in the BabyDiab study, all children had at least one parent with type 1 diabetes, whereas in the DIPP study, the children were selected from the general population based on HLA-conferred genetic risk. Unfortunately, comparison of our findings with those from DAISY, another long-term observational study, is hampered by the fact that the coexistence of diabetes-associated and celiac disease–associated antibodies has so far not been thoroughly presented.

Gluten has been proposed to be a trigger of not only celiac disease but also type 1 diabetes. If that is the case, avoidance of gluten ingestion might delay progression to type 1 diabetes (22,23). Our frequent follow-up of the children with a genetic susceptibility to celiac disease and diabetes indicates that celiac disease–associated autoimmunity often develops at a slightly younger age than diabetes-associated autoimmunity, supporting the hypothesis that a gluten-free diet might indeed prevent or delay diabetes autoimmunity. Interestingly, diabetes-associated autoantibodies developed at a younger

the two types of antibodies usually in a random order within a short time interval. Interestingly, the children with celiac disease–associated antibodies seroconverted to positivity for diabetes-associated autoantibodies earlier than those who did not have celiac disease–associated antibodies. However, overt diabetes and celiac disease were ultimately diagnosed at approximately the same age.

Our results differ clearly from those reported in the BabyDiab study, in which diabetes-associated autoantibodies developed earlier than celiac disease–associated antibodies (12). However, if the analysis was based only on IAA, GADA, or IA-2A and only on TGA, seroconversion to TGA positivity occurred in our DIPP study cohort at 3.0 years and seroconversion to positivity for the bio-

chemical diabetes-associated autoantibodies at 2.5 years. Meanwhile, in the BabyDiab study, the respective seroconversions were seen at 4.9 and 2.3 years. These differences between the two studies are probably explained mainly by the more frequent follow-up in the DIPP study, which permitted more accurate determination of the seroconversion time. Indeed, in the BabyDiab study the samples are collected from antibody-negative children at the ages of 9 months and 2, 5, 8, 11, and 14 years. None of our DIPP study children seroconverted to TGA positivity before age 1 year, although gluten-containing foods were almost without exception introduced between 4 and 6 months of age. However, 23 of the 86 TGA-positive children seroconverted to TGA positivity between 1 and 2 years of age, i.e., during the period when the sam-

Table 1—Median age at seroconversion to positivity for type 1 diabetes–associated and celiac disease–associated antibodies

First seroconversion to positivity for any antibody of the group	n	Age (years)
Celiac disease–associated antibodies: TGA, AGA-IgA, AGA-IgG, EMA, or ARA	88	1.5 (0.5–7.5)
Celiac disease–associated antibodies without AGA: TGA, EMA, or ARA	86	2.5 (1.0–9.0)
Diabetes-associated autoantibodies: ICA, IAA, GADA, or IA-2A	342	3.0 (0.4–11.1)
Biochemical diabetes-associated autoantibodies: IAA, GADA, or IA-2A	146	2.5 (0.5–10.0)
First seroconversion to positivity for each antibody alone		
TGA	86	3.0 (1.0–9.0)
AGA-IgA	50	3.0 (0.6–10.0)
AGA-IgG	78	1.5 (0.5–11.5)
ARA	74	3.0 (1.0–10.5)
EMA	85	3.0 (1.0–9.0)
ICA	342	3.2 (0.4–11.1)
IAA	110	2.0 (0.5–10.3)
GADA	107	3.0 (0.7–10.1)
IA-2A	90	3.0 (0.5–9.8)

Data are n or median (range).

age in children who were positive for both diabetes- and celiac disease–associated antibodies than in children who were positive for diabetes-associated autoantibodies only.

We included in this study all children who developed diabetes-associated and celiac disease–associated antibodies during the follow-up using overt clinical type 1 diabetes as the end point of the study (24). Thus, we have data only until the diagnosis of diabetes from the children who progressed to diabetes, and some children may have developed celiac disease after the diagnosis of diabetes. However, the purpose of this study was to evaluate the early phases of diabetes and celiac disease autoimmunity, not to challenge previous studies analyzing the risk of celiac disease once type 1 diabetes has developed (2,3,6–8).

Our study has some obvious limitations. One is caused by the use of ICA as the primary autoantibody for diabetes autoimmunity screening in children born in 1994–2002, although we also analyzed the three biochemical autoantibodies in all samples drawn from the ICA-positive children. In children born between the beginning of 2003 and the end of the study, all four diabetes-associated autoantibodies were directly analyzed in all samples collected. Our recent study showed that >82% of the samples that

were positive for the first autoantibody were positive for ICA, whereas ICA or IAA accounted for 93% of the positive samples. The sensitivity of our current program when tested using ICA as the marker of commencement of diabetes-associated autoimmunity is 86% (24), and <10% of children with autoantibodies are missed if ICA only is analyzed. We have also shown that 95% of all IAA, GADA, and IA-2A seroconversions occur in young children in a narrow time window (−12 to 8 months) around the time of ICA seroconversion (17). Of the 2,052 children in this cohort, 19 were positive for biochemical diabetes-associated autoantibodies while being continuously ICA negative. Consequently, we probably missed a few children who were ICA-negative but had other diabetes-associated autoantibodies. Defining diabetes autoimmunity as positivity for the biochemical autoantibodies does not eliminate the problems associated with the use of ICA, but it excludes from the study population the children who are positive for ICA only. In any case, defining onset of diabetes-associated autoimmunity by seroconversion to persisting positivity for at least one of the biochemical autoantibodies allows better comparison of our data with those obtained in the BabyDiab study.

Another limitation in our DIPP cohort study is that we used AGA-IgG as one of

the celiac disease–associated antibodies. AGA is highly unspecific, and ~25% of the TGA-negative children with genetic celiac disease susceptibility were AGA-IgG–positive in the DIPP study (data not shown). However, we think that analyzing AGA-IgG together with other celiac disease–associated antibodies is justified, because seroconversion to AGA-IgG positivity may identify the time when the celiac disease process really begins in children who also develop other celiac disease–associated antibodies. AGA-IgG may also be important when celiac disease triggers other than gluten are searched for. We previously also measured antibodies to the deamidated gliadin peptide in part of the currently studied children (25); the findings showed high concordance with the AGA and TGA results.

The follow-up schedules of the children at the three study centers in Finland differed slightly, as the children were seen more frequently in Turku than in Oulu and Tampere (17). Analysis of the data at the three sites slightly postponed the seroconversion ages in Oulu and Tampere for celiac disease–associated antibodies but not for diabetes-associated autoantibodies for unknown reasons (data not shown). However, these changes in the seroconversion ages are minor and do not change the conclusions of our study. On the other hand, the frequent follow-up is also a major strength of our study, permitting rather accurate determination of events contributing to progression to overt clinical diabetes and celiac disease; even the less frequent follow-up schedule is three times more frequent than the follow-up in the older groups in the Baby-Diab study.

In summary, this population-based, prospective follow-up study suggests that celiac disease–associated antibodies often develop earlier than or at the same age as type 1 diabetes–associated autoantibodies in children with a genetic susceptibility to both diseases.

Acknowledgments — This study was supported by the Juvenile Diabetes Research Foundation International (grants 4-1999-731, 4-2001-435, 1-2006-896, and 36-2008-925 to O.S.); Sigrid Juselius Foundation; Academy of Finland; Päivikki and Sakari Sohlberg Foundation; Novo Nordisk Foundation; Jalmari and Rauha Ahokas Foundation; Foundation for Pediatric Research, Finland; Foundation for Diabetes Research, Finland; Signe and Ane Gyllenberg Foundation; Turku University Foundation; Celiac Disease Association, Finland; and Specified Government Transfers to the University Hospitals of Turku, Oulu, and Tampere.

No other potential conflicts of interest relevant to this article were reported.

Parts of the study were presented in abstract form at the 13th International Celiac Disease Symposium, Amsterdam, the Netherlands, 6–8 April 2009.

We are grateful to the families participating in the study, the dedicated staff of the DIPP project, and the personnel at the Departments of Pediatrics, Universities of Turku, Oulu, and Tampere, and at the Departments of Virology and Microbiology, University of Turku, for their support. We acknowledge the contribution of Anne Hekkala, MD.

References

1. Lohi S, Mustalahti K, Kaukinen K, Laurila K, Collin P, Rissanen H, Lohi O, Bravi E, Gasparin M, Reunanen A, Mäki M. Increasing prevalence of coeliac disease over time. Aliment Pharmacol Ther 2007;26: 1217–1225
2. Holmes GK. Screening for coeliac disease in type 1 diabetes. Arch Dis Child 2002; 87:495–498
3. Savilahti E, Simell O, Koskimies S, Rilva A, Åkerblom HK. Celiac disease in insulin-dependent diabetes mellitus. J Pediatr 1986;108:690–693
4. Smyth DJ, Plagnol V, Walker NM, Cooper JD, Downes K, Yang JH, Howson JM, Stevens H, McManus R, Wijmenga C, Heap GA, Dubois PC, Clayton DG, Hunt KA, van Heel DA, Todd JA. Shared and distinct genetic variants in type 1 diabetes and celiac disease. N Engl J Med 2008; 359:2767–2777
5. Simell S, Hoppu S, Hekkala A, Simell T, Ståhlberg MR, Viander M, Yrjänäinen H, Grönlund J, Markula P, Simell V, Knip M, Ilonen J, Hyöty H, Simell O. Fate of five celiac disease-associated antibodies during normal diet in genetically at-risk children observed from birth in a natural history study. Am J Gastroenterol 2007; 102:2026–2035
6. Barera G, Bonfanti R, Viscardi M, Bazzigaluppi E, Calori G, Meschi F, Bianchi C, Chiumello G. Occurrence of celiac disease after onset of type 1 diabetes: a 6-year prospective longitudinal study. Pediatrics 2002;109:833–838
7. Larsson K, Carlsson A, Cederwall E, Jönsson B, Neiderud J, Jonsson B, Lernmark A, Ivarsson SA, Skåne Study Group. Annual screening detects celiac disease in children with type 1 diabetes. Pediatr Diabetes 2008;9:354–359
8. Cronin CC, Shanahan F. Insulin-dependent diabetes mellitus and coeliac disease. Lancet 1997;349:1096–1097
9. Williams AJ, Norcross AJ, Lock RJ, Unsworth DJ, Gale EA, Bingley PJ. The high prevalence of autoantibodies to tissue transglutaminase in first-degree relatives of patients with type 1 diabetes is not associated with islet autoimmunity. Diabetes Care 2001;24:504–509
10. Norris JM, Barriga K, Hoffenberg EJ, Taki I, Miao D, Haas JE, Emery LM, Sokol RJ, Erlich HA, Eisenbarth GS, Rewers M. Risk of celiac disease autoimmunity and timing of gluten introduction in the diet of infants at increased risk of disease. JAMA 2005;293:2343–2351
11. Hummel M, Bonifacio E, Stern M, Dittler J, Schimmel A, Ziegler AG. Development of celiac disease-associated antibodies in offspring of parents with type I diabetes. Diabetologia 2000;43:1005–1011
12. Hummel S, Hummel M, Banholzer J, Hanak D, Mollenhauer U, Bonifacio E, Ziegler AG. Development of autoimmunity to transglutaminase C in children of patients with type 1 diabetes: relationship to islet autoantibodies and infant feeding. Diabetologia 2007;50:390–394
13. Kupila A, Muona P, Simell T, Arvilommi P, Savolainen H, Hämäläinen AM, Korhonen S, Kimpimäki T, Sjöroos M, Ilonen J, Knip M, Simell O, Juvenile Diabetes Research Foundation Centre for the Prevention of Type I Diabetes in Finland. Feasibility of genetic and immunological prediction of type I diabetes in a population-based birth cohort. Diabetologia 2001;44:290–297
14. Nejentsev S, Sjöroos M, Soukka T, Knip M, Simell O, Lövgren T, Ilonen J. Population-based genetic screening for the estimation of type 1 diabetes mellitus risk in Finland: selective genotyping of markers in the HLA-DQB1, HLA-DQA1 and HLA-DRB1 loci. Diabet Med 1999;16:985–992
15. Kukko M, Kimpimäki T, Korhonen S, Kupila A, Simell S, Veijola R, Simell T, Ilonen J, Simell O, Knip M. Dynamics of diabetes-associated autoantibodies in young children with human leukocyte antigen-conferred risk of type 1 diabetes recruited from the general population. J Clin Endocrinol Metab 2005;90:2712–2717
16. World Health Organization/Department of Noncommunicable Disease Surveillance. *Part 1: Definition, Diagnosis and Classification of Diabetes Mellitus and Its Complications.* Geneva, Switzerland, World Health Org., 1999
17. Kupila A, Keskinen P, Simell T, Erkkilä S, Arvilommi P, Korhonen S, Kimpimäki T, Sjöroos M, Ronkainen M, Ilonen J, Knip M, Simell O. Genetic risk determines the emergence of diabetes-associated autoantibodies in young children. Diabetes 2002;51:646–651
18. Simell S, Kupila A, Hoppu S, Hekkala A, Simell T, Ståhlberg MR, Viander M, Hurme T, Knip M, Ilonen J, Hyöty H, Simell O. Natural history of transglutaminase autoantibodies and mucosal changes in children carrying HLA-conferred celiac disease susceptibility. Scand J Gastroenterol 2005;40:1182–1191
19. Ladinser B, Rossipal E, Pittschieler K. Endomysium antibodies in coeliac disease: an improved method. Gut 1994;35:776–778
20. Mäki M, Hällström O, Vesikari T, Visakorpi JK. Evaluation of a serum IgA-class reticulin antibody test for the detection of childhood celiac disease. J Pediatr 1984; 105:901–905
21. Savilahti E, Viander M, Perkkiö M, Vainio E, Kalimo K, Reunala T. IgA antigliadin antibodies: a marker of mucosal damage in childhood coeliac disease. Lancet 1983;1:320–322
22. Norris JM, Barriga K, Klingensmith G, Hoffman M, Eisenbarth GS, Erlich HA, Rewers M. Timing of initial cereal exposure in infancy and risk of islet autoimmunity. JAMA 2003;290:1713–1720
23. Ziegler AG, Schmid S, Huber D, Hummel M, Bonifacio E. Early infant feeding and risk of developing type 1 diabetes-associated autoantibodies. JAMA 2003;290: 1721–1728
24. Siljander HT, Simell S, Hekkala A, Lähde J, Simell T, Vähäsalo P, Veijola R, Ilonen J, Simell O, Knip M. Predictive characteristics of diabetes-associated autoantibodies among children with HLA-conferred disease susceptibility in the general population. Diabetes 2009;58:2835–2842
25. Ankelo M, Kleimola V, Simell S, Simell O, Knip M, Jokisalo E, Tarkia M, Westerlund A, He Q, Viander M, Ilonen J, Hinkkanen AE. Antibody responses to deamidated gliadin peptide show high specificity and parallel antibodies to tissue transglutaminase in developing coeliac disease. Clin Exp Immunol 2007;150:285–293

Inflammatory Tendencies and Overproduction of IL-17 in the Colon of Young NOD Mice Are Counteracted With Diet Change

Catharina Alam,[1] Suvi Valkonen,[1] Vindhya Palagani,[1] Jari Jalava,[2] Erkki Eerola,[1] and Arno Hänninen[1]

OBJECTIVE—Dietary factors influence diabetes development in the NOD mouse. Diet affects the composition of microbiota in the distal intestine, which may subsequently influence intestinal immune homeostasis. However, the specific effects of antidiabetogenic diets on gut immunity and the explicit associations between intestinal immune disruption and type 1 diabetes onset remain unclear.

RESEARCH DESIGN AND METHODS—Gut microbiota of NOD mice fed a conventional diet or ProSobee formula were compared using gas chromatography. Colonic lamina propria immune cells were characterized in terms of activation markers, cytokine mRNA and Th17 and Foxp3[+] T-cell numbers, using real-time PCR and flow cytometry. Activation of diabetogenic CD4 T-cells by purified B-cells was assessed in both groups. Immune tolerance to autologous commensal bacteria was evaluated in vitro using thymidine-incorporation tests.

RESULTS—Young NOD mice showed a disturbed tolerance to autologous commensal bacteria. Increased numbers of activated CD4 T-cells and (CD11b[+]CD11c[+]) dendritic cells and elevated levels of Th17 cells and IL23 mRNA were moreover observed in colon lamina propria. These phenomena were abolished when mice were fed an antidiabetogenic diet. The antidiabetogenic diet also altered the expression levels of costimulatory molecules and the capacity of peritoneal B-cells to induce insulin-specific CD4 T-cell proliferation.

CONCLUSIONS—Young NOD mice show signs of subclinical colitis, but the symptoms are alleviated by a diet change to an antidiabetogenic diet. Disrupted immune tolerance in the distal intestine may influence peritoneal cell pools and B-cell–mediated activation of diabetogenic T-cells. *Diabetes* **59:2237–2246, 2010**

Dietary and microbial factors may be partly responsible for the increase in type 1 diabetes incidence. The intestinal mucosa is constantly exposed to these factors, and it is therefore important to thoroughly understand how these factors affect the intestinal immune system.

Evidence suggesting that gut immune disruptions may trigger type 1 diabetes originated from studies that showed correlations between a high prevalence of cow-milk antibodies, brief breastfeeding in infancy, and an increased risk of type 1 diabetes (1,2). This hypothesis gained further support from the discovery that lymphocytes accumulating in the islets share homing characteristics with gut-associated lymphocytes (3–5). Research in both humans and animals has thereafter lead to an understanding that type 1 diabetes is associated with increased permeability and enteropathy in the small intestine (6–9). The impaired barrier functions of the small intestine may subsequently cause alterations in antigen responses and thus disrupt the immunological homeostasis of the intestine. This in turn could cause intestinal inflammation and induce immune responses that lead to autoimmunity (7,10,11).

Considerably less attention has been paid to the potential role of the large intestinal immune system in type 1 diabetes development. The large intestine differs immunologically in several aspects from the small intestine: The disruptions in small intestinal immunity is linked foremost to ingested antigens or allergens such as insulin from cow milk, cereal-based allergens, and other food derivatives. The most immediate sources of immune disruption in the large intestine, however, are the vast quantities of bacteria residing therein. Moreover, large intestinal lamina propria lymphocytes differ markedly in terms of population dynamics and cytokine expression from the lamina propria lymphocytes of the small intestine (12).

There is some evidence that directly associates immune responses in the large intestine with the pancreas; lymph from the transverse colon has been reported to drain specifically to the pancreatic lymph nodes (13). This could allow innate immune stimuli to interfere with induction of peripheral immune tolerance to antigens. Accordingly, studies in BDC2.5/NOD mice have indicated that dextran sodium sulfate, which disrupts the barrier functions of the colonic epithelium, enhances the activation of islet reactive T-cells in pancreatic lymph nodes of NOD mice (14). It is therefore of interest to further investigate the role of the colonic immune system in type 1 diabetes.

Dendritic cells as well as macrophages play a major part in large intestinal mucosal immune counterbalance. Macrophages and CD11b[−] dendritic cells have been reported to secrete anti-inflammatory cytokines, such as IL-10, while CD11b[+] dendritic cells elicit the production of proinflammatory IL-17 (15,16). Macrophages, which are capable of suppressing dendritic cell-induced IL-17 secretion (17), are reduced in numbers in the lamina propria of mice suffering from colitis, concomitant with a substantial increase of lamina propria CD11b[+] dendritic cells (15). Intestinal macrophages in humans have moreover been

From the [1]Department of Medical Microbiology and Immunology, University of Turku, Turku, Finland; and the [2]Antimicrobial Research Laboratory, National Institute for Health and Welfare (THL), Turku, Finland.

Corresponding author: Arno Hänninen, arno.hanninen@utu.fi.

Received 29 January 2010 and accepted 25 May 2010. Published ahead of print at http://diabetes.diabetesjournals.org on 14 June 2010. DOI: 10.2337/db10-0147.

described as inflammatorily anergic, producing only low levels of proinflammatory cytokines (18).

The cytokine IL-23 has importance in several inflammatory disorders (19). IL-23 is capable of promoting both Th17 and Th1 responses in the intestinal lamina propria, because its absence decreases both Th1- and Th17-type cytokines in the intestine (20). The exact effects of IFN-γ and IL-17 on type 1 diabetes are nevertheless unclear. Though increased production of IFN-γ has been associated with type 1 diabetes, NOD mice lacking IFN-γ or IFN-γ receptor develop type 1 diabetes to a degree equal to wild-type NOD mice (21,22). IL-17 promotes pancreatic inflammation (23) and is upregulated in diabetic mice (24,25). Furthermore, treatment with IL-25, which inhibits the Th17 cell population, and with IL-17 neutralizing antibody, prevent diabetes in NOD mice (26). Treatment with IFN-γ can likewise prevent diabetes in NOD mice, probably by decreasing the production of IL-17 in the spleen and pancreas (27). Th17 cells can moreover transform to Th1-like cells under the influence of IL-12, demonstrating a considerable degree of plasticity between the Th17 and the Th1 cell lineages (28).The results presented in this study indicate that newly weaned NOD mice suffer from a mild level of colitis, which alters the colonic immune cell standing toward a proinflammatory status. This is moreover associated with a disruption of immune tolerance toward autologous intestinal microbiota. As recently reported, NOD peritoneal B cells show a significantly higher efficiency in activating insulin-specific T-cell reactivity than spleen-derived conventional B-cells (29). Remarkably, most of the abnormalities in the colon and peritoneal B-cell antigen-presenting activity of young NOD mice can be abrogated when NOD mice are fed an antidiabetogenic diet from the time of weaning. The substantial effects of the antidiabetogenic diet on the colonic and peritoneal immune system call attention to the importance of colon immune homeostasis in the development of type 1 diabetes in NOD mice.

RESEARCH DESIGN AND METHODS

NOD mice were either on a regular diet (CRM-E, SDS, Tapvei) (hereafter referred to as "NOD" mice) or ProSobee infant formula (Mead Johnson Nutritionals) (referred to as "PNOD" mice). The ProSobee formula was given to the mothers from 2 weeks after giving birth and to the offspring immediately after weaning, and continued throughout the study period. The average weight of 4.5 week old NOD and PNOD mice was not significantly different; NOD, 21.0 g (±1.1 g), and PNOD, 19.6 g (±1.2 g). The diet modifications thus did not impede growth in mice.

Diabetes incidence was assessed through weekly blood tests, and mice were considered diabetic when blood glucose levels exceeded 14 mmol/l on two consecutive measurements. NOD and BALB/c mice originating from commercial breeders have been housed and bred for more than two decades in the central animal laboratory of Turku University. All animal experiments were approved by the National Laboratory Animal Care & Use Committee in Finland and conformed to the legal acts, regulations, and requirements set by the European Union concerning protection of animals used for research.

Cell proliferation in response to commensal bacteria. Fresh fecal pellets were collected from individual BALB/c and NOD mice, incubated in PBS (one pellet/0.1 ml) for 30 min at 37°C, then vortexed and centrifuged to remove undissolved fibrous pieces. The suspension was further incubated for 2 h at 60°C to inactivate the bacteria and sonicated to produce a suspension of dead bacterial components. The bacterial density was adjusted using absorbance measurements relying on a standard curve created on the basis of titration of colony-forming unit values for different absorbance values. Bacterial sonicate was added to cell culture plates containing mesenteric lymph node (MLN) cells (200,000 cells/well) from the same mouse from which the pellets were collected (bacterial sonicate from autologous intestine) or from a littermate (bacterial sonicate from heterologous intestine). The cells were incubated at 37°C for 72 h with the addition of [H³] thymidine (0.4 μCi/ml) during the last 6 h of incubation. Finally, cells were collected using an automatic cell

harvester (Tomtec Harvest 96), and the radioactivity was counted using a beta counter (Wallac). Each experimental condition was performed in triplicate.

Assessment of intestinal histology. For histological studies of the colon, mice were killed at the age of 4.5, 6, or 10 weeks. Colons were excised, washed with PBS, and fixed in 10% buffered formalin. After rehydration, 4–5-μm thick paraffin-embedded sections were stained with hematoxylin and eosin, and hyperplasia was assessed by measuring the thickness of the epithelial crypts using light microscopy (Olympus).

Gas chromatographic analysis of cellular fatty acid profiles of gut bacteria. The intestinal flora of NOD and PNOD mice were assessed for overall differences using gas–liquid chromatography (GLC) techniques. This method allowed computerized profiling of cellular fatty acids of bacteria in NOD and PNOD stool samples. Differing fatty acid profiles correlate to differences in bacterial species because the fatty acid composition is species-specific (30).

To assess the differences in gut flora, stool samples were collected from NOD and PNOD mice and stored at −70°C until processing. Before proceeding to GLC analysis, bacterial mass was separated from other fatty acids present in the feces as described in ref. (31) using sedimentation and centrifugation steps. The bacterial mass was further saponified and methylated, and GLC was run as described in ref. (30).

Isolation of lamina propria lymphocytes and myeloid cells. Colons were excised, washed, and cut into pieces. The pieces were incubated for 3×20 min at 37°C in Hanks' balanced salt solution supplemented with 2% fetal calf serum (FCS) (Life Technologies) and 2 mmol/l EDTA to remove the epithelial layer and intraepithelial lymphocytes.

The colon pieces were then washed with RPMI-1640 (Life Technologies) and digested with Collagenase A (Roche) (0.5 mg/ml) for 1 h at 37°C in RPMI-1640 supplemented with 10% FCS. Undigested pieces were minced and filtered through a nylon mesh. Leukocytes were purified from the resulting cell suspension using Lympholyte-M (Cedarlane) gradient centrifugation (1250 g, room temperature) and thereafter washed twice in culture medium before further use.

Flow cytometry. Anti-CD4 and anti-CD8 conjugated to either fluorescein isothiocyanate (FITC) or phycoerythrin (PE) were used to detect T-cell populations. Cell populations were further stained using PE-conjugated anti-α4 or PE-conjugated anti-CD86 (BD Pharmingen), or FITC-conjugated anti-CD44, PE-conjugated anti-CD69 or FITC-conjugated anti-CD62L (Immunotools).

Peritoneal washout cells were stained with FITC-conjugated anti-CD11b (Immunotools) and allophycocyanin conjugated anti-CD45R (Caltag Laboratories) to identify B1-cells. PE-conjugated anti-CD40 or anti-CD86 (Immunotools) was used for peritoneal B-cell activation marker detection.

Subsets of myeloid antigen-presenting cells were characterized as follows: CD11b⁺ F4/80⁺ macrophages, F4/80⁻CD11b⁺CD11c⁺ myeloid dendritic cells, and F4/80⁻CD11b⁻ CD11c⁺ lymphoid/plasmacytoid DC (all antibodies for this characterization were either FITC or PE conjugated and purchased from Immunotools). The samples were run with FACSCalibur and analyzed using cellQuest software (Becton Dickinson).

Quantitation of colon cytokine gene expression using real-time PCR. Mouse colon samples were cut into pieces and stored in RNA Later (Qiagen). Total RNA was purified with RNeasy Mini Kit (Qiagen). RNA purity and quantity was determined using a Nanodrop spectrophotometer (Nanodrop Technologies). cDNA was synthesized with DyNAmo cDNA Synthesis Kit (Finnzymes), using oligo-dT primers provided with the kit. Levels of cytokine expression in colons of individual mice were evaluated with real-time quantitative PCR using Maxima SYBR Green qPCR Master Mix (Fermentas) and RotoGene cycler (Corbett Research). Ct-values were normalized to the endogenous housekeeping gene GAPDH and are expressed as copy numbers relative to the GADPH copy numbers. Primer sequences are given in supplementary Table 1, available in an online appendix at http://diabetes.diabetesjournals.org/cgi/content/full/db10-0147/DC1.

Analysis of Th17, Th1, and Foxp3 cells in colon lamina propria. Purified colonic lamina propria lymphocytes (LPLs) were incubated in complete RPMI 1,640 (supplemented with 10% FCS, 2 mmol/l L-glutamine, 100 units/ml penicillin, and streptomycin) containing 0.1 μmol/l PMA, 1 μmol/l ionomycin, and 10 μg/ml Brefeldin A (Sigma-Aldrich) for 4 h at 37°C.

Stimulated cells were surface-stained using FITC-conjugated anti-CD4 and allophycocyanin-conjugated anti-CD25. The cells were then fixed with 2% paraformaldehyde and permeabilized with 0.5% saponin. Fc block was used to block nonspecific binding. PE-conjugated anti-IFN-γ, PE-conjugated anti-Foxp3, or PE-conjugated anti-IL-17 and appropriate isotype controls (all reagents from eBiosciences) were used for the intracellular staining.

B-cell antigen presentation capacity. The antigen presentation assay was performed using the same experimental settings as in ref. (29); NOD mice were immunized with 50 μg insulin peptide (Insulin B 9-23, Anaspec) subcutaneously on the hind flank. Ten days later, spleens were collected from these animals and the splenic CD4⁺ T-cells were purified using CD4 MicroBeads (Miltenyi Biotec). These purified T-cells were cocultured (175,000

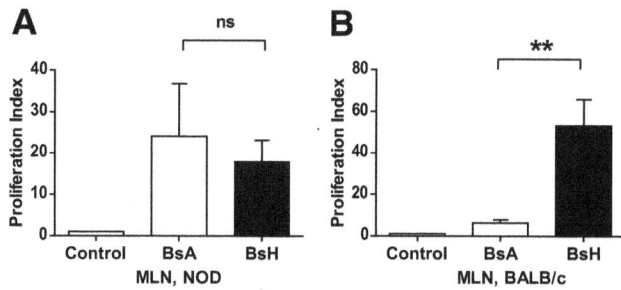

FIG. 1. Lack of tolerance to autologous bacterial flora in NOD. BsA, bacterial sonicate from autologous intestine, BsH, bacterial sonicate from heterologous intestine. *A*: MLN cells from NOD mice; *n* = 10. *B*: MLN cells from BALB/c mice; *n* = 3. **P < 0.01 as calculated using one-way ANOVA and Bonferroni post hoc test. ns, no significant difference.

cells/well) with either NOD or PNOD peritoneal- or splenic B-cells (150,000 cells/well) purified with B220 MicroBeads (Miltenyi Biotech). Purified B-cells (>93% B220$^+$) were irradiated with 3 Gy before adding to cell culture. Additionally, either insulin peptide (4 μmol/l; Insulin B 9-23; Anaspec) or intact insulin (20 μg/ml; σ-Aldrich) was added to the wells in triplicate. The cells were incubated in 37°C for 72 h with the addition of [H^3] thymidine (0.4 μCi/ml) during the last 16 h of incubation. The cells were harvested and analyzed as described above.

RESULTS

Lack of tolerance to commensal bacteria in NOD mice.
MLN cells from NOD mice proliferated vigorously in response to bacterial sonicate from a littermate (heterologous sonicate). Proliferation was, however, at an equal level regardless of whether cells were stimulated with autologous or heterologous bacterial sonicate (Fig. 1*A*). Contrarily, in BALB/c mice, high-level proliferation was observed when the commensal bacteria originated from a heterologous source (littermate), whereas autologous bacterial sonicate failed to induce any significant response (Fig. 1*B*). These results are indicative of a state of inflammation in the NOD colon, because loss of tolerance to autologous commensal bacteria is associated with inflammation and colitis (32,33).

Villous hyperplasia in the colons of NOD mice.
A histological analysis of the colon revealed hyperplasia in the epithelial crypts of NOD mice at 4.5 weeks of age. The crypts of NOD colons were thicker than the crypts of BALB/c colons at 4.5 weeks of age. However, the epithelial layer of the NOD colon was thinner at 6 and 9 weeks of age compared with 4.5 weeks. This was in contrast to the development of BALB/c colons, where a gradual age-dependent thickening was observed (Fig. 2*A*). There were no other signs of frank colitis, such as leukocyte infiltration, goblet cell loss, or crypt abscesses in the NOD colons. When NOD mice were kept on ProSobee diet, hyperplasia was not observed at 4.5 weeks of age, indicating that the occurrence of hyperplasia in newly weaned NOD mice is diet related (Fig. 2*B*).

Differences in NOD and PNOD diabetes incidence and gut flora.
Diabetes incidence was significantly lower in NOD mice that had been fed ProSobee instead of conventional food (Fig. 3*A*). The fatty acid profile of NOD and PNOD did not differ at 3 weeks of age (preweaning). However, at 5 and 10 weeks of age, GLC analysis revealed profound differences in the bacterial fatty acid profiles of NOD and PNOD gut bacteria (Fig. 3*B* and *C*).

Mice within the same age and diet group exhibited consistently similar fatty acid profiles. Moreover, no

significant differences between 5- and 10-week-old NOD mice were observed. PNOD mice, contrarily, showed differing fatty acid profiles at 5 and 10 weeks of age. A summary of *P* values based on these comparisons is provided in Table 1. This data demonstrates that diet has a substantial effect on bacterial species prevalence in NOD mice.

Inflammatory lymphocytes and dendritic cells in NOD colon lamina propria.
Compared with BALB/c mice, NOD mice had a higher proportion of CD4$^+$ T-cells expressing CD44 and CD69 in colon lamina propria. Furthermore, L-selectin was downregulated on the majority of NOD colonic CD4$^+$ T-cells. CD4$^+$ lamina propria cells from NOD mice on ProSobee, in contrast, showed the same level of CD69 and L-selectin expression as BALB/c mice, and intermediary levels of CD44 expression (Fig. 4*A–C*). The colons of NOD mice, moreover, contained an increased fraction of CD11b$^+$CD11c$^+$ (myeloid, inflammatory) dendritic cells and a decreased percentage of macrophages and CD11b$^-$CD11c$^+$ dendritic cells compared with BALB/c mice (Fig. 4*D–F*). PNOD lamina propria contained both less macrophages and CD11b$^+$CD11c$^+$ dendritic cells, but more dendritic cells with the phenotype CD11b$^-$CD11c$^+$. The increase of CD11b$^+$CD11c$^+$ dendritic cells in NOD lamina propria may be indicative of colonic inflammation because these cells have been reported to increase in mice with colitis (15).

Real-time PCR measurement of colonic cytokine expression.
To further elucidate the inflammatory nature of NOD colon immune cells, real-time quantitative PCR was used to measure the expression of different cytokines in BALB/c, NOD, and PNOD colons. Colons from NOD mice showed elevated expression levels of IL-17, IL-23, and IL-10 and decreased expression of TGF-β. IFN-γ expression was also assessed, but all mouse groups only expressed barely detectable levels of it. Foxp3 was also upregulated in NOD colonic cells at 4.5 weeks. This may be a counterbalancing phenomenon to the proinflammatory occurrences. All of the differences observed between NOD and BALB/c mouse cytokine expression leveled out with dietary manipulation (ProSobee diet); PNOD cytokine expression for all of the above listed cytokines was similar to that of BALB/c. (Fig. 5*A–F*).

Intracellular staining of colonic lamina propria CD4$^+$ lymphocytes.
Intracellular staining was performed to confirm that the differences in IL-17 mRNA expression correlated with increased IL-17 production in CD4$^+$ T-cells. The results were similar to RT-PCR; a higher percentage of IL-17 producing CD4 T-cells were present in the colon of 4.5-week-old NOD than in that of BALB/c or PNOD mice (Fig. 5*I* and *J*). The results for IFN-γ and Foxp3 intracellular staining (Fig. 5*G* and *H*, respectively) likewise coincided with the RT-PCR analysis. For IFN-γ intracellular stainings, the percentages of CD4$^+$ IFN-γ$^+$ cells were higher in NOD than in PNOD lamina propria cells. The levels, however, were low (Fig. 5*H*).

Peritoneal B-cell activation markers and antigen-presenting capacity.
NOD peritoneal B1 cells express abnormally high levels of CD40 and CD86, are more effective than splenic B-cells at presenting antigen to diabetogenic T-cells, and migrate at an enhanced rate to the pancreatic lymph nodes (29). The expression of costimulatory molecules CD40 and CD80 is significantly decreased on PNOD peritoneal B1-cells compared with NOD B1-cells (Fig. 6*A* and *B*). Peritoneal and splenic B-cells from NOD and PNOD were next tested in parallel

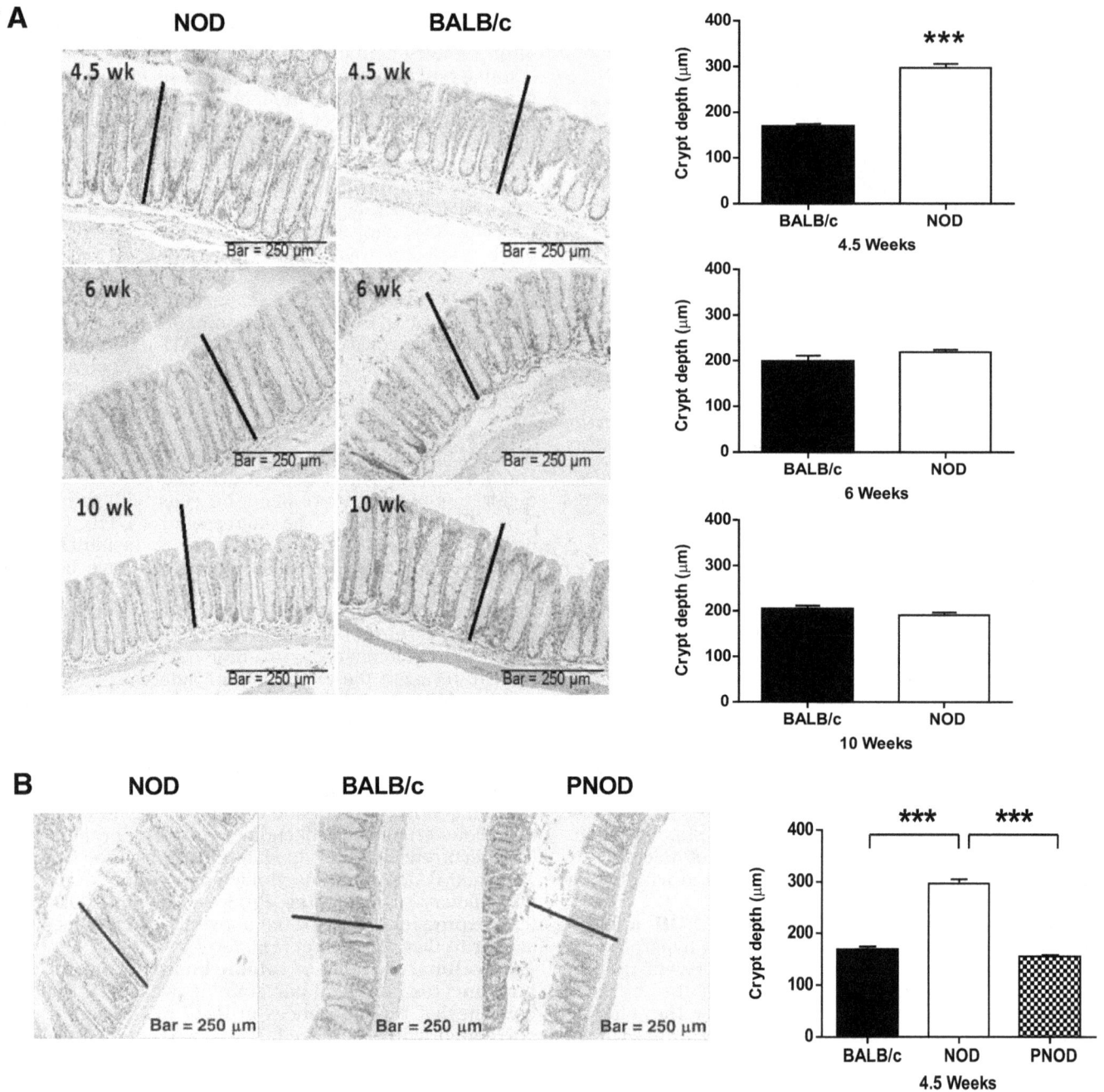

FIG. 2. Colon epithelial layer hyperplasia in young NOD mice. *A* (*Left*): Representative images of longitudinal sections of colons from NOD (*left*) and BALB/c (*right*) mice at 4.5 (*top*), 6 (*middle*), and 10 weeks (*bottom*), stained with hematoxylin and eosin. The black line represents the thickness of the NOD colon at 4.5 weeks. (*Right*): Average crypt depth ± SEM for 4.5-, 6-, and 10-week-old BALB/c and NOD mice. *n* = 4 per group. *B*: Longitudinal sections of colons from NOD, BALB/c, and PNOD mice at 4.5 weeks of age. The black lines represent the thickness of the NOD colon at this age. The bar graph to the right represents average crypt depths ± SEM for NOD, BALB/c, and PNOD at 4.5 weeks. *n* = 4 per group. ***$P < 0.001$ using Student *t* test (*A*) or one-way ANOVA and Bonferroni post hoc test (*B*).

for their antigen-presenting efficiency in presenting insulin or insulin peptide (insulin B9-23) to insulin B9-23 primed NOD CD4 T-cells (Fig. 6*C–F*). In contrast to NOD mice, peritoneal B-cells from PNOD mice were less efficient than splenic B-cells at presenting antigen (Fig. 6*D* and *F*). It is suggested that the decreased expression of CD40 and CD86 and the lessened antigen-presenting capacity in PNOD peritoneal cells is a consequence of lower activation status in the peritoneum, which in turn

is a result of the lower inflammation level in the colon of PNOD mice.

DISCUSSION

The evidence presented herein indicates that young NOD mice suffer from a mild level of colitis, which disrupts the immune homeostasis of the large intestine. Intolerance to autologous microbiota, colonic hyperplasia, increased

A

B

Correlation between groups

C

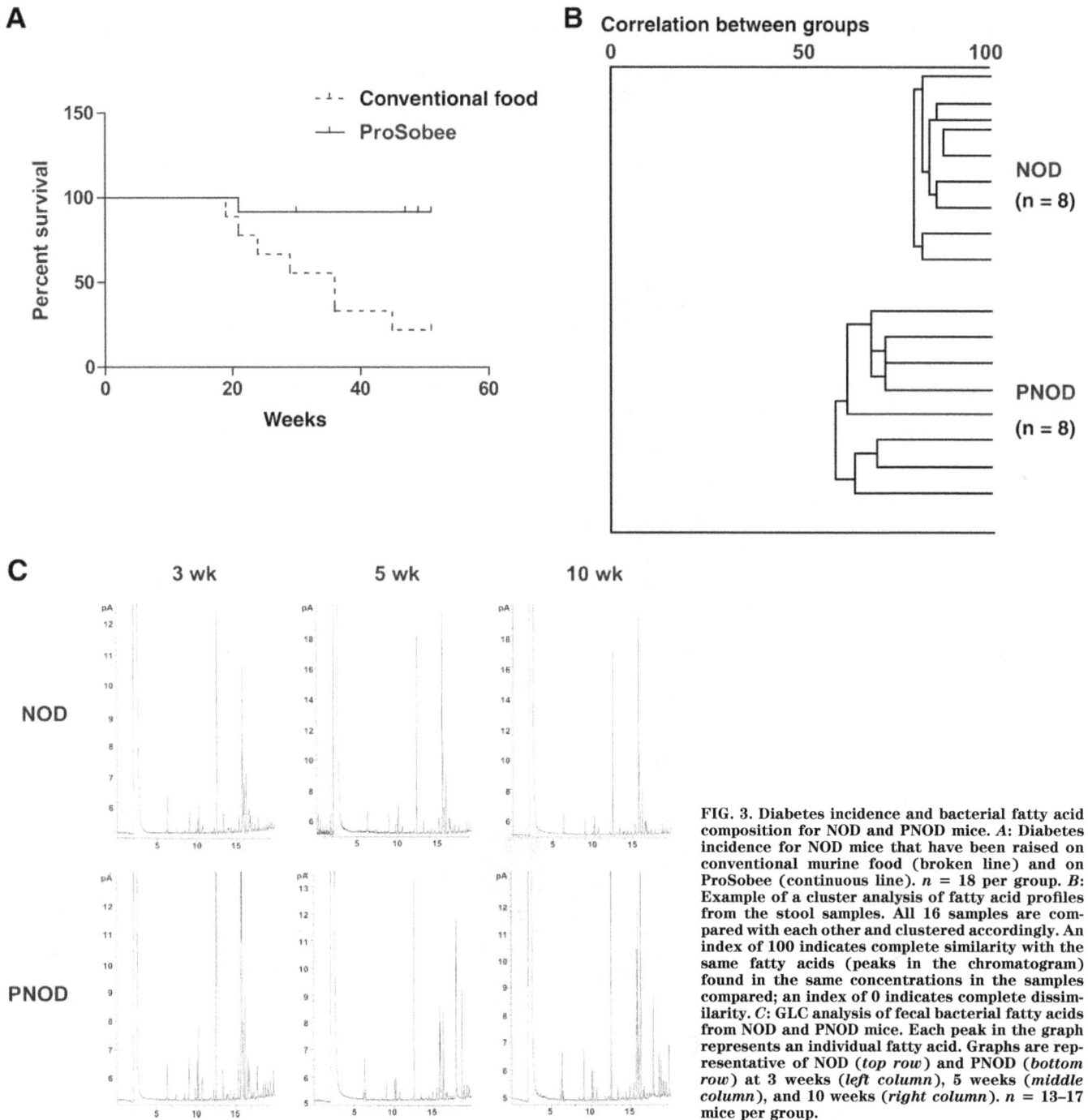

FIG. 3. Diabetes incidence and bacterial fatty acid composition for NOD and PNOD mice. *A*: Diabetes incidence for NOD mice that have been raised on conventional murine food (broken line) and on ProSobee (continuous line). *n* = 18 per group. *B*: Example of a cluster analysis of fatty acid profiles from the stool samples. All 16 samples are compared with each other and clustered accordingly. An index of 100 indicates complete similarity with the same fatty acids (peaks in the chromatogram) found in the same concentrations in the samples compared; an index of 0 indicates complete dissimilarity. *C*: GLC analysis of fecal bacterial fatty acids from NOD and PNOD mice. Each peak in the graph represents an individual fatty acid. Graphs are representative of NOD (*top row*) and PNOD (*bottom row*) at 3 weeks (*left column*), 5 weeks (*middle column*), and 10 weeks (*right column*). *n* = 13–17 mice per group.

numbers of dendritic cells, and increased levels of IL-17 and IL-23 in the NOD colon are all indicative of colonic inflammatory activity. Remarkably, this condition is alleviated if the standard mouse diet is changed to an antidiabetogenic diet (ProSobee) from the time of weaning. With respect to human type 1 diabetic patients, an increased risk of type 1 diabetes in the offspring of mothers diagnosed with ulcerative colitis has been observed (34). Moreover, mucosal inflammation in the small intestine has been associated with type 1 diabetes in humans (35,36). However, a mild and perhaps transient colonic inflammation, like that observed in NOD mice, would easily escape diagnosis in human type 1 diabetic patients.

The increased levels of IL-17 and IL-23 in the colons of 4.5-week-old NOD mice are a clear indication of an inflammatory response. Increased levels of Foxp3 and IL-10, which were also observed, may demonstrate a countereffect to the ongoing inflammation in the colon. A significant increase in IL-10 in inflamed mucosa of patients with ulcerative colitis has in fact already been reported (37). Similarly, the accumulation of naturally occurring T-regulatory cells has been detected in inflamed pancreatic lymph nodes and in the pancreas (38). Increased numbers of Foxp3 T cells have also been detected in the small intestine of children with both celiac disease and type 1 diabetes (39).

TABLE 1
Bacterial fatty acid composition comparisons between NOD and PNOD mice at 3, 5, and 10 weeks

Mice, n	NOD		PNOD		
	5 weeks	10 weeks	3 weeks	5 weeks	10 weeks
NOD					
3 weeks	68.59 ± 16.88***	74.47 ± 14.03***	85.41 ± 17.75, ns	47.73 ± 12.96***	50.21 ± 9.18***
5 weeks		80.89 ± 16.27, ns	34.69 ± 11.62***	49.97 ± 13.38***	52.90 ± 9.95***
10 weeks			39.21 ± 11.87***	56.01 ± 12.21***	56.74 ± 11.10***
PNOD					
3 weeks				53.43 ± 17.10***	69.46 ± 20.42***
5 weeks					62.01 ± 17.54**

Data are expressed as a similarity index of the fatty acid profile of the grouped samples when compared with the fatty acid profile of the grouped samples of the other group $\pm$ SD of individual samples within the group. An index of 100 indicates complete similarity with the same fatty acids (peaks in the chromatogram) found in the same concentrations in the samples compared; an index of 0 indicates complete dissimilarity. n = 13–17 mice per group. **$P < 0.01$; ***$P < 0.001$; ns, not significantly different.

Though antibiotics alleviate intestinal inflammation (40), depleting commensal bacteria by antibiotic treatment has been shown to render the colon more susceptible to chemically induced epithelial injury in mice (41). Proper immune recognition of bacteria, rather than just commensal bacteria per se, is thus considered a critical element in the immune regulation of the colon (41,42). The immune cells in healthy individuals are hyporesponsive to resident bacterial flora, but this immune tolerance is broken in patients suffering from inflammatory bowel disease (32,33). Moreover, disruption of the balance between potentially pathogenic and potentially beneficial commensal bacteria may also underlie inflammatory bowel disorders (43,44). BB diabetes-prone and diabetes-resistant rats differ in the composition of microbial species present in the gut (45). Moreover, it has been reported that *Bacteroides fragilis* has the ability to suppress IL-17 production in a model of *H. hepaticus* induced colitis (44). Recent studies indicate that intestinal Th17 cells are controlled by the specific composition of intestinal microbiota and that the segmented filamentous bacteria with the candidate name Artromitus are particularly potent inducers of Th17 cells (46). Removal of the MyD88 protein moreover protects against diabetes by modulating the composition of gut microbiota (42). It is thus becoming ever more evident that the composition of the bacterial species in the gut

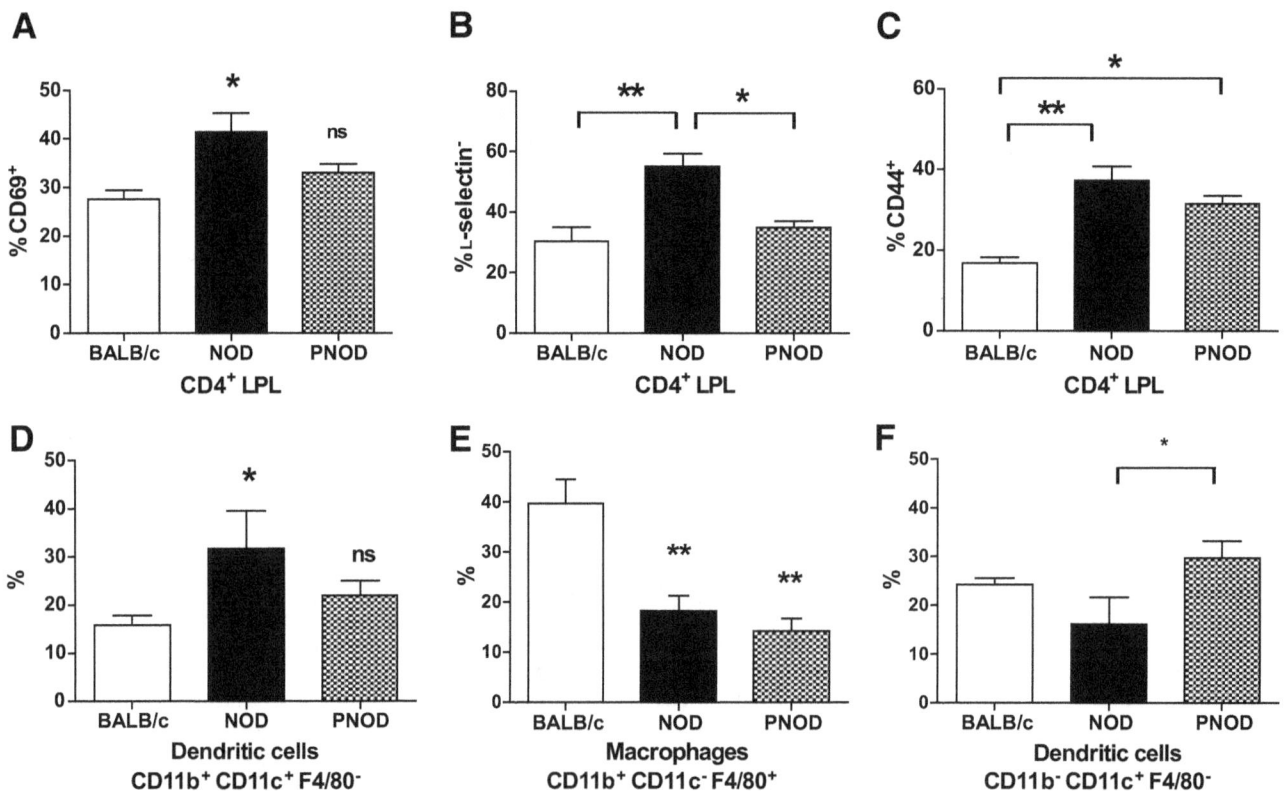

FIG. 4. Colon lamina propria CD4$^+$ T-cell activation markers and lamina propria dendritic cell/macrophage populations in BALB/c (white bars) and (black bars) NOD or PNOD (hatched bars) LPLs. *A*: Percent CD69 positive CD4 LPL. *B*: Percent L-selectin negative CD4 LPL. *C*: Percent CD44 positive CD4 LPL. *D*: Percent CD11b$^+$CD11c$^+$ dendritic cells. *E*: Percent CD11b$^+$CD11c$^-$F4/80$^+$ macrophages. *F*: Percent CD11b$^-$CD11c$^+$F4/80$^-$ dendritic cells. Bars represent means $\pm$ SEM. n = 4–8 mice per group. *$P < 0.05$ and **$P < 0.01$ as calculated using one-way ANOVA and Bonferroni post hoc test.

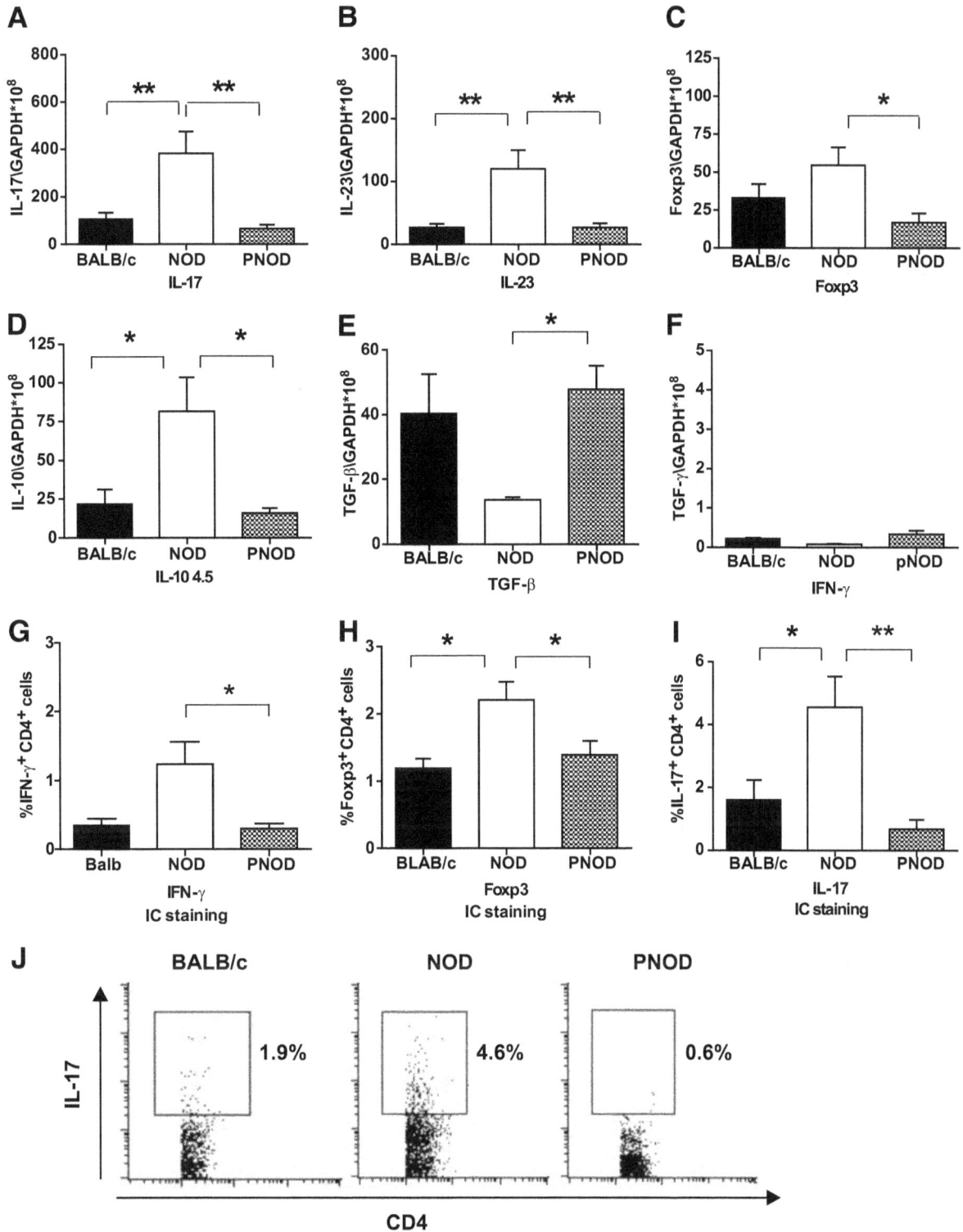

FIG. 5. Colonic cytokine and Foxp3 mRNA and IFNg, Foxp3, and IL-17 protein expression measured with real-time PCR and intracellular staining methods. Colon samples derive from 4.5-week-old BALB/c (black bars) and NOD (white bars) or PNOD (hatched bars). *A–F*: mRNA expression, normalized to GADPH copy numbers, of IL-17, IL-23, Foxp3, IL-10, TGF-β, and IFN-γ. *G–I*: Percent IFN-γ⁺, Foxp3⁺, and IL-17⁺ CD4⁺ cells in colonic lamina propria measured with intracellular (IC) staining of BALB/c, NOD, and PNOD samples. Bars represent mean values ± SEM. $n =$ 4–8 per group. *$P = 0.05$ and **$P < 0.01$ as calculated with one-way ANOVA and Bonferroni post hoc test. *J*: Representative dot plots of intracellular staining for IL-17.

profoundly affects the immune homeostasis of the intestinal immune system.

A wheat-free diet reduces the number of microbes in the intestine (47), and delayed introduction of wheat into the diet has positive long-term effects on diabetes prevention in mice (48). It is thought that the intestinal immune

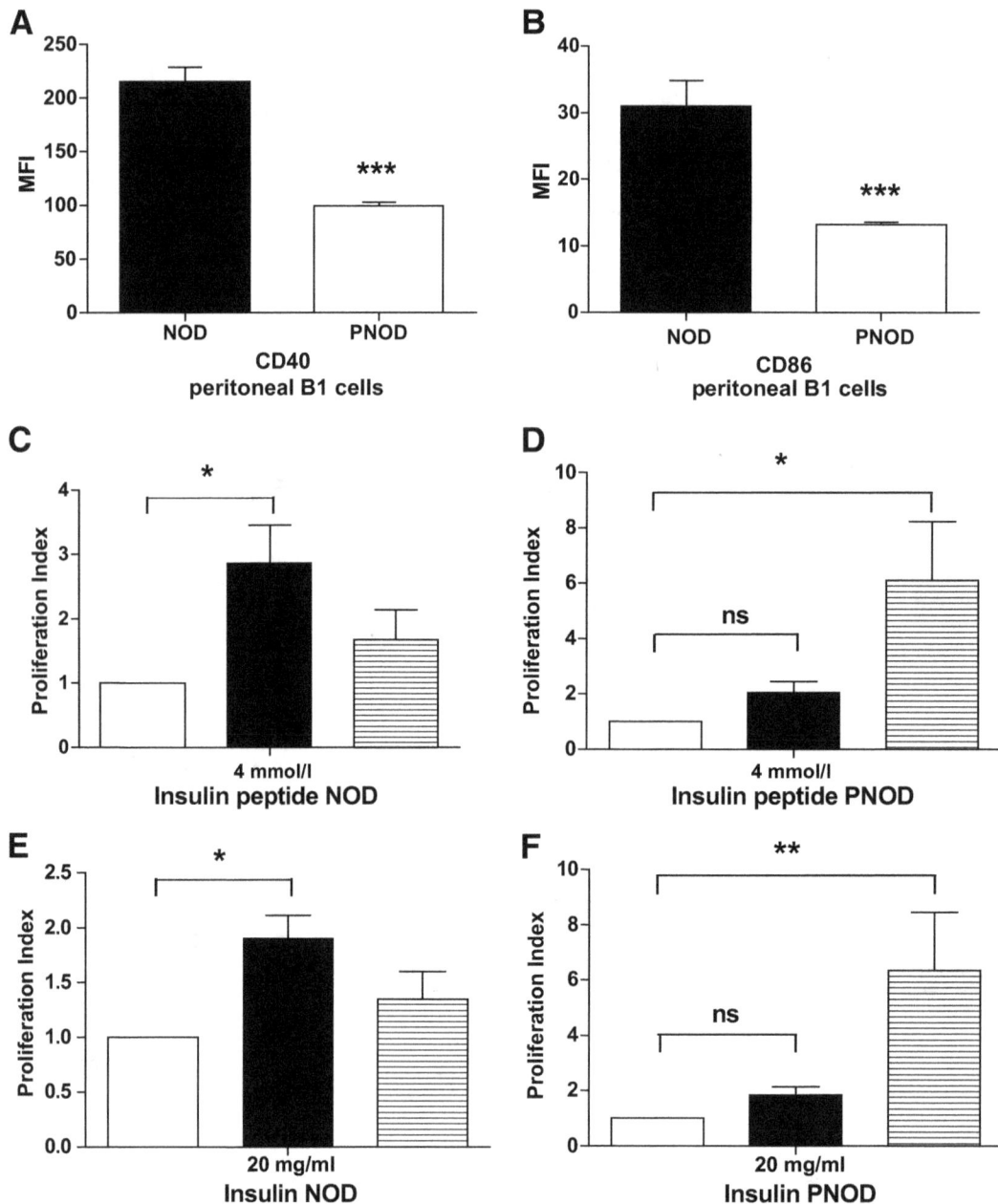

FIG. 6. Peritoneal B-cells' activation markers and antigen-presenting cell (APC) efficiency. *A*: Mean fluorescence intensity (MFI) of CD40 on peritoneal B1-cells from NOD (black bar) or PNOD (white bar). *B*: MFI of CD86 on peritoneal B1 cells from NOD (black bar) and PNOD (white bar). Data represent means ± SEM. ***$P < 0.001$, Student *t* test. $n = 3$–5 per group. *C–F*: Antigen-presenting cell capacity of peritoneal B-cells from NOD and PNOD to 4 μmol/l insulin peptide (*C, D*) and 20 μg/ml intact insulin (*E* and *F*). The graphs show B-cell induced T-cell proliferation using purified NOD (*C* and *E*) or PNOD (*D* and *F*) peritoneal B-cells (black bars) or splenic B-cells (striped bars). White bars indicate control values (relative baseline proliferation of T-cells + B-cells in the absence of insulin/insulin peptide). Baseline counts per min ranged between 50 and 300 cpm. Data present mean values ± SEM. $n = 3$–4 per group. *$P < 0.05$, **$P < 0.01$ as calculated with one-way ANOVA and Dunnet post hoc test. Peritoneal cells were pooled for each experiment from four mice to yield sufficient numbers of purified B-cells. Splenic B-cells were pooled and purified from the same donors.

system of newly weaned individuals may be particularly sensitive to immune disruption due to the yet immature immune system, higher permeability of the intestinal wall, and lower numbers of IgA positive B-cells in infancy (49). The findings presented herein indicate that a diet change from standard murine pellet food to ProSobee infant formula dramatically alters microbial species prevalence in the intestine. The ProSobee diet moreover brings about a decline in colonic proinflammatory cytokine levels and eases the hyperplasia observed in NOD colons. At 6 weeks

of age, differences between BALB/c, NOD, and PNOD had largely leveled out (results not shown), indicating that the changes seen in NOD at 4.5 weeks may be transient. This correlates with the idea that the weaning period is particularly critical for the development of gut immunity, because the mice were weaned at ~3 weeks of age.

It has been proposed that the pancreatic lymph nodes are the primary draining sites for the transverse colon (13). Furthermore, dextran sodium sulfate, which causes colitis, has been reported to promote T-cell activation in the pancreatic lymph nodes (14). Thus, it is possible that a direct connection exists between NOD colonic immune interruptions and the onset of autoimmune events in the pancreatic lymph nodes, which ultimately lead to type 1 diabetes. However, it is also possible that events occurring in the colonic lamina propria may cause a response in the peritoneal immune cell pool. Indomethacine, which disrupts the epithelial barrier mainly in the small intestine, causes rapid changes in the composition of cells in the peritoneum (50). The peritoneal cavity B-cells in turn preferentially migrate to the pancreatic lymph nodes (29) and, hence, may provide the link between gut immune system disruption and type 1 diabetes onset. The elevated expression of activation markers CD40 and CD86 and the enhanced efficiency of NOD peritoneal B-cells to present antigen to diabetogenic T-cells decline when NOD mice are fed ProSobee instead of the conventional diet. The events in the peritoneum of NOD mice thus may be interlinked with intestinal immune regulation.

The evidence brought forward in this study emphasizes the importance of the colonic immune system and the role of microbial prevalence in the development of type 1 diabetes in the NOD model. It is suggested herein that the antidiabetogenic effects of the ProSobee diet derive, at least in part, from its capacity to restore colonic immune homeostasis in NOD, where a proinflammatory bias otherwise prevails. The anti-inflammatory effects of the ProSobee diet also have implications outside of the gastrointestinal immune system, because it changes the properties of the peritoneal B-cells. It can be proposed that the colonic immune imbalance in NOD mice reflects on the peritoneal immune cells, which subsequently aid in initiating an autoimmune response in the pancreatic lymph nodes, triggering type 1 diabetes development.

ACKNOWLEDGMENTS

This work was supported by The Academy of Finland, The Päivikki and Sakari Sohlberg Foundation, Finland and The Finnish Diabetes Research Foundation. No potential conflicts of interest relevant to this article were reported.

C.A. and A.H. researched the data and wrote the manuscript. S.V. and V.P. researched the data. J.J. contributed to discussion. E.E. researched the data and contributed to discussion.

We also thank Jani Jaakkola (Turku University of Applied Sciences) and Seija Lindqvist (Central Animal Laboratory of Turku University) for skillful technical assistance.

REFERENCES

1. Vaarala O, Knip M, Paronen J, Hämäläinen AM, Muona P, Väätäinen M, Ilonen J, Simell O, Akerblom HK. Cow's milk formula feeding induces primary immunization to insulin in infants at genetic risk for type 1 diabetes. Diabetes 1999;48:1389–1394
2. Virtanen SM, Saukkonen T, Savilahti E, Ylönen K, Räsänen L, Aro A, Knip M, Tuomilehto J, Akerblom HK. Diet, cow's milk protein antibodies and the risk of IDDM in Finnish children. Childhood Diabetes in Finland Study Group. Diabetologia 1994;37:381–387
3. Hänninen A, Salmi M, Simell O, Jalkanen S. Mucosa-associated (beta 7-integrinhigh) lymphocytes accumulate early in the pancreas of NOD mice and show aberrant recirculation behavior. Diabetes 1996;45:1173–1180
4. Hänninen A, Jaakkola I, Jalkanen S. Mucosal addressin is required for the development of diabetes in nonobese diabetic mice. J Immunol 1998;160:6018–6025
5. Yang XD, Sytwu HK, McDevitt HO, Michie SA. Involvement of beta 7 integrin and mucosal addressin cell adhesion molecule-1 (MAdCAM-1) in the development of diabetes in obese diabetic mice. Diabetes 1997;46:1542–1547
6. Bosi E, Molteni L, Radaelli MG, Folini L, Fermo I, Bazzigaluppi E, Piemonti L, Pastore MR, Paroni R. Increased intestinal permeability precedes clinical onset of type 1 diabetes. Diabetologia 2006;49:2824–2827
7. Graham S, Courtois P, Malaisse WJ, Rozing J, Scott FW, Mowat AM. Enteropathy precedes type 1 diabetes in the BB rat. Gut 2004;53:1437–1444
8. Maurano F, Mazzarella G, Luongo D, Stefanile R, D'Arienzo R, Rossi M, Auricchio S, Troncone R. Small intestinal enteropathy in non-obese diabetic mice fed a diet containing wheat. Diabetologia 2005;48:931–937
9. Lefebvre DE, Powell KL, Strom A, Scott FW. Dietary proteins as environmental modifiers of type 1 diabetes mellitus. Annu Rev Nutr 2006;26:175–202
10. Vaarala O. Leaking gut in type 1 diabetes. Curr Opin Gastroenterol 2008;24:701–706
11. Vaarala O, Atkinson MA, Neu J. The "perfect storm" for type 1 diabetes: the complex interplay between intestinal microbiota, gut permeability, and mucosal immunity. Diabetes 2008;57:2555–2562
12. Reséndiz-Albor AA, Esquivel R, López-Revilla R, Verdín L, Moreno-Fierros L. Striking phenotypic and functional differences in lamina propria lymphocytes from the large and small intestine of mice. Life Sci 2005;76:2783–2803
13. Carter PB, Collins FM. The route of enteric infection in normal mice. J Exp Med 1974;139:1189–1203
14. Turley SJ, Lee JW, Dutton-Swain N, Mathis D, Benoist C. Endocrine self and gut non-self intersect in the pancreatic lymph nodes. Proc Natl Acad Sci U S A 2005;102:17729–17733
15. Cruickshank SM, English NR, Felsburg PJ, Carding SR. Characterization of colonic dendritic cells in normal and colitic mice. World J Gastroenterol 2005;11:6338–6347
16. Rescigno M, Lopatin U, Chieppa M. Interactions among dendritic cells, macrophages, and epithelial cells in the gut: implications for immune tolerance. Curr Opin Immunol 2008;20:669–675
17. Denning TL, Wang YC, Patel SR, Williams IR, Pulendran B. Lamina propria macrophages and dendritic cells differentially induce regulatory and interleukin 17-producing T cell responses. Nat Immunol 2007;8:1086–1094
18. Smythies LE, Sellers M, Clements RH, Mosteller-Barnum M, Meng G, Benjamin WH, Orenstein JM, Smith PD. Human intestinal macrophages display profound inflammatory anergy despite avid phagocytic and bactericidal activity. J Clin Invest 2005;115:66–75
19. Kobayashi T, Okamoto S, Hisamatsu T, Kamada N, Chinen H, Saito R, Kitazume MT, Nakazawa A, Sugita A, Koganei K, Isobe K, Hibi T. IL23 differentially regulates the Th1/Th17 balance in ulcerative colitis and Crohn's disease. Gut 2008;57:1682–1689
20. Shen W, Durum SK. Synergy of IL-23 and Th17 cytokines: new light on inflammatory bowel disease. Neurochem Res 2010;35:940–946
21. Hultgren B, Huang X, Dybdal N, Stewart TA. Genetic absence of gamma-interferon delays but does not prevent diabetes in NOD mice. Diabetes 1996;45:812–817
22. Serreze DV, Post CM, Chapman HD, Johnson EA, Lu B, Rothman PB. Interferon-gamma receptor signaling is dispensable in the development of autoimmune type 1 diabetes in NOD mice. Diabetes 2000;49:2007–2011
23. Martin-Orozco N, Chung Y, Chang SH, Wang YH, Dong C. Th17 cells promote pancreatic inflammation but only induce diabetes efficiently in lymphopenic hosts after conversion into Th1 cells. Eur J Immunol 2009;39:216–224
24. Srinivasan S, Bolick DT, Lukashev D, Lappas C, Sitkovsky M, Lynch KR, Hedrick CC. Sphingosine-1-phosphate reduces CD4+ T-cell activation in type 1 diabetes through regulation of hypoxia-inducible factor short isoform I.1 and CD69. Diabetes 2008;57:484–493
25. Vukkadapu SS, Belli JM, Ishii K, Jegga AG, Hutton JJ, Aronow BJ, Katz JD. Dynamic interaction between T cell-mediated beta-cell damage and beta-cell repair in the run up to autoimmune diabetes of the NOD mouse. Physiol Genomics 2005;21:201–211
26. Emamaullee JA, Davis J, Merani S, Toso C, Elliott JF, Thiesen A, Shapiro AM. Inhibition of Th17 cells regulates autoimmune diabetes in NOD mice. Diabetes 2009;58:1302–1311
27. Jain R, Tartar DM, Gregg RK, Divekar RD, Bell JJ, Lee HH, Yu P, Ellis JS, Hoeman CM, Franklin CL, Zaghouani H. Innocuous IFNgamma induced by adjuvant-free antigen restores normoglycemia in NOD mice through inhibition of IL-17 production. J Exp Med 2008;205:207–218
28. Bending D, De La Pena H, Veldhoen M, Phillips JM, Uyttenhove C, Stockinger B, Cooke A. Highly purified Th17 cells from BDC2.5NOD mice convert into Th1-like cells in NOD/SCID recipient mice. J Clin Invest 2009, 2 February (Epub ahead of print)
29. Alam C, Valkonen S, Ohls S, Törnqvist K, Hänninen A. Enhanced trafficking to the pancreatic lymph nodes and auto-antigen presentation capacity

distinguishes peritoneal B lymphocytes in non-obese diabetic mice. Diabetologia 2010;53:346–355

30. Eerola E, Lehtonen OP. Optimal data processing procedure for automatic bacterial identification by gas–liquid chromatography of cellular fatty acids. J Clin Microbiol 1988;26:1745–1753

31. Toivanen P, Vaahtovuo J, Eerola E. Influence of major histocompatibility complex on bacterial composition of fecal flora. Infect Immun 2001;69: 2372–2377

32. Duchmann R, Kaiser I, Hermann E, Mayet W, Ewe K, Meyer zum Büschenfelde KH. Tolerance exists towards resident intestinal flora but is broken in active inflammatory bowel disease (IBD). Clin Exp Immunol 1995;102: 448–455

33. Duchmann R, Schmitt E, Knolle P, Meyer zum Büschenfelde KH, Neurath M. Tolerance towards resident intestinal flora in mice is abrogated in experimental colitis and restored by treatment with interleukin-10 or antibodies to interleukin-12. Eur J Immunol 1996;26:934–938

34. Hemminki K, Li X, Sundquist J, Sundquist K. Familial association between type 1 diabetes and other autoimmune and related diseases. Diabetologia 2009;52:1820–1828

35. Westerholm-Ormio M, Vaarala O, Pihkala P, Ilonen J, Savilahti E. Immunologic activity in the small intestinal mucosa of pediatric patients with type 1 diabetes. Diabetes 2003;52:2287–2295

36. Auricchio R, Paparo F, Maglio M, Franzese A, Lombardi F, Valerio G, Nardone G, Percopo S, Greco L, Troncone R. In vitro-deranged intestinal immune response to gliadin in type 1 diabetes. Diabetes 2004;53:1680–1683

37. Matsuda R, Koide T, Tokoro C, Yamamoto T, Godai T, Morohashi T, Fujita Y, Takahashi D, Kawana I, Suzuki S, Umemura S. Quantitive cytokine mRNA expression profiles in the colonic mucosa of patients with steroid naive ulcerative colitis during active and quiescent disease. Inflamm Bowel Dis 2009;15:328–334

38. Tritt M, Sgouroudis E, d'Hennezel E, Albanese A, Piccirillo CA. Functional waning of naturally occurring CD4+ regulatory T-cells contributes to the onset of autoimmune diabetes. Diabetes 2008;57:113–123

39. Vorobjova T, Uibo O, Heilman K, Rägo T, Honkanen J, Vaarala O, Tillmann V, Ojakivi I, Uibo R. Increased FOXP3 expression in small-bowel mucosa of children with coeliac disease and type I diabetes mellitus. Scand J Gastroenterol 2009;44:422–430

40. Videla S, Vilaseca J, Guarner F, Salas A, Treserra F, Crespo E, Antolín M, Malagelada JR. Role of intestinal microflora in chronic inflammation and ulceration of the rat colon. Gut 1994;35:1090–1097

41. Zaph C, Du Y, Saenz SA, Nair MG, Perrigoue JG, Taylor BC, Troy AE, Kobuley DE, Kastelein RA, Cua DJ, Yu Y, Artis D. Commensal-dependent expression of IL-25 regulates the IL-23-IL-17 axis in the intestine. J Exp Med 2008;205:2191–2198

42. Wen L, Ley RE, Volchkov PY, Stranges PB, Avanesyan L, Stonebraker AC, Hu C, Wong FS, Szot GL, Bluestone JA, Gordon JI, Chervonsky AV. Innate immunity and intestinal microbiota in the development of Type 1 diabetes. Nature 2008;455:1109–1113

43. Frank DN, St Amand AL, Feldman RA, Boedeker EC, Harpaz N, Pace NR. Molecular-phylogenetic characterization of microbial community imbalances in human inflammatory bowel diseases. Proc Natl Acad Sci U S A 2007;104:13780–13785

44. Mazmanian SK, Round JL, Kasper DL. A microbial symbiosis factor prevents intestinal inflammatory disease. Nature 2008;453:620–625

45. Roesch LF, Lorca GL, Casella G, Giongo A, Naranjo A, Pionzio AM, Li N, Mai V, Wasserfall CH, Schatz D, Atkinson MA, Neu J, Triplett EW. Culture-independent identification of gut bacteria correlated with the onset of diabetes in a rat model. ISME J 2009;3:536–548

46. Ivanov II, Atarashi K, Manel N, Brodie EL, Shima T, Karaoz U, Wei D, Goldfarb KC, Santee CA, Lynch SV, Tanoue T, Imaoka A, Itoh K, Takeda K, Umesaki Y, Honda K, Littman DR. Induction of intestinal Th17 cells by segmented filamentous bacteria. Cell 2009;139:485–498

47. Hansen AK, Ling F, Kaas A, Funda DP, Farlov H, Buschard K. Diabetes preventive gluten-free diet decreases the number of caecal bacteria in non-obese diabetic mice. Diabetes Metab Res Rev 2006;22:220–225

48. Flohé SB, Wasmuth HE, Kerad JB, Beales PE, Pozzilli P, Elliott RB, Hill JP, Scott FW, Kolb H. A wheat-based, diabetes-promoting diet induces a Th1-type cytokine bias in the gut of NOD mice. Cytokine 2003;21:149–154

49. Vaarala O. Is it dietary insulin? Ann N Y Acad Sci 2006;1079:350–359

50. Ha SA, Tsuji M, Suzuki K, Meek B, Yasuda N, Kaisho T, Fagarasan S. Regulation of B1 cell migration by signals through Toll-like receptors. J Exp Med 2006;203:2541–2550

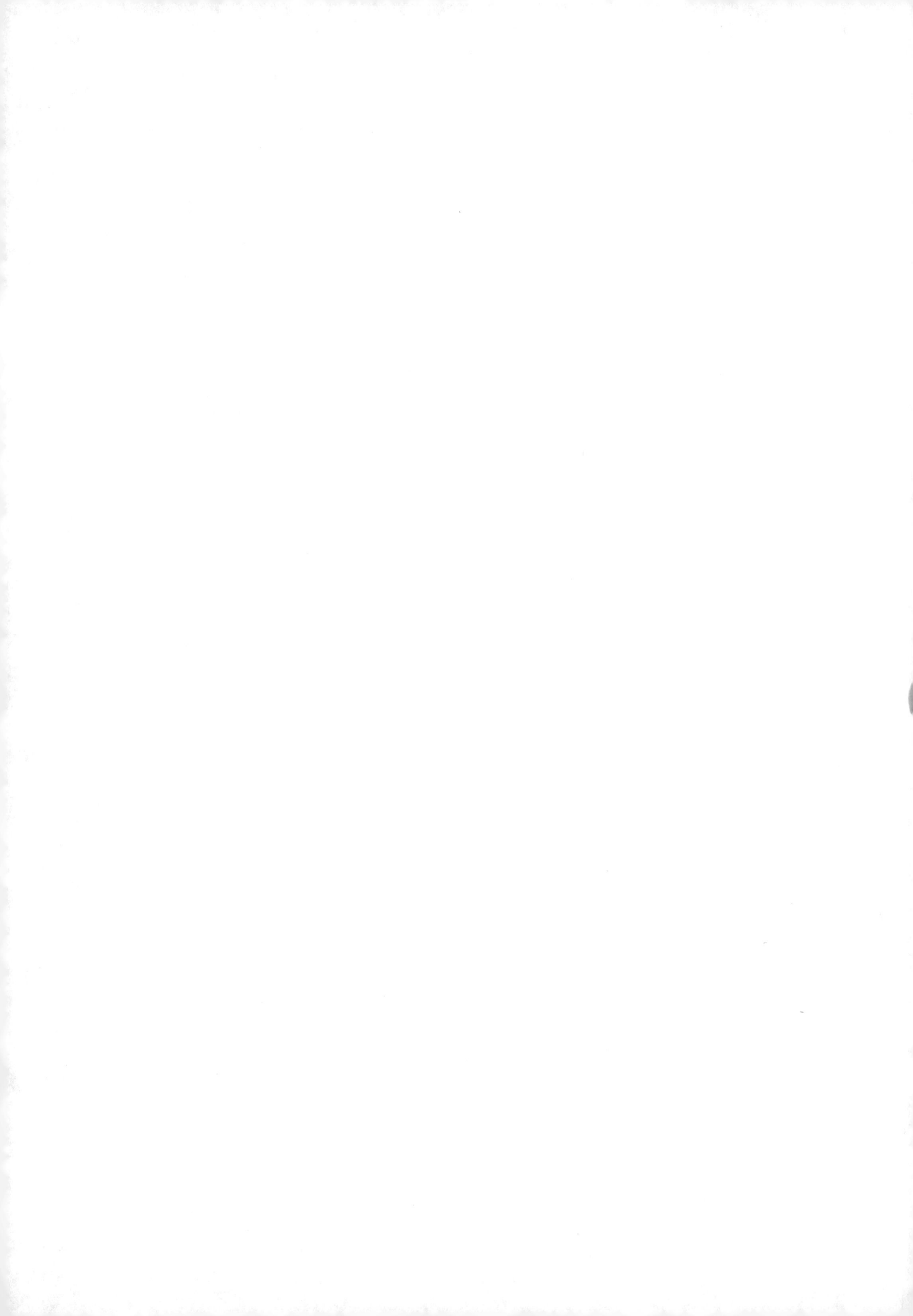

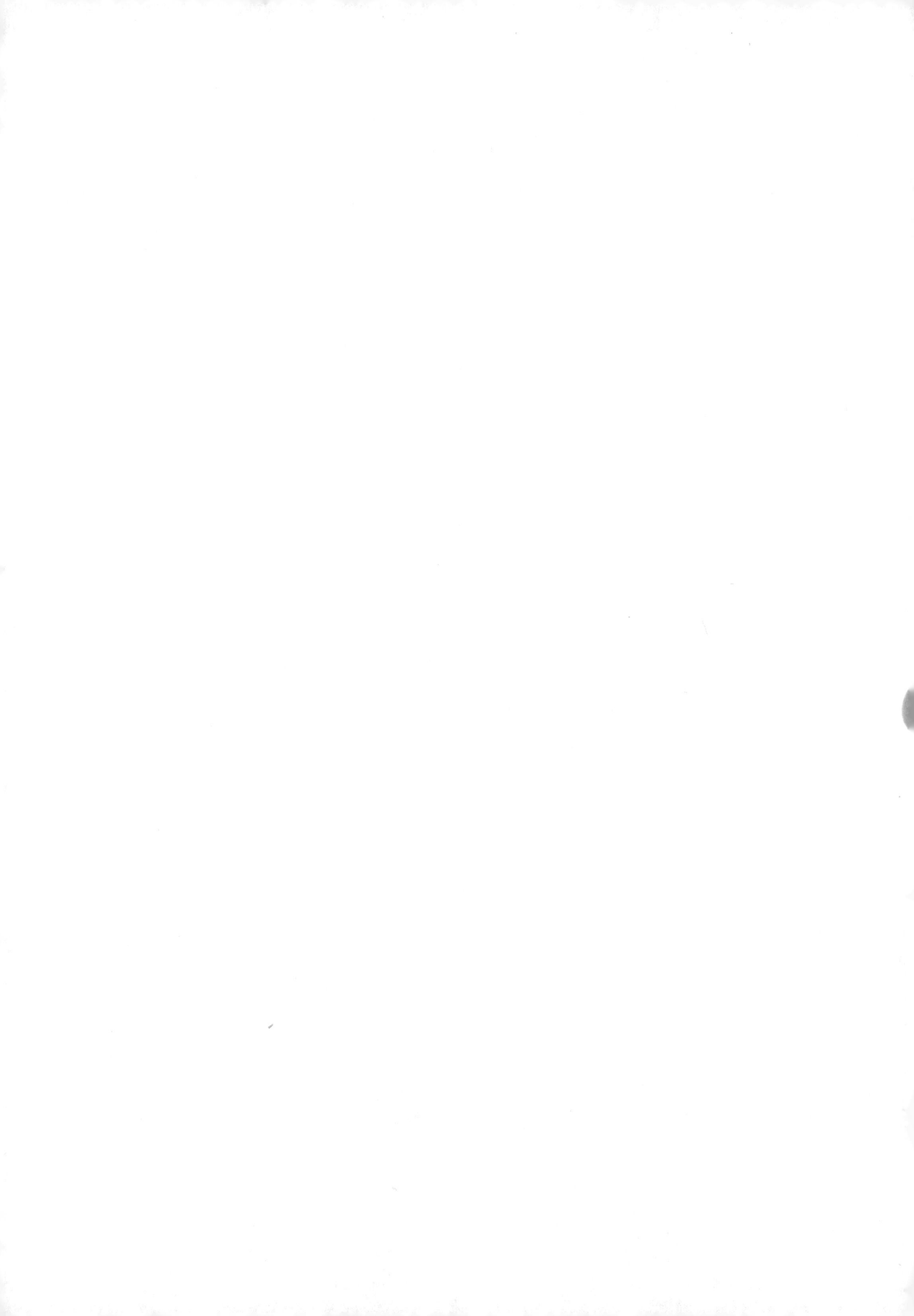

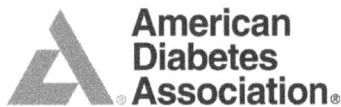

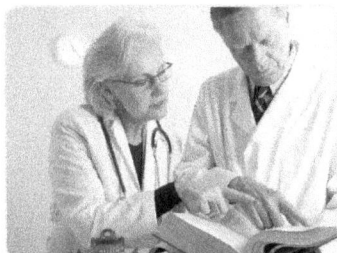

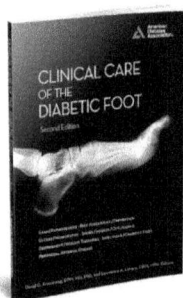

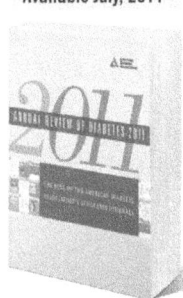

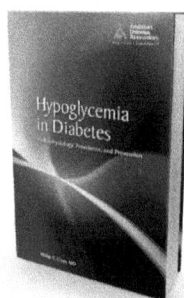

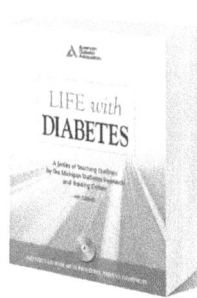

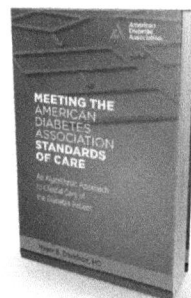

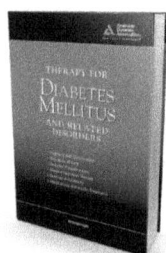

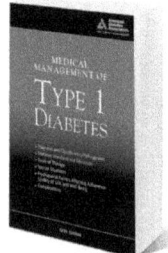

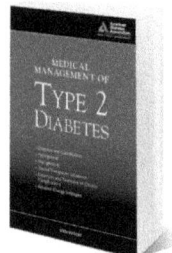

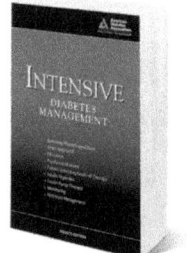

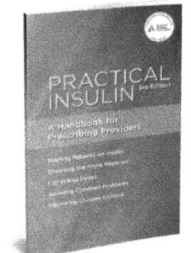

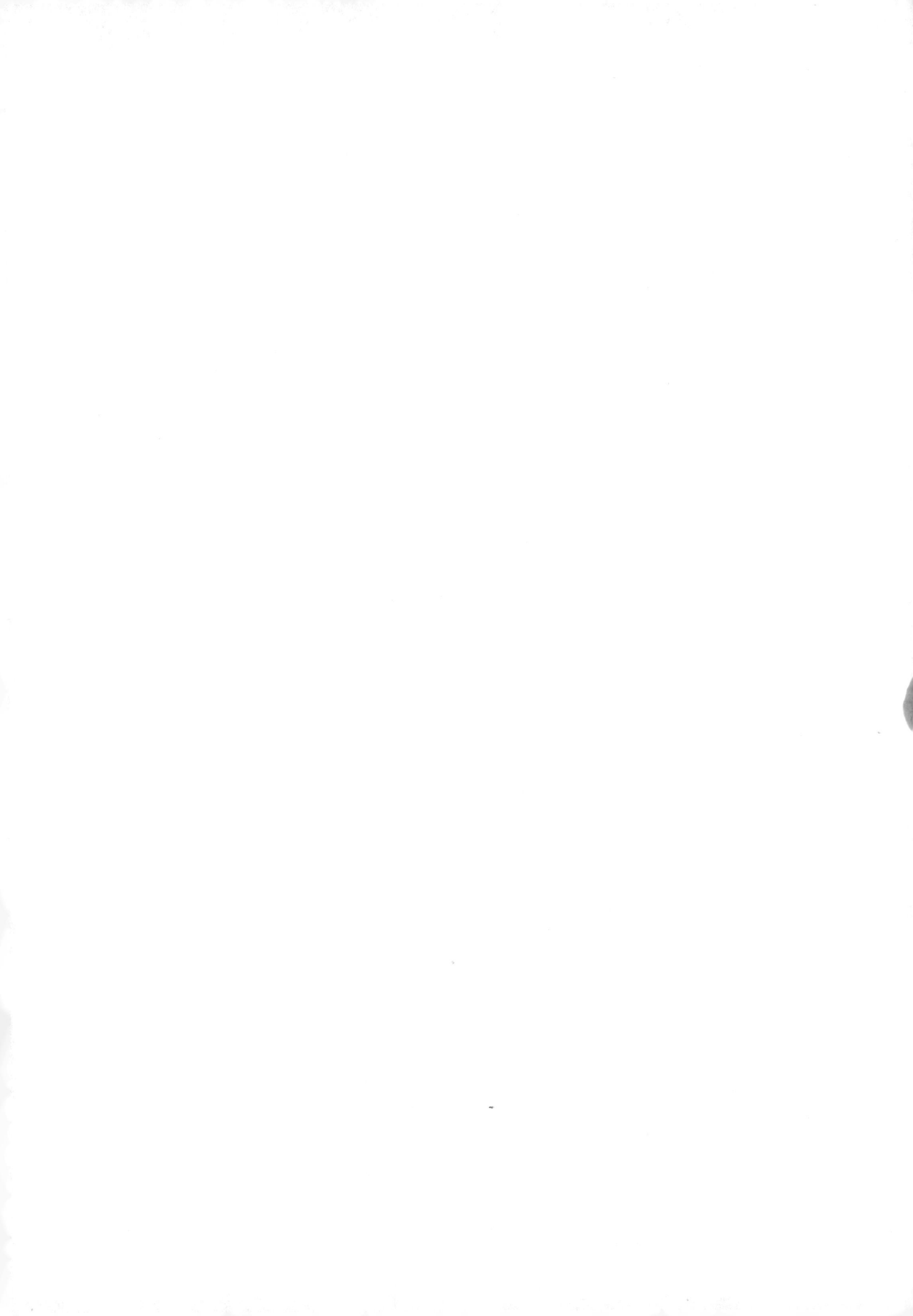

www.ingramcontent.com/pod-product-compliance
Lightning Source LLC
Chambersburg PA
CBHW081427270326
41932CB00019B/3117

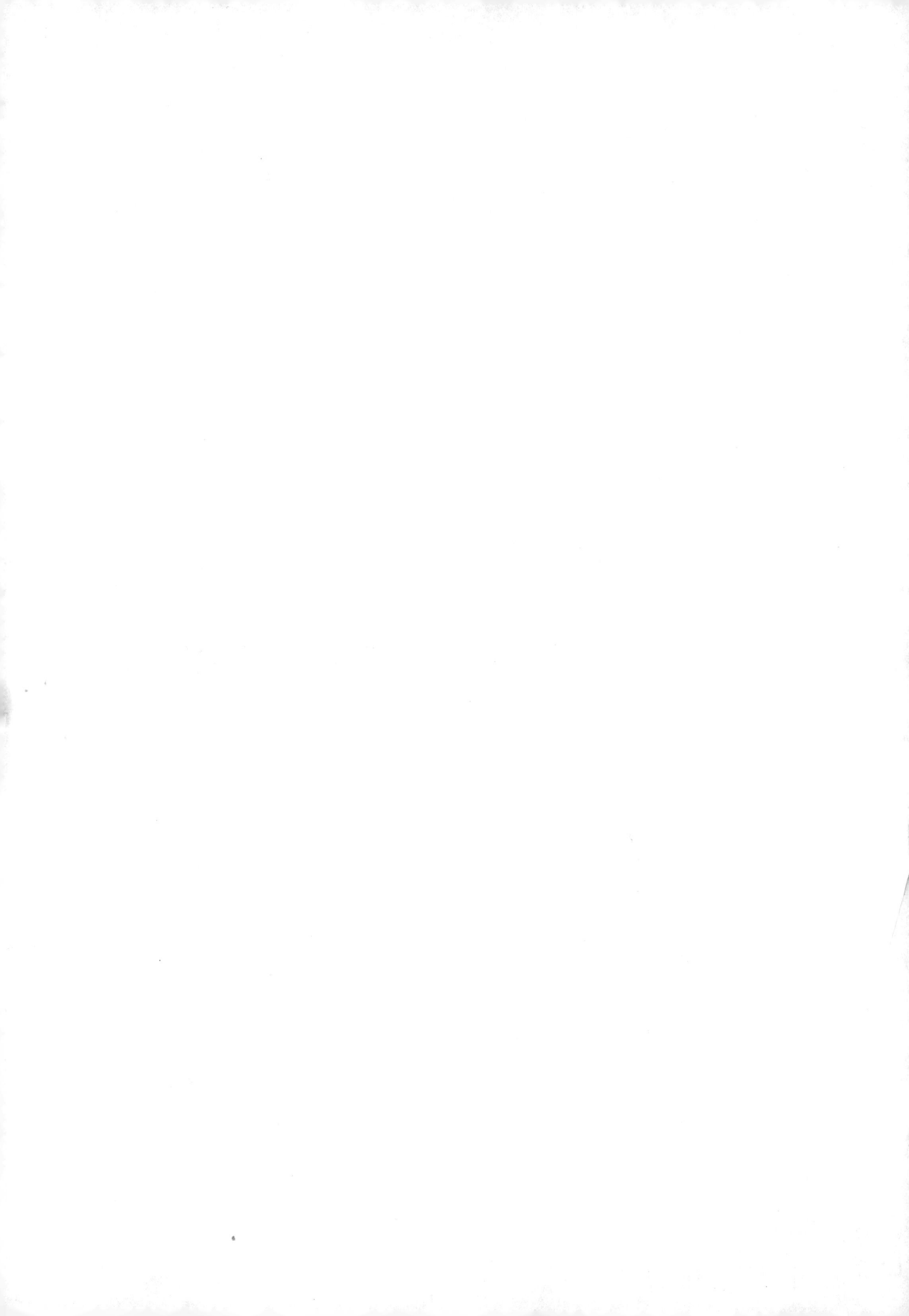